Core Concepts in Health

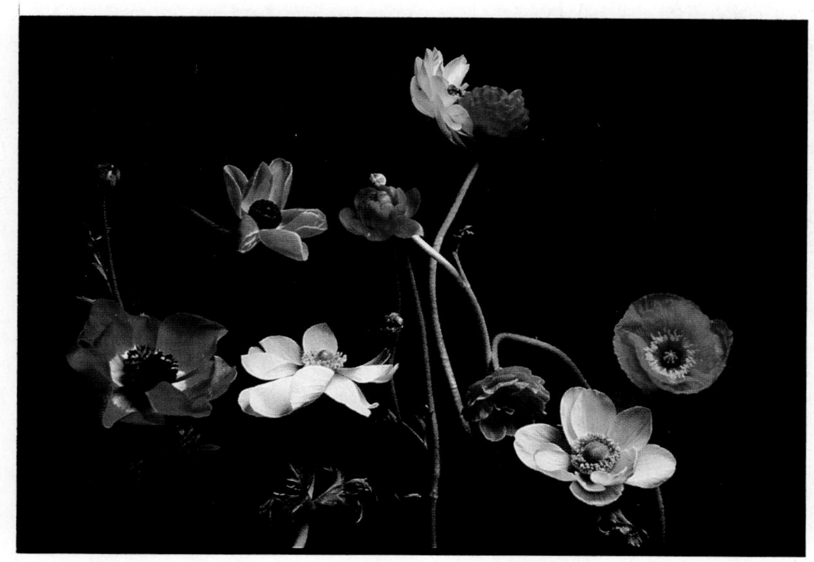

Fifth Edition

Paul M. Insel   Walton T. Roth

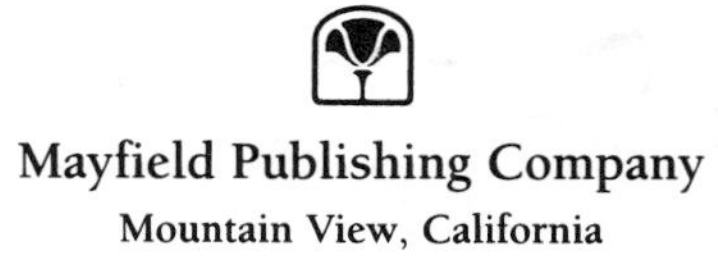

Mayfield Publishing Company
Mountain View, California

Fifth Edition

Library of Congress Cataloging in Publication Data

Core concepts in health.

Includes bibliographies and index.
1. Health. I. Insel, Paul M. II. Roth, Walton T.
[DNLM: 1. Health 2. Hygiene. QT 180 C797]
RA776.C83 1988 613 87-23977
ISBN 0-87484-795-8

Manufactured in the United States of America
10 9 8 7 6 5 4 3

Mayfield Publishing Company
1240 Villa Street
Mountain View, California 94041

Sponsoring editor, James Bull; *developmental editor,* Jan Beatty; *manuscript editor,* Linda Purrington; *production editor,* Helene Harrington; *art director and designer,* Janet Bollow; *cover photograph,* Shotaro Akiyama, © 1987 The Image Bank; *illustrators,* Judi McCarty, Victor Royer, Barbara Barnett

Credits and Sources

Page 3 Donald M. Vickery, *Life Plan for Your Health,* pp. 17, 18. © 1978 by Addison Wesley Publishing Co., Reading, Massachusetts. Reprinted with permission.

Page 9 Joyce D. Nash, *Maximize Your Body Potential,* 1986, pp. 50–51. Reprinted with permission of Bull Publishing Co.

Pages 11–12 From the book *Become an Ex-Smoker* by Brian G. Danaher and Edward Lichtenstein. Copyright © 1978 by Prentice-Hall, Inc. Published by Prentice-Hall, Inc., Englewood Cliffs, NJ 07632.

Page 29 Richard S. Lazarus, "Little hassles can be hazardous to health." Reprinted with permission from *Psychology Today* Magazine. Copyright © 1981 by American Psychological Association.

Page 73 Adapted from *Shyness* by Philip G. Zimbardo, pp. 138–141. Copyright © 1977 by Philip Zimbardo. Reprinted by permission of Addison Wesley Publishing Co., Reading, Massachusetts.

Page 79 External female genitalia from Dienhart, *Basic Human Anatomy and Physiology.* Copyright © 1979 by W. B. Saunders.

Page 94 Reprinted from January 19, 1987 issue of *Business Week* by special permission, copyright © 1987 by McGraw-Hill, Inc.

Page 126 Reprinted with permission from Family Planning Perspectives, Vol. 15, No. 4. The Alan Guttmacher Institute, 1983.

Page 144 From *Our Bodies, Ourselves,* The Boston Women's Health Book Collective. Copyright © 1971, 1973, 1976 by The Boston Women's Health Book Collective, Inc. Reprinted by permission of Simon & Schuster, Inc.

Page 153 Copyright © 1986 by Harper's Magazine. All rights reserved. Reprinted from the July issue by special permission.

Pages 154, 155 From "America's Abortion Dilemma," *Newsweek,* January 14, 1985. The Alan Guttmacher Institute. Copyright © 1985 by Newsweek, Inc. All rights reserved. Reprinted by permission.

Page 184 From "Am I Parent Material?" by Carole Goldman, published by the National Organization for Non-Parents, 806 Reisterstown Road, Baltimore, MD 21208.

Page 185 From "Redefining 'Mother' and 'Father'," by Don Colburn, *Washington Post Health,* February 24, 1987.

Page 225 Reprinted from *Children of Alcoholics: Growing Up Unheard,* copyright © 1986 by Do It Now Foundation, Phoenix, AZ. Used by permission.

Page 241 From "The Valium Habit," *Newsweek,* October 13, 1986. Copyright © 1986 by Newsweek, Inc. All rights reserved. Reprinted by permission.

Page 244 "High Price of Abuse," *Time,* June 2, 1986. Copyright © 1986 by Time, Inc. All rights reserved. Reprinted by permission from TIME.

Page 268 From *Jane Brody's Nutrition Book* by Jane E. Brody. Copyright © 1981 by Jane E. Brody. Reprinted by permission of W. W. Norton & Company, Inc.

Page 300 © 1984 by Family Media, Inc. Reprinted with permission of Ladies' Home Journal and the Diet Center.

Preface

The first edition of *Core Concepts in Health* (published in 1976) was truly an experiment. In it, we shifted away from the commonly held medical model of health to a behavioral one in which the individual becomes an active participant in maintaining his or her health. It worked! Since then, thousands of instructors and hundreds of thousands of students have used our book in their classes, and their feedback indicates that our approach has been gratifyingly successful.

With each succeeding edition, we continue to emphasize the important concepts in this rapidly changing field. The trends now toward behavior and self-care could not be stronger. It is clear that if we want to achieve optimum or exuberant health, we must take charge!

Features of the Fifth Edition

The fifth edition of *Core Concepts in Health* builds on the features that so strongly attracted readers' interest in the previous four editions. We continue to experiment with innovative teaching materials that have been tested and confirmed by gifted teachers in our profession.

A New Chapter on Self-care Western society continues to move further toward an emphasis on self-care. Self-care is a new and daunting role for most of us. We can no longer rely solely on the doctor, but must learn to see him or her as a therapeutic ally.

This trend is taking place not only because we are becoming more enlightened about health, but also because of economic necessity. Health costs continue to soar, forcing us to become more creative and self-reliant in using health care services. Health Maintenance Organizations (HMOs) are springing up everywhere—there, a person or a family pays a fixed monthly fee and receives prepaid medical care. Health insurance companies such as Blue Cross are raising their rates as much as 20 percent to keep up with the spiral. And hospitals are investigating community outreach strategies to stay alive because people are refusing to pay outrageous fees for hospitalization.

We think that the days of centralized, acute care systems are coming to an end. They are being replaced by satellite facilities that can provide emergency and surgical procedures at one-fifth the cost and with significantly more convenience. More importantly, they are being replaced by the health care consumer who has developed medical self-care skills. To help readers become well trained in self-care skills, we have devoted an entire chapter in this edition to medical self-care. It is the longest chapter in the book, and it discusses self-assessment, self-treatment, when to see the doctor, the diagnostic process, medical tests for healthy people, and other self-care concerns.

A New Chapter on Environmental Health By popular demand, we have added a chapter that treats an important health concern—"Environmental Health." It focuses on by-products of our environment, the issues of waste disposal, clean water, insect and rodent control, pollution, radiation, acid rain, and other vital environmental health problems.

A New Chapter on Safety Following the suggestions of hundreds of instructors, we've added a chapter "Safety and First Aid." This chapter discusses the causes of accidents, how accidents affect our lives, accident prevention, rape, and first aid, as well as other safety issues.

A New Chapter on Abortion Realistically, abortion is a health-related issue that most college students will confront; an overwhelming majority know someone either directly or indirectly who has faced the prospect of abortion. To reinforce that abortion is *not* a method of birth control, we've moved the topic out of the chapter on birth control and into its own chapter. Recognizing the controversial nature of abortion, we have taken care to provide an even-handed discussion of the legal and social issues connected with it.

A Completely Reorganized Introductory Chapter The introduction has been incorporated into the first chapter, making a more cohesive opening unit.

An Emphasis on Scientific Accuracy and Documentation The text has been continually updated throughout the revision and production process and reflects the most current knowledge and research available at the time we went to press. Yet health, like other fields, is constantly changing. Yesterday's wild guesses may become today's scientific beliefs. To achieve genuine insight into the human condition, we must have the flexibility to keep an open mind while remaining somewhat skeptical. Fish oil, for example, has been a favorite home remedy for various ills for years, yet the scientific community has regarded it as having little or no health value. It is now recognized that fish oil contains omega-3 fatty acids, which act favorably against heart disease and other problems. Other issues that may have scientific merit—how psychological factors affect physical health, for example—are treated by us as either unproven or unscientific because they are currently unsubstantiated.

In this edition, we have taken pains to provide the sources that inform each chapter in "Selected References" at the end of each chapter.

More Than 70 Percent New Boxed Inserts In an effort to be as current as possible, we've included more new boxes than in any previous edition. Please see the list of boxes, chapter by chapter, that follows the table of contents. Among the topics of current interest: depression, suicide, date rape, surrogacy, child abuse, AIDS, Epstein-Barr virus, acid rain, and the deterioration of the ozone layer.

A Continued, Innovative Use of Color and Graphics Our open, magazine format attracts reader interest and reduces the boredom often elicited by lengthy, uninterrupted text. Our bold and dramatic color illustrations break up the text and express complex ideas vividly. Health and well-being are positive concepts needing expression in illustrations as vibrant and as realistic as possible. Life *is* colorful! We want our text to imitate life, to be challenging and invigorating. We hope the color makes you smile and feel as you think about what the text is saying, for we believe that effective health education touches both our sensibilities and thoughts at once.

A Handy Reference Chart on Emergency First Aid Tips Conveniently located on the inside back cover, this chart offers tips on what to do in a variety of emergency situations.

Chapter Organization To place the focus of each chapter even more strongly on individual responsibility, we've slightly modified the chapter elements in this fifth edition. Our goal is to encourage self-understanding and self-inquiry by bringing together an exploration of values with practical health information.

- *Rate Yourself:* At the beginning of each chapter, the reader is asked to complete a brief assessment of his or her attitudes and behaviors linked to the chapter content. The reader can then find his or her place on a wellness or awareness ladder, which gives a quick sketch of the individual's health and potential for wellness. With this self-assessment in mind, each reader can actively approach the chapter content with an eye toward learning what he or she can do to move higher up the wellness ladder.
- *Exploring Your Emotions:* Throughout the chapter, questions explore emotional issues to highlight awareness of feelings that can affect the cognitive information within each chapter. Because some of us respond more deeply to visual rather than verbal stimuli, the questions accompany our dramatic illustrations; at other times they stand alone.
- *Take Action:* At the end of each chapter, we specify actions each reader might take to improve wellness. We also encourage the keeping of an extended journal to reinforce the self-understanding that should accumulate as the book is read.
- *Behavior Change Strategy:* Models for altering some behaviors that prevent individuals from achieving maximum wellness appear at the end of appropriate chapters.
- *Selected References and Recommended Readings:* Curious readers will find an annotated list of suggestions for further study at the end of each chapter.

Learning Aids To help readers better comprehend what they've read, we've included a number of valuable learning tools.

- Chapter opening outlines
- A running glossary in which terms are defined on the text page where they first appear
- An index, in which page references to glossary items appear in boldface type
- An extended illustration program of provocative and positive full-color images

Supplementary Materials

Instructor's Resource Guide Much more than a collection of test items, the Instructor's Resource Guide provides abundant teaching aids. It includes numerous learning activities that use various teaching techniques—from research projects to group-facilitated discussion topics. A major feature of the Instructor's Resource Guide is its collection of behavioral action handouts (Wellness Worksheets), which supplement material in the text. This edition contains an extensive annotated listing of films, books, articles, and other resources of potential interest to instructors and students. It also includes learning objectives and a full range of test questions for each chapter.

Computerized Test Bank All the test items in the Instructor's Resource Guide are contained in software compatible with major microcomputers. The software allows the instructor to select specific questions, edit existing questions, generate several versions of the same test with answer keys, and enlarge the test item data bank by adding new questions.

Transparencies To help instructors project important concepts, selected illustrations and tables are available as overhead transparencies.

Student Study Guide This guide, prepared by Thomas M. Davis and Dennis Cryer of the University of Northern Iowa, provides students with learning objectives, key terms, major concepts, and sample test questions for each chapter. It is an especially well-written aid for students who want to solidify their understanding of course material.

Computerized Health Risk Appraisal Bound into the study guide is a diskette containing a computerized Health Risk Appraisal that will alert each student to his or her health risks and offer advice about what areas he or she should be particularly aware of. The student, for example, will be able to discover his or her risk of AIDS, of accident or death from riding a motorcycle, and of illness from smoking and other behaviors.

A Note of Thanks

This book represents the combined efforts of more than fifty people. Without their contributions, this book would never have seen publication. To all—contributors, advisors, and reviewers—thank you so very much.

Academic Contributors

Stephen Barrett, M.D., consumer advocate, and Editor, *Nutrition Forum Newsletter*
Nutrition Facts and Fallacies; Choosing Health Care Professionals and Insurance

Boyce Burge, Ph.D., Triton Bioscience, Inc.
Infection and Immunity

Thomas Fahey, Ed.D., California State University, Chico
Exercise for Health and Performance

Michael R. Hoadley, Ph.D., University of South Dakota
Safety and First Aid

Lieselotte Hofmann, B.A., M.A.
Stress and the Social Environment

Marcia Seyler Insel, M. Phil.
Pregnancy, Childbirth, and Parenting; Aging; Dying and Death

Paul Insel, Ph.D., Stanford University
Taking Charge of Your Health; Toward a Tobacco-free Society; Cardiovascular Health; Cancer

Herant Katchadourian, M.D., Stanford University
Sex and Your Body; Sexual Behaviors and Relationships

Bea Mandel, R.N., M.P.H., Seton Medical Center (Director, Education Services)
Sexually Transmissible Diseases

James Olson, San Mateo County Health Department (Public Health Advisor)
Sexually Transmissible Diseases

Walton T. Roth, M.D., Stanford University School of Medicine
Mental Health

James Rothenberger, M.P.H., University of Minnesota
Environmental Health

David Sobel, M.D., M.P.H., Kaiser Permanente Medical Care Program, Northern California Region (Director of Patient Education and Health Promotion)
Medical Self-care: Skills for the Health Care Consumer

Carl Thoresen, Ph.D., Stanford University
Weight Control

Jared R. Tinklenberg, M.D., Palo Alto VA Medical Center and Stanford University
Alcohol; Other Psychoactive Drugs

Mae V. Tinklenberg, R.N., M.S., Fair Oaks Family Health Center
Birth Control; Abortion

Academic Advisors and Reviewers

Daniel D. Adame, Emory University
Evelyn E. Ames, Western Washington University
Rick Barnes, East Carolina University
Stephen Barrett, Editor, *Nutrition Forum Newsletter*
Kenneth H. Beck, University of Maryland
Fay R. Biles, Kent State University (emeritus)
Judith E. Brown, University of Minnesota
Donald G. Carter, Western Kentucky University
David H. Chenoweth, East Carolina University
Michael R. Davey, Western Illinois University
Michael S. Davidson, Montclair State College
Thomas M. Davis, University of Northern Iowa
Judy C. Drolet, Southern Illinois University
David F. Duncan, Southern Illinois University
Patricia C. Dunn, East Carolina University
Richard A. Fee, University of Louisville
Mal Goldsmith, Southern Illinois University, Edwardsville
Michael R. Hoadley, University of South Dakota
Theophanis Hortis, St. Cloud State University

Mark J. Kittleson, Youngstown State University
Tim Knickelbein, Normandale Community College
Jane W. Lammers, University of Central Arkansas
L. Clark McCammon, Western Illinois University
Raymond Meister, California State University, Sacramento
Larry K. Olsen, The Pennsylvania State University
Robert J. Piercy, Indiana University
Marion B. Pollock, California State University, Long Beach (emeritus)
James H. Rothenberger, University of Minnesota
Laurna Rubinson, University of Illinois
Cynthia Smith-Fee, University of Louisville
Richard W. Wilson, Western Kentucky University

Paul M. Insel
Walton T. Roth

Contents

Part Two
Sexuality

Chapter 4
Sex and Your Body 76

Chapter 5
Sexual Behaviors and Relationships 98

Chapter 6
Birth Control 124

Chapter 7
Abortion 148

Boxes

Chapter 1

Contents

Rate Yourself

Your Health Behavior Read the following statements carefully. Choose the one in each section that best describes you at this moment and circle its number. When you have chosen one statement for each section, add the numbers and record your total score. Find your position on the Wellness Ladder.

5 My health is my responsibility.
4 I am the person most responsible for my health.
3 When it comes to my health I depend on others as well as myself.
2 Good health is often determined by finding a good doctor.
1 Good health is a matter of good genes and good luck.

5 I usually think about how diet and lifestyle affect my health.
4 I will usually pass something up if I think it's bad for my health.
3 I pay attention to my health, but only when it is convenient.
2 I only worry about my health when I get sick.
1 It is usually too much work to practice health prevention.

5 In making a decision about my health, I am inclined to get a second or even a third opinion from other health professionals.
4 I would usually get a second opinion if making a critical decision about my health.
3 I am not inclined to get a second opinion about my health.
2 I would rarely get a second opinion about my health.
1 I would never get a second opinion about my health.

5 I wouldn't hesitate to question a doctor's recommendations.
4 I would usually question the doctor if I had doubts about his or her recommendations.
3 I would reluctantly question a doctor's recommendations.
2 I would rarely question a doctor's recommendations.
1 I would never question the doctor if I had doubts about his or her recommendations.

5 I am pretty good at using the health care system.
4 If I have a special health problem, I can usually find out how to take care of it.
3 I ask my doctor about any health problems that arise.
2 I rely on my friends or relatives for health advice.
1 I am usually uncertain about where to go for health advice.

Total Score ______

Taking Charge of Your Health

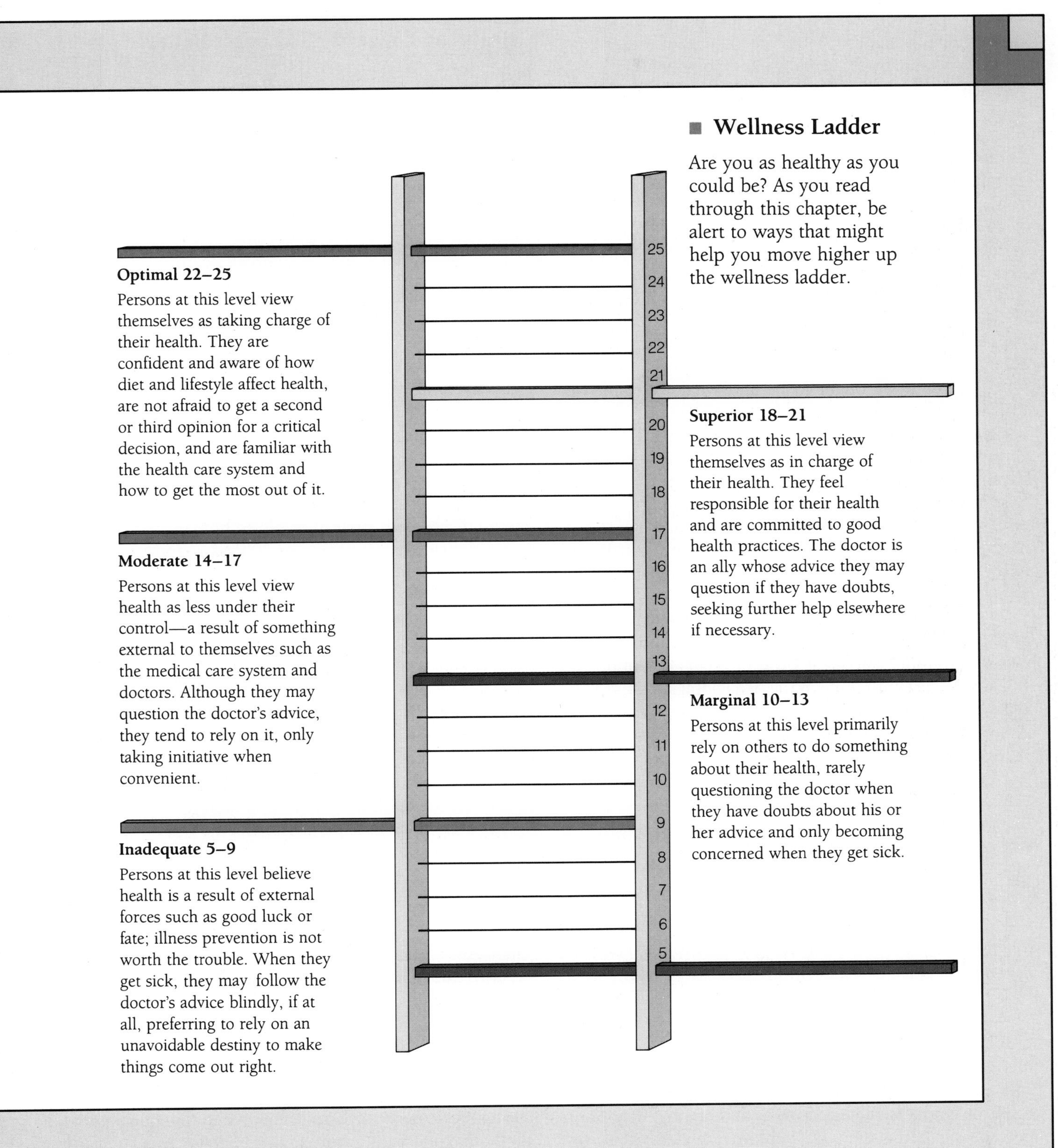

■ Wellness Ladder

Are you as healthy as you could be? As you read through this chapter, be alert to ways that might help you move higher up the wellness ladder.

Optimal 22–25
Persons at this level view themselves as taking charge of their health. They are confident and aware of how diet and lifestyle affect health, are not afraid to get a second or third opinion for a critical decision, and are familiar with the health care system and how to get the most out of it.

Superior 18–21
Persons at this level view themselves as in charge of their health. They feel responsible for their health and are committed to good health practices. The doctor is an ally whose advice they may question if they have doubts, seeking further help elsewhere if necessary.

Moderate 14–17
Persons at this level view health as less under their control—a result of something external to themselves such as the medical care system and doctors. Although they may question the doctor's advice, they tend to rely on it, only taking initiative when convenient.

Marginal 10–13
Persons at this level primarily rely on others to do something about their health, rarely questioning the doctor when they have doubts about his or her advice and only becoming concerned when they get sick.

Inadequate 5–9
Persons at this level believe health is a result of external forces such as good luck or fate; illness prevention is not worth the trouble. When they get sick, they may follow the doctor's advice blindly, if at all, preferring to rely on an unavoidable destiny to make things come out right.

Rejuvenation Making young again.

Superlongevity An excessive increase in life span.

Life span The duration of life, longevity.

The next time you ask someone "How are you?" and get the automatic response "Fine," be grateful. If that person told you how he or she actually felt—you might wish you had never asked. Your friend might be one of the too many people who live most of their lives feeling no better than just all right, or so-so, or downright miserable. Some do not even know what exuberant health is. How many people do you know who feel great most of the time? Do you?

Health is considerably more than the absence of a minor or major illness. It is partly biological status, a matter of how well all the body's component parts are working. It is partly a consequence of behavior, a reflection of our ability to live in harmony with nature and with other people. And it is partly a product of personal and philosophical values, intimately tied to our concept of self—what we think we ought to be and what we think we really are.

Over the last several decades, breakthroughs in biology and medical science have led to exciting, even startling, advances in the battle against disease. Wonder drugs such as penicillin have substantially reduced the impact of some diseases, while at the same time new or improved vaccines have virtually wiped out other problems. Since 1900, deaths from contagious disease in the United States have been reduced by 98 percent.

It is clear, however, that we cannot reasonably expect future technological and biological advances to be of this same magnitude. The great breakthroughs of tomorrow will almost certainly come in the behavioral sphere—that is, in a much expanded understanding of why we behave as we do and, more particularly, how we can go about changing behavior that is harmful to our health.

Exploring Your Emotions

Rate yourself, your family members, and your closest friends for attentiveness and responsiveness to health issues (rate people from 1, indifferent, to 5, responsive). What feelings seem to keep people both attentive and responsive to health information that may involve personal change?

A large percentage of the health problems that pervade this country are self-inflicted. They are rarely inflicted with the aim of self-destruction, but are commonly the result of ignorance and confusion and apathy. The purpose of this book, then, is to inform, to clarify, and to dispel indifference.

Health as Longevity: Is Longer Better?

The impulse to survive is very strong. Hence the possibility of finding a fountain of youth, a definite means of prolonging life, has teased our imaginations for thousands of years. Fountain of youth legends can be traced back to at least 700 B.C. in the fable of Cyavana, an elderly Hindu priest who revealed certain religious secrets to two demigods in exchange for **rejuvenation.** By the time Ponce de Leon accidentally discovered Florida in 1513 while seeking the Fountain of Youth, the superlongevity idea was firmly established in European thought. Carried down to modern times, this myth continues to fuel markets for a wide variety of ineffective rejuvenation aids.

Evidence for the possibility of **superlongevity** is meager. Every animal, including humans, appears to have a maximum **life span** that is extremely difficult to modify. Reports of humans living well into their second century almost always fail to be correct—a reputed 140-year-old becomes 104 on closer examination. About a century ago there was a widespread belief that with the aid of soon-to-be-discovered medical miracles human beings could extend their life span to 150 or 200 years. Today, although some of the public, especially certain types of health faddists, cling to that belief, most knowledgeable scientists see no immediate prospect of appreciably extending our life span.

Perhaps a more important question is "What would superlongevity mean if we had it?" Is a longer life a better life? Clearly this is no certainty, since a long life without the ability to function in a vital way is not a blessing, but one of life's major tragedies. Being alive longer may be an interesting health statistic, but it is not equivalent to good health. In the literature of all ages, merely being alive has often been equated to being in hell. We will have to look elsewhere for the true meaning of health.

Health as Vitality: Becoming More Alive

Health is difficult to define, but it is remarkable how often analysts with widely divergent backgrounds come close to the same definition as they struggle with this concept. More often than not, good health is seen as vitality, as being particularly alive, as being able to function well, as being in tune with nature and humanity. A particularly poignant description of health was given by British author

Ages of Health Advancement

A study of death rates over the last century illustrates the dramatic changes that have taken place in the nature of health problems and solutions to these problems. The figure below shows overall death rates in the United States (age-adjusted) from 1885 to 1985, with the times at which major medical innovations became available.

Burn these facts into your mind:

- Over 70 percent of the decline in death rate between 1885 and 1985 occurred *before* the most significant medical innovations were introduced, in a period dominated by improvements in the environment and in our public health policies.
- The discovery of antibiotics in the 1930s ushered in what might be called the Age of Medicine and did noticeably accelerate the decline in the U.S. death rate. For about 20 years substantial progress was made via the "magic bullet" route.
- The decline slid to a stop in the early 1950s as the problems still responsive to this approach began to disappear. For the next 20 years there was almost no reduction in the death rate or corresponding increase in life expectancy. Ironically, this was the same period in which many of our most expensive medical innovations were introduced—intensive care units, open heart surgery, and all the rest. The cost of medical care rose dramatically in this period.
- Finally, in the early 1970s, death rates again began to decline at a significant rate. This continuing decline reflects a drop in the deaths due to heart attacks and stroke. It coincides with reduced use of tobacco, less saturated fat and cholesterol in the diet, and increased exercise among American adults. This could be called the beginning of the Age of Life-Style in health.

Thus the "miracles of modern medicine" have had little to do with the long-term declines in the death rate. The two things simply do not go together historically. Furthermore, we appear to be in an era where lifestyle, rather than medicine, will be the dominant factor in further gains in health.

SOURCE: Donald M. Vickery, *Life Plan for Your Health*

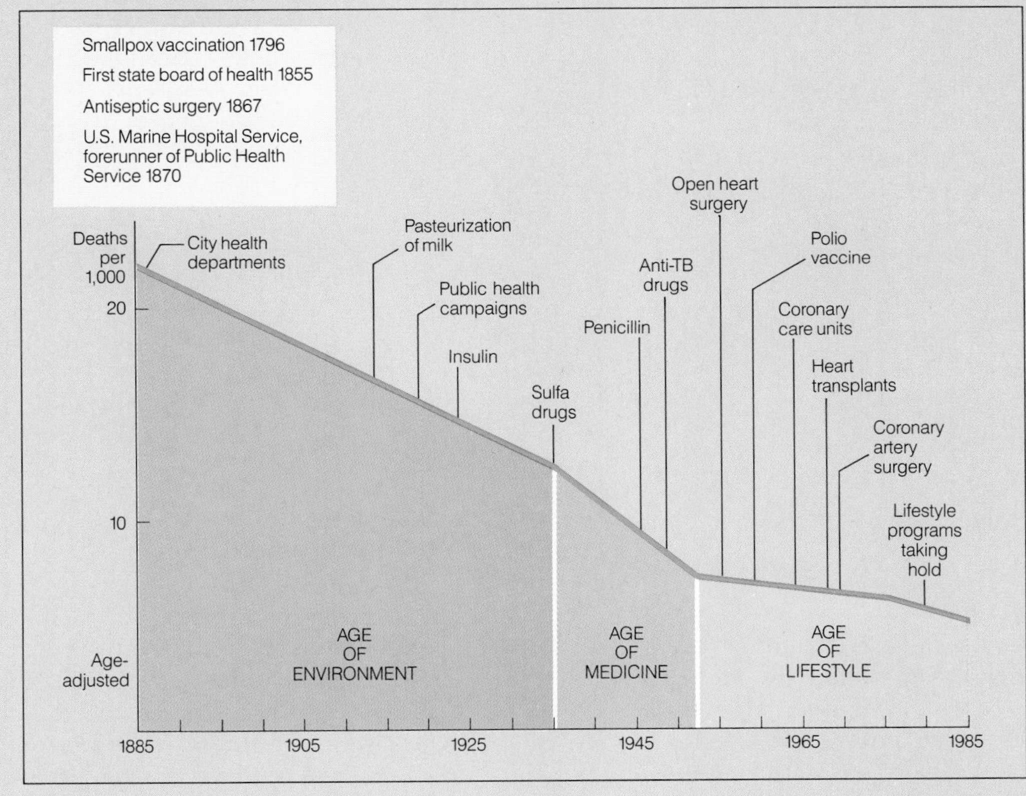

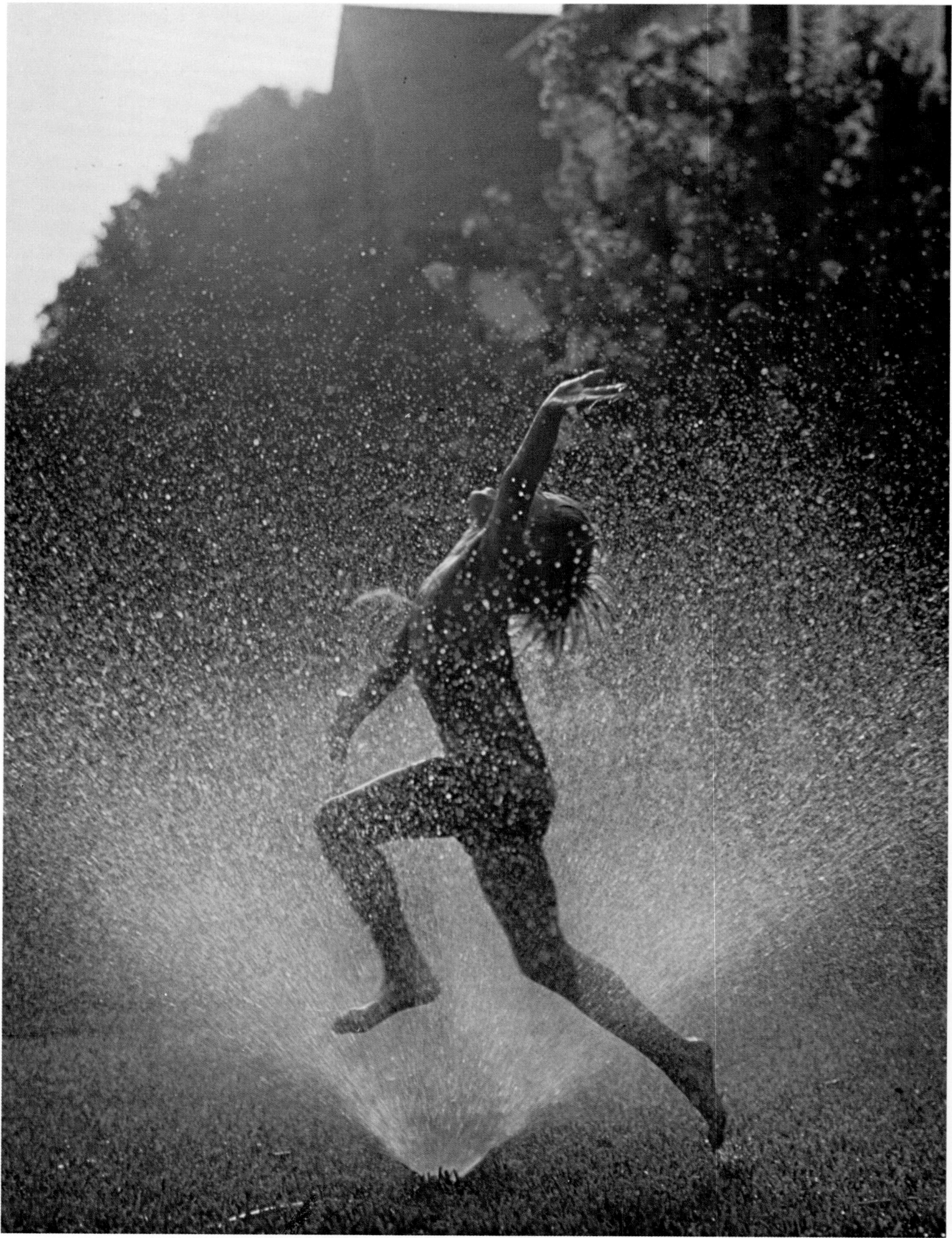

Vitality The ability of an organism to function with vigor.

Lifestyle A consistent and habitual way of life.

Arthritis A painful disease characterized by inflammation of a joint or joints.

Katherine Mansfield, who, when she was dying of tuberculosis, wrote in the final pages of her journal:

> By health, I mean the power to live a full, adult, living breathing life in close contact with what I love—the earth and the wonders thereof—the sea—the sun. . . . I want to be all that I am capable of becoming, so that I may be . . . there's only one phrase that will do—a child of the sun.

Exploring Your Emotions

How might your feelings about your own death illuminate your feelings about and care of your own health?

One of the best-known definitions of health in modern times comes from the World Health Organization, which defines health as "a state of complete physical, mental, and social well-being and not merely the absence of disease or infirmity." In the last few years this idea has been carried a step further, and we are beginning to realize that even disabled people (such as paraplegics or the mentally handicapped) who are achieving the maximum they are capable of are in a sense role models of good health.

In their interesting book *Vitality and Aging* (1981), wellness researchers James Fries and Lawrence Crapo assert that **vitality**, defined as the functioning power of the organism, is in fact the very essence of health. They also argue strongly that vitality is not something available only to the young, but can and will be maintained well into old age, as lifestyles in the United States slowly become more healthful. Maintaining vitality is not automatic, however, but requires attention, vigilance, and effort. And this requirement leads us to another key aspect of health.

Health as Conservation: The Human Spaceship

In the heyday of wonder drugs and magic bullets, it almost seemed as if we could buy health at the drugstore. But those days are gone. The wonder drugs have worked their wonders, reducing the impact of infectious disease by a factor of almost 50:1. More recently, a whole new set of much more difficult health problems has been uncovered.

The health problems that we now face are largely those of chronic disease in a wide variety of forms. These problems do not readily respond to magic bullets and the other tools and techniques available at medical centers. Mainly, these problems are affected by and respond to the **lifestyle** and behavior of each individual.

We must learn to consider our own resources and to rely less on the formal system. Since many of these problems will be around for most or all of our lives, we are, in effect, embarked on a long and somewhat lonesome journey. Each of us has resources that can be partially renewed, but they are not inexhaustible. It is critically important to conserve these resources. Each of us is like a spacecraft, spending long intervals out of the reach of help from our ground support systems and having to rely on ourselves to stay out of trouble, recognize problems, make repairs, and carefully conserve our life support systems.

And there are other important implications of this model. As is true for a spacecraft, each action that we take at a certain point can have consequences far into the future. Many choices can produce irreversible effects and take us down one-way streets on which there is no way back. For example, in most cases alcoholism and other serious addictions produce effects that are never fully reversed. People can be recovering alcoholics for life, but few, once seriously affected by addiction, will ever be able to live as nonaddicts again.

In this era of increasingly important and effective self-care, we have a great opportunity to think about and make wise choices. Perhaps to a larger extent than ever before, the health aspects of our lives are in our own hands. And the choices made in early adult years are perhaps more important than ever before. Health is a process, and the critical time for decisions is yesterday, today, and tomorrow.

Wealthy, Unhealthy Americans

Americans have the highest standard of living in the world in terms of material goods (except for a few very small oil principalities). Yet three major chronic diseases—**arthri-**

Exploring Your Emotions

What makes you feel exuberant?

tis, heart disease, and **diabetes**—partially incapacitate more than 20 million of our citizens. **Atherosclerosis**, a disease almost unknown in some countries, kills some 2,000 Americans every day and sends thousands more to the hospital. Imagine what an uproar would be made if 2,000 people a day were killed in airplane crashes!

Our **infant mortality rate** ranks fifteenth in the world. For men, our life expectancy ranks fourteenth, and for women it is a little better, at sixth. The average U.S. adult is about 20 pounds, or 15 percent, over ideal weight from a health point of view. About one person in six is more than 40 pounds overweight. More than 30 percent of the adult population smokes, in spite of the widespread dissemination of facts on the adverse effects of tobacco use in all its forms. Maybe we are too well off. Clearly, affluence does not equal health.

But there is a bright side to these figures. Many of the trends are favorable. **Coronary heart attack** rates, although still quite high, are down by about 25 percent over the last decade. **Stroke** rates are down by an amazing 40 percent. Average blood pressure levels and average **cholesterol** levels are down by small but significant amounts. Smoking rates are headed down in most segments of the population. (Lung cancer rates are peaking in women, due to the high smoking rates they reached in previous years—one of the unfortunate costs of increasing gender "equality.") These figures indicate that widespread changes in lifestyle have favorably affected health in the recent past and could have even greater positive effects in the years to come.

Other trends, however, are somewhat disturbing. Although the adult population appears to be exercising more and consequently becoming somewhat more fit, fitness in the grade school population appears to be declining, perhaps because children spend too much time in front of the television set. Drug use is rising, and the costs associated with drug use seem to be rising even faster. And of course **AIDS** presents a very difficult problem, unlikely to be fully solved for many years. All these problems, and the favorable trends as well, have a strong behavioral component, and, without question, the direction of the trends in the future is largely in the hands of individuals. With a few exceptions, each individual can be the major factor in his or her present and future health.

Exploring Your Emotions

What kinds of feelings does this picture arouse in you? Can you write a caption for it to suggest its relationship to issues of feeling touched on in this chapter?

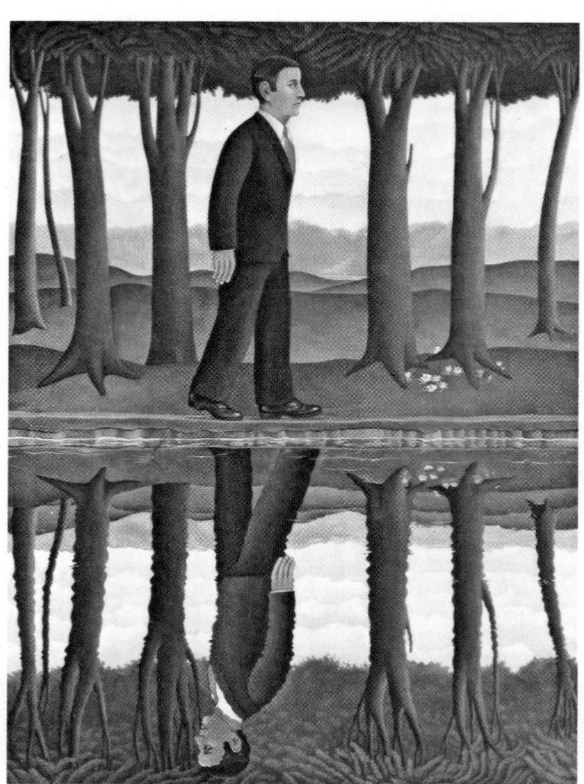

Illustration: Richard Hess

Choosing Optimum Health

Optimum health—you cannot get it from your doctor, your clinic, your astrologist, your lover, a wonder drug, or a miracle diet. You can get it only through what the Chinese call *tzu-li keng-sheng,* or "regeneration through your own efforts." If this effort sounds like too much of a hassle, remember that as you approach optimum health, everything in your life becomes much less trouble. Health is the most important prerequisite for effective functioning.

Given the care it deserves, your body can fully use its remarkable capacity for healing itself and for protecting itself against occasional injuries, and attempted invasions by foreign life forms. It can also give you reserves of energy for peak efforts in the important situations of your life. Perhaps most important, good health will make the sunsets brighter and all the flowers sweeter smelling.

There is no one path to optimum health. Because you are a unique individual, you have unique transactions with both the world that you inherited and the world you are making for yourself. Important results can be obtained only by sustained effort. Become informed, especially about pitfalls. Learn about ways and means. Learn about yourself, your family history, your health strengths and weak-

Diabetes A serious disease characterized by excessive urine output and high blood sugar.

Atherosclerosis A disease in which fatty substances narrow coronary arteries.

Infant mortality rate The number of deaths of infants usually expressed per 100 of live births.

Coronary heart attack A reduction of blood flow to the heart muscle causing damage from lack of oxygen.

Stroke Sudden bleeding in the brain or reduction in blood flow causing brain damage.

Cholesterol The fatty substance implicated in artery disease.

AIDS Acquired immune deficiency syndrome is a fatal disease of the immune system that is caused by a virus and has no known cure.

Emphysema A serious incurable lung disease caused mainly by smoking.

Predisposing factor Usually a hereditary factor encouraging the expression of a trait in a person.

Enabling factor A facilitating or helping factor that influences a person's behavior.

Reinforcing factor A strengthening or supporting factor that influences a person's behavior.

nesses, and your critical health behaviors. True insight can be obtained only by being honest with yourself, by tuning in to what your body is trying to tell you, and by having the wisdom and respect to listen.

What You Don't Know *Will* Hurt You It is important to be informed about the blind alleys and the one-way streets: the pathways from which there is no return. If you ruin your back by age 30, you won't have it to help you at age 40. If you become seriously addicted to alcohol or some other drug, you may possibly become a stable, recovered addict (or you may not) but you probably will never again be able to live as a nonaddict. If you let your bones lose calcium until they break from your own weight, little or nothing can be done. If through smoking or other abuse you develop **emphysema**, you have little hope of reversing a lingering, ten-year decline to death by suffocation.

Modern medical science, in spite of media ballyhoo, has little to offer for these problems after the damage is done. Consider the recent experimentation with artificial hearts in humans. Is this a contribution to the quality of life or a fiasco? Is it something you would like for yourself? It is not possible to buy back health from the drugstore today, and there is no indication that it will be possible within our lifetime. Our best bet is to try to nurture and enhance the very extraordinary human machinery that nature has given all of us.

Being informed is much more important today than it was just ten or twenty years ago, because of the tremendous increase in useful knowledge about wellness and self-care in recent years. Potentially, we have tools in our hands that are very powerful. But to gain the benefit of these tools we have to know about them; we have to be informed about the details of health and what contributes to health.

Moving on to Ways and Means Once you have information to build on, you are ready to look at the behavioral aspects of the problem. Six key steps in the process of health behavior change are discussed one by one in the following sections. Since behavior change is an action-oriented process, actively participate in the procedures discussed by using an example that is meaningful to you.

Organizing for Self-change

To a large extent our health is a direct result of how we live, love, work, and interact with others and with our environment. In short, our health is a reflection or product of how we behave.

All of us behave in some ways that promote our own health and in other ways that put our health at risk. Sometimes we are aware of the implications of what we are doing but too often we are not. While it is very important to be informed about the health benefits or risks inherent in our lifestyles, this is not enough. We also need to understand ourselves and why we behave as we do. The purpose of this chapter is to lay a foundation for understanding how we can maintain the behaviors that contribute to wellness and change behaviors that contribute to health risk.

Changing a health behavior is no simple process. But it gets easier when it is broken into the following six steps.

Exploring Your Emotions

What kinds of behaviors do you want to change to affect your future health? Among your parents' generation, identify some people who are paying the consequences of these same behaviors. How can you use your feelings about such "role models" to change your own behavior?

In this review of behavioral techniques, you will learn how to identify and change **predisposing**, **enabling**, and **reinforcing factors** that may be influencing your behavior. Your likelihood of achieving interesting results and lasting success will be determined by how well you learn and are able to apply these practical self-management techniques.

Internal stimuli Any factor that arouses activity from within the person.

External stimuli Any factor that arouses activity from outside the person.

Why Do You Behave as You Do?

Before you consider ways of changing a particular behavior or habit, first find out all you can about it. Compile information about your behavior. Then analyze the information. What provokes the behavior? When are you most vulnerable? How do outside factors influence your behavior?

Self-monitoring and Data Collection Most behavior change experts ask their clients to begin by keeping careful records of the circumstances that surround a particular behavior. These records are usually kept in a health diary. They provide a practical basis for understanding and analyzing what is going on, since most of us are not fully aware of the situational factors that set our adverse behaviors in motion.

In general, you should include a brief note on what the activity was, when the activity happened, and what your feelings were at the time. In a diary of a weight loss program, for example, you would typically record the amount of food you consumed, the time of day, situation, location, your feelings, and the intensity of your hunger. (See Figure 1-1.) Such health behavior diaries often can provide clues to changes that might improve your behavior patterns. Later in this chapter we will consider ways in which your health diary can lead you to specific self-management strategies.

Select any habit, such as smoking, overeating, poor study habits, shyness, test anxiety, or any other behavior that is creating a problem for you. Keep a diary on this problem for one or two weeks. The object will be to identify the **internal** and **external stimuli** that lead to this particular behavior.

Exploring Your Emotions

How do you think this man got where he is today?

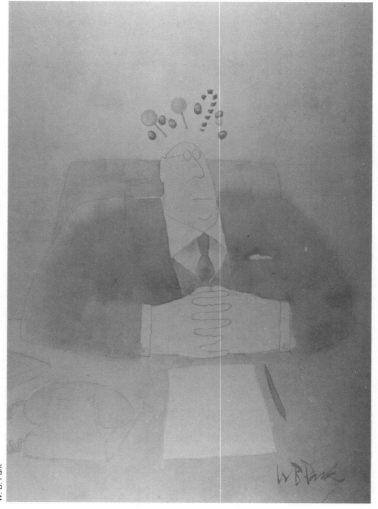

W. B. Park

Figure 1-1 Daily Eating Behavior Record

DATE Sept 23 DAY (M) TU W TH F SA SU

Time of Day	M/S	Food Eaten	Cals.	Hunger Rating (0–3)	Speed (1–4)	Where did you eat?	What else were you doing	How did someone else influence you?	What made you want to eat what you did?	Emotions and feelings?	Thoughts and concerns?
7:30	M	1 oz. shredded wheat ½ c. skim milk	110 40 150	3	1	kitchen	reading paper	eating alone	time for breakfast, shredded wheat has no sugar	a little excited	thinking about project, want to get going
10:20	S	1 peach	40	1	4	office	working	alone	fuzzy, need a break, brought peach to work	slight headache	how to solve problem, puzzled
11:45	M	Tuna melt: 2 sl. bread 3 oz. tuna 2 tsp. mayo 2 oz. cheese 2 tsp. butter 2 glasses of wine, 6 oz. ea.	 140 165 90 200 90 300 985	1	2	restaurant	talking	Pat ordered tuna melt, so I did too!	didn't want to feel left out	excited, happy	anxious to hear latest gossip
4:30	S	5 wheat thins	125	2	2	office	thinking	alone	need break, wheat thins handy	sleepy, mentally tired	what to have for dinner
4:40	S	4 wheat thins	100	0	2	office	still thinking	alone	first one tasted good	still tired	need to cut down on calories
6:30	S	1 glass wine 6 oz.	150	1	1	living room	talking with husband	hubby had drink, so I did too	it's relaxing	drink makes me feel relaxed	talking about vacation plans
9:00	M	Lean Cuisine Salad dressing 1 tbs.	300 35 135 470	3	2	living room	watching TV	he suggested Lean Cuisine	was in freezer	relaxed but getting tired	nothing, just TV show
		Total for day:	2020								

Medications:

Self-assessment and Data Analysis After you have collected data on a particular bothersome habit, analyze the data to identify patterns in stimuli and responses. Perhaps you are especially hungry late in the afternoon. Discover the time of day that hunger strikes. Do you find that you drink more alcohol at a party than anywhere else? That wouldn't be particularly surprising. But do you drink more at certain kinds of parties, or when with certain friends?

Discover how you react to the environment and the personal factors. Do you find that you crave a cigarette more right after dinner than at any other time of day? Do you find that your craving for a cigarette is much stronger when someone else lights up at some especially critical time? Once you have identified the interaction between your feelings and external stimuli such as location, time of day, situation, and actions of significant others, you can design strategies to divert your behavior in new directions.

Implementing a Change

If you've tried the suggested self-monitoring procedures, you may have found a need to modify your health behavior. Using a diary and other self-assessment tools, you have had a chance to identify some of the factors that contribute to the problem. The next steps in the development of your behavior change program include setting goals, making a personal contract with yourself, planning alternative responses, and developing a system of personal incentives and rewards to support your efforts.

Set Specific Goals Assuming that you have a fairly definite idea about where you want to go in changing your behavior, the next question is what route you should take in getting there and how to stay on the track as you proceed. It is helpful to analyze the ultimate goal and break it into several relatively small sequential steps, or "chunks." As you proceed, you will need mileposts to measure your progress just as you would count the miles or cities you pass on a long trip.

For example, if you decide to quit smoking you may want to line up a series of steps to get ready (such as assessing readiness to quit, reasons for quitting, and patterns in your previous attempts to quit), with milestones for each step. If you plan to lose 30 pounds, you will find it easier to accomplish if you proceed in 10-pound stages. Take the easy steps first, then move progressively to what is harder. By carefully setting goals, you can increase the probability of your eventual success.

Make a Personal Contract Once you have set an objective and developed a plan of action, it is a good idea to summarize your plan in a personal contract. A serious personal contract specifies resources, time, energy, and

(continued on p. 13)

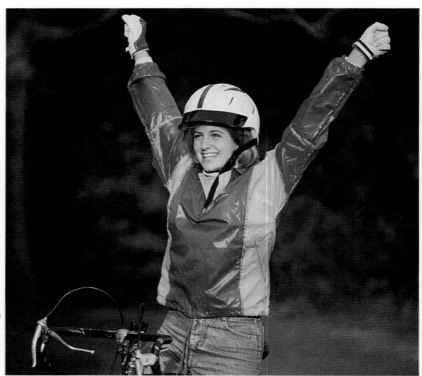

Richard Hutchings

Personal Contracts for Change

All of us are familiar with the power of signed contracts. Documentation in black and white that commits our word, money, and/or property carries a strong impact and results in a higher chance of follow-through than casual, offhand assurances or promises. Contracts can be used to try to change a health behavior if they include the time, date, and details of the change program. Some target behaviors, such as quitting smoking or losing extra pounds, lend themselves to contracts with very specific goals. Often a witness is also asked to sign the contract; this helps to set in motion the support and encouragement of a social network. A recent program in which all participants gave their formal commitment over citywide television resulted in much-higher-than-normal levels of change. Contracts reduce procrastination by specifying the dates and other details of the behavioral tasks and goals. They also act as reminders of a personal commitment to change. Here is an example of a behavioral contract for smoking.

Contract for Stopping by Yourself

Many people can stop smoking with little difficulty. In fact, they may have considerable experience with quitting in the past. If this corresponds to your smoking history, then you should follow the rules presented here.

Rule 1 Set a specific date and time for quitting, and write this in your personal contract. The time could be as early as three days from now or as far away as next week, whichever you prefer. This date and time (early in the morning or in the evening) should be listed in the target date box. Of course, you should follow through with the date, once chosen, and actually stop smoking at that time.

Rule 2 Three days before your target date, you should cut your daily smoking in half. For example, if you smoke 20 cigarettes per day, then you should reduce that total to only 10 cigarettes daily for the three-day period. Do NOT try to gradually reduce your smoking down to zero, however, because this will actually increase the value of each remaining cigarette and make your attempt to quit extremely frustrating. This rule is based on strong clinical evidence, so we urge you not to gradually go to zero cigarettes per day.

Rule 3 When you reach your target date, you may want to throw away all your cigarettes. Some people like to make a ceremony out of this event. If you feel that you will panic unless you have cigarettes available somewhere (even if they are in the garage, the trunk of the car, or the attic), then you should follow your own inclinations. That is particularly true if these methods have been at least temporarily helpful to you in the past.

Rule 4 Try not to make too much out of quitting. Do not magnify it out of proportion because this may make you experience more stress and other withdrawal effects.

Rule 5 Once you have reached your target date and have successfully stopped smoking, remember to continue keeping track of smoking urges in your smoking diary.

Contract for Stopping with Help from Others

The second method for stopping smoking involves arranging a contract with yourself and another person, preferably a trusted friend. The contract would involve a commitment on your part to stop smoking as of a particular date and hour following three days of reduced smoking—half the usual level—as was described in the previous section. In this case, however, you also build in an added incentive—the possible loss of

My Personal Contract for Quitting

I agree to stop all smoking on __________ *at* __________ *. I understand that it*
(target date) *(target time)*
is important for me to make a strong personal effort at this particular time so that I can become a permanent ex-smoker. I sign this contract as an indication of my personal commitment to stop smoking on target.

________________ __________
(your signature) *(date of signing)*

Personal Contracts for Change (*continued*)

money! The contract states that you [deposit a specified sum of money, which you will forfeit] if you fail to stop smoking. But you will receive portions of the deposit back as "payment" if you become an ex-smoker.

This contract arrangement can work without the help of others; you may act as your own banker for the agreement. But many people find that asking assistance of a friend helps them stick to their contract. Of course, it is important that this friend be trusted, because putting up your money and its repayment must be governed strictly by the written contract. This friend, the "banker" in your contract, should not be a smoker and should not attempt to tell you how to quit.

There are several rules for developing a contract with the help of others as a method for stopping smoking.

(*Your copy*)

Two-Party Contract for Quitting

I agree to stop smoking on ________ *at* ________ *. I have given the sum of*
(*target date*) (*target time*)
$ ________ *to* ________ *with the understanding that he/she will send the money*
(*banker's name*)
to ________ *if I am unable to stop smoking according to this agreement. If I am*
(*organization*)
able to stop smoking completely for the first week after the target date specified above, I will at that time receive half of the deposit back. The remaining portion of the deposit will be returned after the second week of nonsmoking (two weeks from the target date).

________ ________
(*your signature*) (*date*)

________ ________
(*banker's signature*) (*date*)

(*Banker's copy*)

Two-Party Contract for Quitting

I agree to stop smoking on ________ *at* ________ *. I have given the sum of*
(*target date*) (*target time*)
$ ________ *to* ________ *with the understanding that he/she will send the money*
(*banker's name*)
to ________ *if I am unable to stop smoking according to the agreement. If I am*
(*organization*)
able to stop smoking completely for the first week after the target date specified above, I will at that time receive half of the deposit back. The remaining portion of the deposit will be returned after the second week of nonsmoking (two weeks from the target date).

________ ________
(*your signature*) (*date*)

________ ________
(*banker's signature*) (*date*)

Rule 1 Risk an amount of money that would hurt you if it were forfeited. Five dollars would very likely be small and insignificant to you if it were lost; $50 or $100 is more significant!

Rule 2 Choose the banker with great care. He or she can be any nonsmoker you trust, who is willing to help by taking responsibility for keeping your deposit.

Rule 3 Once the contract is signed, stick to it. There should be no changes made in the target date and the monetary agreement, because changes undermine the effectiveness of this entire procedure.

Rule 4 Decide with great care what will be done with any forfeited money. The money must *not* go to your banker. Instead, it should be payable to either a favorite charity or, even better, your least favorite organization—one you would hate to see get your good money! Write checks in advance with the name of the least favorite organization for the banker to hold, so that payment is almost automatic if you smoke. These strategies provide a powerful incentive for you to uphold the contract.

Rule 5 Use the contract presented here. One side should be signed by you and become your copy; it remains in this book. The other copy is kept by the trusted banker as his or her copy of the contract.

B. G. Danaher and E. Lichtenstein
Become an Ex-Smoker

Intrinsic rewards Personal satisfaction or benefits achieved as a result of improved behavior.

Incentives Any motive or stimulus that encourages a person to action.

Rebates Money returned from an amount placed in trust after achieving a milestone.

Cost-effective Achieving a maximum result with minimum cost.

---

priorities to reach your goals. The contract should record your commitment, your objective, and the mileposts against which you will measure your progress. To help you begin, the contract should identify exactly what your first step will be and on exactly what day and time it will take place. A useful addition is to have a witness to the contract, who may also be an active participant of some sort, or possibly an umpire or a banker.

You can include other behavior change strategies in your personal contract. How you plan to reorganize your time, rewards for following your plan, support from family and friends, and alternative responses are examples of tactics we shall discuss in further detail. But the important thing for you to remember is that the purpose of the personal contract is to help you be as specific as possible. In essence, you can develop a blueprint or guide for accomplishing change.

You may need a series of small contracts, or one big one with a number of check points. In either case, start by identifying your first goal and then lay out your subgoals. Be sure that your first subgoal includes a starting and completion date and time and a clear description of what you hope to accomplish.

Establish Rewards Think about how you get yourself to tackle any difficult job. What is the long-range payoff? What are the rewards and satisfactions that you get as you go along? Sometimes **intrinsic rewards** for improvement in health behaviors lie too far in the future or are too hard to measure. You can increase the immediate **incentives** by rewarding yourself for good behavior or penalizing yourself for bad behavior.

As you begin a project, decide on a reward you can earn with six months of diligent effort, or the attainment of certain behavioral goals. Note this reward on a piece of paper and put it in your wallet or your project notebook. Your reward could be a new dress or suit to go with a new figure, or it could be a bicycle purchased with money saved by not buying cigarettes. The "grand" prize does not have to be expensive, but it should be personally meaningful.

Some experts like the so-called blackmail approach, where you put a significant amount of dollars or other assets in trust, which will be given to a cause that you hate if you fail to reach your goal. Monetary rewards can be a motivator, such as **rebates** given for successfully completing weight loss or stop-smoking courses. Competition can be a highly effective incentive in several modes: competing against yourself, competing against one or more buddies or running mates, or joining a contest among naturally competitive groups such as departments of an organization.

Think carefully about the criteria for deciding when a reward is due. In most situations, the greatest rewards should be for reaching specific objectives toward improving your vitality. For example, plan to treat yourself to a movie after you have finished your first three-mile race in good time. But also plan to reward good behavior if it is consistent and persistent, because that behavior is moving you toward the vitality goal.

Develop a list of rewarding activities that are inexpensive and preferably unrelated to food or alcohol—activities you can enjoy as much or more than snacking, smoking, or drinking. Treat yourself to a concert, go to the ball game, buy a good record you've been wanting, or a fancy shirt, or whatever. Find out what works for you. Be creative. You can identify and effectively apply reinforcing factors that support your good behavior. Sometimes it is quite helpful to enlist a friend in this process.

Maximize Return on Investment One of the best ways to reward constructive health behaviors is to try to make them **cost-effective.** In a temporary surge of enthusiasm to improve ourselves, we often tend to overdo or to undertake activities where the efforts may outweigh the potential gain. First of all, be sure that the proposed new behavior has a real and lasting value for you personally. Without that ingredient, no behavior change project can be a success.

But there are often many ways to pursue a given goal. Different levels of effort can be used. Usually an effort that is quite moderate but sustained is the best. There are often a large number of mechanisms. Physical fitness can be pursued in many ways, for example. One or two of these are likely to fit your needs and time schedules much better than the others. If you can integrate the new activity smoothly into your existing schedule, you can make a significant gain in cost-effectiveness. Sometimes you can kill more than one bird with the same stone. Exercise may increase physical fitness and help cure mild depression at the same time. Creatively look for ways to move toward your objectives while being economical of your own time and effort. If you create a program that seems cost-effective to you, you have taken a giant step toward success.

Antecedents of health behaviors Preceding events that provide insight into a particular behavior.

Co-factors Related factors that contribute to a certain behavior or event.

Negative reinforcing factors Factors that contribute to unwanted behavior, decreasing the probability of a desired response.

Aerobic exercise Active exercise that conditions the heart and lungs by increasing the body's efficiency of oxygen intake.

Commitment A promise or pledge to achieve something in the future.

Staying on the Track

As you go about making some long-term change in your health behavior, you will want to develop strategies for staying on track. One of the best ways to do so is by a system of periodic checks and activity records that provide a basis for (1) monitoring status and trends and (2) comparing actual results to plans.

Using Your Health Diary The health diary has already been suggested as a way to gain insight into the **antecedents of health behaviors.** However, its value doesn't end there. It can also continue to keep you aware of progress or lack of progress and alert you to weak points in your behavior change program.

Trace the Habit Chain Using the data gathered in the early stages of your program, trace the whole chain of events—for example, from your purchase of snack foods to your consumption of them. At several places along this chain, you can choose an alternative response. What factors triggered the purchase to begin with? Once the snacks were in your home, what situations made them especially attractive? What situations tended to lead to excessive consumption? What **co-factors** were at work that could be changed?

Monitor Your Progress Just as you would check off cities as you pass by them on a long trip, you will want to keep track of your progress toward goals by using the mileposts you have established. The best way to track this information is by keeping a diary or log. Record your daily activities and your weekly progress against your goals. Each week chart your progress on a graph. You may want to track a couple of variables, rather than just a single one. For example, because exercise can be very beneficial in a weight control program, you might want to chart your weekly exercise activity and your weight on the same page. Post your progress graph on your dresser mirror, the refrigerator door, or in some other equally conspicuous place.

Exploring Your Emotions

How do you feel about the self-change strategies presented in this chapter? Which ones appeal most to you? Can you suggest any others that might be added to this list?

Self-management Despite our human frailties and the pressures of stress and other external influences, we all can exert a good deal of control over our lives. Self-management is a skill we can all develop if we allow ourselves to be creative, perceptive, and flexible.

Control Environmental Stimuli At the beginning of a lifestyle change program, you may find yourself especially sensitive to environmental stimuli. If you have just stopped smoking, arrange to spend most of your time in places where smoking is absent or restricted and with nonsmoking friends. Discuss your change program with friends and family and agree ahead of time on the rules of the game. Ask them not to offer you excluded items, and, if they have to snack or smoke or otherwise create bad examples, leave the room until they have finished.

For the first few weeks of a program, you may want to avoid social gatherings where you are likely to be tempted to overindulge. Carefully weigh the roles that sight, smell, mood, situation, and accessibility play in triggering your response. You can control environmental stimuli or **negative reinforcing factors** by arranging to have excluded items out of sight, in highly inconvenient locations, or best of all, out of the house. You also can rearrange the critical situations themselves, breaking up activity patterns that have been leading to the unwanted behavior.

Control Related Behavior Avoid other habits that may be linked to the habit that you are changing. For example, alcohol has the effect of increasing appetite, and people also tend to eat when they drink. Excessive TV watching and eating away from the table are often linked to heavy snacking. When trying to squelch an unhealthy habit, it often helps to substitute something healthy, such as low-calorie (but tasty) snacks for high-calorie ones, or **aerobic exercise** and music for beer, snacks, and TV.

Plan and Rehearse Alternative Responses Try to anticipate temptation and to work out ways to deal with it through practical alternatives. Inevitably, if you recently became an ex-smoker, someone will offer you a cigarette. Mentally rehearse a polite refusal. At a party, plan your drinking ahead of time and switch to a mixer to avoid encouragement to drink more than you feel you want. If you go out to eat, decide ahead of time what you will eat and stick to your decision. Don't be afraid to ask for the food combinations, preparation, dressings, and so on that you want. If you feel that you deserve a special reward or that you must have some relief from an austere program you have set for yourself, go out for it—do it outside your regular environment. Go and celebrate with some ice cream, but don't buy a half gallon to keep in the freezer.

Control Stress in Your Life The stress of heavy efforts, critical events, or even everyday living can derail your change program. Stress rarely is totally absent in modern life. Analyze the present and potential sources of stress that you encounter, and the role that stress may play in the behavior that you are working on. Chapter 2 of this book discusses stress and includes a stress scale that allows you to measure stressful events and their probable intensity in your life.

People often use overeating, drinking, or smoking as techniques for managing stress in their lives. Plan to explore some healthier ways to reduce tension caused by stress. For example, many people find that relaxation and regular exercise are effective ways to manage stress.

Maintaining the Commitment

It is easier to maintain lasting **commitment** to behavior change if you develop positive but realistic expectations at the beginning and get others to support and help you.

Shaping Your Expectations Shakespeare wrote, "There is nothing either good or bad, but thinking makes it so." What we think or expect will happen often does happen. If we are optimistic about our ultimate success, the chances are that this attitude will improve the probability of success. At the same time it is important to be realistic. Lasting behavior change takes time. Being human, we are bound to slip occasionally. But we can learn from our mistakes and from other people with similar problems.

Expect Success Think thin or think of yourself as a nonsmoker. Change your identity from a fat person to a thin person. How would a thin person react to a particular problem situation? Formerly overweight people often carry a fat self-image around for years after they have lost weight. This "fat person" is always eager to say, "I told you so!" Your expectations can have very strong effects on your behavior. Think of yourself as a thin person or a nonsmoker and begin to behave accordingly.

Expect Change to Take Time Fad diets may promise "instant" weight loss. In reality, weight loss and most other significant vitality changes are long-term projects that take many weeks, accomplished one day at a time. Most of the people who have quit smoking did not quit forever on the first try or even the second. Expect change to take time and to have inevitable ups and downs. Expect plateaus, since they are a natural part of all learning processes. If you don't give up on yourself, plateaus can be periods of consolidation and preparation for the next step forward. Plan to be persistent and work your way through the doldrums.

Forgive and Forget Suppose you are losing weight and go on an eating binge. You could then conclude that you are, and always will be, "fat and ugly"—why keep on trying? Or you can look at the binge as a problem to be expected once in a while, try to discover what set it off, and develop a plan to deal with similar situations in the future; a binge is not a catastrophe, but a problem to be solved. Be forgiving of occasional missteps. Observe and analyze them in a nonjudgmental way and avoid the self-destructive effects of guilt.

Use a Role Model Find someone who possesses what you are striving for. This person might be a celebrity, a sports figure, someone in your immediate family or your family tree, or a friend. Why do you admire this person? How would this person respond to the situation you are struggling with? Talk to people you know who have successfully maintained aerobic fitness or weight loss, have stopped smoking, or have broken a serious drug habit. See if you can find someone with a handicap who has achieved a high degree of fitness in spite of problems much more difficult than yours. What strategies have worked for these people? How can you borrow from their experience?

Recruit Support Some people inspire us by their achievements, but others who are not necessarily role models can actively help us reach our goals by their support and assistance. It is somewhat surprising that one of the few things that successful chief executives have in common is a supportive spouse. Similarly, people working on behavior change programs come in all shapes and sizes but they are much more likely to be successful if they have a support person or group.

Exploring Your Emotions

How do you feel about the health risks related to your intended occupation? How could you use those feelings for your future benefit?

Find Yourself a Buddy Using the "buddy system" has many advantages. If you check the people around, you are likely to find someone who wants to make some changes similar to those you are making. You may have to look no further than your roommate, classmate, or family. Recruit one or more friends to participate in your plans for a lifestyle change. Or if that seems impractical, consider joining one or another group that forms a ready-made set of buddies for the problem at hand, such as Weight Watchers.

A buddy can serve as a second set of eyes and ears for learning, a monitor, a sympathetic listener, a running mate (literally), and someone who is interested in your progress. Things tend to go easier when you have a buddy. It's easier to run on a cold morning when you know that someone else will be doing it with you. And a little friendly competition can be fun as long as it isn't taken too seriously. In a crisis situation, you can ask your buddy to help you overcome the urge to smoke, gorge on snacks, take drugs, or whatever. For some problems, such as alcoholism, the buddy system (in the form of Alcoholics Anonymous) is the most successful of all methods that have been tried.

Recruit Support from Family and Friends Since lifestyle is a family affair, it obviously makes sense to encourage your whole family to get into the act. Friends with whom you spend a lot of time are similar sources of support. Ask for specific kinds of assistance. Encourage significant others to be active, interested participants, and to be part of a direct support network. Remind them not to do things that cause you to "break training" and not to be hurt if you have to refuse something when they forget. Properly oriented, your family and other close associates can be a powerful source of reward, encouragement, and objective feedback. By building such a network, you can positively influence the reinforcing factors for the behavior changes that you undertake.

Realistically, it is important to recognize that in some instances a given family member may be totally uninterested in the whole idea of health or, even worse, may have an emotional stake in preserving the behavior that you are trying to change. Solving such a problem is beyond the scope of this book, but obviously such individuals are best left out of your behavior change program until the inherent conflicts can be resolved.

Exploring Your Emotions

Do your concerns for your health and for the health behaviors you want to establish conflict with the general feelings of your friends? How can you handle potential conflicts in this area?

Troubleshooting the Bugs

It is not unlikely that you will encounter various problems on your way to your behavior change goal. Don't be surprised or overly concerned. In fact, it's not a bad idea to expect problems and to schedule an occasional stopping point in your program where you step back, review how you are doing, and make some changes to accommodate the problems that you find.

Identifying and Getting Past Barriers As you review your situation at such a stopping point, you are likely to find that the problems you are having fall into one of the following categories.

Social Influences Social influences are a likely source of problems. While your family and associates can be very helpful when they are "with you," they can also be a part of the problem. Often, they have been part of the problem to start with, and some may not be interested in or willing to change. Look closely at this and consider putting further efforts into network building.

Level of Commitment Be sure that your level of commitment is sufficient. No real progress is likely until you are really convinced that you want to commit to the goal. You may have to wait a while until the problem you are dealing with becomes more oppressive, or you may find that a modified goal has more power to command your sustained interest.

Ineffective Techniques The techniques you are using may not be as suitable as you assumed in your original planning. Review them in the light of experience and make changes where you are having the most trouble. Behavior change is an **empirical** process, and there are usually many ways to move toward your objective.

Level of Effort Consider your level of effort. You may be using techniques that are appropriate but may not be putting in enough effort. The slogan "No gain without pain" may be overdoing it, but in some sense you need to "sweat," to really push toward your goal.

Motivation Levels Examine your level of motivation. You need to have that internal thrust toward action that comes from good motivation. Motivation is a combination of desire, belief in success, and support, so look at these components and try to find ways to build them up if they are a problem.

Procrastination Simple **procrastination** may be part of the problem. One way to get around procrastination is to break the program down into still smaller steps and force

Empirical Describing a process based on observation or experience.

Procrastination Intentionally postponing something that should be done right away.

Rationalization A superficial excuse or explanation for one's behavior.

yourself to take the small steps one at a time. Don't be too perfectionistic. Set firm dates and proceed one day at a time.

Stress Barrier Stress in your life may be a barrier to pursuing the goal. If the stress is temporary, you may want to wait until it has cleared before putting major effort into a change program. If the stress is a more or less permanent feature of your life, it may be necessary to work on your stress management skills as the first step in any program designed to improve your vitality.

Self-deception You may find that you are telling yourself things that don't quite jibe with the facts when you look at them closely. Be sure to do some careful checks of reality and watch out for excuses, excessive "explanations," and other forms of **rationalization.** In self-care, the only one you are fooling is yourself, so anything "won" by deception is a hollow victory indeed.

Blaming Versus Action Excessive blaming is a common form of self-deception. You may find that instead of taking action you are blaming yourself, others around you, handicaps that you have, or the "system." Certainly all these things can be factors for you, as for anyone else. But consider what those far more handicapped than you have done, and think through the problem again, this time with the emphasis on action.

Outside Sources of Help You can probably find substantial resources in your community to provide additional help. On campus, courses in personal health, physical fitness, stress management, and weight control are often available. The student health center or campus counseling center may also be a source of assistance. In most locales, a wide variety of low-cost community services are available through adult education, school programs, health departments, and private agencies. Consult the Yellow Pages, your local health department, or the Referral Service often sponsored by the United Way.

Being Healthy for Life

Your first few improvement projects may be just that, projects. They may not all succeed. But as a few of these projects do succeed and you begin to see progress and changes, something is likely to happen. You will experience new and surprising positive feelings about yourself. You probably will find that you are less vulnerable to stress. You may begin to enjoy new kinds of social activities and friends. You may discover that you have things in common with new groups of people that you haven't thought about very much before. You may find yourself accomplishing things you never thought possible, such as winning a race, climbing a mountain, having muscles that show, and so forth. Enter that race, and wear your T-shirt proudly.

Basically, you can become involved in a new way of life that will help to sustain you for life. Being more healthy takes effort, but it returns energy and an improved ability to function that pays the effort back with interest. It is a lifetime job, so you do need to organize yourself for the long pull.

Plan for a Lifetime Assume that health improvement is forever. Tackle one subject at a time, but make a careful inventory of your health strengths and weaknesses, and lay out a long-range plan. Take the easier problems first, and then use what you have learned to address more

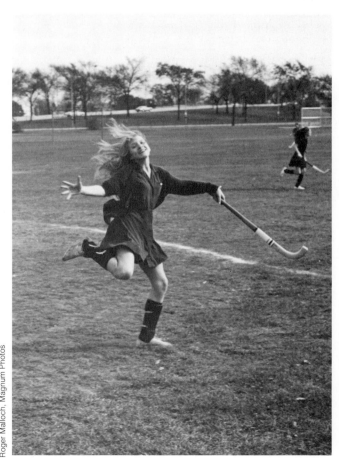
Roger Malloch, Magnum Photos

difficult areas. Maintain vigilance over past problems, continuing to monitor yourself for a long time after the problem has been nominally solved. Knowledge about wellness is progressing rapidly, so try to stay up with trends as they affect things you are interested in. Realize that many of the most important health problems have a mental health component, and become familiar with these aspects of health.

Assume there will be setbacks, and work your way through them. Be careful not to be overzealous and create problems in the process of trying to solve them. Exercise needs particular care. Moderation is the key. There are many ways to improve fitness without injuring yourself. Get familiar with the latest.

Change the Environment Around You Use what you have learned to help create an environment around you that supports a healthy lifestyle. Become an advocate of nonsmoking in public areas, more nutritious food in vending machines, more supportive environments in the workplace, moderate approaches to drug use, and so forth. Persuade your drinking buddies to play more and drink less at the regular Friday night party. Lobby for better facilities, such as a pool, an indoor track, or campus bicycle trails. Get involved in special activities, such as fun runs and health fairs. You will be part of a trend that is likely to have major effects on the American scene in the next couple of decades. And you have the opportunity to truly be one of the "healthy Americans."

Take Action

Your placement level on the wellness ladder will, we hope, encourage you to begin a process of self-exploration and self-discovery that you will continue. Reflect on the entire chapter's content and ask yourself how each point relates to your own life. Then take action:

1. Start a Take Action for Health notebook. List the positive behaviors that have helped to enhance your health. Consider what additions you can make to the list or how you can strengthen or reinforce the behaviors that have helped you. Don't forget to congratulate yourself for these positive aspects of your life. Next list the behaviors that block your achieving wellness. Consider each of these behaviors and decide which ones you can change. Begin with the easiest ones first.

2. Review the general techniques for accomplishing change that were presented in this chapter and discuss them in class or with a close friend. What conclusions can you draw?

3. Find a person (or people) who has the same problem you have (smoking, overweight, and so on). Invite that person to join you in a self-help strategy to deal effectively with the problem. Set specific goals, make a personal contract, and establish rewards.

4. Think about what troubled you most during the past week. In your notebook, write down the names of three or four people who might be able to help you with whatever troubled you. If the problem persists, consider starting at the top of your list and talking to this person about it.

Selected References

Fries, James F., and Crapo, Lawrence M. 1981. *Vitality and Aging*. New York: W. H. Freeman and Co.

Fuchs, Victor. 1974. *Who Shall Live? Health Economics and Social Choice*. New York: Basic Books.

Healthline, A monthly newsletter. 1149 Chestnut St. Suite 10, Menlo Park, Calif., 94025.

Healthy People: The Surgeon General's Report on Health Promotion and Disease Prevention. U.S. Department of Health, Education and Welfare, DHEW Publication No. 79-55071.

Hiatt, Howard H. 1987. *America's Health in the Balance: Choice or Chance?* New York: Harper & Row.

Chapter 2

Contents

Rate Yourself

Your Stress Level Read the following statements carefully. Choose the one in each section that best describes you at this moment and record its score at the right. (For example, "Some stress but coping well" has a score of 4.) When you have chosen one statement for each section, add the numbers and record your total. Find your position on the Wellness Ladder.

5 Free from symptoms of stress
4 Some stress but coping well
3 Slightly uncomfortable stress
2 Fairly heavy stress
1 Severe stress

5 Highly productive
4 Productive
3 Efficient
2 Inefficient
1 Highly unproductive

5 Quickly responsive to change
4 Adaptable to change
3 Tolerant of change
2 Resistant to change
1 Distressed by change

5 Very decisive
4 Decisive
3 Somewhat hesitant
2 Indecisive
1 Very indecisive

5 Regularly enjoys recreation
4 Plans recreation time
3 Has trouble getting away to relax
2 Rarely makes vacation time
1 Seldom enjoys vacations

Total Score ______

Stress and the Social Environment

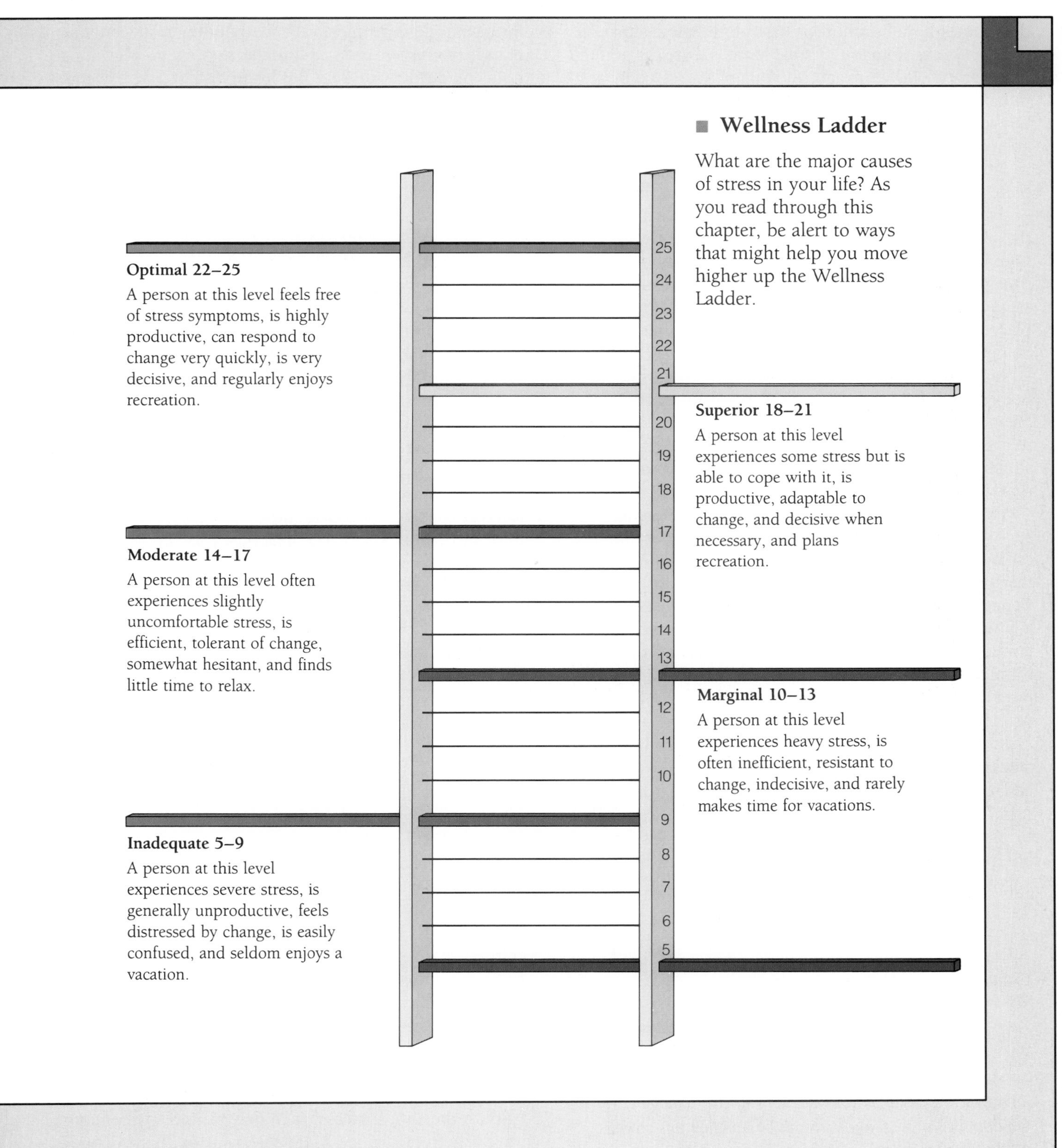

Optimal 22–25

A person at this level feels free of stress symptoms, is highly productive, can respond to change very quickly, is very decisive, and regularly enjoys recreation.

Moderate 14–17

A person at this level often experiences slightly uncomfortable stress, is efficient, tolerant of change, somewhat hesitant, and finds little time to relax.

Inadequate 5–9

A person at this level experiences severe stress, is generally unproductive, feels distressed by change, is easily confused, and seldom enjoys a vacation.

Wellness Ladder

What are the major causes of stress in your life? As you read through this chapter, be alert to ways that might help you move higher up the Wellness Ladder.

Superior 18–21

A person at this level experiences some stress but is able to cope with it, is productive, adaptable to change, and decisive when necessary, and plans recreation.

Marginal 10–13

A person at this level experiences heavy stress, is often inefficient, resistant to change, indecisive, and rarely makes time for vacations.

To be alive is to be under **stress.** Biological stress and psychosocial, or cultural, stress are intertwined and integral to life itself. How we respond to the common and uncommon events and circumstances of our lives largely determines how healthful or destructive these situations will be. As the Roman Emperor Marcus Aurelius pointed out nearly 2,000 years ago, "If you are distressed by anything external, the pain is not due to the thing itself but to your estimate of it. This you have the power to revoke at any time."

Life is dependent, precariously so, on ceaseless **metabolic activity.** The body is constantly subject to the process of change, growth, degradation, and replacement. But, all the while, it tries to maintain a dynamic steady state, or **homeostasis.** Anything, whether internal or external, that disrupts this steady state stresses the organism. If that steady state is to be restored, adaptive reactions must take place. Life is, in a sense, just one adaptation after another. Sometimes the **adaptive reaction**, or defense mechanism, is misdirected; the mind-body signals can misfire. The body's remarkable system of self-regulating checks and balances does not always work perfectly. If our responses to events and circumstances are too weak, it offers inadequate protection; if they are too strong, it overreacts, so that we harm ourselves.

Virtually all of us engage in a daily masquerade, constantly intermeshing with other people's needs, moods, assumptions, bodies, and demands. To be natural, spontaneous, whole, and supportive in our socially conditioned world is hardly easy. Even nonconformists are usually not the free spirits they aim to be: they have merely traded one set of conventions for another, and they conform closely to this new set. And if free spirits are scarce, rarer still are those who can leaven their need for independence with commitment and compassion.

In our society, maintaining social relationships often takes priority over preserving physical health. We tend to behave as though our primary function is to fulfill the social roles that we have chosen or have been compelled to play. Yet the demands of these social roles, and of interpersonal relations, have given rise to some hefty biological challenges.

Exploring Your Emotions

Take a moment to write down the circumstances involved when you last got terribly angry. What caused your distress? What did you do to adjust to this stress? List as many coping techniques that you used as you can remember. Would you say that you successfully handled this stress? What constitutes successful adaptation to stress?

We have no grounds for saying point-blank that life is more stressful now than ever before, yet the fallacy of "the good old days" lives on. Granted, we live in a world of seemingly endless turmoil and inequity, a world in which, for instance, governments spend about the same amount of money every year on children as they spend every two hours on deadly weapons. But history is filled with events and conditions so appalling as to defy our imagination. Many people in the past lived under such stressful circumstances as to make most of our own anxieties and discomforts pale by comparison. Today the mass media instantly and constantly inform us of ills all over the world, and this, added to our personal woes (real or imagined), may well give the impression that life has never before been so stressful.

Is life truly more stressful now than in the past? Why do some individuals become ill under mildly stressful conditions while others seem to thrive under considerable stress and some even seek more stressful situations? When is stress harmful and when is it harmless and even helpful?

These questions do not have conclusive answers. Nevertheless, some of the stress felt in modern society clearly is different in quality and quantity from stress felt in the past, and misdirected adaptations to the social environment can help trigger possibly unhealthful physiological reactions. It is also clear, however, that we can control to a surprising degree our responses to life situations, thereby not only preserving but also, perhaps, enhancing our physical and mental health.

Biological Versus Cultural Evolution

The human being, unlike any other organism, is the product of two evolutionary systems: the biological one, which is inborn, and the cultural one, which is learned. Culture consists not only of ideas, beliefs, and institutions but also of material objects and the know-how and technology to produce those objects.

The machine technology that has so dramatically changed life has appeared only in the last fraction of our history. Biological evolution has moved at an exceedingly slow but fairly steady rate over the eons. But the rate of cultural change, suddenly picking up speed through technological innovations, has accelerated at an astonishing pace in a relatively brief time. Minor and infrequent technological changes can be absorbed rather easily. But the rate of change characteristic of Western technology is so great that our hearts have trouble keeping up with our heads.

With the appearance of each new technology comes a wave of cultural change. Our relationship with the natural environment is affected to various degrees by this change,

Stress The sum of the biological reactions to any stimulus—pleasant or unpleasant; physical, mental, or emotional; internal or external—that tends to disturb the organism's homeostasis.

Metabolic activity Chemical and physical processes that involve the body's use of food to convert nutrients into energy.

Homeostasis A state of stability and consistency in the physiological functioning of an organism.

Adaptive reaction The organism's attempt to readjust its activities and restore homeostasis when the demands of stress have disturbed the body's equilibrium.

Central nervous system The brain and spinal cord; one of the two main divisions of the nervous system, the other being the peripheral system, composed of the autonomic and voluntary systems.

Neuroendocrine systems Networks of interaction between the nervous system and the endocrine system (glands and other structures that secrete hormones into the bloodstream).

Stimulus (plural stimuli) Any action, agent, or condition that causes a physiological or psychological response.

Input overload Excess of stimuli; stimulation to a point where a person can no longer respond to it.

but so too are our health, our belief systems, and our economic, political, and educational institutions. This change is typically uneven, with some parts of the culture altering drastically and others not at all. This cultural lag or unevenness inevitably creates stress and disruption. It undermines the integration any culture needs to function smoothly.

Among the most startling changes of scale in our lives is that of the sheer number of people we either know or know of. With the rare exception of the happy hermit, we humans do not develop well physically or mentally or even remain quite sane unless we maintain close association with other people. But too many contacts can be just as harmful as too few. What is safe depends not only on our genetic makeup and past experiences but also on the traditions, conventions, and values of the groups with which we are most familiar.

We have created a social environment that embodies vibrancy, diversity, and infinite possibilities on the one hand, and frustration, fears, and infinite anxieties on the other. Through our culture, through our attitudes, economics, and technology, we have brought about unprecedented environmental changes. We are faced with trying to adapt to the accelerating stresses we ourselves have generated.

Our Interaction with Our Environment

A constant interaction between an organism and its environment is essential for maintaining life. We exchange energy primarily through the skin, lungs, gastrointestinal tract (stomach and intestinal tract), and kidneys. We acquire information mainly through the sense organs—the organs of vision, hearing, smell, and taste as well as special organs inside the body and within the skin that are receptive to touch, temperature, pressure, spatial orientation, and acceleration. These organs are closely allied with the **central nervous system** and, through it, with the **neuroendocrine systems**. This setup enables us to draw conclusions about aspects of the environment that are removed in time and place. The whole human system becomes involved in adaptive responses to this "environment at a distance," an environment that is largely composed of other people and our social world.

Whenever **stimuli**—sights, sounds, and smells as well as the actions of others—become too profuse or too varied, we are the victims of **input overload** (also called *sensory, psychic, cognitive,* or *stimulus overload*). The human being has a remarkable ability to adjust, biologically and socially, to a vast variety of living conditions, even to apparently incompatible ones. This adaptability is good (it is how the human race has survived), but it is not *all* good. If we passively accept an overdose of stimuli, if we come to regard endless striving and competitive behavior, hostile personal relationships, overcrowding, and poisonous environments as acceptable and unchangeable, we are likely to suffer emotional stunting or warping, physical degradation, and personal and social degeneration.

Whether environmental stimuli intrude directly or indirectly, stress responses invariably will accompany them. Nearly all highly stressful situations throughout most of our history involved physical threats of some kind—hunger, excessive heat or cold, dangerous terrain, hazardous hunting. These threats called for exertion and endurance, and human beings emerged victorious largely because of their superb biological equipment. We are dynamic creatures, designed to be on the move. Now many of the trappings of our future-oriented society, with its large numbers of people, its labor-saving devices, and its comparatively sedentary ways, present unfamiliar challenges to the human organism, although we perceive them as normal rather than novel.

Exploring Your Emotions

How assertively are you seeking solutions to stressful events? For example, think back to the last time you were really bored. Did you go to bed and wait for the boredom to go away? Is such a passive response good for you, or is it a rationalization for avoiding the problem? Did you do something more active? What? Was this act effective in relieving your boredom?

Stressor Any physical or psychological event or condition that produces stress.

Fight-or-flight reaction A defense reaction that prepares the organism for conflict or escape by triggering hormonal, cardiovascular, metabolic, and other changes.

Eustress A stress state believed to be pleasant, even beneficial.

Distress An unpleasant stress state believed to cause illness.

GAS (general adaptation syndrome) A pattern of stress responses described by Hans Selye as having three stages: alarm, resistance, and exhaustion.

Adaptive energy Limited body reserves that are activated when the body feels exhausted.

Hormones Chemical messengers produced in the body and transported by the bloodstream to target cells or organs for specific regulation of their activities.

Autonomic nervous system The branch of the peripheral nervous system that, largely without conscious thought, controls basic body processes; subdivided into the sympathetic and parasympathetic systems.

Sympathetic nervous system A division of the autonomic system that reacts to danger or other challenges by almost instantly putting the body processes in high gear.

Parasympathetic nervous system A division of the autonomic system that tones down the excitatory effect of the sympathetic system, slowing metabolism and restoring energy supplies.

Hypothalamus A part of the brain that activates, controls, and integrates the autonomic mechanisms, endocrine activities, and many body functions.

Clearly, to live in a state of stress is unavoidable and indeed healthful: nonexcessive stress is just as natural as body temperature. Without stress, we would be bored and listless and would lack adequate outlets for our creative and aggressive urges. Boredom can, in fact, be just as stressful as pressure and may have even worse effects. (For example, drug addiction is often the result of an attempt to escape boredom.) Many people whose lives are drab and uneventful are driven to risk-taking activities for the stimuli they offer. And while some people put themselves under extra stress out of vanity, or for kicks, or to prove something to themselves or to others, many thrill-seekers find the exhilaration of a risky venture a means to self-fulfillment. (Mountain climbing, for instance, has been described as providing "elbow room for the soul.")

The stresses imposed by nature are probably less destructive than those we impose on ourselves and on others. As we have seen, our modern world is obviously uniquely difficult in many ways. Yet, in the final analysis, the **stressors** (physical and psychological stress-producing factors) that affect the greatest number of people have remained essentially the same throughout human history. The most common and often most potent stressors of all are interpersonal relations and any changes in personal circumstances. If physical or emotional illness is the reaction to such stressors, the illness itself then becomes a further stressor.

Determine your own stress score from the Student Stress Scale, after first reading "Life Events: An Update" (see Boxes).

The Stress Response

If you slip on a banana peel, watch a horror movie or a comedy, meet a celebrity or a long-absent friend, get a good grade or a mediocre one on an exam, attend a party, get caught in the rain, win or lose a game, run for a bus, or catch a cold, you are likely to experience only a mild, relatively harmless state of stress. If you get fired, discover you have diabetes, flunk four courses, get mugged, or win a million-dollar lottery, you will undergo much greater, potentially damaging stress. Whatever the situation—pleasurable or not, mild or severe—your body initially reacts in the same way the cave-dweller's did when he or she faced a saber-toothed tiger: it interprets the situation as an emergency.

This immediate response which alerts and prepares you for physical action, has been dubbed the **fight-or-flight reaction.** Though often absurdly inappropriate, it is part of our biological heritage. We may mask emotional turmoil in order to be socially acceptable, but our aroused physiological processes are indifferent to such niceties. Fortunately, the body has ways of cushioning this primary response, for if it should continue over a long period or become too generalized, the tissues of the body would be severely damaged, even to the point of death.

How do the body's adaptive defense mechanisms work and when do they stop working? No one has more thoroughly explored the biochemical and environmental facets of stress than Dr. Hans Selye, an endocrinologist and biologist. Selye defines stress as the common denominator of all the body's adaptive reactions; it is "the nonspecific response of the body to any demand." It can be pleasant and curative (**eustress**), or unpleasant and disease producing (**distress**). The totality of changes in the body that help us adjust to constant internal and external changes is what Selye calls the **GAS (general adaptation syndrome)**, or stress syndrome.

The GAS develops in three stages: the alarm reaction, resistance, and exhaustion. Normally active people often go through the first two stages in order to adapt to their various activities and to the demands made on them. During the resistance (or adaptive) stage, the body begins to repair the damage sustained during the alarm reaction, and the stress symptoms diminish or disappear. But if the stress continues and the entire body is affected for a long time, the adaptation is lost. Exhaustion eventually culminates when the body runs out of energy. The effects of exhaustion can usually be reversed, because the body can

Life Events: An Update

In 1967 Drs. Thomas Holmes and Richard Rahe published the Social Readjustment Rating Scale (SRRS) in the *Journal of Psychosomatic Research*. The scale, comprising 43 life events, was thought to have great promise in predicting future illness events and became the basis for hundreds of publications in books, journals, magazines, and newspapers. The concept was intuitively a good one. If a person experiences an event or events that requires a substantial accommodation or readjustment in his or her life, the change may cause that person to be vulnerable to physical or mental disorders.

Holmes and Rahe studied the case histories of numerous patients and extracted 43 events both desirable and undesirable that are likely to be disruptive. Examples of these life events are death of a spouse, divorce, marriage, pregnancy, troubles with the boss, an outstanding personal achievement, and Christmas. The researchers hypothesized that people experiencing one or more of these events in a specified period of time would become ill. And, in fact, many investigators found that when they administered a life events scale to a patient population they indeed obtained higher life events scores than from a "normal" population.

Unfortunately, it was difficult to tell from this type of study whether the patients' illnesses caused them to recall more life events or whether the greater number of life events caused their illnesses. Subsequent prospective studies either failed to predict future illnesses or obtained statistically significant associations that were so small that they could not be interpreted.

Why has an obviously good intuitive idea failed to yield useful results? One answer is that an illness that has psychological antecedents is likely to be more complex than the assumptions leading investigators to expect a strong relationship between life events and illness. We don't know, for example, whether the person would have developed the illness even without experiencing a disruptive life event. Another source of inquiry is the effects of the social environment on the development of physical and mental illness. No study of life events and illness has adequately taken account of the social environment despite the fact that the social environment has been shown to have powerful effects on behavior as well as on immunity to various illnesses. Social support, for example, has been shown to counteract the effects of negative variables.

While the life events methodology has not produced expected results (that is, predictions of future illnesses), mental illness itself successfully predicts future physical illnesses. Results from many diverse studies are remarkably consistent in showing a strong positive association between emotional disturbance and physical illness. Thus the diagnosis of mental illness as a predictor of future physical illnesses has succeeded where the life events methodology has failed.

activate its reserves of **adaptive energy.** But these reserves are limited. If they are spent, there is general exhaustion, and the result may be death. We can restore them to some extent through proper diet and exercise, adequate sleep, and so on, but there is no evidence that we can ever *fully* determine them—indeed, they may be genetically programmed. Clearly, avoiding intense reactions to people and events will help maintain our precious reserves. (Whenever, for instance, we fly off the handle over a trifle, we are, however unknowingly, wasting our resources.) If the body's biological adaptation to stress is unsuccessful, it can develop what Selye calls "diseases of adaptation," which include cardiovascular, kidney, and glandular diseases, ulcers, mental disorders, and possibly cancer.

Whenever we are faced with a real or imagined threat, powerful **hormones,** which act as natural pep pills, are released into the bloodstream, as the **autonomic nervous system** prepares the body for instant action. This nervous system (functioning in many respects independently of conscious thought) controls the organs and glands. It is made up of two parts, the **sympathetic** and the **parasympathetic** branches. When stress stimulates the body, the sympathetic branch mobilizes the body for action by promoting a quick supply of oxygen and energy. Then the parasympathetic branch calms the body down, slowing rapid heartbeat, drying sweaty palms, and adjusting skin temperature. This marvelous system of checks and balances can, however, go awry during prolonged or too-frequent stress.

As soon as the brain signals "Danger!" (anything from an argument to an avalanche), a complex series of chemical reactions takes place. The **hypothalamus,** a remark-

Student Stress Scale

The Student Stress Scale represents an adaptation of Holmes and Rahe's Life Events Scale. It has been modified to apply to college-age adults and should be considered as a rough indication of stress levels and health consequences for teaching purposes.

In the Student Stress Scale each event, such as beginning or ending school, is given a score that represents the amount of readjustment a person has to make in life as a result of the change. In some studies people with serious illnesses have been found to have high scores on similar scales. People with scores of 300 and higher have a high health risk. Subjects scoring between 150 and 300 points have about a 50–50 chance of serious health change within two years. Subjects scoring below 150 have a 1 in 3 chance of serious health change.

To determine *your* stress score, add up the number of points corresponding to the events you have experienced in the past six months or are likely to experience in the next six months.

SOURCE: Adapted from T. H. Holmes and R. H. Rahe, 1967, The social readjustment rating scale, *Journal of Psychosomatic Research* 11:213.

	PAST		FUTURE
1. Death of a close family member	☐	100	☐
2. Death of a close friend	☐	73	☐
3. Divorce between parents	☐	65	☐
4. Jail term	☐	63	☐
5. Major personal injury or illness	☐	63	☐
6. Marriage	☐	58	☐
7. Fired from job	☐	50	☐
8. Failed important course	☐	47	☐
9. Change in health of a family member	☐	45	☐
10. Pregnancy	☐	45	☐
11. Sex problems	☐	44	☐
12. Serious argument with close friend	☐	40	☐
13. Change in financial status	☐	39	☐
14. Change of major	☐	39	☐
15. Trouble with parents	☐	39	☐
16. New girl- or boyfriend	☐	38	☐
17. Increased workload at school	☐	37	☐
18. Outstanding personal achievement	☐	36	☐
19. First quarter/semester in college	☐	35	☐
20. Change in living conditions	☐	31	☐
21. Serious argument with instructor	☐	30	☐
22. Lower grades than expected	☐	29	☐
23. Change in sleeping habits	☐	29	☐
24. Change in social activities	☐	29	☐
25. Change in eating habits	☐	28	☐
26. Chronic car trouble	☐	26	☐
27. Change in number of family get-togethers	☐	26	☐
28. Too many missed classes	☐	25	☐
29. Change of college	☐	24	☐
30. Dropped more than one class	☐	23	☐
31. Minor traffic violations	☐	20	☐

Total ________

able control center nestled in the lower brain and capable of sending messages both to and from the brain, stimulates the **pituitary gland** (the "master gland" at the base of the brain), which in turn releases **ACTH (adrenocorticotropic hormone)** into the bloodstream, which conveys it to the **adrenal glands**, just above the kidneys. The cortex (outer layer) of the adrenal glands, cued by ACTH, then rushes **cortisol** and other "stress hormones" into the bloodstream, while the medulla (inner core), cued by the sympathetic nervous system, releases **epinephrine** (or adrenalin, the "fear hormone") and **norepinephrine** (or noradrenalin, the "anger hormone"). These events, all orchestrated by the hypothalamus, cause various useful changes (see Figure 2-1), including, happily, the release of **endorphins**, which provide relief from pain in case of injury (they act like morphine but are far more potent).

So there we are—all revved up for physical action. The trouble is that in civilized society the tense or competitive situations that so often arise usually cannot be reasonably handled by physical means. (Say you've received what

Pituitary gland The "master gland," closely linked with the hypothalamus, that controls other endocrine glands and secretes hormones that regulate growth, maturation, and reproduction.

ACTH (adrenocorticotropic hormone) A hormone, formed in the pituitary gland, that stimulates the outer layer of the adrenal gland to secrete its hormones.

Adrenal glands Two glands, one lying atop each kidney, their outer layer (cortex) producing steroid hormones such as cortisol, and their inner core (medulla) producing the hormones epinephrine and norepinephrine.

Cortisol A steroid hormone secreted by the cortex (outer layer) of the adrenal gland; also called *hydrocortisone*.

Epinephrine A hormone secreted by the medulla (inner core) of the adrenal gland; also called *adrenalin*, the "fear hormone."

Norepinephrine A hormone secreted by the medulla (inner core) of the adrenal gland; also called *noradrenalin*, the "anger hormone."

Endorphins Opiate-like chemical substances, produced in the brain, that help kill pain and produce sedation and euphoria (sense of well-being).

---

you regard as an unfair grade on a paper. You complain to the professor, who remains unmoved. To take out your anger by socking her would hardly be in your best interests.) The result is frustration and, possibly, disability. If the body's rapid mobilization for combat occurs too often or is too prolonged (sometimes continuing long after the stressor has vanished), serious or irreparable damage can occur.

How do you know when you are "overmobilizing"? Table 2-1 highlights the danger signals of stress. Of course, you don't have to experience them all to realize you're "overstressed." Some of the signals cannot always be dismissed as merely symptoms of stress; they may call for medical attention. In general, though, such signals are distinct warnings about a problem that you can probably handle on your own. To either ignore or just worry about them will only prolong your stress. If your body is trying to tell you something, try to decode the message, act on it, and you may be able to relieve your misery.

Although stress is part of our lives from day one, we have enormous differences in how little or much stress each of us can tolerate. A situation that might be very stressful to you could leave someone else utterly calm. Your tolerance depends largely on your genetic inheritance, your previous experiences, your ability to separate real from imagined or remembered psychosocial assaults, your unique response to stimuli and to the symbols associated with the stimuli, your philosophy of life, and how much social support you have. You might be able to ward off or at least lessen the effects of distress and disease by paying attention to the body's signals and then, whenever necessary, doing something about them.

Figure 2-1 The Body's Response to Stress

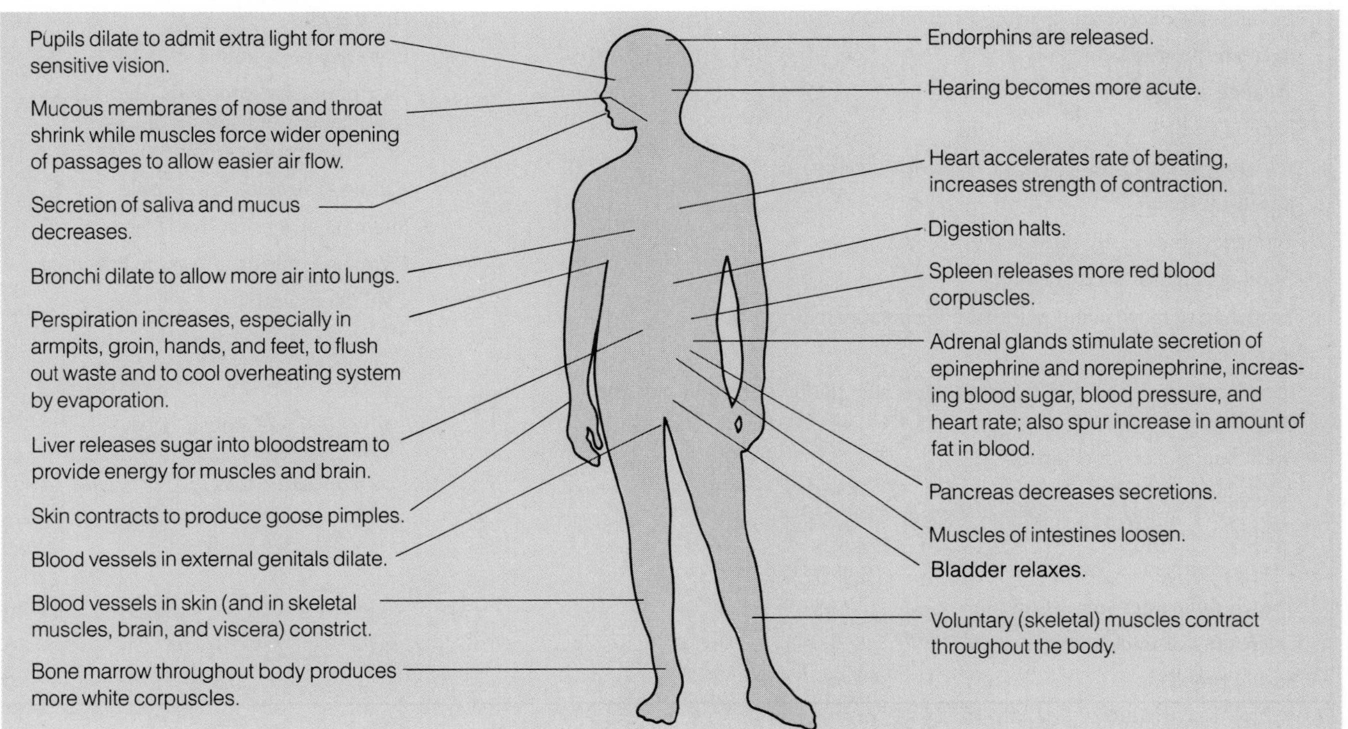

Pupils dilate to admit extra light for more sensitive vision.
Mucous membranes of nose and throat shrink while muscles force wider opening of passages to allow easier air flow.
Secretion of saliva and mucus decreases.
Bronchi dilate to allow more air into lungs.
Perspiration increases, especially in armpits, groin, hands, and feet, to flush out waste and to cool overheating system by evaporation.
Liver releases sugar into bloodstream to provide energy for muscles and brain.
Skin contracts to produce goose pimples.
Blood vessels in external genitals dilate.
Blood vessels in skin (and in skeletal muscles, brain, and viscera) constrict.
Bone marrow throughout body produces more white corpuscles.
Endorphins are released.
Hearing becomes more acute.
Heart accelerates rate of beating, increases strength of contraction.
Digestion halts.
Spleen releases more red blood corpuscles.
Adrenal glands stimulate secretion of epinephrine and norepinephrine, increasing blood sugar, blood pressure, and heart rate; also spur increase in amount of fat in blood.
Pancreas decreases secretions.
Muscles of intestines loosen.
Bladder relaxes.
Voluntary (skeletal) muscles contract throughout the body.

Disorientation Confusion with respect to time, place, or person.

Culture shock Confusion and anxiety on being exposed to a culture or environment that greatly differs from a person's customary one.

Some Common Stressors

Four stressors seem to be most strongly linked to stress: change, frustration, overload, and deprivation. Whatever its virtues, our advanced technological society brings with it high stress levels, and change in these levels is not likely to occur soon. Neither is the adaptation that would be needed to tolerate such levels without ill effects. So we are each largely on our own in undertaking to reduce undue stress. This situation calls for tough self-examination, because each person's circumstances and physical and emotional makeup are obviously different from anyone else's. How do you rate your tolerance of change, disruption, and uncertainty? What are some of the situations that you face now or are likely to face in the future that might require excessive adaptation and be potentially damaging to you?

Social Change Such events as going to college, getting married, changing jobs, and moving to another area are common, but they can provoke considerable stress, especially if several occur at the same time or closely together. The cumulative impact of the pressures, decision making, and insecurities that are part of the normal events of life can have a great effect on health. Changes are often perceived as threatening, not because they are necessarily bad but because people have not learned to adapt to them adequately—that is, they don't know how to cope.

Even seemingly moderate social readjustments may take their toll. For instance, some years ago, when Navajo Indians were moved from their homes and located on reser-

Table 2-1 Signals of Stress

Emotional and Behavioral Signs	Physical Signs
Tendency to be irritable, hyperexcited, or depressed	Pounding heart
Impulsiveness, aggressiveness, emotional instability	Trembling, with nervous tics
Overpowering urge to cry or to run and hide	Grinding of teeth
Inability to concentrate, general disorientation, flight of thoughts	Dry mouth
Accident proneness	Excessive perspiration
Weakness, dizziness, or sense of unreality	Gastrointestinal problems (diarrhea, constipation, indigestion, queasy stomach, perhaps vomiting)
Fatigue and loss of the joy of living	Aching of neck or lower back
"Floating anxiety" (fear without an obvious reason)	Migraine or tension headaches
Keyed-up feeling	Frequent colds or low-grade infections
Tendency to be easily startled by small sounds	Cold hands and feet
Nervous, high-pitched laughter	Allergy or asthma attacks
Tendency to move about or gesture for no apparent reason	
Increased smoking	
Increased use of prescription drugs, especially tranquilizers and pep pills (e.g., amphetamines)	
Addiction to alcohol or drugs	
Addiction to TV	
Frequent feelings of boredom	
Sleep disturbances (insomnia, nightmares) or excessive sleep	
Speech difficulties (e.g., stuttering)	
Overeating or undereating	
Sexual problems	

Source: Partially based on Selye, 1979, pp. 66–68.

The Top Ten Hassles and Uplifts

What are the most common sources of pleasures and hassles in life? It all depends on who you are.

When my colleagues and I asked 100 white, middle-class, middle-aged men and women to keep track of their hassles and uplifts over a one-year period, we got one set of candidates for the Top Ten annoyances and joys. When we asked a group of college students, we got another. Canadian health professionals gave us still another list.

The ten most frequent hassles and uplifts in the middle-aged group were, in order of frequency:

Hassles

1. Concern about weight
2. Health of a family member
3. Rising prices of common goods
4. Home maintenance
5. Too many things to do
6. Misplacing or losing things
7. Yard work or outside home maintenance
8. Property, investment, or taxes
9. Crime
10. Physical appearance

Uplifts

1. Relating well with your spouse or lover
2. Relating well with friends
3. Completing a task
4. Feeling healthy
5. Getting enough sleep
6. Eating out
7. Meeting responsibilities
8. Visiting, phoning, or writing someone
9. Spending time with family
10. Having a home pleasing to you

People differ widely in the problems and pleasures typical of their lives. Only three hassle items—and not a single uplift—rated among the top 10 of all three groups. The big three: misplacing or losing things, physical appearance, too many things to do.

Each group had certain hassles common to its station in life. For the middle-aged, middle-class group, the pertinent theme was economic concern—worries about investments and rising prices. The Canadian health professionals tended to check off hassles that reflect the anxieties and pressures of their careers: too much to do, not enough time to do it all, too many responsibilities, trouble relaxing. Students were most hassled by anxiety over wasting time, meeting high standards, and being lonely.

As for pleasures, there again the groups diverge. The uplifts of the middle-aged are the joys of a homebody: being in good health, enjoying hearth, home, and kin. Students, on the other hand, tend to be more hedonistic; their uplifts include having fun, laughing, entertainment. The only two shared by young and middle-aged alike: completing a task and having good times with friends.

SOURCE: Richard S. Lazarus, 1981 (July), Little hassles can be hazardous to health, *Psychology Today* 15:61.

vations only a few miles away, their death rate from tuberculosis rose alarmingly. The Navajos' food, clothing, and hygiene were unchanged; their new physical setting was virtually the same as their old one. But the social disorganization was enough to overtax the adaptive capacities of many.

Migrants and immigrants of all races and countries are especially vulnerable to psychosocial stress. The rates of psychiatric hospitalization and illnesses among these groups are ordinarily higher than those of other population groups. The risk of mental **disorientation** increases as newcomers experience **cultural shock**—as they are faced with unfamiliar conditions, cultural differences, less social support, and pressures for assimilation, especially when there are no familiar groups to join. Migrants also appear to be more vulnerable to chronic, or recurring, diseases than their contemporaries who stay put; and occupationally and geographically mobile people tend to have a higher incidence of coronary heart disease than more stable populations.

Anything that challenges one's values and beliefs is a source of stress. In recent years, for example, the women's movement has impelled both sexes to reinterpret feminine and masculine roles and interpersonal relations. But the new freedoms and competitiveness of women can be both heady and disturbing to them and potentially threatening to men. As more women enter the work force and more of them occupy executive positions, they are becoming as susceptible to peptic ulcers and cardiovascular disease as men are. (Besides, women haven't actually left their traditional roles of wife and mother to become job-holders; they've just piled them up, impossibly attempting to devote full time to each role while filling all three simultaneously.)

Urban Versus Rural Stress About 75 percent of the people in this country are bunched together on a mere

Social anonymity The state of being unrecognized as an individual by members of society.

1.5 percent of the land. Of those who abandon the cities to take up the truly rural life, many drift back to the cities, perhaps deciding that they have simply traded one set of stresses for another. But quite a few people have found, as we'll see, a happy medium.

Crowding and Urban Life Some individuals feel lost, alienated, and helpless in the urban world of strangers, while others welcome the **social anonymity.** They savor a distinct sense of privacy. Others, paradoxically, feel so hemmed in by people that privacy is regarded as a rarely attained, though blessed, state. As a lonely character in a Jules Feiffer skit grumbles, "If only not being alone didn't depend on other people."

Because they cannot scan, let alone process, the flow of urban stimuli, people attempt to protect themselves from overload by developing adaptive responses that streamline it. For instance, they screen out whatever they find of little personal importance (the drunk—or ill or even dead—person on the sidewalk is ignored; people bumping into each other don't bother to apologize); they shift responsibility to another party ("It's not *my* problem"); and they discourage personal contact (phone numbers are unlisted; phone receivers are left off the hook). But such withdrawal and seeming callousness may cause urbanites to miss out on life-enhancing stimuli and to become geared to a routine existence with little turmoil and many superficial relationships. It is not the stresses themselves that appear to account for the ills of urban living; it is the means people use to try to escape them.

Exploring Your Emotions

Late one night on the way home from the library you are startled by a man's figure in the shadows just off the sidewalk. You hurry on, wondering why your heart is racing. A few yards farther along, you pass a young woman. For a minute you consider warning her about the man who startled you, but then you think you are unnecessarily alarmed and say nothing. The next day you learn that a woman was raped and beaten near the library last night. What would you have done in this situation?

Rural Stress When harassed urbanites begin to think wistfully about rural life, they tend to dwell on the relative quiet, the closeness to nature, the neighborliness, and the farmer's independence. Yet rural life can be just as stressful as urban life, and sometimes even more so. Certain types of mental illness (such as manic-depressive problems) are more rampant in rural than in urban settings, and ulcers are a common occupational hazard of farming. Very small towns are apt to lack stimulation and to exert a stifling social pressure.

For the farmer, every year is a financial gamble: enormous economic stakes can be wiped out if it rains too little, too much, or at the wrong time, if disease or pests attack, if agribusiness (farming run as big business) squeezes out the competition, if the government embargoes overseas sales. And when the small farmer finally sells the products, he or she ends up with only a fraction of the money the consumer pays: wholesalers, transportation, and stores gulp the rest. In addition, there are the long hours—sometimes 16 hours a day. The great outdoors may not seem so great to a farmer who must go out in the freezing rain at four in the morning and work almost without letup until eleven at night or who must tend crops under a merciless sun. And because cows have to be milked, chickens fed, and manure shoveled every day of the year, there's scant chance to get away for long; hiring someone to pinch-hit requires money and trust, both of which may be in short supply. Farmers must face all these situations in relative isolation: they have few community resources and are tied to a strong cultural tradition that makes them reluctant to ask for help or admit to emotional problems. To top it all off, children of farmers often seek greater opportunity in the cities, leaving the farmer with no one to carry on the work on land that may have been in the family for generations. In the mid-1980s, when bankruptcy became commonplace, a rash of suicides occurred when farmers lost everything they had built up over so many years and were forced to leave the soil they cherished.

"Countrified Cities" as a Happy Medium Almost 50 percent of urbanites would rather live in a small town or rural area, according to a 1985 Gallup poll. (The term *town* means different things to different people: inhabitants of New York or Los Angeles might regard Shreveport, Louisiana, and Eugene, Oregon, as small towns, while for Louisianians and Oregonians—residents of largely rural states—they would qualify as cities.) Each year some 40 million Americans change residences. Job transfers, often from one city to another, and changes in personal relationships probably account for most of these moves, but a significant number stem from disenchantment with urban life and a desire for the adventure (and perhaps the risk) of starting anew in the countryside.

For those unwilling to give up the amenities of urban life but longing for a less hectic existence, the small city (population from 25,000 to 100,000) is often a nice compromise—places like Flagstaff, Arizona; Palo Alto, California; and Reno, Nevada. Others prefer even smaller places, "Edens" that could qualify as either "countrified cities" or "citified country towns." Thousands of such towns are scattered across the nation, many of them little known. For a few million Americans, migration to such places seems to be at least a partial solution to undue stress, even if it means taking less prestigious jobs or changing professions.

The Work Environment and Job Choice According to the U.S. Department of Labor, 80 percent of the employees in this country are misemployed, working at the wrong jobs. Some promotions indeed reflect the Peter Principle: employees are promoted from jobs they perform competently to higher positions until they reach a level of incompetence.

In all types of jobs, many employees claim to be *alienated* from their work: They feel trapped, overwhelmed by meaninglessness, self-estrangement, isolation, and powerlessness. Alienation is usually regarded as an affliction of the blue-collar worker, but in recent years thousands of executives have abandoned their jobs for work that may pay less but promises to be more rewarding. For instance, they have become artists, craftworkers, or singers, or have established agricultural communes.

One of the effects of alienation is sheer escapism. Thousands of assembly line workers and an equal number of executives daydream through their work. More than half

Exploring Your Emotions

How do you react to cities? Do you like them? Dislike them? Have you ever lived in a very large city, such as New York, or Chicago, or Los Angeles? How do you feel about this picture, and what do you think it suggests about cities? Can you identify some of the devices the photographer used to build up these images? Give this picture a caption.

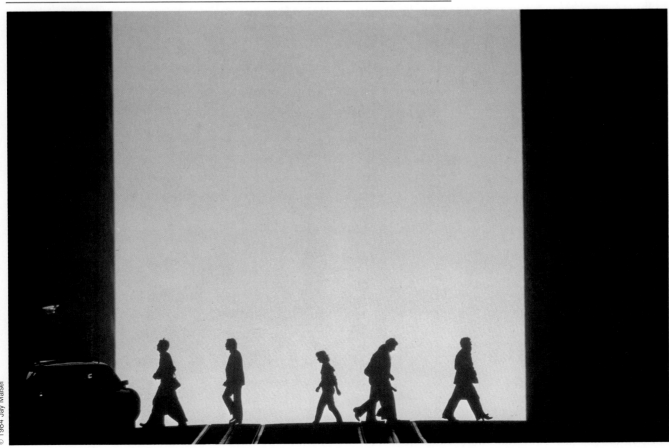

admit they are working at only half their potential. Others escape through drugs and alcohol: Workers in some factories stay high on drugs during their entire shift, and many executives rely on the three-martini lunch to get through the day. In an effort to deal with work alienation, some organizations are embarking on "job enrichment" programs, giving each worker more varied tasks and allowing him or her a greater sense of responsibility for the finished product.

Clearly, excessive stress is the lot of almost every worker at some time. Job dissatisfaction, too little or too much responsibility, conflict with co-workers or with supervisors, lack of support, vague job expectations, and time pressure—all are stressors. When extremely aroused, a person usually cannot do certain kinds of tasks as well as when less aroused. It is hard to do a complicated job, to think creatively, or to learn something new when under excess stress. For example, if you're nervous about an exam, you cannot absorb information as well as you could if you were less anxious. But if you're taking an exam that is not too hard and that you are fairly well prepared for, being slightly "keyed up" will probably be helpful (see box).

Monotony can be just as stressful as excessive activity. Such traditional stressors as heavy workloads, long hours, and critical responsibilities have been found to result in

Exploring Your Emotions

What class do you think she might be studying for? Can you suggest the action from a Gothic movie that this photo might be taken from? How do you think she would react if you tapped her on the shoulder? If you asked her to get you a cup of coffee? If you invited her to a yoga class?

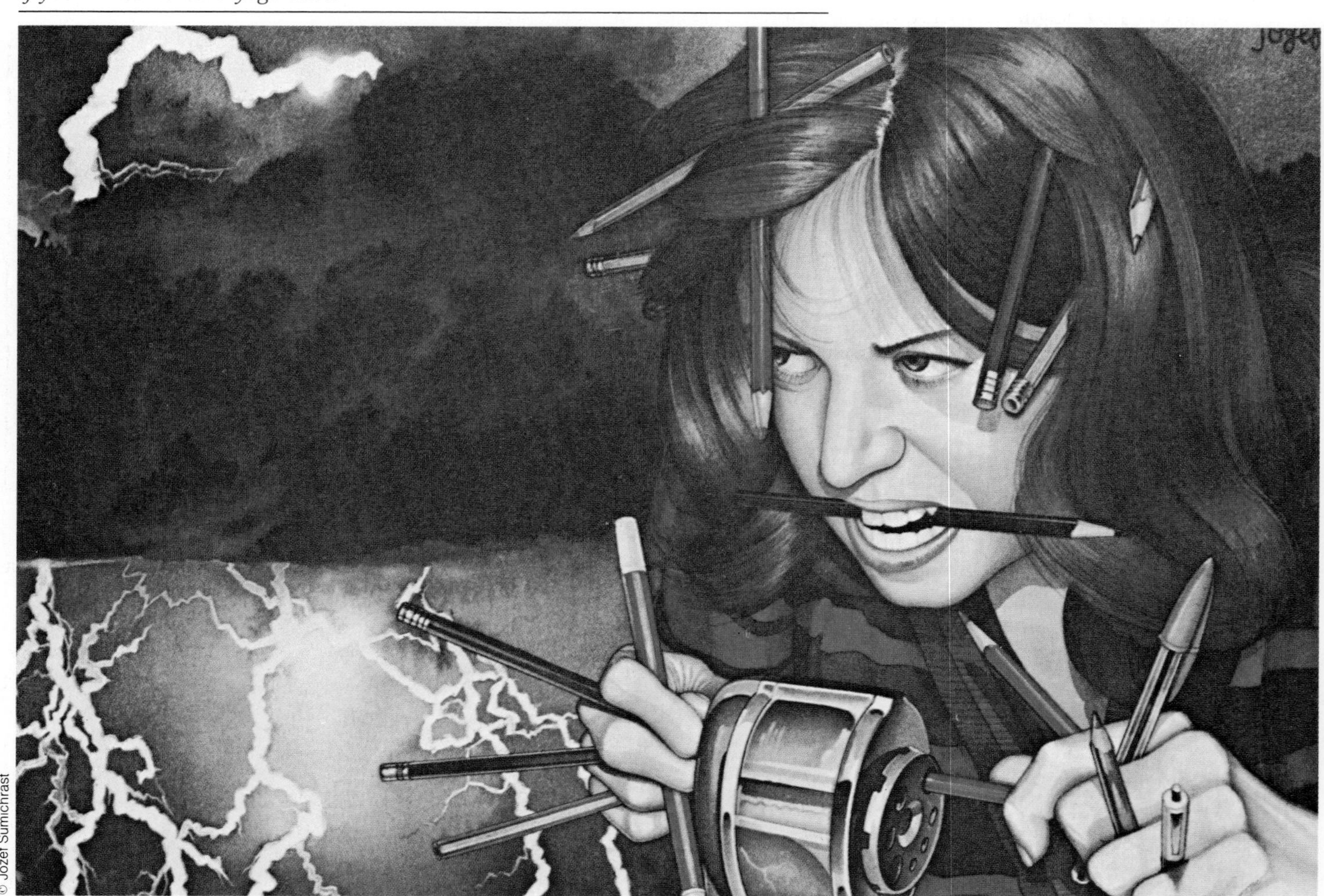

© Józef Sumichrast

Test Anxiety and Stress

Dan Ross is a freshman at California Community College. He has been thinking about the test his history instructor announced last week. Dan can hardly think of anything else. In three days he will be required to take a test for which he feels unprepared. He tries to study the textbook but sees disconnected words rather than concepts. Stray thoughts fill his mind. He realizes he is so worried by the thought of failing the test that he has become paralyzed with fear. With each passing day, he becomes increasingly anxious.

Dan is experiencing *test anxiety*. Anxiety can be defined as a state marked by heightened self-awareness and perceived helplessness. This self-absorption of anxious individuals may be the result of an inability to evaluate when they are prepared and when they are not. Every teacher knows students who are bright, competent, and well prepared but who become paralyzed at exam time.

Each student comes to the test-taking situation with certain assumptions, concerns, and expectations. Regardless of the objective situation, it is the individual's personal interpretation of the situation that may lead to feelings of anxiety and stress. For example, a student who is unaware that he has failed a test may feel unconcerned. Correspondingly, a student who believes she has failed a test, but hasn't, may feel exceedingly distressed.

Students cope with test anxiety and stress in different ways. Some actively deal with the anxiety-arousing situation by talking with the instructor or a counselor or by developing a program of effective study. Others deny the importance of the test or complain about the instructor's teaching ability. Many students respond to test anxiety by worrying excessively about failure or by finding ways to avoid taking action.

Students suffering from test anxiety react to the situation in one or more of the following ways:

1. They see themselves as unprepared or inadequate in taking tests.
2. They view the test situation as difficult, hazardous, and threatening.
3. They concentrate on the negative consequences of failure.
4. Their preoccupation with inadequacy interferes with their ability to mobilize resources to deal with the problem.
5. They expect and anticipate failure, which leads to a self-fulfilling prophecy.

What can Dan and other test-anxious students do to overcome or reduce this problem? One of the most effective techniques has evolved from research aimed at strengthening the student's ability to handle the stress and self-preoccupation associated with the test situation. Briefly, this technique involves the following: (1) The student is educated about the stress response and his or her level of anxiety. (2) The student learns a rehearsal technique that uses physical coping skills, such as relaxation, and specific strategies to defuse the anxiety. (3) During an application phase, the student practices the acquired skills with a real or imagined stress situation. (See *A Computerized Self-program for Coping with Tests,* developed by Health Sciences Software, 1149 Chestnut Street, Suite 10, Menlo Park, California 94025.)

less physical illness, anxiety, and depression than less demanding jobs. Some corporation executives admit to deliberately stressing their employees because this seems, to them, the best way to get a job done. Emotional strain associated with job responsibility does contribute to ill health, however. For example, heart disease or ulcers frequently afflict police officers, firefighters, taxi drivers, air-traffic controllers, and musicians on one-night stands. (A study of 100 police in Cincinnati unexpectedly showed that their most significant stressors were neither life-threatening situations nor the hostility they often encountered; instead, the stressors were those circumstances that undermined their sense of professionalism, such as a reprimand from a superior.)

Some social scientists believe that clerical workers suffer more stress than their bosses. Roughly 85 percent are women, and they have almost twice the incidence of heart disease as do either other working women or housewives. Work overload, low pay, production quotas, monotony, and powerlessness largely account for the high stress rate among secretaries. But computer technology, for all its advantages, has a lot to answer for, too. When, as often happens, their productivity is monitored by computers, secretaries tend to become demoralized and intimidated.

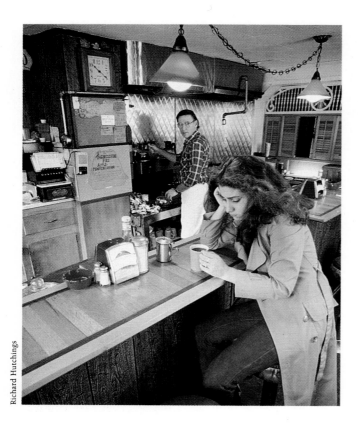

Richard Hutchings

In addition, spending unrelieved hours in front of a video display terminal (VDT) can lead to eyestrain, improper posture, and even fear of radiation. In fact, people who work with VDTs have recently been found to have the highest level of stress among *all* occupations.

But the most telling example of occupational overload is that of psychiatrists and physicians. According to a recent survey, for instance, a third of psychiatrists sometimes do not know how to cope with their own stress—which helps explain a high suicide rate among psychiatrists. As for physicians, day in and day out they deal with matters of life and death, trying all along to maintain a distance between themselves and their work to preserve their sanity. In addition, they are sometimes subjected to two extreme attitudes among their patients: at the one end are those patients who expect doctors to be infallible (which no one can be); and at the other are those who hold doctors in such low esteem that they see them all as impersonal, uncaring money-grubbers.

If you spend a large part of your life doing something that matters to you, you can withstand a good deal of stress. Both your emotional and material needs can be satisfied if your skills and talents are used to their fullest. Whether it is your first job or your next job, you should, if you can, choose to do what you truly think is most suitable for you, basing your judgment on the amount of adaptation you believe will be needed to achieve maximum eustress and minimum distress.

The Role of Stress in Disease

Are in-laws a common cause of the common cold? Yes, according to some researchers. A person frequently catches cold when his or her mother- or father-in-law comes for a visit; and once the visit and the cold are over, just talking about the in-law can renew the cold symptoms. It is increasingly evident that people do get sick when they have to cope with many ordinary life events. When they try to cope with overpowering crises, they may get seriously ill, although no specific event or situation is linked to a specific disease.

Most researchers no longer doubt that psychosocial stress contributes to the occurrence, course, and deadliness of diseases. What puzzles them is why some people become ill under stress and others remain wholly unaffected and healthy, and why the same stress triggers different illnesses in different people. One important clue, some investigators suspect, is that resistance to disease is lowered as the person tries to cope and that resistance becomes even lower when he or she uses faulty coping techniques, techniques not relevant to the problem being confronted. We all have a finite amount of energy. If too much is expended in coping with the environment, there is less reserve for preventing disease. If life becomes too hectic, and our coping attempts fail, we get sick. Although major life events have often been cited as the most important factor in the onset of stress-linked disease, it is possible that the individual's effectiveness or ineffectiveness in adapting to daily, chronic irritants is the overriding factor.

Some doctors estimate that anywhere from 30 to 80 percent of their patients' illnesses are significantly linked to social and economic stresses on the one hand and to personal worries and circumstances on the other. Although the medical profession appears to regard the finding that disease can be socially generated as yet another breakthrough in modern medicine, shamans (medicine men or women) in less sophisticated cultures recognized long ago that physical ailments can be expressions of emotional or spiritual distress or of snags in the web of social contacts. The shaman was, in a sense, the world's first sociologist and its first psychiatrist; he or she did not erect an artificial wall between the social environment and the individual.

The traditional model of disease is that of infection or injury—that is, a single cause for a specific ailment. But more and more scientists are beginning to accept the idea that even susceptibility to infectious diseases can be not merely a matter of exposure to an external source of infection; it has to be a reflection of environmental conditions that culminate in physiological stress. It is not, in other words, simply the germ that causes the disease but our relationship to the germ.

In the current model of disease, illness is regarded as having many causes. Among them are stressful environmental conditions, the person's perception that the conditions are stressful, the relative ability to adapt to them, inherited tendency toward a disorder, the degree of physical fitness, and the presence of a disease agent. In addition, according to one school of thought, unique personality profiles may be connected with such disorders as heart disease, asthma, arthritis, colitis, migraine and tension headaches, and even cancer.

A growing number of stress researchers maintain that, contrary to popular belief, certain types of relationships or situations are not inherently stressful and detrimental to health. For example, they point out that disease epidemics that were expected when Londoners were subjected to the horrors of being bombed during World War II did not materialize. Hardships cannot be unquestionably equated with a state of health. If you stop to think about it, you will realize that most people do not become disabled even when awful things happen to them. So exposure to stressors alone is not usually an adequate explanation for the onset of illness. Their impact seems to depend on three factors: the characteristics of stressful events (their magnitude, intensity, unpredictability, duration, and novelty); the individual's biological and psychological makeup; and the social supports available to serve as buffers.

The Mind and the Immune System When we get sick and/or depressed, it is easy and comforting to think that, after all, we have little control over our body's biochemistry. But we are often more responsible for biochemical changes than we realize. When our emotional reactions to stressful events are too strong or misguided, they trigger biochemical changes that in turn can trigger illness and/or depression. But what we do we can undo. Relaxation and, more important, a different perspective can help prevent or correct such biochemical imbalances.

Even some of the most skeptical scientists and physicians are beginning, however reluctantly, to admit that thoughts and images can activate anatomical and chemical mechanisms that deliver messages from the brain to cells everywhere in the body. In times of stress or disease, the brain sends signals along nerve pathways to help defend against infection and pump out chemicals that enable the body to fight more vigorously against disease. The brain thus talks to the immune system, and (as discussed earlier) during stress the nerves and hormones that carry the brain's message are activated. They can turn the immune system on and off, which helps explain why emotions can alter our susceptibility to disease.

Personality Types Hard as it may be for a student to believe, sometimes a *B* may be preferable to an *A*, and a *C* may be preferable to either of them. People with what cardiologists (heart specialists) call Type A personality suffer from "hurry sickness," which can be an open invitation to hypertension (high blood pressure) and heart attacks. Yet such people are so energetic, mentally alert, and productive, and apparently so rarely depressed, that they give the impression of being unusually healthy. They often hold responsible managerial jobs and engage in a host of community activities. Typically aggressive, competitive, easily angered, impatient, and controlling, Type A's hate to waste a moment. They try to tackle more than one thing at a time; and anything that holds them up—a waiting line, a traffic jam, a slow-moving or slow-talking person—is apt to drive them bonkers.

In contrast, Type B's are low-keyed, relaxed, contemplative. They tend to accomplish things slowly and methodically, to be less concerned with the quantity than with the quality of their output, and to be content with doing a few things really well. Type B women, though not as quick to reach intimacy as Type A's, seem to have more stable and satisfying romances over the long term, no matter what the man's personality; but they tend to have happier marriages if the man is also a Type B. Although Type B's are apt to work fewer hours than Type A's, they seem to win just as many promotions and often are highly successful precisely because they don't waste energy on worry about traffic jams and petty details and because their composure inspires confidence. Yet, despite these positive qualities, the notion persists that Type B's are too laid back and that if Type A's were to modify their behavior, they would lose the drive that makes them successful.

Extensive studies of Type A's suggest, however, that they have heart attacks more frequently and at a younger age than the general population. Their risk of coronary heart disease is apparently high because their behavior leads them into stressful situations to which they react more explosively than is usually justified. They are "hot reactors." Thus, a Type A who seethes in a traffic jam sets off the fight-or-flight response. The blood vessels constrict (narrow) under the influence of norepinephrine (the "anger hormone" described earlier). If the constricted artery is already clogged with a plaque of cholesterol, which can accumulate on the arterial wall as a result of frequent surges in blood pressure and stress hormones, and a piece of that plaque breaks off, a blood clot can form and block the artery (the blood clots more easily, in any case, during acute stress so that a wound can stop bleeding sooner). The result could be a heart attack or stroke.

Critics of the many studies of Type A's contend that so far there is no absolute proof that Type A's are at high risk for heart attacks. The problem is that researchers have tried to identify Type A's through the use of questionnaires, and these are filled out by people who may not want to admit to, or may not recognize, certain aspects of their behavior. So differentiating between Type A's and Type B's is sometimes tricky. The result may be that people mistakenly identified as Type A's may be studied as candidates for heart attacks. Interviews instead of questionnaires appear to assess people more accurately, but even they are not conclusive because the interviewers may not be sufficiently trained or competent.

Nevertheless, researchers have found that heart attacks do seem more frequent among people who display three particular characteristics: self-centeredness, hostility, and cynicism. Dr. Meyer Friedman believes that Type A's are consumed by self-hate and a tendency to self-destruct.

On the basis of controlled experiments with hundreds of Type A's, Friedman is convinced that modifying their behavior can significantly reduce their risk of heart attacks. He claims that his treatment program, which is available in do-it-yourself form, has achieved results far superior to those of any other therapy (diet, exercise, drugs, or surgery). If you suspect you're a Type A, and would like to modify your behavior, see the Behavior Change Strategy at the end of the chapter.

A neat compromise between Type A and Type B is Type C, the "hardy personality," who thrives on challenge, has more drive than Type B's, but, unlike Type A, doesn't go overboard. For more on this type, see page 38.

Social Support Systems and Social Stressors Social support systems consist of the enduring interpersonal ties you have with groups of people—at home, at school, at work, and so on. These are the people you can count on to give you emotional support, feedback, and assistance and resources when needed, and with whom you share values and standards (see the Social Support Scale). We often think of blood ties as the only ones that deserve to be called "familial," but even if your relatives are not your friends and your family is held together only by loveless duty, you can still have a family by turning your friends into relatives.

The social position individuals or groups occupy can measurably affect their experience of stress and, it is assumed, their vulnerability to all sorts of disorders. The effects of exposure to stressful situations may be scaled down for anyone who is well bolstered by support systems, but the effects are ordinarily made worse when these systems are impaired. Three basic impairments in the social network can be singled out: social isolation, social marginality, and status inconsistency.

Social isolation is now believed to be a major factor in increasing the risk of disease. Some examples: disproportionately high rates of physical and psychiatric disorders occur in deteriorating, socially shunned areas of the central city; people who live alone, uninvolved with other people or organizations, are especially vulnerable to chronic disease; institutionalized children, who commonly lack warm relationships with other people, often suffer from "failure to thrive"; and grief may contribute to ill health when social isolation is brought on by loss of a mate.

"Marginal" individuals are deprived of nourishing social contacts for various reasons, such as continuous residential and occupational mobility, isolated living conditions, broken homes, or membership in a minority group that is spurned by the dominant majority. They have an increased vulnerability to ill health and other problems that may take many forms—schizophrenia, tuberculosis, multiple accidents, alcoholism, suicide.

If someone plays two or more distinct social roles involving social expectations that are not compatible, he or she is burdened with status inconsistency and perhaps, as a result, ill health. Such an inconsistency may be, for instance, a discrepancy between education and occupation, between education and income level, or between age or sex and employment. Several studies indicate that extremely healthy workers have social backgrounds, interests, and goals that match their circumstances; and their educational, occupational, and family statuses are also consistent. Workers who are often ill may have an educational or family status that does not match the sort of work they are doing.

The strength or weakness of social supports may figure prominently in rates of disease and of death. Single men (between the ages of 25 and 64) have a significantly higher death rate from heart disease than married men. Married people have lower death rates than single, widowed, or divorced people for a wide range of conditions. The states in this country that have high death rates for one cause appear to have high death rates for almost all causes. Death rates from all causes are low for certain religious groups, such as Mormons (Church of Latter-Day Saints) and Seventh Day Adventists (these groups not only are apt to have especially strong social cohesiveness but also have dietary restrictions and generally do not drink or smoke). Social and cultural mobility tends to result in higher rates of coronary heart disease, lung cancer, depression, and pregnancy difficulties.

Social Support Scale

Social support has been recognized for a long time in the behavioral sciences as an important adjunct to therapy. However, only recently has social support emerged among health care professionals as a moderator of stress, with high social support facilitating the ability to cope with stress and adapt to change and thus placing the vulnerable individual at lower risk for serious illness.

The Social Support Scale (SSS) measures the extent to which a person receives or obtains social and psychological support from community activities, friends, and relatives. The score for the amount of social support obtained is found by adding all the numbers next to the boxes checked plus all the numbers circled. The following totals indicate high, moderate, and low support:

70 or more = *High Support,* which suggests that you have a well-developed social support structure to counter the negative effects of stress.

40 to 69 = *Moderate Support,* which suggests that you have sufficient areas of social support to counter the negative effects of stress.

less than 40 = *Low Support,* which suggests that you lack the minimum support structure to counter the negative effects of stress.

1. Do you belong to any of these kinds of groups? If YES, please indicate how much you take part in group activities. For example, VERY ACTIVE means you attend most meetings; SOMEWHAT ACTIVE means you attend meetings once in awhile; INACTIVE means that you belong, but hardly ever go to meetings.

How Much Do You Take Part?

	DO YOU BELONG?		INACTIVE	SOMEWHAT ACTIVE	VERY ACTIVE
a. A social or recreational group?	1☐ NO	2☐ YES	→1☐	2☐	3☐
b. A labor union, commercial group, or professional association?	1☐ NO	2☐ YES	→1☐	2☐	3☐
c. A political-party group or club?	1☐ NO	2☐ YES	→1☐	2☐	3☐
d. A group concerned with children (such as PTA or Boy Scouts)?	1☐ NO	2☐ YES	→1☐	2☐	3☐
e. A group concerned with community betterment, charity, or service?	1☐ NO	2☐ YES	→1☐	2☐	3☐
Aside from the above groups, do you belong to					
f. A church-connected group?	1☐ NO	2☐ YES	→1☐	2☐	3☐
g. A group concerned with a public issue such as civil liberties, property rights, etc.?	1☐ NO	2☐ YES	→1☐	2☐	3☐
h. A group concerned with the environment, pollution, etc.?	1☐ NO	2☐ YES	→1☐	2☐	3☐
i. A group concerned with self-improvement that meets regularly?	1☐ NO	2☐ YES	→1☐	2☐	3☐
j. Any other groups?	1☐ NO	2☐ YES	→1☐	2☐	3☐

Describe them: ____________________

2. How many close friends (people you feel at ease with, can talk to about private matters, and can call on for help) do you have?

Circle one: None 1 2 3 4 5 6 7 8 9 10 or more

3. How many relatives do you have that you feel close to?

Circle one: None 1 2 3 4 5 6 7 8 9 10 or more

4. How many of these friends or relatives do you see at least once a month?

Circle one: None 1 2 3 4 5 6 7 8 9 10 or more

5. About how often do you see any close relatives or friends?

5☐ MORE THAN ONCE A WEEK 4☐ ONCE A WEEK 3☐ A FEW TIMES A MONTH 2☐ ONCE A MONTH 1☐ LESS THAN ONCE A MONTH

6. How often are you on the telephone with any close relatives or friends?

5☐ MORE THAN ONCE A WEEK 4☐ ONCE A WEEK 3☐ A FEW TIMES A MONTH 2☐ ONCE A MONTH 1☐ LESS THAN ONCE A MONTH

7. How often do you exchange letters with any close relatives or friends?

5☐ ONCE A WEEK OR MORE 4☐ A FEW TIMES A MONTH 3☐ ONCE A MONTH 2☐ A FEW TIMES A YEAR 1☐ ONCE A YEAR OR LESS

Coping

As you can now see, the most potent stressors in your life are not the natural physical demands made on the tissues of your body, including such activities as healing wounds, fighting infections, and restoring lost blood, though these are obviously essential. It is the emotional stimuli you face day in and day out, particularly those that cause distress, that are the chief, potentially harmful, stressors. When you experience anger, fear, frustration, resentment, or envy, these emotional reactions (often unwarranted) evoke physical reactions that can affect you both immediately and, because of their cumulative power, far into the future. But the stressor itself is neutral. The effect of a stressor depends much less on what happens to you or on what you do, than on how you take it.

Exploring Your Emotions

You are one day away from a very important final examination. Although you have not prepared very thoroughly and you are very nervous, you decide to go to sleep early rather than cram all night. You have just made a coping decision. Is it a wise one? How about all those earlier coping decisions that you used to put off course preparation you should have been doing each week?

Of the countless ways of coping with stress, the most effective are those that call for a shift in attitudes and expectations and that make us acutely aware of how intimately our feelings interlock with the body's self-regulating and healing abilities. Among the methods offered here, try to find and stick with the one or more particularly attuned to your needs, taste, and style. Whether your progress is gradual or swift doesn't matter. What does matter is that you'll be learning to listen to your body. That alone should bring you some relief from the very start. And remember that how well you cope is closely linked with how well you *think* you'll cope.

The Three C's Stress survivors have a characteristic that psychologist Suzanne Kobasa calls "hardiness," which she says is even more important than a strong constitution in defusing stress. Even when under extreme stress, hardy people—sometimes called Type C's—remain healthy because they cultivate "the three C's of health," challenge, commitment, and control:

- *Challenge.* See change for what it is: natural and usually stimulating, not a threat or disruption from which you must retreat in dread or helplessness. Be open and flexible toward change. Welcome it as a tonic, an opportunity for growth and learning.
- *Commitment.* Whatever you are doing or whatever you encounter, become really involved. By steering your course with a strong sense of inner purpose, you aren't apt to give up at the first sign of a roadblock. If you really enjoy what you're doing, commitment comes naturally. But be sure not to confuse commitment with overcommitment, the out-of-control response so common to Type A's.
- *Control.* Overeating and the abuse of alcohol and drugs are among the crutches grasped by those who feel at the mercy of every change, be it major or minor. By contrast, people who have control act rather than react; they write their own scripts, instead of following one written by somebody else. Their control does not mean they dominate others. Nor does it mean they do not recognize and accept external things that cannot be changed. Rather, they realize they have the power, the internal means, to control their lives; their positive attitude thus enables them to deal with adversity and to adapt readily to different circumstances. It is unreasonable, then, to regard your fate as controlled by outside forces. Clearly, you can greatly influence the direction of your life by using your skills, knowledge, imagination, and freedom of choice.

Kobasa suggests three ways to promote hardiness:

1. Focus on your body's stress signals and think back to the situations that might have set them off.
2. Re-create a stressful episode. Then write down six ways the outcome could have been different—three of them better, three worse. (Especially note that it truly could have been worse.)
3. Take on a new challenge (for example, learn a new sport, tutor a disabled child) to reassure yourself that you can indeed cope.

Time Management If you're a procrastinator, time management is probably a complete mystery to you. Although occasionally postponement of a task may be defensible, chronic procrastination is self-defeating: it creates stress, which then leads to more procrastination, which leads to more stress. Not only does procrastination cause emotional upsets but it can sabotage personal relationships, college life, and careers (about a quarter of college students are procrastinators, and they often drop out). True, some people refuse to cling to a rigid schedule and work so well under pressure that they can accomplish in a few frantic hours what they couldn't have done as well in a week. But if they gave time management a decent try, even they might find that frenzied last-minute efforts aren't necessarily their key to success.

The reasons for procrastination are as far-ranging and numerous as the excuses made for it (such as "I'll wait until I'm inspired," "What difference will this make in the planetary scheme of things?"). But in general procrastination is a camouflage for self-doubt, for an unreasonable desire for perfection, and for a reluctance to make changes. A primary solution is to stop endlessly thinking or talking about what you're going to do and just do it. How can you prod yourself into doing instead of stewing? Here, in abridged form, are some tips from two psychologists who are reformed procrastinators: "Visualize your progress. Optimize your chances. Stick to a time limit. Don't wait until you feel like it. Watch out for your excuses. Focus on one step at a time. Get beyond the first obstacle. Reward yourself after you've made some progress. Be flexible about your goal. It doesn't have to be perfect."

Time pressures can be stressful, though, even in the unlikely case that you never procrastinate. Depending on your needs, any or all of the following steps should help you manage your time productively and creatively:

- *Set your priorities.* Split your tasks into three groups: essential, important, trivial. Focus only on the first two; ignore the third.
- *Schedule your tasks for peak efficiency.* Distribute your time not only according to your priorities but also in harmony with your body's natural rhythm. You've undoubtedly noticed that you're most productive at certain times of the day (or night). Schedule your tasks for those hours. Remember, no one can work at top capacity all the time.
- *Aim for realistic goals.* Believable goals will continually spur you on. Strive for the impossible, and you'll almost surely give up.
- *Write down your goals.* First make sure your goals aren't merely wishes. Then fully commit yourself to achieving them (a half-baked attitude will get you only halfway there, if that far.)
- *Allow yourself enough time.* It's just wishful thinking to make an unrealistic prediction about how long a project will take. After you've made a reasonable estimate, tack on another 10 or 15 or even 25 percent as a buffer against mistakes or unanticipated problems.
- *Sweeten your long-term goals with short-term goals.* Instead of waiting for and relying on a large block of time, use snatches of time either to start a project or to keep it moving. Say you have a 50-page report to write and are about to panic. You could start by spending just a half hour or so at a time on it, or you could do three to five pages at a time and happily watch the pile of pages grow. In either case, just a bit of progress will make you feel so much better that you'll be stimulated to plow on.
- *Visualize the achievement of your goals.* By mentally rehearsing your performance of a task, you can reach your goal quite smoothly because, after all, you'll have traveled that road before (see p. 41).
- *Sleep on it.* Before you go to sleep, take about five minutes to write down in order of priority the problems you might have the next day. Then ignore them. While you're asleep, your unconscious mind will be hard at work tackling those problems. When you deal with them by rank the next day, you may be surprised at how easily you'll be able to work them out.
- *Delegate responsibility.* If common sense tells you that you need some aid, don't be a martyr. Asking for help isn't a cop-out as long as you don't delegate to others the jobs you know you should do yourself.
- *Say no when necessary.* If the demands made on you don't seem reasonable, just say no—tactfully, but without guilt and endless apologies.
- *Give yourself a break.* Allow time for play—real free time when you ignore the clock and don't compulsively engage in structured activities.

Exploring Your Emotions

How did you react the last time you missed a bus or a plane? Did you get totally disgusted with yourself? Curse your luck? Stew about why you were late or about the mess you caused by missing an appointment? Or did you take advantage of the chance to read, catch up on some work, or observe the people around you (perhaps noting whether they showed signs of stress)? What are some other ways you could have coped?

Relaxation Techniques The goal of all relaxation techniques is to trigger what Dr. Herbert Benson, of Harvard Medical School, has called the relaxation response—a physiological state that is the opposite of the fight-or-flight response. If you decide to try any or all of the techniques we'll be describing, stick with just one for a while. Practice it every day until it becomes natural to you, and then use it whenever you feel the need. Although you may feel calmer and more refreshed after each session, no matter how inept you are, it may take several weeks for subtle changes to occur. If one technique doesn't seem to work well enough for you after you've given it a good try, have a go at another one. After you've mastered deep relaxation, its effects will carry over into everyday life so that, after a while, you'll probably notice that you have fewer hassles, work more efficiently, and have more free time. None of the techniques takes long to do—for instance, just a few minutes away from the television set should do the trick.

Progressive Relaxation Here's a technique that, unlike most of the others, doesn't require imagination, willpower, or self-suggestion to master. Progressive relaxation helps you become aware of and counteract the tenseness that occurs when you're under stress, by enabling you to identify which muscle groups are involved and relaxing them. Other systems of the body then get the message and ease up on the stress response.

Basically, all you do is tense and then relax each part of your body at least twice, tensing up while inhaling and then relaxing completely while slowly exhaling. As a start, for instance, tense and then relax, in turn, the right fist; right biceps (the large muscle at the front of the upper arm); left fist; left biceps; forehead; eyes; jaw. If you want to relax more quickly, just tense and then relax whole muscle groups at one time (for example, both right and left fists and biceps simultaneously). The fastest tension relaxation method of all—and surprisingly effective—isn't progressive but will certainly do in a pinch: simply clench your fists for a few moments and then fully relax them.

Biofeedback Get yourself hooked up to a biofeedback machine and you'll soon have solid evidence that medi-

Exploring Your Emotions

What do you think this person is feeling? What events could have triggered this reaction? If you could speak to this person in private, what would you say? What circumstances might make you feel like this?

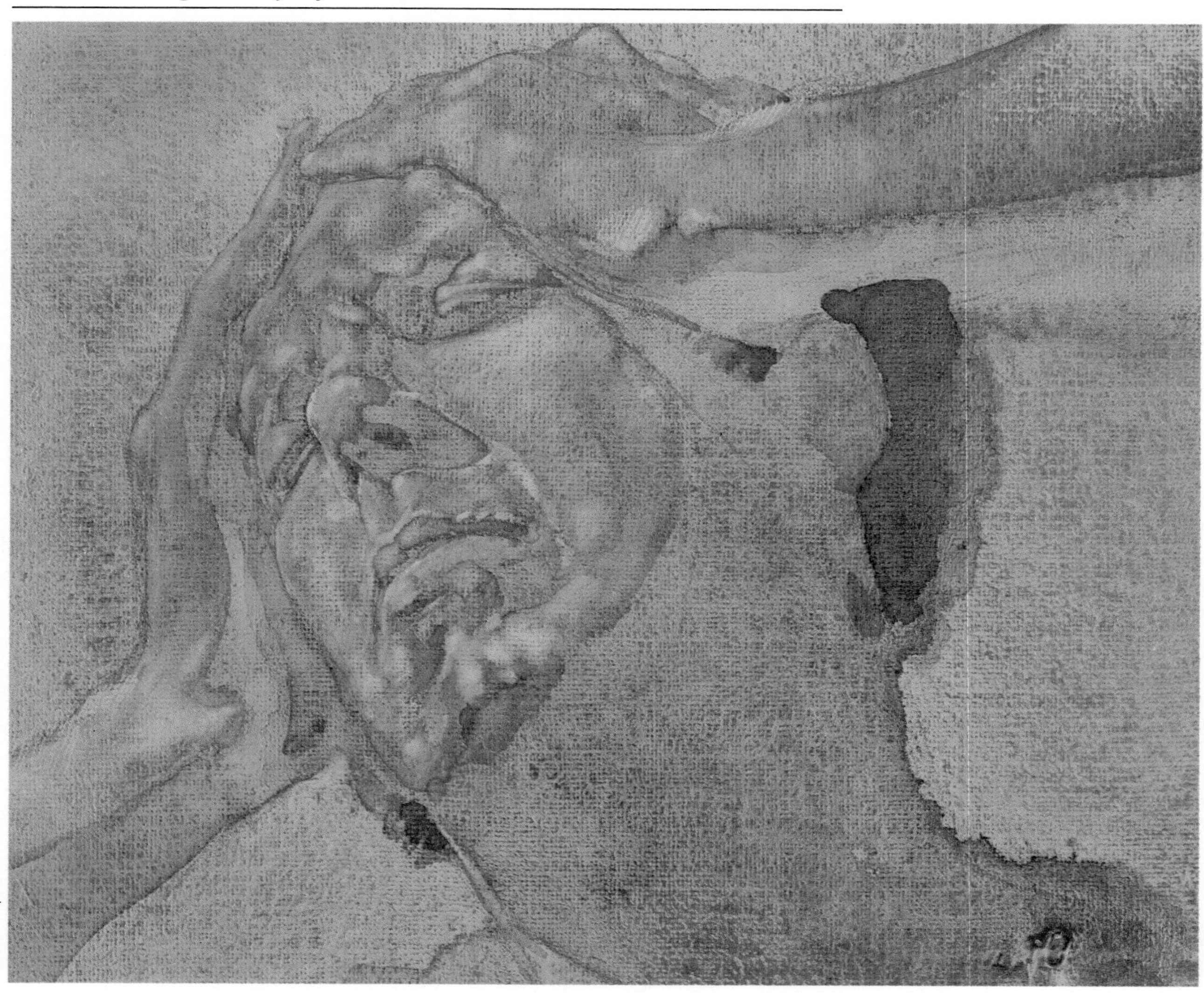

tation, which we'll discuss shortly, actually does result in an altered brain state. When electrodes connected to the machine are attached to a specific system of your body, any internal change immediately generates a signal—a sound, a light, or a meter reading. In this way biofeedback allows you indirectly (through measurements) to see or hear what is going on in your body (such as heart rate, blood pressure, brain wave activity, muscle tension). You become aware of processes you usually don't notice and are guided into gaining voluntary control over them.

Biofeedback does have drawbacks. Its goal is to enable you, at any time, to re-create the relaxation procedure without the machine. But when on their own, most biofeedback trainees eventually stop practicing no matter what gimmicks they use—they seem lost without the expensive gadgetry and the certified trainers to prompt them. Over-the-counter and mail-order versions of the sensitive equipment used are crude and virtually useless.

Imagery When you use imagery, or visualization, you can blissfully daydream—without guilt. With this technique, you visualize a desired change or performance, and your body responds to the image as if it were real. You can use imagery not only to help you relax but also as an aid to healing, to changing habits, and to performing well (for example, before taking an exam, playing a sport, writing a paper, or making a public speech).

Say your back aches or you're at the dentist's. You could try some guided imagery: vividly visualize yourself floating on a cloud, sitting on a mountaintop, or lying in a meadow, and try to involve all five senses (sight, sound, smell, taste, and touch). Or, with eyes closed, imagine your body filled with a deep purple light that you'd like to change to a soothing golden color; then imagine the color changing, and you'll probably feel an easing of your discomfort. If you're worried about doing well at some task, imagine yourself performing it flawlessly.

Meditation Meditation is a way of politely telling the mind to shut up for a while. The need to periodically stop the incessant mental chatter is so great that, from ancient times, hundreds of forms of meditation have been developed in cultures all over the world. Because meditation has been at the core of many Eastern religions and philosophies, it has acquired an "Eastern" mystique that has caused some people to shy away from it. Yet meditation requires no special knowledge or background. We all know how to meditate; we need only discover that we do and to put our knowledge to use. Whatever philosophical, religious, or emotional reasons may be given for meditation, its power derives from its ability to elicit the relaxation responses.

Meditation helps you tune out the world temporarily, relieving you from both inner and outer stresses. It gives you a chance to transcend past conditioning, fixed expectations, and the trivial pursuits of the psyche; it clears out the mental smog. The "thinker" takes time out to become the "observer": calmly attentive, without analyzing, judging, comparing, or rationalizing. Regular practice of this quiet awareness will subtly carry over into your daily life, encouraging physical and emotional balance no matter what confronts you.

Any or all of the relaxation techniques described here should be helpful. Why, then, don't most of them work for long? Because although people might like a certain technique, even become enthusiastic over it, all too often they don't stick with it: after two or three weeks, they slack off, finally abandon it, and resume their seemingly endless search for relief. Most of the methods take time to learn and require a certain amount of discipline, so their appeal tends to fade. Faced with a busy schedule and countless daily hassles, many people find it inconvenient to withdraw, to stop everything while they take time out to practice some form of relaxation. Besides, a few can't seem to relax enough to relax.

So let's consider some other possibilities.

Two Special Helpers Among the great variety of ways to defuse stress, the following two are age-old and nearly universally used.

Music Why is quiet music that you like so calming and healing? Several neurophysiological processes appear to be involved. Such music causes you to breathe more deeply; it directly affects the midbrain network that governs most of the emotions and metabolic responses; and it may trigger endorphins.

At those times when music seems to work especially well for you, concentrate on the sounds and feel the vibrations, which affect the autonomic nervous system, throughout your body—and perhaps you'll know what author Aldous Huxley meant when he wrote, "After silence, that which comes nearest to expressing the inexpressible is music." Try to take the time someday to listen intently to a tape of the poignant songs of whales: it may change forever the way you regard yourself, your troubles, and your place in the world.

As an alternative to just listening to music, playing—or learning to play—an instrument is a time-honored physical and mental diversion (and, because the voice is an instrument, singing is included here). When approached with patience, care, and delight, it gives a sense of fulfillment, engages the mind, and is an almost magical way to iron out woes.

Massage Kneading, pressing, or stroking the muscles has been used for centuries as a way to relax the body, relieve pain, and soothe the mind.

The Relaxation Response

Relaxation and meditation open the gateway to the relaxation response, which is a set of physiological changes that are scientifically measurable (such as slowed brain waves and decreased heart rate, breathing rate, metabolic rate, and blood pressure). These changes occur as the relaxation response blocks the arousal of the sympathetic nervous system. According to recent experiments, the regular practice of a relaxation-response technique produces special benefits that merely sitting still by oneself does not. By countering the destructive cycle of anxiety, the relaxation response tends to banish inner stresses and exert a healing, calming influence. So it not only helps preserve emotional balance in everyday life, but also enhances therapy for a host of illnesses.

The Procedure

Several years ago, Dr. Herbert Benson developed a simple, practical technique for eliciting the relaxation response. Since then, he has found that combining the technique with the "faith factor" can multiply its benefits. Here is the basic procedure Dr. Benson recommends in *Beyond the Relaxation Response* (1984):

1. Select a word or brief phrase that has a deep meaning for you (such as one that reflects your personal philosophy or religious faith).

2. Take a comfortable position in a quiet environment.

3. Close your eyes.

4. Consciously relax your muscles.

5. Breathe slowly and naturally through your nose, silently repeating your focus word or phrase each time you exhale.

6. Keep your attitude passive—disregard thoughts that drift in.

7. Continue for 10 to 20 minutes, once or twice a day.

Suggestions

If, at least at first, you don't care to combine the technique with the "faith factor," you can pick almost any focus word or phrase, such as "one" or a nonsense word or even "Coca Cola" (or, if you prefer, "Pepsi Cola"). In Zen meditation, the word *mu* (literally, "absolute nothing") is often used. Some meditators find it helpful to focus on the breath—in, out, in, out—rather than on a word or phrase. Others prefer to focus on an object such as a candle flame. By contrast, in Zen meditation, the eyes are open to discourage a dreamy state but are not focused on anything.

Passively allow relaxation to occur at its own pace, without trying to force it, without making judgments. Whether you think you're doing well or badly, smilingly dismiss the thought. Don't be surprised if your mind refuses to stop its shenanigans for more than a few seconds at a time. It's nothing to get angry about or think about. The more you ignore the intrusions, the easier it will get to do so.

If you want to time your session, peek at a watch or clock occasionally, but don't set a jarring alarm.

Getting to your feet immediately after a session can make you feel slightly dizzy. Sit quietly for a few moments, with eyes closed at first and then open.

The technique works best on an empty stomach—before a meal or about two hours after eating. And avoid those times when you're obviously tired—unless you want to fall asleep.

Although you'll feel refreshed even after the first session, it may take a month or more to get noticeable results. Be patient. Above all, don't harbor expectations or try to aim at a goal. You'll be achieving your goal just by giving the relaxation response a chance—the process itself is the product. Even if you think all you're doing is chasing your mind around and futilely trying to keep it tied down, the relaxation response will be taking place. And long before you assume you know how to elicit the response, its benefits will start showing up in your daily life. Eventually it will become so much a part of you that it will occur spontaneously, or on demand, when you sit quietly for a few moments.

Variations range from the deep, often painful manipulations of Rolfing and the vigorous approach of Swedish massage, to the more gentle acupressure (finger pressure) therapy of Shiatsu, to the delicate touch of Esalen massage. All forms of massage tend to be both relaxing and invigorating, but the most convenient of all is self-massage, which is easy to learn. For instance, just crossing your arms and then vigorously rubbing your shoulders with your hands can make you feel more relaxed.

Exercise When you experience a fight-or-flight response, your body is telling you that it's all set to move. And there is no more natural way to heed that message than exercise. It not only helps buffer any existing stress but, when done regularly, enhances your physical and emotional strength and gives you the stamina to handle future stress. (For further information about exercises, see Chapter 14.)

Nutrition Neither nutrition nitwits nor nutrition fanatics are apt to handle stress well. At the one extreme, people who have foolish eating habits can, over time, unwittingly contribute to their stress: the malnourishment of careless eaters makes them more prone to illness and less able to deal with stressors in general. At the other extreme are those who are so preoccupied—even obsessed—with nutrition that they worry about every morsel they eat or plan to eat. The stress caused by an occasional dietary lapse pales by comparison with the continual stress generated by overconcern about nutrition.

A sensible diet (see Chapter 12) undeniably helps promote the well-being that enables the body to withstand stress. The basic principles of good nutrition are so easy to learn and to use that their practice can quite rapidly become automatic. The person who is informed and guilt-free about nutrition has an energy bank to draw on whenever stress strikes, as well as a sense of self-control and of self-esteem that is a prime key to managing stress.

Some people react to stress by eating too much, others by eating too little. When you're in deep distress, it may be wise to eat rather lightly, because digestive functions slow or shut down during the stress response (they don't have high priority in the body's attempt to cope).

Although caffeine in small amounts seems to be harmless and definitely provides a mental lift, this stimulant tends to make some persons jittery, irritable, and unable to sleep unless consumed only early in the day. So, when you're under stress, coffee—along with tea, cola, and other soft drinks containing caffeine—may be particularly uncongenial. Eating or drinking chocolate, especially at night, is usually no help either, as it contains the stimulant theobromine.

"Stress vitamins"—high-potency formulations that commonly contain vitamins C, E, and B-complex—are worthless in combatting psychological or emotional stress. In fact, because such supplements may contain up to 80 times the U.S. Recommended Daily Allowance (RDA) for B vitamins and 16 times that for vitamin C, they could even heighten stress through potential side effects (for example, excess vitamin B_6 could lead to neurological disorders). The only usefulness of such supplements might be to provide a boost during periods of *physical* stress (such as during pregnancy, after surgery, or during drug therapy).

Humor Laughter is probably the ultimate stress reliever. A built-in tranquilizer and healer, it is simple and natural and, unlike sex (which can also be an admirable antidote to stress), is always available. You can actually alter your mood if you smile (or frown). A smile or a laugh produces changes in the autonomic nervous system. The result is a reinforcement of your emotion.

A genuine belly laugh stimulates the heart and the glandular system and raises both the pulse rate and blood pressure, but afterward, the heart rate and blood pressure dip below normal and muscles are more relaxed. In addition, laughter aids digestion, eases pain (apparently by releasing endorphins), massages the insides, and dusts off the mind. Therapeutic humor—which does not include ridiculing, cynical, or sarcastic humor—is an appreciation of life's absurdities and paradoxes. Black humor, which is sometimes so gruesome as to be offensive, is an unconscious means of dealing with fears and anxieties. When we joke about serious things (such as dead babies, paraplegics, or concentration camps), we are actually "laughing to keep from crying."

The comic perception offers a respite, however brief, from the tyranny of any situation you may find yourself in. It detaches you from both your situation and yourself. Don't allow yourself to be a slave to all the dramas in your life. Hone the ability to laugh at yourself, and you'll always have on hand a stress reliever that is instantly effective.

A Few Other Suggestions Once you get the knack of dealing with stress, you'll probably devise your own special aids. Here, in the meantime, are some suggestions for defusing stress over both the short and the long term.

Worry Constructively Worrying, someone once said, is like shoveling smoke. Think back to the worries you had last week. How many of them were needless? Worry, if you must, only about things you can control. Try to stand aside from the problem, consider the positive steps you can take to solve it, and then carry them out. You've done what you can; you can quit worrying.

If I Had My Life to Live Over . . .

Looking back over her life, an 85-year-old Nadine Stair of Louisville, Kentucky, recently reflected,

If I had my life to live over, I'd dare to make more mistakes next time. I'd relax. I'd limber up. I would be sillier than I have been this trip. I would take fewer things seriously. I would take more chances. I would take more trips. I would climb more mountains and swim more rivers. I would eat more ice cream and less beans. I would perhaps have more actual troubles, but I'd have fewer imaginary ones.

You see, I'm one of those people who live sensibly and sanely hour after hour, day after day. Oh, I've had my moments and if I had it to do over again, I'd have more of them. In fact, I'd try to have nothing else. Just moments, one after another, instead of living so many years ahead of each day. I've been one of those persons who never goes anywhere without a thermometer, a hot water bottle, a raincoat and a parachute. If I had to do it again, I would travel lighter than I have.

If I had my life to live over, I would start barefoot earlier in the spring and stay that way later in the fall. I would go to more dances. I would ride more merry-go-rounds. I would pick more daisies.

Source: Quoted by Edward A. Charlesworth and Ronald G. Nathan, 1984, in *Stress Management: A Comprehensive Guide to Wellness* (New York: Atheneum), p. 300.

Moderate Expectations Expectations are exhausting and restricting. The fewer expectations you have, the more you can live spontaneously and joyfully. We assume that people expect a lot from us, just as we do from them. Yet the surest road to failure is to try to please everyone—and that is a road you can choose to bypass. In therapist Fritz Perls's memorable words, "I don't exist to fulfill your expectations, and you don't exist to fulfill mine."

If you can't live without expectations, here are two approaches to consider:

- Expect the worst (this is a natural if you're a pessimist). You'll then not be disappointed if things don't turn out well, and pleasantly surprised if they do.
- Expect the unexpected. This realistic outlook can give you the flexibility to adapt readily to changing circumstances.

Weed out Trivia You can burden your memory with too much information. One of the major sources of stress is trying to remember too many things. Forget the unimportant ones (they will usually be self-evident) and keep your memory free for the essential ones.

Live in the Present Do you clog your mind with the debris of past events by reliving them? Clinging to experiences and emotions, particularly unpleasant ones, can be a deadly business. Let them go; keep your mind free and clear for what's happening now. As writer Ernest Hemingway put it, "You don't want to live backwards."

Go with the Flow As we've noted, stress itself is neutral, neither good nor bad; it is our responses to stress that affect our well-being. If we follow the principles of good health, if we see life (and even people, as writer Lawrence Durrell suggested) as an adventure and look forward to the unknowns ahead of us, we should be able to take in stride almost anything that life dishes out, without relying on techniques or gimmicks. The very expression "stress management" can then lose its meaning: we can manage stress automatically, without having to think about it. If we glide along with the flow of life, we don't even need the idea of coping.

When we look at mountains or at shifting clouds, or listen to a bird call or to the rain fall, we are calm, absorbed, choicelessly attentive. We aren't analyzing or judging or fretting. J. Krishnamurti, often called "the intellectual's philospher," urged that we carry over this unforced awareness into our daily life—and then see what happens.

Create Pleasure Pleasure, or joy, is vital for optimum health. But it should not be regarded as simply a reward for something you do, or as a feeling that you can have only occasionally, or as something you must pursue. Rather than take an I'll-be-happy-when attitude (I'll be happy when I graduate, when I fall in love . . .), try to realize that pleasure is integral to being alive and that you yourself can create it every day of your life.

In spite of the flood of self-help books on the market, all of which in one way or another advise you about how to combat stress, there is no procedure manual, no ready-made success formula, that suits everyone. The simplest formula probably ever devised is "roll with the punches."

Take Action

Your answers to the Exploring Your Emotions questions in this chapter and your placement level on the Wellness Ladder at the beginning of this chapter will, we hope, encourage you to begin a process of self-exploration and self-discovery that you will continue. Reflect on the entire chapter's content and ask yourself how each point relates to your own life. Then take action:

1. Dr. Edmund Jacobson of the University of Chicago noted that people tense their muscles when they are stressed but don't realize they are doing it. He reasoned that if they can learn to relax, they can lower the stress they experience.

Think about a specific time when you felt anxious or stressed. Now take your pulse rate and record it in your Take Action notebook. Learn and practice progressive relaxation. (See page 40.) Immediately after relaxing the last muscle group, take your pulse rate and record it in your notebook, indicating the time, date, and conditions after which you took it. Was there any difference in your pulse rate? If so and your pulse rate slowed, you may want to incorporate relaxation as a regular technique in your behavioral approach to stress.

2. Think about the next important test you will be taking. It might be a mid-term, final, or qualifying exam. Do you feel a bit anxious or fearful at the thought of it? If so, plan a systematic attack on the problem. Begin by reviewing the box "Test Anxiety and Stress." Next design for yourself a personal program to reduce your anxiety about the upcoming exam. *Hint:* Are there any exams you don't feel anxious about? Also try combining a relaxation technique with your plan.

3. Think about all the different environments in which you function, including your classrooms, the student union, the dorm, your house. Are some more stressful than others? Make a list of the environments in order of the most stressful to the least stressful. Indicate next to each environment the reasons you think it is stressful or nonstressful. Now start at the top of your list and record three or more ways to reduce the stressful impact these environments have on you.

4. Turn to the Student Stress Scale and determine your score. Distinguish the events you can change from those you cannot change. List the former in your notebook and note how you are going to try to change them.

5. According to some health care professionals, social support can help people cope with stress and thereby lower their risk of serious illness. Find your level of social support on the Social Support Scale. If your score is 40 or higher, congratulate yourself. If it is below 40, think of at least four specific ways in which you can seek increased social support. Then act on those specifics.

6. Fill in the questionnaire in the following Behavior Change Strategy, and if you think you are a Type A, take appropriate action.

Behavior Change Strategy

Type A and Type B Behavior Patterns

On reading the section "Personality Types," you may have wondered whether you are a Type A or a Type B. (It might be helpful to reread that section before continuing.) Although we've noted that questionnaires do not provide conclusive assessments of Type A or Type B behavior, you may nevertheless find it interesting to see which type you seem to be.

Following are 30 items defining Type A and Type B behavior. After you complete the questionnaire, you can score yourself to see what category you fall into. If you appear to be a Type A and wish to become more of a Type B, the suggestions at the end of the questionnaire should help you alter your behavior.

Instructions Read each of the following statements. Then circle one of the numbers *on each line* to indicate whether the statement is true or false *for you*. There are no right or wrong answers.

- If a statement is definitely true for you, circle 1.
- If it is mostly true for you, circle 2.
- If you don't know whether it is true or false, circle 3.
- If it is mostly false for you, circle 4.
- If it is definitely false for you, circle 5.

	DEFINITELY TRUE	MOSTLY TRUE	DON'T KNOW	MOSTLY FALSE	DEFINITELY FALSE
1. I am more restless and fidgety than most people.	1	2	3	4	5
2. In comparison with most people I know, I'm not very involved in my work.	1	2	3	4	5
3. I ordinarily work quickly and energetically.	1	2	3	4	5
4. I rarely have trouble finishing my work.	1	2	3	4	5
5. I hate giving up before I'm absolutely sure I'm licked.	1	2	3	4	5
6. I am rather deliberate in telephone conversations.	1	2	3	4	5
7. I am often in a hurry.	1	2	3	4	5
8. I am somewhat relaxed and at ease about my work.	1	2	3	4	5
9. My achievements are considered to be significantly higher than those of most people I know.	1	2	3	4	5
10. Tailgating bothers me more than a car in front slowing me up.	1	2	3	4	5
11. In conversation I often gesture with hands and head.	1	2	3	4	5
12. I rarely drive a car too fast.	1	2	3	4	5
13. As a young person I preferred work in which I could move around.	1	2	3	4	5
14. People consider me to be rather quiet.	1	2	3	4	5

	DEFINITELY TRUE	MOSTLY TRUE	DON'T KNOW	MOSTLY FALSE	DEFINITELY FALSE
15. Sometimes I think I shouldn't work so hard, but something drives me on.	1	2	3	4	5
16. I usually speak more softly than most people.	1	2	3	4	5
17. My handwriting is rather fast.	1	2	3	4	5
18. I often work slowly and leisurely.	1	2	3	4	5
19. I thrive on challenging situations. The more challenges I have the better.	1	2	3	4	5
20. I prefer to linger over a meal and enjoy it.	1	2	3	4	5
21. I like to drive a car rather fast when there is no speed limit.	1	2	3	4	5
22. I like work that is slow and deliberate.	1	2	3	4	5
23. In general I approach my work more seriously than most people I know.	1	2	3	4	5
24. I talk more slowly than most people.	1	2	3	4	5
25. I've often been asked to be an officer of some group or groups.	1	2	3	4	5
26. I often let a problem work itself out by waiting.	1	2	3	4	5
27. I often try to persuade others to my point of view.	1	2	3	4	5
28. I generally walk more slowly than most people.	1	2	3	4	5
29. I eat rapidly even when there is plenty of time.	1	2	3	4	5
30. I usually work fast.	1	2	3	4	5

Scoring Instructions To find out whether you are Type A or Type B, compare your answers with those on the scoring sheet. Note which of your answers are A's and which are B's. Give yourself plus 1 point for every A item you have circled. Add these pluses for a total A score. Give yourself *minus* 1 point for every B item you have circled. Add these minuses for a total B score. Give yourself *minus* 1 point for every *Don't Know* item you have circled. Divide the *Don't Know* number by 2. The difference between all your plus scores and all your minus scores is your total. Type A's are described as aggressive, ambitious, competitive, restless, and often working against deadlines. Type B's appear to be much more relaxed. They are less aggressive and competitive. Type A's are more vulnerable to heart attacks than Type B's. The following table indicates whether you are an A or a B.

+15 to +30	= Definite A
+ 1 to +15	= Moderate A
0 to −15	= Moderate B
−16 to −30	= Definite B

Here is an example of scoring: If you circled nine A items, you would have a subtotal A score of +9. If you circled fifteen B items, you would have a subtotal B score of −15. If you circled six *Don't Know* items, you would divide −6 by 2, which would give you a subtotal *Don't Know* score of −3. The difference between −18 and +9 is your total, −9. Your score indicates you are a moderate B.

Answers—Scoring Sheet

	Definitely True	Mostly True	Don't Know	Mostly False	Definitely False
1. I am more restless and fidgety than most people.	1=A	2=A	3	4=B	5=B
2. In comparison with most people I know, I'm not very involved in my work.	1=B	2=B	3	4=A	5=A
3. I ordinarily work quickly and energetically.	1=A	2=A	3	4=B	5=B
4. I rarely have trouble finishing my work.	1=B	2=B	3	4=A	5=A
5. I hate giving up before I'm absolutely sure I'm licked.	1=A	2=A	3	4=B	5=B
6. I am rather deliberate in telephone conversations.	1=B	2=B	3	4=A	5=A
7. I am often in a hurry.	1=A	2=A	3	4=B	5=B
8. I am somewhat relaxed and at ease about my work.	1=B	2=B	3	4=A	5=A
9. My achievements are considered to be significantly higher than those of most people I know.	1=A	2=A	3	4=B	5=B
10. Tailgating bothers me more than a car in front slowing me up.	1=B	2=B	3	4=A	5=A
11. In conversation I often gesture with hands and head.	1=A	2=A	3	4=B	5=B
12. I rarely drive a car too fast.	1=B	2=B	3	4=A	5=A
13. As a young person I preferred work in which I could move around.	1=A	2=A	3	4=B	5=B
14. People consider me to be rather quiet.	1=B	2=B	3	4=A	5=A
15. Sometimes I think I shouldn't work so hard, but something drives me on.	1=A	2=A	3	4=B	5=B
16. I usually speak more softly than most people.	1=B	2=B	3	4=A	5=A
17. My handwriting is rather fast.	1=A	2=A	3	4=B	5=B
18. I often work slowly and leisurely.	1=B	2=B	3	4=A	5=A

	DEFINITELY TRUE	MOSTLY TRUE	DON'T KNOW	MOSTLY FALSE	DEFINITELY FALSE
19. I thrive on challenging situations. The more challenges I have the better.	1=A	2=A	3	4=B	5=B
20. I prefer to linger over a meal and enjoy it.	1=B	2=B	3	4=A	5=A
21. I like to drive a car rather fast when there is no speed limit.	1=A	2=A	3	4=B	5=B
22. I like work that is slow and deliberate.	1=B	2=B	3	4=A	5=A
23. In general I approach my work more seriously than most people I know.	1=A	2=A	3	4=B	5=B

	DEFINITELY TRUE	MOSTLY TRUE	DON'T KNOW	MOSTLY FALSE	DEFINITELY FALSE
24. I talk more slowly than most people.	1=B	2=B	3	4=A	5=A
25. I've often been asked to be an officer of some group or groups.	1=A	2=A	3	4=B	5=B
26. I often let a problem work itself out by waiting.	1=B	2=B	3	4=A	5=A
27. I often try to persuade others to my point of view.	1=A	2=A	3	4=B	5=B
28. I generally walk more slowly than most people.	1=B	2=B	3	4=A	5=B
29. I eat rapidly even when there is plenty of time.	1=A	2=A	3	4=B	5=B
30. I usually work fast.	1=A	2=A	3	4=B	5=B

Making Changes

If you think you are a Type A, here are some suggestions from Dr. Meyer Friedman to get you started in modifying your behavior:

- Don't wear your watch.
- Drive only in the right lane all day.
- Cancel an errand and go to the ballet or walk in the woods instead.
- Play a game to lose.
- Quit worrying about numbers, about how fast you get things done.
- Take an interest in the lives of others.
- Be understanding, compassionate, and forgiving when dealing with others.
- Focus on the three P's: people, pets, and plants.
- Keep in mind sayings like Emerson's "For every minute you are angry, you lose 60 seconds of happiness."

If, as a Type A, you want to make an intensive effort to change, you'll find the specifics of a do-it-yourself treatment program in *Treating Type A Behavior—and Your Heart* (Friedman and Ulmer, 1984).

Selected References

Benson, Herbert, with William Proctor. 1984. *Beyond the Relaxation Response*. New York: Times Books.

Borysenko, Joan. *Minding the Body, Minding the Mind*. 1987. Menlo Park, Calif.: Addison-Wesley.

Burka, Jane B., and Lenora M. Yuen. 1983. *Procrastination: Why You Do It; What to Do about It*. Reading, Mass.: Addison-Wesley.

Friedman, Meyer, and Diane Ulmer. 1984. *Treating Type A Behavior—and Your Heart*. New York: Knopf.

Girdano, Daniel, and George Everly. 1979. *Controlling Stress and Tension: A Holistic Approach*. Englewood Cliffs, N.J.: Prentice-Hall.

Kobasa, Suzanne Ouellette. 1982. "The hardy personality: Toward a social psychology of health." In G. S. Sanders and J. Suls, eds., *Social Psychology of Health and Illness*. Hillsdale, N.J.: Lawrence Erlbaum Associates.

Kobasa, Suzanne Ouellette. 1984 (September). How much stress can you survive? *American Health* 3:64–77.

Selye, Hans. 1976. *The Stress of Life*, rev. ed. New York: McGraw-Hill.

Selye, Hans. 1979. Stress: The basis of illness. In Elliot M. Goldwag, ed., *Inner Balance: The Power of Holistic Health*. Englewood Cliffs, N.J.: Prentice-Hall.

Tierney, John. 1987 (May–June). Stress, success, and Samoa. *Hippocrates* 1:74–85.

Wechsler, Rob. 1987 (February). A new prescription: Mind over malady. *Discover* 8:51–61.

Wein, Bibi. 1987 (April). Body and soul music. *American Health* 6:66–77.

Recommended Readings

American Health Magazine, Editors of, with Daniel Goleman and Tara Bennett-Goleman. 1986. *The Relaxed Body Book: A High-Energy Anti-tension Program*. Garden City, N.Y.: Doubleday. *Excellent guide to identifying one's stress spiral and creating a program for handling specific problems.*

Brallier, Lynn. 1982. *Transition and Transformation: Successfully Managing Stress*. Los Altos, Calif.: National Nursing Review. *Thoroughly explains how stress arises and then suggests a practical, holistic path to assessing and managing stress.*

Charlesworth, Edward A., and Ronald G. Nathan. 1984. *Stress Management: A Comprehensive Guide to Wellness. Offers pointers to identifying areas of stress and describes proven techniques (supported by case examples) for handling stress, overcoming fears, and unleashing creative energy.*

Davis, Martha, Elizabeth Robbins Eshelman, and Matthew McKay. 1982. *The Relaxation & Stress Reduction Workbook*. 2nd ed. Oakland, Calif.: New Harbinger Publications. *Step-by-step instructions for a wealth of techniques, supplemented by questionnaires and personal charts (but skip page 181, which contains misinformation on "stress vitamins" and on hair analysis).*

Hanson, Peter G. 1986. *The Joy of Stress*. Kansas City: Andrews, McMeel & Parker. *Engagingly presented, compact, well-tested advice from a Canadian doctor who shows how to turn stress into an ally rather than an enemy.*

Chapter 3

Contents

Rate Yourself

Your Mental Wellness Read the following statements carefully. Choose the one in each section that best describes you at this moment and circle its number. When you have chosen one statement for each section, add the numbers and record your total score. Find your position on the Wellness Ladder.

5 Spontaneous
4 Independent
3 Self-sufficient
2 Dependent
1 Closed-minded

5 Open to new experiences
4 Accessible
3 Informal
2 Formal
1 Hostile

5 Up front/undisguised
4 Honest
3 Trustworthy
2 Deceptive
1 Dishonest

5 Open to criticism
4 Tolerates criticism
3 Resists criticism
2 Offended by criticism
1 Dictatorial

5 Self-confident
4 Secure
3 Stable
2 Insecure
1 Unstable

Total Score ______

Mental Health

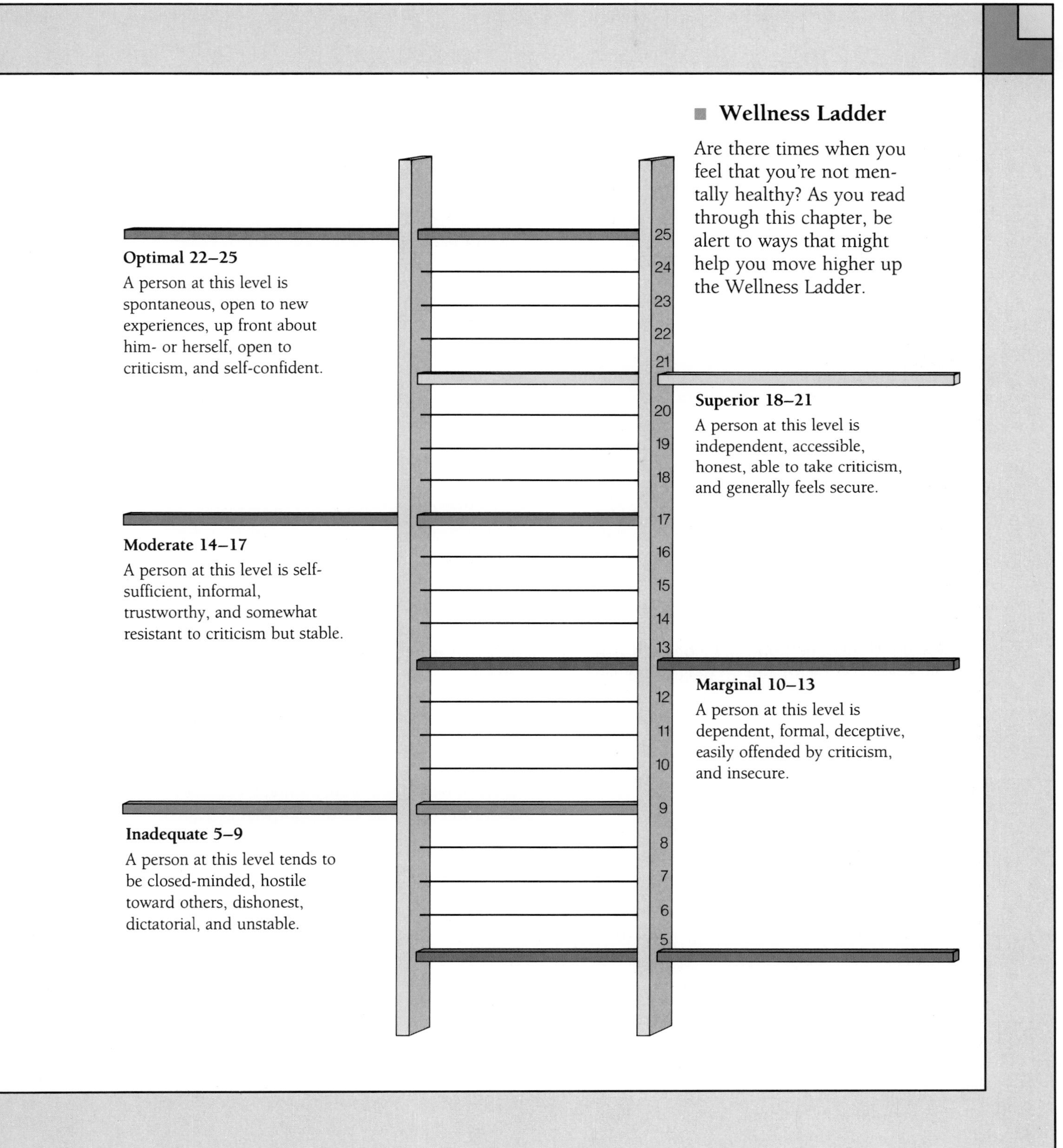

Wellness Ladder
Are there times when you feel that you're not mentally healthy? As you read through this chapter, be alert to ways that might help you move higher up the Wellness Ladder.
25
24
23
22
21
20
19
18
17
16
15
14
13
12
11
10
9
8
7
6
5
Optimal 22–25
A person at this level is spontaneous, open to new experiences, up front about him- or herself, open to criticism, and self-confident.
Superior 18–21
A person at this level is independent, accessible, honest, able to take criticism, and generally feels secure.
Moderate 14–17
A person at this level is self-sufficient, informal, trustworthy, and somewhat resistant to criticism but stable.
Marginal 10–13
A person at this level is dependent, formal, deceptive, easily offended by criticism, and insecure.
Inadequate 5–9
A person at this level tends to be closed-minded, hostile toward others, dishonest, dictatorial, and unstable.

Normality The mental state attributed to the majority of people in a population at a given time.

What exactly *is* mental health? What people think, feel, and do is so varied that it's just about impossible to find clear-cut indications of *mental* health. Some people may try to convince us to live life *their* way, saying that it leads to better mental health than ours does, and they may insult us by calling us "sick" or "crazy" if we refuse. Sometimes lawyers argue that their clients were insane or were "mentally incompetent" when they committed a crime. Conversely, citizens' groups want to illegalize involuntary mental hospitalization or treatment because they feel mental illness is just a "myth" promoted by government or by the mental health "establishment." Many people question the value of dragging mental health into the courts. Expert witnesses often contradict each other, some criminals go unpunished on pleas of craziness, and some innocent people are held in mental institutions for indeterminate periods of time. Mental health issues are battled out at all levels of the legislatures and courts.

We think there *is* such a thing as mental health just as there is physical health (and the two are intertwined). Just as your body can work well or poorly, giving you feelings of pleasure or pain, your mind can also work better or worse, giving you happiness or unhappiness. Is it right to let a depressed person commit suicide on the grounds that humans should have the right to end their lives, for example, when a few weeks of medical or mental therapy might make him or her as eager to live as most of us are? If you answer no to this question, as we do, you believe in the concept of mental health. But it's not easy to define. Here are some possible definitions for you to consider.

What Mental Health Is Not

Mental health is not the same as mental **normality.** Being mentally normal simply means being close to average. We can define a normal body temperature because a few degrees above or below this temperature always means physical sickness. But your ideas and attitudes can vary tremendously without your losing efficiency or feeling emotional distress. And psychological diversity is valuable; living in a society of people with varied ideas and lifestyles makes life interesting. Such a society can respond creatively to unexpected challenges.

Conforming (adjusting) to social demands also is not a mark of mental health. If you always say yes to what is going on around you, you are not all that a human can become. For example, we admire the framers of the U.S. Constitution and the abolitionists, who rebelled against injustices. If conformity were mental health, then political dissent would be mental illness by definition (as some dictators say it is). And Galileo would have been mad for insisting that the earth went around the sun, instead of the reverse.

Never seeking help for personal problems also does not mean that you are mentally healthy, any more than seeking help proves that you are mentally ill. Unhappy people may not want to seek professional help because they don't want to reveal problems to others, may fear what their friends might think, or may lack knowledge about whom to ask for help. People who are severely disturbed mentally may not even realize they need help, or they may become so suspicious of other people that they can only be treated against their will.

And we cannot say people are "mentally ill" or "mentally healthy" on the basis of symptoms alone. Life constantly presents problems. Time and life inevitably change the environment and change our minds and bodies, and changes present problems. The symptom of anxiety, for example, can help us face a problem and solve it before it gets too big. Someone who shows no anxiety may be refusing to recognize problems or refusing to do anything about them. A person who is anxious for good reason is likely to be judged more mentally healthy in the long run than someone who is inappropriately calm.

Finally, we cannot judge mental health from the way people look. All too often a person who seems to be OK and even happy suddenly takes his (or her) own life. Usually such people lack close friends who might have known of their desperation. We all learn early to conceal and "lie." We may believe that our complaints put unfair demands on others. True, suffering in silence can be a virtue sometimes, but it can also block help.

Exploring Your Emotions

Have you ever felt you were going crazy? What made you feel that way? How did you try to cope with the feeling? Were other people helpful to you? What have you learned from the experience?

What Mental Health Is

It is even harder to say what mental health *is* than what it is *not*. Should we think of wellness as much more than just not being sick, or can we just say that mental health

America's Mental Health

The mental health of U.S. citizens is always interesting to scientists. During the past thirty years, four major surveys have estimated the amount of psychological dysfunction in the general population. The estimates varied widely—from 10 to 80 percent—because the investigators defined psychological dysfunction quite differently. In 1979, the National Institute of Mental Health (NIMH) in Rockville, Maryland, began the largest and most systematic survey of psychiatric disorders ever, covering 20,000 households and institutions such as hospitals and nursing homes in five U.S. cities. On the basis of a questionnaire interview, the investigators determined if a person sampled showed any mental disorders as defined by the American Psychiatric Association. A report from three of the [five] sites, published in 1984, challenges some common assumptions about mental illness.

The most surprising finding is that the highest rates for most psychiatric disorders were found among young adults—primarily among those between 25 and 44 years old and secondly among 18- to 24-year-olds. The researchers anticipated that the oldest group (those over 65) would report more illness, having lived more years at risk; but the elderly showed the highest rates only for general intellectual impairment. Most serious psychiatric illnesses—including schizophrenia, panic disorder, obsessive-compulsive disorder, depression, anti-social personality and alcohol dependency—were much more common among younger adults. According to NIMH epidemiologist Darrel A. Regier, a director of the study, these data are difficult to interpret with confidence; they may reflect a sampling bias or the fact that older people fail to report problems more often (perhaps because they forget). However, Regier adds, the data also raise the possibility that a true historical increase in mental illness has taken place over the past few generations.

The scientists also found that the most common problem in U.S. society today is alcohol dependency, which affected one of every seven adults surveyed. This finding runs contrary to the widely held view that depression is the most prevalent psychological disorder. Phobias, too, were found to be somewhat more common than depression, which ranked third and was diagnosed in about 5 percent of the population. Drug abuse was the fourth most prevalent disorder, and not surprisingly, it was found largely among the 18- to 24-year-olds.

The survey data were gathered from interviews with more than 11,000 adults living in Baltimore, St. Louis, and New Haven, Connecticut, by researchers at Johns Hopkins University, Washington University and Yale University, respectively.

The data were remarkably consistent across all three sites. Other findings include the following:

- Men had slightly higher rates of mental illness than did women, contradicting another common view—that women are more susceptible to emotional illness. The survey only included 15 selected disorders, however, so that the prevalence rates may not accurately reflect the total psychiatric disability in the community, the researchers note. As other studies have suggested, women and men suffer from different disorders. Men were five times as likely to have alcohol problems and antisocial personality, where women were twice as likely to be depressed and reported many more cases of phobia—including agoraphobia.
- Blacks and whites had equal overall rates of illness. Blacks had slightly higher rates for drug dependence and phobia; whites had slightly higher rates for anorexia nervosa and depression.
- There was no association between bereavement and depression.
- City dwellers had modestly higher rates of mental illness than did those from rural areas. Those with a college education had modestly lower rates than those without.

Data from an additional 7,000 interviews in Los Angeles and North Carolina, now being compiled, are expected to provide information on distress in Hispanic and rural communities.

SOURCE: Adapted from an article originally appearing in *Science News*.

Myths about Suicide

Many popular statements made about suicide are false or only true in some cases. These statements may be false generalizations from a few atypical cases, wishful thinking, or just ignorance. People often conceal details about suicides, which helps false assumptions such as the following.

Myth People who really intend to kill themselves do not let anyone know about it.

Fact This belief is a convenient excuse for doing nothing when someone says he or she might commit suicide. In fact, most people who eventually commit suicide *have* talked about doing it.

Myth People who made a suicide attempt but survived did not really intend to die.

Fact This may be true for certain people, but people who seriously want to end their life may fail because they misjudge what it takes. Even a pharmacist may misjudge the lethal dose of a drug.

Myth People who succeed in suicide really wanted to die.

Fact We can not be sure of that either. Some people were trying only to make a dramatic gesture or plea for help but miscalculated.

Myth People who really want to kill themselves will do it regardless of any attempts to prevent them.

Fact Few people are single-minded about suicide even at the moment of attempting it. People who are quite determined to take their lives today may change their minds completely tomorrow.

Myth Suicide is proof of mental illness.

Fact Many suicides are committed by people who do not meet ordinary criteria for mental illness, although people with depression, schizophrenia, and other mental illnesses have a much higher than average suicide rate.

Myth Certain groups of the population are immune to suicide: alcoholics because they have alcohol as a crutch, elderly men because they have achieved a stable life adjustment, and black teenagers because they are not achievement oriented.

Fact Certain groups do have low suicide rates, but not these—the first two groups mentioned have much higher than average suicide rates, and the suicide rate for black 15- to 24-year-olds is about the same as for whites of the same age.

Myth People inherit suicidal tendencies.

Fact Certain kinds of depression that lead to suicide can be inherited. But many examples of suicide running in a family can be explained by factors such as psychologically identifying with a family member who committed suicide, often a parent.

Myth All suicides are irrational.

Fact Maybe by some standards all suicides are "irrational." But many people find it at least understandable that someone might want to commit suicide, for example, when approaching the end of a terminal illness or when facing a long prison term.

is the absence of mental sickness (the traditional definition)? Both these ideas are important "*part* truths."

Presence of Wellness Abraham Maslow, an American psychology professor, eloquently described an ideal of mental health in his book *Toward a Psychology of Being* (1968). He was convinced that psychologists were too preoccupied with people who had failed in some way. He studied a group of visibly successful people who seemed to be living at their fullest. Among them were historical figures such as Abraham Lincoln, Henry David Thoreau, and Ludwig van Beethoven; famous people then living, such as Eleanor Roosevelt and Albert Einstein; and some of his own friends and acquaintances. He called these people **self-actualized;** he thought they had fulfilled a good measure of their human potential and suggested that such people all share certain qualities:

- They are able to deal with the world as it is, and don't demand that it should be otherwise.
- They are able to largely accept themselves, others, and nature.
- They experience profound interpersonal relations.
- They have a continuing fresh appreciation for what goes on around them.

The Story of David

When a person begins to act strangely in public or when with friends or family, others rarely reach an immediate consensus about what this behavior means. Different observers form different opinions. These opinions do not just represent different levels of education or sophistication, because conflicts also occur between the best educated and most knowledgeable. Conflicts between models of mental health are not just theoretical but have practical results, as this true case history illustrates. Only his name and a few details have been changed to protect those involved.

David was a twenty-year-old junior at a large and competitive university, majoring in humanities. He had been the best all-around student in his high school class. The principal of the high school remembered him as brilliant and caring. David had maintained his outstanding academic record. Students in his dorm said he was cheerful, outgoing, and "laid back." For six months he had been attending meditation classes, had become a vegetarian, and had started to jog daily. He avoided all drugs including alcohol. Shortly before spring vacation, he told a friend he had been hearing voices and seeing "real" visions. He was convinced that the end of the world—the "Last Judgment"—was coming. He talked of taking his own life because he felt unworthy, and said that his death would help humanity. In contrast to his usual personality, he became withdrawn and isolated. The worried friend called David's father, who lived far away from the university. The father talked to his son several times on the telephone, and arranged to fly up to see him in a week. The day before they were to meet, David jumped off a high bridge and drowned.

How did different people make sense of what happened? In his father's opinion, David's suicide was a result of spiritual striving—a deep interest in Eastern religions—combined with a drive for perfection in everything he attempted. According to his father, David was totally committed in life and in death. The problem his son had faced was trying to live simultaneously in a world of reality and in a world devoted to spirituality.

His friend took a medical point of view. He thought David's visions and voices sounded schizophrenic. The father agreed only partially. From his telephone conversations, he felt that something had temporarily snapped in David's mind. Perhaps a biochemical change had altered his mental state. But during the last telephone call, the day before the suicide, his son seemed to have become completely lucid and calm again. David assured him that he was OK now and that his father could stop worrying. They would see each other soon and be able to hold and love each other. His father found consolation in the thought that his son had found a kind of peace at the end. Yet to many who knew David, the story was only a tragedy—a talented, kind young person with most of his life in front of him died before the seriousness of his problems was recognized and treatment could be begun.

There is a strong temptation to lay blame here. Was his father spiritualizing a schizophrenic disorder? Of all people, the father, who had known his son for all of his twenty years, should have recognized that something was wrong. But his father lived far away, and was merely empathetically supporting his son's spiritual quest. Religious impulses and spiritual crises are usually not crazy; they can have positive outcomes. And why did his friend not intervene more actively? He could have contacted a dean or a professor and insisted that someone in authority should step in. Perhaps his respect and admiration for David made him hesitate. David might have felt betrayed if he had been hospitalized. And what kind of university was it, that a student could become so troubled and so few people noticed it? But many large universities do not watch students very closely, because they believe students should be treated as grown-ups, with rights to privacy and to living under a minimum of rules and social requirements. Troubled students often keep to themselves; it would be enforcing conformity not to allow them to do so.

Thus, we cannot convincingly lay blame, but we can hope that in the future better informed students, parents, and college administrators will be more sensitive to serious danger signs such as the ones in this case: hearing voices and seeing visions, a major and sudden change in personality, suicidal thoughts, and the ominous false calm that can follow a firm decision to commit suicide.

Self-actualized Describes a person who has achieved the highest level of growth in Maslow's hierarchy.

Authenticity Genuineness.

Other-directed Describes a person who looks to others for guidance in how to behave.

Inner-directed Describes a person who has an inner set of rules about how to behave.

Emotional intimacy A closeness between people that includes a mutual awareness and influence of feelings.

- They are able to direct themselves, rather independently of culture and environment.
- They trust their own senses and feelings.
- They are creative.
- They are democratic in their attitudes.

Let's look at these qualities in a little more detail, using the ideas of Maslow and other theorists.

First, mentally healthy people are realistic. If you are realistic, you know the difference between what is and what you want. You also know what you can change and what you cannot. Unrealistic people often get stuck on their idea of what should be. This habit makes them unable to accept what is, so they spend a great deal of energy trying to force the world and other people into their ideal picture. Realistic people accept evidence that contradicts what they want to believe, and if it is important evidence, they modify their beliefs.

A key factor in your mental wellness is self-concept. Mentally healthy people like themselves; in current jargon, they have a positive self-concept or self-image, or appropriately high self-esteem. They have positive but realistic mental images and positive good feelings about themselves, about what they are capable of, and about what roles they play. People who feel good about themselves are likely to live up to their positive self-image and enjoy a success that in turn reinforces these good feelings. A good self-concept is based on a realistic view of personal worth. It does not mean being egocentric or "stuck on yourself."

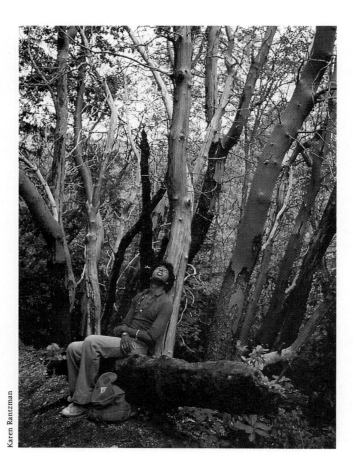

Karen Rantzman

According to Maslow, being free and autonomous is another characteristic of mentally healthy people. Freedom is more than simply not being physically controlled by something or someone outside the self. Many people, for example, shrink from being themselves and from expressing their own feelings because they fear disapproval and rejection. They are unable to act freely and respond only to what they feel as outside pressure. Such behavior is **other-directed.** In contrast, **inner-directed** people find guidance from within, from their own values and feelings. They are not afraid to be themselves. Mentally free people act because they choose to, not because they are driven or pressured.

Mentally healthy people can be comfortable both with silence and with being alone. Maslow believed that mentally healthy people periodically make time for solitude and silence to refresh and renew themselves. Such time seems to help many of these people welcome the stimulation of company and activity when they return. (In contrast, some people feel they must have a radio or stereo going constantly to drown out the silence. Others cannot stand to be alone and feel they must always be surrounded by people. Still others always require definite signs of human life—lights, hamburger joints, gas stations, anything—to keep feelings of loneliness at bay. These people are likely to be running away from something within themselves that they do not want to face.)

Exploring Your Emotions

When you were a child, who was in charge of defining your fears as realistic or unrealistic? Did differences of opinion arise? How do you feel "realistic fear" should be defined? Do you have any fears that you think few people share? Do you feel they are realistic? Why or why not?

Being free can give healthy people certain childlike qualities. Very small children have a quality of being "real." They respond in a genuine, spontaneous way to whatever happens. When you are genuine, you need no pretenses. You are not phony, and you do not always need to censor your words or actions. You don't plan out what you will say or how you will act in order to get approval or to make an impression. Instead, you are unselfconsciously yourself, here and now. This quality is sometimes called **authenticity**; such people are *authentic,* the "real thing."

Mentally healthy people are aware of their own feelings and can express them. One reason why small children often seem so real is that they instantly express how they feel—sometimes to the embarrassment of their parents! Adults and older children have been taught to hide their feelings. Indeed, in most cultures, learning to hide feelings is considered part of growing up. But it would really be healthier for us as individuals to recognize, handle, and express our emotions in appropriate ways. Of course, we must temper emotional self-assertion by considering its effects on others and on ourselves. Expressing anger is not the same as acting it out, for example.

Healthy people are capable of physical and **emotional intimacy.** They can expose their senses, feelings, and thoughts to other people. They are open to the pleasure of intimate touching and to the risks and satisfactions of being close to others in a caring, sensitive way. Intimate touching may mean "good sex," but it also means something much more—intense awareness of both your partner and yourself in which contact becomes communication.

Mentally healthy people take responsibility for their own feelings and actions. They do not blame others for what they do or feel. For example, it is both more responsible and more honest to say, "I'm feeling rattled," than

Exploring Your Emotions

What do you feel the photographer is suggesting by floating the artist in the air? How would you describe the personality of this artist, and what clues are you following in doing so? Describe how you would photograph yourself to present the same sort of patterned hints to your own personality.

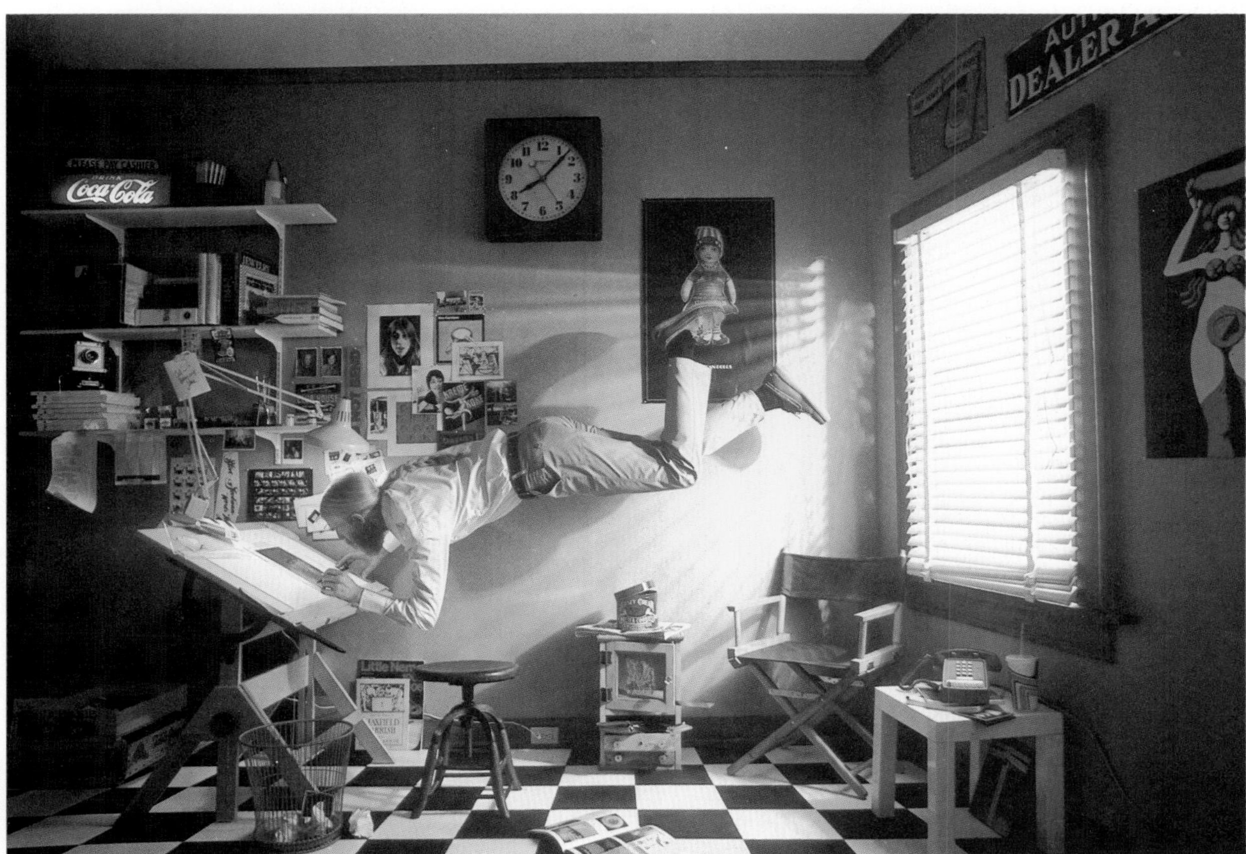

Don Carstens

Exploring Your Emotions

What do you feel is being said or suggested about people? If you were here, how would you be feeling?

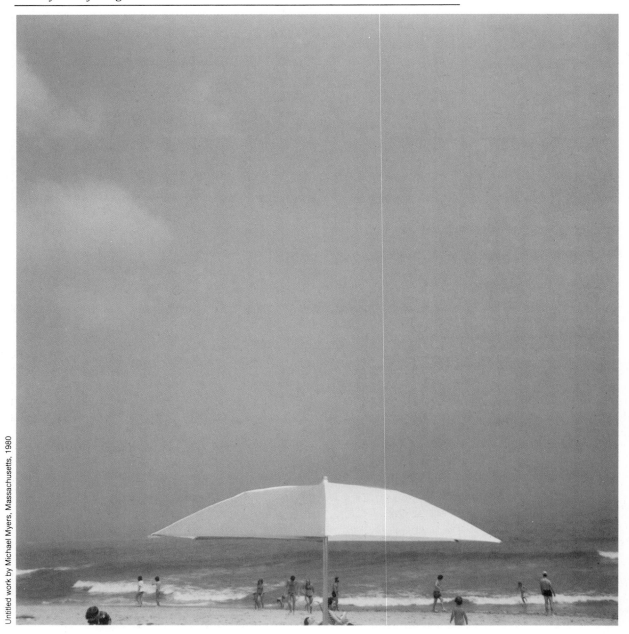

Untitled work by Michael Myers, Massachusetts, 1980

Schizophrenic disorders Mental disorders that involve a disturbance in thinking and in perceiving reality.

Hallucination False perception.

Delusion Firmly held false belief not shared by other members of a person's social group.

to say, "You're trying to confuse me." A person who no longer says, "He made me do it," or "It was all her fault" is moving toward personal responsibility.

Maslow also saw creativity and boldness as characteristic of the group he studied. Mentally healthy people are not necessarily great poets, scientists, or musicians, but they do live their everyday lives in creative ways. "A first-rate soup is more creative than a second-rate painting." Creative people seem to see more and to be open to new experiences; they don't fear the unknown. And they don't need to reduce uncertainty or avoid it, but actually find it attractive.

How did Maslow's group achieve their exemplary mental health, and (more importantly) how can *we* attain it? Maslow does not really answer that question. Undoubtedly it helps to have been treated with respect, love, and understanding as a child, to have experienced stability and been given a sense of mastery. As adults, we probably should concentrate on specific difficulties that block our path to this ideal, as discussed later. For most of us, achieving mental health does not take superhuman effort; usually it's more a matter of relaxing, letting our best self emerge.

Absence of Sickness The idea of mental health as being the *absence* of mental illness is more narrow and more negative than Maslow's concept. In the most extreme form of this definition, anyone is mentally well who is not one of those few people in every society who are severely mentally disturbed. Wherever you go, you will find some people who have occasional or permanent problems in behavior, thinking, or feelings, problems so severe (or so difficult for others to empathize with) that such people can't function adequately at home, school, or work. Some of these people have specific groups (syndromes) of symptoms that suggest biological disturbances, as we discuss later.

There are a number of arguments in favor of defining mental health as the absence of illness. A broad concept of mental wellness could lead us to ignore serious mental suffering and to pretend that we or our own loved ones could never have those problems. Or we could use it as an excuse to spend society's resources only on the well, not on the sick. In addition, mental wellness is too vague and moralistic an idea on which to base criminal law. Maslow's ideal is based on certain humanistic values that are governed more by philosophy or religion than by science. And his description of the ideal self is derived from Western cultural ideals and is not truly universal. However, it is probably also short-sighted to focus entirely on a negative definition of health. A positive vision of mental health can make you aware of human potential in yourself that you might want to develop.

Models of Human Nature

How and what people see is shaped largely by the model—the picture—of reality they carry in their minds. Many models of human nature have been suggested, four of which we discuss here: the biological, behavioral, cognitive, and psychoanalytic models. Each model implies its own kinds of therapy. These models are not exclusive: concepts from each can help you understand and cope with specific challenges in living.

The Biological Model The biological model emphasizes that human beings, like other animals, have an evolutionary history that has shaped not only our anatomy and physiology but also our behavior and emotions. The mind's activity depends completely on an organic structure, the brain, whose composition is determined by genes. This structure can be damaged by infectious agents such as viruses or bacteria, or by physical trauma such as that which sometimes accompanies birth. Such damage can produce mental abnormalities. Chemical compounds introduced into the body can both induce abnormal mental states similar to certain natural mental diseases, as well as partially *reverse* such mental symptoms.

Certain differences among people in abilities and personality, just as in hair color, may stem from genetic differences present at birth. Evidence shows a link between genes and certain kinds of schizophrenia and depression. Studies of identical and fraternal twins, especially when they have been raised apart, have contributed to that evidence. Genetic explanations of behavior, however, do not mean that the environment has no influence. The effects stress has on you, for example, depend both on your genes and your environment, which includes your own behavior. Stress can produce changes in your brain chemistry that result in abnormal thinking, attention, mood, sleep, and other mental functions, just as it may cause the arteries supplying your heart to become clogged.

The biological model is used less in the mental health context than in the mental illness context. For example, **schizophrenic disorders** are a group of related mental conditions that have many possible symptoms. Common ones are auditory **hallucinations** (false perceptions) and **delusions** (firmly held false beliefs). We describe these diseases and their symptoms in more detail near the end of this chapter.

Although the outward symptoms of schizophrenia are psychological, they are usually thought of as caused by a biological brain disorder. The chief reason for this idea is not that schizophrenics show a specific biological abnormality, but that drug treatment—which changes specific chemical processes in the brain—has been shown to be an essential part of the most effective therapy. Nonbiological treatments alone are less effective, especially in severe cases.

Certain **affective disorders** (disorders of mood or emotion) are also often thought of as fitting the biological model for the same reason as for schizophrenic disorders: biological treatments are relatively effective. Severe depressions, especially in middle age, and cyclic shifts in mood from depression to euphoric and hyperactive highs (**mania**) are examples of affective disorders. (We describe depression in more detail later in the chapter.) Both these disorders often respond to antidepressant medications. Lithium carbonate, a salt, taken daily can prevent excessive mood swings in patients with cyclic affective disorders.

Panic disorder also may fit the biological model, partly because the anxiety attacks that define it are often unrelated to the patient's current life and partly because drugs can block the attacks. The chief symptom is sudden surges in anxiety, accompanied by symptoms such as rapid and strong heartbeats, shortness of breath, loss of physical equilibrium, and a feeling of losing mental control. Such attacks usually begin in the early twenties, and can lead to **phobias**, or unfounded fears of specific things. Panic patients often have phobias of being in crowds or closed places, or of driving or flying. It is surprising that antidepressants can block these attacks as effectively as antianxiety drugs.

Although the evidence available today does not firmly prove the correctness of biological models for any mental health problem, such models have been useful in many ways. Some people feel consoled by believing that they have a biological rather than a psychological problem. Somehow that idea relieves them of the tendency to blame themselves or their parents. Biological models have motivated scientists to develop new drugs for treating symptoms such as the ones discussed. These drugs have been immensely helpful, but it is important not to forget that all drugs have side effects, some of which can harm the patient. Thinking that is too narrowly focused on biology can result in doctors overprescribing antianxiety drugs. Ordinary anxiety can prompt you to learn better and more mature coping skills. Although antianxiety drugs are seldom physically addicting, they can become a psychologically addictive substitute for more effective ways of dealing with anxiety.

Biological models can also be misused in other ways. Some people promote treatment of mental disease with special diets or vitamins without any scientific evidence that these treatments work. Others try to achieve mental health through drugs such as LSD or mescaline, in spite of the fact that the insights thus produced may prove empty on return to normal consciousness or the risk that fear and paranoia will result. Finally, biological models (like other models discussed later) may be falsely used to excuse people for antisocial acts or to deprive them of their civil rights.

The Behavioral Model The behavioral model focuses on what people do—on their overt behavior—rather than on brain structures and brain chemistry. Russian physiologist Ivan Pavlov laid the groundwork for the behavioral model in the late nineteenth century when he found that he could train (condition) dogs to salivate in response to various signals. Later, about sixty years ago, in his book *Psychological Care of Infant and Child* (1928), the American psychologist John Watson argued that human psychology also should focus on behavior: "The time has come when psychology must discard all reference to consciousness. . . . [Psychology's] sole task is the prediction and control of behavior."

The behavioral model regards psychological problems as "maladaptive behavior"—bad habits. When and how the person learned that behavior in the past is not important, because that is irrelevant to planning how to change it now. Behaviorists have built their treatment methods on studies of how animals learn. They analyze learning in terms of **stimulus**, **response**, and **reinforcement**. One (of two) kinds of learning takes place when a stimulus becomes associated with a response. For example, if a student (let's call him Joe) once became anxious when giving a talk in class, perhaps because he was poorly prepared and gave a faltering delivery, that anxiety response can become conditioned to stimuli that preceded it, such as being in a certain classroom, looking at notes prepared for speaking, or seeing a group of students waiting to hear the speech. The next time he encounters these stimuli, Joe may feel anxious even if he is well prepared.

The second kind of learning explains why a person may repeat a response or not. If a certain response, such as standing up and giving a speech, is followed by a reward (positive reinforcement) such as a good grade or compliments, it is more likely that the student will repeat the response in a classroom or in another context. However, if punishment follows the response (negative reinforcement)—in this case, fear or negative feedback about a poor performance—the response is more likely to *extinguish* (disappear). In other words, negative reinforcement leads the person to avoid certain places and actions.

Affective disorders Disorders of mood or emotion.

Mania An elated or irritable, hyperactive state of mind.

Panic disorder A syndrome of severe anxiety attacks accompanied by physical symptoms.

Phobias Unfounded fears of specific things.

Stimulus Anything that causes an organism to respond.

Response An organism's reaction to a stimulus.

Reinforcement Reward or punishment; consequence.

Desensitization A technique that reduces fear by gradually increasing exposure to the thing that is feared.

Exposure Direct contact or experience.

Behavior therapy consists of learning new adaptive responses and unlearning old maladaptive responses. People might learn not to be afraid if they routinely returned to feared situations, but often they just avoid such situations and they never unlearn their fear response. Behavioral therapies put people back in the feared situation long enough and often enough that the fear disappears. Two important methods are **desensitization** and **exposure.** Desensitization is useful for phobias (excessive fear) of, for example, snakes or spiders. A person who has a phobia of snakes is first taught to relax and then to begin imagining a small, harmless snake in a secure container some distance away. When the person can imagine this without fear, he or she goes on to imagine more frightening snakes while remaining relaxed. Therapy thus progresses to a point where the person can handle live snakes calmly.

Exposure therapy does not begin with relaxation or imagined situations, but encourages people to immediately expose themselves to real situations that they fear. Joe, who has become phobic to giving talks in class, would develop with his therapist a program in which he would expose himself, step by step, to ever more frightening speaking situations. For example, he might begin by briefly contributing to class discussions, then making longer statements, then volunteering to lead discussions, and finally giving a formal presentation. For someone who has become afraid of going shopping because of previous panic attacks in that situation, the sequence of assignments might be (1) going into small stores with a friend, (2) going into small stores alone, (3) going into larger stores with a friend, (4) going into larger stores alone when they are not crowded, and finally (5) going into crowded stores alone. Therapists can have various roles: they help set up the assignments, accompany patients on their assignments, and organize groups of patients to do their assignments together.

Behavioral models can also be useful in taking care of institutionalized people. A mentally retarded person or severe schizophrenic may not respond to verbal requests or instructions. Analyzing such behavior in terms of response and reinforcement can give the institution staff ideas for promoting cleanliness, appropriate eating behavior, nonaggressive social interactions, and simple work assignments. First the desired behavior is defined very concretely, and a system of reward and nonreward is set up. For example, washing hands before meals might be rewarded by dessert; doing assigned work might carry the reward of going for a walk outside. Whether it is ever right to use such punishments as electric shocks to change behavior has raised sharp ethical controversy.

The Cognitive Model The cognitive model emphasizes the effect of ideas on behavior and feelings. Human beings differ from other animals in thinking and expressing themselves in complex ways. In humans (say the cognitive therapists) behavior results from complicated attitudes, expectations, and motives rather than from simple, immediate reinforcements. Perhaps we should talk about cognitive models, *plural,* because cognitive theorists disagree about the relationship between ideas and other aspects of behavior, and about how to change behavior by changing ideas.

One theory is that automatically recurring false ideas produce feelings such as anxiety and depression. Thus identifying and exposing these ideas as false should relieve these painful emotions. When you are anxious, the idea behind your anxiety is "Something bad is going to happen and I won't be able to handle it." Of course, each anxious person has his or her own versions of this basic idea. The therapist challenges such ideas in three ways: (1) showing that there isn't enough evidence for the idea, (2) suggesting different ways of looking at the situation, and (3) showing that no disaster is going to occur. The therapist does not just *state* his or her position, but encourages clients to examine the logic of their own ideas, and then to test the truth of the ideas. "Of course, sometimes bad things do happen, and sometimes you can't handle them, at least alone. Life is not simple, and some fear is realistic."

Our student (Joe) who was afraid to give oral reports in class probably harbored ideas such as "If I begin to speak, I'll say something stupid; if I say something stupid, the teacher and my classmates will lose respect for me; and then I will get a low grade, my classmates will avoid me, and life will be hell." In cognitive therapy, this student would be taught to examine these ideas critically. If Joe prepares for the presentation, how likely is it that he will sound stupid? Does Joe actually believe that everything he is going to say will be stupid, or is he really aiming for an impossible perfection, every sentence exactly correct and beautifully delivered? Will people's opinion of Joe be completely transformed by how he does in one presentation? Do his classmates even care that much about how well he does? And why does *he* care so much about what *they* think? Joe will be taught to notice thoughts that automatically attack him in feared situations, and to substitute more realistic ideas for them. The therapist will advise him to speak in front of class again and to test his assumptions.

The Psychoanalytic Model The psychoanalytic model, like the cognitive model, emphasizes thoughts, but it says that false ideas cannot be fought directly because they are fed by other ideas that are **unconscious.** Sigmund Freud, a Viennese neurologist, developed these revolutionary theories around 1900. He discovered that certain paralyses that had no apparent physical basis and certain losses of sensory function (such as some cases of blindness) were better understood in terms of the patients' hidden (unconscious) wishes than in terms of nerve pathways. The ideas that were disturbing behavior were at first hidden from both patient and therapist, but gradually surfaced in dreams, slips of the tongue, and the patient's behavior toward the therapist. Freud removed the moral stigma from such behavior by saying that patients had no conscious intention to deceive. In fact, such behavior was medical disorder appropriately studied and treated by physicians. Freud also refused to make any sharp distinction between the mentally healthy and the mentally ill. We all have irrational ideas, which may emerge suddenly and demonstrate convincingly that we can't consciously control all of our own acts.

Therapies based on Freud's ideas imply that symptoms cannot be changed in a thorough and lasting way without changing the client's personality as a whole. Furthermore, to know that personality in depth takes much work by both client and therapist. Secret loves and hates, wishes, and emotions are hidden by active **defenses** that keep them unconscious. Sometimes it is so difficult to face the truth that people can both lie to themselves and conceal from themselves that they have lied. The concealed truth often turns out to be socially and personally unacceptable sexual and aggressive impulses. For example, the master defense of **repression** allows us to push down, to forget what we don't want to remember. What was once conscious now becomes unconscious—but not inactive or without influence. In the defense of **projection,** we conveniently attribute our unacceptable impulses to others: "I am a gentle, loving person, but X is a real pig, and I'm afraid of him." In **reaction formation,** we conceal unconscious destructive impulses behind exaggerated concern for another person's well-being. And **displacement** shifts our impulses to safer but unsatisfying substitutes, as if a person were to say, "If I cannot be angry at my mother, I'll be angry at my sister instead."

In the last few decades, psychoanalytic theorists have studied how people form basic concepts about themselves and about others. These concepts become an important part of our personalities, and profoundly influence our interpersonal relations. A person who lacks a stable self-concept is open to startling shifts of self-esteem. At times the person regards him- or herself as good, capable, and lovable (an ideal self), and at other times as bad, incompetent, and unworthy of love. While at the first pole, someone may develop such an inflated ego that he or she totally ignores other people's needs. Such a person may see others only as instruments for fulfilling his or her desires. At the other pole, someone may feel so small and weak that he or she runs for protection to another person who seems powerful and caring. At neither extreme does the person see him- or herself or others realistically, so his or her personal relationships with real people are filled with misunderstandings and ultimately conflict. These theorists also point out that we can take in images from our mothers or fathers and incorporate them into our self-

Exploring Your Emotions

What kind of personality has the author sketched, and what visual clues have been given? What kind of therapy would you recommend, and why?

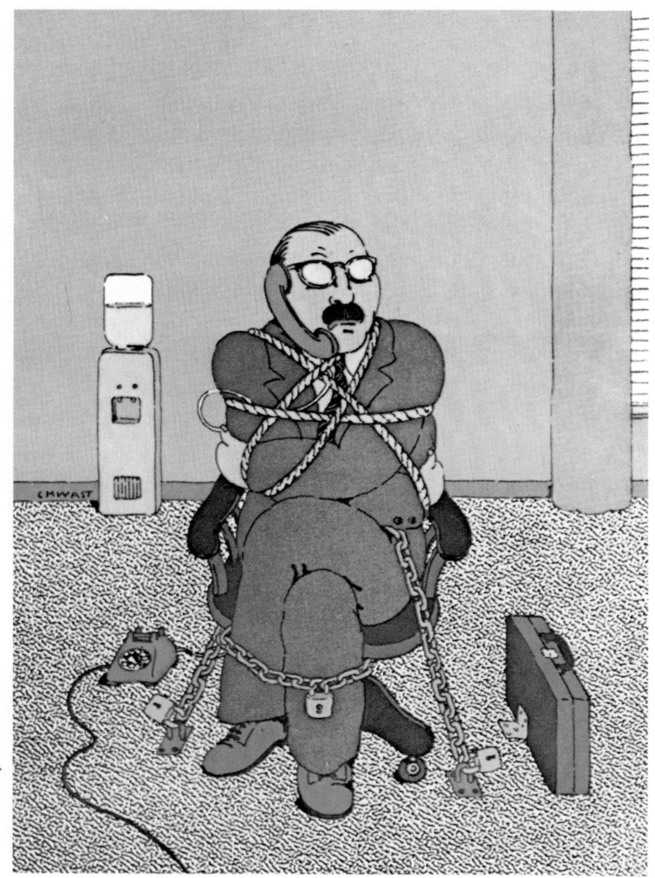

Illustration: Seymour Chwast

Unconscious Whatever is in the mind but out of the awareness.

Defenses Mental devices for controlling anxiety.

Repression A psychological defense that allows us to forget disturbing ideas.

Projection A psychological defense that allows us to attribute our unacceptable impulses to others.

Reaction formation A psychological defense that turns feelings into their opposites. For example, we conceal from ourselves hostile impulses toward another person behind exaggerated concern.

Displacement A psychological defense that allows us to shift our impulses to safer but less satisfying substitutes.

Psychotics People who do not recognize reality.

Neurotics People who recognize reality but who have irrational thoughts and feelings.

Obsessive Referring to irrational, repetitious thoughts or behavior.

Compulsive Referring to irrationally repetitive, forced behavior.

---

concepts without really making them our own. We are startled when we suddenly catch ourselves acting like one of our parents, especially if we always objected to such behavior in that parent.

Modern psychoanalytic therapists often pride themselves on allowing their clients to express themselves as freely as possible in therapy. The therapist is nondirective and tries not to impose his or her own values or ideas about morality or human nature on a client. Some therapists are influenced by the existential philosophers, who believe that humans are free to decide what they will be. Such therapists often adopt ideals of positive mental health, in contrast to ideas that define mental health as the absence of illness.

If Joe, the speech-phobic student, received psychoanalytic or other nondirective therapy, he might learn some startling things about himself. He might discover, for example, that his anxiety in speaking was part of a more general problem of low self-esteem. Standing up in front of others and letting them see him might make him feel attacked. For example, he might fear others would notice unpleasant traits he thought he had. Finally, Joe might recall childhood experiences related to his current difficulties, such as being ridiculed by a parent for a lisp, and in doing so he might learn to distance himself from childish ways of thinking and reacting, such as a panicky avoidance of all public speaking.

Implications of the Four Models The people who believe in the four models we've just described argue out their disagreements. Behaviorists accuse supporters of the biological model of getting stuck in medical ways of thinking and of thus endangering their patients with drug side effects and dependence. Professional rivalries fuel this accusation because behavioral therapists are usually not licensed to prescribe drugs. Behaviorists attack psychoanalytic and other nondirective psychotherapists for making a patient pay for endless, ineffective therapy. Psychoanalytic therapists accuse behaviorists of simplistic (or simple-minded) thinking, of regarding human beings as behavior machines, with no human rights or responsibilities.

We think these fights are mistaken and not helpful, because each model represents certain truths about human beings. Each model can help people dealing with specific types of human problems. When two therapies compete to solve the same problem, scientific studies should be conducted to measure rival claims. At present, strong evidence suggests that therapy is better than no therapy. Showing effectiveness is hardest for therapies that do not focus on specific problems or symptoms, because measuring the changes that occur is difficult, and differences in the therapists' skills may make the difference. There are important practical considerations too. Some people and some problems cannot wait long enough for slowly acting treatments to work.

Exploring Your Emotions

Do you feel attracted to one model of mental health more than to the others? If you had an episode of severe depression, what model would you prefer your therapy to be based on, for example? What do you think is the basis for your preference?

Human Problems

Psychological problems vary greatly in degree and kind. Traditionally, psychologists and psychiatrists have classified problems as either psychotic or neurotic. **Psychotics** are so mentally disturbed that they are unable to test their perceptions and beliefs against reality. Hallucinations and delusions are hallmarks of psychosis. **Neurotics** recognize reality but act irrationally or have irrational thoughts or feelings, which they themselves recognize as irrational but cannot easily correct. Some examples of neurosis are having persistent fears or depression without good reason, having **obsessive** thoughts, or performing **compulsive** rituals such as repeatedly checking whether the oven has been turned off, or becoming blind or paralyzed without a neurological reason. In its widest sense, any self-defeating behavior or irrational feeling is neurotic. So if we are honest, each of us must admit to being a little neurotic.

Assertiveness Expressing wishes forcefully, but not necessarily hostilely.

Classifying people or behaviors as psychotic, neurotic, and normal has been criticized as too vague. All people, patients or nonpatients, show a mixture of these behaviors. The latest diagnostic manual of the American Psychiatric Association has dropped the terms *neurotic* and *psychotic* in favor of a classification based on specific symptom patterns. For example, the manual distinguishes between schizophrenic disorders, depressive disorders, anxiety disorders, and so on. Although this new system is reliable, it only roughly outlines human problems, compared to any of Freud's case histories or to a well-written biography. Furthermore, many important human psychological problems are either so universal or considered to be so trivial, that they never appear in diagnostic classifications. Among the many such possibilities, we will discuss three very common problems of daily living, and two more serious mental health problems.

Poor Communication It can be very frustrating for us and for people around us if we cannot communicate what we want and feel. Others can hardly respond to our needs if they don't know what those needs are. The first step is for us to realize what we want to communicate and then to express it clearly. For example, how do you feel about going to the party instead of to the movie? Do you care if your roommate types a paper late into the night? Some people know what they want others to do, but don't state it clearly because they are afraid that the request or themselves will be rejected. Such people might benefit from **assertiveness** training. They need to learn to insist on their rights and to bargain for what they want. Assertiveness includes being able to say no or yes depending on the situation.

Because expressing feelings has become so central to pop psychology, many misconceptions have arisen. Neither "sharing" feelings with everyone on every occasion, nor letting feelings alone guide important decisions, are legitimate mental health goals. The word *feel* has at least two fairly distinct meanings in English: compare "I feel sad" and "I feel that I should stay home tonight." The first sentence expresses an emotion; the second, a politely worded intention, or an intuition of need or duty. To tell people you are sad can imply various things and have various effects: they may feel closer to you and express an intimacy of their own, they may feel guilty because they may feel you are implying that they have caused your sadness, or they may feel angry because they feel forced to help cheer you up. Depending on your intention and prediction of how your statement will be taken, you may or may not want to make it. To say that you feel like staying home can also have a variety of implications according to the context. You may be politely saying, "Don't bother me," opening a negotiation about what you will do with someone that evening, or expressing your demoralization. Good communication means saying things clearly when you intend to do so. You don't need any special psychological jargon to communicate clearly.

Insomnia To a sound sleeper, not being able to fall asleep may sound like a minor human problem. But to an insomniac, twisting and turning and dreading exhaustion the next day, sleep is a precious necessity that some unexplainable poverty keeps snatching out of reach. Before gulping a sleeping pill, however, the poor sleeper should consider other help.

First, do you get up at the same time every day and avoid naps during the day? A regular 24-hour rhythm of being awake and asleep promotes alertness during the day and sleepiness at night. Getting up at a regular time is more powerful in setting up that rhythm than going to bed at a regular time. Some insomniacs fall into a cycle of sleeping during the day to make up for lack of sleep at night. Even after a sleepless night, it is important to keep busy and carry on with your normal activities.

Second, are you preparing for sleep properly? Avoid caffeine-containing beverages and alcohol for several hours before bedtime. Alcohol may push a person into sleep, but such sleep is not normal in quality or duration. Exercise or exciting discussions before bedtime can delay sleep.

Third, has bed become a place for worry instead of sleep? Some insomniacs spend a lot of their time in bed worrying—often about not sleeping. If you are not sleepy, stay up a little longer. If you go to bed and cannot fall asleep after half an hour, get up and read for a while. In this way, you begin to associate bed with sleep instead of with worried wakefulness.

Demoralization Ideally, as children grow up they develop positive feelings about themselves based on their experiences within the family and outside it. They develop a sense of being loved, and of being able to give love and to accomplish their goals—in other words, a positive self-image. Sometimes, however, less favorable experiences produce a less positive or stable self-concept.

As adults, most of us run into situations that challenge our self-concepts: people you care about may tell you that they do not love you or feel loved by you, or your attempts to accomplish a goal may end in failure. You can react to such challenges in several ways. The best way is to acknowledge that something has gone wrong and to try again, adjusting your goals to your abilities without radically revising your self-concept. A less good reaction is to deny that anything went wrong or to blame someone else. Defense or projection may preserve a good self-concept temporarily, but they keep you from coping in the long run. The worst reaction is to become demoralized, to develop a negative self-concept in which you feel bad, unloved, and ineffective. Instead of coping, the demoralized person gives up, which reinforces the negative self-concept. Thus, a vicious circle of bad self-concept and failure is set in motion. In people who are biologically predisposed to depressions, demoralization can progress to additional symptoms, discussed in the next section.

Cognitive psychotherapists recommend fighting demoralization (and depression) by recognizing and testing your negative thoughts and assumptions about yourself and others. The first step is to note exactly when an unpleasant emotion—feeling worthless, wanting to give up, feeling depressed—occurred or got worse, to identify the events or daydreams that triggered that emotion, and to observe whatever thoughts came into your head just before or during the emotion. It is helpful to keep a systematic daily record of such events.

Let's consider the example of Jane, a student who went to the college counseling center because she had been feeling "down" lately. Her social life had not been going well, and she had begun to think that it never would—that she was basically just an unattractive person. Asked to keep a daily record, she wrote in it that she felt let down and discouraged when a boyfriend who promised to meet her at 7:30 in the evening was 15 minutes late. The kind of thoughts that occurred to her were "He's not going to come. It's my fault. He has more important things to do. Maybe he's with another girl. He doesn't like me. Nobody likes me because I'm not pretty. What if he got in a car accident?"

People who are demoralized tend to use all-or-nothing thinking: things are either black or white, but never in between. They overgeneralize from negative events. They selectively see the negative and overlook the positive. They jump to negative conclusions. They minimize their own successes and magnify the successes of others. They take responsibility for unfortunate situations that are not their fault. Jane realized that the minute her boyfriend was late she jumped to the conclusion he was not coming. She immediately blamed herself. Then she jumped to more negative conclusions and more unfounded overgeneralizations.

Jane needs to develop more rational responses. For Jane, more rational thinking could be "He's a little late so I'll have time to reread the study questions." If he had not come after 30 minutes, Jane might have called him to see if something was holding him up, without jumping to any conclusions about the meaning of his lateness. At first it may be hard to figure out a rational response until hours or days after the event, but once you get used to the way your mind works, you may be able to catch yourself thinking negatively and change it while it's happening.

This approach is not the same as positive thinking—substituting a positive thought for a negative one. Instead, you simply try to make your thoughts as logical and accurate as possible. If Jane continues to think she's unattractive, she should try to collect evidence to prove or disprove that. If she has exaggerated her cosmetic defects, as do many demoralized people, her investigations may prove her wrong. For example, she might ask her friends their candid opinions about her appearance, or she can observe if any men come up to talk to her at parties. It is possible that she harbors the false assumption that if she is pretty, everyone must find her pretty. This assumption would mean that if she could find one person who did not treat her as if she was attractive, she could continue her belief. Demoralized people can be so tenacious about their negative beliefs that they make them come true in a self-fulfilling prophesy. Jane might conclude that since she is so unattractive no one will like her anyway, so she need not bother to comb her hair carefully or to keep her clothes clean. This behavior could help her negative belief become reality.

Depression Depression comes in many kinds and degrees. Demoralization is usually part of depression, but it's not the whole story. The following description of severe depression, or what psychiatrists call a "major depressive episode," shows what depression can include:

- A feeling of sadness, hopelessness, and sometimes also irritability
- A loss of interest or pleasure in usual activities and pastimes
- Poor appetite and weight loss
- Insomnia, especially early morning awakening
- Restlessness or, alternatively, slowing down in movement and speech (lethargy)
- Loss of sexual drive
- Fatigue
- Thoughts of worthlessness and guilt, sometimes to a delusional degree
- Inability to think or concentrate
- Thoughts of death and suicide

Not all these features are present in every depressive episode. Sometimes instead of poor appetite and insomnia, the opposite occurs—eating too much and sleeping too long. In some cases, depression is a clear-cut reaction to specific events, such as the loss of loved ones and failing in school or work, while in other cases no trigger event is obvious.

(continued on p. 68)

Beck Depression Inventory

This questionnaire contains groups of statements. Please read each group of statements carefully. Then pick out the *one* statement in each group that best describes the way you have been feeling the *past week, including today*. Circle the number beside the statement you picked. If several statements in the group seem to apply equally, circle the highest number. *Be sure to read all the statements in each group before making your choice.*

1. 0 I do not feel sad.
1 I feel sad.
2 I am sad all the time and I can't snap out of it.
3 I am so sad or unhappy that I can't stand it.

2. 0 I am not particularly discouraged about the future.
1 I feel discouraged about the future.
2 I feel I have nothing to look forward to.
3 I feel that the future is hopeless and that things cannot improve.

3. 0 I do not feel like a failure.
1 I feel I have failed more than the average person.
2 As I look back on my life, all I can see is a lot of failures.
3 I feel I am a complete failure as a person.

4. 0 I get as much satisfaction out of things as I used to.
1 I don't enjoy things the way I used to.
2 I don't get real satisfaction out of anything anymore.
3 I am dissatisfied or bored with everything.

5. 0 I don't feel particularly guilty.
1 I feel guilty a good part of the time.
2 I feel quite guilty most of the time.
3 I feel guilty all the time.

6. 0 I don't feel I am being punished.
1 I feel I may be punished.
2 I expect to be punished.
3 I feel I am being punished.

7. 0 I don't feel disappointed in myself.
1 I am disappointed in myself.
2 I am disgusted with myself.
3 I hate myself.

8. 0 I don't feel I am any worse than anybody else.
1 I am critical of myself for my weaknesses or mistakes.
2 I blame myself all the time for my faults.
3 I blame myself for everything bad that happens.

9. 0 I don't have any thoughts of killing myself.
1 I have thoughts of killing myself, but I would not carry them out.
2 I would like to kill myself.
3 I would kill myself if I had the chance.

10. 0 I don't cry any more than usual.
1 I cry more now than I used to.
2 I cry all the time now.
3 I used to be able to cry, but now I can't cry even though I want to.

11. 0 I am no more irritated now than I ever am.
1 I get annoyed or irritated more easily than I used to.
2 I feel irritated all the time now.
3 I don't get irritated at all by the things that used to irritate me.

12. 0 I have not lost interest in other people.
1 I am less interested in other people than I used to be.
2 I have lost most my interest in other people.
3 I have lost all my interest in other people.

13. 0 I make decisions as well as I ever could.
1 I put off making decisions more than I used to.
2 I have greater difficulty in making decisions than before.
3 I can't make decisions at all anymore.

14. 0 I don't feel I look any worse than I used to.
1 I am worried that I am looking old or unattractive.
2 I feel that there are permanent changes in my appearance that make me look unattractive.
3 I believe that I look ugly.

15. 0 I can work about as well as before.
1 It takes an extra effort to get started at doing something.
2 I have to push myself very hard to do anything.
3 I can't do any work at all.

16. 0 I can sleep as well as usual.
1 I don't sleep as well as I used to.
2 I wake up 2–3 hours earlier than usual and find it hard to get back to sleep.
3 I wake up several hours earlier than I used to and cannot get back to sleep.

17. 0 I don't get more tired than usual.
1 I get tired more easily than I used to.
2 I get tired from doing almost anything.
3 I am too tired to do anything.

18. 0 My appetite is no worse than usual.
1 My appetite is not as good as it used to be.
2 My appetite is much worse now.
3 I have no appetite at all anymore.

19. 0 I haven't lost much weight, if any, lately.
1 I have lost more than 5 pounds.
2 I have lost more than 10 pounds.
3 I have lost more than 15 pounds.

I am purposely trying to lose weight by eating less
____ yes ____ no

20. 0 I am no more worried about my health than usual.
1 I am worried about physical problems such as aches and pains; or upset stomach; or constipation.
2 I am very worried about physical problems, and it's hard to think about anything else.
3 I am so worried about my physical problems that I cannot think about anything else.

21. 0 I have not noticed any recent change in my interest in sex.
1 I am less interested in sex than I used to be.
2 I am much less interested in sex now.
3 I have lost interest in sex completely.

Add the numbers of the separate items selected. Do not score weight lost on purpose (Item 19). A score of 0–9 would be considered in the normal range, 10–15 would suggest mild depression, 16–23 would be consistent with moderate depression, and a score of 24 or more suggests marked depression.

Anyone who scores between 10 and 23 should repeat the test in two weeks. If the score is still between 10 and 23, and particularly if it has risen, a doctor should be consulted for an evaluation. If the score is greater than 23, a prompt evaluation is certainly indicated. If the score is less than 10 but other indications of depression exist, evaluation is also wise.

It is important not to depend too heavily on any one measure of depression. The subjective experience of depression is highly variable. Some people with normal scores on a depression questionnaire are severely depressed and respond dramatically to treatment.

SOURCE: Aaron T. Beck, 1972.

One of the principal dangers of severe depression is suicide. Although suicide can happen unpredictably, and even in the absence of depression, the more severe and numerous are the symptoms just listed, the greater is the risk for suicide. Additional danger signals are

- Expressing the wish to be dead, or revealing contemplated methods
- Increasing social withdrawal and isolation
- A sudden, inexplicable lightening of mood (which can mean the person has finally decided to commit suicide)

Risk factors increase the likelihood of suicide. Some risk factors are

- A history of previous attempts
- A suicide by a family member or friend
- Readily available means such as guns or pills
- Addiction to alcohol or drugs
- Serious medical problems

If you are severely depressed or know someone who is, expert help from a mental health professional is essential. Don't try to do it all yourself. If you suspect one of your friends is suicidally depressed, try to get him or her to see a professional. If that fails, you might try to contact your friend's relatives and tell them that you are worried. If the depressed person is a college student, you may need to let someone in your college administration know your concerns. Finally, most communities have emergency help available, often as a suicide prevention agency that has a hot-line telephone counseling service (check the yellow pages).

Treatment for depression depends on its severity and on whether the depressed person is suicidal. The basic treatment is usually some kind of psychotherapy, which may be combined with drug therapy especially if the depression is severe enough to disturb sleep or appetite. "Uppers" such as amphetamines are not good antidepressants. More effective are special drugs that work over a period of two or more weeks. Therefore, when suicidal impulses are too strong, hospitalization for a week or so may be necessary.

Schizophrenia Schizophrenia can be one of the most severe and debilitating of the mental illnesses, or it can be quite mild and hardly noticeable. Although people are capable of diagnosing their own depression, people usually don't diagnose their own schizophrenia, because schizophrenics often can't see that anything is wrong. This disorder is not rare: one out of 100 people has a schizophrenic episode sometime in his or her lifetime. However, people who are directly and indirectly affected do not like to talk about it. Also, schizophrenics tend to withdraw from society when they are ill.

Schizophrenia has so many forms that the official psychiatric classification refers to "schizophrenic disorders" rather than "schizophrenia." Some general characteristics of these disorders are as follows:

- *Delusions.* These include, for example, thinking your mind is controlled by outside forces, that people can read your mind, that you are a great person like Jesus Christ or the President of the United States, or that you are being persecuted by a group such as the CIA.
- *Auditory hallucinations.* For example, you might hear people talking about you or to you when no one is present.
- *Disorganized thoughts.* Sometimes a schizophrenic expresses thoughts with unusual words, or mixes words together in a way that is hard for the listener to follow.
- *Inappropriate emotions.* Sometimes all emotion (affect) seems to be absent, and at other times emotions are strong but inappropriate.
- *Deteriorating social and work functioning.* Social withdrawal and increasingly poor performance at school or work may be so gradual that they are hardly noticed at first.

As with severe depression, a schizophrenic person needs help from a mental health professional. Schizophrenia may or may not be accompanied by some form of depression, but in either case suicide is a definite risk. People suffering from schizophrenia may kill themselves to escape from anxiety, confusion, and failure, or to obey inner voices. Expert treatment can reduce the risk of suicide and can minimize the social consequences by shortening the period when symptoms are active.

Exploring Your Emotions

In society as a whole, people who seek help for personal difficulties are often disparaged or discredited, while people who seek help for medical problems usually are not. Do you feel this difference in attitude is warranted? Why or why not? For example, would you feel more comfortable voting for a presidential candidate who had had an episode of schizophrenia or one who had had an episode of cancer?

Treating milder cases of schizophrenia does not require hospitalization. The keystone of successful treatment is antipsychotic medication, taken regularly. Medication is especially useful at the onset of the disease and whenever thoughts and emotions become unbearably frightening. At such times, medication for schizophrenia is like insulin for diabetes—it makes the difference between being able

Choosing Therapy and a Therapist

Faced with the bewildering array of therapies and therapists, how can people choose the best kind of therapy for their problems and the best person to administer it? There are no hard-and-fast answers, but the following dialogue may be helpful.

Q: How do I know if I need therapy?
A: Let's answer that question with other questions. Are you often unhappy? Do you have problems making and keeping close relationships? Do you have trouble doing schoolwork or holding a job? Do irrational fears get in the way of your daily life? Has there been a big change in your habits—sleeping too much or not enough, overeating or losing your appetite, losing interest in activities and people you used to enjoy? Do you think about suicide? Do you generally feel out of control of your life? If you have problems like these, it's time to speak to a therapist.

Q: How do I start?
A: With a thorough physical examination, since some emotional problems are related to physical health. Your family doctor may be able to recommend a therapist. Someone you know who has had a good therapeutic experience can give you a name. You could go to your college's counseling/psychological service. Check the yellow pages to find a family service agency or a mental health center. Or you could contact the closest school of medicine or major teaching hospital that has an outpatient psychiatric clinic. Such clinics often offer psychological testing, diagnostic screening by psychiatrists, and the ongoing services of psychologists and social workers.

If you go first to a interdisciplinary team, you'll find out whether your problems are physically caused, you'll have access to professionals qualified to prescribe medication, and you'll reap the benefits of several heads.

Q: How can I tell whether a particular therapist is right for me?
A: Only through a personal meeting. Besides checking out a therapist's basic professional qualifications, you'll know whether you feel comfortable with his or her personality, values and belief systems, and psychological orientation. Does she or he seem like a warm, intelligent person who would be able and interested in helping you? Is she or he willing to talk about the techniques she or he uses? Does she or he make sense to you?

If you get good vibrations from the first therapist you see, there's no need to shop around. If you feel at all uncomfortable, however, it's worthwhile setting up one-shot consultations with one or two others before you make up your mind. The therapist's attitude toward your interest in talking to someone else may be the first barometer of his or her suitability. If you are not in need of emergency care, be prepared to spend at least as much time shopping for a therapist as you would for a new car. This decision may have lifelong ramifications, and it pays to invest time and money to make it as wisely as possible.

Q: How much will I have to spend?
A: As of this writing, costs for therapy vary from no fee on up to $100 per 45-minute session. Therapists in private practice charge more than those affiliated with centers or large institutions, and psychiatrists usually charge more than psychologists, who charge more than social workers. Many therapists charge on a sliding scale based on what the client can afford, and many health insurance plans cover the costs.

Q: What should I do if I start with a therapist and then decide that she or he is not helping me?
A: First, ask yourself whether you're displeased because your therapy is raising difficult, painful issues that you don't want to deal with. Then express your dissatisfaction to your therapist and deal with it in your sessions. Finally, if you are convinced that your therapy is either ineffective or harmful, find another therapist (*not* one referred by your current therapist!)

to function and not. When schizophrenic symptoms get out of control, hospitalization is helpful to find the proper dose and type of medication quickly, to prevent self-destructive acts, and to relieve family and friends from responsibility for restraining the erratic behavior. In some cases, for reasons still unknown, schizophrenia takes a downward course to where sustained independent living cannot be maintained. Such people must then be found half-way houses and institutional settings in which they can live.

Getting Help

An intelligent way to begin solving a personal problem is to find out what you can do on your own. This book gives some guidelines about what to do for specific problems. Behavioral and some cognitive approaches are especially useful for self-help. Books are available in the psychology or self-help sections of your college library or bookstore.

Often self-help is not enough—help is needed from someone else. Talking to friends can be useful, but sometimes a person needs more objective, more expert, or more discreet help. Many people have trouble accepting the idea of outside help to handle personal problems, and often the people who most need help are the most unwilling to get it. You may find yourself someday having to overcome your own reluctance toward seeking help or the reluctance of a friend for whom you want to get help.

It is impossible to state firmly the exact signs of needing outside help except, of course, when the problems are extremely severe or obvious. Clearly, if a person begins to fail all across the board in school or work because of emotional problems, he or she should find help. A person who cannot keep from thinking about suicide should refer him- or herself to a mental health professional, and should be referred by anyone else who is aware of the situation.

Of course, some people are just interested in improving their mental health in a general way by going into individual or group therapy to learn more about themselves and about how to interact with others. Certain therapies teach people how to adjust the effect of what they say and do on people around them. Clearly, seeking help for these reasons is optional, not necessary. Interpersonal friction among family members or between partners often falls in the middle between necessary and optional. Successful help with such problems can mean the difference, for example, between a painful divorce and a satisfying relationship.

The college student is usually in a good position to find inexpensive expert guidance toward mental health. Larger colleges have both health services that employ psychiatrists and psychologists, and counseling centers staffed by professionals and students (peer counselors). Psychology departments and education departments sometimes offer student counselors. University medical centers often have low-fee clinics where psychiatrists in training treat patients. Student newspapers may announce "sensitivity training groups" or other self-awareness groups sponsored by student organizations. Smaller colleges offer fewer of these services on campus, but generally provide referrals to outside help.

Exploring Your Emotions

Suppose you have gone to a therapist for six weeks now, and you feel (rather reluctantly) that the therapist really doesn't take you seriously. But when you suggest looking for another therapist, he (or she) says you are hiding from your own problems and need two years of therapy. In addition, the therapist raises the fee, "so that you will really value your work here." How do you feel about all this? What will you do?

Communities also offer help. Family physicians, clergy, or family service agencies may be able to help you choose from the lists of psychologists, marriage counselors, or psychiatrists in the telephone book. Financial considerations are important, too. Be sure to check whether your health insurance or prepaid medical care plans provide mental health benefits. If you're not covered, don't let that stop you from getting help; investigate low-cost alternatives.

Whomever you choose to help you, respect your own judgment as to whether you are actually being helped. Although too much "shopping around" may be a way of avoiding resolving problems, you certainly have the right to change therapists if therapy is not helpful after a reasonable period of time.

Take Action

Your answers to the Exploring Your Emotions questions in this chapter and your level on the Wellness Ladder will, we hope, encourage you to begin a process of self-exploration and self-discovery. Reflect on the entire chapter's content and ask yourself how each point relates to your own life. Then take action:

1. Most students have had the experience of writing lengthy papers on various topics. One topic they rarely write about is themselves. Yet this is a good way to explore feelings and attitudes and gain insight into aspects of yourself you rarely think about. Write your personal biography. Let your mind freely wander. Continue writing until the well runs dry. Write anything you want to as long as it relates directly to you and your innermost feelings. When you finish, consider showing it to a close friend or someone whose reactions might be valuable.

2. Answer each of the following questions in three sentences or fewer: Who am I? Who would I like to be? What are the similarities between the person you perceive yourself to be and the person you would like to be? What are the differences? What conclusions can you draw from this assignment?

3. List the positive behaviors that help you adapt to change and remain open. Also list those behaviors that block your openness and adaptation to change. Consider how you can strengthen your existing positive behaviors and reduce the blocking behaviors. Don't forget to congratulate yourself for positive behaviors.

4. Read the following Behavior Change Strategy, and take the appropriate action.

Behavior Change Strategy

Shy and Lonesome: Social Anxiety

Many people experience significant personal difficulty in getting along with others—particularly members of the opposite sex. This problem is usually referred to as *shyness* or *loneliness,* but researchers have coined several other labels such as *social inhibition, heterosexual anxiety, social anxiety,* and *interpersonal anxiety.*

College-student dating has been given the greatest amount of research attention probably because of the easy access to likely clients who are experiencing acute difficulties initiating new friendships. In collecting questionnaire data from 479 students enrolled in an introductory psychology course at Stanford University, Horowitz and French (1979) found that 5 percent of the sample, or about 25 students, could be classified as lonely. The researchers found that the most common problem for these lonely college students was inhibited sociability. A more specific listing of the statements of lonely students is presented in the list on p. 73.

Of course, it should come as no surprise that physical appearance plays a major role in terms of friendship development—but looks are often given too much credit or blame in this regard. A variety of subtle social skills is needed to initiate and then sustain human relationships. These skills include appropriate eye contact, sense of humor, reflection, facial expression, initiating topics in conversation, maintaining the flow of conversation by asking questions, and so on.

One general plan of treatment assumes a *skills-deficit perspective,* and it teaches college students how to use interpersonal skills to greater personal advantage by means of videotape feedback and modeling (practice exercises). Practice-dating programs in which both partners know that their interaction has been scheduled for practice and self-improvement help extend modeling well beyond the clinic into "real world" social settings.

A slightly different approach stems from the perspective that people know well enough what to do to make and keep friends—the problem of social inhibition comes from the anxiety that reduces a person's ability to perform key social skills. Reduced performance produces even greater self-doubt and anxiety, which only interferes further with later performance to produce a vicious circle of damaging experiences. With this approach, people for whom anxiety plays a key role receive special training in relaxation skills and other stress management strategies—perhaps in conjunction

(continued on p. 73)

The Social Disease Called Shyness

We rather admire a touch of arrogance, a self-assured demeanor. Shyness is not a part of the American Dream. It may be surprising to learn, therefore, that over 40 percent of adults in the United States suffer from shyness. But apparently almost all of us are shy in certain situations.

Shyness is a form of social anxiety, a fear of what others will think of our appearance or our behavior. The accompanying feelings of self-consciousness, embarrassment, and unworthiness can be overwhelming. The distressing telltale symptoms include cold sweats, clammy hands, trembling hands and legs, butterflies in the stomach, pounding heart, nausea, a sinking sensation, blushing, and an urgent need to evacuate the bowels.

Philip Zimbardo, Stanford University psychologist, believes that shyness is increasing in the population: "Shyness is an insidious personal problem that is reaching such epidemic proportions as to be justifiably called a social disease." Research on shyness has boomed in the past few years, as experts try to pin down the cause of shyness. Three major theories have emerged from various studies: shyness is an inherited personality trait; shyness results when effective social skills are not learned; and shyness is the result of social programming. Evidence suggests that all three premises may be true.

At Harvard University a study being conducted by Jerome Kagan indicates that when faced with the unknown, shy infants and toddlers withdraw. They become reserved and silent, and their heart rate pattern alters. Infants and toddlers who are not shy do not grow wary when presented with unfamiliar stimuli, nor does their heart rate pattern change. By the time the children in this study had entered kindergarten, none of the nonshy children had become shy. About a third of the shy ones had become less shy; and these, interestingly, were mostly boys. The two-thirds who remained shy still responded to mild stress with apprehension as well as with the increased heart rate they had demonstrated four years earlier. Apparently, the no-longer-shy had been encouraged by their parents to become more assertive and more confident, qualities valued in our society. And those who remained shy probably will always be so. Kagan states, "You begin to get significant predictive correlations to adult behavior around age 5 or 6. Beginning at that time, a boy who is, say, one of the most aggressive in a group of 100 children is likely to be one of the more aggressive adults in that group."

Most shy adults probably were not shy infants. When a schoolchild's self-esteem is battered by family or peers, the child becomes shy. It doesn't take much to make a young person shy, and that shyness emerges in adulthood whenever related situations arise. Adults are shy if they learned early to be uncertain about their looks, say, or their intelligence. They may also become shy when confronted by social groups of a higher or lower class than they were raised in. Also, being surrounded by better-educated people or working alongside more skillful people can bring back shyness.

To define shyness as a fear of social rejection is correct, but it isn't enough. Shyness also includes an exaggerated sense of self, a very real concern with one's outward behavior, physiological symptoms, and feelings of self-consciousness. Shy people tend to be self-absorbed. They typically are anxious about their effect on others and about how others will view them. They often fear that other people will be contemptuous toward them. Generally, shy people are worried about themselves; the feelings of others don't touch them.

Shyness is the opposite of self-confidence. Shy persons believe that others are confident in all arenas of society. And yet, very few adults have confidence in their attractiveness to others *and* their social skills *and* their job competence *and* their knowledge *and* their grace and dexterity *and* their techniques in bed. Most of us experience the discomfort of shyness in certain situations.

While the social scientists continue their research, and many important studies are going on right now, shy people are taking a pragmatic approach. Some of them are fed up with shortchanging themselves and are reaching out to community center shyness classes, assertiveness training groups, and public speaking clinics.

Lynne Henderson, director of the Palo Alto Shyness Clinic, in Palo Alto, California, states that most of her patients come to the clinic because they are tired of being lonely or they feel limited at work. Meeting in small groups, the patients receive training in social and cognitive skills and in assertiveness. The emphasis is on changing behavior and learning how to negotiate so that everybody wins.

Shy people may always be shy, but with professional help they can learn behavior that benefits their personal and work lives. And they can learn to tolerate and to modify their physiological symptoms. Many are doing just that. The rest are still sweating it out.

SOURCE: L. F. Jacobson, 1985 (July), The social disease called shyness, *Healthline*.

Indications of Shyness

Behavior

Avoidance of social gatherings

Inability to make eye contact

Speaking in a low voice

Reluctance to return an item to a store

Reluctance to complain about poor service in a restaurant

Inability to make suggestions to sex partner

Never volunteering

Inability to make a speech

Feelings

Embarrassment

Self-consciousness

Feeling inadequate

Feeling inferior

Wanting to get out of a situation

Physiological Symptoms

Blushing

Increased pulse

Pounding heart

Dry mouth

Perspiration

Shaky hands

Butterflies in the stomach

Trembling

SOURCE: Philip G. Zimbardo, 1977, *Shyness* (Menlo Park, Calif.: Addison-Wesley.)

with the more complex and time-consuming anxiety-reduction procedure known as *systematic desensitization*.

In most cases shyness and loneliness are not unidimensional, not easily diagnosed as being only a problem of skills or a problem of anxiety. Most programs assume that *both* skills and anxiety play a role, and these programs provide a comprehensive treatment that includes modeling, structural practice, and stress management components.

Programs usually begin with a self-monitoring phase in which all facets of a person's daily routine are noted in a diary format. The Social Activity Diary (Figure 3-1) shows how a coding scheme (noted in the key) can be used to help keep track of the pattern of social contacts, the amount of time spent in effective

Statements Identifying Lonely College Students

It is a common problem for me to . . .

- □ Make friends in a simple, natural way.
- □ Introduce myself to others at parties.
- □ Make phone calls to others to initiate social activity.
- □ Participate in groups.
- □ Get pleasure out of a party.
- □ Get into the swing of a party.
- □ Relax on a date and enjoy myself.
- □ Be friendly and sociable with others.
- □ Participate in playing games with others.
- □ Get buddy-buddy with others.

SOURCE: Adapted from L. M. Horowitz and R. de S. French, 1979, "Interpersonal Problems of People Who Describe Themselves as Lonely," *Journal of Consulting and Clinical Psychology* 47:762–64.

Figure 3-1 Social Activity Diary

	DATE:	11/16	DATE:		DATE:	
	AM	PM	AM	PM	AM	PM
12		I, I, W				
1		A, W				
2		S				
3		S				
4		S				
5		I, I				
6		W				
7		W				
8		S				
9		S P, P				
10	I, I, S	S				
11	S	W				

KEY
P = Social phone call
I = Social interaction (at least 5 minutes)
A = Social activity
S = Study time
W = Wasted time

studying, and the amount of time wasted each day. These patterns are monitored for at least one week so that general trends can be identified.

Depending on the particular program, the shy person is then told to make better use of "wasted time" and to begin to practice some of the skills he or she has learned in the class or clinic in the least troublesome (anxiety-producing) situations. This tactic might be translated into an assignment (and behavioral contract) to initiate brief, nonthreatening conversations with same-sex classmates on an academic topic (the upcoming midterm or the homework assignment, for example). Once these conversations are successfully accomplished, then the next phase of the program could encourage practice of discussions that involve more personal subjects (personal opinions about nonacademic topics). Later assignments might involve members of the opposite sex. The individual steps would form a type of hierarchy, incorporating topics, people, and places, from least to most difficult. The person would accomplish these steps by using a consistent theme of practice, modeling, and stress management skills while moving up the hierarchy.

One final point is in order regarding the role of a person's living situation. Research has shown that students—both male and female—who live off campus may well have to take a more assertive role in initiating social contacts and developing friendships than students who live on campus. This is because living off campus is often more isolated than the highly concentrated social environment on campus.

Selected References

American Psychiatric Association. 1987. *Diagnostic and Statistical Manual of Mental Disorders* (DSM-III-R), 3rd ed. revised. Washington, D.C.: American Psychiatric Association Press.

Beck, A. T., A. J. Rush, B. F. Shaw, and G. Emery, 1979. *Cognitive Therapy of Depression: A Treatment Manual.* New York: Guilford.

Berger, P. A., and H. K. H. Brodie, (eds.). 1986. *American Handbook of Psychiatry.* Vol. 8: *Biological Psychiatry.* New York: Basic Books.

Hatton, C. L., and S. M. Valente, (eds.). 1984. *Suicide: Assessment and Intervention.* 2nd ed. Norwalk, Conn.: Appleton-Century-Crofts.

Hauri, P. J., and M. J. Sateia, 1985. Nonpharmacological treatment of sleep disorders. Chapter 29 in R. E. Hales and A. J. Frances (eds.), *Psychiatry Update: American Psychiatric Association Annual Review* 4:361–78 (published by the American Psychiatic Press, Washington, D. C.)

Hersen, M., and A. S. Bellack, (eds.). 1985. *Handbook of Clinical Behavior Therapy with Adults.* New York: Plenum Press.

Kohut, H. 1971. *The Psychology of the Self.* New York: International Universities Press.

Lazare, A. 1973. Hidden conceptual models in clinical psychiatry. *New England Journal of Medicine* 288:345–51.

Maslow, A. H. 1968. *Toward a Psychology of Being.* 2nd ed. Princeton, N.J.:Van Nostrand-Reinhold.

Regier, D. A., J. K. Myers, M. Kramer, L. N. Robins, D. G. Blazer, R. L. Hough, W. W. Eaton, and B. Z. Locke, 1984. The NIMH Epidemiologic Catchment Area Surveys. *Archives of General Psychiatry* 41:934–42. (Also see other articles on pp. 942–78 of the same volume.)

Recommended Readings

Agras, S. 1985. *Panic: Facing Fears, Phobias, and Anxiety.* San Francisco: Freeman. *This popular book explains the nature of fears and phobias and how to overcome them.*

Andreasen, N. C. 1984. *The Broken Brain: The Biological Revolution in Psychiatry.* New York: Harper & Row. *Here is a clear, simple presentation of the biology of mental illness.*

Brenner, C. 1957. *An Elementary Textbook of Psychoanalysis.* Garden City, N.Y.: Doubleday. *Brenner gives an authoritative and moderately detailed account of Freudian theory and therapy.*

Sarason, I. G., and B. R. Sarason. 1987. *Abnormal Psychology: The Problem of Maladaptive Behavior,* 5th ed. Englewood Cliffs, N.J.: Prentice-Hall. *This up-to-date textbook is a good place to look for more detailed discussions of topics in this chapter.*

Zimbardo, P. G. 1977. *Shyness—What It Is. What to Do about It.* Reading, Mass.: Addison-Wesley. *Students and their interpersonal problems are the focus of the research and therapy techniques reported in this book.*

Chapter 4

Contents

Rate Yourself

Your Sexual Awareness and Health Read the following statements carefully. Choose the one in each section that best describes you at this moment and circle its number. When you have chosen one statement for each section, add the numbers and record your total score. Find your position on the Wellness Ladder.

5 Very satisfied sexually
4 Satisfied sexually
3 Somewhat satisfied sexually
2 Rarely satisfied sexually
1 Frustrated sexually

5 Consider partner's needs before my own
4 Am sensitive to partner's needs
3 Am sensitive to partner's needs most of the time
2 Am rarely sensitive to partner's needs
1 Am insensitive to partner's needs

5 Can openly discuss my sexual needs
4 Can discuss sexual problems with my partner
3 Am embarrassed by frank sexual discussion
2 Am reluctant to discuss sexual problems
1 Am unable to discuss sexual problems

5 Enjoy sex as part of a total relationship
4 Prefer intimacy to an exclusively sexual relationship
3 Am affectionate with sexual partner
2 Have frequent sexual encounters
1 Have unsatisfactory sexual encounters

5 Can communicate sexual pleasures to partner
4 Can reveal sexual preferences to partner
3 Am easily aroused
2 Seek immediate sexual gratification
1 View myself as sexually inadequate

Total Score ______

Sex and Your Body

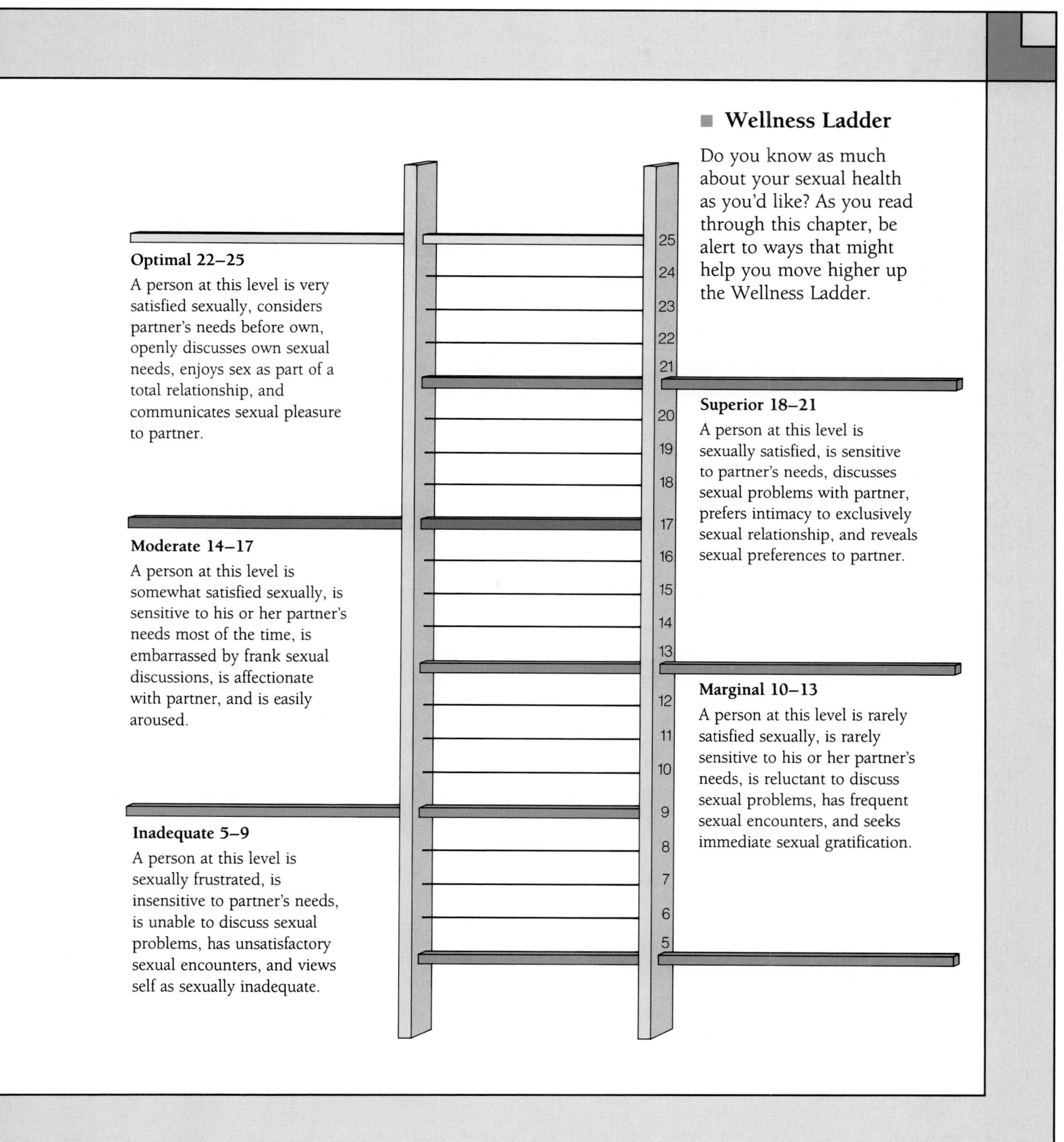

Wellness Ladder
Do you know as much about your sexual health as you'd like? As you read through this chapter, be alert to ways that might help you move higher up the Wellness Ladder.
Optimal 22–25
A person at this level is very satisfied sexually, considers partner's needs before own, openly discusses own sexual needs, enjoys sex as part of a total relationship, and communicates sexual pleasure to partner.
Superior 18–21
A person at this level is sexually satisfied, is sensitive to partner's needs, discusses sexual problems with partner, prefers intimacy to exclusively sexual relationship, and reveals sexual preferences to partner.
Moderate 14–17
A person at this level is somewhat satisfied sexually, is sensitive to his or her partner's needs most of the time, is embarrassed by frank sexual discussions, is affectionate with partner, and is easily aroused.
Marginal 10–13
A person at this level is rarely satisfied sexually, is rarely sensitive to his or her partner's needs, is reluctant to discuss sexual problems, has frequent sexual encounters, and seeks immediate sexual gratification.
Inadequate 5–9
A person at this level is sexually frustrated, is insensitive to partner's needs, is unable to discuss sexual problems, has unsatisfactory sexual encounters, and views self as sexually inadequate.
25
24
23
22
21
20
19
18
17
16
15
14
13
12
11
10
9
8
7
6
5

Gonads Ovaries and testes, primary reproductive organs that produce germ cells and sex hormones.

Ovaries Paired female gonads, produce ova and secrete estrogens and progestins.

Testes Paired male gonads, produce sperm and secrete androgens.

Germ cells Sperm and ova.

Sex hormones Chemical substances that stimulate and promote the development of sex characteristics.

Ovum (plural, *ova*) Mature egg cell.

Sperm (spermatozoa) Male germ cell.

Genitals External sex organs.

Penis The male organ of copulation or urination.

Scrotum The loose sac of skin and muscle fibers that contains the testes.

Glans Rounded head of the penis or of the clitoris.

Prepuce Foreskin.

Sexuality is part of all our lives from birth to death. In one form or another, we reflect our sexuality in our thoughts and feelings, dreams and longings, fears and frustrations.

Sex can mean many things. Biologically, it refers to whether you are male or female, as determined by your reproductive function. Culturally, it means taking on masculine and feminine roles or behaviors. You can express sexual behaviors in a wide variety of fantasies and activities. And social judgments on such behaviors reveal an equally broad range of attitudes and values. All these biological, psychological, and social forces interact. Without a body, you couldn't engage in sexual behavior; yet "purely physical" sex doesn't exist. In the next chapter we discuss the psychological and relational aspects of sexual behavior. Here we describe the sexual organs and how they work.

Sexual Anatomy

In spite of their different appearance, the sexual organs of men and women fulfill similar functions. Each person has a pair of **gonads: ovaries** are the female gonads, **testes** are the male gonads. The gonads produce **germ cells** and **sex hormones.** The female germ cells are **ova** ("eggs"); the male germ cells are **sperm.** Ova and sperm are the

Figure 4-1 The reproductive organs: (a) male external organs; (b) male internal organs; (c) female external organs; (d) female internal organs.

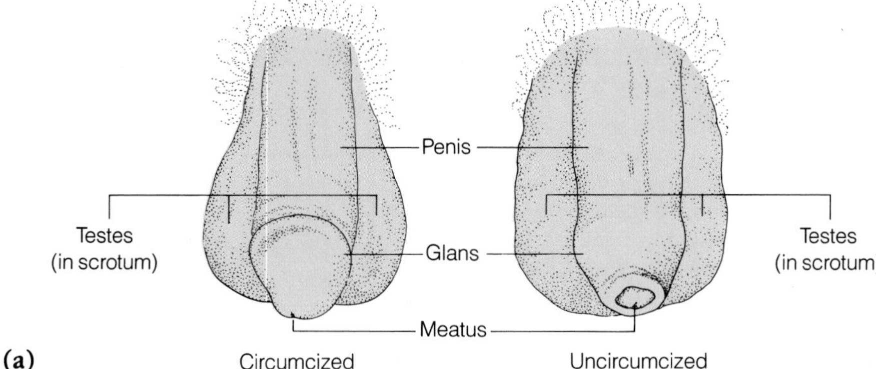

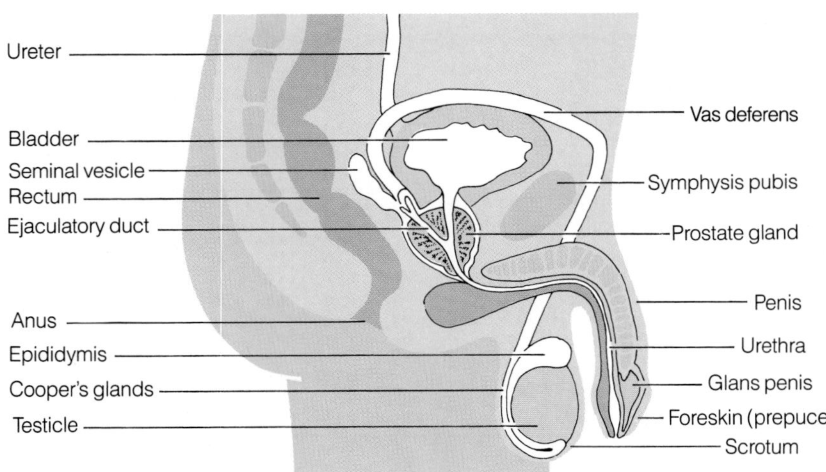

Urethra A tube that carries urine in the female, urine or semen in the male.

Semen Seminal fluid. Thick, whitish fluid containing sperm and nutrients, ejaculated during orgasm, hence also known as the *ejaculate*.

Meatus Opening of the urethra to outside the body.

Sphincter Muscular ring around a body opening or tube.

Seminiferous tubules Convoluted thin tubes, packed in the testes, that produce and transport sperm.

Epididymis Tubal structure that stores and transports sperm from the testis to the vas deferens.

---

basic units of reproduction. Their union initiates the creation of a new life.

Male Sex Organs A man's external sex organs, or **genitals**, are the **penis** and the **scrotum** (see Figure 4-1a and b). The penis consists of spongy tissue that becomes engorged with blood during sexual excitement, causing the organ to enlarge and become erect. The scrotum is a pouch that contains a pair of testes. In response to cold, to sexual arousal, and to some other stimuli, the scrotum contracts and pulls the testes closer to the body.

The smooth, rounded tip of the penis is the **glans.** It is the most sensitive part of the penis and an important source of sexual arousal. It is partially covered by the foreskin, or **prepuce**, a retractable fold of skin that is sometimes removed by circumcision.

Through the entire length of the penis runs the **urethra,** which can carry both urine and **semen** to the opening at the tip of the glans called the **meatus.** Although urine and semen share a common passage, they are prevented from mixing together by muscular **sphincters** that control their entry into the urethra.

The testes contain tightly packed **seminiferous** ("sperm-bearing") **tubules** within which sperm are produced. These tubules end in a maze of ducts that flow into a single storage tube called the **epididymis,** on the surface of each

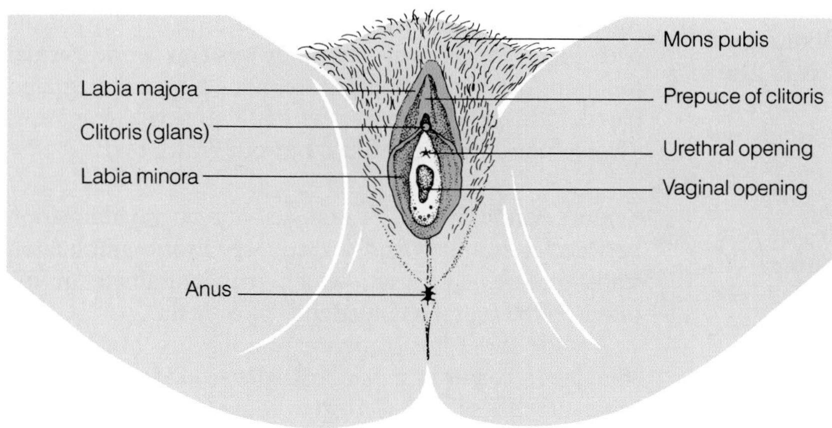

(c)

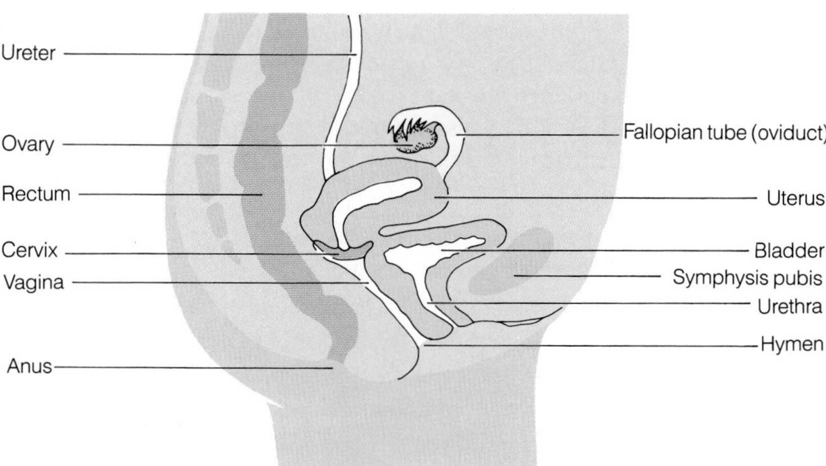

(d)

Vas deferens (plural *vasa deferentia*). Tubal structures that carry sperm from the epididymis.

Prostate gland Male accessory gland, the secretions of which contribute to the seminal fluid.

Seminal vesicles In the male, paired organs secretions contribute nutrients to semen.

Ejaculatory ducts Paired tubes that carry sperm from the vas deferens and fluid from the seminal vesicles into the urethra.

Cowper's glands Paired glands that produce pre-ejaculatory fluid during sexual excitement.

Vulva Female external genitals.

Mons pubis Rounded mass of tissue in the female, covered with pubic hair and located above the genitalia.

Labia majora Two folds of skin that enclose the labia minora, vaginal and urethral openings, and the clitoris.

Exploring Your Emotions

How do you feel about your own sexual organs and those of the opposite sex? Do you find them attractive? Repelling? How might you have developed such feelings? Where have you learned what you already know about these organs and from whom?

testis. This tube leads to the **vas deferens,** two tubes that rise into the abdominal cavity and enter the **prostate gland.** This gland produces some of the fluid in semen that nourishes and transports sperm.

The prostate gland contains the ducts of the two **seminal vesicles,** whose secretions also provide nutrients to semen. The tubes of the seminal vesicle and the vas deferens on each side lead to the **ejaculatory duct,** which joins the urethra. The **Cowper's glands** (bulbourethral glands) are two small structures flanking the urethra. During sexual arousal, these glands secrete a clear, sticky fluid that appears at the tip of the penis. This pre-ejaculatory fluid may contain some stray sperm.

Female Sex Organs The external sex organs, or genitals, of the female are called the **vulva** ("covering"). Its most prominent part is the **mons pubis,** a rounded mass of fatty tissue over the pubic bone that becomes covered with hair during puberty. Beneath it are two paired folds of skin called the **labia majora** and the **labia minora.** Enclosed within are (1) the **clitoris,** (2) the opening of the vagina, and (3) the opening of the urethra. The clitoris is highly sensitive and plays an important role in female sexual arousal. The glans of the clitoris is its most prominent part, outside the prepuce of the clitoris.

The female's urethra leads directly from the bladder and opens to the outside between the clitoris and the opening of the vagina. Unlike the male's urethra, it's independent of the genitals.

The vaginal opening is partially covered by the **hymen** (which exists only among humans and serves no known physiological function). This membrane is usually stretched or torn when a woman has sexual intercourse for the first time.

The **vagina** is the canal that leads to the internal reproductive organs. Its soft, flexible walls are normally in contact with each other. A ring of muscles surrounds the vagina. During sexual excitement, the tension in these muscles increases and the **bulbs of the vestibule** swell with blood.

The **cervix** leads out of the upper part of the vagina up into the pear-shaped **uterus.** The uterus, which slants forward above the bladder, is where the fertilized egg implants itself and grows in the uterine wall.

The pair of **Fallopian tubes** (or oviducts) leads out from the top of the uterus. The fringed end of each tube surrounds an ovary and guides the mature ovum down into the uterus after the ovum bursts through the ovary wall.

Sexual Physiology

Anatomy is concerned with structure; physiology deals with function, the way that body systems work. Sexual functions don't take place in isolation; they are integrated parts of the body's whole operation. Our sexual responses involve not only our genitals but our entire body.

Sexual Stimulation Sexual activity is an interaction between a stimulus and a response. Erotic stimulation leads to sexual arousal, which may culminate in the intensely pleasurable experience of **orgasm.**

A wide variety of stimuli can arouse us. Much erotic stimulation comes from various sights, sounds, and smells. Most often these sexual triggers come from other people. But we may also be aroused by books, photographs, or films.

Erotic thoughts may be linked to an imagined external source, such as a person we find sexy, or a past erotic experience we want to repeat. The sexual experience we fantasize may also be purely imaginary, involving activities that we may or may not wish to actually experience.

Exploring Your Emotions

Is the prospect of sexual arousal and orgasm a source of pleasant anticipation for you, or does it prompt feelings of uneasiness, fear, and shame? To what extent do you feel sexual functions are a natural part of being a man or a woman? How do you feel they should be controlled, if at all?

Labia minora Two hairless folds of skin enclosing the urethral and vaginal openings.

Clitoris Erectile female genital tissue. Highly sensitive.

Hymen A thin membrane partially covering the vaginal opening.

Vagina A female organ of copulation.

Bulbs of the vestibule Two bodies of spongy tissue around the vaginal opening.

Cervix The part of the uterus projecting into the vagina.

Uterus Pear-shaped female reproductive organ that houses the developing fetus.

Fallopian tubes Pair of tubes within which fertilization normally takes place; oviducts.

Orgasm Discharge of accumulated sexual tension with characteristic genital and bodily manifestation and a subjective sensation of intense pleasure.

All sensory stimulation ultimately has a physical basis which is given meaning by the brain. But to help us understand our sexual experiences, it is useful to differentiate between physical and psychological forms of sexual stimulation.

Physical Stimulation The most obvious and effective physical stimulation involves touching. Even though culturally defined practices vary and individual people have different preferences, most sexual encounters eventually involve some form of touching with hands, lips, and body surfaces. This is why we often kiss, caress, fondle, and hug in sexual encounters, as well as to simply express affection.

The most intense form of stimulation by touching involves the genitals. The clitoris and the glans penis are particularly sensitive to such stimulation. Other highly responsive areas are the vaginal opening, the nipples, the

Exploring Your Emotions

How does this picture make you feel? What might this man be feeling or thinking in an imaginary movie? How would you include him as a character in a script that expresses your feelings about sexuality?

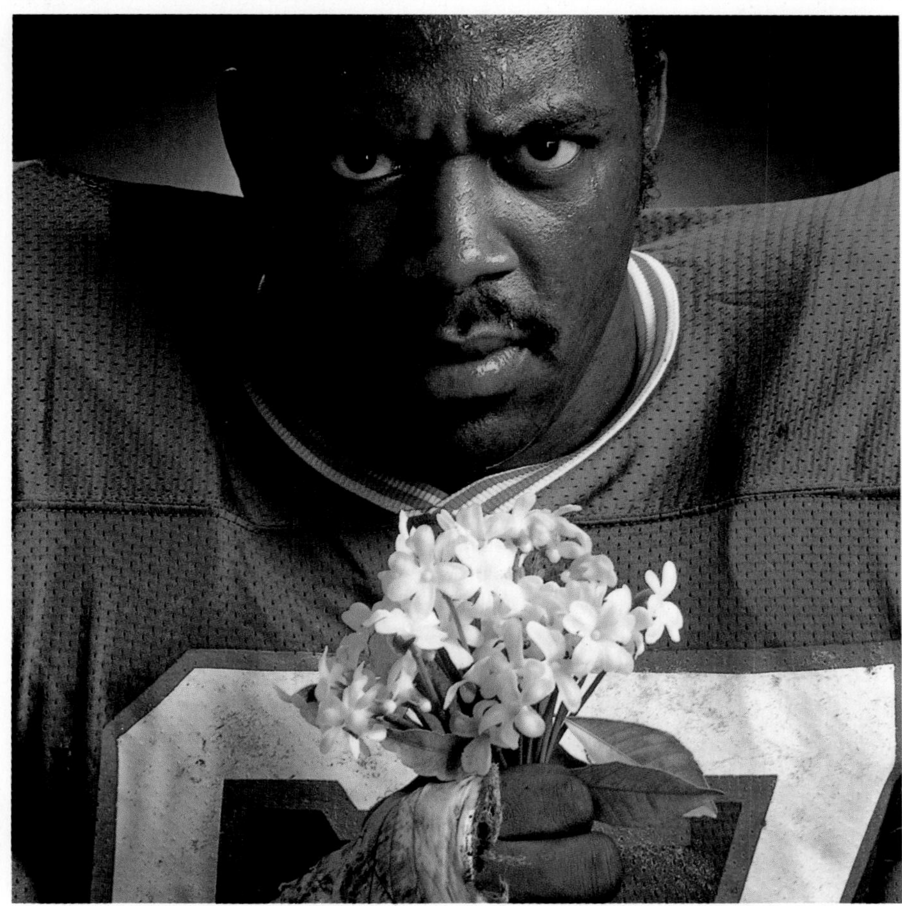

© Turnau 1979

Pheromones

The term **pheromone** (from the Greek, "to transfer excitement") was coined in 1959 to describe chemical sex attractants in insects, the existence of which had been known since the nineteenth century. These are remarkably potent substances; the minute amount of pheromone that exists in a single female gypsy moth is enough to sexually excite more than a billion males from as far as two miles away. In a number of insect species, the males in turn produce "aphrodisiacs" to induce the female to copulate. In the male cockroach this is an oily substance whose consumption induces the female into the coital posture.

There are numerous examples of the influence of pheromones in mammalian reproductive and social behavior: housing female mice together inhibits their ovarian cycles; exposure to a male or just his urine will revive the cycles; the odor of male mice accelerates puberty of young female mice; the introduction of a male from a foreign colony suppresses the pregnancy of mice who have mated with their own males.

The menstrual cycles of women show a similar tendency to be influenced by the odors of other women without their being conscious of it. For example, women who live together in college dormitories or other close quarters often begin to menstruate close to the same time. When a "donor" woman wears cotton pads under her arms for a 24-hour period and other women are then exposed to her armpit odor, the menstrual periods of the recipient women shift to become closer to the periods of the donor. There is also some evidence of male influence. In one study, women who seldom dated had longer cycles; those who dated more often had shorter and more regular cycles.

What are the substances that cause such curious effects? Some investigators have reported the presence of volatile fatty acids ("copulins") in vaginal secretions of rhesus monkeys in midcycle that stimulate male sexual interest, mounting, and ejaculation. Similar compounds have been identified in human vaginal secretions that peak at midcycle, but this does not seem to be the case for women on the pill. But other investigators have failed to confirm these findings. Hence, the role of such human "copulins" is currently unclear.

Vaginal secretions moreover need not be the primary source of erotic scent signals. Our body is studded with odor-producing glands, and despite our scrupulous efforts to eliminate and conceal them, they well may still be part of the "silent language" of sex. One perfume company at least is counting on that by marketing a fragrance that contains *alpha androstenol,* a synthetic chemical similar to a substance in human perspiration (and a powerful pheromone produced by boars, which makes the sow adopt the mating posture) even though there is no scientific evidence of its sexual effect on people.

Source: Herant Katchadourian, 1985. *Fundamentals of Human Sexuality,* 4th ed. (New York: Holt, Rinehart & Winston), p. 101.

breasts, the inside of the thighs, the buttocks, the anal region, the scrotum, the lips, and the ear lobes.

Such erotic areas, or **erogenous zones,** are especially susceptible to sexual arousal for most people, most of the time. This is useful to know as long as it doesn't lead to a push-button mentality. Often it's not *what* is touched but how, for how long, and under what circumstances (by whom, for example) that determines the response.

Exploring Your Emotions

How do you both control and express your sexual urges? Do you always recognize and satisfy them? Why not?

Under the right circumstances, touching any part of the body can arouse someone sexually.

Psychological Stimulation Sexual stimuli that depend on sights, sounds, and smells are strongly colored by psychological considerations. Each person must give a physical stimulus its psychological meaning in order to find it sexually arousing.

Your emotions powerfully influence your sexuality. How you feel about a person, and how he or she feels about you makes a tremendous difference in how sexually responsive you are likely to be. Even the most direct forms of physical stimulation carry emotional overtones. Kissing, caressing, and fondling express affection and caring. Hence, the emotional charge they impart to a sexual inter-

Erogenous zones Regions of the body highly responsive to sexual stimulation.

Pheromones Chemical substances that stimulate other animals through their sense of smell; presence in humans is uncertain.

Vasocongestion Accumulation of blood in tissues and organs.

Myotonia Increased muscular tension.

Excitement phase First stage of sexual response cycle, characterized by vasocongestion and myotonia.

Plateau phase Second stage of the sexual response cycle, characterized by high and sustained level of excitement.

Orgasmic phase Third phase of the sexual response cycle when myotonia culminates in orgasm.

Resolution phase Fourth and last phase of the sexual response cycle, during which vasocongestion and myotonia subside.

Ejaculation Expulsion of semen during orgasm.

Skene's glands Paraurethral glands in the female that are the homolog of the male prostate gland; produce ejaculatory fluid in some women.

Grafenburg spot (G-spot) The region of the anterior vaginal wall overlying Skene's glands. Reported to be highly responsive to stimulation.

Refractory period Obligatory period of rest following male orgasm.

Spinal cord Part of the central nervous system that runs through the vertebral column.

Reflexive Involving an involuntary response elicited by a specific stimulus.

---

action is at least as significant to sexual arousal as the purely physical stimulation achieved by touching. These issues are discussed further in the next chapter.

Sexual Response In response to effective sexual stimulation, the body shows a predictable set of reactions (see Figure 4-2). Physiologically, these reactions are the same regardless of the nature of the erotic stimulus—whether they are brought about by fantasy, masturbation, or sexual intercourse. But these experiences may feel quite different subjectively.

Two physiological mechanisms explain most of the genital and bodily reactions of men and women that become manifest during sexual arousal and orgasm. These mechanisms are **vasocongestion** and **myotonia.** Vasocongestion is the engorgement of tissues when more blood is flowing into an organ than is flowing out. Thus, the penis becomes erect on the same principle that a garden hose becomes stiff when the water is turned on. Myotonia is increased muscular tension, which culminates in the rhythmical muscular contractions during orgasm.

Four stages characterize the sexual response cycle. In the **excitement phase**, the penis becomes erect by becoming congested with blood. The testes expand and are pulled upward within the scrotum. In women, the clitoris and the labia are similarly congested with blood and the vaginal walls become moist with lubricant fluid.

The **plateau phase** is an extension of the excitement stage. Reactions become more marked: the penis becomes harder, the testes larger; the lower part of the vagina swells up, while its upper end expands, and vaginal lubrication becomes more profuse.

In the **orgasmic phase**, rhythmical contractions occur along the man's penis, urethra, the prostate gland, and seminal vesicles. Identical contractions occur in the lower part of the woman's vagina and the uterus. The muscles in the pelvic region as well as the anus respond similarly.

In the **resolution phase**, all the changes initiated during the excitement phase are reversed. Excess blood drains from tissues, the muscles in the region relax, and the genital structures return to their unstimulated state.

More general bodily reactions accompany the changes in the genital organs in both sexes. Beginning with the excitement phase, the nipples of both sexes become erect, the woman's breasts begin to swell, and in both sexes the skin of the chest becomes flushed; all these changes are more marked among women. The heart rate doubles in the plateau phase, and respiration becomes faster. During orgasm, breathing becomes irregular and the person may moan and cry out. The feeling of warmth leads to increased sweating during the resolution phase. Deep relaxation and well-being pervade the body and the mind.

There are a few differences between the male and the female reactions during the sexual response cycle. Generally, the male pattern is more uniform, while the female pattern is more varied. For instance, the female excitement phase may lead directly to orgasm, or orgasmic and plateau phases may be fused.

Male orgasm is marked by the **ejaculation** of semen. Women may also emit some fluid during orgasm through the urethra. This fluid is produced by the female counterpart of the male prostate gland (called **Skene's glands**). The region of the front vaginal wall that overlies the glands is known as the **Grafenburg spot** (G-spot) and has been reported to be erotically highly sensitive. After ejaculation, men enter a **refractory period**, a time of obligatory rest, during which they cannot be restimulated to orgasm. Women do not have a refractory period, so they can more readily have a number of orgasms in succession.

Sexual stimulation relies on the same set of sensory nerves that transmit impulses from the surface of the body. There are no special nerves for conveying sexual sensations. However, specialized nerve centers in the lower portions of the **spinal cord** regulate the mechanisms of erection and ejaculation. Their actions are **reflexive**, they do not need to be learned (although learned responses may inhibit them).

The ultimate control of sexual functions rests in the

Figure 4-2 Stages of Sexual Response

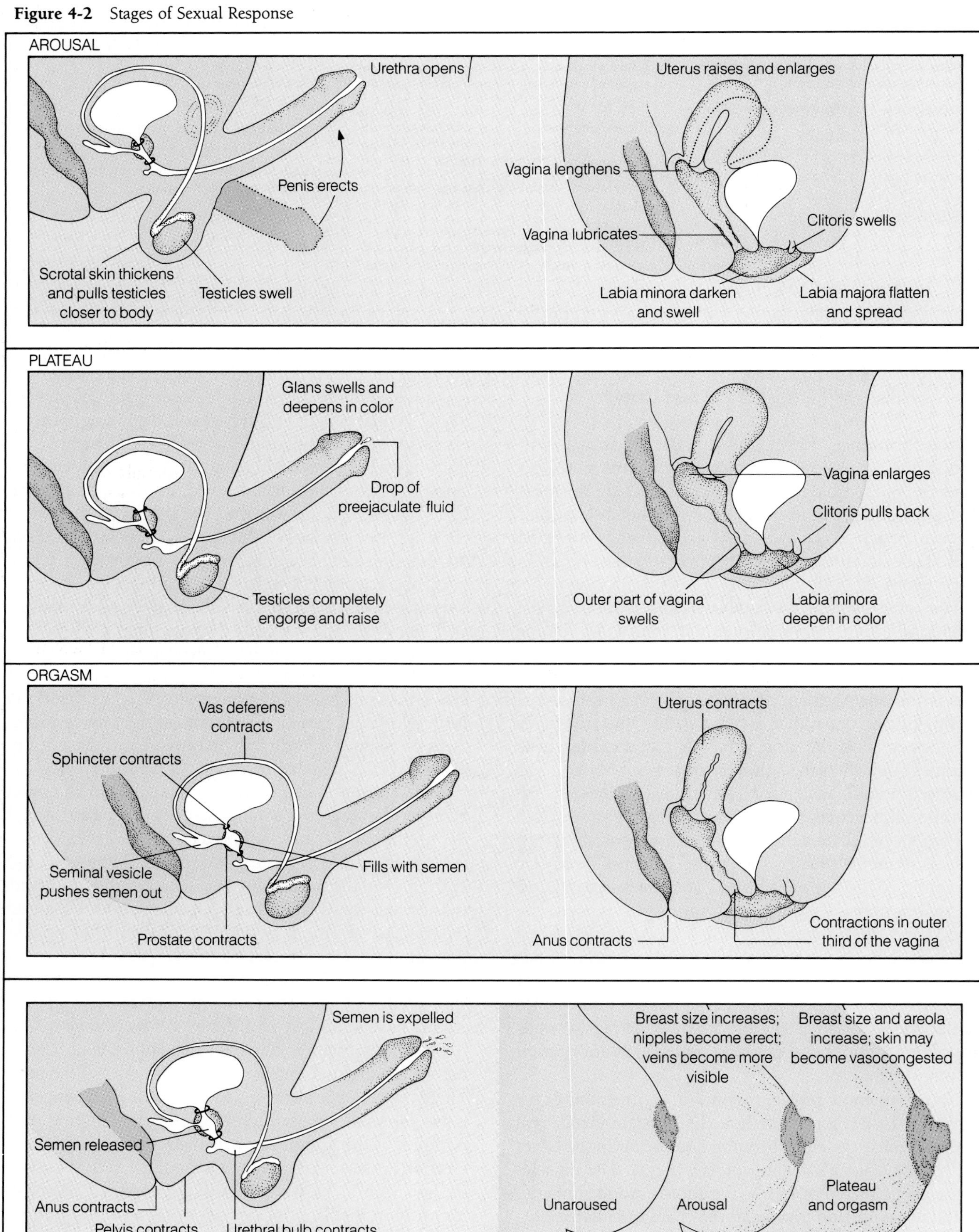

Myths About Sex

Myth Bigger the man, bigger the penis; larger the nose, larger the penis; men with bigger penises are more virile and make better lovers.

Fact There is no known correlation between the size of the penis and body build. Nor does the size of the penis determine the capacity to enjoy or provide sexual pleasure.

Myth The correct fit between vagina and penis is important for satisfactory sexual relations.

Fact The vagina expands to accommodate the penis, whatever its size. It is the fit between the sexual partners rather than the organs that counts.

Myth Men have a stronger sex drive than women.

Fact Men generally engage in more sexual activity and a greater variety of sexual behaviors, but within a satisfying sexual relationship women are no less interested in sex than men and are capable of attaining more orgasms during a sexual encounter.

Myth Ancient cultures had secret potions to enhance the sexual drive.

Fact So they believed, as many cultures still do. But there is no evidence that sexual stimulants (aphrodisiacs) work other than by suggestion.

Myth A woman who does not reach orgasm does not get pregnant.

Fact Female orgasm is not necessary for pregnancy.

Myth Alcohol makes people want sex, and marijuana makes sex better.

Fact Alcohol removes inhibitions and makes people behave in ways they would not otherwise. But it does not as such enhance sexual arousal. In excess, it is certain to interfere with sexual function. Similarly, marijuana may alter the perception of the experience without necessarily improving performance.

Myth If you have a lot of sex when you are young, you will run out of steam when you get older.

Fact On the contrary, men and women who are sexually active as young adults are more likely to remain so in their older years.

Myth Sex interferes with athletic performance.

Fact Not so. Baseball manager Casey Stengel may have said it best when he told his players, "Going to bed with a woman never hurt a ballplayer. It's staying up all night looking for them that does you in."

Myth Men are physically superior to women.

Fact It depends on how superiority is assessed. Men are generally stronger and can out-perform women in strenuous physical activities. But women outlive men in every decade of life, and the capacity to survive is the more important criterion of fitness.

Myth Masturbation is an unnatural, immature act that can cause blindness, insanity, and numerous other ailments.

Fact Masturbation is a natural function. People in most cultures masturbate, many of them throughout their lives. Many sexually active people with available partners masturbate as an additional gratification. There is no evidence that masturbation impairs physical or mental health.

Limbic system A set of structures in the brain regulating motivational-emotional behaviors, including some aspects of sexual activity.

Endocrine glands Glands that produce hormones.

Steroids A class of chemicals that includes the sex hormones.

Adrenal glands Endocrine glands, located over the kidneys, that produce androgens (among other hormones).

Pituitary gland Endocrine gland at the base of the brain, which produces gonadotropic (FSH and LH) and other hormones.

Androgens Male sex hormones produced by testes and the adrenal glands.

Testosterone Male sex hormone.

Hypothalamus A region of the brain above the pituitary gland whose hormones control the secretions of the pituitary. Also involved in the nervous control of sexual functions.

Chromosomes The genetic material within the cell nucleus.

Sex chromosomes The X and Y chromosomes, which determine the sex of the individual.

Puberty Period of biological maturation during adolescence.

Gonadotropin-releasing hormone (GnRH) Hypothalamic hormone that controls the release of gonadotropic hormones from the pituitary gland.

---

brain. As in the lower spinal centers, specific regions in the **limbic system** of the brain control the various aspects of sexual arousal and orgasm. Far less understood is the way the brain regulates the subjective experience of sexual arousal and the state of altered consciousness we experience during orgasm.

Sex Hormones

Hormones are chemicals that are secreted directly into the bloodstream by **endocrine glands** and specialized cells. The sex hormones greatly influence the development and functions of the reproductive system as well as sexual behavior.

The sex hormones belong to a group of compounds called **steroids.** The sex hormones of the male are called **androgens** (the most important of which is **testosterone**); the female sex hormones belong to two groups—**estrogens** and **progestins** (the most important of which is **progesterone**). In addition to the estrogens and progestins produced by the ovary and testosterone from the testes, the cortex of the **adrenal glands** (located at the top of the kidneys) also produces androgens in both sexes.

The hormones produced by the testes, the ovaries, and the adrenal glands are regulated by the hormones of the **pituitary gland,** located at the base of the brain. This gland in turn is controlled by hormones produced by the **hypothalamus** in the brain.

Developmental Effects of Hormones Sex hormones exert their primary developmental influences first in the embryo and later during adolescence.

Differentiation of the Embryo The sex of the individual, as male or female, is determined by the fertilizing sperm at the time of conception. All human cells normally contain 23 pairs of **chromosomes,** including a pair of **sex chromosomes,** which have an XY configuration in the male, XX in the female. The germ cells are the only exception—they have 23 *single,* not paired, chromosomes. All ova carry an X chromosome; some sperm carry an X, other sperm carry a Y chromosome. When a sperm carrying an X chromosome fertilizes an egg, the baby will be a girl; if it carries a Y-chromosome, the baby will be a boy. The Y chromosome is responsible for initiating the process of sexual differentiation of the reproductive system. Until the sixth week of embryonal life, the reproductive system is undifferentiated. Both sexes have a set of gonads, two sets of tubes, and other related structures.

Under the influence of the Y chromosome, the undifferentiated gonads begin to develop into testes. The embryonal testes in turn produce two hormones. The first hormone, testosterone leads to the further development of male reproductive organs. The second hormone inhibits the rest of the undifferentiated structures from developing into female organs. This results in a normal set of male genital organs.

In the absence of a Y chromosome, the undifferentiated set of gonads becomes an ovary. The embryonal ovaries do not need to produce female hormones to prompt development of the female reproductive system. If no testosterone is present, the developmental process leads naturally to normal female genital organs. In other words, without testosterone we would all develop female reproductive organs regardless of our genetic makeup.

The common embryonal origin of male and female systems means that every structure in one sex has its developmental counterpart in the other. Thus, the penis corresponds to the clitoris; the scrotal sac to the labia majora, and other male parts have their female counterparts. Thus the reproductive system of male and female are built on the same basic plan.

Reproductive Maturation at Puberty Although babies are sexually fully differentiated at birth, their bodies are not significantly different until **puberty.** At puberty the reproductive system matures, secondary sexual characteristics (such as pubic hair) develop, and the bodies of male and female appear more distinctive (see Figure 4-3).

The changes of puberty are initiated by the **gonadotropin-releasing hormone (GnRH)** of the hypothalamus under whose influence the anterior pituitary gland increases the production of its two **gonadotropic hormones.** These are the **follicle-stimulating hormone (FSH)** and the **luteinizing hormone (LH).**

In the female, FSH stimulates the immature ovarian

Gonadotropic hormones Follicle-stimulating hormone (FSH) and luteinizing hormone (LH) produced by the pituitary gland in both sexes.

Follicle-stimulating hormone (FSH) Pituitary hormone that stimulates maturation of the ovum in the female and sperm production in the male.

Luteinizing hormone (LH) Pituitary hormone that stimulates the production of progestins in the female and androgens in the male.

Estrogens A class of female sex hormones, produced by the ovaries, that bring about sexual maturation at puberty and maintain reproductive functions.

Progestins A class of female sex hormones, produced by the ovaries, that sustain reproductive functions.

Menstrual cycle Monthly ovarian cycle that leads to menstruation in the absence of pregnancy.

Menarche The first menstrual period.

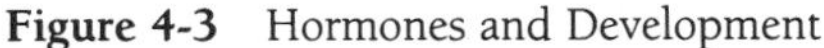

follicles to mature. The cells of the maturing follicle in turn produce **estrogens.** Under the effect of LH, the follicular cells also produce **progestins.** These two hormones are responsible for the **menstrual cycle** (see box).

The first menstrual period, or **menarche,** occurs at the average age of 12.8 years, but it may also normally start several years earlier or later. The age at menarche has steadily gone down, but it has stabilized over the past several decades. In the United States girls now reach puberty at about the same age as did their mothers.

Menarche is typically not the first sign of puberty. The first visible sign is breast development, followed by the growth of pubic hair. These and related changes in the reproductive system and the rest of the body transform the immature girl into a young woman capable of reproducing. Although pubescent girls usually become fertile after menarche, they may not begin ovulating regularly for a year or more. However, this irregularity does not provide a teenage girl contraceptive security.

Reproductive maturation of boys lags a year or two behind that of girls. Enlargement of the testes, development of pubic hair, growth of the penis, the onset of ejaculation (usually at about age 11 or 12), deepening of the voice, and the appearance of facial hair complete the transformation of boys into young men.

The hormonal basis for these changes is quite similar

Figure 4-3 Hormones and Development

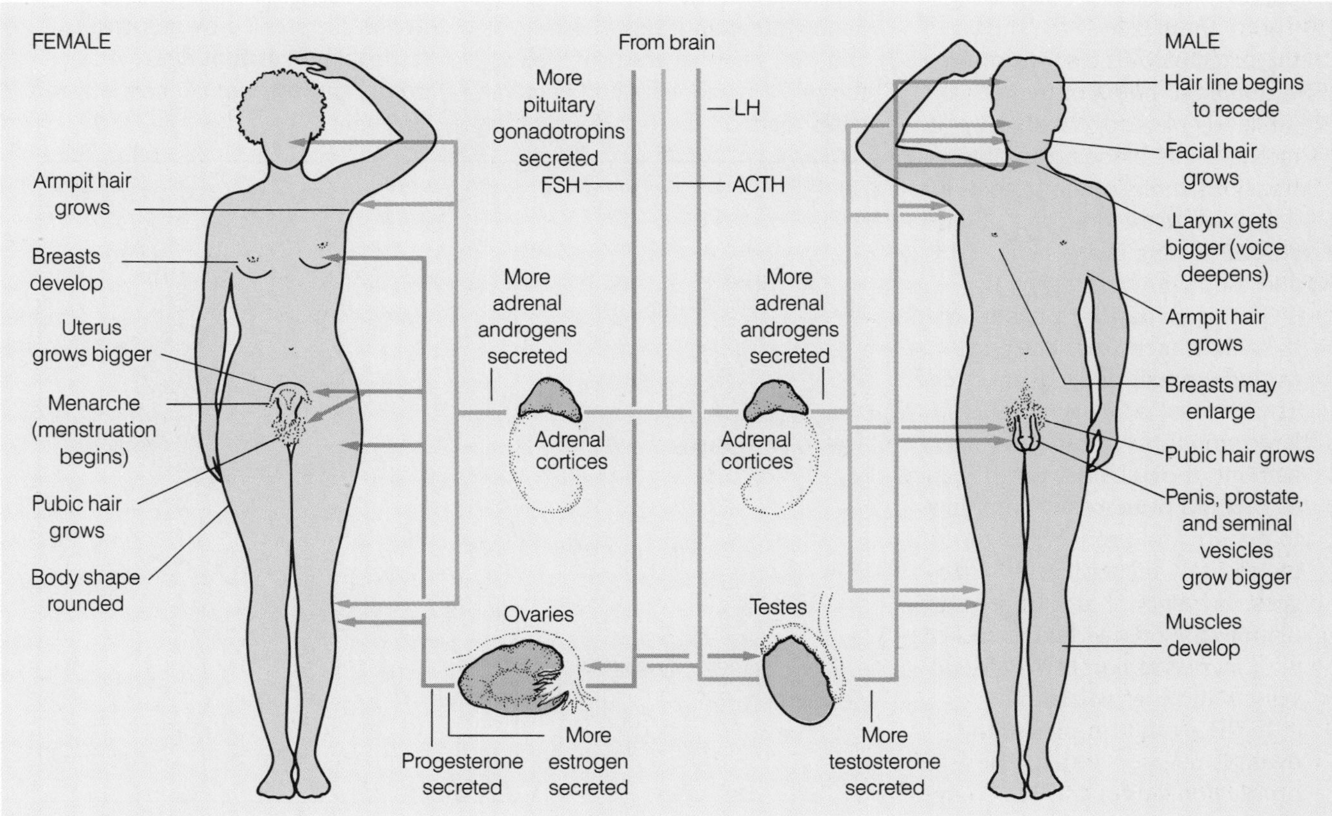

The Menstrual Cycle

The menstrual ("monthly") cycle is one of the key physiological functions of the female body. An ovarian, or **estrus,** cycle is characteristic of all female mammals but **menstruation,** periodic uterine bleeding that accompanies the ovarian cycle, occurs only in women, in female apes, and some monkeys.

The average length of the menstrual cycle is 28 days, although somewhat longer and shorter cycles are also quite common and normal. Because the onset of bleeding is easier to note than its gradual cessation, the day that bleeding starts is counted as the first day of a given cycle.

The menstrual cycle is controlled by neuroendocrine mechanisms involving hypothalamic, pituitary, and ovarian hormones. The cycle has (roughly) four phases. The changes that occur during these phases are shown in the diagram with respect to the endometrial lining of the uterus, the levels of estrogens and progesterone in the bloodstream, the transformations of the ovarian follicle, and the blood levels of follicle-stimulating hormone (FSH) and lutinizing hormone (LH).

The **preovulatory phase** starts as soon as menstrual bleeding from the previous cycle has ended. The anterior pituitary produces large amounts of FSH and a small amount of LH. Under the influence of FSH, an ovarian follicle begins to mature and produces in turn increasingly higher level of estrogens. In response to estrogen stimulation, the uterine lining thickens with increased numbers of blood vessels and uterine glands.

In the **ovulation phase,** the ovum is released at midcycle as LH production surges and FSH output decreases. Gonadotropic hormones that control the output of ovarian hormones are in turn regulated by the level of ovarian hormones, through a negative feedback mechanism. Thus, the increased level of estrogens depresses FSH production. Following ovulation, the follicle transforms into the **corpus luteum** ("yellow body"), which produces progesterone.

In the **post-ovulatory phase,** the secretion of progesterone begins to rise. Under the combined influence of estrogens and progesterone, the endometrium continues to develop and the uterine glands secrete nutrient materials. The endometrium is now ready to receive and sustain the fertilized ovum if fertilization has occurred. The levels of ovarian hormones then remain high and the uterine lining is maintained intact through pregnancy. In the absence of pregnancy, the high levels of estrogens and progesterone gradually fall as the body metabolizes and eliminates them.

Below a certain level of hormonal support, the uterine lining can no longer be maintained and begins to slough off, initiating the final **menstrual phase** of the cycle. As levels of ovarian hormones drop, their inhibiting effect on the pituitary gonadotropins is lifted. FSH and LH production now begins to rise, and a new cycle starts.

When pregnancy occurs, the hormone **human chorionic gonadotropin (HCG)** sustains the corpus luteum in maintaining high levels of estrogens and progestins. Hence, the uterine lining (which now houses the embryo) does not slough off and the pregnant woman misses her period.

Birth control pills (see Chapter 6) consist of synthetic estrogens and progestins. Because the pills maintain high blood levels of these hormones, gonadotropin production is suppressed by negative feedback. Ovulation does not occur, and the woman cannot get pregnant.

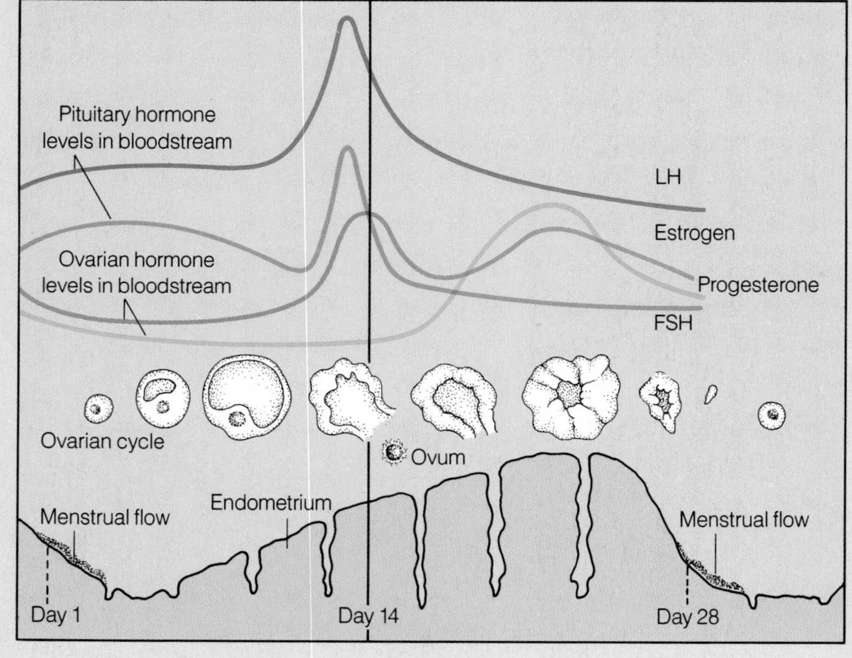

Estrus The period of maximum sexual receptivity among female animals; associated with ovulation; being "in heat."

Menstruation The normal bleeding phase of the menstrual cycle of women; a woman's "period."

Preovulatory phase The phase of the menstrual cycle that starts with the end of menstrual bleeding and leads to ovulation.

Ovulation phase The release of the egg from the ovary; occurs at midpoint of the menstrual cycle.

Corpus luteum The part of the ovarian follicle left after ovulation; secretes hormones during the second half of the menstrual cycle.

Postovulatory phase The phase of the menstrual cycle that follows ovulation and ends with the onset of menstrual bleeding.

Human chorionic gonadotrophin (HCG) Hormone produced by developing placenta; sustains the functions of the corpus luteum during pregnancy.

---

to that of the female. Hypothalamic hormones trigger the anterior pituitary to produce gonadotropins. FSH promotes the maturation of sperm; LH stimulates testicular cells to produce testosterone, which brings about most of the male changes of puberty.

Although both sexes show a rapid growth in height, weight, and physical development throughout puberty, boys register greater gains than girls in muscular development and in their capacity to exert strenuous physical effort. There is a fourteenfold increase in the number of muscle cells among boys and a tenfold increase among girls. Blood volume, hemoglobin level, and the number of red blood cells show greater increases in the male, as does respiratory capacity. As a result of these factors, males in general have a greater exercise capacity than females.

These physiological sex differences are real. But they have been greatly exaggerated by cultural expectations that men expand their physical potential at work and in

Exploring Your Emotions

Write a short sketch of a movie in which this photo is one image; what character is being portrayed here, and what action might involve such a character? What role would you write for yourself in such a movie to interact with this character?

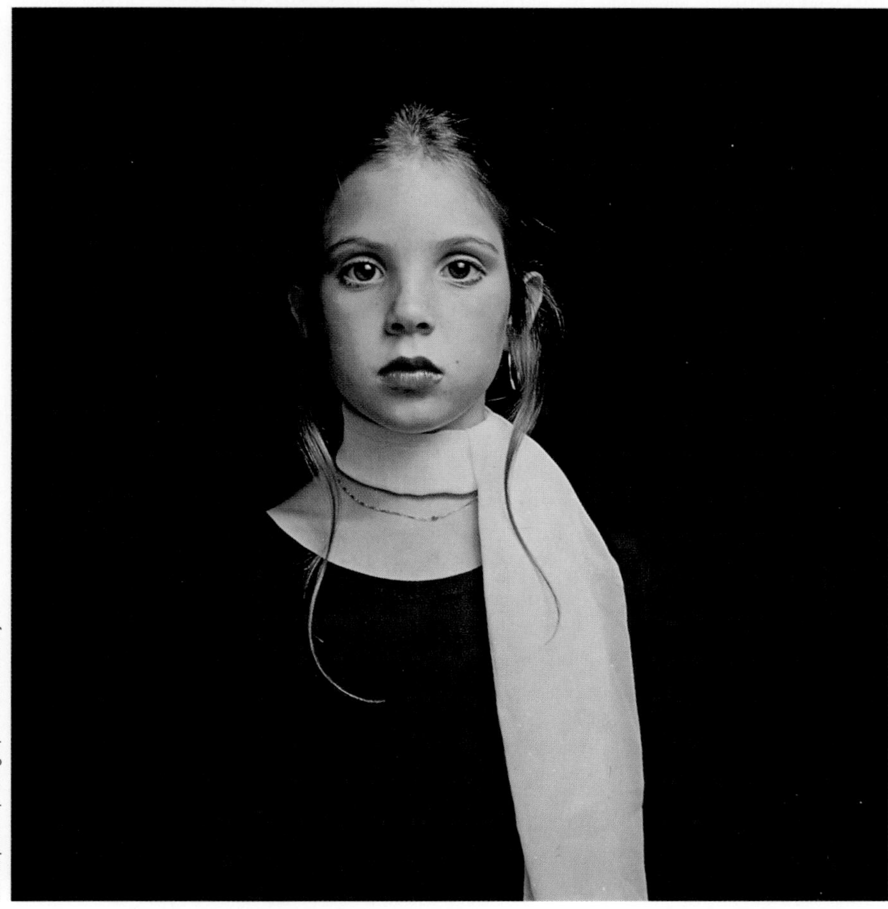

Concept and photograph: Alan Dockery

Menopause Cessation of menstruation in middle-aged women.

Gender identity The personal sense of masculinity and femininity.

Masculinity Culturally defined characteristic of being male.

Femininity Culturally defined characteristic of being female.

Trichomoniasis Vaginal infection caused by the organism *Trichomonas vaginalis*.

Candidiasis Vaginal infection caused by the organism *Candida albicans*.

Cystitis Infection of the urinary bladder.

Dysmenorrhea Painful menstrual periods.

Premenstrual syndrome (PMS) Physical symptoms and psychological distress experienced by some women for a few days before menstruation.

Prostaglandins Chemicals produced by the uterine lining that cause dysmenorrhea (they are also produced by the prostate and other tissues and have numerous other effects).

Edema Swelling.

Diuretics Chemicals that increase the output of urine.

Analgesics Painkillers.

Hot flashes A wave of warmth; common menopausal symptom.

---

sports more than women. Women who are physically fit can readily outperform men who are less fit in most physical activities.

Hormones and Sexual Behavior The exact role of hormones in establishing and maintaining sexual behaviors among humans is not clear. Animal models show that sex hormones influence behavior at two levels, organizational and activational. The organizational effects of hormones involve the differentiation of those portions of the brain that deal with sexual behavior. Just like the reproductive system, the undifferentiated brain becomes "sexualized" and develops in a male or female direction. Once again, the primary factor is testosterone: in its absence, all animals develop female-type sexual behavior, just as they develop female-type genitalia.

The organizational effect of hormones occurs shortly before or around the time of birth during a critical period, when the brain is particularly susceptible to such influences. After the brain has been "primed," the influence of hormones shifts to their activational effects, which make possible the initiation and maintenance of sexual behavior. In this sense, hormones act like a "sex fuel" to keep the machinery going.

The fact that there is an upsurge in sexual interest and activity at puberty suggests that sex hormones play a similar activational role among humans, which also presupposes the presence of an earlier organizational role. When men suffer a significant loss in testosterone production, their sex drive and ability to have erections and orgasm suffer markedly over a period of time. If treated with testosterone, their sexual functions improve.

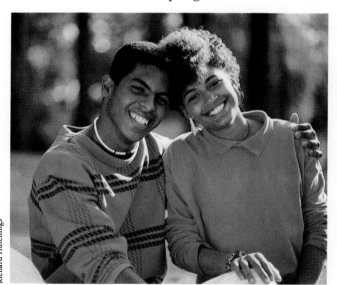

Richard Hutchings

The situation is more complicated with women. The production of estrogens and progestins drops sharply as women enter **menopause.** Although after menopause women can no longer bear children, they do not typically lose sexual interest or the ability to reach orgasm. Nor does the administration of these hormones (such as in birth control pills) necessarily enhance sexual drive or performance. Women have different concentrations of sex hormones during the menstrual cycle, but their level of sexual interest does not seem to consistently shift with the various phases of their monthly cycle. It is possible that the hormones responsible for female sexual function are androgens, which continue to be produced by the adrenal cortex throughout female adult life.

Whatever the role of sex hormones on behavior, it is clear that human sexual behavior is largely shaped by cultural factors. Thus, although hormones make it possible for us to act sexually and may predispose us to act in one way or another, how (and whether) we engage in sexual behavior is greatly influenced by our culture and our sexual upbringing.

Hormones and Gender Identity The possible role of sex hormones in determining **gender identity** is even more problematic. Whereas *sex* refers to being biologically male or female, *gender* defines **masculinity** and **femininity.** Men and women are expected to perceive themselves as masculine or feminine, in culturally prescribed ways, and to behave accordingly.

Female children born with ambiguous-looking genitals (due to hormonal abnormalities) have been raised as girls in some cases, and as boys in others. In these situations, the person's sense of gender identity seems to be determined by rearing. Those raised as girls think of themselves as female, those raised as boys think of themselves as male (even though biologically female).

Other evidence points to the possible influence of hormones in determining gender-related behaviors. For instance, female babies who have been exposed to abnormal levels of masculinizing hormones before birth (either due to hormonal abnormalities or in drugs taken by the mother) are more likely to manifest "tomboyish" behavior by acting more like typical boys, even though they have been brought up as girls. Hence, how biological factors interact with cultural forces in shaping our sexual and gender behaviors currently remains unclear.

Sexual Health and Dysfunction

The human body is a superbly designed living system, more intricate and efficient than any machine, but it requires proper care and maintenance to work well. Furthermore, considerations of psychological health are inseparable from physical health. This unity is particularly important with respect to sexual functions, which are highly influenced by psychological factors, interpersonal relationships, and cultural attitudes.

Common Complaints A number of common problems, although part of normal functions (such as menstruation), may cause discomfort and occasionally lead to further complications.

The greater vulnerability of women to genitourinary problems is due to the anatomical and hormonal characteristics of their reproductive organs. Women have a more "open" system, which allows micro-organisms to grow in the vagina, producing the irritating discharges associated with **trichomoniasis** and **candidiasis.** More importantly, since the Fallopian tubes open into the abdominal cavity, they provide an avenue for infections to spread inward, causing pelvic disorders. Women are also more vulnerable to bladder irritation and infection (**cystitis**).

Menstrual Distress Menstruation is a normal process but it entails considerable discomfort for at least one out of ten women. This usually takes the forms of **dysmenorrhea** ("painful menstruation") or **premenstrual syndrome (PMS).**

Dysmenorrhea is typically manifested by cramps in the lower abdomen, bloating, backache, headache, nausea, vomiting, diarrhea, and loss of appetite. These symptoms are attributed to uterine spasms caused by **prostaglandins**, chemicals released from the uterine lining shed during menstruation. Hence, drugs that counteract the effects of prostaglandins are quite effective in preventing and treating dysmenorrhea.

Symptoms of premenstrual tension are less well defined, and their causes are less clear. The more common symptoms are **edema** (swelling) of the legs, weight gain, bloated feeling in the abdomen, tenderness in the breasts, headache, and various psychological symptoms such as anxiety, depression, irritability, insomnia, and difficulty in concentration and forgetfulness.

Some of these physical symptoms are due to fluid retention but the causes of the mental symptoms are obscure. Premenstrual tension may be helped by **diuretics** (which rid the body of excess fluid), by **analgesics** (which ease pain) and psychological support.

Menopause As a woman approaches 50, her ovaries gradually cease to function and she enters the menopause ("stopping of menses"). The associated drop in hormone production causes a set of symptoms that are troublesome for some women.

The most common physical symptom of the menopause are **hot flashes** (or flushes), experienced by three out of four women. They consist of a sensation of warmth rising to the face from the upper chest with or without perspiration and chills. Other symptoms include headaches, dizziness, palpitations, and joint pains. The bones become more porous (osteoporosis) making older women more liable to suffer fractures. Some menopausal women become moody, even markedly depressed. They also complain of tiredness, irritability, and forgetfulness. Estrogen replacement significantly improves some of these symptoms.

As a result of the drop in estrogen production, the vaginal walls become thinner and the lubricatory response to sexual arousal is diminished. As a result, sexual intercourse may become painful. Hormonal treatment or the use of lubricants during coitus eliminate these problems.

Most women do not lose sexual interest at this time, and many take menopause in stride. Women who become excessively preoccupied with aging and who associate menopause with losing sexual attractiveness have a more difficult time adjusting.

Exploring Your Emotions

If a classmate snaps at you and later explains that she has her period, how would you respond? Would you feel sympathetic? Annoyed? Awkward? How often does PMS affect your interactions?

Problems of Midlife in Men Men do not experience a comparable drop in hormone production in midlife, although testosterone levels gradually decline with age. Nonetheless, the pattern of male sexual response definitely changes. As they get older, men depend more on direct physical stimulation for sexual arousal. They take longer to get an

Making Allowances for Premenstrual Stress

One or two weeks a month of misery, of tears and tension and temper is the lot of the millions of women who suffer from premenstrual syndrome (PMS).

The emotional and physical symptoms that precede menstruation may dominate their lives. One PMS sufferer avoided planning social engagements or trips during that time because she would be too cranky and depressed to enjoy them.

Another woman, Karen Owen, 38, had bouts of overwhelming fatigue, insomnia, crying fits, and a feeling she was shrouded in a fog. Like other victims, she resigned herself to withdrawing from life for nearly half of each month.

Finally, she found herself as a patient in a research project at Johns Hopkins University in Baltimore. Owen, a nutritional biochemist, is now part of the research team.

Women aren't the only victims of PMS. Their families suffer too. Ask any husband who monthly has to cope with his wife's mood swings.

Premenstrual syndrome has even been used as a defense in a Brooklyn, New York, case of child abuse, and in England as a mitigating circumstance in two murder cases.

Though 70 percent of women may have some premenstrual symptoms, such as breast tenderness, bloating, acne, or a craving for sweets, about 10 percent have symptoms severe enough to require treatment.

Dr. Susan Lark, director of the PMS Self-Help Center in Los Altos, California, and a veteran with 10 years experience in the field, reports that more than 150 symptoms have been identified as associated with PMS. Some of the less common ones are arthritis, heart palpitations, and visual changes.

Ten to 12 of the most common symptoms turn up again and again. They are anxiety, irritability, mood swings, a craving for carbohydrates, headaches and dizziness, bloating, swelling, breast tenderness, depression, insomnia, acne, and oily skin and hair.

All those symptoms might be associated with other ailments, but there's one characteristic that marks them as related to PMS. They occur on a cyclical basis and disappear as soon as menstruation starts.

For that reason, a key part of any treatment plan is to have women with PMS chart a daily record for several months, rather than trust their subjective recollections.

Premenstrual syndrome usually appears in women from their thirties on and may grow worse until menopause. Pregnant women never have PMS.

PMS frequently is confused with another syndrome, called dysmenorrhea—the cramps and back pain that occur during menstruation. For years patients with dysmenorrhea and PMS were thought to have psychological problems. Doctors tended to brush away women's complaints with the implication, "It's all in your head."

Research, however, has pinpointed the cause of dysmenorrhea, and sufferers now can be treated successfully with medication.

PMS hasn't advanced to that point yet, although researchers are actively trying to discover first the cause and then an effective cure.

A British gynecologist, Dr. Katherine Dalton, labeled the syndrome in the 1950s, bringing it that much closer to its recognition as a genuine disease.

Dalton advocated treating PMS with large doses of progesterone, a hormone produced by women during part of the menstrual cycle and during pregnancy. The theory was that women suffering from PMS had a deficiency of progesterone. The "cure" was to give them large doses of the hormone.

In the United States PMS didn't become well known until the early 1980s, when the media devoted a great deal of attention to it.

Clinics opened across the nation to treat PMS sufferers. Some of these clinics were legitimate; others were not.

The U.S. Food and Drug Administration (FDA) didn't approve the use of progesterone for treating PMS, but this hormone was available for other FDA-approved uses, and it was frequently given to PMS patients.

PMS also got caught up in the growing self-help trend in medicine, which focuses on diet and exercise. Liberated women wanted to take responsibility for themselves, and women with PMS had an even greater motivation.

Dr. Lark believes that premenstrual syndrome doesn't take just one form, but that there are different types, each with a different cause.

The symptoms and their causes are:

- Anxiety, irritability, and mood swings caused by an imbalance of estrogen and progesterone during the second phase of the menstrual cycle.
- A craving for carbohydrates, marked by headaches, heart pounding, dizziness, and a desire for sweets. The problem is caused by a deficiency of magnesium and B vitamins. One possible reason why many PMS sufferers crave chocolate is that it contains magnesium.
- Depressive symptoms, crying, forgetfulness, and insomnia, which are caused by changes in hormone levels.
- Fluid retention and weight gain, which are due to an increase in total body fluid caused by increases in sodium chloride (salt) and water retention.

Dr. Lark urges PMS sufferers to give up their morning coffee, cut out salt and sugar, and stay away from chocolate. Instead, they should eat complex carbohydrates such as whole grains, vegetables, legumes, and fruits. Poultry and fish are preferable to red meat. Women with PMS are also encouraged to exercise and to guard against overwork, fatigue, and insufficient sleep. Positive results from this regimen often occur within three to six months.

The Johns Hopkins method, used by Karen Owen, offers similar guidelines.

"PMS is similar to diabetes in that we don't know exactly what is the cause and we don't have a cure," Owen says. "But by treating the symptoms, people can live a normal life."

Dr. Lark believes that diet is the most effective method of controlling symptoms and that it "should be the core of any home treatment program. It takes away about 75 percent of the symptoms. Then exercise can finish the job."

Many women who have turned to diet and exercise had tried progesterone but became disenchanted with the idea of drug therapy. Progesterone is not a cure, and they did not like the prospect of having to take the medicine for 20 years or more. But other women would rather take progesterone than give up coffee and sugar.

In the future PMS sufferers may have better means of treatment, so that they will not have to make the tough choice between long-term drug therapy and a strict diet.

Though some doctors still shrug off complaints of premenstrual tension, more and more members of the medical community are taking a serious look at the syndrome. Slowly but surely answers are coming in.

The National Institute of Mental Health (NIMH) is engaged in an extensive study of PMS. Researchers are exploring the biological factors that turn a calm, rational woman into an irritable, tense shrew one or two weeks a month. Researchers believe neurotransmitters—brain hormones that carry signals from one nerve to another—may be involved. The NIMH program is also testing a range of treatments, including progesterone and vitamin B6.

A team of researchers at the University of California, San Diego, recently made an interesting discovery in a study based on evidence of a relationship between PMS and ovarian function.

Eight women in the study were given a medication that had the effect of a medical ovariectomy. It was as if their ovaries had been removed surgically; their ovaries ceased to function and thus cut off the cyclical hormonal changes of the menstrual cycle. The change was reversible, and the women's ovaries returned to normal function when they stopped taking the medication. The treatment markedly reduced PMS symptoms.

The researchers aren't certain how the medication works. And they don't know yet whether long-term use at a low dosage would be safe, or if only short-term therapy might work. More research is needed.

These advances may be a slight comfort to the woman who is dreading the next attack of PMS. But it may give her a lift to know that somewhere down the road there is an effective treatment and that it's getting closer to reality every day.

Source: Mary T. Fortney, Premenstrual syndrome, *Healthline,* March, 1985.

Impotence Is More Treatable than You Think

Nobody wants to talk about it, but impotence afflicts one man in 10. Stress or fatigue can cause difficulty getting or keeping an erection, and when those conditions pass, the problem becomes only a troubling memory. But if the problem continues for months, it's time to see a doctor. "Diagnosis and therapy for impotence have improved tremendously in the last three or four years," says Dr. Jacob Rajfer, who teaches urology at UCLA's medical school.

You can find one of numerous urologists who now specialize in impotence through your family doctor, a teaching hospital, or county medical society. After your medical history is taken, you will get a physical that often includes special tests to gauge hormone levels, penile circulation, and nocturnal erections. Expect to be asked about possible psychological causes. Until recently, experts felt that most impotence had mental roots—now they believe that 60 percent of all cases have physical origins.

The culprit may turn out to be smoking, drinking, hardening of the arteries, or some other medical condition. It could even be a drug you're taking for another ailment.

Treatment may be as simple as giving up smoking or changing medication. Or your doctor may prescribe one of the standard therapies: injection of a drug called papavarine into the penis (which can be done at home), suction and blood-entrapment devices, or a surgical implant. The substantial cost of an implant—up to $10,000—is usually covered by insurance if the problem is organic.

If the cause is emotional, treatment may range from a few visits to a counselor to long-term therapy. Dr. Richard E. Berger, chief of urology at Harborview Hospital in Seattle, often recommends counseling in tandem with other forms of treatment.

Self-Help Group

Whatever therapy is prescribed, make sure your partner knows all about it and feels involved: it helps both the treatment and the relationship. Recovery of Male Potency, a self-help group affiliated with 23 hospitals, offers informational meetings and literature. Write to R-Center, Grace Hospital, 18700 Meyers Rd., Detroit, Mich. 48235 (313 966-3219 or 800 835-7667).

More information? Send a stamped, self-addressed envelope to Impotents Anonymous, 119 S. Ruth St., Maryville, Tenn. 37801 (615 983-6064). Recommended reading: *Lifelong Lover,* by Marvin and Sally Brooks ($8.95), available at bookstores or from Doubleday & Co., 245 Park Ave., New York, N.Y. 10167.

Source: Teresa Carson, 19 January 1987, Impotence is more treatable than you think, *Business Week,* p. 106.

erection and find it more difficult to maintain. Orgasmic contractions are less intense.

At the same time, many men go through a period of reassessment and readjustment in middle age ("midlife crisis"), which may have repercussions on their sexuality.

Exploring Your Emotions

In what ways do you find yourself sexually vulnerable? Do any aspects of your sexual interactions interfere with your desires and your partner's satisfaction? How would you like to overcome such interference?

As with women, there is no reason why sexual activity cannot continue to be a source of pleasure and satisfaction for men as they grow older. When problems do arise they are more often due to psychological reactions to bodily changes than to the physical changes themselves.

Overcoming Sexual Dysfunction **Sexual dysfunction** entails disturbances in sexual desire, performance, or satisfaction. Although a wide variety of physical conditions and drugs may interfere with sexual functions (for instance, diabetes may interfere with the blood and nerve supply to sex organs), sexual dysfunctions more often result from psychological causes and problems in intimate relationships.

The same two mechanisms—vasocongestion and

Sexual dysfunction Disturbances in sexual desire, performance, or satisfaction.

Impotence Failure to get an erection.

Premature ejaculation Involuntary orgasm before or shortly after the penis enters the vagina. Ejaculating before one wishes to.

Delayed ejaculation Inability to ejaculate when one wishes to during coitus.

Sex therapy Treatment of sexual dysfunction.

Sexually transmissible diseases Infectious diseases spread by sexual contact.

---

myotonia—that form the bases of the sexual response cycle also explain the main forms of sexual disturbance: inability to become aroused and problems with orgasm.

In the male, the inability to become aroused is manifested by **impotence**, the failure to attain or maintain an erection. Orgasmic problems involve either **premature ejaculation** or **delayed ejaculation.** The first, which is far more common, occurs when a man involuntarily ejaculates before he wants to. This reduces the period of time he can engage in sexual intercourse to his and to his partner's satisfaction. Delayed ejaculation is the opposite; in these cases a man has difficulty reaching orgasm when he wants to.

In the female, the inability to become sexually aroused may not preclude her engaging in sexual intercourse but prevents her from experiencing sexual pleasure and orgasm. Women are also far more vulnerable than men to pain during sexual intercourse. The pain may be due to physical causes (such as pelvic infections) or to psychological factors, such as anxiety, that cause muscular spasm in the vaginal opening.

Most forms of sexual dysfunction can be treated. The first step is to treat any underlying medical condition. Then, new methods of **sex therapy** seek to modify the behavior patterns that interfere with satisfactory sexual relationships.

Some of the most important health consequences of sexual activity are **sexually transmissible diseases.** Because of their particular significance, they are discussed separately in Chapter 19.

Take Action

Your answer to the Exploring Your Emotions questions in this chapter and your placement on the Wellness Ladder at the beginning of this chapter will, we hope, encourage you to begin a process of self-exploration and self-discovery that you will continue. Reflect on the entire chapter's content and ask yourself how each point relates to your own life. Then take action:

1. Place sex in perspective. Sexual responsiveness is a relative matter; there is no absolute standard of normalcy against which to compare yourself. What counts most is the extent to which your sexual responsiveness fulfills *your* expectations of what role sex should play in your life. Make a list of your sexual expectations. Over the next few weeks, evaluate your list and change it accordingly.
2. Sexual myths and misconceptions abound in our culture. Create your own list of myths you've heard. Find out the facts by consulting books and pamphlets mentioned here or available through your school health center.
3. Ask an intimate friend to rate you on the Rate Yourself statements at the beginning of the chapter. Compare his or her rating with your own. Discuss any discrepancies you discover in a nondefensive way.
4. Read the following Behavior Change Strategy and take any appropriate action.

Behavior Change Strategy

Sexual Dysfunction

Most people will experience sexual dysfunction sometime in their lives. This often involves difficulty in becoming aroused or reaching orgasm. William Masters and Virginia Johnson, in *Human Sexual Response* (1970), estimate that approximately half of all married couples in the United States have experienced some form of sexual dysfunction. Single people have an even higher rate, a fact that is usually attributed to insecurity in their relationships and less familiarity with their partner's sexual preferences.

Male sexual dysfunctions include ejaculatory incompetence (difficulty in reaching orgasm); premature ejaculation (ejaculation earlier than desired); and erectile dysfunction, also known as impotence (the lack of a sustained erection for intercourse). Female dysfunctions include vaginismus (involuntary contraction of vaginal muscles that prevents entry by the penis); primary orgasmic dysfunction (a woman has never reached orgasm and is unable to do so); situational orgasmic dysfunction (a specific situation, partner, etc., prevents orgasm). Women with orgasmic dysfunction may be very sensitive, concerned, and frustrated; there should be no implication that they are "frigid" or uninterested in sex.

Sexual dysfunction may be caused by physical or psychological factors. Approximately 10 to 20 percent of all sexual dysfunctions stem from disease. Diabetes and heart disease, for example, may be an underlying cause of erectile dysfunction. Fatigue can cause problems that are temporary unless one becomes overly anxious about future performance. Drugs, especially depressants such as alcohol, may also inhibit sexual responses. People experiencing sex difficulties should have a thorough physical examination.

Psychosocial causes of dysfunction include troubled relationships, lack of sexual skills, irrational attitudes and beliefs, anxiety, and psychosexual trauma. One outmoded traditional attitude holds that sex is an undesirable duty for women and pleasurable only for men. This kind of stereotypical thinking can create such anxiety for a woman that she cannot enjoy coitus and may, in turn, cause erection or ejaculation problems for the man.

Like other skills, sexual competence is learned. We learn what makes us and others feel good by talking with them about sex, reading about it, watching films, and experimenting. Many people, however, do not acquire sexual skills because they lack the opportunity to experiment or because even the thought of violating traditional mores creates overwhelming anxiety for them.

Sex Therapy The behavioral treatment of sexual dysfunction concentrates on reducing performance anxiety, changing self-defeating expectations, and learning sexual skills or competencies. Masters and Johnson offer a two-week treatment program for couples, who live in residence at their clinic. Included in the program is "bibliotherapy" or treatment through the reading of self-help manuals. Examples of other techniques that have been effective follow.

A man who is unable to attain an erection learns to relax and receive sexual stimulation. The partners first massage each other without touching the genitals, using verbal instructions and guiding each other's hands in order to communicate. Genital manipulation follows after a few sessions. When erection is reliably attained, the couple does not immediately attempt intercourse because performance anxiety might develop. Instead, the partners follow a series of sexual activities that ultimately ends in intercourse. Masters and Johnson report that erectile dysfunction has been reversed in 72 percent of the couples treated.

Premature ejaculation is often treated by the "squeeze technique" in which the tip of the penis is squeezed when the man feels he is about to ejaculate. This technique is learned from a sex therapist. Gradually, the man learns to prolong intercourse without ejaculating. Masters and Johnson report that this technique is successful in 90 percent of the men treated.

Primary orgasmic dysfunction frequently occurs among women who feel that sex is dirty and may have been taught never to touch themselves. They are anxious about their sexuality and have not had the chance to learn through trial and error what types of sexual stimulation will excite them and bring them to climax. Most sex therapists prefer the use of masturbation to treat this problem. Masturbation provides women with a chance to learn about their own bodies and to give themselves pleasure without depending on a sex partner. Masturbation programs first teach women about their own anatomy by means of reading, discussion groups, and the use of a mirror. They experiment with self-caresses at their own pace, learning gradually to bring themselves to orgasm. The behavioral approach uses the reward or pleasure principle to counter negative or anxiety-provoking situations. Once a woman can masturbate to orgasm, she may need additional treatment to transfer this learning to sex with a partner.

Selected References

Bancroft, J. 1983. *Human Sexuality and Its Problems*. Edinburgh: Churchill Livingston.

Bermant, G., and Davidson, J. M. 1974. *Biological Bases of Sexual Behavior*. New York: Harper & Row.

Kaplan, H. S. 1974. *The New Sex Therapy*. New York: Brunner-Mazel.

Masters, W. H., and Johnson, V. E. 1966. *Human Sexual Response*. New York: Little, Brown.

Meyer-Bahlburg, H. F. L. (ed.). 1984 (October). Gender development: Social influences and prenatal hormone effects. *Archives of Sexual Behavior* 13:391–93.

Money, J., and Erhardt, A. A. 1972. *Man and Woman, Boy and Girl*. Baltimore: Johns Hopkins University Press.

Tanner, J. M. 1978. *Fetus to Man*. Cambridge, Mass.: Harvard University Press.

Recommended Readings

Belliveau, F., and Richter, L. 1970. *Understanding Human Sexual Inadequacy*. New York: Bantam. *Popularized rendition of Masters and Johnson's approach to sex therapy.*

Brecher, R., and Brecher, E. 1966. *An Analysis of Human Sexual Response*. New York: New American Library. *A nontechnical summary of the manifestations of the sexual response cycle.*

Budoff, P. W. 1980. *No Menstrual Cramps and Other Good News*. New York: Putnam's. *Cause and treatment of menstrual distress.*

Katchadourian, H. 1977. *The Biology of Adolescence*. San Francisco: Freeman. *The changes of puberty and their underlying hormonal mechanisms.*

Katchadourian, H. 1985. *Fundamentals of Human Sexuality*. 4th ed. New York: Holt, Rinehart & Winston. *A comprehensive college textbook. Chapters 2–7 cover the biological aspects of sexuality.*

Chapter 5

Contents

Rate Yourself

Your Attitudes about Sexual Behavior and Intimacy Read the following statements carefully. Choose the one in each section that best describes you at this moment and circle its number. When you have chosen one statement for each section, add the numbers and record your total score. Find your position on the Awareness Ladder.

5 Seeks both emotional and physical intimacy
4 Tends to emphasize one form of intimacy over the other
3 Would rather keep emotional and physical intimacy separate
2 Can deal with only one form of intimacy
1 Avoids any form of intimacy

5 Expresses inner feelings freely
4 Expresses inner feelings cautiously
3 Can express inner feelings but would rather not
2 Has difficulty expressing inner feelings
1 Is incapable of expressing inner feelings

5 Easily responsive to the needs of others
4 Capable of meeting others' needs when wants to
3 Reluctant to respond to others' needs
2 Has much difficulty responding to others' needs
1 Uninterested in others' needs

5 Seeks the partner's best interest, as well as own
4 Will compromise readily
3 Willing to negotiate
2 Yields to the partner's wishes with much reluctance
1 Must have his or her way all the time

5 Has a realistic sense of the assets and liabilities of oneself and the partner and is eager to help oneself and the other to grow in the relationship
4 Is quite satisfied with how things are but unwilling to exert much effort to make them better
3 Interested in closeness if the personal investment required is not high
2 Unrealistically intent on reforming the partner, and to a lesser extent the self
1 Involvement of differences, unwilling to compromise, blind to own shortcomings

Total Score ______

Sexual Behaviors and Relationships

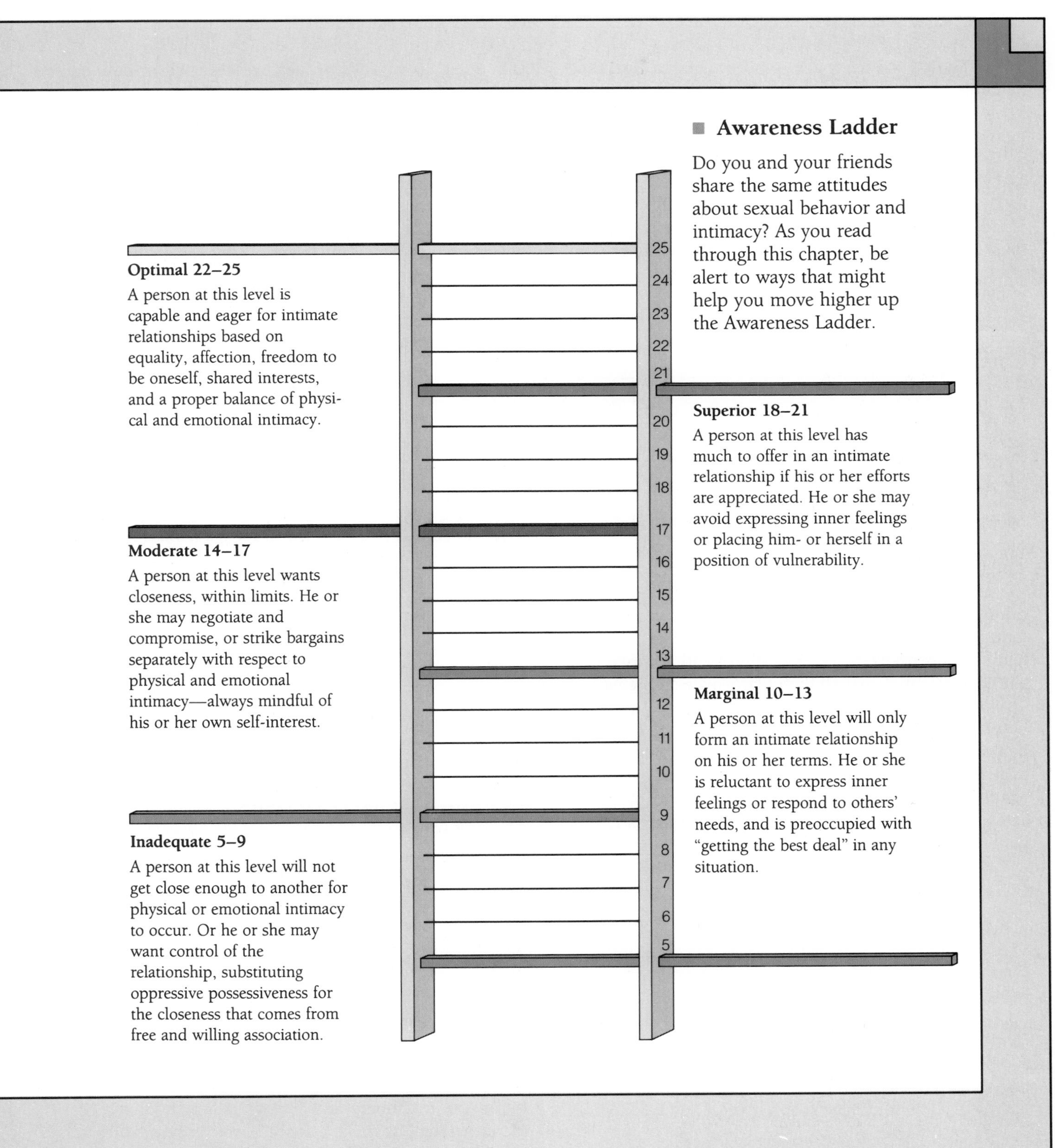

Optimal 22–25
A person at this level is capable and eager for intimate relationships based on equality, affection, freedom to be oneself, shared interests, and a proper balance of physical and emotional intimacy.
Moderate 14–17
A person at this level wants closeness, within limits. He or she may negotiate and compromise, or strike bargains separately with respect to physical and emotional intimacy—always mindful of his or her own self-interest.
Inadequate 5–9
A person at this level will not get close enough to another for physical or emotional intimacy to occur. Or he or she may want control of the relationship, substituting oppressive possessiveness for the closeness that comes from free and willing association.
25
24
23
22
21
20
19
18
17
16
15
14
13
12
11
10
9
8
7
6
5
Superior 18–21
A person at this level has much to offer in an intimate relationship if his or her efforts are appreciated. He or she may avoid expressing inner feelings or placing him- or herself in a position of vulnerability.
Marginal 10–13
A person at this level will only form an intimate relationship on his or her terms. He or she is reluctant to express inner feelings or respond to others' needs, and is preoccupied with "getting the best deal" in any situation.

Awareness Ladder

Do you and your friends share the same attitudes about sexual behavior and intimacy? As you read through this chapter, be alert to ways that might help you move higher up the Awareness Ladder.

Reproduction Generating offspring; having children.

Instinct Unlearned goal-directed motivational force.

Drive Innate behavioral motive.

Conditioning A basic form of learning that establishes acquired responses.

Social learning Acquisition of personal and social behavior through learning.

Sexual scripts Socially learned patterns of sexual behavior.

We all know what sex is about, but we have a hard time defining it. As W. C. Fields put it, "Sex isn't the best thing in the world, or the worst thing in the world—but there's nothing else quite like it."

Broadly defined, *sexual behavior* refers to all activities that lead to sexual arousal, with or without orgasm. Although a variety of behaviors are sexual, four aspects of such behaviors are particularly important: reproduction, erotic pleasure, gender identity and behavior, and affection and aggression.

Components of Human Sexuality

The association of sexual activity and **reproduction** is crucial for preserving our species, but it is not necessary or desirable that every person should reproduce. Furthermore, reproductive intent accounts for only a small measure of why people engage in sexual behaviors. Most people usually engage in sexual activity because it is pleasurable.

The associations of sex with gender, affection, and aggression may be less obvious than its links with reproduction and erotic pleasure, but they are no less important. We defined gender identity as the self-perception and social expectation of masculinity and femininity—the characteristics that go with being male and female.

No matter what culture we belong to, we can't possibly behave sexually without simultaneously acting as a man or a woman, even though behavioral distinctions between male and female are blurring in the United States. But gender expectations still influence what form of sexual activity we engage in, how often, for what purposes, and with what consequences.

The link between sex and gender works both ways. Gender not only influences sexual behavior but also is influenced *by* it. Thus, if men are expected to be more active and women more passive in sexual encounters, similar expectations are also likely to influence how men and women relate to each other in the workplace and other nonsexual contexts.

As we express by the term "making love," we usually assume or hope and expect that sexual relationships will have a measure of affection and love. But the two do not always go together. Many forms of affection are not erotic in intent. And sex does not always seem to require affection.

A good deal of sexual activity is also used to assert dominance and express aggression. In some sexual behaviors, such as rape, the primary motivation is not sexual pleasure or reproduction but the humiliation of the victim. Even in less extreme forms, the issue of dominance often colors sexual interactions between people.

Exploring Your Emotions

How aware do you feel you are of your own sexual wishes and preferences? Do you feel that your sexual impulses are healthy and desirable, or do you feel you harbor them "in spite of yourself"? Do you feel safe with your sexual fantasies, confident that you control your sexual behavior?

Sexual Drive and Learning

Why do so many of us seem to have a deep impulse to act sexually? Various theories have tried to answer this question on the basis of a sexual **instinct** or **drive:** They presuppose the presence of some innate force (called *libido* in psychoanalytic theory) that impels us to seek sexual satisfaction even against considerable obstacles.

The concept of a sexual instinct presupposes a biological process. Yet the role of biology in human sexual motivation is not agreed on. Students of animal social behavior see the patterns of human sexual behavior as predetermined by evolution. Like a role of exposed camera film, the images are already there. Society then acts like the "developer fluid" that brings out these images in the form of sexual behaviors.

Behavioral scientists place much greater emphasis on the role of learning. In their opinion, various forms of **conditioning** and **social learning** shape our sexual behaviors. One model of social learning is embodied in the concept of **sexual scripts.** Such scripts, like the text of a play, are learned during development and act like a blueprint, influencing why, with whom, how, and under what circumstances one has sexual relations.

A more integrative approach explains sexual behavior as the outcome of interacting biological and psychosocial factors. In this view, neuroendocrine processes maintain the sexual machinery and biological factors predispose the individual, or make it more likely for him or her to behave in a certain way. These predispositions are then

Three Couples

Couples on today's college campuses show a wide range of orientations toward love and sex. In a study of 231 student dating couples, three types of couples were identified. For *sexually traditional couples,* love alone is not a sufficient justification for sexual intercourse—the more permanent commitment of marriage is a necessary prerequisite. For *sexually moderate couples,* sex is considered permissible if a man and woman love each other; in this view, sex is an expression of love and caring. For *sexually liberal couples,* sex is acceptable even without love; sex is considered an enjoyable activity to be valued for its own sake.

The following are examples of each of the three types of couples:

A Sexually Traditional Couple: Paul and Peggy

Peggy believes that intercourse before marriage is wrong. She explained that "even if I were engaged, I wouldn't feel right about having sex." Many of Peggy's girlfriends are having sexual affairs, which Peggy accepts "for them." It's not right for Peggy, however, and she believes that Paul respects her views. For his part, Paul indicated that he would like to have intercourse with Peggy, but he added that intercourse "just isn't all that important for me."

A Sexually Moderate Couple: Tom and Sandy

Three weeks after their first date, Tom told Sandy that he loved her. She was in love, too, and their relationship grew quickly. In a few months they were spending weekends together at one of their dorms. They slept in the same bed but did not have intercourse. Although Tom was very attracted to Sandy, he was slow to initiate intercourse. "I didn't want to push it on her," he said. "I felt that we shouldn't have sex until our relationship reached a certain point. [Sex] is something I just can't imagine on a first date." Tom and Sandy first had intercourse with each other just before becoming engaged. For Tom, "Sex added another dimension to our relationship; it's a landmark of sorts."

A Sexually Liberal Couple: Diane and Alan

About two weeks after they started dating, Alan asked if Diane would like to make love. She declined, saying she wasn't ready yet, but implying that she would be soon. Since they were alone in Alan's apartment, she jokingly suggested that he go "exhibit himself" across the room so she could get used to his body. They spent the weekend together, and by Sunday Diane felt ready for intercourse. Diane told us that she and Alan were not in love when they first had intercourse. Nonetheless, she enjoyed the sex and felt it was "part of our getting to know each other. It led to an obvious closeness."

The central distinction between these three orientations concerns the links between sexual intimacy and emotional intimacy. For traditionalists, emotional intimacy develops in the context of limited sexual activity; sexual intercourse is tied not only to love but to a permanent commitment, as well. For moderates, emotional intimacy sets the pace for sexual intimacy. As feelings of closeness and love increase, greater sexual exploration is possible. For liberals, sexual intimacy and emotional intimacy need not be related. Sex can be enjoyed in its own right, or sexual intimacy can be a route to developing emotional intimacy.

As you may have noticed, in all three of the couples the man was the one who took the lead in increasing sexual intimacy, while the woman played a more passive or limit-setting role. In all types of couples—traditional, moderate, and liberal—aspects of the sexual double standard . . . live on.

Source: Rubin/McNeil 1985
The Psychology of Being Human (New York: Harper & Row), p. 532.

Autoerotic play Self-exploration and genital manipulation in childhood.

Masturbation Self-stimulation to obtain sexual arousal and orgasm.

Sociosexual play Sexual activity between children.

Nocturnal emission Orgasm during sleep accompanied by ejaculation (wet dream).

Autoerotic behavior Activities aimed at sexual self-stimulation.

Sociosexual behavior Sexual activities involving other people.

Sexual orientation Preference for opposite-sex or same-sex partners.

Erotic fantasy Sexual thoughts or daydreams.

Sexual intercourse Heterosexual relations involving genital union. Also called *coitus* or *making love,* and by various colloquial names.

Coitus Heterosexual intercourse.

Foreplay Sexual stimulation preparing for coitus.

Cunnilingus Oral stimulation of the female genitals.

Fellatio Oral stimulation of the penis.

Exploring Your Emotions

Do you remember specific events from your childhood that clearly defined for you what it meant to be a member of your sex? When did you first start to accept different behaviors for each sex? In raising your own children, how would you handle their acquisition of gender roles? What disadvantages would your children have if they were raised without any clearly described gender roles?

---

further elaborated and given meaning by cultural forces. Our actual behavior is shaped by the interplay of our predispositions and our learning experiences throughout life.

Development of Sexual Behavior

Our capacity to respond sexually is present at birth. In fact, ultrasound studies suggest that boys experience erections in the womb. After birth, both sexes have the capacity for orgasm, even though only some babies may actually experience it. As we grow, more of us discover this capacity through self-exploration.

Childhood Sexual Behavior Sexual behaviors gradually emerge in childhood in the form of self-stimulating play. Self-exploration and touching the genitals are the most common forms of such play (observed among infants as young as 6 months). They gradually lead to more deliberate forms of **masturbation** with or without orgasm.

Children simultaneously engage in sexual play with others by exploring their playmates' genitals. These activities are often part of games like "playing house" or "mommy and daddy." By age 12, 40 percent of boys have engaged in sex play; the peak age for girls is age 9, by which time 14 percent have had similar experiences.

Children are actively taught and socialized by their parents and teachers. But in our culture this task is largely avoided with respect to sexual learning, or it is carried out in indirect ways. Our society also forbids any direct sexual interaction between adults and children.

Adolescent Sexuality A person who has gone through puberty is biologically an adult. But in psychological and social terms, it takes five to ten more years before we attain full adult status. This discrepancy between biological and social maturity creates much confusion over what constitutes appropriate sexual behavior during adolescence.

Most teenage boys and somewhat fewer girls masturbate more or less regularly. Once puberty is reached, orgasm among boys is accompanied by ejaculation. Occasionally, teenage boys also have **nocturnal emissions** ("wet dreams"). Girls also have orgasmic dreams. Although masturbation no longer carries the social stigma and the false fears of former times, adolescents (and some adults, too) are often still embarrassed by it.

Sexual interaction in adolescence usually takes place between peers in the form of dating, which fulfills a variety of other social functions as well. Sexual intimacy takes place in such relationships through petting and necking, which involve kissing, caressing, and stimulating the breasts and the genitals. These activities lead to sexual arousal but may or may not culminate in orgasm.

Many American teenagers now also engage in premarital sex. About 35 percent of women aged 15 to 19 and a presumably higher proportion of males are sexually active. Rates for premarital sex vary considerably from one group to another, however, based on ethnic, educational, religious, geographic, and other factors.

Many factors influence when a person engages in coitus for the first time: moral considerations, psychological readiness, fear of consequences, being in love, going steady, peer pressure, trying to act adult, gaining popularity, rebelliousness, and a host of other factors. Some of us make thoughtful decisions, and others take the plunge recklessly.

Adolescent sexual behaviors are not confined to heterosexual relationships. Beginning with childhood, sex play involves members of one's own sex as well as of the opposite sex. Homosexual attractions, with or without sexual encounters, are likewise quite common in adolescence. For many, these are passing episodes but for others they become the basis of adult **sexual orientation.** Most adult gay men and women trace back their sexual preferences to their early years.

Varieties of Sexual Experience

Sexual behaviors may be **autoerotic** (such as masturbation) and aimed at self-stimulation or **sociosexual** (such as coitus) and involve direct sexual interaction with others. Sociosexual behaviors may be further differentiated by sexual partner or object and by sexual aim (what one wishes to do with the sexual partner). Sexual behaviors are also judged according to medical, moral, and legal standards as to whether or not they are healthy, ethical, or lawful.

Autoerotism The most common sexual activity is **erotic fantasy.** It may range from fleeting thoughts to elaborate scenarios replaying past sexual experiences or expressing unfulfilled wishes. Such erotic imaginings may be engaged in for their own sake or may accompany masturbation, coitus, or some other activity.

Fantasies may substitute for what is not attainable at the time. They may also enhance sexual arousal during sexual encounters. Some sexual fantasies may be frightening or offensive, but in most instances they are not acted out even if the person has an opportunity to do so.

The term *masturbation* refers to any sexual activity that depends on physical self-stimulation. Typically it involves manually stimulating the genitals, rubbing the genitals against objects (such as a mattress or pillow), and (less often) using special devices such as vibrators.

Although commonly associated with adolescence, masturbation remains a frequent sexual outlet throughout adult life. It may be used as a substitute for coitus or some other sociosexual behaviors, or engaged in for its own sake or as part of sexual activity with a partner. Masturbation allows the person to obtain sexual release and pleasure at his or her own choosing, time, place, and pace. Most men and women masturbate. Two out of three college students masturbate a few times a week on average, others do it more or less frequently, and some don't do it at all.

Exploring Your Emotions

If you could change any present social attitudes toward any aspect of sexuality, what would you change? Why?

Sexual Intercourse For most adults, most of the time, sexual intercourse is what having sex is all about. Men and women engage in **coitus** or make love to fulfill sexual as well as psychological needs. The term *sexual intercourse* includes the whole experience in making love, while *coitus* ("to link together") may be more narrowly applicable to penile-genital interactions.

In addition to various types of **foreplay,** couples may use genital stimulation by the mouth (oral sex) to heighten arousal or reach orgasm. About 90 percent of married couples below age 25 reportedly engage in oral stimulation both of the female genitals (**cunnilingus**) and of the penis (**fellatio**). Some partners, however, object to such activities.

Exploring Your Emotions

Touching can be sexually arousing. But touching can also soothe, comfort, and calm.

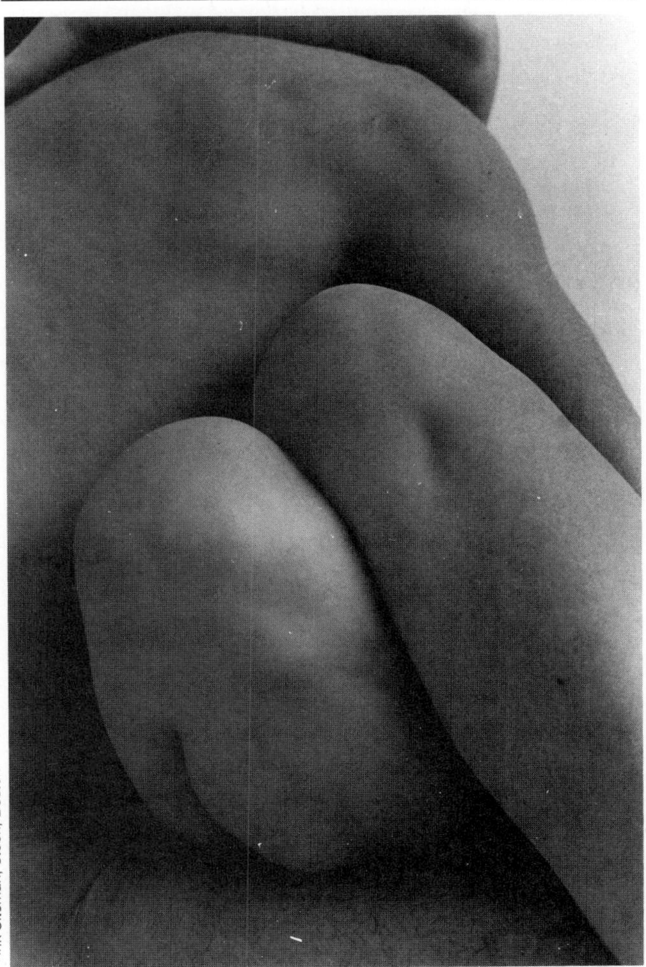

Frank Siteman, Stock, Boston

How Liberal or Conservative Am I? The Sexual Attitude Scale

This questionnaire is designed to measure the way you feel about sexual behavior. It is not a test, so there are no right or wrong answers. Answer each item as carefully and accurately as you can by placing a number beside each one as follows:

1. Strongly disagree
2. Disagree
3. Neither agree nor disagree (undecided)
4. Agree
5. Strongly agree

	SD	D	U	A	SA
1. I think there is too much sexual freedom given to adults these days.	1	2	3	4	5
2. I think that the increased sexual freedom seen in the past several years has done much to undermine the American family.	1	2	3	4	5
3. I think that young people have been given too much information about sex.	1	2	3	4	5
4. Sex education should be restricted to the home.	1	2	3	4	5
5. Older people do not need to have sex.	1	2	3	4	5
6. Sex education should be given only when people are ready for marriage.	1	2	3	4	5
7. Premarital sex may be a sign of a decaying social order.	1	2	3	4	5
8. Extramarital sex is never excusable.	1	2	3	4	5
9. I think there is too much sexual freedom given to teenagers these days.	1	2	3	4	5
10. I think there is not enough sexual restraint among young people.	1	2	3	4	5
11. I think people indulge in sex too much.	1	2	3	4	5
12. I think the only proper way to have sex is through intercourse.	1	2	3	4	5
13. I think sex should be reserved for marriage.	1	2	3	4	5
14. Sex should be only for the young.	1	2	3	4	5
15. Too much social approval has been given to homosexuals.	1	2	3	4	5

Much has been written on how to enhance pleasure through various coital techniques, postures, and the like. From a woman's perspective, the key factor in terms of physical readiness for coitus is adequate vaginal lubrication. But she should also feel receptive for the act. For a man, conditions must arouse him to attain and maintain erection.

Although personal preferences vary, most people prefer a safe, private setting. Candlelight and music, for example, can further enhance the mood of the occasion.

Knowledge of sex techniques is useful, yet psychological factors and the quality of the relationship of the couple are more important in sexual satisfaction. Sexual intercourse works best among equals who are willing to share their bodies freely. It matters little who does what to whom as long as it is mutually enjoyable and safe. People need to be willing to express wishes as well as to be sensitive to the desires of their sexual partners. We feel strongly that coitus should not be a power struggle, endurance contest, or occasion for martyrdom but a joyous, carefree, and fulfilling experience between two consenting partners in a context of affection and trust.

Homosexuality A minority of men and women are sexually and romantically attracted only to members of their own sex. Except for that fact, they are no different from

16. Sex should be devoted to the business of procreation.	1	2	3	4	5
17. People should not masturbate.	1	2	3	4	5
18. Heavy sexual petting should be discouraged.	1	2	3	4	5
19. People should not discuss their sexual affairs or business with others.	1	2	3	4	5
20. Severely handicapped (physically and mentally) people should not have sex.	1	2	3	4	5
21. There should be no laws prohibiting sexual acts between consenting adults.	1	2	3	4	5
22. What two consenting adults do together sexually is their own business.	1	2	3	4	5
23. There is too much sex on television.	1	2	3	4	5
24. Movies today are too sexually explicit.	1	2	3	4	5
25. Pornography should be totally banned from our bookstores.	1	2	3	4	5

To determine your score on the Sexual Attitude Scale, reverse the scores for Statements 21 and 22 in the following way: 1 = 5, 2 = 4, 4 = 2, 5 = 1. For example, if you wrote 1 for Statement 21 ("There should be no laws prohibiting sexual acts between consenting adults"), change that number to 5 for scoring purposes. Reverse score Statement 22 similarly.

Add the numbers you assigned to each of the 25 statements. Your score may range from a low of 25 (strongly disagreed with all items: 1 × 25 = 25) to a high of 125 (strongly agreed with all items: 5 × 25 = 125). If you scored between 25 and 50, you might be regarded as a high-grade liberal, between 50 and 75, a low-grade liberal. If you scored between 100 and 125, you might be regarded as a high-grade conservative; between 75 and 100, a low-grade conservative.

In this scale a liberal is one who feels that the expression of human sexuality should be open, free, and unrestrained. A conservative is one who feels that sexual expression should be considerably constrained and closely regulated.

Knox, *Human Sexuality,* pp. 123–25.

heterosexuals. A larger number of bisexuals are sexually attracted, to various degrees, to both men and women.

Currently, most homosexual men prefer to be called gay, and women lesbian. Their sexual behaviors and lifestyles have received a good deal of public attention that has helped to dispel some of the prejudices against them. Homosexuality is no longer classified formally as a psychiatric disorder, although it has not received the societal approval that heterosexuality has.

The sexual practices of gay men and women are quite similar to their heterosexual counterparts except for coitus. In addition to kissing and other types of foreplay, gay sex relies more heavily on mouth-genital stimulation as a means of attaining orgasm. Some gay men also engage in anal intercourse. Contrary to common misconceptions, gay partners do not consistently assume "active" or "passive" roles.

Much of the sexual lifestyle of gays depends on whether they are overt or covert homosexuals. Those who feel forced to be secretive about their sexual preference may lead double lives, a public and a private life. Those who have "come out" participate more or less actively in the gay subculture.

About 30 percent of lesbians and 17 percent of gay men form close and stable ties. Others, particularly gay men, interact with a large number of sexual partners whom

The Roots of Sexual Orientation

Why is it that some people are heterosexual and others homosexual? A short answer is that we don't know. Despite much study and speculation, when, how, and why we develop our sexual orientation is still unclear.

Studying the roots of sexual orientation would be the most appropriate way to understand the choice between heterosexuality and homosexuality. Yet research in this area usually has been aimed at discovering the causes of homosexuality because it traditionally has been assumed to be an abnormality and because scientists often investigate what is unusual.

Because exclusive homosexuality precludes reproduction, it is biologically maladaptive for human societies as a whole, although not necessarily for individuals. But the same concern with reproduction does not apply to bisexuality. In fact, one wonders why we aren't sexually attracted equally to men and women. After all, we love members of both sexes, and love and sexuality often go together.

It has long been argued that homosexuality is "unnatural," biologically aberrant, and therefore morally reprehensible. However, if by "natural" we mean what exists in nature, that position is not tenable. Same-sex interactions (genital stimulation, mounting, thrusting) can be observed among various species of monkeys. Whether homosexuality is socially acceptable or not, homosexual behavior has been present for centuries in almost every culture.

Much research about biological determinants of homosexuality has focused on genetic and hormonal factors. Studies have found that the brothers of gay men are more likely to be homosexuals than the brothers of straight men, especially if they are twins. But in such studies, genetics, heredity, and common patterns of upbringing cannot readily be sorted out. Other studies have shown gay men to have lower testosterone levels than their heterosexual counterparts, whereas lesbians have higher-than-average levels of the male hormone. Investigators have also noted differences between physical structures, blood chemistry, and metabolic processes of homosexuals and heterosexuals. Yet inconsistencies in methodology and outcomes make these studies inconclusive.

The search for psychosocial determinants likewise has failed to reveal consistent patterns. Psychoanalysts have pointed to parental relationships as a basis for growing up to be gay. Typically, gay men report having detached and hostile fathers and seductive and domineering mothers. Social learning theorists have also pointed to poor peer relationships, atypical sexual experiences, and homosexual seduction in childhood as factors in homosexuality. One can find cases to fit any theory, but none can be generalized as a sole cause of homosexuality.

Nonetheless, some interesting patterns in sexual development cast some light on this matter. By the time boys and girls reach adolescence, their sexual preferences are already largely set. Romantic attraction to the same sex is present several years before any homosexual activity takes place. Adolescents who become gay are not particularly lacking in heterosexual experience—they just don't find such experiences as gratifying. Gender nonconformity—effeminate boys and tomboyish girls—is strongly linked to the development of homosexuality.

These findings indicate once again the futility of trying to understand sexual orientation and behavior outside of the broader context of gender identity and personality development. Sex should be considered an integral part of life.

Source: A. P. Bell, et al., 1981. *Sexual Preferences: Its Development in Men and Women* (Bloomington: Indiana University Press).

Exploring Your Emotions

Suppose a close friend told you that he or she was homosexual. How would you react? Would you feel threatened? Would your friendship undergo any changes? Would you still talk about the same things with your friend? Could you talk freely about sexual behavior with your friend?

Homosexuality Romantic and sexual attraction to members of the same sex. Male homosexuals are now usually called *gay;* females, *lesbians.*

Premarital sex Coitus before marriage.

Extramarital sex Coitus between a married person and someone other than his or her spouse.

Incestuous relations Sex between close relatives, such as siblings or parents and their children.

Prostitute A person who provides sexual services in exchange for money or goods.

Paraphilias Sexual behaviors involving a variant choice of sexual partner for means of gratification.

Sex offenders Those who engage in sexual behaviors prohibited by law.

Pedophilia Sexual contact between adults and children.

Zoophilia Sexual contact between humans and animals; bestiality.

Fetishism Sexual attachment to inanimate objects or body parts.

Transvestism Getting dressed in the clothes of the opposite sex; cross-dressing.

Transsexual A person who rejects his or her assigned gender and feels trapped in the wrong-sex body.

Gender dysphoria Mismatch between biological sex and gender identity.

---

they meet in gay bars, baths, and other locations. Such gay men face serious health hazards from sexually transmitted diseases especially due to the threat of AIDS. Such behavior currently appears to be on the decline.

Socially Problematic Behaviors Certain sexual behaviors are condemned not because of the sexual activity involved but because of the social relationship between the sexual partners. Thus, **premarital sex, extramarital sex, incestuous relations,** and sex with **prostitutes** all are condemned by broad segments of U.S. society.

Other behaviors are socially problematic because the nature of the sexual activity violates moral and legal codes, offends the public sense of decency, or threatens others. Some sexual behaviors, such as rape, are so patently offensive that they are generally unacceptable. But the condemnation of other forms of behaviors tends to be more arbitrary. Such judgments may also vary over time. Thus, homosexual relations have recently become more acceptable, or at least better tolerated, in our society, and our attitudes toward premarital sex have become far more permissive than even a few decades ago.

Socially problematic behaviors such as voyeurism or exhibitionism typically fall within the category of **paraphilias,** which are defined as psychological disorders. A few of them reflect deep-seated psychological disturbances; mostly they are the more exaggerated versions of quite common behaviors. For instance, many of us are interested in nudity, but only voyeurs will peek through bedroom windows. To qualify as a paraphilia, the behavior must be a repeatedly preferred or exclusive method of obtaining sexual gratification in the presence of other legitimate outlets. Those who engage in paraphilic behaviors are legally defined as **sex offenders.**

Virtually all sex offenders are men. This is partly because of the way such behaviors are socially perceived. For instance, if a man stands nude at a window and a woman sees him, he may be considered an exhibitionist. If a woman exposes herself to a man in a similar situation, the man may be considered a voyeur.

Men are also generally more aggressive than women. Because paraphilias often have a thinly veiled hostile element to them, they become vehicles for more aggressive aspects of male sexuality.

Attempts to find genetic and hormonal causes for such behaviors have not been successful. According to psychoanalytic theory, the paraphilias represent residues of unresolved immature sexual impulses from childhood. Other theorists explain these behaviors on the basis of social learning.

Variant Choices of Sexual Partners Adults who are sexually attracted to and interact with children for sexual gratification are called **pedophiles.** Most pedophiliacs are male and are typically interested in prepubescent girls or boys. In most cases, the pedophile is a relative, family friend, or someone known to the child. Sexual contacts are typically brief and consist of genital manipulation; genital intercourse is rarely attempted. How traumatic the experience proves to the child depends on the circumstances under which the sexual encounter occurs and the consequences of discovery. When the pedophile is a close relative, such as the father, the effects are apt to be far more serious for the child and disruptive to the family relationships.

Sexual contact with animals, **zoophilia** or **bestiality,** has been known since ancient times. The practice is usually restricted to some young men who live close to farm animals. At the level of fantasy, men and women may have erotic thoughts involving animals.

In **fetishism,** the object of erotic interest is an inanimate object or body part. It is quite common to be more attracted to certain parts of the body than to others. It is also fairly common practice to wear articles of clothing (such as fancy underwear) to be sexually provocative. But with a fetishist, a woman's breasts, legs, feet, or panties become more important than the woman herself. Furthermore, "hard" fetishes, such as black leather garments, spike-heeled shoes, chains, whips, and the like are often associated with practices involving pain and humiliation.

Transvestism or **cross-dressing** involves wearing the clothes of the opposite sex. **Transsexuals** should not be confused with transvestites. Transsexualism is a gender disorder or **gender dysphoria,** whereby the person feels

Voyeur A person who observes people who are undressing, nude, or engaging in sex as a preferred form of sexual activity; "peeping Tom."

Exhibitionist A person who exhibits his genitals to shock women and children; "flasher."

Sexual sadism Inflicting pain to obtain sexual enjoyment.

Sexual masochism Suffering pain to obtain sexual enjoyment.

Dominance Exerting control and authority over others.

Agression Use of force; hostile action.

Sexual pressuring The persistent use of unwanted sexual advances.

Sexual harrassment Sexual pressuring of someone in a vulnerable position.

Sexual assault Use of force to gain sexual access to someone.

Rape Coercing a person into having sex under the threat or the use of force.

Statutory rape Sex with someone below the legal age of consent.

---

trapped in a body of the opposite sex. Thus when a biologically male transsexual dresses up as a woman, he is dressing up consistently with his own female gender identity.

Variant Choices of Sexual Means In these cases, the sexual partner may be an adult member of the opposite sex but rather than engaging in coitus, the person chooses some other means of sexual gratification as a repeatedly preferred or exclusive method of obtaining sexual gratification.

The **voyeur** ("peeping Tom") is sexually aroused by secretly watching a woman undress, bathe, or engage in sex. To be sexually exciting, the act must be forbidden—a voyeur gets no special enjoyment from observing his own wife undressing or from being in a nudist club. Violating a woman's privacy and doing a forbidden act arouse the voyeur.

The **exhibitionist** ("flasher") is motivated by similar impulses but instead of viewing others, he exhibits his genitals to them. Typically, he does so in a relatively isolated area, such as a park, but he may also do so on an uncrowded bus or subway. The victims are women and children. Their shocked reactions are what the exhibitionist is after. Telling unwelcome dirty jokes, using sexual innuendos to embarrass others, and making obscene telephone calls similarly use sex to shock.

Voyeurs and exhibitionists usually do not physically molest their victims unless they are confronted and provoked. They masturbate during or soon after the act, as a sexual release.

Sadomasochism Pinning the partner down and causing mild pain through biting and scratching may be part of a couple's sexual repertory. Some sexual partners tie each other down to the bed, and use various paraphernalia in their lovemaking. Fantasies of being coerced into sex, being subdued by multiple partners, and similar activities are not uncommon among ordinary men and women.

As a paraphilia, **sexual sadism** entails inflicting physical and psychological suffering on another person. **Sexual masochism** is the erotic enjoyment of one's own suffering. Sadomasochism (S-M) is typically engaged in by men with the aid of (often hired) female partners who dress up in fetishistic clothing and "dominate" them, whip them, and act out various other sadomasochistic rituals. Other men restrict their involvement to reading S-M magazines that depict women as being gagged, bound, humiliated, beaten up, and sexually abused.

Sadomasochism clearly demonstrates the role of **dominance** and **aggression** in sexual interactions. In its most vicious form, sadism inflicts humiliation, pain, and suffering on an unwilling victim, and may lead to murder and mutilation.

Coercive Sex The use of force and coercion in sexual relationships is one of the most serious problems in human interactions. Its most extreme manifestation is rape, but in many other forms of sexual coercion as well one person is forced to submit to another's sexual desires.

Sexual Harassment A common attitude, not only in our culture, is that men push for sex and women resist but eventually yield, or that women say no even if they mean yes. As a result, **sexual pressuring** has been considered somewhat legitimate even when women have clearly felt annoyed and humiliated by it. Women are now less willing to put up with such unwelcome advances, and men are becoming more aware of their feelings in this regard.

When sexual pressuring involves someone in a vulnerable position (such as an employee pressured by the boss, or a student by a professor) then it constitutes **sexual harassment.** Men are usually, but not always, the offenders because they are more often in positions of power, and this sort of predatory behavior is more typically male. There is nothing inherently wrong in fellow workers being sexually interested in each other, although romantic and sexual entanglements with colleagues tend to complicate professional relationships. But the abuse of power for sexual gain is clearly unacceptable.

Sexual Assault Sexual coercion that relies on the threat and use of physical force, or takes advantage of circumstances that render a person incapable of giving consent (such as when drunk) constitutes **sexual assault** or **rape.** When the victim is below the legally defined "age of consent," then the act constitutes **statutory rape**, regardless of the issue of coercion.

In most cases, women are raped by men. Some men are raped by other men, and very rarely by women. In a given year, over 80,000 cases of rape are reported in the United States. But half of all rapes may go unreported, and the true incidence may be five to twenty times the official figures. Women of all ages and backgrounds may be victims of rape. Middle-class women who are raped are the victims of friends and acquaintances in almost half such cases. Perhaps as many as one in ten wives are raped at some time by their husbands.

Rapists fall into a number of categories. Some are amoral, aggressive young men who take by force what they cannot have otherwise. A second type is the sexually inadequate man who is unable to obtain satisfaction otherwise. The more hostile and sadistic rapists are not primarily interested in sex but in hurting and humiliating a particular woman, or women in general.

Victims of rape are currently less likely to be blamed for their traumatic experience than was the case even in the recent past. Nonetheless, much can be gained by being aware of risk factors and by learning how to deal with such situations. Rape prevention programs in colleges and communities can provide practical guidance.

Date Rape Most college women are in much less danger of being raped by a stranger in a dark alley than of being sexually abused by men they date. The use of force for sexual purposes is already part of the dating interactions of high school students and follows certain patterns. Some boys feel (mistakenly) justified in forcing a girl to have sex if they were engaged sexually and then she refused to "go all the way." This disregard is especially common if the girl is known to have slept with other boys or showed up at a party where she knew there would be drinking and drugs.

That coercion is already accepted by at least some adolescents in mainstream American society points to a serious problem in their socialization. Sex and violence are so linked in history that no simple solutions are likely. But at least among well-educated and responsible young men and women, much of the difficulty may be resolved by a few basic changes in attitudes.

So the use of pressuring and force in sexual interactions, *under any circumstance* is not acceptable. Whatever the relationship, when a woman says no, a man must stop. Although he may feel frustrated, let down, or betrayed, he should use talk, not force, to express his feelings.

Sex and Intimacy

There is far more to sex than physical pleasure. Sexual relationships are also an important way to express affection and love. Those two aims are mutually reinforcing. Sharing sexual pleasure brings a couple closer together; intimacy and affection make sex more fulfilling. Physical intimacy can include touching each other, allowing one's body to be seen, and various sexual interactions, including intercourse. Emotional intimacy, in a sexual sense, requires sharing erotic thoughts and personal feelings. Emotional intimacy usually seeks expression through physical intimacy. Yet a couple may be very much in love but not become physically intimate. Conversely, some people engage in primarily physical encounters with an acquaintance, or prostitute, with no pretense of becoming emotionally intimate with the person.

Intimate Relationships A truly intimate loving relationship is a priceless benefit to health and happiness. Intimate relationships provide us with a human context in which to live our lives. Intimate relationships can offer

Exploring Your Emotions

How would you describe the relationship shown in the painting? Would you like to have such a relationship? How would you imagine this relationship might change over the next five years?

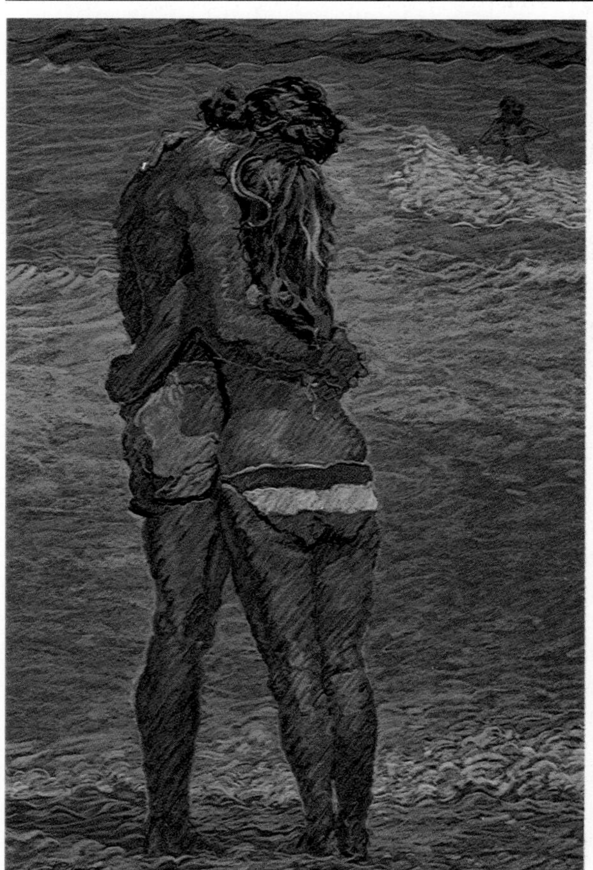

Illustration by Bill James

Date Rape

According to a Cornell University study, as many as one fifth of all college women have experienced forced sex. A similar survey at North Carolina State University recently showed that as many as 27 percent of the undergraduate women who were interviewed had experienced what is known as "date rape" or "acquaintance rape."

It is known that about 70 percent of all reported rapes are committed by men who know their victims. An estimated 80 percent of these rapes take place in the man's home or apartment, and drinking or drug use is common. Rarely is a weapon or even a direct, overt threat part of the scenario.

Many women are uncertain of their rights in a potential date-rape situation. Lisa Ramsour, a victims' advocate at the Turning Point, a multi-service agency in Greensboro, North Carolina, said women must understand they retain the right to say no to their date no matter how long the relationship has continued.

Jane M. Alford, a social worker at the Veterans Administration Hospital in Topeka, Kansas, feels the American system of dating, which puts women in the position of sexual objects to be "purchased" by men, is to blame for the high incidence of date rape.

Alford believes the social games men and women play contribute to misinterpretations that can have serious consequences. But how can these misunderstandings lead to such differing views on whether a crime has been committed?

Researchers at Kent State University recently surveyed more than 7,000 students at 35 schools on the issue of sexual victimization. That survey uncovered facts that help explain the discrepancy in understanding.

According to the survey, one man in twelve admitted to having fulfilled the prevailing definition of rape or attempted rape at least once, but hardly any men identified themselves as rapists.

As for women, the Kent State survey also revealed that one out of eight women was raped according to the legal definition, yet nearly three quarters did not identify their experience as rape.

If any common denominator among victims of date rape exists, it may be their lack of sophistication about men, experts have said. The average age of date rape victims is 18, according to several studies. A report on campus gang rape, conducted by the Association of American Colleges' Project on the Status and Education of Women, states that college women may be particularly unaware of date rape because they are emotionally vulnerable. They are away from home, usually for the first time, and are often unsure how to handle themselves in new situations.

The stereotypical, nightmarish image of the unknown rapist doesn't apply in the case of the date rapist. Alford said the date rapist will wine and dine his intended victim with the expectation that she owes him sexual repayment, and when she refuses his advances, he continues anyway.

These men are remarkably adept at determining the kind of weaknesses that will allow them to force themselves on a woman, Alford said.

Because they can be charming, they can be difficult to spot, especially for a young woman unskilled in sexual interpersonal relations. Alford advises young women to be wary of forming relationships with men they don't know. It is often in such relationships that the date rapist misinterprets the cues women give.

A man who often speaks of violence or use of force to get his way or refers to abuse within his family might be a potential date rapist. Also, a man who has trouble getting along with women in relationships or who displays a great deal of anger against women in general could be a problem.

The date rapist usually doesn't believe in his own manliness, and an athlete who rapes might be attempting to maintain his manly image and releasing the anger he feels over the constant pressure to perform—both on the field and off.

Having identified the potential problem date, what should a woman do to prevent herself from being a victim? Again, most date rapists normally won't use violence to have their way, and a forceful "no" early on will often prevent a date rape. But before it gets to that point, rape counselors say women must be more careful of the men they date and be clear about what they want from a relationship.

Source: *National Association of Social Work News*, Vol. 31, No. 8, (September 1986), pp. 5–6.

Falling in Love

Love carries many meanings from the casual to the lofty. It is a feeling, or emotional state, with regard to another person that arises from recognizing attractive qualities in that person, or from parent-child relationships. Love is shown by concern and caring for the loved person, delight in his or her presence, and the desire for approval and reciprocal affection.

Being in love is a special case. Unlike parental love, which is "given," and the love of friends, which develops over time, "falling in love" is sudden ("love at first sight"), and compounded by a sense of inevitability and involuntariness.

Some physicians even consider the experience as a transient illness ("lovesickness") because of its predictable course, physical features, and emotional upheaval.

People fall in love in many ways, but they all show certain basic signs. They are preoccupied with the loved person. Their longing for return of feelings makes them highly susceptible to ecstasy and despair, depending on the beloved's behavior. The person who is in love develops an extraordinary ability to dwell on what is admirable and to deny what is not. Love is blind: idealization makes a crooked nose look straight and "crystallization" makes the nose look cute.

The fear of rejection induces uncertainty, anxiety, and shyness. "Heartache," palpitations, flushing, and weakness accompany states of doubt. But when love is reciprocated, the person in love is exhilarated ("walking on air").

People in love are particularly vulnerable to pangs of *jealousy* that arise from intense feelings of possessiveness. Jealousy may range from reasonable self-interest in safeguarding the affections of the beloved to the intense suspiciousness that makes the lover highly intolerant of any other person's interest in and intimacy with the beloved. Jealousy is a destructive emotion that often leads to alienation or even violence.

An episode of being in love may last from a few weeks to many years. The relationship may end in a sudden and explosive breakup, or it may gradually wind down as one or the other partner becomes disenchanted with the other. Compatible couples who develop intimate relationships gradually shift into more sedate and enduring forms of affection.

Source: Dorothy Tennov, 1979. *Love and Limerance* (New York: Stein and Day).

adult counterparts of security and support provided by parents in our childhood. In turn they can provide the most secure foundations for raising children.

Intimacy with another person can allow us to grow, to expand our inner horizons, to learn, and to understand ourselves. Shared thoughts can take on added meaning; shared feelings can grow deeper. Sex within an intimate relationship can be more secure, less riddled with anxiety, endowed with more meaning.

Some of us find it harder to form intimate relationships than do others, but no one finds it easy. First we must choose a partner thoughtfully, and work together to develop and sustain the relationship over time.

Intimate relationships have both a personal and an institutional or social side. The personal part is our private dealings with each other; the sort of companionship we develop, the agreements we negotiate, the satisfactions and dissatisfactions about each other that we harbor within ourselves. The institutional side of intimacy defines the social setting and commonly agreed-on reciprocal rights and responsibilities within a given relationship. The institution of marriage in many forms has defined one such relationship over thousands of years.

How to Select a Compatible Intimate There are no set rules for choosing intimates, whether in a nonsexual ("platonic") relationship, a love affair, or marriage. In fact, some people feel that deliberately choosing a partner sounds cold-blooded. Westerners often like to think in more romantic terms: the right person will somehow arrive unexpectedly, and we will fall in love, marry, and live happily ever after.

But choosing intimates is neither random nor mysterious. At least more mature women and men select partners for stable relationships quite carefully and through a fairly predictable process.

In principle, we are free to be intimate with or to marry anyone we wish. The pool of potential candidates is huge. But look around you; notice that most people pair up with those who are quite similar in racial and ethnic background, social class, lifestyle, physical attractiveness, and other traits. Most of us hope to get the "best" person we

(*continued on p. 115*)

Compatibility Quiz

How compatible are you and your prospective mate? To find out, take this quiz and let your spouse-to-be do the same. Then compare your answers.

According to psychologist Karen Shanor of Washington, D.C., who helped put this quiz together, the more areas of agreement here, the less possible conflict in marriage.

However, she says, it is no fun to be married to a clone, so it is OK to have some disagreement—provided that you are able to compromise or, at least, agree to disagree.

This quiz is not meant to be a valid scientific measure of your compatibility. It was put together as an exercise to get you thinking about situations that can be difficult and cause stress in marriage.

The issues were chosen because they have specifically been mentioned by various couples who have sought counseling from Shanor.

This quiz can be taken by anyone, but it was primarily designed for those going into a first marriage, and for that reason, you'll find no questions referring to children and/or former marriages.

1. How many of the 10 items on this list do you have in common with your prospective mate: religion, career, same home town or neighborhood, friends, education level, income level, cultural pastimes, sports/recreation activities, travel, physical attraction?
- a. Almost everything on the list.
- b. Quite a few.
- c. A few.
- d. Almost none.

2. Would you prefer a relationship that is
- a. Male-dominated.
- b. Female-dominated.
- c. A partnership.

3. What banking arrangement sounds best after marriage?
- a. Separate account.
- b. Joint account.
- c. Joint account, but some cash for each of you to spend as you please with no accounting.

4. If you share an account, whose responsibility should it be to balance the checkbook and pay bills?
- a. The man in the family.
- b. The woman in the family.
- c. Whoever is better at math and details.

5. If you inherited $10,000, would you prefer it to be:
- a. Saved toward a major purchase.
- b. Spent on something you could enjoy together such as a vacation.
- c. Spent on luxury items you could enjoy individually, such as a fur coat or golf clubs.

6. Where do you think you should spend major holidays?
- a. With his family.
- b. With her family.
- c. Alternating with his and her family.
- d. At your place and inviting the relatives.
- e. Just the two of you at home, or with friends, or off on vacation.

7. How frequently do you want to see your in-laws if they live in the same town?
- a. Only on special occasions and holidays.
- b. Twice a month.
- c. At least once a week.

8. How frequently do you enjoy talking with your own parents?
- a. Every day.
- b. Once a week.
- c. Once a month or less.

9. If you both have careers, what will be your priority?
- a. Marriage before career.
- b. Marriage equally important to career.
- c. Career before marriage; my spouse is going to have to be understanding.

10. If you are offered a career promotion with a hefty raise making your income much more than your spouse's but involving a move out of state, would you
- a. Expect your mate to be agreeable to relocation.
- b. Try a commuter marriage; only seeing each other weekends or occasionally.
- c. Say no rather than move, money isn't everything.

11. If your new spouse sets aside one evening a week to go out with a friend or friends of his or her same sex would you feel
- a. Jealous of the time away from you.
- b. Happy that he or she has friends.
- c. This should not go on; let your feelings be known.

12. If you've had a bad day at the office and come home feeling moody, would you prefer that your mate
- a. Back off, get out of the way.
- b. Act sympathetic, be a good listener.
- c. Discuss the events that led to your mood, perhaps offering some alternative suggestions for dealing with the peo-

ple or problems that made you unhappy.

13. If your mate does something that makes you extremely angry, are you most likely to

a. Forgive and forget it.
b. Hurl insults.
c. Mention you are angry at an appropriate time, preferably when the anger is first felt and explain why without making derogatory accusations.

14. If you can't stand his or her friends and he or she can't stand yours, how will you deal with this after marriage? (You may choose more than one.)

a. Cultivate new friends that you both can enjoy.
b. See your friends by yourself and let him or her do the same.
c. Phase out the friends you knew before marriage; expect your partner to do the same.

15. If you and your spouse-to-be are different religions, would you expect to

a. Convert before marriage.
b. Have him or her convert before marriage.
c. Take turns attending each other's place of worship.
d. Observe religious days separately.
e. Not worry about it; religion is not an issue in your relationship.

16. When do you want to start a family?

a. As soon as possible.
b. After you have spent a few years enjoying your relationship as a couple.
c. As soon as careers are firmly established.
d. Never.

17. What is your attitude about housework? (You may check more than one.)

a. It is unmasculine for a man to do it. A woman should do all of it even if she chooses to have a career.
b. It is fine for a man to help, but only with certain tasks, such as mowing the lawn or taking out the trash.
c. If a woman works outside the home, cleaning should be shared.
d. Even if a woman does not work outside the home, cleaning should be shared.
e. Hire a maid, regardless if it fits the family budget.

18. Before marriage, you go out as a couple several times a week. A few months after marriage, you realize that you are going out a lot less. Would you consider this

a. OK. The pace was exhausting.
b. Dull. You worry that you are being taken for granted.
c. Not OK. You and your mate should make plans for some evenings out or evenings at home with friends.

19. You need to buy a new suit. Your spouse wants to come along. Would you see this as a sign of

a. Interest in spending time with you.
b. Crowding your relationship.
c. Watch-dogging your taste or pocketbook.

20. How would you prefer to spend your annual vacation? (Check as many as apply.)

a. On a trip by yourself.
b. On a trip with your mate.
c. On a trip with your mate and another couple.
d. Visiting your relatives or in-laws at their homes.
e. At a beach relaxing.
f. Engaged in an active sport such as skiing, tennis camp, or hiking/camping.
g. Traveling to another city for sightseeing/shopping.
h. At home catching up on repairs, appointments, books, visits with friends.
i. I would rather take a vacation less frequently than once a year and spend this money on rent or mortgage, enabling us to live in a more convenient or prestigious neighborhood.

21. If you were hunting for a place to live, would you prefer being in

a. The country.
b. The suburbs.
c. The city.

22. If your spouse-to-be had many loves before he or she met you, would you prefer that he or she

a. Keep the details to himself or herself.
b. Tell you everything.
c. Answer truthfully, but only the questions you ask, such as what broke up each relationship.

23. If your new spouse is in a romantic mood and you are not, how would you be most likely to respond?

a. Communicate your mood; suggest another time.
b. Pretend you are feeling romantic.
c. Invent an excuse rather than communicate your mood.

Compatibility Quiz (*continued*)

Psychologist Karen Shanor Explains

1. The more you have in common, the more of your life you can share and enjoy together.

2. Research and experiences of many couples have shown that the equal relationship is most successful.

3 and 4. There is no one right answer. Decide what works best for you and creates the least tension in your relationship.

5. We've all learned early in life to spend our limited money in certain ways. For some, it's on clothes; for others, it's on home or travel. Unless we understand our priorities and communicate them to our partner, we can find ourselves in great financial conflict and tension.

6. Very often we expect others to celebrate holidays as we do and give them the same sense of importance as the family in which we grew up. This isn't always so. Be able to compromise on this one.

7 and 8. Some are happy going for years at a time without seeing relatives. Others intentionally buy the house next door and want to drop in every day. Most important here is to let your spouse know that he or she comes first before parents and in-laws.

9. Talk about career and marriage priorities. Can you be accepting of your spouse's choice if he or she considers time spent on work more important right now than time spent with you?

10. There is no one right answer. Decide what works best for you and creates the least tension in your relationship.

11. It's healthy to have friends. You can't realistically expect your mate to spend 24 hours around the clock with you. If you or your mate go off for a time with friends, it wouldn't be too mushy to kiss, hug, or otherwise reassure your mate by words or actions that he or she is still first in your life. A spouse needs to hear this.

12. There are times when answer A would be best; other occasions call for B or C. Be sensitive to your mate's mood. If you are the one in the bad mood, don't expect your mate to read your mind as to whether you need space, sympathy or discussion. Clue him or her in.

13. Answer C is best. Somewhere along the way, people have to learn how to express anger constructively.

14. Be careful here. If you make his or her old friends feel left out or unimportant, they could work on your prospective mate to break up your relationship.

15. If you have major differences on this one, you may want to consider terminating the relationship instead of committing to marriage.

16. It's impossible to have half a child. Compromise won't work on this one, so it is best to speak your mind before marriage.

17. The most successful marriages are the ones in which men and women do not limit themselves in the traditional masculine-feminine roles. The sharing of responsibility heightens a sense of trust, caring and cooperation.

18. Sometimes the pace during dating is frantic. It is nice to calm down, but not nice to settle down to the point that each of you is taking the other for granted. Marriage requires continual work if you are going to keep adventure and interest in the relationship.

19. Whether you see it as interest, crowding, or distrust, communicate your feelings to your mate. If you'd rather shop alone, let that be known too.

20. Agree upon your needs in advance of the annual vacation, or what should be a time of relaxation away from the daily grind will turn into a source of tension and arguments. There is nothing wrong with separate vacations if one of you wants to fish on the lake and the other enjoys sightseeing.

21. If you are set on a particular style of living and not willing to change it after marriage, speak up before you say, "I do."

22. In general, it is not a good idea to go into great detail about past relationships because they are not totally relevant to your current one. However, trust and honesty are very important. If your partner asks a question, answer honestly but think very carefully. If you are the one doing the questioning, ask yourself, "Do I really want to hear this?"

23. There are times in your relationship when you may not want to go along with your spouse's romantic feelings, but it is generally best to communicate in a nice way without making him or her feel rejected or unloved that you simply are not in the mood. Do suggest another time.

Engagement Provisional agreement to get married.

Homogamy Marriage between people of similar traits and backgrounds.

can, but the rules of supply and demand and our preferences lead to the general rule of **homogamy**: like usually marries like.

First attractions are based on easily observable characteristics—looks, dress, social status, and the other person's apparent interest in us. As we become better acquainted, personality traits and more private behaviors become more significant. We each now begin to get a better sense of the other's capacity for closeness and his or her readiness for forming an intimate relationship with us. Self-revelation gradually deepens our understanding of each other. The emphasis shifts to basic values such as religious belief, political persuasion, sexual attitudes, and future aspirations with regard to family and children. At some point each partner decides that the relationship feels right (or that this is the best he or she could hope for) and the couple formalizes their union.

In Western society, courtship during a period of **engagement** has traditionally provided a socially approved means of getting to know each other. At present, dating, going steady, and sometimes living together for a while may precede engagement or substitute for it. Many couples, particularly young ones, try to settle down before true intimacy has developed.

In choosing a compatible intimate, we can't act like an employer assessing job applicants. Nonetheless, we can use some standards for evaluating possibilities:

1. *Tolerance for differences.* A tolerance for differences in other people is more important than and overrides many of the following variables. Tolerance brings us a long way toward coping with differences of background, viewpoint, interest, and energy level. If you are able to grant your would-be partner a lot of leeway, and if that person can do the same for you, you will have plenty of freedom to be yourself and retain your identity.
2. *Educational level.* College graduates have lower divorce rates than nongraduates, perhaps because they marry later and have had more time to compare choices. They also earn more money, which makes life easier. Great differences in educational levels may mean great differences in dealing with people, in power, in knowledge. (In the past men usually received more education than women did; fortunately that is changing.) However, if both partners are committed to grow, they may be able to solve problems of educational differences.
3. *Socioeconomic background.* Lifestyle depends partly on socioeconomic background. What are your and your potential intimate's attitudes toward money, social position, family background? Flexible people may be able to adapt to differences in types of neighborhoods, housing, clothes, transportation, recreation, and so on, but a big difference in socioeconomic background can make adjustment—either up or down—very difficult.
4. *Values and taste.* How do your values and tastes compare in terms of religion, politics, music, art, types of people? If either of you is not very tolerant, having similar values and tastes is a necessity.
5. *Self-esteem.* Do you respect and like yourself? What about your intended partner? The more one is at ease with oneself, the more nourishment one can offer to another person and to an intimate relationship.
6. *Commitment to growth.* Commitment to growth is reflected in a willingness to expand your world, to learn more about yourself, others, new ideas, and new activities. Without a commitment to growth, both the partners and the relationship can grow stale and stagnate. There is some risk in continuing growth because two people can grow apart. But growing apart is most likely when there is a big difference in interest and commitment to consider new ideas and experiences.
7. *Authority.* Do you and/or your would-be partner insist on making the final decision or having the last word? Collaboration works best. Although authority is almost never shared equally, it is probably best divided according to time and talent. Can the two of you do that?
8. *Energy level.* How do your energy levels compare? Do you like to laze around in the house while the other person wants to be on the go constantly? A significant difference in energy levels can strain a relationship.
9. *Communication skills.* People are not mind readers. How are you at sharing when you are anxious and irritable? Can you say unpleasant things that need to be said? What about the other person? Can the two of you communicate positive feelings of praise, support, and empathy? Most important, can you really listen to each other? Communication skills are essential to a healthy relationship.
10. *Tolerance of intimacy.* Are you or the other person embarrassed or anxious about expressing your feelings and thoughts? Must you defend yourselves against closeness with jokes, teasing, planning escape routes through activities? What do the two of you really want and expect of a relationship with each other?

Building an Intimate Relationship Making the right choice is crucial. But even relationships and marriages made in heaven require care and maintenance once they get down to earth. Ideally an intimate relationship evolves through mutually sharing inner feelings. Its strength derives from a constancy of affection, trust, acceptance, dependability, respect, willingness to make oneself available, understanding and avoiding unrealistic expectations. Intimates can reveal themselves without fear of being hurt. You may not always agree with each other, but you can try to understand each other and work together toward mutual goals.

Frequently, people don't achieve these ideals because they have different personalities and expectations. No relationship means the same thing to both people. Everyone has different needs, and everyone has different expectations of an intimate relationship. The relationships that have the best chance of surviving are those in which the partners become aware of their expectations and limitations and share them openly with each other. Worthwhile relationships recognize and protect the rights of both parties. They allow two people with equal rights to grow and share a view of the world that is greater than either person sees alone.

Intimacy is not fusion. Each person in a meaningful relationship must allow the other person freedom in which to grow. Mutual respect and helping a partner to develop her or his full potential actually strengthens a relationship.

Exploring Your Emotions

What advantages come with marriage and other intimate relationships? What proportion of these advantages come only from your own thinking and emotions? What proportion come from parental and societal expectations? Is there anything inappropriate about accepting traditional marriage roles?

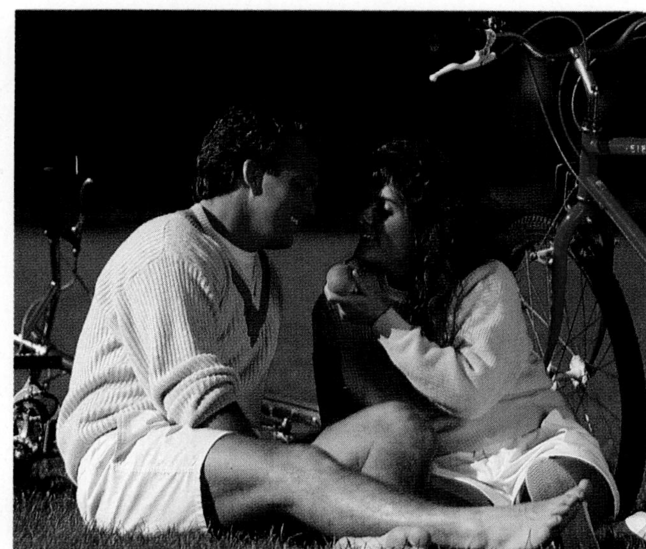

Tim Davis

Successful intimate relationships help preserve certain other individual rights. Among the most important is the right to be yourself. If you demand that the other change to keep the relationship alive, it is likely to become further undermined. People change themselves; no one can make another person change, and trying to do so usually provokes resentment. Each partner has the right to respect. Showing respect for an intimate means that you listen to the other person and share his or her triumphs and problems.

Partners in a relationship also have the right to privacy. Everyone needs time and space to be alone, to sort out thoughts and feelings, to organize oneself, to tap one's own resources. Other rights are honesty and trust. Self-disclosure by partners is essential, but it must not jeopardize them. Not being able to share attitudes and emotions closes off intimacy, but the matter of trustworthiness is fragile and, if betrayed, often can't be fully repaired.

In intimate relationships, as in all other human interactions, rights go hand in hand with responsibilities. Healthy relationships require that men and women take responsibility for their own self-development, quality of life, and personal identity. Passive partners who do not take responsibility for themselves pose a burden to their partners. They let others make decisions for them; they protect themselves by never taking a position, never giving a response that is truly their own. There is a price for yielding responsibility. If you regularly surrender your responsibilities to another person, you yourself become less of a person, and you undermine the relationship itself. You hold the other person liable for your losses, and your resentment eventually eats you up.

A truly intimate relationship is a celebration of life. Nevertheless, no one can make you feel truly complete but yourself. No relationship, no matter how deep and satisfying, can avoid all hurts or ward off all loneliness. In a sense, we are each ultimately alone, but less so if we are part of a truly intimate relationship.

Ending Intimate Relationships Intimate relationships may begin with all good intentions but they may not last. Ending an intimate relationship is never easy. But you can do it with tact and compassion instead of harshly and hurtfully. The consequences of a breakup also depend on the circumstances; the ending of a two-month affair is different from the breakup of a 20-year marriage.

Relationships can end because a couple was mismatched to start with, or because the association did not evolve and thrive over time—usually some of both. It's tempting to consider relationships that fail as mistakes. But sometimes a perfectly good relationship at the time may outlive its usefulness if partners grow apart from each other.

Sometimes it's hard to know where you stand in a relationship. Consider your partner's words as well as

Breaking Up Is Hard To Do

In our study of student dating couples, my coworkers and I investigated some of the factors that lead people to take the "exit" route (Hill, Rubin, and Peplau, 1976). Over a two-year period, about half of the couples in our sample stayed together and the other half broke up. We found that the people who stayed together tended to be more similar to each other in age, intelligence, career plans, and physical attractiveness than the people who broke up. In addition, when people who had broken up were asked to explain why the relationship had ended, they frequently mentioned differences in interests, backgrounds, sexual attitudes, and ideas about marriage. It seems that similarities between people not only lead to attraction in the first place but also encourage the continuation of relationships. Partners who have serious differences or disagreements are likely to end up going their separate ways.

Our study also found that relationships were most likely to end if one of the partners was considerably more involved in the relationship than the other. Of the couples in which both members initially reported that they were equally involved in the relationship, only 23 percent broke up during the subsequent two-year period. But among those couples in which one partner was more involved than the other, 54 percent broke up. There seems to be an inherent lack of stability in relationships in which one partner is more invested than the other. In such a relationship, the more involved partner may feel overly dependent and exploited, while the less involved partner may feel restless and guilty. "Commitments must stay abreast for a love relationship to develop into a lasting mutual attachment," writes sociologist Peter Blau (1964). "Only when two lovers' affection for and commitment to one another expand at roughly the same pace do they tend mutually to support their love" (p. 84).

The ending of a close relationship often leads to feelings of pain and distress, similar to the symptoms of loneliness. These feelings are likely to be most acute for the partner who was broken up with (assuming that the ending was not completely mutual), but they affect the partner who wanted to break up as well. There is also evidence that the more satisfying the relationship had been in the past, the longer it takes for the couple to break up and the more acute the partners' distress over the breakup (Lee, 1984).

But in spite of the pain involved, the ending of close relationships can teach us valuable lessons. By experiencing firsthand the difficulties of close relationships, we are likely to learn more about our own interpersonal needs, preferences, strengths, and weaknesses. These lessons can be of value to us as we enter new relationships. After the ending of her relationship with David, for example, Ruth told an interviewer, "I don't regret having the experience at all. But after being in the supportive role, *I* want a little support now. That's the main thing I look for" (Hill, Rubin, and Peplau, 1976, p. 156). And after his breakup with Kathy, Joe indicated that he would exercise greater caution in future relationships. "If I fall in love again," he said, "it might be with the reservation that I'm going to keep awake this time" (p. 155). Breakups are most valuable if they take place before marriage. . . . As an anonymous wise person once said, "The best divorce is the one you get before you get married."

Source: Rubin/McNeil, 1985. *The Psychology of Being Human*, New York: Harper & Row.

deeds, in making an assessment. Intimacy implies trust but neither blind trust nor a compulsive need for absolute certainty work well. Make your feelings known, and expect reciprocal openness. Beyond that, nagging attempts to extract confessions of love, for example, merely drive a partner away. When ethical, emotional, and practical considerations suggest a parting of the ways, bear in mind the following:

1. Give the relationship an honest decent chance before you break it up. You can then make a cleaner break, have fewer doubts, and feel less guilt.
2. Be fair and honest. You owe it to yourself and to your friend, lover, or spouse to learn something from the experience so you don't repeat the same mistakes in the next relationship.
3. Be tactful and compassionate. Your freedom from a burdensome relationship need not be gained at the cost of damaging another person's self-esteem. Rather than dwelling on the partner's shortcomings, emphasize your mutual lack of fit and admit your own contributions to the problem.
4. If you are the rejected one, give yourself time to resolve the bitterness you are apt to feel. Then be forgiving.

As in response to other losses, you will need to go through a process of "mourning." You may first feel disbelief ("This can't be happening to me"), then anger, then sadness, and finally acceptance. Despite all the romantic talk about "one and only" loves, you actually have many potential candidates with whom you can establish intimate relationships.

Marriage and Its Alternatives

Intimate relationships that last long enough usually become formalized around a living arrangement. In our culture, that has typically taken the form of monogamous marriage and still does for well over 90 percent of the population. Even though a number of alternatives to marriage, such as living together, have lately become more common, such associations either lead to marriage or fulfill comparable functions.

Because so many marriages break up and so much conflict troubles even those marriages that survive, why do so many people still get married? Marriage fulfills a number of basic needs, and its long history has made it an integral part of our culture. There are many important social, moral, economic, political, and other aspects of marriage. But we shall be concerned with its more personal face.

Marriage, Intimacy, and Sex Living together is the best setting for developing intimacy. Daily interactions between husband and wife leave little concealed. Similar interests

Exploring Your Emotions

What is the artist suggesting by forming faces out of the growth rings of a tree trunk? How are these faces relating to each other? To their environment? Are there any other cues to the visual/emotional statement? How would you phrase what the author is saying?

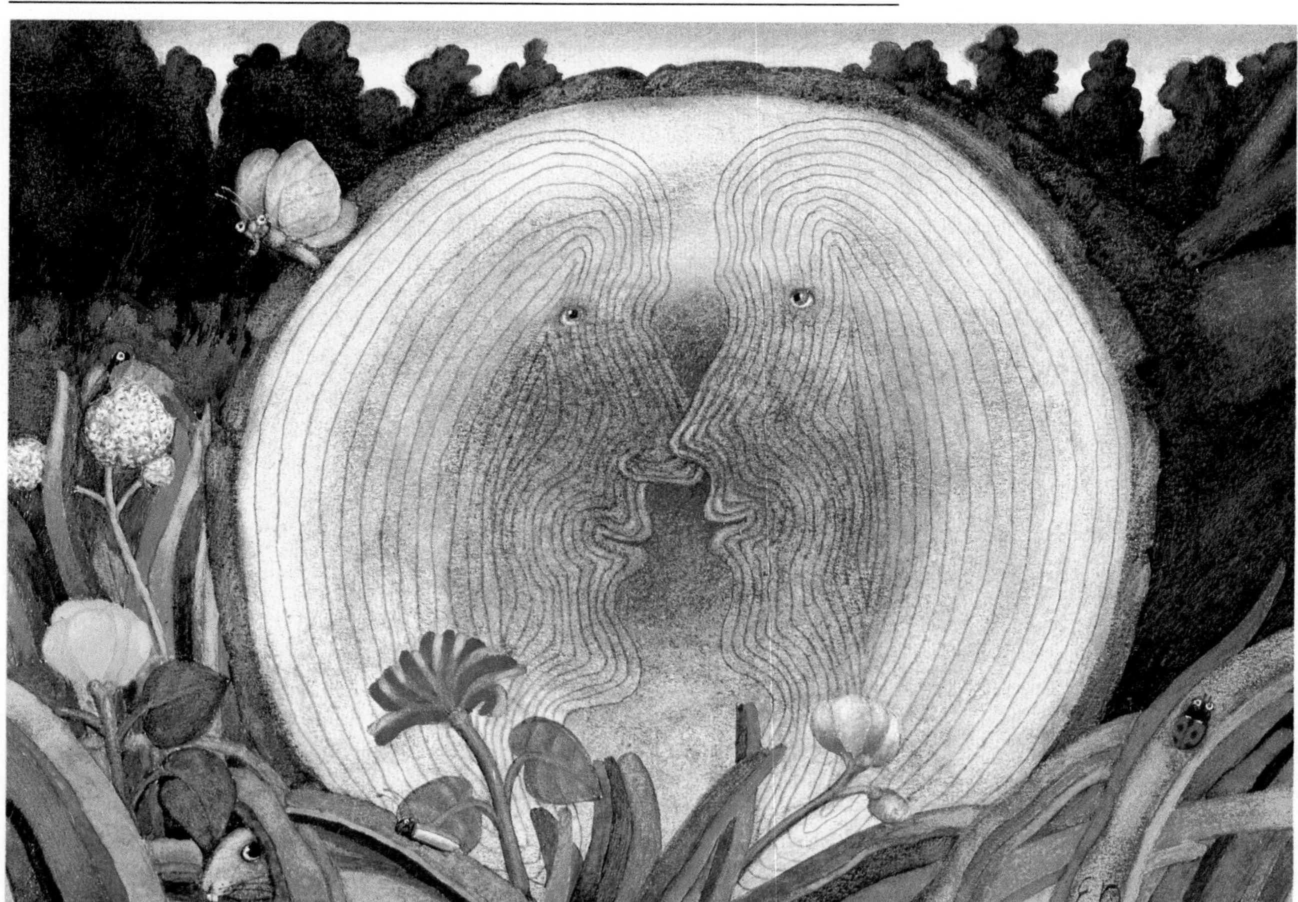

Illustration by Etienne Delessert

Conflict Management: Learning to Fight

Conflicts in intimate relationships may result from differences in emotional and sexual needs, or tastes in music, political views, or even degrees of neatness. So you cannot entirely avoid frustration and anger in intimate relationships. This is not something to feel guilty about, but rather an indication that strong feelings of dissatisfaction need to be worked out. Expressing dissatisfaction usually does not mean you do not care for your partner. (If lack of caring is the real message, actions will show it and arguing won't help.)

Women, in particular, have been taught to deny their aggressive feelings. But now many therapists are recognizing the value of expressing anger and conflict. They are training clients in conflict management, a skill everyone needs. This does not mean that you are entitled to have a temper tantrum at any time over any issue. To be constructive, the amount of anger must fit the problem at hand, and you must keep your anger within reasonable bounds. Physical violence is always and completely unacceptable.

The point of a fruitful argument is not to insult or demean your partner but to discuss or explain whatever is bothering you, to give the other person an opportunity to explain and make amends, thereby clearing the air and improving your mutual understanding. The aim is not victory for one and defeat for the other, but some reasonable compromise. Here are some suggestions for managing conflict:

1. Try not to start an argument unless you know what you are angry about. If you are jealous, don't pretend your anger is about not taking out the garbage. And don't argue just to get attention.

2. Try to determine whether your feelings and their intensity are appropriate to the issue. Don't dramatize.

3. Know what you want to accomplish. Are you just letting off steam? Just making a point? Will you insist on behavior change? Settle for compromise? State your complaint and your desires simply and clearly. Then wait for a response.

4. Allow enough time. Avoid jumping into an argument five minutes before you are scheduled to go out for a night on the town or if you are expecting company. Pick a time and place where you can both be open without embarrassing each other. That will give you time to cool off and to think through the problem.

5. Try not to lay on the guilt. Relating what you feel—anger, hurt—is more effective than blaming and accusing. And don't leave in the middle of an argument.

6. Do not let the situation overwhelm you. If you feel overpowered by the other person, say so and ask for the courtesy of speaking your mind without interruption. If you feel intimidated, say so. Remember, you are supposed to be equals.

7. Listen. See if your partner has acceptable reasons for her or his actions. Laziness, greediness, and selfishness are not good reasons. If you are the defendant, acknowledge what you hear by repeating the accusation to make sure you heard it clearly.

8. Try corresponding by mail. Personal feelings can sometimes be more easily influenced by logic and rational thought with some emotional distance.

9. If you are the one confronted, do not immediately try to defend yourself or feel righteously indignant. Let the other person vent his or her wrath. Don't crumble in guilt or defensiveness. Don't close yourself off angrily. Don't deny the conflict.

10. So far as possible, focus on the particular issue at hand. Deal with one problem at a time. Criticize your partner's behavior but do not attack his or her personality. Stick to concrete actions, avoid abstractions.

and objectives draw them together. Having children bonds a couple further together and raising children calls for close collaboration and sharing.

A long-term marriage both fulfills immediate needs and provides security for the future. By committing themselves to stick together through good and bad times, married men and women count on not being abandoned in sickness or other troubles, or in old age. They also hope to share the positive aspects of aging.

Similar advantages accrue sexually. Having a desirable mate living under the same roof provides a ready and willing sexual partner. This allows far more sexual activity to take place between ordinary married couples than if they were single.

Moreover, as they get to learn about each other's likes and dislikes, spouses need to spend little time in figuring out what to do when they go to bed. They don't need to prove themselves. Their bodies work in harmony, they communicate well, their affection fills emotional needs, and commitment keeps rivals at bay.

For most people, marriage entails some loss in personal freedom. Your movements become tied to those of another person. Where and how you live must be negotiated. Your time is no longer entirely your own, and your friendships and other relationships (even with your parents) are no longer entirely your own business.

Marriage also entails a potential loss in personal identity, especially for women. Traditionally, they have acquired new names in becoming wives. They have been expected to subordinate their personal and professional aspirations to the service of their families. And those who have maintained or begun careers usually do the housekeeping and are primary caretakers of the children as well.

Marriages may prove unworkable because couples may expect too much of each other, or their needs and aspirations may be incompatible. They may lack the ability to solve problems and make compromises. Bearing and rearing children places enormous additional demands on parents.

In marital conflicts, sex is one of the earliest casualties; conversely, sexual incompatibilities often lead to marital problems. Among couples who are sexually unhappy, men tend to lose interest in their wives as sexual partners. Monogamy proves too restrictive for a man who gets a reaffirmation of his masculinity and potency with each new sexual partner. Those who engage in extramarital relations often admit that coitus with their wives is more satisfying yet they continue to pursue other women because of the excitement of the chase.

Women in monogamous relationships may also miss the variety and reaffirmation of new partners. But they are more apt to be unhappy with their husbands' lack of affection and romance. Sex becomes routinized; a wife may merely serve her husband's sexual needs, getting little satisfaction herself. At best such women are taken for granted, and at worst they are sexually used, abused, and brutalized through marital rape.

So marriage is a high-gain, high-risk proposition. For most couples, it offers a reasonable framework in which to face the ups and downs of life.

Exploring Your Emotions

How do you feel about marriage for yourself? For others? Do you think marriage is dying out as an institution? Why or why not? How does marriage relate to sex?

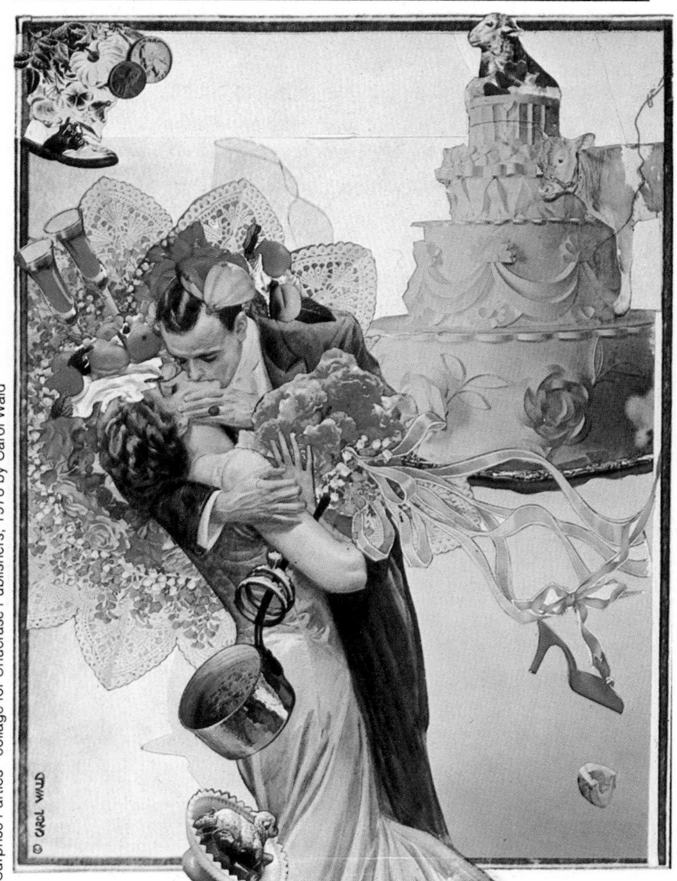

''Surprise Parties'' collage for Unucrase Publishers, 1978 by Carol Wald

Alternatives to Marriage Much current dissatisfaction with marriage has to do with its traditional forms. The most serious concerns relate to the respective roles that men and women have been expected to fulfill as spouses. The traditional pattern, where the husband is the sole breadwinner and the wife takes care of home and children, is no longer the standard in our society. However, although there has been a tremendous shift of women into the labor force, only a few men have taken on major housekeeping roles. In addition, men are not the head of household or the breadwinner in one-third of U.S. families.

Other challenges deal with marital intimacy and fidelity. Some partners agree to have social and even sexual interactions with others as long as they do not compromise the primacy of their marital relationship. An even greater proportion of married men and women engage in extramarital affairs without the spouse's consent. Most but not all such involvements disrupt the primary relationship.

Cohabitation In an attempt to establish relationships based more on companionship than on formal ties, an estimated 2 million couples (4 percent of single adults) now live together as unmarried couples. These couples tend to be younger adults with no children or older couples whose

Cohabitation Living together in an intimate and sexual relationship.

Marital contract An agreement drawn between a couple, specifying their mutual rights and responsibilities in their marriage.

Group marriages A stable living arrangement where several men and women have sexual access to one another.

---

incomes would suffer were they to marry. For most younger couples, cohabitation is either temporary or the prelude to marriage. Only a minority find **cohabitation** a satisfactory long-term alternative to marriage. And they must still deal with some of the same issues inherent in any stable and exclusive relationship.

Living together without legal or religious sanction can give people a greater sense of autonomy. One does not have to be bound by the social rules and expectations of the institution of marriage. The woman finds it easier to keep her identity and more of her independence. The man, in turn, does not incur the same set of obligations that he does by getting married.

Yet living together has its own liabilities. For instance, such arrangements do not provide the legal protections of marriage. This consideration can become particularly serious when the couple has children.

Marital Contracts Marriage is a legally binding union that is only available in our society to monogamous heterosexual couples. In addition to, or instead of, the basic legal agreement, some couples now draw up their own **marital contracts** specifying their respective rights and obligations. Such documents may be quite useful in setting forth the financial terms of a couple's relationship or specifying other aspects of living together that can be stated in concrete terms. But beyond that, such agreements are not likely to prove any more effective than traditional marital vows.

Gay Unions About 28 percent of lesbians and 10 percent of gay men live together as close couples, in gay unions. Their relationships are in many ways quite similar to cohabiting heterosexuals.

Gay couples may not get legally married, although some religious organizations will solemnize their union. If the law allowed homosexual marriages, a significant proportion of those living together would presumably get married, more or less for the same reasons that heterosexuals marry.

Group marriages Living arrangements based on threesomes, sharing spouses by couples, and small communities have been tried on and off without gaining wide acceptance. Public awareness of **group marriages** was heightened during the 1960s because of hippie communes. But such arrangements, whereby a group of people live together and have sexual access to each other, go back, in the recent past to certain utopian communities of nineteenth-century America.

Divorce The divorce rate, which has been generally going up for the past 60 years, rose very sharply after World War II. Marriages ending in divorce then skyrocketed from 14 percent in 1940–1945 to 45 percent by 1975–1980 for white women; for black women, the rates are even higher. Divorce rates are highest in the 25 to 29-year-old group for both sexes.

From a health perspective, divorce means a series of stressful events: the decision by one of the partners to dissolve the marriage and his or her announcement of that intent; the awkward period of living together after the announcement but before the separation; the separation; the legal procedures, and the granting of the decree. The impact divorce has on human health is only hinted at in Table 5-1, which lists common symptoms of people going through a divorce.

More general reactions include anxiety, depression, grief, hostility, loneliness, and a sense of failure. The divorced person is likely to feel emotionally bruised and in need of nurturing. How these needs are met can have a considerable effect on the success of the person's re-entry into the "single" world, and a common reaction is to seek refuge in another marriage. All too often this solution merely recycles the original problem.

Being Single The most obvious alternative to marriage is being single. Only one person out of 20 men and women has never married by age 50 (and such people are unlikely to do so thereafter). But a more substantial segment of the population is divorced or widowed. For instance, in the 45- to 54-year age group, 11 percent of women and 9 percent of the men are divorced; 6 percent of the women and 1 percent of the men are widowed.

There are many reasons for being single. Some men and women choose not to marry. Others cannot find a

Table 5-1 Common Symptoms of People Experiencing a Divorce

Symptom	Percent of people experiencing symptom at Decision	Separation	Decree
Sleep loss	16	27	11
Diminished health	15	26	12
Loneliness and melancholy	11	29	12
Decreased work efficiency	8	16	11
Decreased memory	6	11	6
Increased smoking	4	11	6
Increased drinking	1	5	4

desirable spouse, a problem that is more serious for older women (because there are fewer older men, and they tend to remarry younger women).

Being unmarried is not a dismal prospect. Countless single women and men, with or without children, now make fulfilling, happy lives for themselves. Being single does not mean being lonely. It is possible to have friendships and intimate relationships, with or without a sexual component, without marriage. There is no need to feel like "half a person" without a spouse; in fact, some people only feel whole when single.

Ultimately we stand or fall on the basis of who we are, not because of who sustains us. To be able to be intimate with another, we need to be capable of being intimate with ourselves. Once that task is accomplished, it becomes both easier to establish meaningful intimate relationships with others and also to do without them.

Take Action

Your answers to the Exploring Your Emotions questions in this chapter and your placement level on the Awareness Ladder at the beginning of this chapter will, we hope, encourage you to begin a process of self-exploration and self-discovery that you will continue. Reflect on the entire chapter's content and ask yourself how each point relates to your own life. Then take action:

1. To what extent are the difficulties in intimacy your own doing, and to what extent are you a victim of your culture's expectations? For example, as a man, do you really want to dominate women, or do you do so because you think that is the way "real men" are supposed to behave? As a woman, is passive dependency what you want, or is that your idea of being "feminine"? The times are changing. Take a fresh look and make up your own mind as to what the changes mean to a man or a woman in an intimate relationship. Make a list of those changes and how they affect you.

2. Intimate relationships are like living beings—they change constantly. Keep attuned to the changes you and your partner may be undergoing. List the behaviors or attitudes that block your getting the most out of your relationship. Consider each one carefully and decide which you can change.

3. Read the box "Three Couples" on page 101. Interview three older students about their attitudes toward the different couples. Contrast their attitudes with those of three much younger students. Are there significant differences? If so, what do you think accounts for the differences? Do you believe a "sexual double standard" lives on?

4. Take the Compatibility Quiz on page 112. Then read the psychologist's comments following it. In your notebook write down what you have learned that you were unaware of before.

5. Review the statements in the Rate Yourself section at the beginning of this chapter. Have your feelings or values changed? Do you think you now are better prepared to handle the problems and the rewards associated with intimate relationships?

Selected References

American Psychiatric Association. 1980. *Diagnostic and Statistical Manual of Mental Disorders* (DSM-III). 3rd ed. Washington, D.C.: American Psychiatric Association.

Bell, A. P., Weinburg, M. S., and Hammersmith, S. K. 1981. *Sexual Preference—Its Development in Men and Women.* Bloomington: Indiana University Press.

Carroll, J. L., Volk, K. D., and Hyde, J. S. 1985 (April). Differences between males and females in the motives for engaging in sexual intercourse." *Archives of Sexual Behavior* 14(2):131–39.

Kanin, E. J. 1985 (June). Date rapists: Differential sexual socialization and relative deprivation. *Archives of Sexual Behavior* 14:219–31.

Reiss, I. L. 1980. *Family Systems in America.* 3rd ed. Holt, Rinehart & Winston.

Symons, D. 1980. *The Evolution of Human Sexuality.* 3rd ed. New York: Holt, Rinehart & Winston.

Recommended Readings

Buscaglia, L. 1985. *Loving Each Other: The Challenge of Human Relationships.* New York: Holt, Rinehart & Winston. *Guide to intimate relationships by a highly popular author.*

Comfort, A. 1972. *The Joy of Sex.* New York: Crown. *A sophisticated and attractively illustrated sex manual.*

Goode, W. J. 1982. *The Family.* 2nd ed. Englewood Cliffs, N.J.: Prentice-Hall. *A sociological overview of the family.*

Katchadourian, H. 1985. *Fundamentals of Human Sexuality.* 4th ed. New York: Holt, Rinehart & Winston. *Chapters 8 to 14 deal with sexual behaviors and relationships.*

Tennov, D. 1979. *Love and Limerance.* New York: Stein and Day. *A study of the experience of falling in love.*

Chapter 6

Contents

Rate Yourself

Your Attitudes about Birth Control Read the following statements carefully. Choose the one in each section that best describes you at this moment and circle its number. When you have chosen one statement for each section, add the numbers and record your total score. Find your position on the Awareness Ladder.

5 Well educated about birth control
4 Knowledgeable about birth control
3 Familiar with birth control methods
2 Unfamiliar with many birth control methods
1 Ignorant of birth control methods

5 Openly discusses birth control methods
4 Discusses birth control methods with partner
3 Resists discussions of birth control
2 Avoids discussions of birth control
1 Resents discussions of birth control

5 Takes responsibility for contraception
4 Shares responsibility for contraception
3 Shares costs of contraception
2 Resists responsibility for contraception
1 Takes no responsibility for contraception

5 Prefers inconvenience of contraception to risk of pregnancy
4 Sacrifices convenience to avoid an unwanted pregnancy
3 If contraception is inconvenient, will sometimes risk pregnancy
2 Believes the female should be responsible for birth control
1 Risks unwanted pregnancy for the sake of convenience

5 Educates others about birth control
4 Discusses contraceptives with pharmacist
3 Is uncomfortable buying contraceptives
2 Avoids buying contraceptives
1 Refuses to buy contraceptives

Total Score ______

Birth Control

Awareness Ladder

Do you know the pros and cons of available birth control methods? As you read through this chapter, be alert to ways that might help you move higher up the Awareness Ladder.

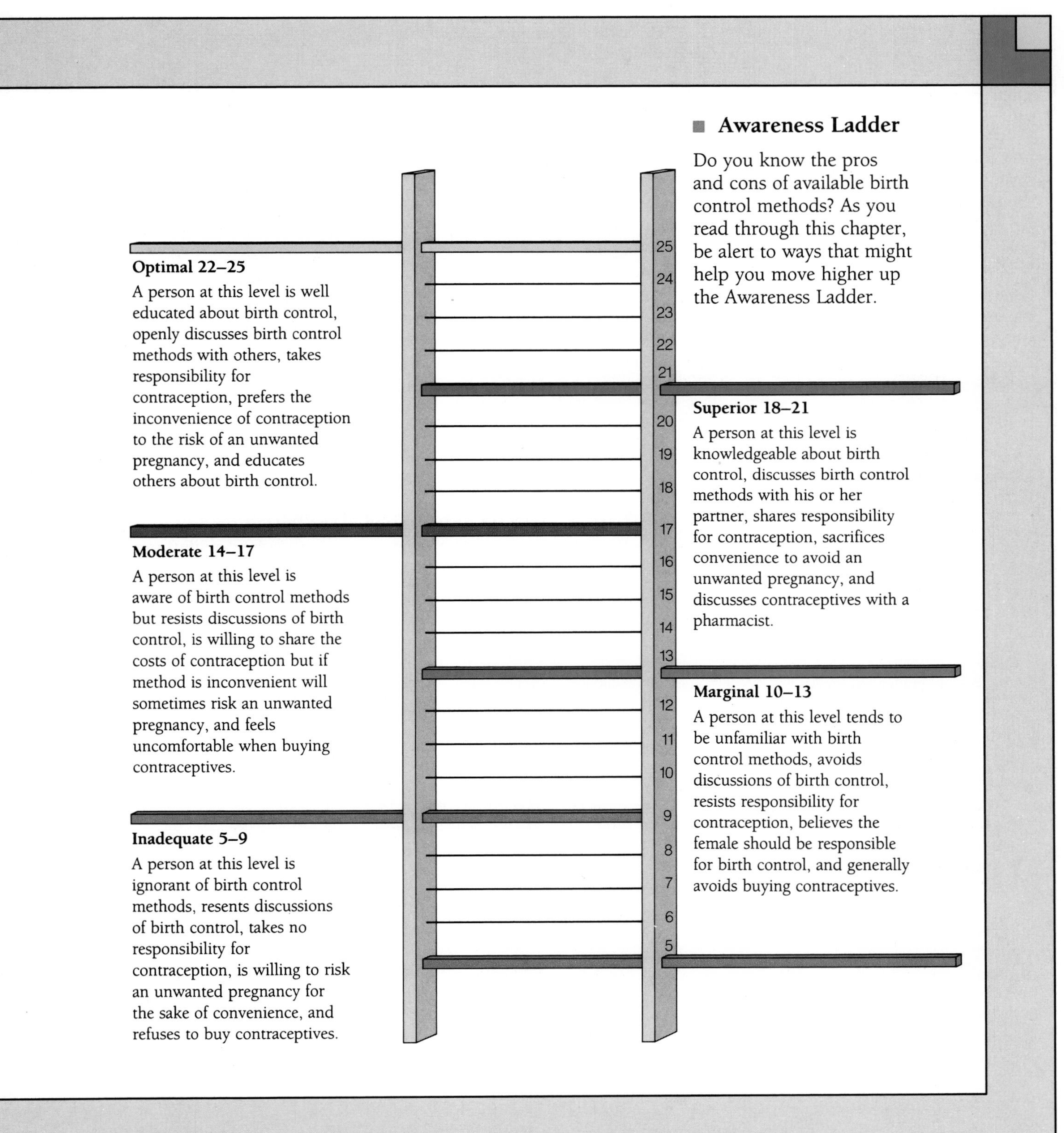

Optimal 22–25

A person at this level is well educated about birth control, openly discusses birth control methods with others, takes responsibility for contraception, prefers the inconvenience of contraception to the risk of an unwanted pregnancy, and educates others about birth control.

Superior 18–21

A person at this level is knowledgeable about birth control, discusses birth control methods with his or her partner, shares responsibility for contraception, sacrifices convenience to avoid an unwanted pregnancy, and discusses contraceptives with a pharmacist.

Moderate 14–17

A person at this level is aware of birth control methods but resists discussions of birth control, is willing to share the costs of contraception but if method is inconvenient will sometimes risk an unwanted pregnancy, and feels uncomfortable when buying contraceptives.

Marginal 10–13

A person at this level tends to be unfamiliar with birth control methods, avoids discussions of birth control, resists responsibility for contraception, believes the female should be responsible for birth control, and generally avoids buying contraceptives.

Inadequate 5–9

A person at this level is ignorant of birth control methods, resents discussions of birth control, takes no responsibility for contraception, is willing to risk an unwanted pregnancy for the sake of convenience, and refuses to buy contraceptives.

Contraceptive Any agent that can prevent conception. Condoms, diaphragms, intrauterine devices, and oral contraceptives are examples.

Conception The fusion of ovum and sperm, resulting in a zygote (fertilized egg).

Ovulation The release of the egg (ovum) from the ovaries.

Corpus luteum A gland in the ovary that forms after ovulation; secretes progesterone. If the ovum is not fertilized, the corpus luteum degenerates each month (menstruation).

Progesterone A hormone produced by the corpus luteum and, during pregnancy, by the placenta. Used in oral contraceptives to prevent ovulation.

Estrogen A hormone produced by the ovaries. An active ingredient in birth control pills.

Oral contraceptive (OC) Any of various hormone compounds in pill form taken by mouth. Oral contraceptives prevent conception by preventing ovulation.

People have always searched for ways to prevent unwanted pregnancy. The writings of Plato, Aristotle, and the physician Hippocrates in the fourth century B.C. mention the use of sponges, douches, and crude methods of abortion. Other materials listed in the literature of that time as potential contraceptives include seaweed, lemon juice, parsley, camphor, opium, olive oil, copper sulfate—and foam from a camel's mouth! The underlying principle of these trial-and-error methods, although not clearly understood at the time, was basically the same as that of the more effective **contraceptives** used today: the female's ovum (egg) is blocked from uniting with the male's sperm (**conception**), thereby preventing pregnancy.

Contraception

Although the principle of most contraceptives, old and new, is simple, the actual experience of choosing and using a method is more complex and can vary greatly. Each couple and individual must consider many variables in deciding which method is most acceptable and appropriate for them. Some important considerations include individual health risks of each method in terms of personal and family medical history, implications of unwanted pregnancy and therefore the importance of effectiveness, convenience and comfort of the method as viewed by each partner (see Table 6-1), the ease and cost of obtaining and maintaining each method, and the method's acceptability in terms of religious or other philosophical beliefs.

To make a wise contraceptive choice, you will need a core of information about each available option. We hope this chapter will provide a basic framework of facts and figures. Once you have chosen a method, obtain more detailed descriptions of use instructions, possible side effects, and potential danger signals from your health care provider, and read these descriptions carefully.

Oral Contraception—The Pill A century ago or more, a researcher made a key observation: **ovulation** does not occur during pregnancy. Further research showed that ovulation is controlled by the **corpus luteum,** a gland that in nonpregnant women appears and disappears with

Table 6-1 Estimated Number and Percentage Distribution of U.S. Women Aged 15–44 Who Are Exposed to the Risk of Unintended Pregnancy, by Method of Contraception Currently Used, According to Age Group

Method	Number (in 1000s)							Percent						
	Total	15–19	20–24	25–29	30–34	35–39	40–44	15–19	20–24	25–29	30–34	35–39	40–44	Total
Total	36,478	3,563	7,848	7,853	7,144	5,795	4,263	10	22	21	20	16	12	100
Sterilization	11,643	*	468	1,942	3,039	3,578	2,616	*	4	17	26	31	22	100
Tubal	(6,783)	(*)	(278)	(1,135)	(1,809)	(2,063)	(1,498)	(*)	(4)	(17)	(27)	(30)	(22)	100
Vasectomy	(4,860)	(*)	(190)	(807)	(1,230)	(1,515)	(1,118)	(*)	(4)	(17)	(25)	(31)	(23)	100
Pill	9,996	1,539	3,958	2,664	1,191	446	199	15	40	27	12	5	2	100
IUD	2,307	102	479	602	632	334	158	4	21	26	27	15	7	100
Condom	4,475	726	986	962	876	469	456	16	22	22	20	10	10	100
Spermicides	1,463	260	267	270	279	178	211	18	18	18	19	12	14	100
Diaphragm	1,908	39	546	573	471	168	112	2	29	30	25	9	6	100
Withdrawal	930	176	258	225	113	95	63	19	28	24	12	10	7	100
Rhythm	553	13	74	114	104	167	83	2	13	21	19	30	15	100
Other	150	66	7	11	47	10	9	†	†	†	†	†	†	100
None	3,053	642	823	490	392	350	356	21	27	16	13	11	12	100

*Less than 500 or less than 0.5 percent.

†Total *N* too small to distribute.

SOURCE: J. D. Forrest and S. K. Henshaw, 1983 (July–August), What U.S. women think and do about contraception, *Family Planning Perspectives* 15(4):163. Updated figures will next be available in spring 1989.

Myths About Birth Control

Myth Taking borrowed birth control pills for a few days before having sexual relations gives reliable protection against pregnancy.

Fact Instructions for taking birth control pills must be followed carefully to provide effective contraception. With most pills, this means starting them with a menstrual period and then taking one every day.

Myth Pregnancy never occurs when unprotected intercourse takes place just before or just after a menstrual period.

Fact Menstrual cycles may be irregular, and ovulation may occur at unpredictable times.

Myth During sexual relations, sperm enter the vagina only during ejaculation and never before.

Fact The small amounts of fluid secreted before ejaculation may contain sperm.

Myth If semen is deposited just outside the vaginal entrance, pregnancy cannot occur.

Fact Sperm can live up to six or seven days within the woman's body, and are capable of traveling through the vagina and up into the uterus and tubes.

Myth Douching immediately after sexual relations can prevent sperm from reaching and fertilizing an egg.

Fact During ejaculation (within the vagina), some sperm begin to enter the cervix and uterus. Since they are no longer in the vagina, it is impossible to remove them by douching after sexual relations.

Myth If a woman doesn't have an orgasm, pregnancy is unlikely to occur.

Fact The sperm and the egg can travel and unite to begin a pregnancy with or without orgasm.

Myth A woman who is breastfeeding does not have to use any contraceptive method to prevent pregnancy.

Fact Frequent and regular breastfeeding may at times prevent ovulation, but does not do so in a consistent, reliable fashion.

Myth Women can't become pregnant the first time they have intercourse.

Fact *Any time* intercourse without protection takes place, sperm may unite with an egg to begin a pregnancy. There is nothing unique about first intercourse to prevent this.

Myth A pill is readily available as postcoital contraception.

Fact "Morning after pills" are not available in most U.S. clinics, as they have not been approved by the Food and Drug Administration.

each new menstrual cycle. It forms in the ovary after ovulation and then degenerates at the end of the cycle and is absorbed into the system. In pregnant women, however, the corpus luteum remains and continues to secrete a hormone called **progesterone.**

To test the theory that progesterone prevents ovulation, extracts of progesterone were given to animals that were not pregnant. Ovulation did not occur in most cycles. Researchers later found that when **estrogen,** a hormone produced in the ovaries, was given along with progesterone, ovulation was prevented more consistently. Estrogen, progesterone, and certain closely related laboratory-made compounds are the active ingredients in birth control pills.

In addition to preventing ovulation, the birth control pill also has other backup contraceptive effects. It hampers the movement of sperm by thickening the cervical mucus, alters the rate of ovum transport by means of its hormonal effects on the Fallopian tubes, and may inhibit implantation by changing the lining of the uterus, in the unlikely event that a fertilized ovum reaches that area.

Exploring Your Emotions

What division of responsibility do you feel men and women should take for contraception, if any? Has it worked out like that for you? What difficulties might arise from requiring equal responsibility always? From requiring complete control by one or the other partner? What would be your ideal division of responsibility in your ideal marriage?

The **oral contraceptive** (OC) most commonly used today is the combination pill. Each one-month packet contains three weeks of pills that combine varying types and amounts of estrogen and progesterone. Most packets also include one week of inactive pills to be taken following the hormone pills; others instruct the woman to simply take no pills at all for one week before starting the next cycle. During the week in which no hormones are taken, a light menstrual period occurs. Because many dif-

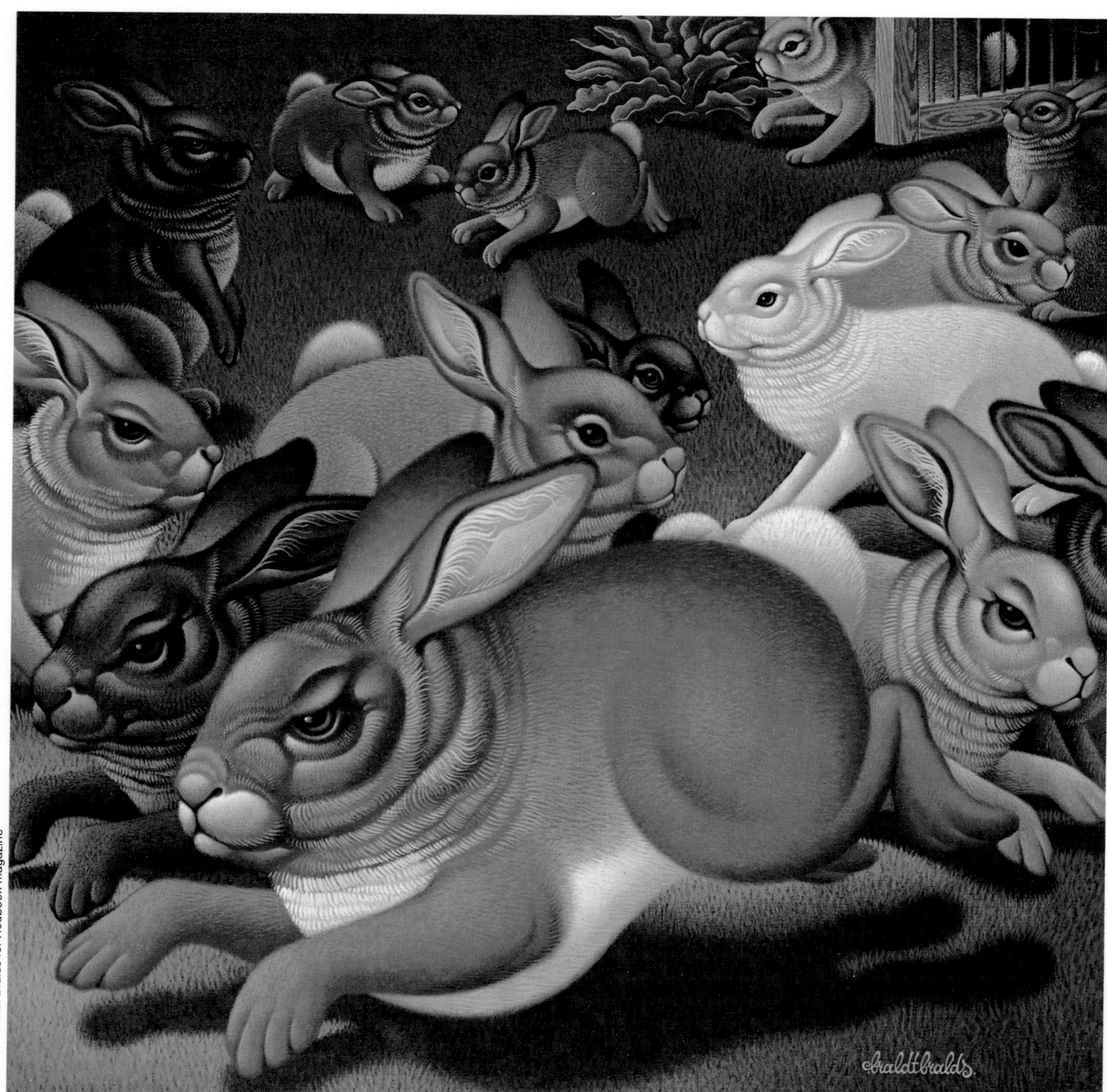

Illustration: Braldt Bralds for *Redbook* magazine

Exploring Your Emotions

Rabbits are prolific reproducers—as Australian ranchers have reason to know. How do you feel about human reproduction capacity and the size of the world? What issues are involved? How have these issues already touched your own life?

Fertility The state or condition of being able to reproduce.

ferent types of combination pills are available today, if minor problems occur with one brand, women can switch to another. The overall trend has been toward lower-dose pills (those with 50 micrograms or less of estrogen), which offer the same high effectiveness rate with fewer unwanted side effects.

A second, much less common, type of OC is the "minipill," a small dose of a synthetic progesterone taken every day of the month. The minipill has fewer side effects, but it also carries a higher risk of pregnancy and irregular bleeding.

Users must start the first cycle of the birth control pill with a menstrual period (the first day, the fifth day, or the following Sunday, depending on the instructions given with each specific pill); this procedure eliminates the possibility of beginning pills during an unsuspected pregnancy and will most effectively prevent ovulation the first month of use. Thereafter, users must take each cycle completely and according to instructions. A few pills taken before sexual relations will not prevent pregnancy.

During the first cycle or two when hormonal adjustment is occurring in the body, slight bleeding may occur between periods. This spotting is considered normal, and users should continue the daily intake of one pill. During the first month, when maximal levels of hormones have not yet been reached, full effectiveness cannot be guaranteed and using an additional backup method, such as foam and/or condoms, is recommended. Similarly, if users forget any pills, effectiveness decreases and backup contraception should be used for the rest of that particular cycle. Pregnancy is practically impossible if a pill has been taken every day according to instructions. Women who did not take a pill every day in the last series and find no period occurs, or if periods fail to occur more than one time, should consult a doctor.

Pill use in the United States reached an all-time high in the mid-1970s and then declined rather rapidly between 1975 and 1977, following intense publicity regarding possible health risks. In recent years, however, many of those risks have been reduced by using lower-dosage pills and by clarifying the personal factors that place a specific woman in a high-risk category. Currently, the pill is again the birth control method of choice for many U.S. women, especially those in the younger age groups. A marked decline in pill use has occurred among women who have been married more than ten years, with the main challenge coming from the increasingly popular method of surgical sterilization. Among couples in whom neither partner has been sterilized, however, no other birth control method comes close to the birth control pill in popularity.

Exploring Your Emotions

Do you have religious or philosophical objections to contraception? If so, how do you prefer to deal with questions of overpopulation, crowding, pollution, exhaustion of natural resources, and so forth? Suggest a solution that recognizes this very public dilemma while also recognizing the privacy of individual lives and ideals.

Advantages The main advantage of the oral contraceptive is its high degree of effectiveness in preventing pregnancy. Nearly all unplanned pregnancies result because the user did not take the pill as directed. The pill is relatively simple to use and does not require any mood-destroying interruptions that could hinder sexual spontaneity. Most women also enjoy the predictable regularity of periods, as well as the decrease in cramps and other premenstrual symptoms. For young women, its reversibility is especially important; **fertility** (ability to reproduce) returns after the pill is discontinued, although not always immediately. The medical advantages include a decreased incidence of the following conditions: benign breast disease, iron-deficiency anemia, pelvic inflammatory disease (PID), ectopic pregnancy, uterine cancer, and ovarian cancer. Women who have never used the pill are twice as likely to develop uterine or ovarian cancer as users who have taken it for at least 12 months.

Disadvantages The hormones in birth control pills influence all tissues of the body, and they can lead to a variety of minor disturbances, and for some women, to serious side effects. Symptoms of early pregnancy—morning nausea, weight gain, and swollen breasts, for example—may appear during the first few months of oral contraception. They usually disappear by the fourth cycle. Other complaints include depression, nervousness, changes in the sex drive, dizziness, generalized headaches, migraine headaches, bleeding between periods, and changes in the lining of the walls of the vagina, with an increase in clear or white discharge from the vagina. Chloasma, or "mask of pregnancy," sometimes occurs, causing brown "giant freckles" to appear on the face. Acne may develop or worsen, but in most women, using the pill causes acne to clear up, and it is sometimes prescribed for young women for that purpose.

Yeast fungus infections are more common among women who are taking the pill. These infections are not serious, but the itchiness and increased discharge in the vagina that accompany them are often extremely uncomfortable.

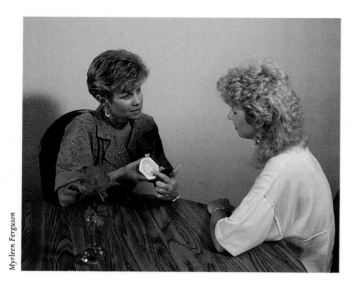
Myrleen Ferguson

Medical treatment, usually in the form of vaginal creams, gives prompt relief most of the time.

Serious side effects of pill use have been reported in a small number of women. These include blood clots, stroke, heart attack, and benign tumors of the liver that may bleed and rupture. Pill users also show a slight increase in the incidence of high blood pressure, which is usually quickly reversed on discontinuation of the pill, and of gall bladder disease.

Most investigations regarding oral contraceptive use and breast cancer have shown no increased risk among users. A few reports suggested that certain subgroups of women might be at higher risk (women with a history of benign breast disease or a family history of breast cancer, and women who started the pill at a very young age and/or before their first pregnancy). However, no such links have been found in more recent, large-scale studies. Similarly, no causal relationship has been established between pill use and cervical cancer. Although some investigations have indicated a slightly increased risk following prolonged pill use, these changes may be related more closely to other behavioral characteristics of pill users, such as sexual relationships at an earlier age and with a greater number of partners.

Avoidance of oral contraceptives is generally recommended for women who have or have had blood clots in any part of the body, stroke, heart disease or defect, severe endocrine disorder, recurrent jaundice of pregnancy, markedly impaired liver function, any form of cancer, or abnormal genital bleeding from unknown causes. The pill is not recommended for women over 35 years old, especially if they are smokers. (Cigarette smoking adds an additional increase to the risk of heart attack, stroke, and other blood clot problems at any age, and markedly so after age 35.)

Many health care professionals also advise women with present or previous high blood pressure not to use oral contraceptives. Physicians usually give more frequent follow-up appointments when oral contraceptives are prescribed for women who smoke, have or have had high blood pressure, varicose veins, migraine headaches, diabetes, asthma, epilepsy, fibroid growths of the uterus, significant psychiatric problems, gall bladder disease, sickle-cell disease, nonmalignant breast disease, or irregular menstrual cycles. When women with any of these conditions or with a family history of cancer, high blood pressure, or diabetes do choose to use the pill, preliminary tests and careful follow-up examinations are important. For women who have or have had liver disease, kidney disease, or mild endocrine disorders, successful treatment of those conditions is usually required before starting oral contraception.

In trying to decide whether to use oral contraception, an attempt must be made to weigh the benefits against the risks for each individual woman. For most women, the known, directly associated risk of death from use of the pill is much lower than the risk of death from pregnancy. This is especially true as newer, low-dose combinations become available. However, many long-term effects are still not completely understood and thereby complicate the decision-making process. Nevertheless, there are many important actions that the potential user can take to make the most informed decision possible. She can discuss and evaluate with a health care professional the risk variables that are known and that apply to her; request a low-dosage pill; stop smoking; carefully and consistently follow the pill-taking instructions; be alert to preliminary danger signals (severe headaches, problems with vision, severe pain in the abdomen, chest, or legs); have regular checkups of her blood pressure, weight, and urine, and an annual examination of the thyroid, breasts, abdomen, and pelvis. By following these measures, women can better evaluate and actively affect the benefit-risk ratio of pill use.

Effectiveness Contraceptives can be evaluated according to either of two standards: theoretical effectiveness or use effectiveness. **Theoretical effectiveness** is the failure rate of a contraceptive when it is "taken as directed." It cannot be accurately measured, but it is inferred from studying the most successful users. For the combination pill, the theoretical effectiveness is one pregnancy per 1,000 women during one year of use.

Use effectiveness is the failure rate of a contraceptive when it is used under average conditions by average people. This measurement includes pregnancies that result from erratic pill taking, as well as those that occur when a woman stops taking pills and fails to use another method of contraception. When these pregnancies have been taken

Theoretical effectiveness The failure rate of a contraceptive when it is "taken as directed."

Use effectiveness The failure rate of a contraceptive when used under average conditions by average people.

Continuation rate The percentage of women who continue to use a particular contraceptive after a specified period of time.

Diethylstilbestrol (DES) A synthetic hormone that produces the effects of natural estrogen. DES is not considered safe.

Intrauterine device (IUD) A plastic device inserted into the uterus as a contraceptive.

into account, the use effectiveness of the combination pill has been reported to be as low as ten pregnancies per 1,000 women during one year of use. This figure will differ markedly, as it depends on numerous patient and program variables. Again, it is critical that the woman become thoroughly informed in regard to all aspects of pill use and that she follow all guidelines carefully.

Effectiveness is also measured by the **continuation rate**—the percentage of women who continue to use the method after a specified period of time. The continuation rate for oral contraceptives has also varied considerably from one group of users to another, with the range being 50 to 75 percent after one year.

The "Morning After" Pill A "morning after" pill containing large doses of **diethylstilbestrol (DES)**, a synthetic preparation of estrogen, was approved by the FDA in the mid-1970s as a postcoital contraceptive. In recent years, however, DES has been used infrequently, because it has been linked to cervical and vaginal cancers in daughters of women who had taken the drug to avoid miscarriage (a common practice from 1945 to 1960). If a pregnancy does result after DES use, a therapeutic abortion should be considered because of possible damage to the fetus.

Another "morning after" pill, a combination of estrogen and progesterone, was recently approved in western Europe for emergency situations (most frequently, rape). It has not been approved for postcoital use in the United States, however, and probably will not be in the near future. Postcoital contraception is often seen as controversial, not only because of its potential health risks, but also because its opponents see it as an agent that causes abortion rather than prevents pregnancy.

Exploring Your Emotions

Because women take the major responsibility for contraception, women also experience most of the unwanted side effects, including those of many inadequately tested drugs. How would you devise a system to share responsibility for such side effects among those involved: the women affected, their partners, the drug companies, government, society as a whole, and so on? What does your system show about how you feel on this issue?

Intrauterine Devices (IUDs) Placing objects inside the uterus is one of the oldest methods of birth control. Over two thousand years ago, Hippocrates, the Greek physician, described various devices, including one that was inserted into the uterus through a piece of lead tubing. Another example, perhaps more familiar, is the method used by camel owners who insert small stones into the uterus of the camel before a long desert trip. The possibility of intrauterine methods of birth control was almost ignored in modern times until E. Grafenberg, a German physician, reported his use of an intrauterine ring of silkworm gut and silver in 1930. Grafenberg's ring did not work because of flaws in design and insertion techniques. Improvements in materials, design, and insertion techniques greatly increased the acceptability of the **intrauterine device (IUD)**, and in the United States there was a sharp increase in its use between 1965 and 1973.

By 1976, however, there was a slight decline, which was probably related to the publicity about the dangers of the widely used Dalkon Shield and its withdrawal from the market. Currently, an even greater decline in IUD use is likely to result from the 1985–1986 decisions to discontinue U.S. marketing of the Lippes Loop, the Copper 7, and the Copper T, the IUDs used by most women. The companies manufacturing these IUDs decided to stop U.S. distribution, not because of new findings of increased medical risk, but due to the financial risk of ongoing lawsuits. Current users should discuss with their physicians whether to continue using these IUDs. One IUD, the hormone-releasing Progestasert, is still available to U.S. women.

No one knows exactly how IUDs work. They may cause biochemical changes in the uterus, such as the production of specific cells that destroy the egg and/or sperm; they may immobilize sperm in the uterus or shorten the normal travel time of the egg in the Fallopian tube; or they may interfere with the implantation of eggs in the uterus. Progestasert acts primarily by slowly releasing the hormone progesterone, which makes the uterine lining unsuitable for implantation. The amount of progesterone released is very small and does not change hormone levels in the bloodstream.

Before an IUD is inserted, a medical history and a gynecological examination should be completed to rule out the presence of pregnancy, infection, anatomical abnormalities, or other potentially complicating conditions. If none of these complications exists, the IUD is threaded

Pelvic inflammatory disease (PID) An infection that progresses from the vagina and cervix and eventually moves into the pelvic cavity.

Spontaneous abortion A miscarriage; the premature expulsion of a nonliving fetus.

Condom A sheath, usually made of thin rubber, designed to cover the penis during sexual intercourse. Used for contraception and to prevent disease.

Sexually transmissible diseases (STD.) Any of several contagious diseases such as syphilis and gonorrhea contracted through intimate contact.

Ejaculation An abrupt discharge of semen from the penis after sexual stimulation.

---

into a sterile inserter, which is then introduced through the cervix until it reaches the lowermost portion of the uterus. The plunger pushes the IUD into the uterus, and the inserter is withdrawn. The threads protruding from the cervix are trimmed so that only 1 to 1½ inches remain in the upper vagina. These are unnoticeable during coitus. (See Figure 6-1.)

The best time for insertion of the IUD is during the menstrual period because the cervical canal is most open during that time and there is the least possibility of an unsuspected pregnancy.

IUDs with nylon threads can usually be removed by pulling on the threads. Only a trained professional should undertake this process, however, because the cervix might have to be expanded, or dilated. Timing of removal can be crucial; some unwanted pregnancies have resulted when sperm have survived from intercourse that took place a couple of days before the IUD was removed.

Advantages Intrauterine devices are highly reliable (second only to the pill) and are simple to use, requiring no attention except for a periodic check of the string position. They do not require the user to anticipate or interrupt sexual activity. Usually IUDs have only localized side effects, and in the absence of complications, such as infection, their effects are considered fully reversible. In most cases fertility resumes as soon as the IUD is removed. IUDs also have a low long-term cost.

Figure 6-1 An IUD (Progestasert) properly positioned in the uterus. The attached threads that protrude from the cervix into the upper vagina allow the woman to check to see that the IUD is in place.

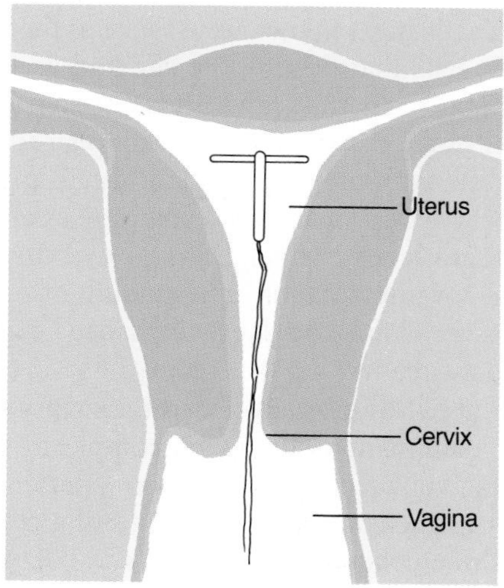

Disadvantages Most side effects of IUD use are limited to the genital tract. By far the most common complaint is abnormal menstrual bleeding. The menstrual flow tends to appear sooner, last longer, and become heavier after insertion of an IUD. Bleeding and spotting between periods may also occur. Another common complaint is pain, particularly uterine cramps and backache, side effects that seem to occur most often in women who have never been pregnant. Uterine cramps that accompany insertion usually disappear after a few days, but in some cases they are severe enough to require the removal of the device.

Spontaneous expulsion of the IUD happens in 5 to 15 percent of all users within the first year after insertion. If a woman does not notice that she has lost it, an unwanted pregnancy may result. Most expulsions occur during the first months after insertion, usually but not always during the menstrual period, so checking tampons or menstrual pads for the device is a wise precaution. It is also a good idea to check occasionally that the device is in place by locating the threads, particularly prior to sexual activity. Expulsion after the first year is uncommon. If one IUD is expelled, the risk of expelling another IUD becomes two to three times greater, although about one-half of all women who experience a first expulsion eventually retain the device. The older the woman is and the more children she has had, the less likely she is to expel the device.

A serious complication sometimes associated with IUD use is **pelvic inflammatory disease (PID).** Many research studies indicate that this condition occurs most commonly during the first two weeks following insertion, with an incidence of 1 to 5 percent during the first year of use. However, the actual incidence of PID may be higher because pain and bleeding are often reported as the chief reasons for removal rather than the infection, which also may have been present. The risk of infection is markedly increased when women have multiple partners. Most pelvic infections among IUD users are relatively mild and can be treated successfully with antibiotics. However, early and adequate treatment is critical, for a smoldering infection can lead to tubal scarring and subsequent infertility.

In about one of 2,000 insertions, the IUD punctures the wall of the uterus and migrates into the abdominal cavity.

No evidence has been found that IUDs cause cancer in women, but the long-term effects are not well known.

Most doctors advise against the use of IUDs by young women who have never been pregnant because of the increased incidence of side effects in this subgroup of women and the risk of infection with the possibility of subsequent infertility. The IUD is not recommended for women of any age who have a history of pelvic infection, suspected pregnancy, large tumors of the uterus or other anatomical abnormalities, irregular or unexplained bleeding, history of ectopic pregnancy, rheumatic heart disease, or diabetes.

Early IUD danger signals that the user should be alert for are abdominal pain, fever, chills, foul vaginal discharge, irregular menstrual period, and other unusual vaginal bleeding. An annual checkup is important and should include a Pap smear and a blood check for anemia if menstrual flow has increased. (And in the case of Progestasert use, the IUD must be replaced every twelve months.)

Effectiveness The use effectiveness rate of IUDs is about 50 pregnancies per 1,000 women during the first year of use. Many of these pregnancies are due to undetected partial or complete expulsion of the device. For all types the failure rate tends to decline rapidly after the first year. Because most pregnancies occur in the first few months after IUD insertion, some doctors advise using an additional method of contraception during that time. Regular checking of the cervix to verify the presence of thread and absence of the IUD stem is also recommended.

Pregnancy may occur with the device in place. If the patient wishes to maintain the pregnancy, the IUD should be removed. Following removal, there is a 25 percent chance of a **spontaneous abortion** (miscarriage). Birth defects are no more common among babies born of such pregnancies than among other babies. Pregnancy with an IUD left in place may lead to fatal infection, bleeding, and has a 50 percent chance of ending in miscarriage.

The continuation rate of IUDs is 70 to 85 percent after one year of use.

Assessing Risks

Activity	Chance of Death in a year
Motorcycling	1 in 50
Smoking, 1 pack per day	1 in 200
Horse racing	1 in 750
Automobile driving	1 in 6,000
Power boating	1 in 6,000
Rock climbing	1 in 7,500
Playing football	1 in 25,000
Canoeing	1 in 100,000
Using tampons	1 in 350,000
Using Rely tampons	1 in 50,000
Using birth control pills (nonsmoker)	1 in 63,000
Using birth control pills (smoker)	1 in 16,000
Using IUDs	1 in 100,000
Using diaphragm, condom, or spermicide	None
Using fertility awareness methods	None
Undergoing sterilization:	
laparoscopic tubal ligation	1 in 10,000
hysterectomy	1 in 1,600
vasectomy	None
Pregnancy:	
continuing pregnancy	1 in 10,000
illegal abortion	1 in 3,000
legal abortion:	
before 9 weeks	1 in 400,000
before 9–12 weeks	1 in 100,000
before 13–16 weeks	1 in 25,000
after 16 weeks	1 in 10,000

SOURCE: R. A. Hatcher, 1982. *It's Your Choice* (New York: Irvington), p. 7.

Condoms In the sixteenth century, the Italian anatomist Fallopius described the use of linen sheaths worn over the penis as a protection against **sexually transmissible diseases** (STDs). By the eighteenth century the contraceptive function of the **condom** had been recognized, and the French and English used condoms made of sheep gut or the amniotic membrane of newborn lambs. Sheaths of skin were too expensive for most people, but the vulcanization of rubber in 1844 made a less expensive condom possible. Since the early 1900s, "rubbers" have, by and large, replaced animal skin condoms.

The condom is still one of the most popular contraceptives in North America. In recent years, its sales have increased dramatically, partly due to fear of sexually transmissible diseases, particularly AIDS and herpes. Of all condoms purchased, at least one-third are bought by women. Every year, 800 million to a billion are sold in Canada and the United States. Currently, condom use is the third most popular of all birth control methods used in the United States and is exceeded only by the pill and sterilization. (See Figure 6-2.)

The user or his partner must put on the condom before the penis is inserted into the vagina, as the small amounts of fluid secreted prior to **ejaculation** often contain sperm capable of causing pregnancy. The rolled-up condom is placed over the head of the erect penis and unrolled down to the base of the penis, leaving a half-inch space (without air) at the tip to collect semen. If the user has not been

circumcised, he must first pull back the foreskin of the penis. He and his partner must be careful not to damage the condom with fingernails, rings, or other rough objects.

Some condoms are sold already lubricated. If the users wish, they can lubricate their own condoms with vaginal foam, cream, or jelly, or other nongreasy jellies. Vaseline or any other kind of petroleum jelly or oil should never be applied to rubber condoms: rubber dissolves in petroleum.

When the male loses his erection after ejaculating, the condom loses its tight fit. To avoid spilling semen, the condom must be held around the base of the penis as the penis is withdrawn. If any semen is spilled on the vulva, the sperm may easily find their way to the uterus.

A new type of condom already popular in England and several European countries has recently been introduced in the United States. The lubricant on this condom contains the same spermicidal agent found in many of the contraceptive foams and creams that women use. Since this agent kills many of the sperm soon after ejaculation, its addition may significantly decrease contraceptive failure associated with breakage and the spilling of semen and may be used to replace the recommended combination of foam and condom use.

Advantages Condoms are easy to purchase and are available without prescription or medical supervision. They are simple to use and allow increased male participation in contraception. Condoms do not require daily use during intervals of sexual inactivity, and their effects are immediately and completely reversible. In addition to being free of medical side effects (other than occasional allergic reactions), condoms help to protect against sexually transmissible diseases (including herpes and AIDS), which in turn may diminish the likelihood of cervical cancer in some women.

Exploring Your Emotions

Would you feel comfortable buying condoms from a drugstore clerk? Could you ask the clerk what brand is best? Would you prefer to put your purchase in a "brown paper bag" before leaving the store? Why might you (and many other people) feel uncomfortable making such a purchase? Can you suggest any ways to ease that problem?

Disadvantages The two most nearly universal complaints about condoms are that they diminish sensation and interfere with spontaneity. Although some people find these drawbacks serious, others consider them only minor disadvantages. It is hard to think of a human activity in which losing sensation and spontaneity would be less welcome than in coitus. Many couples, however, learn to creatively integrate condom use into their sexual activities. Indeed, it can be a way to improve communication and add shared responsibility to the relationship.

Effectiveness Condoms, when used exactly as directed during each act of intercourse, have a theoretical effectiveness of 30 pregnancies per 1,000 women during one year of use. In actual use, however, the failure rate is considerably higher, reaching approximately 100 pregnancies per 1,000 women during one year of use. At least some of these pregnancies happen because the condom

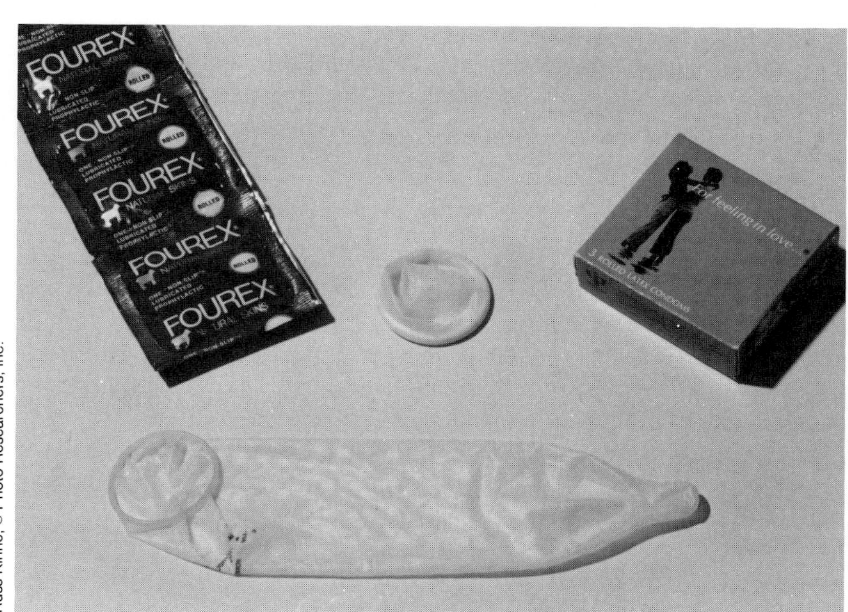

Russ Kinne, © Photo Researchers, Inc.

Figure 6-2 A sample of condoms presently available. The elongated tip on the unrolled condom (*bottom*) is a reservoir to collect semen.

Circumcise To remove the foreskin of the penis.

Spermicide An agent that kills sperm.

Diaphragm A contraceptive consisting of a flexible, dome-shaped cup that covers the cervix. The diaphragm prevents sperm from entering the uterus.

is carelessly removed after ejaculation. Some may also happen because of a break or a tear, which is estimated to occur once in every 150 to 200 instances. (Since heat destroys rubber, condoms should not be stored for long periods in a wallet or in the glove compartment of a car.) If either type of accident occurs, the risk of pregnancy can be reduced somewhat by the prompt use of a vaginal **spermicide** (a preparation for killing sperm). The use effectiveness of the condom can be greatly improved, to approach that of the pill, by using a spermicidal foam, inserted just *before* intercourse, along with a condom.

The most common cause of pregnancy with condom users is "taking a chance"—that is, not using a condom at all—or waiting to use it until after pre-ejaculate fluid (which may contain some sperm) has already entered the vagina.

Diaphragms and Jelly Before oral contraceptives were introduced, about one-fourth of all U.S. couples who used any form of contraception relied on the **diaphragm.** Many former diaphragm users have been won over to the pill or to IUDs, but the diaphragm continues to offer advantages that are important to certain couples.

Wilhelm Mensinga, a German physician, invented a rubber diaphragm in the late 1800s, and there have been few changes in design since. The diaphragm is a dome-shaped cup of thin rubber stretched over a collapsible metal ring. When correctly used with spermicidal cream or jelly, the diaphragm covers the mouth of the cervix, blocking sperm from entering the uterus.

Diaphragms can be obtained only by prescription. Because of individual differences in women, a diaphragm must be carefully fitted to ensure that it will be both effective and comfortable, and only a trained person can make these adjustments. The fitting should be checked with each routine annual medical examination, as well as after childbirth, abortion, or a weight change of more than 10 pounds.

Before inserting the diaphragm, the woman should spread about a tablespoon of spermicidal jelly or cream over the surface of the dome that will be against the cervix. The diaphragm is easiest to insert if the user squats, lies down, or stands with one foot raised. The user squeezes the diaphragm into a long narrow shape with one hand. She holds the labia apart with the other hand and pushes the diaphragm up along the back wall of the vagina as far as it will go, keeping it behind the cervix. She then tucks the front rim up behind the pubic bone. (See Figure 6-3.) Because the vagina tilts backward, a user who inserts the diaphragm while she is standing up must insert it almost horizontally.

After the diaphragm is inserted, its position should be checked. The cervix should be located and felt through the dome of the diaphragm to make sure that it is com-

Figure 6-3 Use of the diaphragm: (a) spermicidal jelly is placed in the concave side of the diaphragm, and the diaphragm is pressed firmly between the thumb and forefinger; (b) diaphragm is inserted in the vagina; (c) diaphragm is checked for correct position against the cervix.

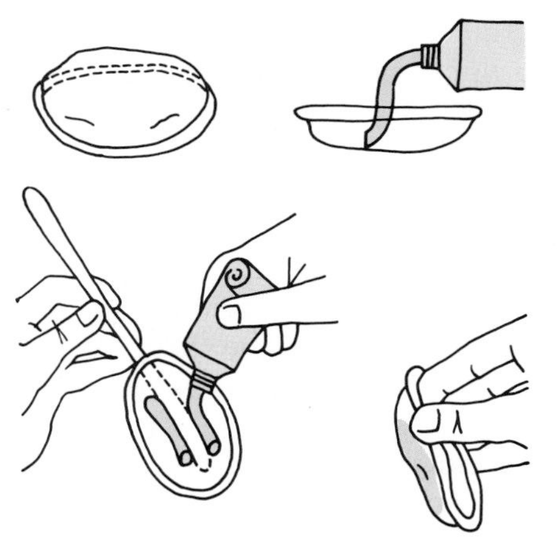
(*a*)

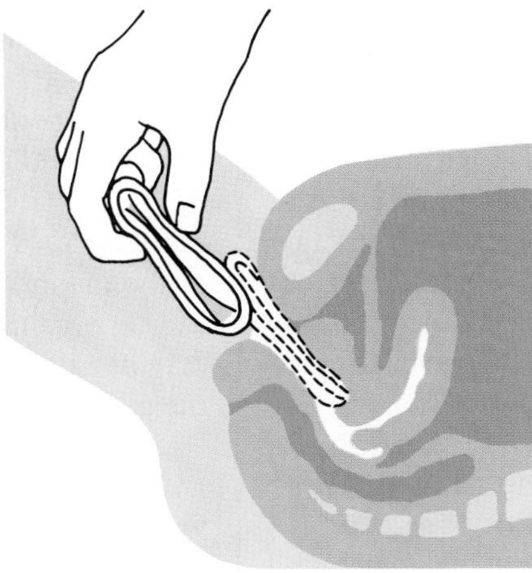
(*b*)

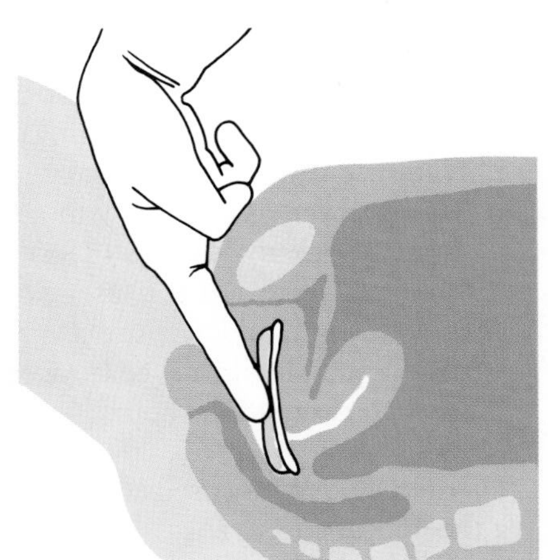
(*c*)

pletely covered and that the front rim of the diaphragm is pushed up behind the pubic bone.

The diaphragm must not be inserted more than six hours before intercourse. If the time between insertion and coitus is longer than six hours, an applicatorful of spermicide should be inserted into the vagina, or the diaphragm should be taken out and spermicide freshly applied before it is reinserted. Additional cream or jelly should also be inserted into the vagina before any additional act of coitus. The diaphragm must be left in place for at least six hours after the last act of coitus to give the spermicide enough time to kill all the sperm.

To remove the diaphragm, the user simply hooks the front rim down from behind the pubic bone with one finger. After the diaphragm is removed, it should be washed with mild soap and water, rinsed, and patted dry. It should then be examined for holes or cracks. Defects are mostly likely to develop near the rim, and they can usually be spotted by looking at the diaphragm in front of a bright light. After the diaphragm is inspected, it can be dusted with cornstarch (*not* talcum powder, which may damage the diaphragm and irritate the vagina) and stored in its case.

Advantages Diaphragm use destroys spontaneity less than the condom does because a diaphragm can be inserted up to six hours before intercourse. Its use can be limited to times of sexual activity only, and allows for immediate and total reversibility. The diaphragm is free of medical side effects (other than rare allergic reactions). When used along with spermicidal jelly or cream, it offers some protection against gonorrhea and probably other sexually transmissible diseases (such as herpes, chlamydia, and AIDS).

Disadvantages Diaphragms must always be used with a spermicide, and therefore a user must keep both of these somewhat bulky supplies with her whenever she anticipates sexual activity. Diaphragms require extra attention, since they must be cleaned and stored with care to preserve their effectiveness. Some women cannot wear a diaphragm because of their anatomy. In other women, diaphragm use can cause an increase in bladder infections. It has also been associated with a slightly increased risk of **toxic shock syndrome (TSS)**, an occasionally fatal disease related to tampon use. To diminish the risk of TSS, women should not use a diaphragm during menstruation and should never leave the device in place for more than twenty-four hours.

Effectiveness When used consistently, the diaphragm has a theoretical effectiveness of twenty to thirty pregnancies per 1,000 women during one year. In actual practice, women rarely use the diaphragm correctly every time they have intercourse. Use effectiveness of the diaphragm is 130 pregnancies for 1,000 women during one year. The main causes of failures are inaccurate fitting and incorrect insertion. Sometimes, too, the vaginal walls expand during sexual stimulation, allowing the diaphragm to be dislodged. This displacement seems to happen most commonly with the woman-on-top position.

Cervical Cap The **cervical cap** is a thimble-shaped rubber or plastic cup that fits snugly over the cervix and is held in place by suction. It is used in a manner similar to the diaphragm, a small amount of spermicide being placed in the cup before each insertion. Use of the cervical cap in the United States remains limited. Since they are not currently approved for marketing, these devices can be acquired only at clinics that are carrying out FDA-approved studies on safety and efficacy.

Advantages Advantages of the cervical cap are similar to those associated with diaphragm use. In addition, it can be used as an alternative for women who have anatomical features that preclude diaphragm use, such as very lax vaginal tone, pressure symptoms, or recurrent urinary infections with diaphragm use.

Disadvantages Along with most of the disadvantages associated with the diaphragm, difficulty with insertion and removal is a more common problem for cervical cap users. Cervical irritation may also be associated with prolonged cap use.

Effectiveness Studies completed thus far indicate that cervical cap effectiveness is within the same range as that of the diaphragm.

The Sponge The **sponge**, a more recent addition to the barrier methods, is a round, absorbent device about 2 inches in diameter with a polyester loop on one side (for removal) and a concave dimple on the other side, which helps it fit snugly over the cervix. Most sponges are made of polyurethane and are presaturated with the same spermicide that is used in contraceptive creams and foams. The sponge acts as a barrier, as a spermicide, and as a seminal fluid absorbent.

Advantages The sponge offers advantages similar to those of the diaphragm and cervical cap. In addition, sponges can be obtained without a professional fitting, and they may be safely left in place for twenty-four hours without the addition of spermicide for repeated intercourse.

Disadvantages Reported disadvantages include difficulty with removal and an unpleasant odor if left in place for more than eighteen hours. Allergic reactions, such as irritation of the labia, are more common with the sponge than with other spermicide products, probably because the overall dose contained in each sponge is significantly

Toxic shock syndrome (TSS) A disease whose major symptoms include high fever, vomiting, diarrhea, headache, sore throat, and rash. Although primarily associated with menstruating women who use tampons, the disease has also been reported in men. It is usually caused by the bacterium *Staphylococcus aureus.* Mortality rate has decreased from 10 to 15 percent to 3 percent or less due to earlier recognition and treatment.

Cervical cap A thimble-shaped cup that fits over the cervix, to be used with spermicide.

Sponge A contraceptive device about 2 inches in diameter that fits over the cervix and acts as a barrier, spermicide, and seminal fluid absorbent.

Douche To apply a stream of water or other solutions to a body part or cavity such as the vagina; not a contraceptive technique.

higher than that used with the other methods. (It contains 1 gram of spermicide compared to the 60–100 mg present in one application of other spermicidal products.) Because the sponge has also been associated with toxic shock syndrome, the same precautions must be taken as described for diaphragm use. A sponge user should be especially alert for symptoms of TSS when the sponge has been difficult to remove or was not removed intact. We do not know how much spermicide is absorbed through the vaginal walls with this device, or what possible effects are caused by recurring, extended exposure.

Effectiveness The use effectiveness of the sponge is similar to that of the diaphragm (130 pregnancies for 1,000 women during one year) for women who have never experienced childbirth. For women who have had a child, however, sponge effectiveness is significantly lower than diaphragm effectiveness. One possible explanation is that the one size now marketed may be insufficient to adequately cover the cervix after childbirth. To ensure effectiveness, the user should carefully check the expiration date on each sponge, as shelf life is limited.

Vaginal Spermicides People have used barrier methods for thousands of years. In recent years spermicidal compounds developed for use with a diaphragm have been adapted for use without a diaphragm by combining them with a bulky base.

Foams, creams, jellies, and vaginal suppositories are all available. Foam is sold in an aerosol bottle or a metal container with an applicator that fits on the nozzle. Creams and jellies are sold in tubes with an applicator that can be screwed onto the opening of the tube. (See Figure 6-4.)

Foams, creams, and jellies must be placed deep in the vagina near the cervical entrance and must not be inserted more than one-half hour before intercourse. After an hour, their effectiveness is drastically reduced, and a new applicatorful must be inserted. Another application is also required before each repeated act of coitus. If the woman wants to **douche**, she should wait for at least eight hours after the last coitus to make sure that there has been time for the spermicide to kill all the sperm.

In recent years the spermicidal suppository has become widely marketed and publicized in the United States. It is small and easily inserted like a tampon. Because body heat is needed to dissolve and activate the suppository, it is important to wait at least ten minutes after insertion before having intercourse. The suppository's spermicidal effects are limited in time, and coitus should take place within one hour of insertion. An additional suppository is required for each additional act of intercourse.

The latest addition to the vaginal spermicides is the vaginal contraceptive film, a thin, semitransparent 2-inch-square of film that incorporates the same spermicide as the preceding methods. It is folded over one or two fingers and placed high in the vagina, as close to the cervix as possible. In about ten minutes the film dissolves into a gel that exerts a contraceptive effect against sperm for around 1½ hours. An additional film must be inserted each time intercourse is repeated.

Advantages The use of vaginal spermicides is relatively simple and can be limited to times of sexual activity. They are readily available in most drugstores and do not require a prescription or a pelvic examination. Spermicides allow for complete and immediate reversibility; the only known medical side effects are occasional allergic reactions. Protection against some sexually transmissible diseases is offered by vaginal spermicides, although it may be less than when a diaphragm is used in addition to the spermicide.

Figure 6-4 Application of spermicidal jelly, cream, or foam.

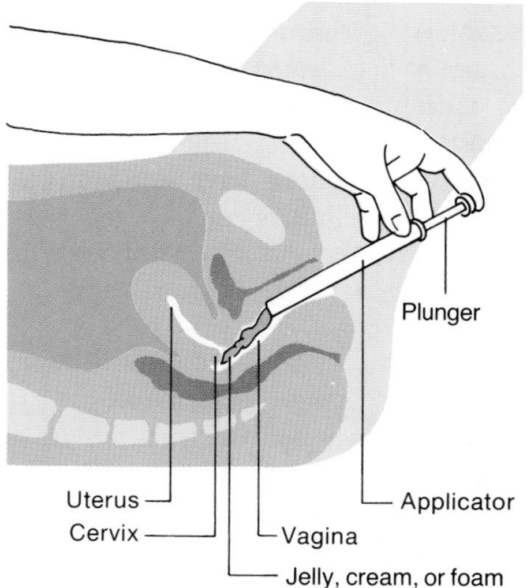

Planned Parenthood

"Every child a wanted child": since its stormy beginnings over 60 years ago, Planned Parenthood Federation of America has sought to end compulsory parenthood by making birth control devices accessible to all who want them. Taking up their cause in local communities and courtrooms throughout the nation, Planned Parenthood has committed itself to making all Americans aware of the problems caused by unrestrained population growth, both here and abroad.

Planned Parenthood's educational goals are equally far-reaching. In the offices of all of its affiliates, basic birth control information is provided through films, group discussions, and individual counseling sessions. In addition, many affiliates offer special discussion groups for young people, where participants can talk about their anxieties, ask their questions, and share their problems in a supportive environment.

All the agency's affiliates also provide educational services within the community. Its trainers prepare teachers, social workers, nurses, and clergy to educate others in matters related to human sexuality and birth control.

Since Margaret Sanger, the agency's founder, began her courageous fight for voluntary parenthood, Planned Parenthood has actively opposed state and federal laws that interfere with parenthood by choice. In 1969, the agency published the nation's first county-by-county study of birth control needs and services among low-income women. This study was probably the single most important piece of research leading to the Family Planning Services and Population Research Act of 1970. With the passage of this act, the federal government for the first time authorized funds ($225 million) for birth control research, expanded family planning services, and the creation of the Office of Population Affairs within the Department of Health, Education, and Welfare.

Planned Parenthood's activities literally span the globe. The International Planned Parenthood Federation (IPPF) is the world's largest voluntary family planning organization. Dedicated to the formation and support of national family planning associations throughout the world, it assists in developing programs to educate people about the personal, social, and economic benefits of family planning. IPPF also provides technical information to several agencies of the United Nations and gives national associations financial support and technical assistance.

Disadvantages All vaginal spermicides when used alone must be inserted shortly before intercourse, so their use may be seen as an annoying disruption. Some women find the slight increase in vaginal fluids after spermicide use unpleasant, but for most this effect is negligible.

Some studies have indicated that spermicide use around the time of conception may be associated with a higher rate of miscarriage, low birth weight, and certain birth defects. Other investigations have not found any such relationship, and no definitive conclusion can be made at this time. Similarly, the effects on the user herself of extended exposure to spermicide are unknown at present.

Effectiveness The reported failure rates of vaginal spermicides cover a wide range, again depending partly on how consistently and carefully instructions are followed. The actual failure rate is estimated to be 180 pregnancies per 1,000 women during one year of use. Of the various types of spermicides, foam is probably the most effective, because its effervescent mass forms a more dense and evenly distributed barrier to the cervical opening. Creams and jellies give only minimal protection unless used with diaphragms or cervical caps. Vaginal spermicides are used by many couples in combination with condoms or as a backup with other birth control methods.

Abstinence, Fertility Awareness, and Withdrawal Millions of people throughout the world do not use any of the methods we have described. Either they will not because of religious conviction or cultural prohibitions or they cannot because of poverty or ignorance. If they use any method at all, they are likely to use one of the following.

Abstinence **Abstinence**, the decision not to engage in sexual intercourse for a chosen period of time, has been followed by human beings throughout history for a variety of reasons. Until relatively recently, many people abstained because they had no other birth control measures. Today, abstinence is being chosen by individuals who do have other means of pregnancy prevention, as well. To some people, all other methods simply seem unsuitable. Concern regarding possible side effects, sex-

Abstinence Avoidance of sexual intercourse. This is one method of birth control.

Fertility Awareness Method (FAM) A method of preventing conception based on avoiding coitus during the fertile phase of a woman's cycle.

Billings, or mucus, method A method of predicting the fertile period in a woman's cycle by means of the texture, color, and amount of cervical mucus.

Withdrawal Sexual intercourse purposely interrupted by withdrawing the penis before ejaculation (to avoid conception).

---

ually transmissible diseases, and unwanted pregnancy may be factors. Or intercourse may be temporarily avoided because of medical reasons such as recent illness or surgery. In other cases, abstinence may be seen as the wisest choice in terms of personal emotional needs. A period of abstinence may be chosen as a time to focus energies on other aspects of interpersonal or personal growth. Religious and cultural beliefs are sometimes motivating factors. For a variety of reasons, what may seem "right" and highly desirable for one person may be unacceptable for another. External pressure alone, either from individuals or from society at large, is being recognized as an unsatisfactory reason to engage in intercourse.

Many couples who do choose to abstain from sexual intercourse in the traditional penis-in-vagina sense turn to other mutually satisfying alternatives. When open communication between partners exists, many new avenues may be explored. These may include dancing, massage, hugging, kissing, petting, masturbation, and oral-genital sex. Sexual feelings may be expressed and satisfied through a wide range of activities and intimacy, in diverse interactions.

Fertility Awareness Method (FAM) **FAM** is based on avoiding coitus during the fertile phase of a woman's menstrual cycle. Ordinarily only one egg is released by the ovaries per month, and it lives about 24 hours unless it is fertilized. Sperm deposited in the vagina are apparently on the average capable of fertilizing an egg for about 48 to 72 hours; so conception theoretically can only occur during four days of any cycle. Predicting *which* four days these are is difficult. It is done either by the calendar method or by the temperature method. Recent information on cyclical changes of the cervical mucus has also been helpful in determining the time of ovulation. The calendar method is based on the knowledge that the average woman releases an egg 14 to 16 days before her next period begins. Few women menstruate with complete regularity, so a record of the menstrual cycle must be kept for 12 months, during which time some other method of birth control must be used. The first day of each period is counted as Day 1. To determine the first fertile, or "unsafe" day of the cycle, subtract 18 from the number of days in the shortest cycle. To determine the last unsafe day of the cycle, subtract 11 from the number of days in the longest cycle. The calendar method is illustrated in Figure 6-5.

A woman's body temperature drops slightly just before ovulation and rises slightly after ovulation. This fluctuation is the basis for the temperature method. A woman using the temperature method records her basal, or resting, body temperature (BBT) every morning before getting out of bed and before eating or drinking anything. Once the temperature pattern can be seen (usually after about three months), the period unsafe for coitus can be calculated as the interval from Day 5 (Day 1 is the first day of the period) until three days after the rise in BBT. To arrive at a shorter unsafe period, some women combine the calendar and the temperature methods, calculating the first unsafe day from the shortest cycle of the calendar chart and the last unsafe day as the third day after a rise in the BBT.

Also useful in predicting the fertile period are changes in the cervical secretions throughout the menstrual cycle. During the preovulatory phase, cervical mucus increases and is clear and slippery. At the time of ovulation some women can detect a slight change in the texture of the mucus and find that it is more likely to form an elastic thread when stretched between thumb and finger. After ovulation these secretions become cloudy and sticky and decrease in quantity. Infertile, safe days are likely to occur during the relatively dry days just before and after menstruation. (See Figure 6-6.) This is called the **Billings,** or **mucus, method.** These additional clues have been found helpful by some couples who rely on the Fertility Awareness Method (FAM). One possible problem that may interfere with this method is that vaginal infections or vaginal products or medication can also change cervical mucus.

FAM is not recommended for women who have very irregular cycles—about 15 percent of all menstruating women. Any woman for whom pregnancy would be a serious problem should not rely on the FAM alone, because the failure rate is high—150 to 300 pregnancies in 1,000 women during one year.

Withdrawal Probably the oldest known method of contraception, **withdrawal** is mentioned in the Book of Genesis. In this method, the male removes his penis from the vagina just before he ejaculates. This method has three advantages: it is free, requires no preparation, and is always available. For many people, these advantages are far outweighed by the disadvantages: the male has to overcome a powerful biological urge. The fear that withdrawal may

Figure 6-5 The Fertility Awareness Method (FAM) of contraception—how to calculate the "safe" and "unsafe" days for coitus.

Length of shortest cycle	First "unsafe" day after start of any menstrual period	Length of longest cycle	Last "unsafe" day after start of any menstrual period
20 days	2nd day	20 days	9th day
21 days	3rd day	21 days	10th day
22 days	4th day	22 days	11th day
23 days	5th day	23 days	12th day
24 days	6th day	24 days	13th day
25 days	7th day	25 days	14th day
26 days	8th day	26 days	15th day
27 days	9th day	27 days	16th day
28 days	10th day	28 days	17th day
29 days	11th day	29 days	18th day
30 days	12th day	30 days	19th day
31 days	13th day	31 days	20th day
32 days	14th day	32 days	21st day
33 days	15th day	33 days	22nd day
34 days	16th day	34 days	23rd day
35 days	17th day	35 days	24th day
36 days	18th day	36 days	25th day
37 days	19th day	37 days	26th day
38 days	20th day	38 days	27th day
39 days	21st day	39 days	28th day
40 days	22nd day	40 days	29th day

Prediction of "safe" and "unsafe" days for a woman whose menstrual cycle varies from 25 to 31 days over a 12-month period.

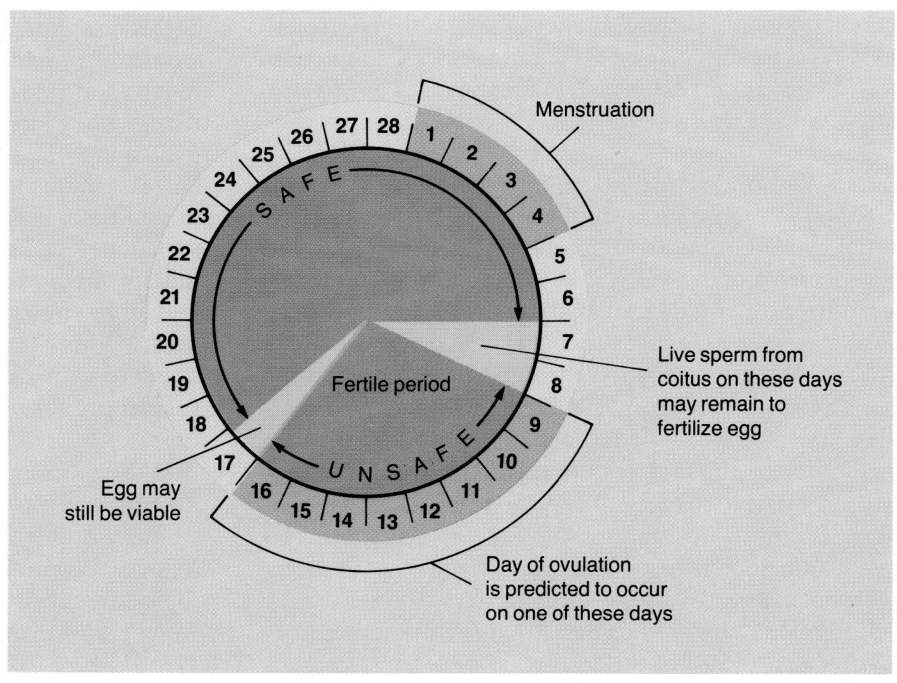

be too late can wreck sexual pleasure for both partners. Also, since in many societies a woman takes longer than a male does to reach orgasm, withdrawal before the woman's orgasm is likely and can leave the woman frustrated if she relies on coitus for satisfaction. And most important, the failure rate for withdrawal is very high: 200 to 300 pregnancies per 1,000 women during one year. One key factor in this high failure rate is the degree of self-control necessary. In addition, pre-ejaculatory fluid, which may contain viable sperm, is commonly secreted before actual ejaculation occurs.

Factors That Contribute to Failure Rates Over half of the pregnancies that occur in the United States are unintended. Many women who are at risk of unintended pregnancy use no contraception of any type. The percentage of those using no method is highest among teenagers who are sexually active and then decreases with age. Also important, however, is the fact that many couples who do practice contraception do not use the most effective methods or use them inconsistently (see Figure 6-7). For a listing of suggestions as to what the user can do to improve contraceptive effectiveness rates, see Table 6-2.

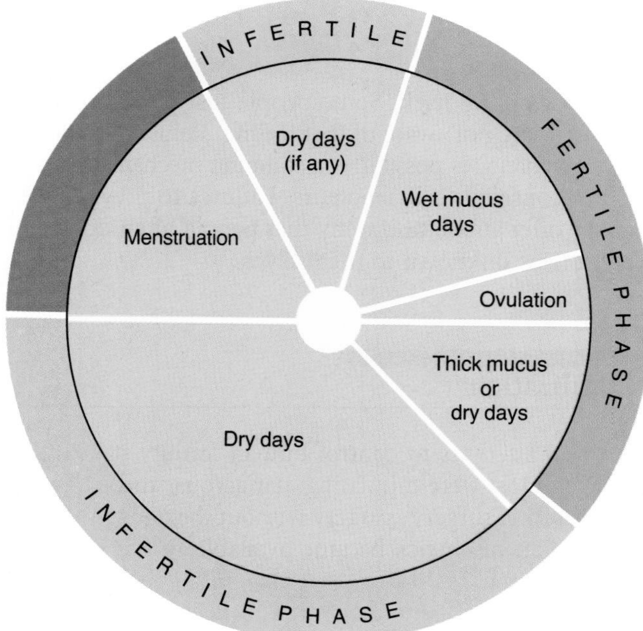

Source: Human Life and Natural Family Planning Foundation.

Figure 6-6 The Billings method relies solely on the presence and quality of cervical mucus to indicate fertile and infertile periods of the menstrual cycle. The beginning of the fertile period is indicated by the onset of mucus flow. The day of the "peak mucus symptom" is the last day of wet, slippery mucus, after which mucus thickens and disappears. The fertile period is presumed to last until four days after the peak symptom.

Table 6-2 What the User Can Do to Improve Contraception Effectiveness Rates

Method	Suggestions
Combination oral contraceptive	Follow pill-taking instructions carefully and consistently. Use a backup method such as foam or condoms during the first month.
IUD	Have IUD inserted by experienced clinician. Frequently check for IUD's position during the first few months. (User should feel thread in cervical opening but not the stem of the IUD.) Use a backup method such as foam or condoms during the first three months and, if desired, at mid-cycle thereafter.
Condom	Use with every act of intercourse. Put condom on penis before *any* penis-vagina contact. Leave space in tip of condom for semen. Remove carefully to avoid spillage. Avoid damage to condom; handle carefully. Avoid heat and Vaseline or other petroleum jelly. Do not use after two years. Buy a good brand (ask your pharmacist). Use foam along with condom.
Diaphragm and jelly	Use with every act of intercourse. Ask for thorough instruction with initial fitting. Have diaphragm fit checked every one to two years by an experienced clinician. Always use ample amounts of jelly or cream; add as necessary. Check position after insertion. Front rim must be behind pubic bone, and dome must cover cervix. Inspect regularly for defects or holes. Avoid use of Vaseline or perfumed powders, including talcum powder, as they can damage the latex and irritate the vagina.
Vaginal spermicides	Use with every act of intercourse. Follow instructions regarding time limits of effectiveness. Use ample amounts. When using foam, shake vigorously before use. Use condoms along with spermicide.
FAM	Combine calendar, temperature, and mucus methods.
Withdrawal	Avoid penis-vagina contact during secretion of pre-ejaculatory lubricating fluid (very difficult to detect). Use foam along with coitus interruptus.

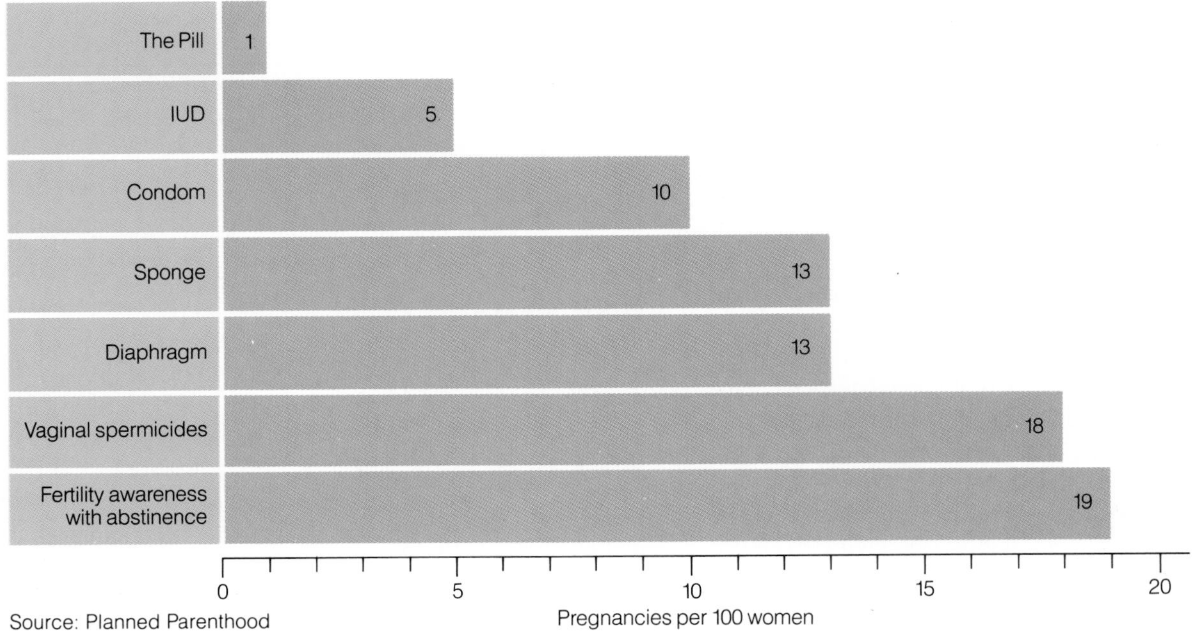

Figure 6-7 Relative use effectiveness of nonsurgical means of birth control.

Causes of failure to prevent unintended pregnancy seem to fall into two groups. The causes in the first group are related to the effectiveness of the method, what the user knows about the method, how he or she feels about it, the strength of motivation, and religious belief. The second group consists of more subtle psychological causes. People who say they do not want pregnancy often act in ways that seem designed to produce "accidents." Some teenagers may be motivated by a wish to use pregnancy and marriage as a springboard out of unpleasant home situations. Some people equate love with self-sacrifice and risk taking. For some people, fertility is a symbol of virility or femininity. For others, getting pregnant is a way of acting out unconscious hostility toward oneself or toward others. The wish to conceive sometimes seems to be part of the sex drive itself. Some people just plain want children but are not aware of that feeling. Refusing to believe that pregnancy is possible is a common mechanism among the unconscious self-saboteurs. Failures to prevent pregnancy offer ample testimony that people often do act out of motives unknown to themselves.

Exploring Your Emotions

Do you want to have children, or want to have more children? How strongly do you feel about this? What experience do you have with child care? What preparations do you consider necessary for someone planning to be (or willing to be) a parent?

Sterilization

Surgical attempts to control human fertility have a long history. Most were mutilating, dangerous, and ineffective until aseptic surgery (surgery without the danger of infection) and anesthetics became available in the late nineteenth century.

Sterilization is permanent, and it provides complete protection, with no further action needed at any time. For these reasons, it is becoming an increasingly popular method of birth control. At present it is the most commonly used method in the United States. It is especially popular among couples who have been married ten or more years, as well as among couples who have had all the children they intend.

An important consideration in choosing sterilization is that, in most cases, it cannot be reversed. Although the chances of restoring fertility are being increased by mod-

Sterilization Surgically altering the reproductive system to prevent pregnancy. Vasectomy is the procedure in males, tubal sterilization or hysterectomy in females.

Vasectomy Surgical severing of the ducts that carry sperm to the ejaculatory duct.

Vasa deferentia (*Vas deferens,* singular form) The two ducts that carry sperm to the ejaculatory duct.

---

ern surgical techniques, such operations are costly and pregnancy can never be guaranteed. Some couples choosing male sterilization are using sperm banks as a way of extending the option of childbearing.

Although some doctors will perform surgery for sterilization on request, most require a thorough discussion with both partners before the operation. Most doctors also recommend that people who have religious conflicts, psychiatric problems related to sex, or unstable marriages not be sterilized. Young couples with one or two children, who might later change their minds and want more, are also frequently advised not to undergo sterilization.

Male Sterilization or Vasectomy **Vasectomy** involves severing the **vasa deferentia,** two tiny ducts that transport sperm from the testicles to the seminal vesicles. The testicles continue to produce sperm, but the sperm are absorbed into the body. Since the testicles contribute only about one-tenth of the total seminal fluid, the actual quantity of ejaculate is only slightly reduced. Hormone output from the testicles apparently continues with very little change and secondary sex characteristics are not altered.

Vasectomy is ordinarily done in the doctor's office and takes about 30 minutes. The patient is instructed to present himself with all pubic hair shaved. After the scrotal region is washed with a surgical cleanser, a local anesthetic is injected into the skin of the scrotum and about the vasa. Small incisions are made at the upper end of the scrotum where it joins the body, and the vas deferens on each side is exposed, severed, and closed off. The incisions are then closed with sutures, and a small dressing is applied. (See Figure 6-8.)

As the local anesthetic wears off, the patient feels a dull ache in the surgical area and often in the lower abdomen. Pain and swelling are usually slight and can be relieved with an ice bag, aspirin, and use of a scrotal support. Bleeding and infection occasionally develop but are in most cases easily treated. Most men are ready to return to work in two days.

Men can have sex again as soon as they feel no further discomfort; for most men this means after about a week. Another method of contraception must be used for the first few weeks after vasectomy, however, because sperm produced before the operation may still be present in the semen. To make sure that sperm are no longer in the ejaculate and that another method of contraception is no longer necessary, a semen specimen should be examined under a microscope.

Recent investigations do not support an earlier hypothesis that a vasectomy may accelerate atherosclerosis (the formation of fat deposits that clog arteries). In fact, one very large-scale study found no long-range complications of any type following vasectomy and actually found lower death rates from cancer and heart disease among vasectomized men when comparing them to matched controls who had not been sterilized. The researchers concluded that perhaps the vasectomized men were healthier to start with in some way.

In about 1 percent of vasectomies, a severed vas rejoins itself, and sperm can again travel up through the duct and be ejaculated in the semen. Because of this possibility, some doctors advise that a semen specimen be examined yearly.

Although some surgeons report pregnancy rates of about 80 percent for partners of men who have their vasectomies reversed within ten years of the original procedure, most studies report considerably lower rates. In at least 50 percent of vasectomized men the process of absorbing sperm (instead of ejaculating it) results in antisperm antibodies that may interfere with later fertility. Other factors, such as length of time between the vasectomy and the reversal surgery, may also be important predictors of reversal success.

Figure 6-8 Vasectomy is a comparatively simple surgical procedure.

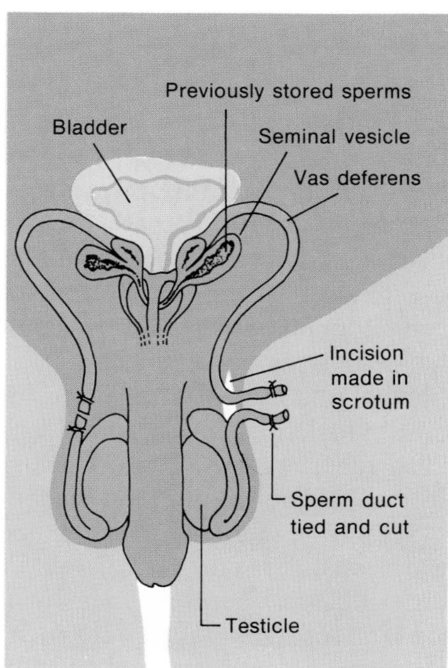

Attitudes Toward Birth Control

Here are some of the personal reasons why we [women] sometimes have trouble using birth control or don't even use it at all:

- We are embarrassed by, ashamed of, confused about our own sexuality.
- We cannot admit we might have or are having intercourse because we feel (or someone told us) it is wrong.
- We are romantic about sex—it has to be a passionate, spontaneous sharing, and birth control seems too premeditated, too clinical, and often too messy.
- We hesitate to inconvenience our sex partner.
- If we are using natural birth control, we sometimes have a hard time abstaining during our fertile days because we fear our partner will get angry and find sex elsewhere.
- We feel, "It can't happen to me. I won't get pregnant."
- We have questions about birth control and sex and don't know whom to talk with.
- We hesitate to go to a doctor or clinic and face the hurried, impersonal care or, if we are young or unmarried, the moralizing and disapproval that we feel likely to receive.
- We don't recognize our deep dissatisfactions with the method we are using and begin to use it haphazardly.
- We want a baby and can't admit it to ourselves. Or we feel tempted to get pregnant just to prove to ourselves that we are fertile, or to try to improve a shaky relationship.

What Can We Do?

Facing these many obstacles to our using birth control effectively, what can we do? First, we can learn for ourselves and teach one another about the available methods. By speaking openly and by carefully comparing experiences and knowledge, we can guide each other to competent doctors and reasonable methods. We can learn to recognize when a doctor is not sufficiently thorough in examinations or explanations, and support each other to ask for the attention we need. By talking together we can also get a better handle on the more subtle personal hassles we have with birth control. We can begin the long but worthwhile process of talking with men about birth control, so that they can no longer comfortably ignore their share in the responsibility. We can learn to be more accepting of our sexuality and join proudly together to insist that legislatures, courts, high schools, churches, doctors, research projects, clinics and drug companies change their attitudes and practices so that we can enjoy our sexuality without becoming pregnant. We can work to create self-help clinics and other alternative health care institutions where our needs for information, discussion and personal support in the difficult choice of birth control will be better met.

The Boston Women's Health Book Collective
Our Bodies, Ourselves

Female Sterilization The most common method of female sterilization involves severing or in some manner blocking the Fallopian tubes, thereby preventing the egg from reaching the uterus and the sperm from entering the tubes. Ovulation and menstruation continue, but the unfertilized eggs are released into the abdominal cavity and absorbed. Hormone production by the ovaries and secondary characteristics are not affected.

One method of **tubal sterilization** is accomplished by making a small incision in the abdominal wall, locating each Fallopian tube, bringing it into view, severing it, removing a small section, and tying or stapling shut the two ends. (See Figure 6-9.) Another method involves making the incision through the vaginal wall, an approach that leaves no visible scar but is associated with a higher complication rate. Also, some conditions such as obesity or recent pregnancy make this method difficult or impossible. Either a regional or a general anesthetic can be used with these two types of tubal sterilization, and the operation takes about thirty minutes. If no complications occur, many hospitals allow the patient to return to her home the same day. The operation can be performed shortly after a normal delivery, or in the case of Caesarian section immediately after the incision in the uterus is repaired.

Female sterilization by the standard abdominal or vaginal procedure is riskier than male sterilization. About 7 percent of the patients experience problems after the operation. Such problems arise mainly from the wound, infection, or bleeding. Serious complications are rare, and the death rate is low—especially when regional rather than general anesthesia is used.

An increasing number of tubal sterilizations are being done by a method called **laparoscopy**. A laparoscope, which is a tube containing a small light, is inserted through a small abdominal incision, and the surgeon looks through it to locate the Fallopian tubes. Instruments are passed

Tubal sterilization Severing or in some manner blocking the oviducts. This prevents ova (eggs) from reaching the uterus.

Laparoscopy Examining the internal organs by inserting a tube containing a small light through an abdominal incision.

Hysterectomy Total or partial surgical removal of the uterus.

either through the laparoscope or through a second small incision, and the two Fallopian tubes are cauterized (sealed off) by electrocautery. Either a regional or general anesthetic can be used, but a general anesthetic is more common. The operation takes 15 minutes and can be done without overnight hospitalization. Most women leave the hospital two to four hours after surgery. Complications, such as bowel injury and hemorrhage, occur in 0.1 to 7 percent of laparoscopic sterilizations. This figure varies widely depending on the experience of the surgeon and type of equipment available. The mortality rate is low.

Laparoscopy has approximately the same failure rate as standard tubal ligations: about 3 out of every 1,000 cases. Reversibility rates are 50–70 percent for all methods.

Complaints of long-term abdominal discomfort and menstrual irregularity have been reported following female sterilization, but these have been difficult to interpret. Most women are satisfied. The number of women who feel regret varies in follow-up studies, and this fact, too, is difficult to interpret. Regret, when it does appear, seems to be related to previous difficulties, initial doubts and reservations, feelings of being pressured by the spouse, or changes in marital and family circumstances.

Hysterectomy, removal of the uterus, is the preferred method of sterilization for only a small number of women, usually women with pre-existing menstrual problems. Because of the risks involved, hysterectomy is not recommended unless the patient has serious gynecologic problems such as disease or damage of the uterus and future surgery appears inevitable.

Figure 6-9 Tubal sterilization is more complex than vasectomy.

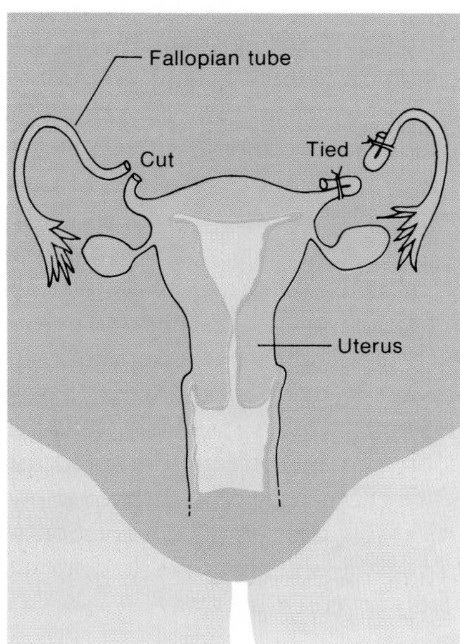

New Methods of Contraception

Even with all the improvements of recent years, the best of the present methods of birth control have drawbacks. The search still continues for the ideal method, the one that will be more effective, safer, cheaper, easier to use, more readily available, and acceptable to more people.

Many people place a high priority specifically on an increase in the male contraceptive alternatives. Throughout history, the responsibility for birth control has been assumed predominantly by women, partly because women have greater personal investment in preventing pregnancy with its many risks and the greater demands that childrearing places on women. Some women in some settings see complete control as crucial. More birth control options have been available for female use, because there are more ways to intervene in the female reproductive system. Another factor may be the continuing underrepresentation of women in medicine, scientific research, pharmaceutical management, the FDA, and other political forces. Participation by women and the expression of their needs regarding birth control has been limited in these areas.

Some new methods are currently considered very promising. Two methods, injection and implant, have actually been approved and made available for public use in several countries around the world. However, it appears unlikely that U.S. manufacturers will introduce any new methods in the near future, partly because preclinical safety testing is so expensive and because the number of liability claims is skyrocketing.

Long-acting Injectables Injections of progestin, a laboratory-made progesterone, every ninety days are almost 100 percent effective in preventing pregnancy. Progestins have several contraceptive effects: cervical mucus becomes thick and hampers the movement of sperm; transport of the egg through the tubes may be slowed down; changes in the uterine lining may prevent implantation; and subtle hormonal shifts may result in the inhibition of ovulation. This method still has disadvantages, however, including irregular menstrual bleeding patterns in the uterus and long delays (12 to 21 months) in the return of ovulatory cycles after injections are stopped. Less frequent injections of higher doses are also being tested.

Prostaglandins Naturally occurring chemicals, two of which induce abortion of the embryo or fetus when injected into the amniotic sac or inserted into the uterus.

Luteinizing Hormone-Releasing Hormone (LHRH) A naturally occurring compound in both sexes, triggers release of pituitary hormones that figure in ovulation and sperm formation.

Implants Two to six capsules that are 1 inch long and spaghetti-width are filled with progestin and inserted under the skin of the inner arm or thigh. They can provide protection for up to five years. Side effects are similar to those of long-acting injectable progestins. Fertility quickly returns, however, on implant removal.

Menstruation-inducing Pills The most developed of these pills is one known as RU 486, a drug that is expected to be approved for clinical use in Europe within a few years. RU 486 must be taken within ten days after a missed period to be effective. It works by preventing the uterus cells from absorbing progesterone. With the progesterone blocked, the uterus sheds its lining as it would with a normal period, and any fertilized egg is expelled along with the menstrual flow.

Vaginal Ring The vaginal ring resembles the rim of a diaphragm and is molded with a mixture of progestin and estrogen. The woman inserts the ring herself and wears it for three weeks, during which time the hormones are absorbed into her bloodstream, preventing ovulation. Menstruation follows removal, and then a new ring is inserted.

Chemical Contraceptives for Men Male and female hormones can interfere with sperm development in the male in a way similar to ovulation suppression in the female. However, effectiveness of these hormones is often unpredictable and side effects may include both the loss of libido (sex drive) and the development of female secondary sex characteristics, for example, enlarged breasts.

Gossypol, a derivative of cottonseed oil used for several years in China, also results in very low sperm counts. Reported side effects include disturbances in potassium metabolism and general weakness. Also, U.S. animal studies indicate that it may be carcinogenic.

Contraceptive Immunization Immunity to fertility has—rarely—occurred because a man has been (nonexperimentally) sensitized to his own sperm cells. He then produces antibodies that inactivate sperm as if they were a disease. Similarly, a woman could be sensitized against her own egg cells or against her partner's sperm cells. Experimentally, at least, the theory works, but widespread human testing cannot begin until several questions have been answered. How long the immunity lasts and how to control it are not yet known, and serious allergic reactions could be a life-threatening problem.

Reversible Sterilization Present methods of sterilization of both men and women are reversible 50–70 percent of the time. Several new techniques of sterilization are being studied in the hope that restoring fertility can be made easier and more predictable.

Female sterilization has been attempted by injecting liquid silicone into the Fallopian tubes, where it solidifies and forms a plug. In animal experiments, however, such plugs have been readily dislodged by normal muscle activity, so this method is not likely to be very effective.

In men, totally blocking sperm flow with removable clips and with various plugs has been tried, but both clips and plugs damaged the vasa, making restoration of fertility less likely. Recanalization of the vas, a phenomenon in which the sperm make a new path around the plug, has also occurred with plugs. Some of the plugs tested contain a tiny valve that can be opened manually or magnetically.

Even when tissue damage and recanalization can be prevented, researchers face another problem: some vasectomized men develop antibodies to their sperm, which may persist after vasectomy reversal.

Prostaglandins A new and promising use of **prostaglandins** is their application to tampons, which are inserted to bring on menstruation shortly after a period is missed. Prostaglandins tampons used regularly at the end of each cycle could induce menstruation each time whether or not the cycle had been fertile.

Luteinizing Hormone-Releasing Hormone (LHRH) LHRH, a naturally occurring compound in both men and women, acts on the pituitary gland, triggering the release of its hormones, which in turn play an essential role in sperm formation and ovulation. Synthetic analogs of LHRH, which are over 100 times as powerful as natural LHRH, are currently available. After these analogs are administered, the levels of pituitary hormones rise sharply, followed by a drop to subnormal levels, probably because the pituitary gland is overstimulated and exhausted. Once the low levels are established, it appears that in women (on whom most of the studies thus far have been completed) the pituitary-ovary cycle is effectively disrupted, and ovulation and menstruation stop temporarily. No immediate side effects have been detected. However, many questions regarding this complex interaction and its long-term effects remain, and any possible clinical application is undoubtedly several years away.

Take Action

Your answers to the Exploring Your Emotions questions in this chapter and your placement on the Awareness Ladder will, we hope, encourage you to begin a process of self-exploration and self-discovery that you will continue. Reflect on the entire chapter's content and ask yourself how each point relates to your own life. Then take action:

1. Consider the different methods of contraception. In your Take Action notebook, rank the methods according to how they best suit your particular lifestyle. Take into account such considerations as how often you have sexual intercourse, cost requirements, and convenience.
2. Consider what health risks you or your partner takes (or would take) by using a particular form of birth control. For example, if you smoke and are female and are taking the pill, you are running increased risk of a future heart attack or stroke. Make a list of the different birth control methods, and indicate whether they carry any additional risk for you or your partner. Don't forget to include the risk of pregnancy. Compare this list with your list in Item 1.
3. List the positive behaviors and attitudes that help you adhere to your beliefs about birth control. How can you strengthen those behaviors? Also list behaviors and attitudes that block your beliefs and actions. Consider each of these behaviors and attitudes and decide which ones you can change in order to improve.
4. Before leaving this chapter, review the statements that open the chapter. Have your feelings or values changed? Are you now better equipped to handle the complex and very human problems associated with birth control?

Selected References

Atkinson, L. E., R. Lincoln, and J. D. Forrest. 1986 (January–February). The next contraceptive revolution. *Family Planning Perspectives* 18(1):19–26.

The Cancer and Steroid Hormone Study Group. 1986 (August 14). Oral contraceptive use and the risk of breast cancer. *New England Journal of Medicine* 315(7):405–11.

Darney, Philip D. 1984 (June). What's new in contraception? *Contemporary OB/GYN* 23(6):117–37.

DeStefano, F., J. A. Perlman, H. B. Peterson, and E. L. Diamond. 1985 (August). Long-term risk of menstrual disturbances after tubal sterilization. *American Journal of Obstetrics and Gynecology* 152(7):835–41.

Edelman, D. A., S. L. McIntyre, and J. Harper. 1984 (December 1). A comparative trial of the Today contraceptive sponge and diaphragm. *American Journal of Obstetrics and Gynecology* 150(7):869–76.

Forrest, Jacqueline D. 1986 (March–April). The end of IUD marketing in the United States: What does it mean for American women? *Family Planning Perspectives* 18(2):52–57.

Huezo, Carlos. 1985 (December). Oral contraceptives and cancer of the reproductive organs. *International Planned Parenthood Federation Medical Bulletin* 19(6):3–4.

Population Information Program—The Johns Hopkins University. 1985 (May). Minilaparotomy and laparoscopy: Safe, effective, and widely used. *Population Reports,* Series C, No. 9, p. 148.

Recommended Readings

Boston Women's Health Book Collective. 1984. *The New Our Bodies, Ourselves.* New York: Simon & Schuster.
Comprehensive paperback, written from a woman's viewpoint. Broad coverage of many women's health concerns, with an emphasis on psychological, as well as physical factors. A favorite for many years. Periodically updated.

Family Planning Perspectives (journal published bimonthly). New York: Alan Guttmacher Institute.
An excellent journal focused entirely on family planning issues. A good source for latest research findings. Some articles are quite technical (science based and statistics oriented), but all are very readable.

Hatcher, R. A., F. J. Guest, F. H. Stewart, G. K. Stewart, J. Trussell, S. Cerel, and W. Cates. 1986. *Contraceptive Technology 1986–1987.* New York: Irvington.
A compact, reliable source of up-to-date information on contraception, with a focus on the technological aspects, rather than the psychological. The information is somewhat geared toward health care providers, but suitable for all readers. Many references and sources of information are included. Updated every two years.

Chapter 7

Contents

Rate Yourself

Your Attitudes about Abortion Read the following statements carefully. Choose the one in each section that best describes you at this moment and circle its number. When you have chosen one statement for each section, add the numbers and record your total score. Find your position on the Awareness Ladder.

5 Well educated about abortion laws
4 Knowledgeable about abortion laws
3 Knows that abortion is legal
2 Unfamiliar with abortion laws
1 Believes that abortion is unlawful

5 Openly discusses abortion
4 Discusses abortion with friends
3 Avoids discussing abortion
2 Resists discussing abortion
1 Resents discussing abortion

5 Can argue both sides of the abortion issue
4 Has bias for one side but is sympathetic to the other
3 Has bias for one side and is unsympathetic to the other
2 Feels strongly there is only one right position to take about abortion
1 Feels angry toward those who take an opposite position

5 Considers abortion a very serious issue
4 Considers abortion a serious issue
3 Considers abortion a political issue
2 Doesn't consider abortion to be an issue worth considering
1 Gives little or no thought to abortion

5 Educates others about abortion issues
4 Would vote on abortion, given the opportunity
3 Would leave abortion to the legislators
2 Would spend little or no time dealing with abortion issues
1 Abortion issues are near the bottom of priorities

Total Score ______

Abortion

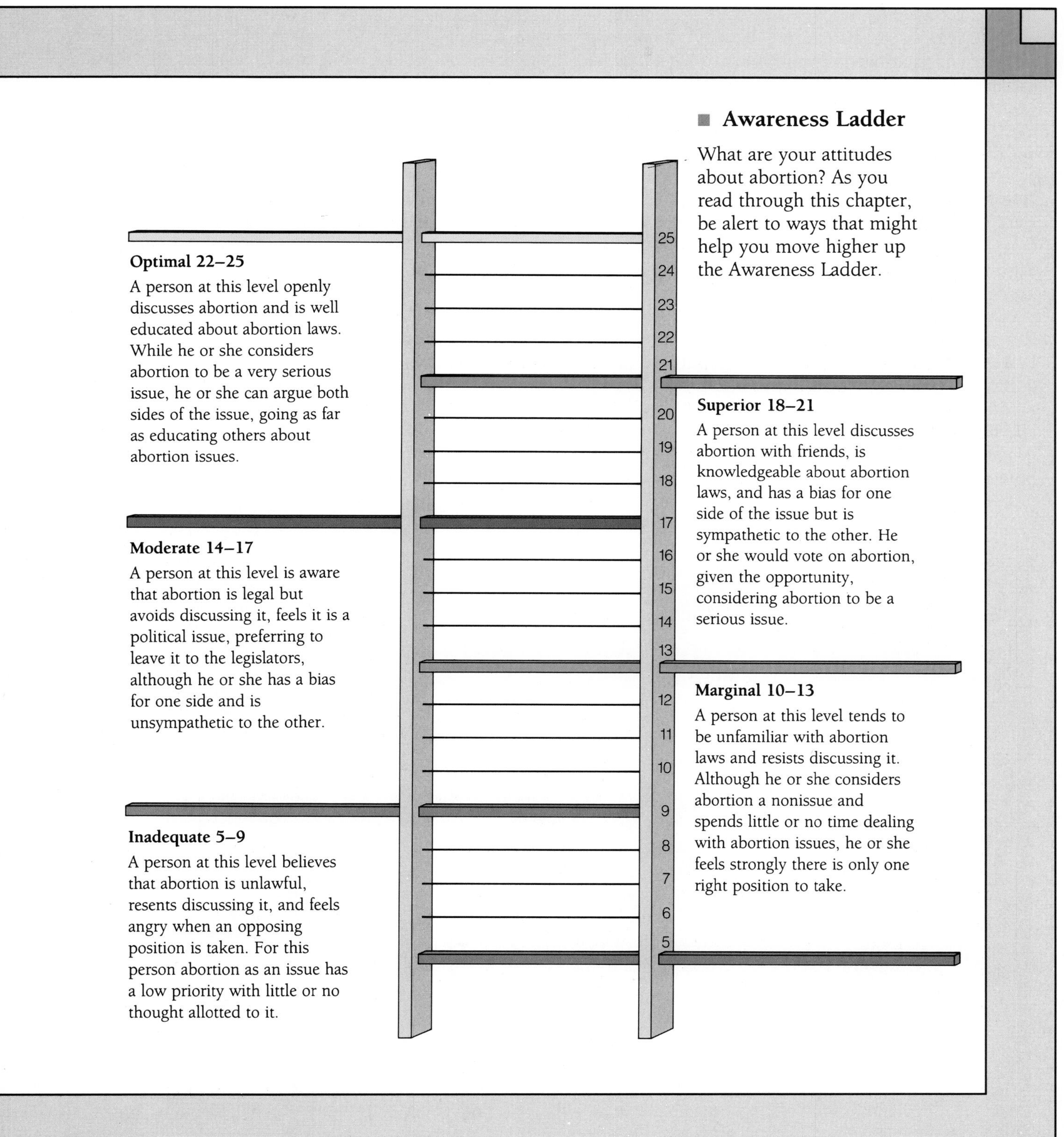
Awareness Ladder
What are your attitudes about abortion? As you read through this chapter, be alert to ways that might help you move higher up the Awareness Ladder.
Optimal 22–25
A person at this level openly discusses abortion and is well educated about abortion laws. While he or she considers abortion to be a very serious issue, he or she can argue both sides of the issue, going as far as educating others about abortion issues.
Superior 18–21
A person at this level discusses abortion with friends, is knowledgeable about abortion laws, and has a bias for one side of the issue but is sympathetic to the other. He or she would vote on abortion, given the opportunity, considering abortion to be a serious issue.
Moderate 14–17
A person at this level is aware that abortion is legal but avoids discussing it, feels it is a political issue, preferring to leave it to the legislators, although he or she has a bias for one side and is unsympathetic to the other.
Marginal 10–13
A person at this level tends to be unfamiliar with abortion laws and resists discussing it. Although he or she considers abortion a nonissue and spends little or no time dealing with abortion issues, he or she feels strongly there is only one right position to take.
Inadequate 5–9
A person at this level believes that abortion is unlawful, resents discussing it, and feels angry when an opposing position is taken. For this person abortion as an issue has a low priority with little or no thought allotted to it.
25
24
23
22
21
20
19
18
17
16
15
14
13
12
11
10
9
8
7
6
5

Abortion The premature expulsion or removal of an embryo or fetus from the uterus.

In the United States today, few issues are as complex and emotion-filled as abortion. The subject is not only complicated and controversial from a legal or a moral perspective, but it is often even more of a dilemma for the woman or couple considering it in a personal sense. For most people, many serious questions arise about abortion, questions that have no objective and easy answers.

Current Views on Abortion

The following paragraphs present various perspectives on abortion. The word **abortion**, by official or strict definition means the expulsion of a fetus from the uterus before it is sufficiently developed to survive. As commonly used, however, *abortion* refers only to those expulsions that are artificially induced by mechanical means or drugs, and *miscarriage* is the word generally used for a spontaneous abortion, one that occurs naturally with no causal intervention. In this chapter, the word *abortion* will be used to mean a deliberately induced abortion.

Legal Status Abortion has been the center of continual legal debate since 1973 when the U.S. Supreme Court made abortion legal in the landmark case of *Roe vs. Wade*. To replace the restrictions most states imposed at that time, the justices devised new standards to govern abortion decisions. They divided pregnancy into three parts, giving a pregnant woman less choice about abortion as she advances toward full term. In the first trimester, the abortion decision must be left to the judgment of the pregnant woman and her physician. During the second trimester, similar rights remain but a state may regulate factors that protect the health of the woman, such as type of facility used. In the third trimester, when the fetus is viable (capable of survival outside of the uterus), a state may regulate and even bar all abortions except those considered necessary to preserve the mother's life or health.

Since 1973, various campaigns have been waged to overturn the Supreme Court decision and to ban abortions by amending the U.S. Constitution. In addition, many other forms of increased abortion regulation have been introduced into legislative bodies at the local, state, and

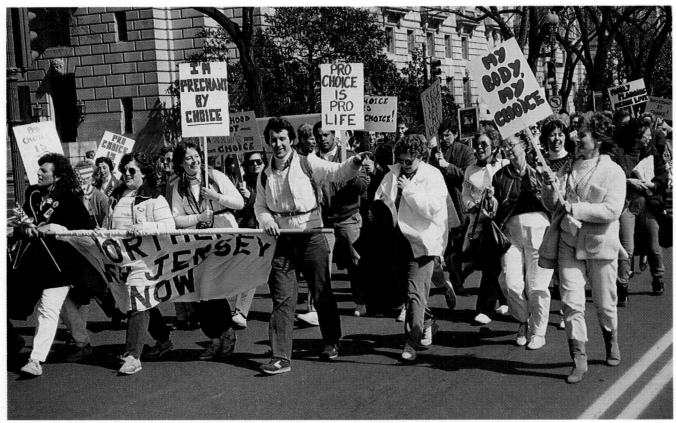

Paul Conklin

national levels. Many states have imposed regulations to restrict governmental funding of abortions, but most other regulations (such as those that would require waiting periods, detailed descriptive information, and parental or spousal consent) have been considered repeatedly and rejected in the majority of cases. The U.S. Supreme Court, which has heard arguments on abortion cases nearly every year, has continued to uphold its 1973 decision. With the presidential appointments of conservative justices in the mid-1980s, however, the Court's vote in favor of abortion rights, originally seven to two in 1973, has dwindled to a probable five-four lineup. Significant legal changes may well be in store.

Moral Positions Along with the legal debates has been an ongoing controversy between "pro-life" and "pro-choice" groups regarding the ethics of abortion, what is right and what is wrong in a moral sense. Central to the pro-life position is the belief that the fertilized egg must be valued as a human being from the moment of conception, and abortion at any time is equivalent to murder. This group holds that any woman who has sexual intercourse knows that pregnancy is a possibility, and should she willingly have intercourse and get pregnant she is morally obligated to carry the pregnancy through. Pro-life followers encourage adoption for women who feel they are unable to raise the child, and point out how many couples are seeking babies for adoption. Pro-lifers do not see the availability of legal abortion as essential to women's well-being, but view it instead as having an overall destructive effect on our traditional morals and values.

By contrast, the pro-choice viewpoint holds that distinctions must be made between the stages of fetal life and that preserving the fetus of early gestation is not always the ultimate moral concern. Members of this group maintain that women must have the freedom to decide whether and when to have children; they argue that pregnancy can result from contraceptive failure or other factors out of a woman's control. When pregnancy does occur, pro-choice individuals believe that the most moral decision possible must be determined according to each individual situation, and that in some cases greater injustice would result

Exploring Your Emotions

What kinds of restrictions, if any, would you place on the availability of abortions? What kinds of moral and ethical considerations do you feel must be weighed and balanced?

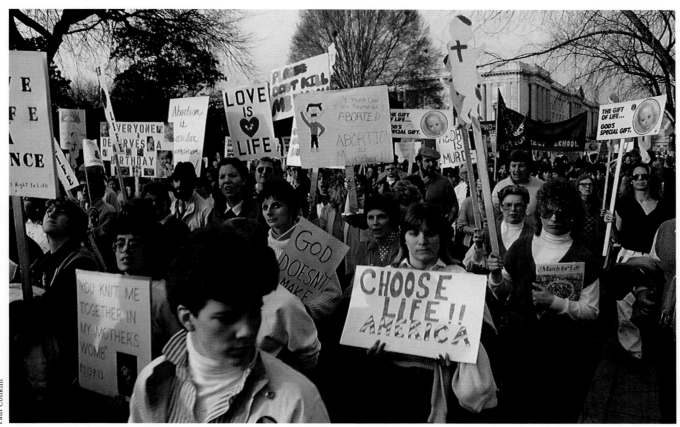

Paul Conklin

Amniocentesis Withdrawal of fluid from the amniotic sac.

if abortion were not an option. If legal abortions were not available, pro-choice supporters say, "back-alley shops" with their many health risks, as well as the births of unplanned children, would again grow in number.

Some individuals strongly identify exclusively with either the pro-life or the pro-choice stance, but many people have moral beliefs that are blurred, less defined, and in some cases a mixture of the two. A common assumption is that all religious organizations and individuals adhere to the pro-life position. This notion can be misleading. Although some generalizations can be made, moral positions regarding abortion can vary widely among religious believers just as they can differ markedly among individuals who consider themselves nonreligious.

Public Opinion In general, U.S. public opinion on abortion is somewhat flexible and seems to change depending on the specific situation. Many individuals approve of legal abortion as an option when destructive health or welfare consequences could result from continuing pregnancy, but they do not advocate abortion as a simple way out of an inconvenient situation. Overall, most U.S. adults continue to approve of legal abortion; surveys indicate little change since 1972. A spectrum of 1985 polls also gives a general indication of approval. (See Figure 7-1.) But this public support does not extend to all circumstances; the wording of the poll takers' questions seems crucial. Many people feel some cases are ambiguous.

For example, people who feel that abortion should be available in early pregnancy often question at which stage in later pregnancy the fetus's rights should take precedence over the woman's rights. The 1973 U.S. Supreme Court decision considered viability the key criterion in establishing the point beyond which a woman's right to choose abortion becomes markedly restricted. In 1973, viability was generally considered to be about twenty-six to twenty-eight weeks. Today it is about twenty-four weeks, with isolated cases of survival at twenty-three weeks. As neonatal intensive care units continue to advance technologically, the point at which viability is common may be lowered still further (although with diminished quality of life in some cases). Thus questions that center on the timing of fetal rights may need to be re-evaluated.

Other individuals associate fetal rights not with viability but with earlier developmental characteristics such as onset of heartbeat, brain size, and nervous system maturity. *The Silent Scream,* a widely shown film that used computer-enhanced ultrasound images, purports to depict a twelve-week-old fetus "screaming in pain" during an abortion procedure, attributing a fully human response to the fetus. Critics contend that the film was manipulated, with portions of the footage being sped up to project the illusion of a fetus thrashing in terror. Experts in fetal medicine have refuted the film's medical premises, stating that at twelve weeks fetal responses are simply reflex activity and that brain and nervous systems are insufficiently developed to feel pain.

Still other individuals argue that the embryo becomes a human being at the point of individuation or twinning, which occurs two to three weeks after conception. (Before that time, the embryo has not yet differentiated into either a single or an identical twin pregnancy.) Others believe that the moment of conception is the only critical point to consider. For them, all other developmental stages are irrelevant to the abortion debate. As can be seen from such wide variation of opinion, objective measures of humanness and clear-cut guidelines regarding fetal rights are elusive, and decisions ambiguous.

Although opinions vary as to whether, or when, in pregnancy, abortion rights should be tightly regulated by law, most people agree that abortions done later in pregnancy present more difficulties in personal, medical, philosophical, and social terms. Who are the women who have late abortions? Of all abortions done after the twenty-first week of gestation, 44 percent are performed on teenagers. Possible explanations include teenagers' ignorance, denial, fear, and lack of supportive family or friends. Other typical recipients of late abortions include poor women who may have more difficulty finding suitable facilities as well as necessary funds, and premenopausal women who fail to recognize a delayed period as pregnancy. Another small group of women who may seek late abortion are those who have learned through **amniocentesis** (the withdrawal and analysis of amniotic fluid) that the fetus is suffering from a specific abnormality, such as Down's syndrome. Because the results of this test are not available until the nineteenth or twentieth week of pregnancy, abortion, if chosen, is necessarily delayed. (Chorionic villi biopsy, a genetic diagnosis technique that can be performed in the first trimester, may become available soon. However, this technique does not diagnose neural tube defects and also carries more risk for the fetus.)

Personal Considerations For the pregnant woman who is considering abortion, the usual legal and moral arguments may sound quite meaningless as she attempts to weigh the many short- and long-term ramifications for all lives directly concerned. If she chooses abortion, can she accept that decision in terms of her own religious and moral beliefs? What are her long-range feelings likely to be regarding this decision? What are her partner's feelings regarding abortion, and how will she deal with his

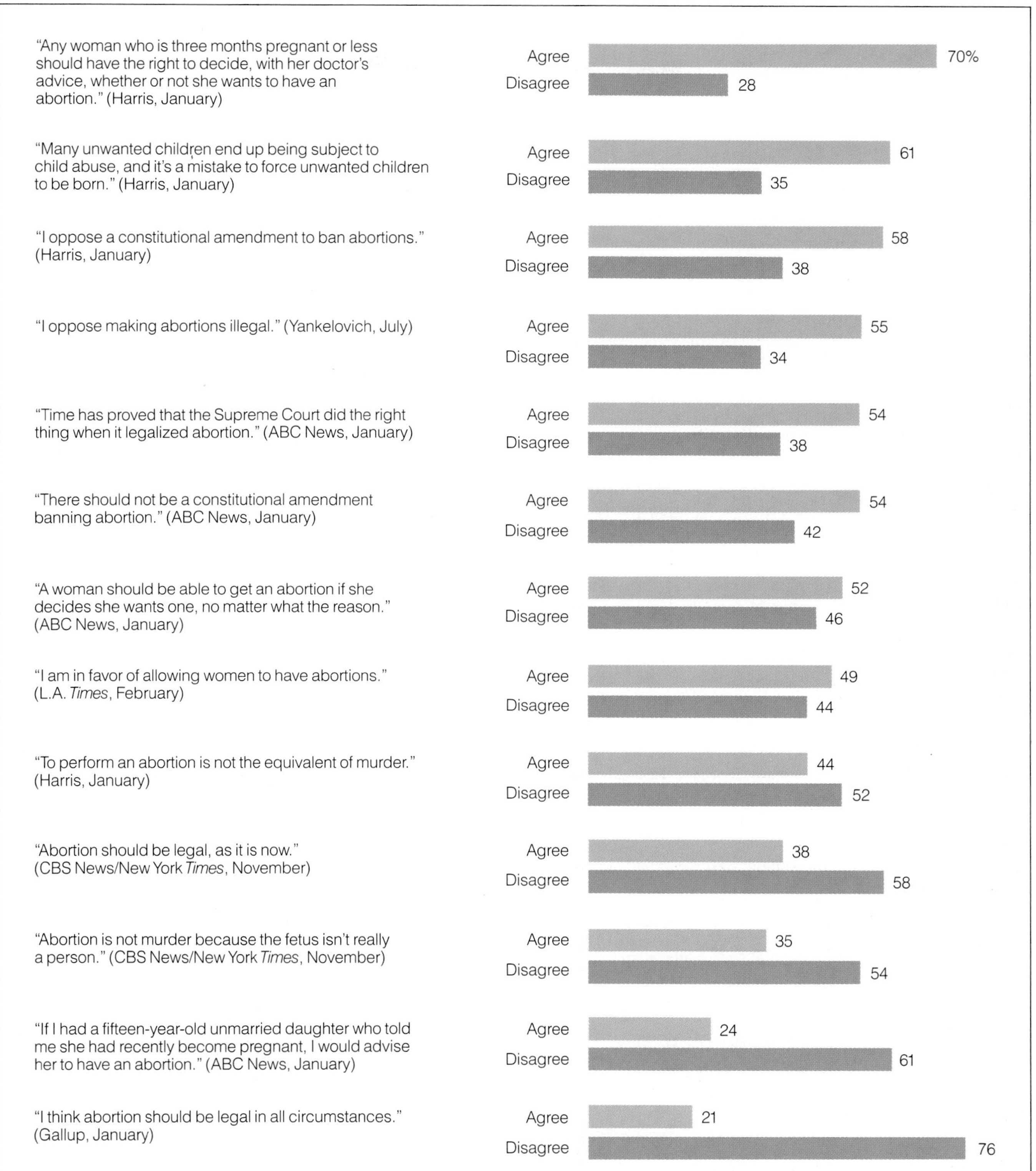

"Any woman who is three months pregnant or less should have the right to decide, with her doctor's advice, whether or not she wants to have an abortion." (Harris, January)
Agree 70%
Disagree 28
"Many unwanted children end up being subject to child abuse, and it's a mistake to force unwanted children to be born." (Harris, January)
Agree 61
Disagree 35
"I oppose a constitutional amendment to ban abortions." (Harris, January)
Agree 58
Disagree 38
"I oppose making abortions illegal." (Yankelovich, July)
Agree 55
Disagree 34
"Time has proved that the Supreme Court did the right thing when it legalized abortion." (ABC News, January)
Agree 54
Disagree 38
"There should not be a constitutional amendment banning abortion." (ABC News, January)
Agree 54
Disagree 42
"A woman should be able to get an abortion if she decides she wants one, no matter what the reason." (ABC News, January)
Agree 52
Disagree 46
"I am in favor of allowing women to have abortions." (L.A. *Times*, February)
Agree 49
Disagree 44
"To perform an abortion is not the equivalent of murder." (Harris, January)
Agree 44
Disagree 52
"Abortion should be legal, as it is now." (CBS News/New York *Times*, November)
Agree 38
Disagree 58
"Abortion is not murder because the fetus isn't really a person." (CBS News/New York *Times*, November)
Agree 35
Disagree 54
"If I had a fifteen-year-old unmarried daughter who told me she had recently become pregnant, I would advise her to have an abortion." (ABC News, January)
Agree 24
Disagree 61
"I think abortion should be legal in all circumstances." (Gallup, January)
Agree 21
Disagree 76

Figure 7-1 Abortion: The Spectrum of Opinion, 1985

responses? Does she have a supportive relative or friend who will help her through this time of emotional adjustment? Which medical facility offering abortions would be most suitable for her? What about transportation and costs? (See Figure 7-2 for a profile of women who choose abortion.)

For the woman who decides against abortion and chooses instead to continue the pregnancy, there are other questions. If she decides to raise the child herself, will she have the critical resources to do it well? Is a supportive, lasting relationship with her partner likely? If not, how does she feel about being a single parent? Are family members available to help with the many demands of child rearing? If she is young, what will the effects be on her own growth? Will she be able to continue with her educational and other personal goals? What about the ongoing financial responsibilities?

If the pregnant woman considers adoption, she will have to try to predict what her emotional responses will be throughout the full-term pregnancy and the adoption process. What are her long-range feelings likely to be? What is the best setting for her during her pregnancy? How can she best maintain continuity with the rest of her life and her long-term goals? Which adoption facility is likely to make the most suitable arrangements for her and her baby? A public or a private agency? Is anonymity between the adoptive parents and herself desirable or not? Does she have someone she trusts to help her with these difficult decisions?

Current Trends

Clearly, all responses to unintended pregnancy can be difficult, including abortion, and especially late abortion. Fortunately, with the increased accessibility to legalized abortion, the rate of late abortions has dropped steadily in recent years. At present, fewer than 1 percent of all abortions are performed at more than twenty weeks and fewer than 9 percent at more than twelve weeks. Also, the overall abortion rate, which rose during most of the 1970s and leveled off around 1979, fell significantly between 1982 and 1984 (see Figure 7-3). With greater public interest and attention, the need and demand for abortions could be decreased much more.

We hope the recent surge of public interest in sexual behavior (largely due to fear of sexually transmitted diseases) will lead to more open discussion regarding sexuality and the wide variety of human responses to this basic drive. With more communication and broader understanding of personal needs (including needs for intimacy and closeness), individuals and couples could perhaps choose more wisely the social and sexual behavior

Figure 7-2 What Kind of Women Choose to Have Abortions: A Social and Economic Profile. When the time comes to make the decision, the social and economic experience of the mother may well be the primary factor in her choice. One of the most complicated and disturbing questions raised in the raging national debate is which women with unwanted pregnancies would suffer most under a strong antiabortion law.

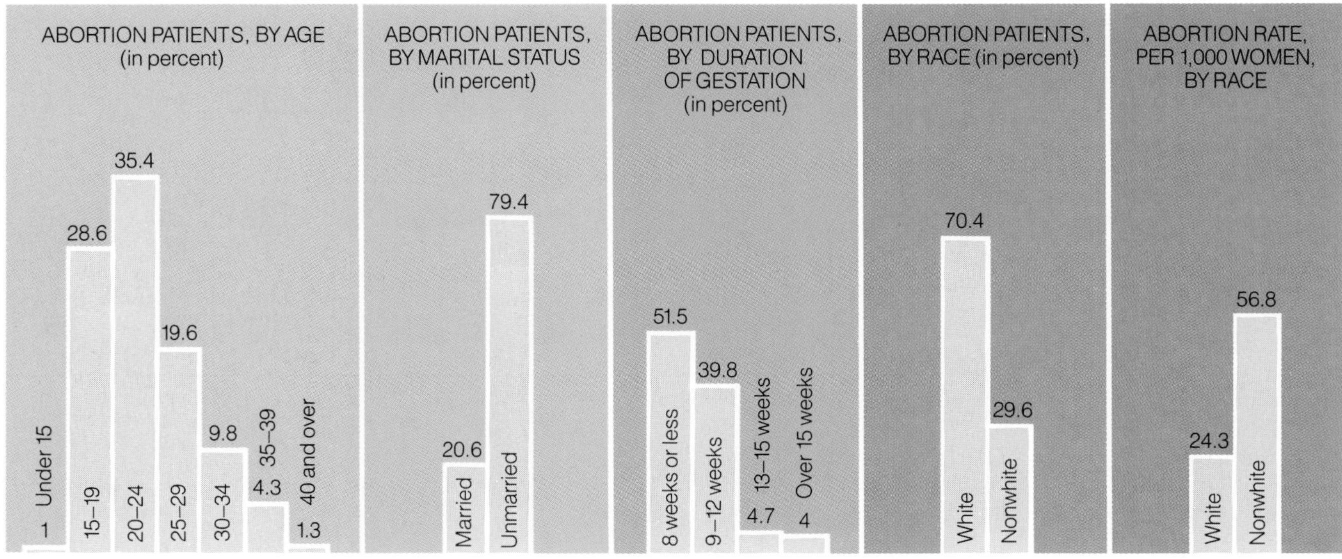

Abortifacients Agent or substance that produces abortion.

Menstrual extraction The vacuum aspiration of uterine contents shortly after a missed period.

Vacuum aspiration Also called *suction curettage,* this procedure involves removal of the embryo or fetus by means of suction.

Dilation and curettage (D & C) Dilation of the cervix and scraping of the uterus to remove the embryo or fetus or for other medical conditions of the uterus.

that would meet those needs most positively, both in the short and the long run. For those who choose to include sexual intercourse as part of their relationships, birth control should be effectively used (see Chapter 6).

Methods of Abortion

"Morning after" pills and IUDs inserted immediately after unprotected sexual relations are generally not considered **abortifacients** (agents that produce abortion) from a medical viewpoint, because they act before implantation of the fertilized egg, should one be present. Therefore, these topics are not discussed here, but are covered in Chapter 6.

Menstrual Extraction **Menstrual extraction** (or regulation), developed in the early 1970s, is the vacuum aspiration of uterine contents shortly after a missed period. It was originally defined as a procedure to be done up to the forty-second day after the last menstrual period and before the absence or presence of a pregnancy was confirmed. Initially, menstrual extraction was seen as safe, cost effective, and as especially suitable for those women uncomfortable with the notion of abortion. Complication rates, including incomplete evacuation, infection, and continuing pregnancy, were higher than expected, however, and menstrual extraction is now rarely performed in the United States. Also, today's pregnancy tests are accurate at a much earlier time, with some blood tests being reliable even before a missed period.

Vacuum Aspiration **Vacuum aspiration** (also called suction curettage), first developed in China in 1958, has rapidly become the preferred method for abortions up to the twelfth week of pregnancy. It can be done quickly, and the risk of hemorrhage or other complications is small. It is usually done on an outpatient basis.

A sedative may be given, along with a local anesthetic. A speculum, a device used to open the vaginal entrance, is inserted into the vagina, and the cervix is cleansed with a surgical solution. The cervix is dilated and a suction curette—a specially designed hollow tube—is then inserted into the uterus. The curette is attached to the rubber tubing of an electric pump, and suction is applied. (See Figure 7-4.) In about 20 to 30 seconds the uterus is emptied. Moderate cramping is common during evacuation. To ensure that no fragments of tissue are left in the uterus, the doctor usually scrapes the uterine lining with a metal curette, an instrument with a spoonlike tip. The entire operation takes only five to ten minutes.

After a few hours in a recovering area, the woman can return home. She is usually instructed not to douche, have coitus, or use tampons for the first week or two after the abortion, and to return for a two-week postabortion examination. This examination is important to verify that the abortion was complete and that no signs of infection are present.

Dilation and Curettage In **dilation and curettage** (commonly called **D & C**) the embryo and placenta are removed by surgical instruments rather than by suction. After the cervix is dilated, a curette is used to scrape the tissues from the wall of the uterus; an ovum forceps, a long grasping instrument, is also used. Because a D & C

Figure 7-3 A Decade of Choice
Ten years after abortion on demand became legal, the number of procedures had begun to level off.

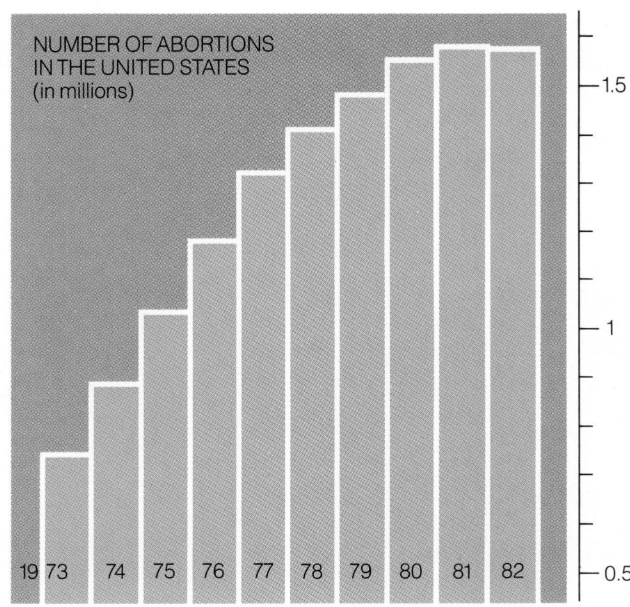

Dilation and evacuation (D & E) The method of abortion most commonly used between 13 and 15 weeks of pregnancy. Following dilation of the cervix, both vacuum aspiration and instruments are used as needed.

Amniotic sac/Amniotic fluid The bag of watery fluid lining the uterus, which envelops and protects the fetus.

Hysterotomy A modified Caesarean section in which the fetus is removed.

Caesarean section A surgical incision through the abdominal wall and uterus; performed when vaginal delivery of a baby is not advisable.

---

takes longer, causes a greater loss of blood, and requires a longer recovery period, it has been largely replaced by vacuum aspiration.

Dilation and Evacuation **Dilation and evacuation** (often referred to as **D & E**) is the method most commonly used between thirteen and fifteen weeks of pregnancy and is now preferred by some physicians up to and past twenty weeks. This procedure combines and extends both vacuum aspiration and D & C, using greater cervical dilation, larger suction curettes, and heavier forceps as required. Intravenous fluid that includes a medication to increase uterine contractions and thus limit blood loss is often given during or after the procedure. Either local or general anesthesia is used. Both the time required for the D & E and the recovery time are slightly longer than for vacuum aspiration.

Medical Methods After the fifteenth week of pregnancy, one of the following medical methods is used in many centers because suction becomes more difficult. With saline instillation, the oldest of these methods, a local anesthetic is given, and a long needle is inserted through the abdominal and uterine walls into the **amniotic sac. Amniotic fluid** is drained from the sac and replaced with an equal amount of 20 percent salt solution. The injection must be made slowly and with great care to avoid introducing the solution into the woman's circulation. The woman must be fully awake to report pain or other symptoms.

The death of the fetus, which occurs immediately due to the disruption in chemical balances essential to life, is followed by labor and delivery within a day or two. The uterus is scraped to reduce chances of infection or hemorrhage. The recovery period is slightly longer than for suction (vacuum) curettage, and complications are more frequent.

Prostaglandins, a group of naturally occurring chemicals, also bring on abortion, apparently by stimulating contractions of the uterus. They can be injected into the amniotic sac or inserted through the cervical canal into the uterus. Their major shortcoming is their effect on the muscles of the digestive tract, which produces nausea, vomiting, and diarrhea. Refined prostaglandins have fewer side effects than natural ones. Another chemical, urea, is often used in combination with prostaglandins to facilitate labor.

Hysterotomy Abortion by **hysterotomy** is a major surgical procedure (a modified **Caesarean section**) usually performed under a general anesthetic, although a spinal anesthetic may be effective. Incisions are made in the walls

Figure 7-4 Vacuum aspiration takes only five to ten minutes and can be performed up to the twelfth week of pregnancy.

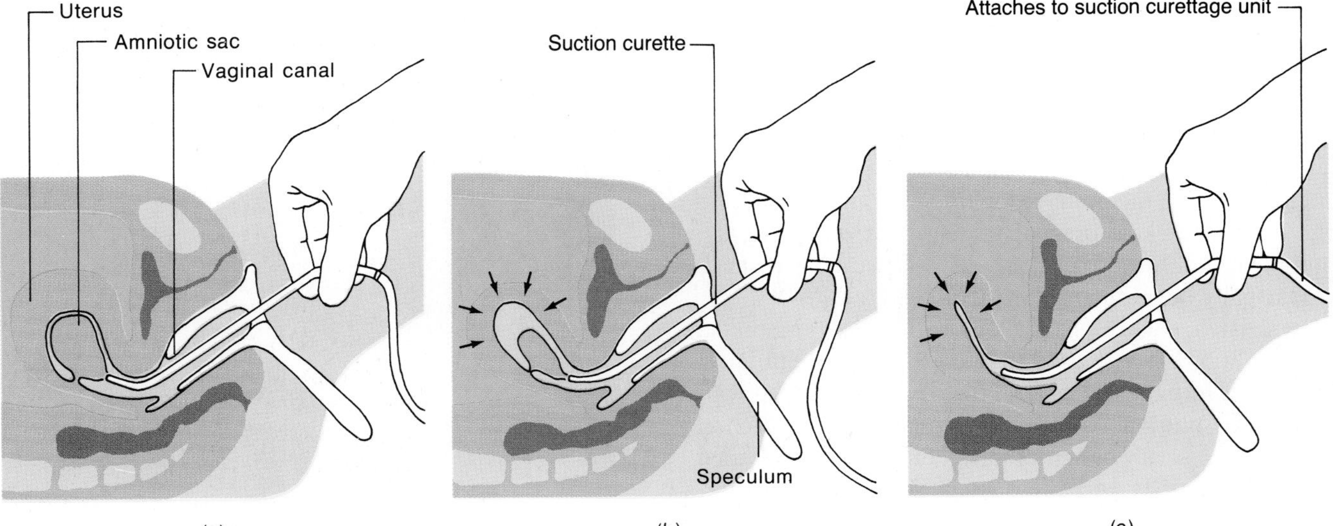

Personal Decisions about Abortion

When unintended pregnancy occurs, decisions regarding the best possible solution will vary according to each personal and social situation. The following examples show how some women in a variety of circumstances responded.

Stephanie

Stephanie hadn't been careless—the contraceptive device she'd used had failed. "I want a baby in what I think is a healthy circumstance," she said. "I don't have a husband. I don't have a man who really wants this child. Russ will see me through an abortion, but he's walking out of my life when it's over."

After the abortion: "I felt abandoned. I wanted a lot of hugging and to know that somebody cared." The father had offered to accompany her to the clinic where she had her abortion and to spend the weekend with her, but he didn't behave lovingly. "Russ couldn't deal with the experience and was quite cruel, really. I suppose he was frightened, but that didn't make it any easier for me. He stayed with me, but when I wanted to be held, he said, 'Don't hug me; we're just friends.' Considering I'd just gone through an abortion in order not to have this person's child, I thought that was a ludicrous thing to say."

Maggie

Maggie said she felt like a "bad girl" when she found out she was pregnant and didn't know which of two men was the father. "I guess my religious background came through. I felt that I was being punished for having sex even though I didn't rationally believe my behavior was wrong. The guilt was pretty bad, and I really needed someone to tell me I was all right."

Maggie's closest girlfriend went to the clinic and stayed with her after the abortion. Like all women who have had abortions, Maggie was in need of comforting. "Eventually that 'bad girl' feeling wears off, but it takes time."

Karen

Karen chose not to have an abortion, but to give her baby up for adoption. When the Bakerfields arrived at the hospital and walked down the corridor, Karen held out her baby to them. The baby was wearing a T-shirt with the inscription, "I love my Mommy and Daddy!" Then the Bakerfields and Karen prayed together, and Karen formally relinquished her child to their care.

"I was so happy to give life to someone else to start a family," Karen said. "That excited me. It still excites me." Karen has told her story to a number of high school audiences, and generally they are puzzled about her decision. What Karen tries to communicate is that love motivated her.

"I never had a father, really, growing up," she said. "By giving my baby to the Bakerfields, I gave her a father. She needed that."

Laura

After eight pregnancy tests and eight personal denials, my father confronted me by asking if I was pregnant, I answered, scared, "yes."

My father gave me an ultimatum: to have an abortion or leave the family. I chose to leave.

Knowing I had to leave the house I went to the crisis pregnancy center. They took care of me.

I am currently at home again with my three-month-old boy. I am now engaged and looking forward to having my own family soon.

Laurie

"At first, Mark didn't want to talk about my pregnancy. Finally he said 'It's totally up to you. If you want to have the baby, I'll stay with you, and if you want to get married, I'll probably marry you. I don't really care, but it's not going to be any different from the way it is now. I won't turn into the president of IBM. You have to decide.' "

Mark is not financially secure; Laurie is a freelance writer with a fluctuating income. She chose not to have the child, "because parenthood would have been entirely my responsibility—Mark wouldn't have supported us—and I don't have the resources to cope with that. It was the first time I'd been pregnant and maybe my last chance. At thirty-nine, how many more opportunities are you going to have?"

Susan

Susan was a freshman in college and was very caught up in her new academic and social activities. Bill (another student) and she had been dating for about three months, when one evening she decided to "take a chance" since she had just finished her menstrual

(continued on next page)

Personal Decisions about Abortion, continued

period. When her next period was two weeks overdue, she had a pregnancy test. It was positive.

When Bill first learned of the pregnancy, he became distant, but he did agree to help pay for an abortion. Soon, however, he withdrew completely and had no further contact with Susan. The hardest time for Susan was before the abortion when she found herself crying frequently. She talked a lot with her close girlfriends, who comforted her. After the abortion, she felt very strongly that she had made the best decision, but she did occasionally wonder how she would feel in future years. After meeting a new boyfriend with whom she could talk openly, Susan felt more certain than ever that she had made the right choice.

Helen

Helen was attending a junior college along with working part-time when she found out she was pregnant. Both Mike and she came from very religious backgrounds, and, for them, marriage was the only acceptable solution. They had met just a couple of months before the pregnancy, and it was only after marriage that they got to know each other well. Now, twelve years later, they have two children and a reasonably stable life together. Although both feel that their relationship lacks closeness, deriving little joy or satisfaction from their times together, they are certain that the decision they made was the best one for them.

Exploring Your Emotions

How does the value you place on human life relate to the issue of abortion? What factors influence this value?

of the abdomen and the uterus and the fetus and placenta are removed. Many doctors insist that Caesarean section be used for all subsequent deliveries to avoid the risk that the uterus will rupture during labor contractions. The saline and prostaglandin methods have largely replaced hysterotomy.

Abortion Complications

Along with questions regarding the actual procedure of abortion, many individuals have concerns regarding possible aftereffects. Over the past years, several detailed and long-term studies have focused on both physical and psychological concerns; slowly, more information is being gathered on this important subject.

Table 7-1 Danger Signs after Abortion

- Fever (temperature 100.4°F or more)
- Abdominal pain or cramps (severe or increasing)
- Abdominal tenderness with pressure, walking, coughing
- Bleeding that is heavy or lasts longer than 3 weeks
- Foul-smelling vaginal discharge
- Rash, hives, asthma (possible medication reaction)
- Normal menstrual period has not begun within 6 weeks

Source: R. A. Hatcher, 1986, *Contraceptive Technology 1986–1987* (New York: Irvington), p. 274.

Possible Physical Effects The incidence of immediate problems following abortion (infection, bleeding, trauma to the cervix or uterus, and incomplete abortion requiring repeat curettage) varies widely. The overall incidence is significantly reduced with good patient health, early timing of abortion, use of the suction method and local anesthesia, performance by a well-trained clinician, and availability and use of prompt follow-up care.

Problems related specifically to infection can be decreased through pre-abortion testing and treatment of asymptomatic gonorrhea and other infections. Also, some clinicians routinely give antibiotics after abortion, while others treat only those patients who have a history of or current symptoms of pelvic infection. All patients should thoroughly understand the postabortion danger signs (see Table 7-1) and should not hesitate to report any concerns.

Excessive bleeding during or after abortion is rare with early vacuum aspiration. In later pregnancies, the use of uterus-contracting medications reduces the risk significantly. Again, early reporting and treatment of any heavy bleeding are very important.

Cervical trauma or laceration and uterus perforation are uncommon as well, especially in early abortion with a well-trained clinician. In more advanced pregnancies, slow and careful dilation of the cervix before abortion can diminish these risks.

Incomplete abortion means that some pregnancy tissue has remained in the uterus. With this condition, or when blood clots form in the uterus shortly after abortion, severe

Immune globulin A sterile solution of specific proteins that carry many antibodies normally present in human blood; a passive immunizing agent derived from adult human blood. One type of immune globulin carries antibodies to the Rh factor in the blood.

cramping and signs of infection often occur and a repeat vacuum aspiration is usually needed. On rare occasions, a pregnancy may continue after incomplete abortion. The recommended two-week postabortion exam is important to establish that the abortion was complete.

Studies on long-term complications (subsequent infertility, spontaneous second abortions, premature delivery, and low-birth-weight babies) have not been conclusive. The risk of postabortion infertility seems to be very low, especially when any signs of infection are reported and treated promptly.

Also, there is apparently no effect on outcome of future pregnancies when an early vacuum aspiration is performed with minimal cervical dilation; with later abortions and with repeated or multiple abortions, there is only a slight risk, if any. One recent study suggests that "neither single nor multiple induced abortions as now performed are likely to increase the risk of miscarriage in subsequent pregnancies." The same study indicated that when two or more abortions were performed *before* 1973, the odds ratio for subsequent miscarriage rose to 2.6. The authors concluded that after the legalization of abortion in 1973, improved techniques have resulted in decreased cervical trauma and thereby greatly diminished any risk of future miscarriages. For Rh-negative women, dangerous sensitization (the buildup of antibodies) can be minimized by an injection of Rh-**immune globulin** given within 72 hours of the procedure.

The risk of death with early, legal abortion is low, as shown in the following estimations: before nine weeks, 1 in 400,000; between nine and twelve weeks, 1 in 100,000; between thirteen and sixteen weeks, 1 in 25,000; and after sixteen weeks, 1 in 10,000. By comparison, the death risk of continuing pregnancy is 1 in 10,000, and that of illegal abortion, 1 in 3,000.

Possible Psychological Effects Psychological side effects of abortion are less clearly defined. Responses vary and depend on the individual woman's psychological makeup, family background, current personal and social relationships, surrounding cultural attitudes, and many other factors. A woman who has specific goals with a somewhat structured life pattern may incorporate her decision to abort as the unequivocally "best" and acceptable decision more easily than a woman who feels uncertain about her future.

Although some women experience great relief after abortion, and virtually no negative feelings, most go through a period of ambivalence. Along with relief, they often feel a mixture of other responses, such as guilt, regret, loss, sadness, and/or anger. When a woman feels she was pressured into sexual intercourse or into the abortion, she may feel bitter. If she has strongly believed abortion to be immoral, she may wonder if she is still a good person. Many of these feelings are strongest immediately after abortion, when hormonal shifts are occurring; such feelings often pass quite rapidly. Others take time and fade only slowly. It is important for a woman to realize that such a mixture of feelings is natural, enabling her to accept all her reactions and to share them with others.

For women who do experience painful feelings, talking freely with a close friend or family member who is understanding and trustworthy can be very helpful. Supportive people can help her feel positive about herself and her decision. Although a legal and common procedure in the United States, abortion is still treated very secretively in most of our society, so it is easy for a woman to feel unique, isolated, and alone. Some women may specifically seek out other women who have had an abortion. Many clinical centers that offer abortions make such peer counseling available. Other women find they can identify with case histories in books written on abortion, which can help them deal with their own reactions. In a few cases, unresolved emotions may persist, and a woman may need more professional counseling, and should seek it.

Decision Making and Unintended Pregnancy

The decision-making process when facing an unintended pregnancy can differ greatly from woman to woman and circumstance to circumstance. Unprotected sexual intercourse may be followed immediately by a vague sense of anxiety. When symptoms of pregnancy appear, some women (especially young women) respond with denial,

Exploring Your Emotions

If you were to find out that your unborn child had Down's syndrome, do you feel you would want an abortion? Why might you not want an abortion? (Consider the time period in pregnancy when amniocentesis is done in your answer.)

How to Help Your Girlfriend or Wife after an Abortion

Your Feelings about the Situation

You can help your partner by first helping yourself. Tune in to your own feelings as well as your thoughts. What are you feeling about the situation? Are you feeling guilty? Rejected? Resentful? Angry? Helpless? Sorry? Scared? Concerned? Numb? These are just some of the possible feelings you may be experiencing; considering the broad range of feelings that accompanies a life crisis. Identify what it is *you're* feeling. Then share your feelings about the situation with your partner. All too often, men try to mask their real emotions, thinking they have to be strong for their woman in her time of distress. Most women want to know how their man is feeling and are disappointed when all they see is cool logic with no show of emotion.

Your Feelings about the Relationship

Do tell her how you feel toward *her* as well as what you feel about the situation. If you feel loving and caring, that's wonderful. But even if you feel like breaking up, be honest with her instead of letting her anxiety and stress build, as she wonders what your intentions are. Don't just vanish into thin air without expressing why. You may need to know what *her* intentions are regarding the relationship. It is no more fair for you to be left dangling than for her to be. Remember: Some couples have said the abortion experience opened communication that brought them closer together. Others have found that the abortion experience was the last straw in an already rocky relationship. One or both of you may decide that the relationship is a dead end and choose to move on. Although endings can be scary and sad, endings also provide the opportunity for beginning anew.

Affection and Sex

If you genuinely feel loving and caring, *do* be affectionate. If she backs away from your affectionate gestures, try to be patient and communicate with her. What does she want from you? Some women want to be held and touched *affectionately* but not *sexually* after an abortion. Some may be completely turned off to sex for a while after an abortion, having been "burned" once. If you notice disinterest or hesitancy, don't push. Talk to her. Find out how she's feeling. You may feel rejected. If so, express it, but remember that this behavior is a fairly common reaction after an abortion, and it usually passes in time. Everybody is different, though, so find out how *she* feels!

Sometimes it will be you who won't feel like touching after an abortion. This may be due to the same fear of having been "burned." Or you may be feeling so guilty, believing that *you* got her into the awful situation that you may be punishing yourself by refusing the comfort of touching. If this is your case, remember that it took two to make the pregnancy. It wasn't any *one* person's fault. Responsibility for what happened should be shared.

Showing that You Care about Her Emotionally and Physically

Do ask her how she is feeling periodically, but don't be a mother hen, clucking and fussing and worrying about her every little move. Showing concern is desirable; overdoing it isn't. Most women appreciate their man doing something very special for them,

ascribing the delayed menstruation, and so on, to other causes. Several days or weeks may elapse before the woman finally has the pregnancy confirmed (a major cause of late abortions). After a positive test, women often feel a mixture of anxiety, depression, guilt, and anger, sometimes tinged with some anticipation and delight. The actual decision making can vary widely. Some women calmly and resolutely make a choice within a very short time, while others, feeling panic and chaos, wrestle with the decision for several weeks. For some women, it is the first time in their lives that they feel unable to find a "right" answer, and instead must settle for a "best" but difficult solution.

The response of a woman's partner can have a significant influence on how she experiences an unintended pregnancy. Men's emotional reactions can vary considerably. Some withdraw and choose to remain completely detached; others simply press for the most expedient solution (abortion). Still others feel very emotionally involved and wish to play an active role in decision making. Partners can be very helpful, both in weighing important considerations and in actually helping with the chosen course such as giving them flowers. You could take her out to dinner or buy her a little present. Use your imagination to make whatever you do special for her. These actions show concretely that you care and can have an amazing impact on boosting her spirits, which in turn will probably boost yours too.

Do read the postabortion after-care instructions. In order to prevent an infection, she will need your cooperation in abstaining from sexual intercourse for two weeks following the abortion. You can also be involved in the after-care by encouraging her to have the two-week checkup, providing the transportation to the clinic or doctor's office. If there is a fee, you could offer to pay part or all of it. These are all ways of showing that you care about her physical welfare.

If She Feels Guilty or "Low"

Many women do *not* feel guilty after an abortion, so don't assume. However, if your partner indicates that she is feeling guilty or if she is criticizing herself, do let her know that she has very good, lovable, and loving qualities. Help her focus on her positive characteristics. In this important way, you will help bolster her sagging self-respect; and there are few things in life that are as essential as one's self-respect.

If You're Feeling Guilty

If you are feeling guilty, and SHE isn't, don't try to make her feel guilty too, or expect that she should feel the same as you do! It is certainly OK for you to express your feelings to her. However, if the majority of your interaction with her is laden with guilt or grief, she probably won't desire your company as much as before. Therefore, it would be worth your while to talk over your own feelings with either a good friend or with a counselor from the abortion clinic or other agency. Men certainly can have as much or even more emotional investment in an abortion experience as a woman, and your feelings are valid and important.

In Conclusion . . .

Remember, there is no right or wrong way to feel after an abortion. Some people feel relieved and happy that it's over, that she is safe and well, and that they can continue their lives the way they were before the pregnancy crisis occurred. Others feel remorseful, sad, guilty, angry, or rejected for a variety of reasons. And still others experience a mixture of feelings.

Therefore, some of what has just been discussed [here] may prove very helpful to you, while some of it may not apply in your case. Take what you need and leave the rest. Hopefully you have gained something that will help you understand and handle your own feelings and those of your partner regarding the abortion experience. And remember for the future, with your involved concern in the area of birth control, you can help to prevent another unplanned pregnancy. We all make mistakes, and the best we can do is learn from them.

Source: Anne Baker, 1981, After her abortion, pp. 5–9. The Hope Clinic for Women Ltd., 1602 21st Street, Granite City, IL. 62040.

of action. Similarly, parents can be important. However, when there are marked disagreements, a stressful situation can become even more difficult. According to current laws, the woman, who is the one most directly affected by unintended pregnancy, has the final rights in the decision.

No matter which of the available options to unintended pregnancy is chosen, a series of questions are likely to arise that must be addressed (see the section on personal considerations). Although a prompt decision carries critical advantages, careful consideration is important. If there are strong feelings of uncertainty or ambivalence, hasty action should be avoided.

Having a supportive confidant, such as male partner, other close friend, or family member, can be very important in sorting out complex feelings. Along with listening and offering understanding and perspective, supportive people can help find suitable medical personnel and plan financial arrangements. Once a course of action has been chosen, a sense of moving ahead usually follows and the next step toward resolution can occur.

Take Action

Your answers to the Exploring Your Emotions questions in this chapter and your placement level on the Awareness Ladder will, we hope, encourage you to begin a process of self-explorations and self-discovery that you will continue. Reflect on the entire chapter and ask yourself how each point relates to your own life. Then take action:

1. In your notebook, list and describe the feelings you might have in confronting the decision to have an abortion, and then the feelings you might have after you had made your decision one way or another, at one-month, six-month, one-year, three-year, and twenty-year follow-ups. Project the consequences of your decision into the future. Explain any changes in feeling that time might produce.

2. Reread Chapter 6 and consider how your feelings about abortion might affect your feelings about contraception. Make any changes you feel are necessary in your use of contraceptive methods.

3. Write a letter stating your feelings about abortion and send it to two or three groups and/or newspapers in your community. You need not take an either-or position, but do clearly outline your criteria for supporting or not supporting current abortion legislation. Suggest legislative changes that you feel are necessary or would be beneficial, on the topic of abortion.

4. Interview (confidentially and sensitively) a woman who has had an abortion; a person who believes that he or she might not now be alive if abortion had been readily available at the time around his or her birth; a man who failed in an attempt to block an abortion in which he thought himself to be the father; or a woman who was denied an abortion she felt she needed. How do your feelings about each case differ from those of the person you interviewed?

5. Outline a semester course (say, 20 hours of work) that could help clarify students' feelings about abortion. Include readings, field trips, specific essay assignments, and one community intern project. Give a copy of your course outline to the departments at your college that offer or might consider offering such a course.

6. Before leaving this chapter, review the Awareness Ladder at the beginning of this chapter. Have your feelings or values changed? Are you now better equipped to consider the complex and very human issues associated with abortion?

Selected References

Abortion: The spectrum of opinion. 1985. 1986 (July). *Harper's Magazine,* p. 42.

Brahams, D. 1983 (May 7). The postcoital pill and intrauterine device: Contraceptive or abortifacient? *Lancet* 1(8332):1039.

Dunn, P. M., and Stirrat, G. M. 1984 (March 10). Capable of being born alive? *Lancet,* 1(8376):553–54.

Hatcher, R. A. 1982. *It's Your Choice.* New York: Irvington.

Henshaw, S. K., Binkin, N. J., Blaine, E., and Smith, J. C. 1985 (March–April). A portrait of American women who obtain abortions, *Family Planning Perspectives* 17(2):90–96.

Kline, J., Stein, Z., Susser, M., and Warburton, D. 1986 (June). Induced abortion and the chromosomal characteristics of subsequent miscarriages (spontaneous abortions), *American Journal of Epidemiology* 123(6):1066–79.

Romney, S. L., Gray, M. J., Little, A. B., Merrill, J. A., Quilligan, E. J., and Stander, R. 1975. *Gynecology and Obstetrics: The Health Care of Women.* New York: McGraw-Hill, p. 578.

Seligmann, J., Witherspoon, D., Gosnell, M., Shapiro, D., and King, P. 1985 (January 14). The medical quandary, *Newsweek,* pp. 26–27.

Smith, T. W. 1985 (August). National Opinion Research Center, unpublished tabulations from the 1982, 1983, and 1985 General Social Surveys.

U.S. Supreme Court. *Jane Roe et al. vs. Henry Wade.* U.S. Supreme Court, Opinion No. 70–18, 22 January, 1973.

Recommended Readings

Castadot, R. G., 1986 (January). Pregnancy termination: Techniques, risks, and complications and their management, *Fertility and Sterility* 45(1) 5–17.
Summary article on the medical aspects of abortion. Good for technical details.

Mohr, J. C. 1978. *Abortion in America: The Origins and Evolution of National Policy, 1800–1900.* New York: Oxford University Press.
A historical perspective of views on abortion within American society. Includes a discussion on the powerful role that physicians played in the formation of public opinion and related legal decisions.

Chapter 8

Contents

Rate Yourself

Your Attitudes about Being a Parent Read the following statements carefully. Choose the one in each section that best describes you at this moment and circle its number. When you have chosen one statement for each section, add the numbers and record your total score. Find your position on the Awareness Ladder.

5 Enjoys children
4 Feels comfortable around children
3 Doesn't mind looking after children
2 Feels uncomfortable around children
1 Dislikes children

5 Knows how to plan for pregnancy
4 Knows about hereditary factors
3 Is familiar with the nutritional requirements of pregnancy
2 Is unfamiliar with nutritional requirements of pregnancy
1 Is ignorant about planning a pregnancy

5 Knows how to plan for childbirth
4 Is familiar with routine delivery procedures
3 Is willing to learn about childbirth
2 Is uninterested in childbirth information
1 Is ignorant about childbirth procedures

5 Understands the benefits of breastfeeding
4 Favors breastfeeding
3 Is unfamiliar with the benefits of breastfeeding
2 Dislikes breastfeeding
1 Disapproves of breastfeeding

5 Recognizes that parents are models for children's behavior
4 Respects the rights of children
3 Views children as extensions of parents
2 Has little respect for children's rights
1 Dominates children

Total Score ______

Pregnancy, Childbirth, and Parenting

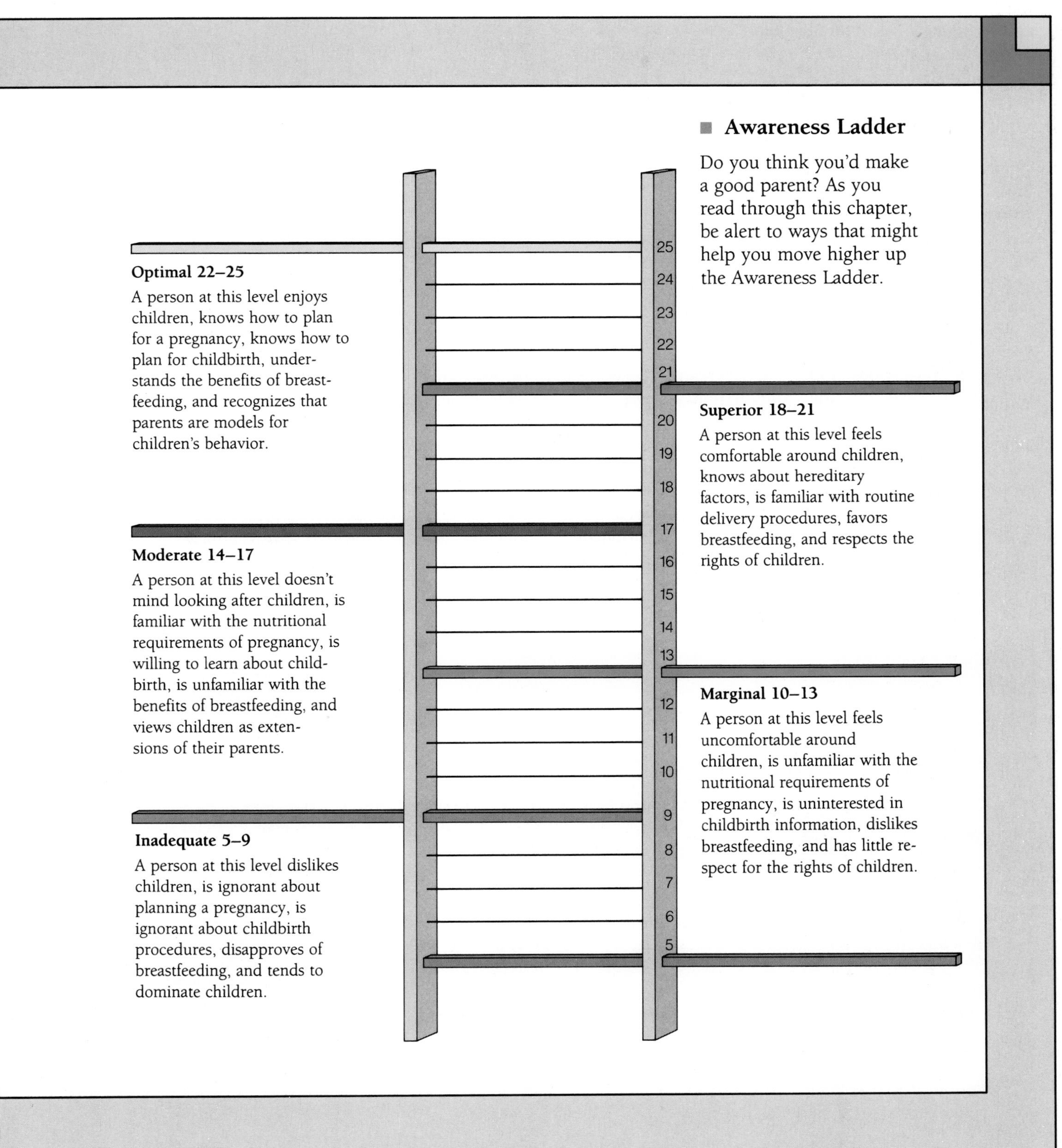

■ Awareness Ladder
Do you think you'd make a good parent? As you read through this chapter, be alert to ways that might help you move higher up the Awareness Ladder.
Optimal 22–25
A person at this level enjoys children, knows how to plan for a pregnancy, knows how to plan for childbirth, understands the benefits of breastfeeding, and recognizes that parents are models for children's behavior.
Superior 18–21
A person at this level feels comfortable around children, knows about hereditary factors, is familiar with routine delivery procedures, favors breastfeeding, and respects the rights of children.
Moderate 14–17
A person at this level doesn't mind looking after children, is familiar with the nutritional requirements of pregnancy, is willing to learn about childbirth, is unfamiliar with the benefits of breastfeeding, and views children as extensions of their parents.
Marginal 10–13
A person at this level feels uncomfortable around children, is unfamiliar with the nutritional requirements of pregnancy, is uninterested in childbirth information, dislikes breastfeeding, and has little respect for the rights of children.
Inadequate 5–9
A person at this level dislikes children, is ignorant about planning a pregnancy, is ignorant about childbirth procedures, disapproves of breastfeeding, and tends to dominate children.
25
24
23
22
21
20
19
18
17
16
15
14
13
12
11
10
9
8
7
6
5

Our changing attitudes toward nature are nowhere more apparent than in our changing attitudes toward birth. Only a few decades ago, most people had an unqualified faith that whatever the rest of nature could do, human science and technology could do better.

That faith has begun to fade, and people in the medical profession, like many other people, are having second thoughts. Natural childbirth may not be the answer for every mother, but more and more women are requesting it. At the same time, some doctors are pointing out that drugged childbirth may harm both baby and mother. Breastfeeding is increasingly viewed as beneficial in all ways to both mother and baby. The practice of forcing labor is being challenged, as is routine circumcision of male babies. The father, once virtually ignored and excluded, is now often brought into the labor and delivery rooms to take part.

More and more parents are insisting on their right to decide how their children will be born. Some mothers want to be unconscious or numb. Others want to be aware, to experience the birthing. The current emphasis on awareness reflects a basic change in cultural values. The pendulum of change is swinging in both directions. For example, bottle-feeding first became popular in the upper economic classes, because it freed mothers to do other things. Its popularity is still growing, especially in the South and Southwest, former strongholds of breastfeeding, and in the lower economic classes, because bottle-feeding allows mothers to work outside the home. At the same time, college-educated women and those who are wealthier are choosing to breastfeed because of the significant advantages for their child's health.

Still another change in attitudes is reflected by a greater public understanding that early life events strongly influence a baby's growth and development. Very young babies whose mothers spend much of their waking hours singing to them and practicing a great deal of eye contact with them are less afraid of strangers. And the more their fathers care for them and play with them, the more they relate to their fathers in a close and satisfying way. Babies who do not crawl enough to develop good hand-eye coordination seem to have trouble developing verbal skills when they go to school. Babies who do not receive a lot of touching and other forms of sensory stimulation are more likely to develop severe psychological problems. Stimulation is clearly essential for growth.

Exploring Your Emotions

Does it frighten you to think a tiny child may (or does) depend on you for food, clothing, a home, emotional support, and almost constant attention, at least for a few years of your life? Can you support a child emotionally? If so, how? If not, why not?

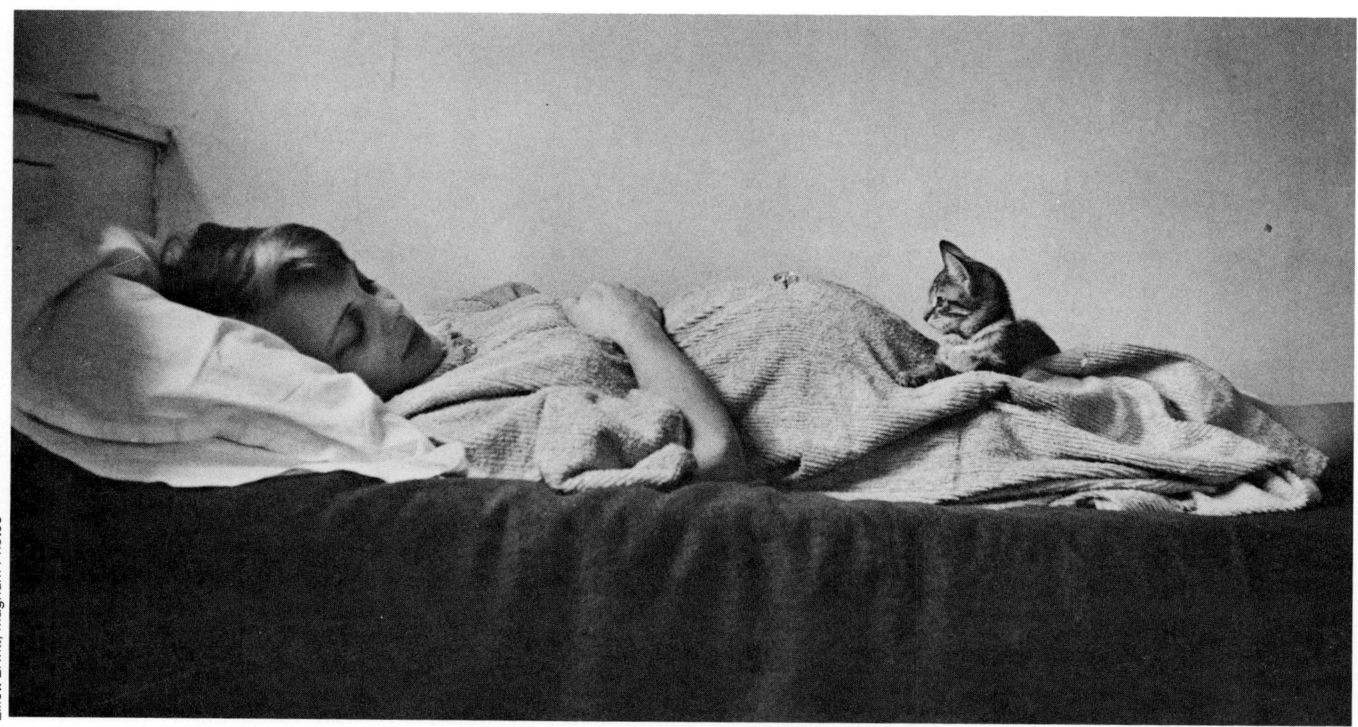

Elliott Erwitt, Magnum Photos

Ovary One of the two female reproductive glands in which the ova (eggs) and hormones are formed.

Follicles The thousands of protecting, enclosing spherical bubbles in the ovaries in which the ova mature. Each follicle contains a liquid supplied with estrogen.

Oviducts (Fallopian tubes) The two passages through which ova travel from the ovaries to the uterus; "normal" place for fertilization.

Uterus The hollow, thick-walled, muscular organ in which the egg develops into a child; located directly above the vagina; the source of menstrual flow; the womb.

Fertilized egg The egg after it has been penetrated by a sperm; a zygote.

Sperm cell A mature male germ cell that serves to impregnate the ovum.

Fertilization The initiation of biological reproduction, as, for example, when the sperm and ovum unite to form a zygote (fertilized egg).

Genetic code Blueprint specifications directing the body's growth and cell differentiation, contained in the structure of DNA (deoxyribonucleic acid), the chemically active ingredient in the chromosomes.

Embryo The developing cluster of cells from the end of the first week to the end of the eighth week following conception.

Trimester One of the three 13-week periods of pregnancy.

Fetus The name given to the embryo from the end of the eighth week after conception to the moment of birth.

The Reproductive Process

Every month during a woman's fertile years, her body prepares itself for childbearing. In one of her **ovaries**, an egg ripens and is released. It bursts from its **follicle.** The egg is then drawn into an **oviduct** (or **Fallopian tube**) through which it travels to the uterus. The journey takes three to four days. The lining of the **uterus** has already puffed out to accept the implanting of a **fertilized egg**. An unfertilized egg lives about twenty-four hours and then disintegrates. It is expelled along with the uterine lining during menstruation.

Each egg is about the size of a pinpoint, 1/250 inch in diameter, and about a half million eggs are in a girl's ovaries at birth. Only about 500 will ripen and be released during her lifetime.

Sperm cells are about 1/32 the size of an egg cell (1/8,000 inch in diameter). They are also much more plentiful; an average ejaculation contains about 400 million. During ejaculation, sperm cells travel from the testicles, where they develop, through two ducts (vasa deferentia) and the seminal vesicles, pouches where they are temporarily stored. At the prostate gland, they enter the urethra, through which they are propelled with great force during orgasm into the woman's vagina. A sperm cell—unless it fertilizes an egg—lives at most about 48 to 72 hours. Many sperm cells do not survive the acidic environment of the vagina. Those that do quickly migrate to the cervix, the "neck" of the uterus, where secretions are more alkaline and thus more hospitable. Once through the cervix and into the uterus, many sperm cells are diverted to the wrong oviduct or get stuck along the way. Those that enter the tube that harbors the traveling egg face one more obstacle: the egg is encased in a tough skin. However, each sperm cell that touches the egg deposits an enzyme that dissolves parts of the membrane. The first sperm cell that bumps into a bare spot on the egg cell can swim into the cell to merge with the nucleus, and thus **fertilization** occurs. The sperm's tail, its means of locomotion, gets stuck in the outer membrane and drops off, leaving the sperm head inside the egg. Now no more sperm can enter the egg, possibly because once it has been fertilized it may release a chemical that makes it impregnable.

The ovum (egg) carries the hereditary characteristics of the mother and her ancestors; sperm cells carry the hereditary characteristics of the father and his ancestors. Together they contain the **genetic code,** a set of instructions for development. The parent cells—egg and sperm—each contain 23 chromosomes, each of which in turn contains at least 1,000 genes, so small that they cannot be seen through a microscope. These genes are packages of chemical instructions for designing every part of a new baby. They specify that the infant will be human; what its sex will be; whether it will tend to be (depending also on its environment) short, tall, thin, fat, healthy, or sickly; and how intelligent it can be.

About 30 hours after the egg is fertilized, the cell inside the membrane reproduces itself by dividing in half. Both cells then divide again about 10 hours later. This process repeats many times, cell size decreasing with each division. They are held together by a clear membrane and look like the facets of a raspberry. This cluster continues to float down through the oviduct. By the time it reaches the uterus—three to four days later—it has multiplied to about 36 cells. It attaches itself to the lining of the uterus and remains attached until birth. One week after conception the cells number over 100, and the cluster is now considered an **embryo.**

Fetal Development

Fetal development, described chronologically, can be roughly divided into three periods of 13 weeks each, called **trimesters.**

First Trimester During the first trimester, the embryo develops into a **fetus** about 4 inches long and weighing 1 ounce. All its parts are developed; its sexual organs are well formed, and it has a whole range of nerve and muscle

Conception The formation of a zygote (fertilized egg); the cell resulting from the fusion of ovum and sperm, and in normal conditions capable of survival and maturation in the uterus.

Blastocyst A stage of human development, lasting only from about Day 6 to Day 14, during which the cell cluster divides into the embryo and the placenta.

Endometrium The mucous membrane that forms the inner lining of the cavity of the uterus.

Chorionic villi Threadlike blood vessels that sprout from the blastocyst into the mother's vessels to draw out blood and nourishment.

Placenta The organ connected to the fetus by the umbilical cord and attached to the wall of the uterus; the organ through which the fetus receives nourishment and empties waste into the circulatory system of the mother. After birth, the placenta (or "afterbirth") is expelled.

Amniotic sac The bag of watery fluid that lines the uterus and surrounds and protects the fetus.

Specialized cells Cells differ in their particular and special functions: some become blood cells, bone cells, or muscle cells.

Umbilical cord The cord that connects the fetus with the placenta.

Sucking reflex Involuntary sucking behavior of a fetus exhibited before and after birth.

---

responses. In fact, the timetable for the formation of the body is so consistent that at any time during the first forty-eight days of life an embryologist can look at an embryo and tell its exact age from its body formation.

First Month As the cluster of cells drifts down the oviduct after **conception,** some cells divide faster than others, and several different kinds of cells emerge. The entire genetic code is passed to every cell, but new cells do not follow the entire instruction or there would be no different organs or parts of the body. For example, all cells carry genes for hair color and eye color, but only the cells of the hair follicles and irises respond to that information.

On about Day 4 of its journey, the cluster, now about thirty-six cells and hollow, arrives in the uterus. In this form, it is known as a **blastocyst.** On about Day 6 or 7, the blastocyst burrows into the uterine lining, usually along the upper curve. (See Figure 8-1.) The cells begin to draw nourishment from the **endometrium,** the uterine lining.

About this time, the spherical cluster collapses in on itself, and the inner cells now transform themselves to become the embryo from which the baby forms. The inner cells separate into three layers. One layer composes the inner body parts, the digestive and respiratory systems; another layer becomes the skin, hair, and nervous tissue; and the middle layer becomes muscle, bone, marrow, blood, kidneys, and sex glands.

The outermost shell of blastocyst cells becomes the placenta, umbilical cord, and amniotic sac. A network of roots called **chorionic villi** sprouts from the blastocyst

Figure 8-1 A cross section of the uterus in pregnancy.

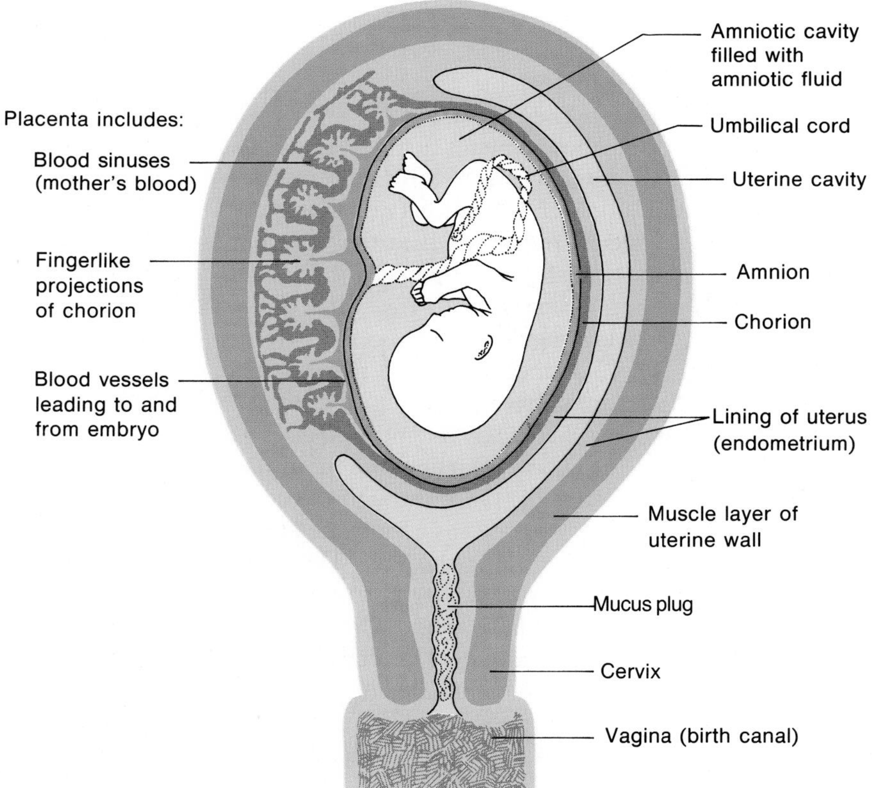

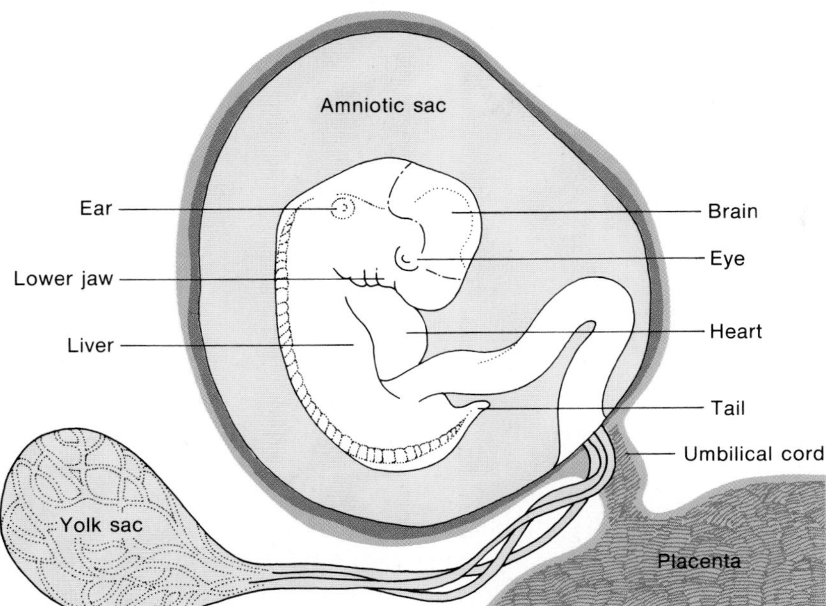

Figure 8-2 The early embryo (about 28 days) in the amniotic sac. At this stage the yolk sac aids in nourishing the embryo, but later it degenerates as the placenta takes on the nourishment function.

and eventually forms the **placenta.** Tapping the small blood vessels in the endometrium, the villi firmly implant the cell cluster and draw nourishment from the mother's blood through a thick, spongy layer into the embryo's blood. They remove waste products by the same route.

Inside this placenta is the **amniotic sac,** or bag of waters. This sac cushions and insulates the embryo.

By the third week, the embryo is 1/10 inch long, and the brain has two lobes. By Day 17, young blood cells appear—the first **specialized cells**. Soon afterward, blood vessels begin to form, and blood flows through them. By the fourth week the embryo is almost 1/2 inch long, is about one-third head, and has a trunk and visible arm buds. The nervous system appears as a hollow tube by Day 24, the same day the tubular heart begins to beat slowly. After a few days of practice, it pumps 65 times a minute to circulate newly formed blood.

By the end of the first month, the embryo also has simple kidneys, liver, digestive tract, and umbilical cord. The embryo is 10,000 times as large as the fertilized egg was and is a finely structured although incomplete body. (See Figures 8-2 and 8-3a.)

Second Month In the fifth week, the arm buds subdivide into hand, arm, and shoulder. By the sixth week, the eyes appear, partly closed. The inner ear is nearly complete, and the outer ear is starting to form. The nose is fully formed. The embryo has a reptilelike head and tail and complete skeleton of cartilage. (See Figure 8-3b.)

By the seventh week, the embryo has a recognizable face with eyes, ears, nose, lips, tongue, and even milk-teeth buds in the gums. The body is padded with muscles and covered by thin skin. The arms have hands with budding fingers and thumbs. The legs, which develop more slowly than the arms until after two years, have knees, ankles, and toes. The tail has begun to shrink, and bone has begun to replace cartilage in the skeleton.

In the eighth week, the embryo is about 1.25 inches long and weighs 1/30 ounce. Almost all internal organs have begun to develop. The brain is beginning to coordinate the functioning of the other organs. The heart beats steadily, and blood circulates. The stomach produces some digestive juices. The liver manufactures blood cells. The kidneys extract some uric acid from the blood. The **umbilical cord** joins the embryo's circulatory system to the placenta, where nutrients and wastes are exchanged with the mother's circulatory system.

The embryo now has a complete body. It is now considered a fetus, and all further changes in the body will be enlargements and refinements. (See Figure 8-3c.)

Third Month: A Fetus The fetus, now 3 inches long and weighing 1 ounce, begins to be quite active. By the end of the month, it can kick, make a fist, turn its head, squint, frown, and open its mouth. The **sucking reflex** begins to appear. The fetus hears the mother's heartbeat and voice, as well as outside noises. Internal organs have begun to function.

Around the eighth or ninth week, female and male embryos have the same sex gland and the same genital—a vertical slit with a swelling on either side and a small rounded bud at the top of the slit. In the female, the bud becomes the clitoris, and the swellings become the labia. In the male, the bud grows into a penis. The testicles

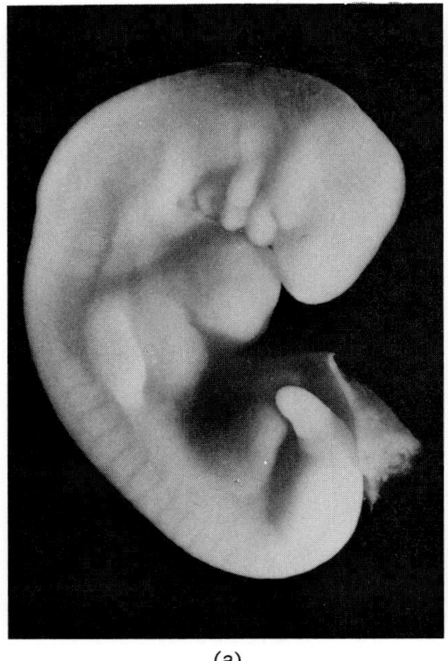

(a)

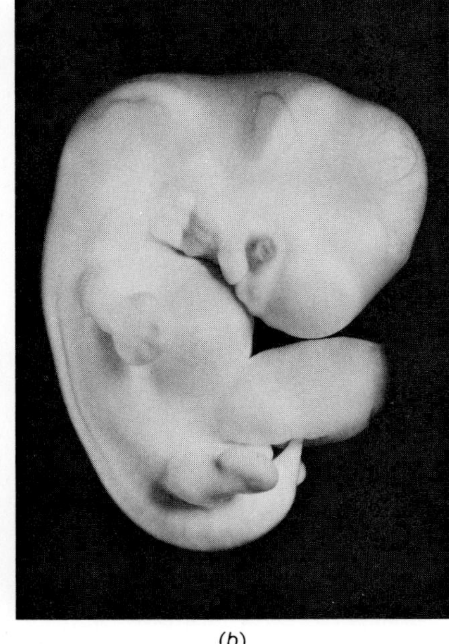

(b)

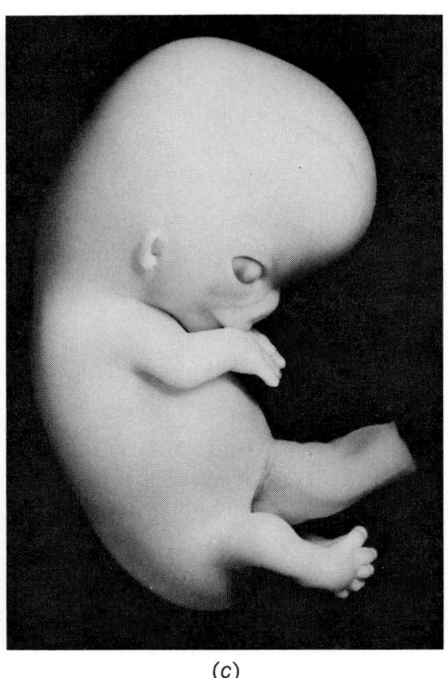

(c)

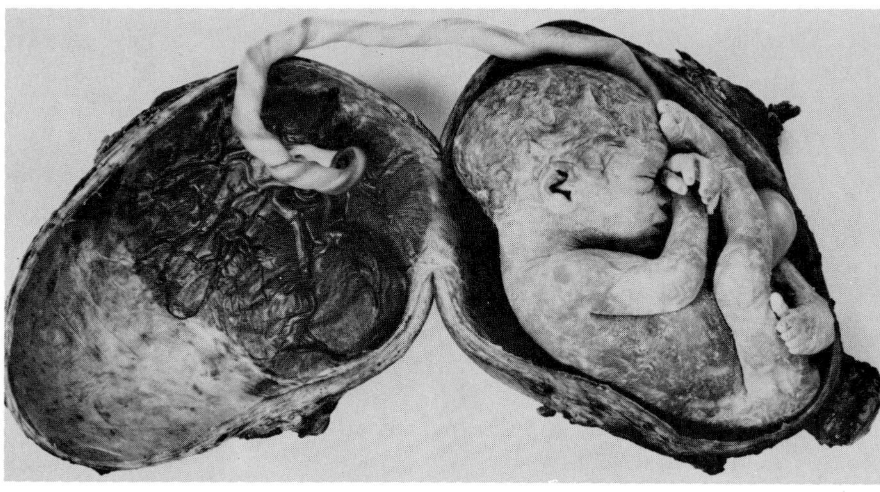

(d)

Figure 8-3 Stages in fetal development: (*a*) about 4 weeks; (*b*) about 6 weeks; (*c*) about 9 weeks; (*d*) 24 to 26 weeks.

descend from the abdomen into the scrotum at about the seventh month. The internal reproductive organs become well formed and already contain some egg or sperm cells.

In the first trimester, the fetus is extremely vulnerable to viral infections, radiation, and drugs. They can cause malformations. The most susceptible parts of the body are the parts growing most rapidly at the time. German measles, for example, can easily cause a **congenital malformation** of a delicate system such as the eyes or ears. Another danger is extended high fever in the mother, which could cause premature labor. The effects of drugs and alcohol are dangerous throughout the entire pregnancy.

Second Trimester During the second trimester, the fetus grows to about 14 inches and 2 pounds. The body grows faster than the head.

Fourth Month In the fourth month, the fetus grows to a height of 10 inches and a weight of 6 ounces. To achieve this growth, the fetus must have large amounts of food, oxygen, and water, which come from the mother through the placenta. (See Figure 8-1.) The placental system is so efficient that within an hour or two the fetus receives any substance entering the mother's bloodstream, including not only nutrients but also drugs, alcohol, and medications.

Fifth Month The fetus grows to be 1 foot long and weighs 1 pound. Much of the skeleton hardens.

The heartbeat gets loud enough to be heard with a stethoscope. Muscles become much stronger, and the fetus begins definite kicking and turning, the first movements that can be perceived by the mother. It can move freely within the amniotic sac, surrounded by a quart of fluid

Congenital malformation A physical defect existing at the time of birth, either inherited or caused during gestation.

that is changed at the rate of 6 gallons per day. The fetus may suck its thumb. It can be startled by noises.

Sixth Month The fetus grows to 14 inches and 2 pounds. It might now be able to breathe regularly for twenty-four hours if it is born prematurely, which means that it might survive premature birth. See Figure 8-3d.

Third Trimester In the last three months, the third trimester, the fetus grows to 20 inches and gains most of its birth weight: about 1 pound in the seventh month and 2 pounds in each of the eighth and ninth months. Some of this weight is fatty tissue under the skin that serves as insulation and food supply and gives the baby its characteristic chubbiness. (The baby may be too fat, however, if the mother overeats during this time.)

The fetus must obtain large amounts of calcium, iron, and nitrogen from the food the mother eats. Some 85 percent of the calcium and iron she consumes goes into the fetal bloodstream.

Although the fetus is able to live if it is born during the seventh month, it needs the fat layer acquired in the eighth month and time for the organs, especially the respiratory and digestive organs, to develop. It also needs the immunities the mother supplies in the last three months. Her blood protects the fetus against all the diseases to which she has acquired immunity. These immunities wear off within six months after birth, but they can be replenished by the mother's milk if the baby is breastfed.

Changes in the Pregnant Woman's Body

During the first trimester, the mother's uterus enlarges about three times the size it was when she was not pregnant, but it still cannot be felt in the abdomen. The mother experiences relatively few bodily changes and some fairly common symptoms.

The second trimester is generally the most peaceful time of pregnancy, with the fewest complications. If the mother experienced nausea and morning sickness, these usually subside, and she gains weight. Some women report feeling healthy and energetic and having a sense of well-being. Some feel prettier. These feelings are governed by physical changes as well as the mother's feelings toward having a child.

The third trimester is the hardest for the mother. She must breathe, digest, excrete, and circulate blood for two people. The weight of the fetus, its pressure on her own body organs, and its increased demands on her own system cause discomfort and fatigue. As a result, the mother may become increasingly lethargic. During the last weeks, she may worry about her own safety and well-being and that of her child, and she may worry that the child will be abnormal.

The Signs and Symptoms of Pregnancy Early recognition of pregnancy is very important, especially for women with physical problems and nutritional deficiencies. The pregnancy symptoms described here are not absolute indications of pregnancy as such. Other far more reliable methods of determining pregnancy are available through the medical professionals. It is best for a woman to visit a gynecologist after missing two menstrual periods.

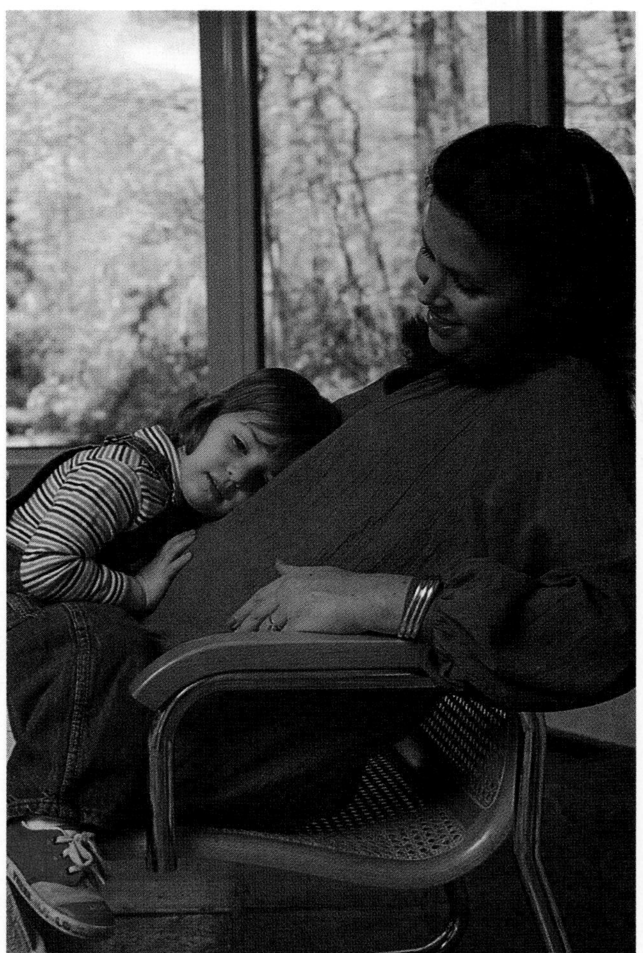
Erika Stone

Amenorrhea The absence or abnormal stoppage of menstrual periods.

Hormones Chemical substances secreted into the body fluids by the endocrine glands.

HCG, human chorionic gonadotrophin A hormone found only in pregnant women; its presence is the basis for pregnancy testing.

Colostrum The thin, milky fluid secreted by the mammary glands around the time of childbirth until milk comes in, about the third day.

Amenorrhea If the uterine lining is retained, then of course no menstrual period occurs. This condition, called **amenorrhea,** is one of the first signals of pregnancy.

Slight Bleeding During early pregnancy, slight bleeding may follow the implanting of the fertilized egg in the uterine wall. Because it happens about when a period is expected, this bleeding is sometimes mistaken for menstruation. The bleeding usually lasts only a few days.

Nausea One of the first noticeable symptoms of pregnancy is nausea, which about two-thirds of pregnant women experience. It has been called "morning sickness," but some women have it throughout the day. Nausea is probably a reaction to increased progesterone and other **hormones** produced during pregnancy. Nausea frequently disappears by the twelfth week.

Sleepiness, Fatigue, and More Frequent Urination Sleepiness and fatigue also result from hormonal changes. The expanding uterus presses against the bladder, causing the need to urinate more often. After the twelfth week, the uterus rises higher in the abdomen, away from the bladder, and the urination rate returns to normal. In the third trimester, urination again becomes more frequent.

General Weepiness Women are likely to experience rapid and unpredictable emotional changes during major variations in their hormone levels—at puberty, menopause, before menstruation, and during pregnancy and immediately after birth. Even a mother who has planned the pregnancy and wants the child may be delighted one moment and upset the next.

Need for Affection and Support Much of the pregnancy experience is beyond the mother's total control—her energy level, her changing appearance, her variable emotions. She must absorb and adjust to many new feelings and ideas, and therefore usually needs extra support and affection.

Changes in Sexual Activity Sexual activity often changes during pregnancy. Varying hormone levels affect the mother's sexual desire. Some women are less interested in sexual intercourse; others are more interested, especially during the fourth to sixth month, when the pelvic area is newly swollen and sensitive but not so large as to make close physical contact awkward.

Both responses are common and are influenced by the partners' attitudes toward sexuality during pregnancy. If an overprotective partner fears that intercourse is harmful, the woman may infer that he does not find her attractive. If he is insensitive to her fears or shows hesitation or lack of interest in intercourse, she may feel he does not value her feelings. Communicating freely with each other and even with a counselor can help. Late in pregnancy, intercourse becomes physically awkward, but new positions can satisfy both people.

Home Pregnancy Test Kits Some women wish to know immediately whether or not they are indeed pregnant. They can test for pregnancy with home testing kits sold over the counter in drugstores. These kits detect a hormone found only in pregnant women. Within about eight days of conception, the placenta produces **human chorionic gonadotrophin (HCG),** a hormone that prevents menstruation and supports the pregnancy. HCG is found in saliva, urine, and secretions of the mother.

Home test kits come equipped with a small sample of red blood cells (usually from a sheep) coated with HCG antibodies, to which the user can add a small amount of her own urine. If the concentration of HCG is great enough, it will clump together with the HCG antibodies, indicating that the user is pregnant.

These home tests are 85 to 95 percent reliable. If used too early in the pregnancy, the HCG concentration is not great enough to cause clumping. Other conditions that can produce a false negative include an unclean test tube, vaginal or urinary infection, presence of some drugs or oral contraceptives, and moving the test while it's working. False positives can occur when the user is near menopause, has uterine cancer, has recently been pregnant, or waits too long to read the results.

Changes That Continue Throughout Pregnancy The mother's body continually prepares the way for the fetus. Her ribs flare out long before the uterus needs the room to expand. Her uterus and the amniotic sac expand long before the fetus needs room. The metabolism of the mother becomes more efficient, to help provide a good nutritional balance for both her and the fetus. The following specific changes occur in the mother's body. (See Figure 8-4.)

Bone and Muscle Structure Beginning early in pregnancy, the muscles and ligaments attached to bones such as the pelvis begin to soften and stretch. The joints between the pelvic bones, which are normally solid, loosen and spread, and become movable by the tenth to twelfth week. This change may be caused by the hormone relaxin. It makes having a baby easier, but makes walking more difficult.

Reproductive Organs By the sixth week, the cervix softens. During the first three months, the uterus enlarges to three times its nonpregnant size. By the fourth month, the uterus is large enough to make the abdomen protrude. By the seventh or eighth month, the uterus pushes up into the rib cage, which makes breathing slightly more difficult. The breasts enlarge and are sensitive by the eighth week, and may tingle or throb. The pigmented area around the nipple, the areola, darkens and becomes broader. After the tenth week, **colostrum**—a thin milky fluid—may be squeezed from the mother's nipples, but actual secretion of milk is prevented by high levels of estrogen and progesterone.

Circulatory System During pregnancy, the mother's blood takes up more oxygen in the lungs, and nutrients are held longer in the bloodstream. Both oxygen and nutrition can then be more readily given to the fetus through the placenta. The increased efficiency of the mother's circulatory system results from about a 50 percent increase in blood plasma and an 18 percent increase in blood cells. Heart output increases by midpregnancy from 9 to 12 pints per minute. Circulation is also more rapid. Most of the increased blood flow goes to the uterus and placenta and to the kidneys.

Lungs Because the mother needs more oxygen during pregnancy, she inhales up to 40 percent more air. The widening of her rib cage permits the greater intake.

Kidneys During pregnancy, kidneys become highly efficient. They must remove the waste products from fetal circulation, which pass into the mother's bloodstream through the placenta. Hormonal changes cause a pregnant woman to retain more water, and by midpregnancy the kidneys can produce prodigious amounts of urine. In late pregnancy, however, this capacity drops below normal level.

Skin When skin is stretched, as in pregnancy or weight gain, small breaks occur in the elastic fibers of the lower layer of skin. The breaks remain as "stretch marks," narrow, shiny streaks on hips, breasts, abdomen, or thighs.

Figure 8-4 Physiological changes during pregnancy: *(left)* the female body at the time of conception; *(right)* development after 30 weeks of pregnancy.

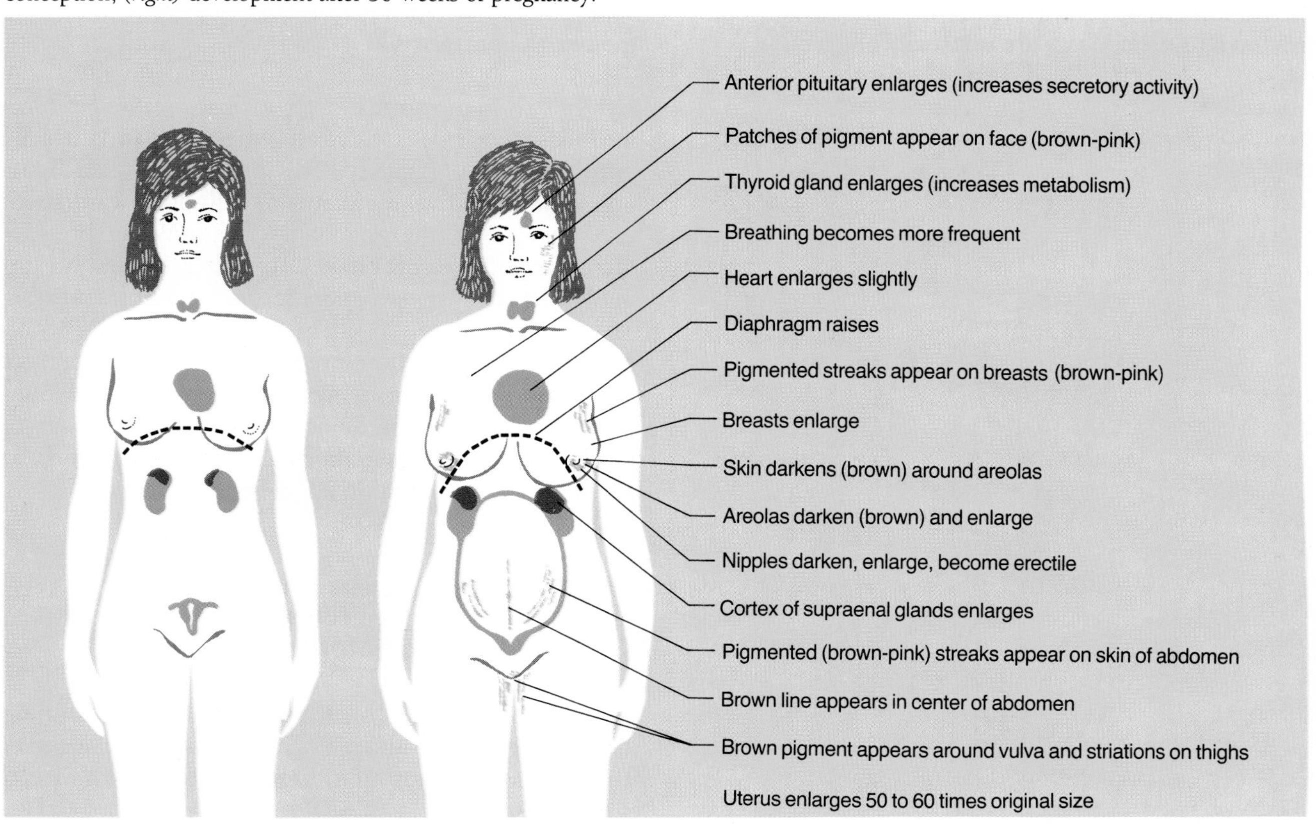
Anterior pituitary enlarges (increases secretory activity)
Patches of pigment appear on face (brown-pink)
Thyroid gland enlarges (increases metabolism)
Breathing becomes more frequent
Heart enlarges slightly
Diaphragm raises
Pigmented streaks appear on breasts (brown-pink)
Breasts enlarge
Skin darkens (brown) around areolas
Areolas darken (brown) and enlarge
Nipples darken, enlarge, become erectile
Cortex of supraenal glands enlarges
Pigmented (brown-pink) streaks appear on skin of abdomen
Brown line appears in center of abdomen
Brown pigment appears around vulva and striations on thighs
Uterus enlarges 50 to 60 times original size

Toxemia of pregnancy A series of metabolic disturbances characterized at first by a rise in blood pressure, excess albumin in the urine, and fluid retention. More severe symptoms follow in the second stage and without appropriate medical attention can cause death.

Diuretic An agent that promotes urine excretion.

Lightening A labor process in which the uterus sinks downward about 2 inches because the baby's head, or other body part, settles far down into the pelvic area

Labor The act or process of giving birth to a child, expelling it with the placenta from the mother's body by means of uterine contractions.

False labor Rather intense and painful contractions of the uterus that do not actually thin the cervix or make obvious progress toward delivery.

Increased pigment production darkens the skin in 90 percent of pregnant women. The darkening appears especially in places that have stretched, as well as in nipples, vulva, moles and scars, and in the *linea nigra* (dark line), which develops during pregnancy and runs from the pubic bone up to above the navel. Ultraviolet radiation also stimulates pigment production, and women who do not want their skin to darken should avoid exposure to sunlight.

Changes and Complications in the Later Stages of Pregnancy By the sixth month, the increased needs of the fetus for oxygen, nutrition, and excretion increase the burden on the mother's lungs, heart, and kidneys. Her legs swell, and fetal activity sometimes makes it hard for her to sleep. To maintain balance while standing, she must throw her shoulders well back.

Figure 8-5 shows the position of the fetus and uterus at the seventh or eighth month of pregnancy.

Heartburn, constipation, and occasionally leg cramps occur, especially in the late months of pregnancy. Although these conditions are hard on the mother, in fact both digestion and metabolism are unusually efficient.

Figure 8–5 Position of the uterus and fetus after 32 weeks of pregnancy.

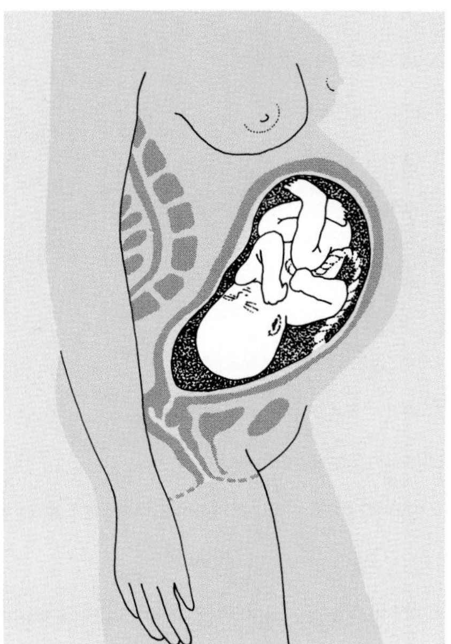

The body retains more water. Normal swelling can mean retaining up to 3 extra quarts of liquid. Some women also swell in the face, hands, ankles, or feet because the kidneys absorb even more water, sodium, and chlorides. If rings that normally fit the fingers become too tight, the swelling may predict a problem.

Toxemia of Pregnancy Sometimes swelling signals **toxemia of pregnancy**, a potentially dangerous condition that develops in three stages. In the first stage, blood pressure rises, there is too much protein in the urine, and face, hands, and legs swell. In the second stage, vision blurs, and the head aches continually. The third stage can bring convulsions and coma. *Any woman who notices such swelling should go immediately to a doctor*. Malnutrition is strongly suspected as a major factor in toxemia of pregnancy, and diet is crucial in controlling it. Salty foods and other sources of sodium are forbidden. Bed rest often helps, and **diuretic** foods and drugs are sometimes prescribed to increase the flow of urine, though their use is controversial. Toxemia usually does not appear until after the twenty-fourth week.

Lightening In the ninth month, the baby settles far down into the pelvic bones, its head—the part that is usually born first—fitting snugly. This process is called **lightening,** and it allows the uterus to sink downward about two inches and the abdomen to fall. Pelvic pressure increases, and pressure on the diaphragm reduces. Breathing becomes easier; urination becomes more frequent.

False Labor Throughout pregnancy, the uterus practices contracting. Near the delivery date, these contractions become more vigorous. Sometimes they are mistaken for true **labor** pains. **False labor** pains are usually irregular and short and stop within a few hours, however.

The Importance of Prenatal Care for Baby and Mother

While a baby's brain, bones, lungs, and eyes are forming, they are extremely vulnerable. If they don't receive exactly the right kind of nutrition through the mother's diet, or

Rh Blood Factor

When a fetus inherits an Rh blood factor that differs from the mother's, medical attention is required to offset the effects. For example, a woman with Rh-negative blood can build up immunity to her child's Rh-positive blood if it enters her own bloodstream during delivery. Exposure to the "foreign" blood of her fetus causes the mother's natural defense mechanism to produce antibodies to it. The antibodies act to neutralize the Rh-positive blood exactly as if it were harmful bacteria.

These antibodies increase with each succeeding pregnancy, and they attack the blood of the fetus in subsequent pregnancies. The blood corpuscles of the fetus are destroyed, and the baby is born with various degrees of anemia and jaundice.

This once dreaded problem is now almost entirely preventable through the use of a special gamma globulin called Rhogam, which is rich in anti-Rh antibodies. Rhogam attaches to and eliminates Rh-positive fetal cells in the maternal circulation before they can sensitize the mother. A first dose is usually given at twenty-eight weeks' gestation and a second larger dose within seventy-two hours after birth, miscarriage, or abortion—the sooner the better. It is beneficial only to those Rh-negative women who show no evidence of having already formed antibodies.

if they receive harmful drugs, even drugs normally not harmful (such as in some cough syrups and cold remedies), the child's body systems may be impaired for life. Special attention to the mother's health and diet during pregnancy is one of the best investments parents can make, because they produce lifelong benefits.

Early advice from health educators, midwives, obstetricians, and teachers of childbirth and baby care can be invaluable. Professionals can offer nutritional and physical fitness guidance and suggest what is harmful to the fetus. A doctor or midwife will advise against X-rays, smoking and even breathing in a smoky room, drinking almost any alcohol, and all drugs (if possible).

In the first prenatal visit, the mother will be asked for lots of information about her general health, diseases, operations, menstrual history, and record of previous pregnancies and abortions. The doctor or midwife will examine the mother's eyes, ears, nose, throat, chest, breasts, and abdomen, and will do a pelvic exam to feel the size, shape, and position of the uterus. He or she will probably do a Pap smear and take pelvic measurements. Urine will be checked for urinary tract infections. The mother will be weighed to begin tracking weight gain, and she will be informed about appropriate diet. Blood pressure will be measured for comparison in later pregnancy, when toxemia can develop.

Detecting Sexually Transmissible Disease Although sexually transmissible disease (STD) can be transmitted from mother to baby in pregnancy, early proper treatment can prevent devastating consequences to the child. Some of these diseases totally lack symptoms, so they require testing. A blood sample will be checked for a variety of conditions, including STDs: herpes, syphilis, gonorrhea, chlamydia, and blood type, anemia, and Rh incompatibilities. If discovered early, these conditions can be compensated for or cured so that the baby is not affected. Professional prenatal care reduces the chances of poor maternal health during and after pregnancy and increases the chances of a healthy baby born well.

If a pregnant woman has AIDS, there is a high probability that she will pass it on to her infant and that the child will develop this fatal disease. Doctors are now recommending that all women with increased risk of AIDS infection be tested before getting pregnant.

Exercise and Work Physical activity is particularly valuable during pregnancy. It contributes to mental as

Exploring Your Emotions

Your sister is seven months pregnant. She has not visited a doctor because she does not consider pregnancy an illness. She wants to deliver her child at home but has not found a physician or midwife willing to attend. How do you feel about her position? What would you counsel her to do?

Natural childbirth Childbirth without the use of painkillers for the mother or tools such as forceps to deliver the baby.

Lamaze method A method of natural childbirth that prepares the parents psychologically and the mother physically for delivery.

Contraction (uterine) A shortening of the uterus that reduces its size and eventually expels the fetus.

well as physical well-being. The prospective mother should continue all reasonable exercising that she is accustomed to—tennis, swimming, low-impact aerobic classes, gardening, dancing—until her stomach inhibits movement. The amniotic sac protects the fetus so that normal activities will not harm it. More strenuous activities that could result in a fall—skiing or skating, for example—are best delayed until after the birth.

Childbirth preparation classes often teach exercises for the body muscles involved in birth. Toned-up muscles aid delivery and help the body readjust to its normal shape afterward.

Working can help keep a prospective mother's mind off the symptoms and anxieties of pregnancy. Many women whose jobs are not too physically demanding work through their seventh or eighth month.

Preparing for Childbirth

In the 1920s Grantly Dick-Read, an English doctor, noted that women in so-called primitive societies had a less difficult time birthing than did women in highly civilized, technological societies. He concluded that fear, especially fear of the unknown, is responsible for much of the pain women suffer. The more the woman tenses up to avoid or block pain, the more unbearable the pain is and the more she obstructs the natural birth process. Dick-Read devised a training system called **natural childbirth**. Several similar methods of childbirth training are also in use now—psychoprophylaxis, the Bradley method, and the Lamaze method—all designed to ease birth by offering knowledge of the birth process and physical conditioning.

The **Lamaze method** is probably the most commonly used in the United States. As practiced here, the Lamaze method emphasizes not so much the mother's performance as her attitude in childbirth. During pregnancy, the mother works toward getting her body into peak physical condition for delivery, and she is trained to regard labor as a time of work, concentration, and confidence rather than of helplessness and suffering. The father is trained to take part, coaching the mother to relax, massaging her, giving moral support, monitoring her breathing, and keeping her informed of her progress. It is an important time for the parents to be together.

Exploring Your Emotions

If you plan to have children, do you want to be present or awake at childbirth? Why or why not?

Labor and Delivery

Just before birth, the uterus is stretched to its limits. The baby's head is about 4¼ inches in diameter, a tight fit for the pelvic bones through which it must pass. The baby's skull does have some "give," however.

Birth is never easy for the baby, and it may last many hours. Average duration of birth is 14 hours for a first baby, 8 hours for following ones. (See Figure 8-6.)

No one knows exactly what triggers birth, but the placenta and the muscles of the uterus seem to play a part. The uterus is the largest human muscle, and its size increases 50 to 60 times during pregnancy. Muscle fibers in the upper portion can contract and then relax to a shorter length than they were originally, without a change in tension. The uterus becomes gradually smaller so that it can continue to supply the force necessary to complete delivery. **Contraction** of the uterus eventually closes off each channel of blood flow between mother and baby, and during the third stage of labor, the placenta is expelled.

While the upper portion of the uterus thickens during labor, the lower portion—the cervix—must enlarge so that the baby's head can pass through. It thins out and lengthens as a result of labor contractions. Contractions are hard work for the mother. Each contraction normally supplies a 55-pound push, and "birthing" the baby's head requires a 100-pound push.

Contractions vary in intensity. They are slight to begin with, but as they travel downward from the top of the uterus, they become more intense. Over a cup of blood is expelled from the uterus with each push, under tremendous pressure. The mother feels pain—not from the contraction but from the grinding pressure of the baby's presenting part—usually the head—against the cervix and the pelvic structures. At their very worst, contractions cause an extremely intense grinding type of pain, lasting about 50 seconds to a minute at the most. This pain can be considered an integral part of giving birth, signaling that all is well. However, the pain can be heightened needlessly by tensing and attempting to block it.

First Stage of Labor The first stage of labor lasts an average of 13 hours for the first birth, and at the end the cervix is fully dilated, opened to about 4 inches. At this point, the head is usually midway down the mother's pelvis, and from now on she usually needs birthing assistance from a midwife or doctor or other experienced practitioner. See Figure 8-6b.

During the first stage of labor, the contractions usually last 25 to 35 seconds and come every 15 to 20 minutes at first, more often later. The mucus plug, which has closed off the cervical canal during pregnancy to keep out infection, is expelled. Its expulsion is a sure sign that labor has begun.

For first births, the obstetrician or midwife should be notified when pains occur about every 6 minutes and last for 30 seconds. A woman in labor should not eat or drink anything, because food stays undigested in the stomach.

In about 20 percent of women, the amniotic sac ruptures during a contraction, and the fluid rushes or trickles out. This action speeds up labor, and usually indicates that the second stage is about to begin. If the sac has not ruptured by the time the cervix dilates about 2 inches, the attendant will probably rupture it, improving the effectiveness of contractions and shortening labor.

Second Stage of Labor The second stage of labor begins when the cervix is completely dilated and the baby's head is in the birth canal (Figure 8-6c); it ends with delivery

Figure 8–6 The birth process: *(a)* full-term fetus before labor begins; *(b)* early stages of labor; cervix begins to dilate; *(c)* second stage of labor; cervix completely dilated; baby's head begins turning toward mother's back; *(d)* late stage of labor; baby's head is completely turned; head begins to emerge.

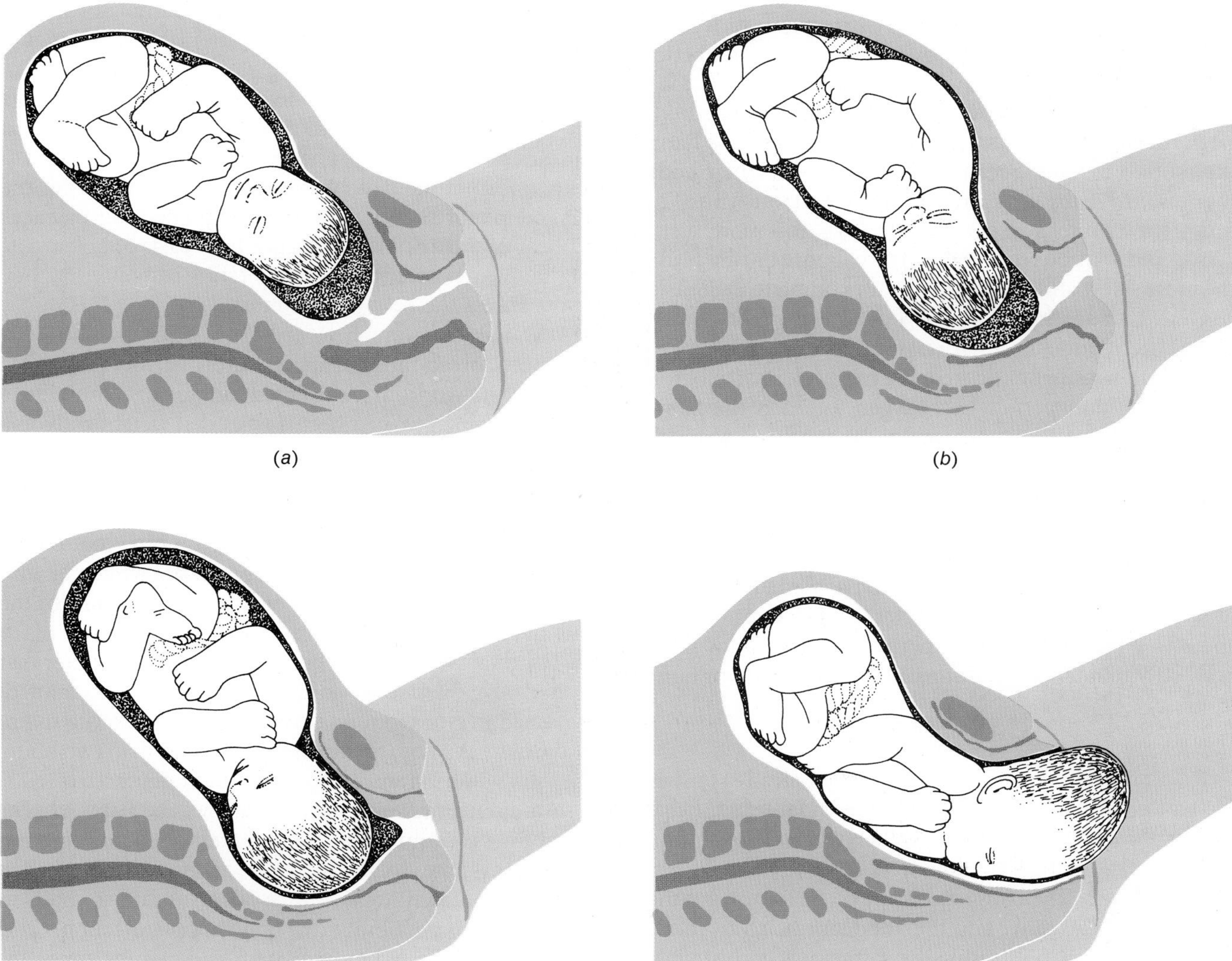

Caesarean section A surgical incision through the abdominal walls and uterus; performed to extract a fetus.

Episiotomy A surgical incision in the vulva to widen the birth canal.

General anesthetic An agent that usually produces unconsciousness to relieve pain.

Regional or local anesthetic An agent that blocks the nerves that carry pain signals from the pelvic area to the brain, while leaving the mother alert to follow instructions and witness the birth.

---

of the baby. It lasts from about 30 minutes to two hours for a first baby, and from 10 to 30 minutes in subsequent deliveries. If the mother cannot supply the 100 pounds of force needed to birth the head, the doctor can help with forceps or deliver the baby by **Caesarean section,** a procedure that involves cutting the abdomen and uterus open and removing the baby by hand. The position of the baby or the narrowness of the mother's pelvic opening may make a Caesarean necessary.

When the head appears, it stretches the perineum, the tissue between the vagina and the rectum, and may tear it. To avoid a jagged tear, which takes longer to heal, the attendant often cuts the tissue. This operation, called **episiotomy,** is usually done with local anesthesia.

Use of Anesthetics During Labor Of many controversies concerning childbirth, that over the use of anesthetics during labor has been one of the most intense. Many people feel that drugs given to the mother during childbirth harm the baby to some degree and sometimes harm the mother as well. Because of differences in their body weights, the baby gets proportionately about 15 to 20 times the mother's dosage. In general, the more alert, active, and vigorous the mother and baby are during birth, the more safely and competently they complete their task.

General anesthesia is not widely favored because it makes the mother unconscious during the birth experience. Such anesthetics depress the mother's physiological functioning and permit less oxygen to reach the baby. The baby's respiratory functions can be depressed so much that it may have trouble taking its first breaths. **Regional or local anesthetics** can relieve pelvic muscle pain without disturbing the baby's oxygen intake. Spinal blocks, used for awake Caesareans, are regional anesthetics.

Many doctors, midwives, and laypeople believe that a healthy woman who understands the mechanics of labor and is well prepared for the experience will, with any luck, need only minor amounts of pain-relieving drugs or none at all.

Birth A final push "crowns" the baby's head—pushes the widest part into the vulva. The attendant then helps deliver the baby, telling the mother when to push and when to pant or breathe quietly as the baby slowly and gently emerges. The baby's head appears, face toward the mother's back usually, and the attendant helps to rotate it to one side to avoid tearing the soft tissues of the vulva. (See Figure 8-6d.) As soon as the head is delivered, the attendant feels for a loop of umbilical cord around the neck, and if there is one he or she either disentangles or cuts it. After the shoulder can be seen, the attendant waits about 30 seconds to give the uterus time to retract and get smaller. Another half-minute is allowed after the shoulder is delivered before the rest of the body is slowly pulled out by the shoulders. The cord is then squeezed to strip the blood back into the infant, adding about 2.5 ounces of blood to the baby's bloodstream. After the crowning of the head, birth is completed in two to three minutes. (See Figure 8-7.)

The cord is tied and cut. Nature seals it with a jellylike substance that swells up on exposure to air and squeezes the embedded blood vessels shut. The resulting buildup of carbon dioxide in the baby's blood stimulates the respiratory center of the brain, and the baby takes its first breath and cries.

The first breath requires five times as much effort as an ordinary breath because thousands of tiny uninflated air sacs of the lungs must be expanded—like blowing up thousands of little balloons. Breathing is irregular for the first couple of days; it takes that long for the air passages to clear of mucus. The early cries help clear out obstructing fluids. Those cries may be a reflex response, or they may express the baby's discomfort.

The baby has much to cry about. He—or she—has just been forced through an incredibly narrow tunnel. He has lost the world that sustained him for his entire life, a world in which he had been suspended weightlessly in a warm, living, pulsating sea, and in which all sounds were muffled and the light if any, was dim. The light is blinding. Every sound is sharp and terrifyingly loud. It is cold—25°F colder than in the uterus. Gravity pins him down. There is a sudden frightening freedom of movement, and those reassuring walls he has been tapping against for the last five months have disappeared.

For the first time ever, he is in contact with matter that is not alive. He is put on a table, wiped off, examined, wrapped in cloth, put in a box, and left in a sterile room. If the baby is a boy, then perhaps no more than two hours later he will be strapped to a tray and circumcised.

An attendant weighs and measures the baby, checks heart rate, breathing, muscle tone, reflex irritability, skin, lungs, eyes, nose, palate, abdomen, and rectum. The baby's eyes are routinely treated with silver nitrate solution to prevent any possibility of gonorrheal infection, and vitamin K is injected to regulate blood-clotting time.

Medical Procedures Some Parents Would Like to Change

Routine Prepping Prepping, shaving the mother's pubic hair when she is ready to deliver, may contribute to a sterile environment for emergency surgery, but appears unnecessary for most births.

Routine Enemas Enemas are often given to the mother about to deliver to guarantee that the delivery bed will not be made unsterile when she is pushing hard and cannot always control her bowels. However, an enema given while a woman is in intense labor causes great physical and mental discomfort.

Routine Episiotomy Routine episiotomies are not necessary because the vagina can often stretch sufficiently during birth without tearing. Episiotomies may be necessary if a baby's head is so large or its birth position is such that it would tear the mother's flesh badly.

Routine Delivery in the Supine Position Mothers usually lie in a supine position (on the back) during hospital deliveries in the United States. In other cultures and times, women often have delivered sitting in a labor chair. An upright sitting position or a semisitting position may be the most comfortable one for delivery and is probably the safest position, partially because it allows gravity to help the mother push out the baby.

Caesarean Sections Caesarean section is delivery of a child through an incision made in the abdominal wall and through the uterus. Usually the mother is given a regional anesthetic of the spinal type so that she will not feel pain and yet can be awake when the baby is delivered. Both incisions are stitched up after the baby and placenta have been removed. Caesarean sections are performed when hard labor does not sufficiently open the cervix or when the mother's pelvic structure is too small to allow the baby to move through the birth canal. They are also performed if the placenta or cord are in the baby's way or if excessive bleeding occurs.

Caesarean delivery is not as safe for the mother or baby as is a normal delivery because it is a major abdominal operation and carries with it the risk that any major operation involves. They should be performed only in case of complications during labor to save the life of either the mother or the child. Yet the number of these operations is increasing with the threat of malpractice suits.

All parents should consider the possibility of a Caesarean and hope they will never have to use it. The best way to avoid an unnecessary C-section is to choose a doctor carefully, perhaps with the advice of a family doctor or a hospital staff member who could find out the prospective obstetrician's C-section rate and general reputation. The parents can interview obstetricians to find out when and why they consider a Caesarean necessary, how many hours they consider an adequate test of labor, whether they use sonograms, amniocentesis, and X-rays to check a baby's progress before making a decision, and how long their Caesarean patients stay in the hospital. It is important to know beforehand if the doctor suspects there will be complications during delivery, so that one can prepare psychologically for it. Doctors frequently keep such information from the parents for fear of scaring them.

Inducing Labor Inducing labor is a deliberate attempt to start labor. This can be done by rupturing membranes or by using chemical substitutes for hormones present in natural labor. Although it may make scheduling a birth more convenient, it presents risk to both child and mother. When induced, labor contractions are usually more painful and more intense than ordinary ones, and the intravenous oxytocin drip must be carefully and wisely monitored to avoid potentially fatal complications. Too heavy a dose can cause the uterus to rupture, maternal blood pressure to rise, and the umbilical cord to prolapse.

More important, if contractions are too intense and too frequent, as they often are during induction, the baby registers a dangerous decrease in heart rate. It has insufficient time to recover enough oxygen between contractions, and the reduced heart rate indicates fetal distress. Consequently, fetal heart monitors are used almost routinely on women in labor. Sensors are placed on the mother's abdomen and a tape constantly records the heartbeat of the unborn infant. The continual monitoring reveals fetal distress that might not even be noticed if the mother were simply checked intermittently with a stethoscope. For women who show some abnormality, a more obtrusive monitor places a catheter

(continued on next page)

Medical Procedures Some Parents Would Like to Change (*continued*)

inside the uterus (through already ruptured membranes) alongside the fetal head, to measure uterine contractions. In addition, a small electrode is attached to the baby's scalp to record the electrocardiogram and heart rate. The intrauterine catheter can provide an entry for infection and should be used only when abnormalities are evident.

Use of both the oxytocin drip and the intrauterine catheter introduces new risks as well as possible advantages to the birth process. Some hospitals do not permit induction for convenience, but the practice of inducing labor is becoming more common nevertheless.

Circumcision Circumcision is a surgical procedure in which part of the penis's foreskin is cut off. Usually an obstetrician does it shortly after a boy's birth. But the disadvantages of circumcision outweigh advantages.

The pain of circumcision, small but real possibilities of infection and bleeding, and (rarely) complications from the procedure, plus the possibility that circumcision desensitizes the penis are reasons enough to dissuade increasing numbers of parents from circumcising their children.

Nationwide, the number of boy babies circumcised has dropped from over 90 to about 72 percent. In most of the modern world, circumcision is the exception rather than the rule. In England, where 80 percent of male babies were circumcised in the 1940s, numbers dropped to 0.5 percent when the National Health Service stopped paying for it in 1950.

Third Stage of Labor After the birth, continuing contractions force the placenta out. Usually the attendant helps by applying pressure on the abdomen just above the pubic bone and gently pulling on the cut cord. Expelling the placenta ordinarily takes from five to fifteen minutes.

The attendant sews up the episiotomy and massages the uterus as it becomes smaller. The mother usually relaxes and sleeps for a while after birth.

The Puerperium

The **puerperium** is the time after childbirth during which the mother's sex organs, especially the uterus, slowly return to the nonpregnant state. This return takes six to eight weeks. Following normal childbirth, women who chose to deliver in the hospital stay only two to three days to make sure all is well, and they need not stay in bed if they don't feel tired. Women who birthed by Caesarean section stay longer while the incision heals.

Postpartum Depression During the first week or so after childbirth, some women are emotionally explosive. A few experience some **postpartum depression**, which may be caused largely by the great drop in hormone levels in the first days after birth. These women vacillate between highs and lows and seem to overreact. General bodily discomfort and discomfort from stitches and sore breasts contribute to feelings of annoyance. Frustration and boredom with a hospital stay are common reactions.

A more critical postpartum depression, which can last for years, affects a small number of women, usually those who have shown previous tendencies toward depression. Women who become suspicious, confused, or incoherent and have real troubles with insomnia should consult their physicians for help, both for their own good and for their child's. Postpartum depression can be treated successfully, and these women can and often do become perfectly competent mothers. And if they become mothers again, the chances are great—80 to 90 percent—that they will not suffer a repetition of this postpartum depression.

Breastfeeding After the child is born, the mother's pituitary gland releases the hormone prolactin, which stimulates milk secretion. In most cases, the advantages of breastfeeding far outweigh the disadvantages. No other food is quite so good for the child as the mother's milk. It is sterile and contains **antibodies** that help protect the child against diseases the mother has had. It is better for humans than cow's milk, parts of which are difficult for humans to digest. It has more milk sugar, more vitamins, and a better balance of minerals than cow's milk.

Breastfeeding usually gives the baby a sense of security and is generally comforting to the mother as well. Female animals show a significant reduction in stressful responses to situations while they are nursing their young. Infants,

Puerperium The period of about six to eight weeks after labor during which the mother's reproductive organs, particularly the uterus, return to the nonpregnant state.

Postpartum depression An emotional low experienced by the mother following childbirth; infrequently intensifies until medical attention is necessary.

Antibodies Proteins in the blood that are generated in reaction to foreign proteins, producing immunity from them.

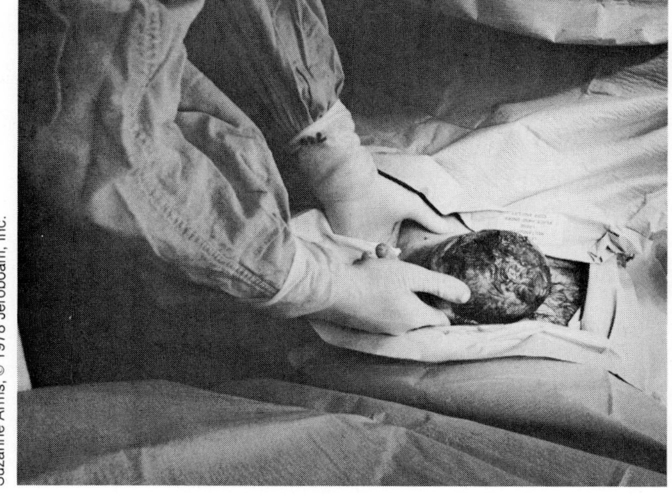

Suzanne Arms, © 1978 Jeroboam, Inc.

(a)

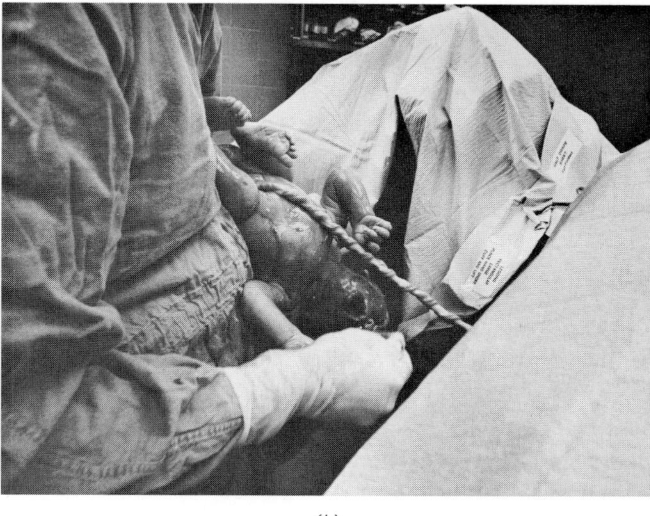

(b)

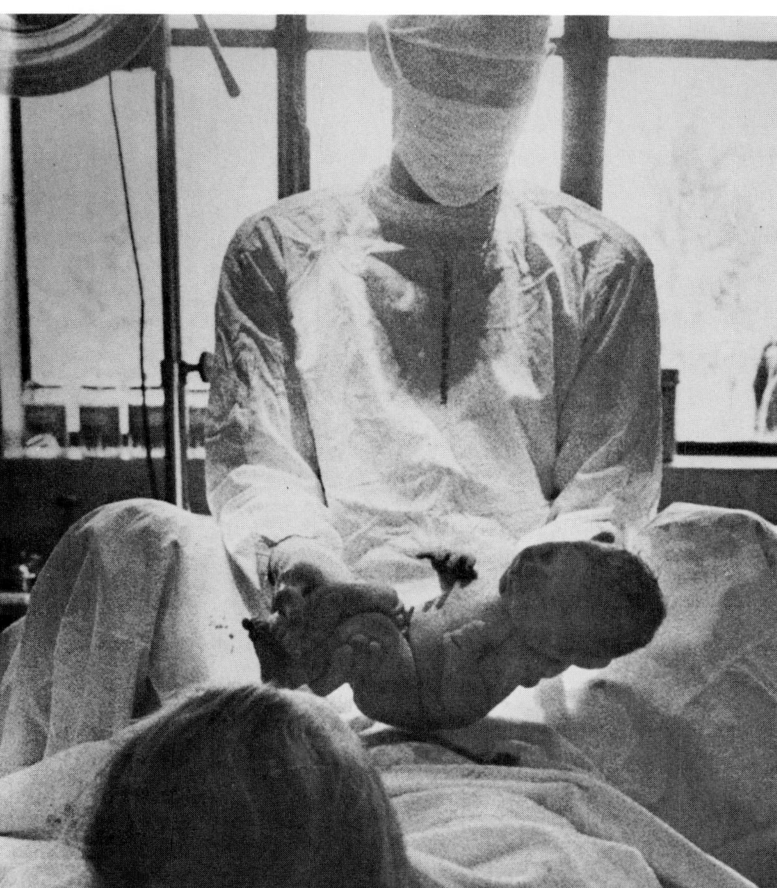

Eve Arnold, Magnum Photos

(c)

Figure 8–7 The sequence of birth after the baby's head emerges: (a) assistance from the doctor; (b) the newly born infant; (c) the mother's first sight of her baby.

Lochia A vaginal discharge occurring for several weeks after childbirth

who are especially sensitive to their mothers' emotional states, benefit from the calm that the nursing mother communicates. Parents are spared the bother of sterilizing bottles and preparing formulas. Bleeding stops sooner, and the uterus and other tissues recover their normal state more rapidly when the mother nurses. (A nursing mother may feel somewhat confined, and an early return to work may complicate breastfeeding. It is possible to express milk from the breast, freeze it, and later bottle-feed it to the baby.)

A very few mothers do not have enough milk to feed the child. Breast size has nothing to do with the amount of milk produced; small breasts can produce as much milk as large ones. The nursing mother must also continue to eat as much as she did during late pregnancy.

Uterine Shrinkage By the end of the second week after birth, the uterus can no longer be felt in the abdomen; in four or five weeks, it returns to normal. For several weeks there is a discharge called **lochia**, a mixture of blood from the site in the uterus where the placenta was attached and from the crumbling of the uterine lining. Exercise helps restore the abdomen to its original size, shape, and muscle tone.

Exploring Your Emotions

Do you like children, on the whole? How do you feel about this one? How do you think he or she feels about life? Write, in this child's words as you imagine them, some advice for parents.

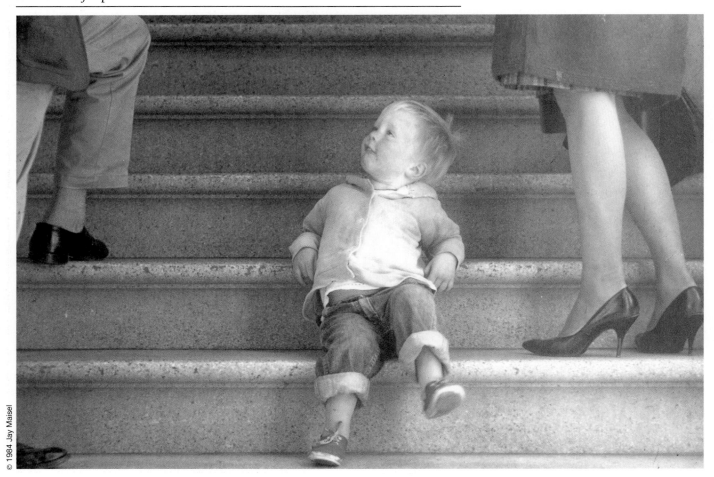

Am I Parent Material?

These questions are posed to you as you consider the most important decision you will ever make—whether or not to have a child. The decision to have a child is one that you will have to live with for the rest of your life. The responsibility of a new life is awesome. These questions are designed to raise ideas that you may not have otherwise considered. There are no "right" answers and no "grades." You must decide for yourself what your answers reveal about your aptitude for parenthood.

You *do* have a choice. Exercise that choice with knowledge and careful thought. And then do what seems right for you.

Is My Lifestyle Conducive to Parenting?

1. Would a child interfere with my educational plans? Would I have the energy to go to school and raise a child at the same time?

2. Would a child restrict my individual growth and development?

3. Could I handle children and a career well? Am I tired when I come home from work, or do I have lots of energy left?

4. Does my job or my partner's job require a lot of traveling?

5. Am I financially able to support a child? Am I prepared to spend about $100 a week to rear my child to age 18? Or over $80,000, not including one partner's income loss if he or she would choose to remain at home?

6. Do I live in a neighborhood conducive to raising a child? Would I be willing to move?

7. Would I be willing to give up the freedom to do what I want to do, when I want to do it?

8. Would I be willing to restrict my social life? Would I miss lost leisure time and privacy?

9. Would my partner and I be prepared to spend more time at home? Would we have enough time to spend with a child?

10. Would I be willing to devote a great part of my life, at *least* 18 years, to being responsible for a child? And spend my entire life being concerned about my child's welfare?

11. Would I be prepared to be a single parent if my partner left or died?

Am I Ready to Raise a Child?

1. Do I like children? Have I had enough experiences with babies? Toddlers? Teenagers?

2. Do I enjoy teaching others?

3. Do I communicate easily with others?

4. Do I have enough love to give a child? Can I express affection easily?

5. Would I have the patience to raise a child? Can I tolerate noise and confusion? Can I deal with disrupted schedules?

6. How do I handle anger? Would I abuse my child if I lost my temper?

7. What do I know about discipline and freedom? About setting limits and giving space? Would I be too strict? Too lenient? Am I a perfectionist? How do I deal with change?

8. Do I know my own values and goals yet? Could I help my child develop constructive values?

9. What kind of relationship did I have with my parents? Would I repeat the same mistakes my parents made or would I overindulge or restrict my child in an attempt not to repeat my parents' mistakes?

10. How much would I worry about my child's health and safety? Would I be able to take care of a hurt or sick child?

11. What if my decision to have a child turns out to have been wrong for me?

What Do I Expect to Gain from the Parenting Experience?

1. Do I enjoy child-centered activities?

2. Do I think that having a child would show others I am a mature person?

3. Would I want my child to be a miniature version of me? Would I be willing to adopt a child?

4. Would I feel comfortable if my child had ideas different from mine? How different?

5. Would I expect my child to make contributions I wish I had made in the world?

6. Would I expect my child to keep me from being lonely in my old age?

7. Would I be prepared emotionally to let my child leave when he or she grows up?

(continued on next page)

Am I Parent Material? (*continued*)

8. Would I expect my child to fulfill my relationship with my partner?

9. Do I need parenthood to fulfill my role as a man or woman?

10. Do I need a child to make my life meaningful?

11. Would I feel strongly about wanting my child to be a boy or girl? What if I didn't get the one I wanted?

Have I Adequately Discussed the Parenting Question with My Partner?

1. Does my partner want to have a child? Is he or she willing to ask these questions of himself or herself? Have we adequately discussed our reasons for wanting a child?

2. Do my partner and I understand each other's feelings about religion, work, family, child raising, future goals? Are our feelings compatible? Are they conducive to good parenting?

3. Would both my partner and I contribute our fair shares in raising the child?

4. Could we provide a child with a really good home environment? Is our relationship stable? Do we have a good sexual relationship?

5. After having a child, would my partner and I be able to separate if we should have unsolvable problems? Or would we feel obligated to remain together for the sake of the child?

6. Would we be able to share each other with a child without jealousy?

7. Do we want to bring a child into today's overpopulated world to face the social problems of our times?

8. Does my partner or do I have a hereditary abnormality we might pass on to a child? Could I emotionally and financially deal with having a physically or mentally handicapped child?

9. Suppose one of us wants a child and the other doesn't. Who wins?

10. Which of the questions in this [questionnaire] do we really need to discuss before making a decision?

Carole Goldman

Return of Menstruation When a mother does not nurse, menstruation usually recurs within ten weeks. Breastfeeding can prevent the menstrual period from returning for as long as six months. The hormone prolactin, which is involved in milk production, suppresses hormones vital to the development of the corpus luteum and mature eggs, and the ovaries produce less estrogen and progesterone. However, ovulation—and pregnancy—can occur before the return of menstruation. If the mother becomes pregnant during nursing, she should stop nursing, to ensure good nutrition for the unborn child.

Exploring Your Emotions

What did your parents know about raising children? What do you know about parenting? Did you learn what you know from your parents? Can you learn anything about disciplining, encouraging, loving, teaching, and tolerating children from courses and textbooks? From observing and thinking about other families?

Prospective Parents as Medical Consumers

As consumers, prospective parents can demand satisfaction from hospital and medical professionals or deprive them of business. Equipped with adequate information about obstetrical care, parents have the power to change hospital birth procedures.

Informed Decisions about Birth Procedures Parents have objected to routines performed to maintain the sterile environment necessary for surgery even though childbirth procedures do not usually require such rigor. Many doctors formerly insisted on enemas and shaving the pubic hair for the mother, kept the father out of the delivery room, and separated the baby from its parents immediately after birth. Some physicians routinely anesthetize the mother, induce labor, use forceps and fetal monitoring, deliver by Caesarean section, and generally manipulate the birth process for their own convenience, occasionally to the detriment of both mother and child.

All these procedures may be necessary at certain times, but decisions to use them are controversial even among

Redefining 'Mother' and 'Father'

More than a contract dispute, even more than a custody fight, the Baby M case is a clash of values—and yet another ethical conundrum posed by the steady advance of medical technology. What the birth control revolution did for sex without babies, artificial insemination and related techniques have done for babies without sex.

Surrogacy arises because of two "very normal" desires, according to Dr. Nancy Dickey, a Houston family practitioner who chairs the American Medical Association's Council on Judicial and Ethical Affairs. One infertile woman wants a child that is her own or as nearly her own as possible in a society with a shortage of babies available for adoption, and another woman who is fertile wants to bear the child for a fee.

In the Baby M case, Mary Beth Whitehead signed a contract with William and Elizabeth Stern, and agreed to bear their child for a $10,000 fee after being artificially inseminated with Mr. Stern's sperm.

Experts voice two main concerns about surrogate motherhood: the difficulty of evaluating potential surrogates to minimize the physical and psychological risk, and the potential for exploitation of poor women who become surrogates merely to earn the customary fee of at least $10,000.

Few observers of the Baby M trial have failed to note the contrast between Elizabeth Stern, an affluent 41-year-old professor of pediatrics and Mary Beth Whitehead, 29, a high school dropout who married at 16.

"In real life," columnist Ellen Goodman has pointed out, "the wealthy don't become surrogates and the poor do not buy surrogates, and the hired matchmakers do not work for love."

The composite portrait of the typical surrogate mother that emerged from a study of 125 surrogate mothers is a 25-year-old woman with two previous pregnancies. Nearly 90 percent were married, 80 percent had at least a high school education. Just over half were Protestant, just under half were Catholic, and none were Jewish.

That a surrogate mother might have second thoughts about giving up her baby is no surprise. Any doctor who has practiced obstetrics, Dickey said, knows how common it is for a woman facing an unplanned pregnancy to undergo a gradual change of attitude and become totally committed to the pregnancy as it develops.

"I only signed on an egg, I never signed on the life of a child," Whitehead said last August.

In a brief opinion issued 18 months ago, the AMA's ethics council neither endorsed surrogate motherhood nor called for its prohibition. The panel concluded that because of "inadequate answers to a number of social, psychological and ethical problems," surrogacy did not yet offer the best solution to infertility, Dickey said.

The American College of Obstetricians and Gynecologists has expressed "significant concern" about unresolved issues in surrogate mothering, which it said tends to "depersonalize the reproductive process." The American Fertility Society last fall expressed "serious ethical reservations" about surrogate motherhood, saying it should remain legal but experimental.

Physicians are divided on the issue, though only a small number have dealt directly with surrogacy cases, Dickey said. One group sees the dilemmas as too intense and too close to the social taboo against child-selling for society to solve. Another group believes the benefits of enabling infertile couples to have children far outweigh the considerable risks involved in surrogate mothering.

Dickey said the "vast majority of professionals" are somewhere in between—uncertain, worried, wary.

The Baby M case is symptomatic of the development of a whole range of "nonstandard human reproduction." Ranging from artificial insemination to gestation in a host uterus, these methods challenge traditional notions about parenthood and individual rights. Even language itself becomes problematic: the New Jersey case, in one sense, is an effort to define for Baby M the words "mother" and "father."

Last February, the Kentucky Supreme Court ruled that a surrogacy contract does not violate a state law against baby selling. The ruling gave the surrogate mother five days after the birth to change her mind about giving up the baby.

State adoption laws typically give a woman 30 days after birth to change her mind about giving up a child for adoption. States currently do not regulate surrogate motherhood, though baby selling, like sale of transplantable organs, is illegal.

The public, though ambivalent, is generally supportive of surrogate motherhood. In a recent Newsweek-Gallup national poll, 60 percent of Americans said they would

(continued on next page)

Redefining "mother" and "father" (*continued*)

not consider contracting with a surrogate mother to bear a child even if health or fertility problems were a factor. But 63 percent approved of a woman making use of a surrogate mother if she is unable to conceive.

But is the benefit worth the physical, emotional and legal risk? To the relatively small but growing number of infertile couples who have become parents through the pregnancy of a surrogate, the answer is obvious. But many experts wonder.

SOURCE: Don Colburn, 1987, *Washington Post Health*, February 24.

Six Ways to Start a Family

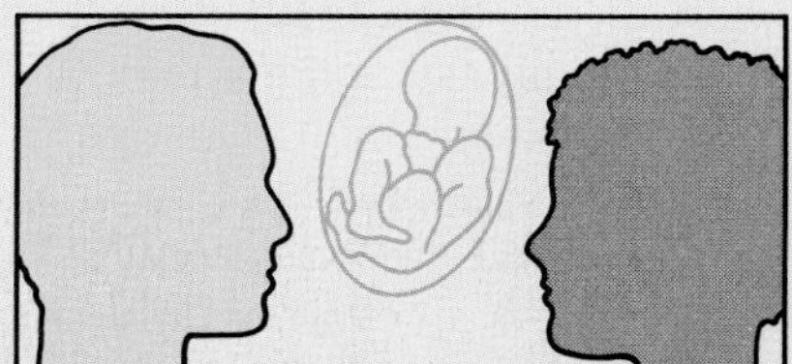

Traditional

1. Couple conceives child.
2. The child stays with the couple, who are its genetic and legal parents.

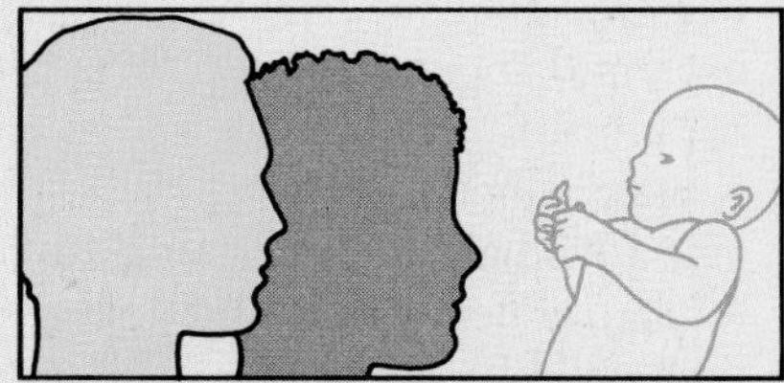

Adoptive

1. Couple is unable to conceive, or chooses not to.
2. An adoption agency matches the couple with child to be adopted.
3. Adoption papers are signed. Couple accepts parental responsibilities but has no genetic link to the child.

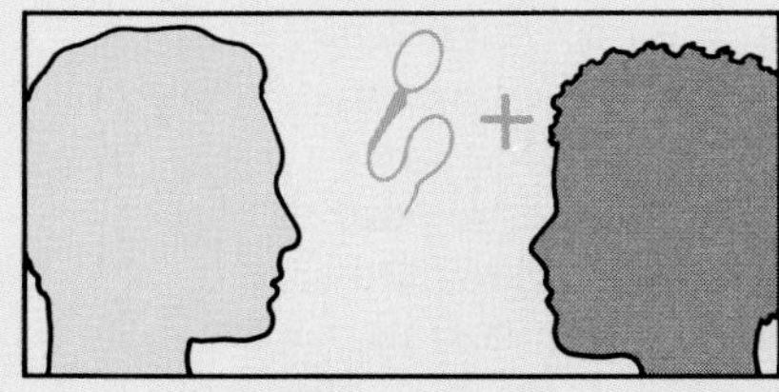

Donor Sperm

1. Couple is unable to conceive because male is infertile.
2. Sperm purchased from a sperm bank is used to impregnate the woman by artificial insemination.
3. The child is genetically linked to the mother but not the father. The sperm donor—the biological father—has no legal link to the child.

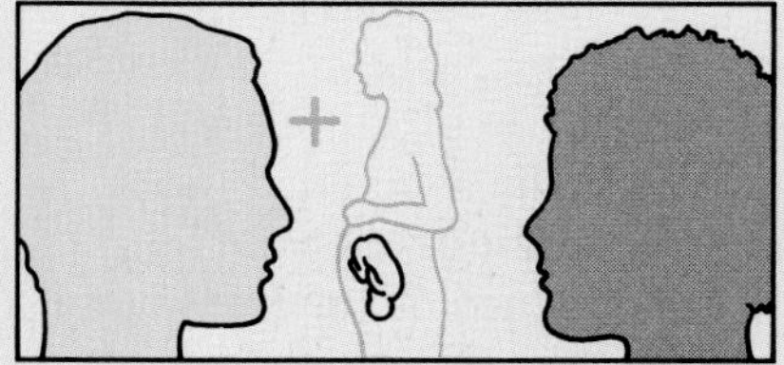

Surrogate Mother (the Baby M case)

1. Couple is unable to conceive because the female is infertile or pregnancy would be too risky.
2. A second woman is selected to be inseminated with the father's sperm. She signs a contract agreeing to bear the child and give it up after birth, usually for a sum of money.
3. Shortly after birth, the child is given to the couple. The child is genetically linked to the father but not to the mother. Whether the woman who bore the child—the biological mother—has the right to change her mind and keep the child is now being considered in court.

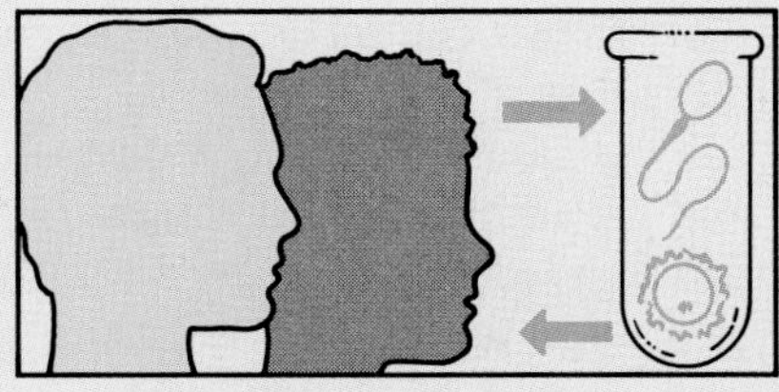

Test-Tube Baby

1. Although male and female produce sperm and eggs, the couple is unable to conceive.
2. Sperm and egg are combined in a laboratory.
3. The fertilized egg is implanted back into the woman.
4. The child stays with the couple, who are its genetic and legal parents.

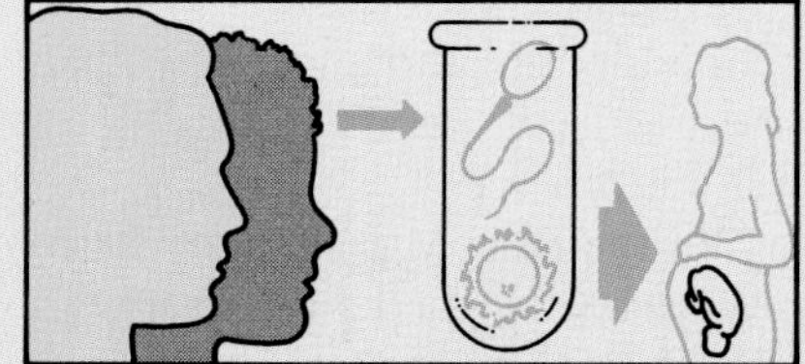

Host Uterus

1. Although male and female produce sperm and eggs, they are unable or unwilling to have a pregnancy.
2. Sperm from the male and egg from the female are combined in a laboratory.
3. The fertilized egg is implanted into a second woman, who agrees to bear the child and give it up, usually for a sum of money.
4. Shortly after birth, the child is given to the couple. Although brought to term in the uterus of another woman, the child's genes all come from the couple.

doctors. Some medical professionals and state governments are recognizing childbirth as a natural and healthy process. They are attempting to break down rigid hospital routines in the delivery room and to offer parents a variety of options. Fathers are often allowed in the delivery room, there is more emphasis on keeping mother and child together, rooming-in is now routine, and in some hospitals fathers even spend the night.

Although parents may not have sufficient knowledge to decide the advisability of performing a Caesarean section or inducing labor, they can choose a doctor who will use such procedures in extraordinary rather than ordinary cases. Through interviews and advice from other doctors and hospital staff members, they can choose a doctor who offers options for treatment—up to the limit of medical safety—to control their own pregnancy and childbirth.

The Alternatives Many families are turning to alternative settings and methods of childbirth to avoid the impersonal environment, imposing equipment, technology, and higher costs of the hospital, even though the risk to life during emergencies is greater.

Home Births During the last fifteen years or so, an increasing number of Americans have chosen to have their children born at home. About one of every ten California babies is born at home.

Midwives Home births create a demand for midwives to assist in pre- and postnatal care and delivery. The medical establishment, after several centuries of outlawing midwives, is finally allowing them a useful role complementary to its own. Some states are certifying nurses to become

Exploring Your Emotions

What feelings do these pictures evoke in you? How do you feel these parents feel about their children? What aspects of the parenting you received as a child would you want to pass on to a child of your own? What aspects would you rather not pass on?

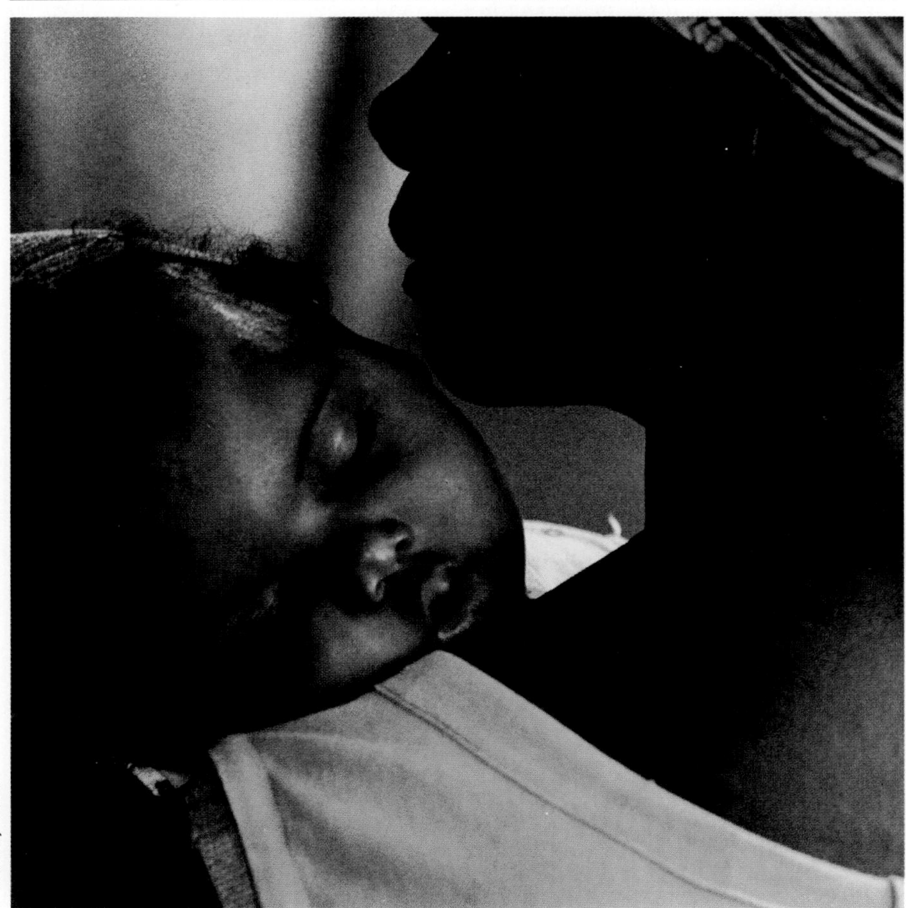

© 1984 Jay Maisel

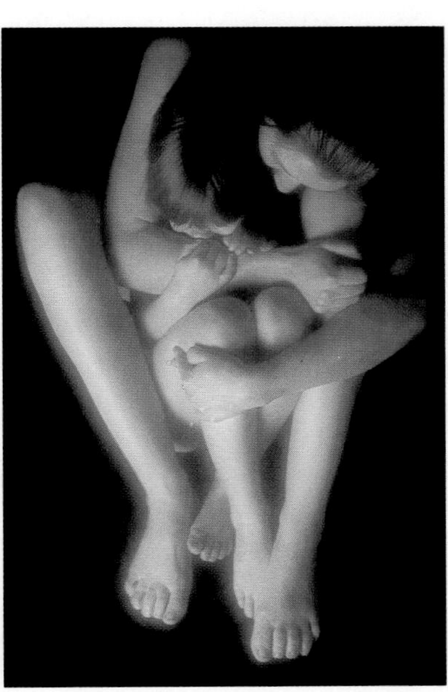

Jim Sadlone/Light Language

Who's Minding the Kids?

In the recently released study, "Who's Minding the Kids?," its most detailed on child care so far, the U.S. Census Bureau estimates that care givers mind about 26.5 million of the kids aged 14 and under, out of 52 million such children in the nation.

- Among children under five years old, an estimated three million are cared for in other people's homes. That accounts for the biggest share, 37 percent, of the nation's preschoolers.
- An estimated 2.5 million preschoolers are cared for in their own homes, nearly half by their fathers.
- Organized day care centers watch about 1.8 million preschoolers, nonrelatives outside the home tend another 1.8 million, and relatives in their own homes watch 1.2 million.
- Some 663,000 preschoolers are cared for by mothers who work at home or take their children with them to their jobs.
- Of children aged five to 14, 13.7 million, or 75.2 percent, attend kindergarten or grade school while their mothers work. Of those, about one million look after themselves after school.
- An estimated 2.1 million school-age children are watched at home by relatives and nonrelatives, about half of them by their fathers.
- Some 782,000 school-age children are watched in other people's homes, 523,000 in professional day care facilities, 581,000 by mothers who work at home or take their children with them to work.
- An estimated 488,000 children care for themselves without supervision.

The Census Bureau said that finding care givers for the youngest children presents the biggest problem, because formal day care facilities often exclude infants and toddlers. Of children less than a year old, 1.7 million, or 78 percent, were cared for at home or in other people's homes.

What criteria can parents use to evaluate people entrusted with the physical, mental, and emotional development of babies?

The best choice for the child, other than having one of the parents, is usually a qualified person who can come into the home—a nanny. This, of course, is also the most expensive. The next best option is a neighborhood family day care in which a well-trained and credentialed individual takes in a maximum of three or four children. Such individuals are often hard to find, because of long waiting lists. Most working parents simply can't afford these two choices. People who *must* work to sustain the family have the least choice in finding quality care for their children.

In many of the subsidized centers, the employees are overworked, poorly paid, and often are not very interested in children. It is important to thoroughly check out anyone before leaving your child in his or her care. So what should you look for, in whatever type of care you may choose?

All caretakers should genuinely like babies and small children, besides being well trained in child care and development. When you bring a sitter into your home, make sure the person can feel caring for the entire family, and not compete with parents for the child's attention. He or she should *want* to follow the parent's directions. The advantages of in-the-home care are less disruptions for the child, and a better chance of screening, getting references, and selecting a person who's sensitive to your child. Also, if your child is sick, you can still go to work.

The next category to consider is the family day care. Find out why this person (usually a mother) is taking in children by the day. If to be at home with her own child, that's a good reason. Watch how she interacts with her child and how the others are allowed to compete with that child. Can she adapt to each child's needs? If so, this can be rated as a warm, responsive environment for your child.

Day care centers should be carefully evaluated. Cleanliness and safety are important, but not the only things you would want to consider. Are parents welcome to drop in at any time of the day? If not, this may be a warning signal. Are the personnel well trained? Do they really care for children, and will they treat each one as an individual? What is the ratio of adults to children? There should be not less than one adult per three or four babies, or one adult per four or five toddlers.

Finding the best affordable child care goes a long way in resolving the conflict all working parents go through, and helps make parenthood a joyful, rewarding experience.

Sources: Deborah Kaplan, 1987, "The Care Tax on Mom's Pay," *The Detroit Free Press,* May 25, pp. B1–2; and Joyce Tintjer, March 1987, "Who Will Take Care of Your Baby When You Go Back to Work?" *Healthline,* pp. 3–4.

midwives, establishing programs to train them, and specifying the conditions under which they can practice. In California, an extra twelve to eighteen months of training for midwife certification is required in addition to the nursing degree. Usually midwives first work in conjunction with a physician and then move into obstetric clinics and private practice.

The procedure often follows this order: if a woman is classified as a low-risk patient at her initial pregnancy examination by a doctor, after considering her health and record of past births, the doctor may recommend that she be attended by a midwife. About three-fourths of all expectant mothers could be so categorized.

The nurse midwife administers all prenatal care and, barring complications, also performs the delivery and subsequent treatment. The midwife can devote time to the psychosocial aspects of routine births, including mental and physical conditioning, long natural labors, and family counseling. It has been convincingly shown that women administered to by a midwife are more likely to adhere to pre- and postnatal treatment than are those who see a doctor.

Alternative Birth Centers In response to the increase in the number of home births, some hospitals are introducing *alternative birth centers (ABCs)* to alleviate some of the criticisms of traditional hospital routines. ABCs have evolved for prospective parents who train toward natural childbirth and who are expected to have low-risk, uncomplicated births. The centers are alternatives to both home birth, where emergencies might not be adequately handled, and to traditional hospital birth, where procedures sometimes seem too impersonal and technological. ABCs attempt to provide a supportive environment to meet emotional needs; because they are located in a hospital, scientific know-how and equipment are available. The cost is substantially lower than that of a regular hospital birth.

Parenting

When the anticipation and anxiety of pregnancy and delivery are over, the joy and anxiety of parenting begin. Many attitudes of parents toward their children are related to how the parents accept and react toward themselves. People who can rejoice in themselves and tolerate their own foibles find it much easier to appreciate the uniqueness and understand the strengths and weaknesses of others.

One important but difficult thing for parents to realize is that their children are separate and potentially independent beings. Parents who have insights into their own needs and desires and who have a healthy respect for the rights of their children develop long-term positive relationships with them. How do such parents behave toward their children? First, they recognize the difference between nurturing and domineering. They tend to use praise and attention to reinforce their children's appropriate behavior. They teach personal responsibility, value orientations, and personal hygiene skills. They recognize that parents tend to be models for their children and try to act accordingly. They pay attention to their children and are patient with them.

Too often parents see their children as extensions of themselves. Such parents attempt to "achieve" through their children, foisting on them their own desires and goals. An early possessive behavior on the part of parents encourages an unhealthy dependence on the part of a child. In later years, usually during adolescence, the dependent child often must turn away from the parents—reject or rebel against them—just to find out who he or she is. For both the parents and the child, this rift is painful and may never be healed.

Exploring Your Emotions

Will or do you treat your children differently from the way your parents treated you? Will you require more work of them? Teach them more things? Spend more time with them? Let them find out that experience is the best teacher?

Exploring Your Emotions

If you do not have children, how do you think you will feel later in life—when you are 30? 40? 50? 60?

Parenting well does not come automatically. Good parents are not just born that way: they work at it and evolve. And it is hard work. Educating ourselves about the best methods of behavior and care during pregnancy and childbirth reduces pain and increases the safety and pleasure of those important events. The same careful preparation toward parenting will yield similar results. Parents can learn much about what to expect from children and from themselves as parents. Observing other children, comparing ideas with other parents, reading about childhood development and behavior, and attending classes on parenting can all contribute to the joys of parenting and reduce the frustrations and anxieties.

Child Abuse

The National Center on Child Abuse and Neglect, a federal agency set up within the U.S. Children's Bureau, finds that approximately one million children are maltreated by parents each year. Dr. Vincent J. Fontana, medical director of New York Foundling Hospital and chairman of the Mayor's Task Force on Child Abuse and Neglect in New York City, has estimated that at least 3,000 children are killed each year by their parents or parent surrogates. He believes child battering has become an "insidious epidemic" and considers it a "national disgrace."

Records indicate that most of the severely injured children are under age three, and that the heaviest concentration of fatalities occurs in the newborn-to-one-year age group.

What impels adults—parents or guardians—to abuse or ignore their offspring to the point of harm? Studies show that most child battering is done by apparently "normal" people in a critical period. Generally, abusive parents, overwhelmed by their life circumstances, strike out because of rage, resentment, or sheer ignorance.

Multiple factors may be at work. Some parents begin abusing their children as a reaction to stress and strain caused by family troubles such as marital discord, financial hardship, and mental illness. Where there is violence within the family, the typical pattern shows the husband hitting the wife, the wife hitting a child. When there is abuse in a family with a number of children, it is likely to be centered on one child. And some children pose more stress to parents and are more vulnerable to beatings or other abuse: low-birth-weight babies, children who are colicky, those who are more difficult to toilet train, and physically handicapped or mentally retarded children.

Incidents of abuse and neglect often happen in families that are socially isolated, without continuing relationships with friends or sympathetic relatives. Then there are parents, perhaps of borderline intelligence, who lack understanding of a child's physical, emotional, and psychological needs, who ignore a child's crying, or who react with impatience.

Also, maltreatment has been traced to compulsive disciplinarians who live by the dictum "spare the rod and spoil the child." A typical instance is that of a young boy who breaks a rule, is beaten by his stern father, and sustains bleeding lacerations on his back and face. The father's defense: "He's my kid and if he does something wrong I have the right to punish him."

Many abusive parents were themselves beaten as children and they repeat the cycle. Some child advocates find an entrenched pattern of violent child-rearing in our country. And abuse begets abuse.

The following questions can serve as guidelines to spot possible abuse or neglect:

- Does the child show signs of repeated skin or other injuries? Does the child appear markedly undernourished or unduly afraid of his or her parents?
- Is the child described by the parents as "bad"? Is he or she obviously destructive?
- Does the parent seem to be a loner, with no one to appeal to at times of overwhelming stress?
- Has the parent made no attempt to explain the child's noticeable injuries, offered absurd excuses, or brushed off the gravity of the child's condition?
- Does the parent show lack of control? Does he or she seem to be drinking heavily or misusing drugs?
- Do you find the parent's behavior generally irrational or possibly cruel and sadistic?

If you suspect abuse or would like further information, contact one of the following agencies:

- Community agencies are listed in the yellow pages of the telephone book under the heading "Social Services Organizations." Most of these will have a name that includes such words as "Family," "Families," "Parents," "Child," or "Children." Parents seeking help should check for names such as "Family Stress Center" or "Parental Stress Hotline."
- The American Humane Association is a national federation of individuals and agencies working toward prevention of abuse and exploitation of children. For information, write American Humane Association, Child Protection, 9725 E. Hampden, Denver, Colorado 80231.
- The Child Welfare League of America is the national standard-setting organization for public and voluntary child welfare agencies in the United States and Canada. Their address is 67 Irvine Place, New York, New York 10003.
- The National Center on Child Abuse and Neglect (NCCAN) serves as the focal point for federal activities related to child abuse and neglect. For information, including the resource center in your area, write to:

Child Abuse (*continued*)

National Center on Child Abuse and Neglect, P.O. Box 1182, Washington, D.C. 20013.

- The National Committee for Prevention of Child Abuse is a volunteer network dedicated to involving citizens to actively prevent child abuse. For information, write to The National Committee for Prevention of Child Abuse, 332 S. Michigan Avenue, Suite 1250, Chicago, Illinois 60604.
- Parents Anonymous is a nationwide organization with local chapters where groups of parents meet with the aim of changing their behavior by understanding and rechanneling destructive attitudes and actions. For information, write Parents Anonymous, 22330 Hawthorne Blvd., Suite 208, Torrance, California 90505.

SOURCE: "To Combat and Prevent Child Abuse and Neglect," Theodore Irwin, Public Affairs Pamphlet #588.

Take Action

Your answers to the Exploring Your Emotions questions in this chapter and your placement level on the awareness ladder will, we hope, encourage you to begin a process of self-exploration and self-discovery that you will continue. Reflect on the entire chapter's content and ask yourself how each point relates to your own life. Then take action:

1. Volunteer to baby-sit for friends or relatives. Take along a copy of the Family Planning Potential Scale and rate yourself during the evening. If you are feeling venturesome, baby-sit with a child who is under two years of age.
2. Visit a hospital and ask to observe the delivery of a baby as part of a health class project. Alternatively, interview an expectant mother and an expectant father. What emotions or attitudes do they share? Which are clearly different?
3. Visit a Lamaze class. Observe the participants and imagine yourself in their place.
4. Carry with you an uncooked egg in its shell for 1 week. Keep it warm. Never leave it alone except for two one-hour naps daily. If you must leave it for a time, arrange for an egg sitter.
5. Answer the questions in the Box entitled "Am I Parent Material?" What do your answers reveal about your aptitude for parenthood?
6. Before leaving this chapter, review the statements that open the chapter. Have your feelings or values changed? Are you now better equipped to handle the complex and very human problems associated with pregnancy, childbirth, and parenting?

Selected References

Eisenberg, Arlene, Heidi Eisenberg Murkoff, and Sandee Eisenberg Hathaway, RN. 1984. *What to Expect When You're Expecting*. New York: Workman Publishing.

Feinbloom, Richard I., M.D., and Betty Yetta Forman, Ph.D. 1985. *Pregnancy, Birth, and the Early Months*. Menlo Park, Calif.: Addison-Wesley.

Hannon, Sharron. 1980. *Childbirth: Source Book for Conception, Pregnancy, Birth and the First Weeks of Life*. New York: Evans.

Rinzler, Carol Ann. 1984. *The Safe Pregnancy Book*. New York: New American Library.

Scher, Jonathan, M.D., and Carol Dix. 1983.*Will My Baby Be Normal: How To Make Sure*. New York: Dial Press.

Shapiro, Howard I., M.D. 1983. *The Pregnancy Book for Today's Woman*. New York: Harper & Row.

Recommended Readings

Kenny, James, and Mary Kenny. 1982. *Whole-life Parenting*. New York: Continuum.

Emphasizes character development, parental strategies and techniques; developmental stages in attaining adulthood.

Main, Frank, Ed.D. 1986. *Perfect Parenting & Other Myths*. Minnesota: CompCare Publications.

Realistic guidance in lowering expectations and dealing with the confusion and complexities of family life.

Sears, William, M.D. 1982. *Creative Parenting*. New York: Everest House.

From conception through birth to early adolescence, this book deals with all aspects of practical childcare.

White, Burton L. 1980. *A Parent's Guide to the First Three Years*. Englewood Cliffs, N.J.: Prentice-Hall.

A mine of carefully researched advice on child rearing.

Chapter 9

Contents

Rate Yourself

Your Tobacco Use and Attitudes Read the following statements carefully. Choose the one in each section that best describes you at this moment and circle its number. When you have chosen one statement for each section, add the numbers and record your total score. Find your position on the Wellness Ladder.

5 Never smoked
4 Quit smoking over one year ago
3 Quit smoking recently
2 Smokes occasionally
1 Smokes regularly

5 Objects to smoking environments
4 Avoids smoking environments
3 Tolerates smoking environments
2 Is sensitive to nonsmokers' complaints
1 Ignores no-smoking signs

5 Discourages smoking in others
4 Discourages teenagers from smoking
3 Complains about smoking around children
2 Defends smoking habit
1 Denies any health consequences of smoking

5 Views smoking as a serious health problem
4 Views smoking as unattractive
3 Finds cigarette ads distasteful
2 Is somewhat influenced by cigarette ads
1 Is strongly influenced by cigarette ads

5 Supports no-smoking ordinances
4 Would vote for no-smoking ordinances
3 Occasionally complains to friends about their smoking
2 Talks about quitting
1 Has smoker's cough

Total Score ______

Toward a Tobacco-free Society

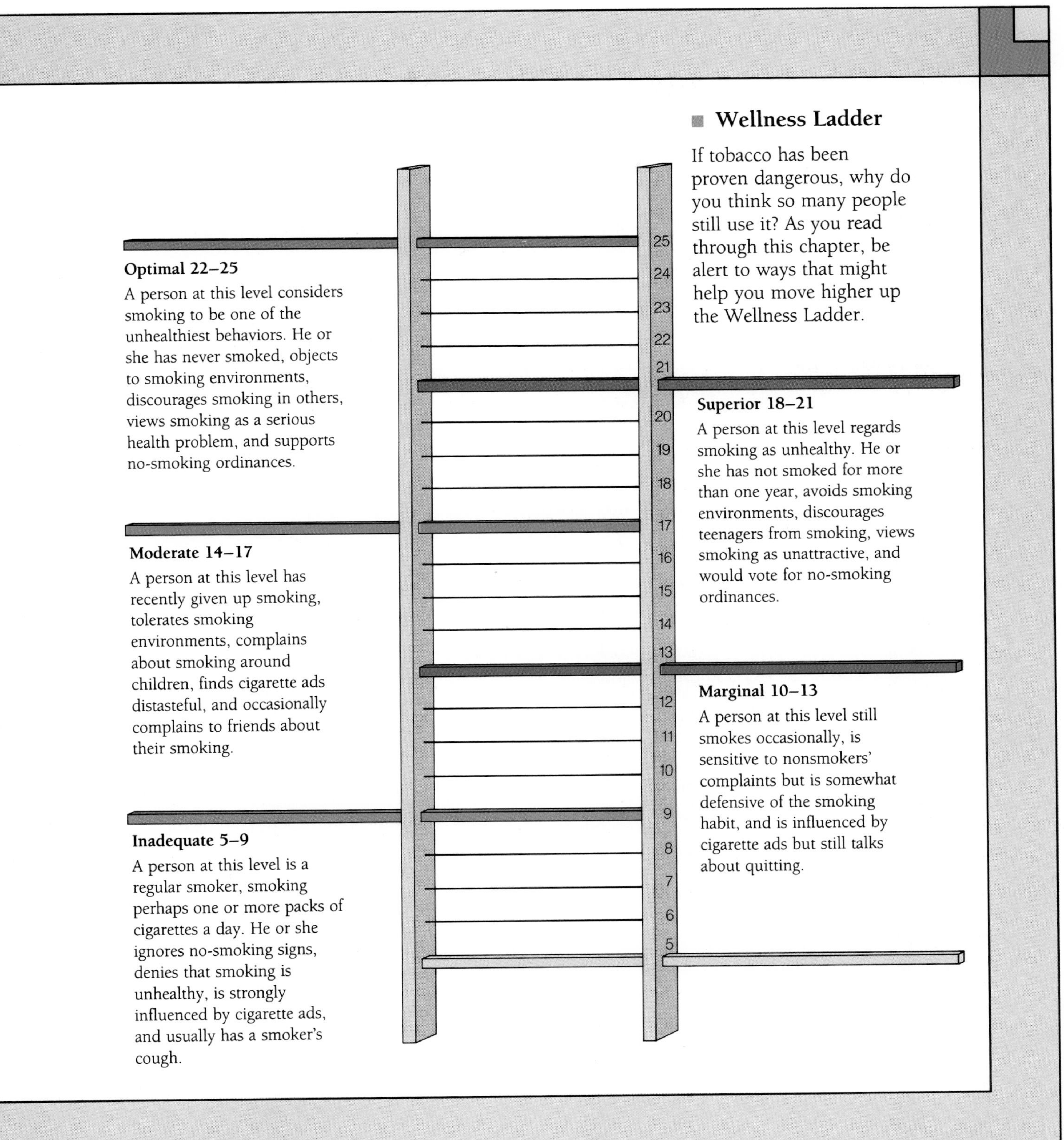

Wellness Ladder

If tobacco has been proven dangerous, why do you think so many people still use it? As you read through this chapter, be alert to ways that might help you move higher up the Wellness Ladder.

Optimal 22–25
A person at this level considers smoking to be one of the unhealthiest behaviors. He or she has never smoked, objects to smoking environments, discourages smoking in others, views smoking as a serious health problem, and supports no-smoking ordinances.

Superior 18–21
A person at this level regards smoking as unhealthy. He or she has not smoked for more than one year, avoids smoking environments, discourages teenagers from smoking, views smoking as unattractive, and would vote for no-smoking ordinances.

Moderate 14–17
A person at this level has recently given up smoking, tolerates smoking environments, complains about smoking around children, finds cigarette ads distasteful, and occasionally complains to friends about their smoking.

Marginal 10–13
A person at this level still smokes occasionally, is sensitive to nonsmokers' complaints but is somewhat defensive of the smoking habit, and is influenced by cigarette ads but still talks about quitting.

Inadequate 5–9
A person at this level is a regular smoker, smoking perhaps one or more packs of cigarettes a day. He or she ignores no-smoking signs, denies that smoking is unhealthy, is strongly influenced by cigarette ads, and usually has a smoker's cough.

Nicotine A poisonous substance found in tobacco and responsible for many of the effects of tobacco.

Smoking causes more ill health than any single behavior or combination of behaviors affecting health. Each year more than 350,000 Americans die prematurely from the effects of smoking. Millions more are incapacitated, with crippled lungs and damaged hearts. More than 30 percent of all deaths from coronary heart disease (CHD) and 30 percent of all cancer deaths can be attributed to cigarette smoking. A study by the U.S. Congress Office of Technology Assessment estimates the cost of smoking to the economy to be $65 billion per year. Smokers are three times more likely to die of cancer than nonsmokers. Smoking is the primary cause of lung cancer; more than 85 percent of deaths in this category are due to cigarette smoking. Smoking is also a primary cause of chronic obstructive lung disease and a variety of cancers. (See Table 9-1 for a list of diseases associated with smoking.) Smoking remains the largest preventable cause of illness and death in the United States, according to the U.S. Sur-

Table 9-1 Risks of Smoking (and Benefits of Quitting)

Risks of Smoking	Benefits of Quitting	Relative Risks: Filter-tipped, Low Tar and Nicotine (T/N) Brands
Shortened life expectancy. 25-year-old 2-pack-a-day smokers have life expectancy 8.3 years shorter than nonsmoking contemporaries. Other smoking levels: proportional risk.	**Reduces risk of premature death** cumulatively. After 10–15 years, ex-smokers' risk approaches that of those who've never smoked.	**Reduced risk of death** from certain diseases (see below) implies increased life expectancy.
Lung cancer. Smoking cigarettes "major cause in both men and women."	Gradual decrease in risk. **After 10–15 years, risk approaches that of those who never smoked.**	**Filter tips reduce risk,** but it is still 5 times that of nonsmokers. Low T/N brands reduce male risk by 20 percent, female risk by 40 percent.
Larynx cancer. In all smokers (including pipe and cigar) it's 2.9 to 17.7 times that of nonsmokers.	**Gradual reduction of risk** after smoking cessation. **Reaches normal after 10 years.**	**Filter tips reduce risk 24 to 49 percent.**
Mouth cancer. Cigarette smokers have 3 to 10 times as many oral cancers as nonsmokers. Pipes, cigars, chewing tobacco also major risk factors. Alcohol seems synergistic carcinogen with smoking.	Reducing or eliminating smoking/drinking reduces risk in first few years; **risk drops to level of nonsmokers in 10–15 years.**	No identified benefit.
Cancer of esophagus. Cigarettes, pipes, and cigars increase risk of dying of esophageal cancer about 2 to 9 times. Synergistic relationship between smoking and alcohol.	Since risks are dose related, reducing or eliminating smoking/drinking **should have risk-reducing effect.**	No identified benefit.
Cancer of bladder. Cigarette smokers have 7 to 10 times risk of bladder cancer as nonsmokers. Also synergistic with certain exposed occupations: dyestuffs, etc.	**Risk decreases gradually to that of nonsmokers over 7 years.**	No identified benefit.
Cancer of pancreas. Cigarette smokers have 2 to 5 times risk of dying of pancreatic cancer as nonsmokers.	Since there is evidence of dose-related risk, reducing or eliminating smoking should have risk-reducing effect.	No identified benefit.

geon General. These facts have been documented by thousands of carefully executed studies.

The minute you stop smoking, your body goes to work to repair the damage inflicted on it. Giving up smoking, however, can be extremely difficult. Most smokers have filled their daily activities with cues that continue to say, "Time to light up." And when smokers feel the urge to light up, they can think of a thousand reasons to do so, no matter how strong their resolve to quit. In addition, the aspiring ex-smoker must be able to see through the advertising assault by the tobacco companies, which attempt to link smoking to friendship, sex, glamor, athletic prowess, and being "cool" or "in." Smokers themselves often don't know their real reasons for smoking—reasons that may include wanting to reduce stress, relieve boredom, get the ritualistic pleasure from lighting and handling cigarettes, use a social prop, or satisfy urges for oral stimulation. Of course, the primary reason people continue to smoke despite the evidence that it is harmful is that they have become addicted to a powerful drug found in tobacco—**nicotine.** Like alcoholics and heroin addicts, smokers who stop experience strong withdrawal symptoms.

Tobacco has some adverse effects on health in whatever form it is used. Although low-tar or low-nicotine cigarettes may reduce risks, it is likely that some smokers who switch to low-tar or low-nicotine brands will actually smoke more cigarettes to achieve their previous absorption levels of nicotine. Researchers warn there is no such thing as a

Table 9-1 Risks of Smoking (and Benefits of Quitting) *(continued)*

Risks of Smoking	Benefits of Quitting	Relative Risks: Filter-tipped, Low Tar and Nicotine (T/N) Brands
Coronary heart disease. Cigarette smoking is major factor; responsible for 120,000 excess U.S. deaths from coronary heart disease (CHD) each year.	**Sharply decreases risk after one year.** After 10 years ex-smokers' risk is same as that of those who never smoked.	**Low T/N male smokers had 12 percent lower CHD rate,** female low T/N smokers 19 percent lower than high T/N smokers.
Chronic bronchitis and pulmonary emphysema. Cigarette smokers have 4–25 times risk of death from these diseases as nonsmokers. Damage seen in lungs of even young smokers.	**Cough and sputum disappear** during first few weeks. **Lung function may improve** and rate of deterioration slow down.	No identified benefit.
Stillbirth and low birthweight. Smoking mothers have more stillbirths and babies of low birthweight—more vulnerable to disease and death.	Women who stop smoking before 4th month of pregnancy **eliminate risk of stillbirth and low birthweight** caused by smoking.	No identified benefit.
Children of smoking mothers are smaller, underdeveloped physically and socially, seven years after birth.	Since children of nonsmoking mothers are bigger and more advanced socially, inference is that **not smoking during pregnancy might avoid such underdeveloped children.**	No identified benefit.
Peptic ulcer. Cigarette smokers get more peptic ulcers and die more often of them; cure is more difficult in smokers.	Ex-smokers get ulcers but these are **more likely to heal rapidly and completely** than those of smokers.	No identified benefit.
Allergy and impairment of immune system.	Since these are direct, immediate effects of smoking, they are obviously **avoidable by not smoking.**	No identified benefit.
Alters pharmacologic effects of many medicines and diagnostic tests and greatly increases risk of thrombosis with oral contraceptives.	**Majority of blood components elevated by smoking return to normal after cessation.** Nonsmokers on Pill have much lower risks of thrombosis.	

SOURCE: American Cancer Society, Dangers of Smoking, Benefits of Quitting & Relative Risks of Reduced Exposure, rev. ed., pp. 8–9.

Trends in U.S. Cigarette Smoking, 1925–1985

Each year cigarette smoking causes the deaths of more than 300,000 Americans, principally from heart disease, cancer, and chronic obstructive lung disease. It can legitimately be termed the most devastating epidemic of disease and premature death this country has ever experienced.

The epidemic began some seventy-five years ago. In 1915, most tobacco was used for pipes, cigars and chewing tobacco, and fewer than 20 billion cigarettes were smoked. Lung cancer, the disease most closely associated with cigarette smoking, was virtually unknown; as late as 1935, there were fewer than 5,000 deaths from this disease. Today Americans smoke 600 billion cigarettes each year, and 120,000 men and women die of lung cancer.

The epidemic of cigarette smoking reached its peak in 1963 and is now receding. The percentage of smokers in the population is falling, per capita consumption is down to the levels of the 1940s, and deaths from cigarette smoking are beginning to fall. However, some 52 million adults and as many as 2 million teenagers continue to smoke.

SOURCE: Smoking, Tobacco, and Health (Washington, D.C.: U.S. Department of Health and Human Services, Public Health Service, Centers for Disease Control, Center for Health Promotion and Education, Office on Smoking and Health)

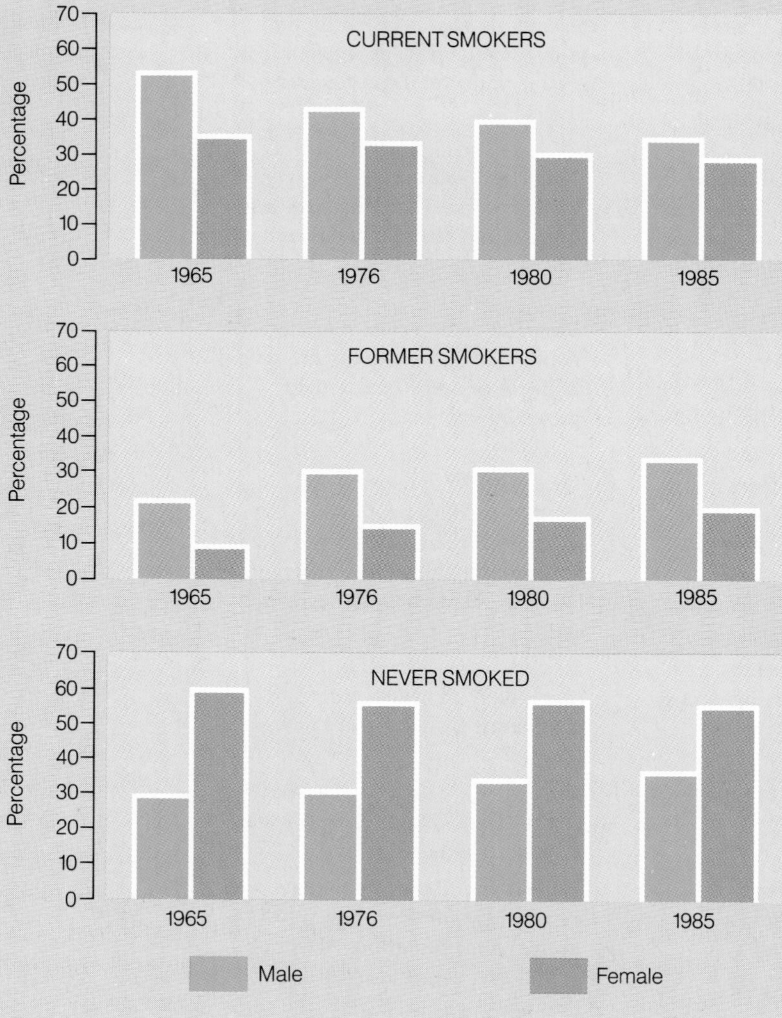

Carcinogenic Cancer causing.

Cocarcinogen A substance that works with a carcinogen to produce a cancer.

Psychoactive drug A drug that affects the brain or nervous system.

Catecholamines Hormones secreted by the adrenal glands, especially during stress.

"safe" cigarette (see Table 9-2). Many smokers have switched from cigarettes to other forms of tobacco use such as cigars, pipes, clove cigarettes, and smokeless tobacco such as snuff and chewing tobacco. However, each of these alternatives is far from safe.

Tobacco Smoke

Tobacco smoke contains hundreds of damaging chemical substances. Smoke from a typical unfiltered cigarette contains about 5 billion particles per cubic millimeter—50,000 times as many as are found in an equal volume of polluted urban atmosphere. The particles in tobacco smoke are made up of several hundred different chemicals, many of them toxic. These particles, when condensed, form the brown, sticky mass called *cigarette tar*.

Some chemicals in tobacco tar are **carcinogenic**; that is, they cause cancer. Other chemicals in tobacco tar are **cocarcinogens**; they do not themselves cause cancer but combine with other chemicals to stimulate the growth of certain cancers, at least in laboratory animals. The phenols present in tar, for example, although not particularly carcinogenic themselves, greatly increase the carcinogenic potency of benzopyrene, a substance also contained in tar. Still other compounds, which may not directly cause cancer, irritate the tissues of the respiratory system and damage the respiratory cilia, which operate to keep the air passages free of mucus and dust.

Smoking interferes with the functioning of the respiratory system and often leads rapidly to the conditions called smoker's throat, smoker's cough, and smoker's bronchitis. Table 9-3 lists some of the common physical complaints of smokers. These conditions usually disappear in people who stop smoking.

Nicotine is the predominant **psychoactive drug** in tobacco. When a person inhales smoke, the nicotine in it passes through the membrane of the lung tissue and rapidly enters the bloodstream. The heart pumps about 15 percent of the nicotine directly to the brain, which absorbs all of it. This process takes about 7 seconds. When the nicotine hits the brain, the brain signals the release of chemicals called **catecholamines.** Both blood pressure and heart rate go up. This change in the body's metabolism is the "lift" that smokers crave. For every puff, the smoker gets a "shot" or "fix" of nicotine. Throughout the day, smokers automatically and unknowingly maintain

(Text continues on p. 200)

Table 9-2 Cancer Death Ratios Among Men Who Smoked Cigarettes (compared with a risk of 1.0 for men who never smoked regularly)

	Age 45–64	Age 65–79
Total Cancer	**2.14**	**1.76**
Lung	7.84	11.59
Mouth, pharynx	9.90	2.93
Larynx	6.09	8.99
Esophagus	4.17	1.74
Bladder	2.00	2.96
Kidney	1.42	1.57
Prostate	1.04	1.01
Pancreas	2.69	2.17

SOURCE: American Cancer Society Survey, 1986

Table 9-3 Physical Complaints of Smokers and Nonsmokers

Complaint	Cigarette Smokers (percent)	Non-smokers (percent)	Ratio (smokers to non-smokers)
Cough	33.2	5.6	5.9
Loss of appetite	3.3	0.9	3.7
Shortness of breath	16.3	4.7	3.5
Chest pains	7.0	3.7	1.9
Diarrhea	3.3	1.7	1.9
Easily fatigued	26.1	14.9	1.8
Abdominal pains	6.7	3.8	1.8
Hoarseness	4.8	2.6	1.8
Loss of weight	7.3	4.5	1.6
Stomach pains	6.0	3.8	1.6
Insomnia	10.2	6.8	1.5
Difficulty in swallowing	1.4	1.0	1.4

SOURCE: E. Cuyler Hammond, 1962 (July), "The Effects of Smoking," *Scientific American*, p. 49.

Exploring Your Emotions

You have just met a very attractive person of the opposite sex, whom you like more and more as the conversation continues. You agree to get together again, and on the second meeting you discover that he or she is a heavy smoker. Does this discovery affect your feelings? How will you handle your feelings?

Clove Cigarettes

Would you guess that cocoa, licorice, caramel, or clove oil could be dangerous? Perhaps not when they are eaten. But when burned and inhaled, any of them can poison you. And all of them have been widely used as additives in conventional tobacco cigarettes.

Clove cigarettes, called *kreteks,* are a fad in the United States, especially popular among teenagers and young adults. Since 1980, when 16 million were imported from Indonesia, imports have increased to over 150 million annually.

Many clove smokers believe they are using a safe, mild cigarette. Since cloves are a flavorful, apparently safe, and widely used spice, people assume that cloves in cigarettes cannot be dangerous. But nothing could be further from the truth.

Clove cigarettes are composed of 60 percent tobacco and 40 percent ground cloves, clove oil, and other additives. But the Indonesian tobacco can have nearly twice the tar and nicotine of moderate tar-containing American cigarettes. And clove cigarettes produce levels of tar, nicotine, and carbon monoxide similar to all-tobacco cigarettes.

Clove cigarettes are at least as hazardous to health as conventional cigarettes. The user can become addicted to the nicotine, just as with conventional cigarettes.

Worse, several deaths, as well as a dozen cases of serious illness, have been linked to the smoking of clove cigarettes. Clove cigarette smokers develop symptoms rarely seen in other young people: coughing up blood, nosebleeds, severe sore throats, shortness of breath and severe—potentially fatal—lung infections.

Cloves have long been used medicinally as mild anesthetics. But their numbing capabilities are dangerous when combined with the other poisons in cigarettes. Inhaled, clove smoke makes the lungs less responsive to the irritation of the smoke. Unfortunately, that numbing effect masks the elevated levels of tar and nicotine. And the mild anesthetic effect makes the throat tingle and hides the warning signal of a scratchy throat. This soothing effect allows smokers to deeply inhale poisons from the cigarettes. But the worst effect may be caused by the clove oil (eugenol) itself. It is suspected of causing cancer when burned and inhaled.

Why are people attracted to clove cigarettes? Well, *kreteks* have an exotic aroma and are advertised as herbal, low-tar alternatives to conventional cigarettes. Their exotic brand names—Djarum, Bima, Krakatoa—entice the unsophisticated buyer. And they are sold in convenience and liquor stores, as well as in tobacco stores. Fortunately, they are rather expensive, and sell for $1.50 to $3.00 for a pack of ten.

What can you do to stop the use of clove cigarettes?

1. Help get the facts out. People with good information are more likely to make good decisions.
2. Ask merchants to stop selling clove (and tobacco) cigarettes voluntarily. Insist that they comply with laws prohibiting the sale of tobacco to minors.
3. Support legislation requiring tobacco companies to disclose the identity and potential health hazards of additives used in cigarettes.
4. And don't smoke them yourself—or any other kind of cigarette. There is no such thing as a safe cigarette.

SOURCE: American Cancer Society, 1986 (November), Smoking, *Healthline.*

Smokeless Tobacco

In February 1986, President Reagan signed the Comprehensive Smokeless Tobacco Health Education Act, which requires manufacturers of chewing tobacco and snuff to include health warning labels on packages.

The warnings, which will be emphasized by arrows and circles, will read:

- This product may cause mouth cancer.
- This product may cause gum disease and tooth loss.
- This product is not a safe alternative to cigarettes.

Chewing tobacco and snuff contain tobacco leaf and a variety of sweeteners, other flavorings, and scents. In chewing tobacco, the leaf may be shredded (loose-leaf),

Smokeless Tobacco (*continued*)

pressed into bricks or cakes (plugs), or dried and twisted into ropelike strands (twists). A portion is either chewed or held in place in the cheek or between the lower lip and the gum. The two categories of snuff, dry and moist, are made from powdered or finely cut tobacco leaves. In some countries, dry snuff is sniffed through the nose, but in the United States both dry and moist snuff are "dipped" by tucking a small amount (pinch) between the lip or cheek and the gum. Nicotine from the tobacco is absorbed into the bloodstream and produces mental effects described by users as relaxing or stimulating.

Last year an expert panel assembled by the National Institutes of Health concluded that despite their hazards, smokeless tobacco products have been gaining rapidly in popularity—especially among teenagers. The panel estimated that at least ten million Americans had used smokeless tobacco products within the previous year, with three million users under the age of 21. Another national study found that 16 percent of male youths 12 to 17 years old had used some form of smokeless tobacco during the previous year, while a local study found that tobacco chewing and snuff dipping had tripled between 1976 and 1982 among boys ages 12 to 14.

The rise in popularity is obviously related to advertising that associates chewing and dipping with "macho" images and athletic prowess. Ads for smokeless tobacco have appeared mainly in male-oriented outdoor publications such as *Field and Stream, Outdoor Life,* and *Sporting News.* U.S. Tobacco Company's Skoal has been a major sponsor of Atlanta Braves baseball telecasts. The company also promotes its products through scholarship offers to rodeo riders. Race car driver A. J. Foyt, four-time winner of the Indianapolis 500, races automobiles bearing bold logos for Copenhagen Snuff. Prominent baseball and football players have appeared in testimonial ads.

Rep. Henry Waxman (D-Calif.), who played a major role in passage of the new law, hopes the warning labels will make it obvious to children that "smokeless tobacco products are not bubblegum." The law also bans radio and television advertising of the products and requires manufacturers to reveal to the U.S. Department of Health and Human Services what additives and flavorings they contain.

Last year, nationwide attention was focused on the problem of smokeless tobacco by a *Reader's Digest* article about Sean Marsee's gruesome death from mouth cancer at the age of 19. Sean, a star high school athlete from Oklahoma, had used snuff daily since age 12 despite warnings from his mother. According to the article, Sean refused to believe that sports stars would sell snuff on TV if it hurt people. His mother sued the U.S. Tobacco Co., producer of 90 percent of the snuff sold in the United States, but the jury ruled that the company should not be held responsible for Sean's behavior.

Chemical analysis of various smokeless products has found three types of chemicals known to produce cancer: polycyclic aromatic amines, nitrosamines, and polonium 210, which is radioactive. Dr. Gregory Connolly, director of the dental division of the Massachusetts Department of Public Health, calls smokeless tobacco use "a chemical time bomb ticking in the mouths of hundreds of thousands of boys in this country."

The risk is not confined to oral cancer. Smokeless tobacco can cause tooth decay, gingivitis (inflammation) and recession of the gums, especially where the tobacco is habitually placed. Epidemiological data on the incidence of heart disease in smokeless tobacco users have not yet been collected. But it is known that chewing and dipping produce blood levels of nicotine similar to those in cigarette smokers that elevate blood pressure, heart rate and blood levels of certain fats. Other chemicals in smokeless tobacco are believed to pose risks to developing babies in pregnant female users.

Because of its nicotine content, smokeless tobacco is also highly addicting. Some users even keep it in their mouth while sleeping. Psychologist Elbert Glover of East Carolina University has reported that only one out of 41 participants at recent quit-smokeless-tobacco clinics was able to stop for more than four hours.

SOURCE: Stephen Barrett, 1986 (December), Smokeless tobacco is dangerous, *Healthline.*

Cerebral cortex The outer layer of the brain, which controls the complex behavior and mental activity of human beings.

Secondary reinforcers Stimuli that are rewarding not because they are pleasurable in themselves, but because they have been associated with other stimuli that are pleasurable.

the nicotine level in their brains by varying the number of cigarettes they smoke and by the way they inhale. In this way, they sustain the "lift" effect without inducing the unpleasant side effects of smoking, such as becoming nauseated and dizzy.

Cigarette smoke also contains carbon monoxide, the deadly gas in automobile exhaust, in concentrations 400 times greater than is considered safe in industrial workplaces. Not surprisingly, smokers often complain of breathlessness when they require a burst of energy to run across campus for their next class. Carbon monoxide displaces oxygen in red blood cells depleting the body's supply of life-giving oxygen for extra work. Carbon monoxide also impairs visual acuity, especially at night.

All smokers absorb some gases, tars, and nicotine from cigarette smoke, but smokers who inhale bring most of these substances into their bodies and keep them there. In one year, a typical one-pack-per-day smoker takes in 50,000 to 70,000 puffs. Smoke from a cigarette, pipe, or cigar directly assaults mouth, throat, and respiratory tract; the nose—which normally filters out about 75 percent of foreign matter in the air we breathe—is completely bypassed.

In a cigarette, the unburned tobacco itself acts as a filter. As a cigarette burns down, there is less and less filter. Thus, more chemicals are absorbed into the body during the last third of a cigarette than during the first. A smoker can therefore cut down on absorption of harmful chemicals by not smoking cigarettes down to short butts. Of course, any gains made will be offset if he or she smokes more cigarettes, inhales more deeply, or puffs more frequently.

Immediate Effects of Smoking

The beginning smoker often has symptoms of mild nicotine poisoning: dizziness, faintness, rapid pulse, cold clammy skin, and sometimes nausea, vomiting, and diarrhea. The seasoned smoker occasionally suffers these effects of nicotine poisoning, particularly after quitting and returning to a previous level of consumption. The effects of nicotine on smokers vary, depending greatly on the size of the nicotine dose and on how much tolerance previous smoking has built up. Nicotine can either excite or tranquilize the nervous system, depending on dosage. Generally the smoker feels stimulated first. This stimulation gives way to feeling tranquil and then depressed.

Exploring Your Emotions

Are you currently smoking? If so, how is your self-concept affected by your smoking? Have you ever tried to quit and failed? How did that make you feel?

Nicotine has many other effects. It stimulates the part of the brain called the **cerebral cortex.** It also stimulates the adrenal glands to discharge adrenalin. And it inhibits the formation of urine, constricts the blood vessels, especially in the skin, increases the heart rate, and elevates blood pressure. Higher blood pressure, faster heart rate, and constricted blood vessels require the heart to pump more blood. In healthy people, the heart can usually meet this demand, but in people whose coronary arteries are damaged so as to interfere with the flow of blood, the heart muscle may be strained.

Frequently, people who smoke do not feel as hungry as people who do not. There are several reasons for this. Smoking depresses hunger contractions. It also causes the liver to release glycogen, which slightly raises the level of sugar in the blood. Smoking also dulls taste buds, so food does not taste as good. People who quit smoking usually notice how much better food tastes.

Creating a Smoking Habit

Regular cigarette smoking is not just a psychological habit but a classic case of physical dependence or addiction to nicotine. Addicted smokers must keep a continuous amount of nicotine circulating in the blood and going to the brain. If that amount falls below a certain level or if they stop smoking, they experience withdrawal symptoms. In one experiment, subjects were given cigarettes that tasted and looked exactly the same but varied in how much nicotine they contained. Although they did not know how much nicotine they were getting, the subjects automatically adjusted their rate of smoking and depth of inhalation to ensure that they absorbed their usual amount of nicotine. In other studies, heavy smokers were given nicotine without their knowing it—and they cut down on their smoking.

These unconscious adjustments made by many smokers may explain why low-nicotine cigarettes are as harmful as high-nicotine ones. Using these cigarettes, many smokers merely puff more frequently, inhale more deeply, smoke down to a shorter butt, or smoke more cigarettes

Why College Women Take Up Smoking

College women are more likely than college men to smoke cigarettes, suggesting that the tobacco industry is successfully linking female smoking with an image of glamour and success, according to a federal study released yesterday.

"The cigarette companies emphasize two major themes in getting women to smoke: One is trying to associate smoking with being liberated and the other is more subliminal, but not very subtle, and that is that women should smoke to stay thin," said one of the researchers, social psychologist Lloyd D. Johnston of the University of Michigan.

The typical cigarette advertisement aimed at women features "very long, slender models and very long, slender cigarettes," Johnston said.

Johnston was a director of the study conducted for the National Institute on Drug Abuse by the University of Michigan's Institute for Social Research.

Among college women, 18 percent said they smoked daily last year, compared with 10 percent for men.

The study did not say how much college women smoke. Past studies indicate that more women than men fall into the "moderate-to-light smoker" category.

"It appears the tobacco industry's expensive and long-term effort to associate smoking with liberation and success among women has paid off, at least for the industry," Johnston said. "The payoff for those young women who bought the message is quite another matter."

About 350,000 Americans die prematurely each year from lung cancer, heart disease, emphysema and other illnesses because of smoking, according to the U.S. Public Health Service.

Scott Stapf of the Tobacco Institute, a trade organization, called the report's conclusions "complete baloney." He said that "peer pressure and the role of parents and elders generally," not advertising, are the main factors in a person's decision to become a smoker.

The study grew out of a ten-year series of surveys of drug use by high school seniors and interviews with about 1,100 college students each year from 1980 to 1985. The results have a margin of error of less than three percentage points.

Johnston said that smoking tends to be highly related to grades and to school performance. "The smarter kids are less likely to get hooked on cigarettes," he said.

The researchers also found that 20.7 percent of those not planning to attend college said that they smoked at least half a pack of cigarettes a day, compared with 6.5 percent of the college-bound.

SOURCE: Associated Press, 1986 (July 8), *San Francisco Chronicle.*

and thus expose themselves and those around them to a greater total amount of smoke.

Like other drug addicts, the chronic smoker who stops may suffer severe physiological withdrawal symptoms. Sudden abstinence can change brain waves, heart rate, and blood pressure. People who quit suddenly are often irritable and complain of insomnia, muscular pains, headache, nausea, and other discomforts. They are easily distracted and perform poorly on objective tests that require sustained attention. Most heavy smokers continue their addiction not for pleasure but because they are unwilling to go through the uncomfortable withdrawal process.

Exploring Your Emotions

How would you feel if your child had just started smoking? What would you do about it? Would you feel responsible if you were smoking yourself? If you were not smoking?

Why Do People Smoke?

Why do smokers have such a hard time quitting even when they want to? Various social and psychological forces combine with physiological addiction to maintain the tobacco habit. Many people, for example, have established habits of smoking while doing something else—smoking while talking, smoking while working, smoking while drinking, and so on. Such people find it difficult to quit smoking because the activities they have associated with it continue to trigger their urge for a cigarette. Psychologists call such activities **secondary reinforcers.** These cues act together with the physiological addiction to keep the smoker dependent on tobacco.

Most people start smoking as teenagers or young adults. Research studies have identified certain behavioral pat-

Coronary heart disease (CHD) Heart disease caused by hardening of the arteries that supply oxygen to the heart muscle.

Atherosclerosis Heart disease caused by the deposit of fatty substances in the walls of the arteries.

Plaque A deposit on the inner wall of blood vessels. Blood can coagulate around a plaque and form a clot.

Angina pectoris Chest pain due to heart disease.

Myocardium The muscle of the heart.

Myocardial infarction Heart attack caused by plaque that completely blocks a main coronary artery.

High-density lipoprotein (HDL) Blood fats that help keep cholesterol in a watery state and thus are protective against heart diseases.

Stroke An impeded blood supply to some part of the brain, resulting in the destruction of brain cells (also called cerebrovascular accident).

Aortic aneurysm A blood-filled bulge in the aorta due to a weakening in its walls.

Pulmonary heart disease A disorder of the right side of the heart caused by changes in the blood vessels of the lungs.

---

terns in these people. Smoking at an early age is often linked to curiosity, low self-esteem, and status seeking. The urge to imitate close friends, older siblings, and parents is very important. Most teenage smokers report that their best friends and parents are smokers. For many teenagers, the choice to smoke or not revolves around their desire to conform to a particular group. Older teenagers tend to report their smoking behavior in more personal terms—stimulation, pleasure, or alleviation of unpleasant moods such as anxiety or depression. Despite their keen awareness of the health hazards of smoking, they often defend their behavior with rationalizations like "My grandmother smoked and lived to be 80" or "You can get killed just by crossing the street."

Different people may smoke for different reasons, but underlying psychological or physiological processes may be associated with all drug dependence or addiction. People who smoke, for example, are also more likely to drink coffee, alcohol, and use other psychoactive drugs. Some studies have found that over 90 percent of heroin addicts and 80 percent of alcoholics are heavy cigarette smokers. Both coffee and alcohol are synergistic with smoking. That is, coffee and alcohol both enhance withdrawal effects and thus encourage the smoker to light up. However, no single factor has yet been found to predict who will smoke and who will quit. No personality measures can successfully identify which people will respond to stop-smoking programs. Some demographic variables are correlated with smoking. Wealthier, more educated people are less likely to start smoking and are somewhat more successful in their efforts to quit. Since the U.S. Surgeon General's initial report on the health hazards of smoking, physicians and other health professionals have stopped smoking at a higher rate than have most other professionals. However, such statistics are not very useful in predicting an individual's behavior.

Health Hazards of Smoking

Beginning in 1964, the U.S. Surgeon General's office issued a number of reports evaluating three major types of evidence linking smoking with disease. The first type of evidence was based on animal studies: nicotine and other chemicals in tobacco smoke were given to animals, and damage to their tissues was measured. The second type of evidence was gathered from clinical and autopsy studies of tissue damage occurring most often in smokers. The third type of evidence came from two kinds of population studies: (1) studies of the past smoking habits of people with a particular disease and (2) studies that followed groups of smokers and nonsmokers over a period of years to record the occurrence and progress of certain diseases, including chronic cough and sputum production—sure signs of bronchitis. These studies also compared death rates and causes of death for the two groups.

A great deal of scientific evidence now indicates that the total amount of tobacco smoke inhaled is a key factor contributing to disease. People who smoke more cigarettes per day, inhale deeply, puff frequently, smoke cigarettes down to small butts, or begin smoking at an early age run a greater risk of disease than do those who behave more moderately or who do not smoke at all. Many diseases have been linked to smoking. And as more time passes and more research is done, more diseases associated with smoking are being uncovered. The most costly ones, to society as well as to the individual, are cardiovascular diseases, respiratory diseases such as emphysema and lung cancer, and other cancers. Although cancer tends to receive the most publicity, **coronary heart disease (CHD)** is actually the most widespread single cause of death for cigarette smokers.

Cardiovascular Disease Cigarette smoking is strongly related to various cardiovascular disorders that involve the heart and blood vessels. CHD is one type and often results from a disease called **atherosclerosis**, in which fatty deposits called **plaques** form on the inner walls of heart arteries, causing them to narrow and stiffen. The crushing chest pain of **angina pectoris**, a primary symptom of CHD, results when the heart muscle or **myocardium** does not get enough oxygen. Sometimes a plaque forms at a narrow point in a main coronary artery. If the plaque completely blocks the flow of blood to a portion of the heart, that portion may die. This type of heart attack is called **myocardial infarction.** CHD can also interfere with the normal electrical activity of the heart, resulting in disturbances of the normal heartbeat rhythm. Sudden and unexpected death is a common result of CHD, particularly among smokers. (See Chapter 17 for a more extensive discussion of cardiovascular disease.) Deaths from CHD associated with cigarette smoking are most common in people 40 to 50 years old. This age bracket is almost twenty years younger than the age at which people are most likely to die from lung cancer caused by smoking. Cigar and pipe smokers run a lower risk than do cigarette smokers.

We do not completely understand how cigarette smoking increases the risk of CHD. However, researchers are beginning to shed light on the process. Smoking reduces the amount of **HDL** cholesterol (**high-density lipoprotein,** the "good" cholesterol) and thus promotes plaque formation and speeds blood clotting. Smoking may also increase tension in the heart muscle walls, speed up the rate of muscular contraction, and increase the heart rate. The workload of the heart thus increases, as does its need for oxygen and other nutrients. Carbon monoxide produced by cigarette smoking combines with hemoglobin in the red blood cells, displacing oxygen and thus providing less oxygen to the heart. Carbon monoxide may also contribute to the development of heart disease.

As suggested earlier, the risks of CHD decrease rapidly when the person stops smoking. This is particularly true for younger smokers whose coronary arteries haven't yet been extensively damaged. Cigarette smoking has also been linked to other cardiovascular diseases, including

1. **Stroke,** a sudden interference with the circulation of blood in a part of the brain.
2. **Aortic aneurysm,** a bulge in the aorta caused by weakening in its walls.
3. **Pulmonary heart disease,** a disorder of the right side of the heart, caused by changes in the blood vessels of the lungs.

Exploring Your Emotions

How do you feel about this person? Write a caption for this photograph (write several captions, if you have different and perhaps conflicting feelings to express).

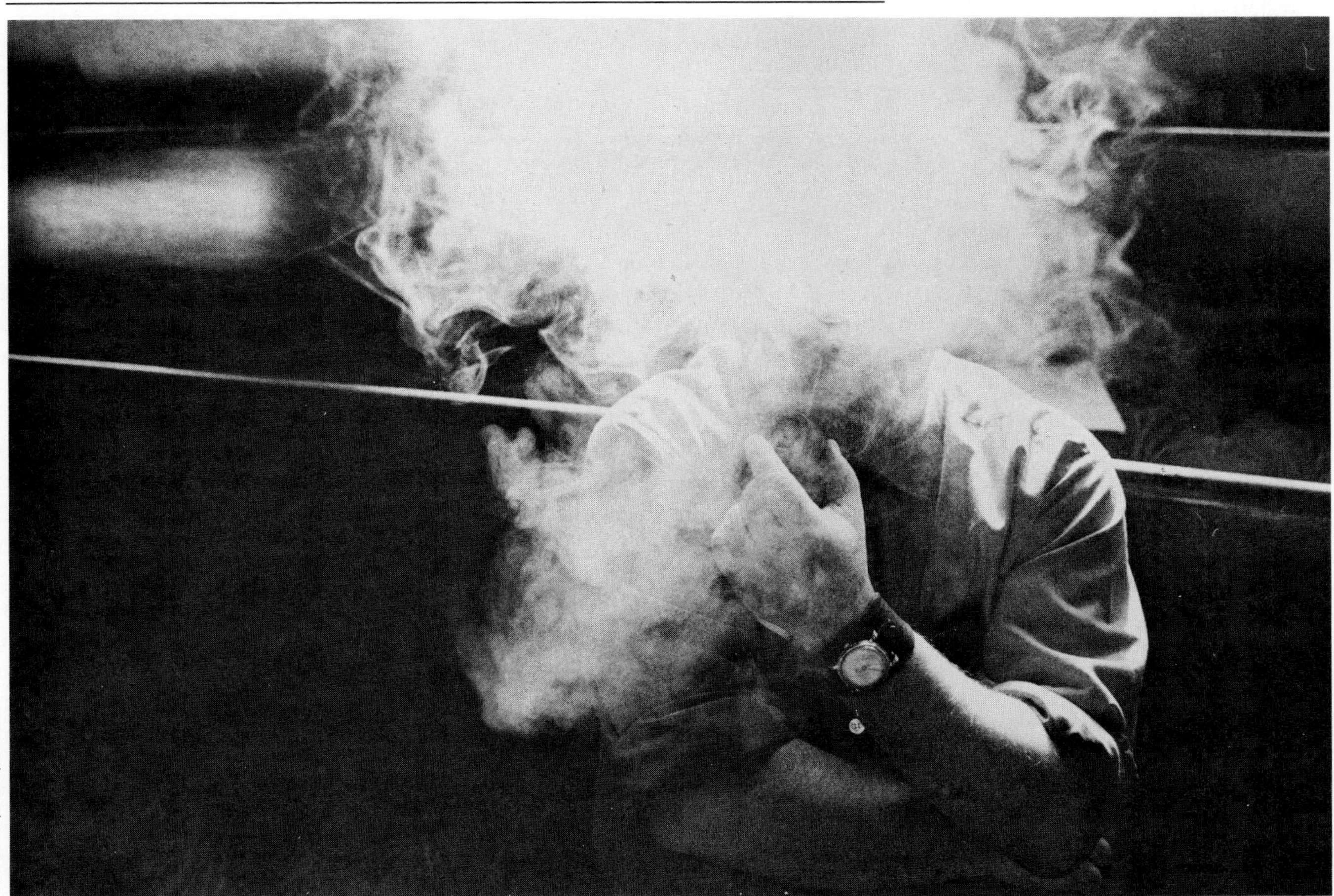

Peter Simon, Stock, Boston

Improving Your Chances

When you stop smoking, you automatically reduce your chances of dying from a smoking-related disease. The longer you abstain, the less likely you are to succumb, until after about fifteen years of nonsmoking your chances of unnecessary early death are just about the same as for someone who has never smoked. How long you smoked makes little difference to the general trend, so it is *always* worth giving up. The graph (right) shows how the average smoker's chances of dying from lung cancer (compared to a nonsmoker) decrease from the time he or she stops smoking. This tendency, though less marked than for lung cancer, applies to all the illnesses associated with smoking.

SOURCE: Kunz and Finkel, eds., 1987, *The AMA Family Medical Guide* (New York: Random House), p. 42.

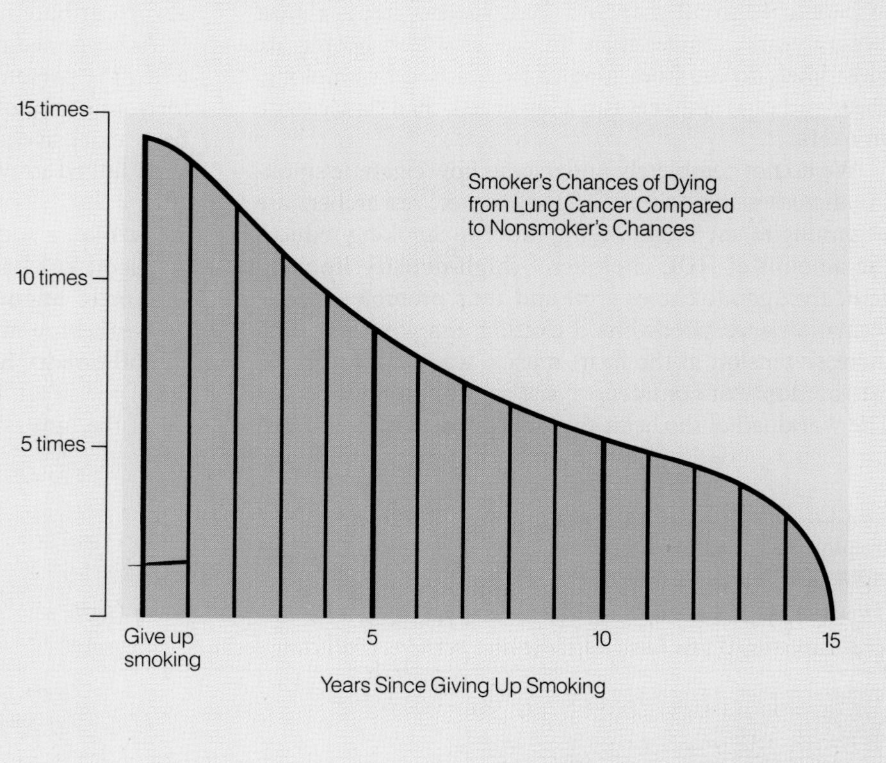

Lung Cancer Cigarette smoking is the primary cause of lung cancer. The risk of developing lung cancer increases with the number of cigarettes smoked each day, the number of years smoking, and the age at which the person started smoking.

Cigar and pipe smokers do run a higher risk of lung cancer than nonsmokers, but that risk is lower than for cigarette smokers. Smoking filter-tipped cigarettes slightly reduces health hazards, unless the smoker compensates by smoking more, as is often the case.

The evidence suggests that after a year without smoking the risk of lung cancer decreases substantially. After ten years, the incidence of lung cancer among ex-smokers approaches the incidence of those who never smoked. If smoking is stopped before cancer has started, lung tissue tends to repair itself, even if changes leading to cancer are already present.

Research has also linked smoking to cancers of the mouth, pharynx, esophagus, pancreas, and bladder.

Exploring Your Emotions

All your life you have urged a certain older friend or relative to quit smoking. Now he or she is dying of lung cancer. How do you feel, and how will you handle your feelings most constructively?

Emphysema Smoking is a primary cause of **emphysema**, a particularly disabling condition. The walls of the lung air sacs lose their elasticity and are gradually destroyed. The lungs' ability to obtain oxygen and remove carbon dioxide is impaired. A person with emphysema becomes breathless and feels as if he or she were drowning. The heart must pump harder and may become enlarged. The person frequently dies from a damaged heart. There is no known way to reverse this disease. In its advanced stage, the victim is bedridden and severely disabled.

Other Respiratory Diseases Cigarette smoking is linked to other diseases of the respiratory system, especially chronic bronchitis. Chronic bronchitis is a persistent, recurrent inflammation of the bronchial tubes. When the cell lining

Emphysema Loss of lung tissue elasticity and breakup of the many small air sacs in the lungs so that fewer, larger, and less elastic air sacs are formed. The progressive accumulation of air causes difficulty in breathing.

Macrophages Large cells in the body that absorb dead tissue and dead cells.

of the bronchial tubes is irritated, it secretes excess mucus. Bronchial congestion is followed by a chronic cough, which makes breathing more and more difficult.

Cigarette smokers are up to eighteen times more likely to die from emphysema and chronic bronchitis than are nonsmokers. If smokers have chronic bronchitis, they face a greater risk of lung cancer, no matter how old they are or how many (or few) cigarettes they smoke. Chronic bronchitis seems to be a shortcut to lung cancer.

Even smokers of high school age show impaired respiratory functioning, compared with nonsmokers of the same age. Although pipe and cigar smokers are more likely to die from respiratory disease than are nonsmokers, they face a smaller risk than do cigarette smokers (Figure 9-1).

The risk of developing respiratory diseases rises with the number of cigarettes smoked and falls when smoking is stopped.

For most people in the United States, cigarette smoking is a more important cause of respiratory disease than atmospheric pollution. But exposure to both atmospheric pollution and cigarette smoking is more dangerous than exposure to either by itself.

Even when the person shows no signs of respiratory impairment or disease, cigarette smoking damages the respiratory system. Normally the cells lining the bronchial tubes secrete mucus, a sticky fluid that collects particles of soot, dust, and other substances in inhaled air. Mucus is carried up to the mouth by the continuous motion of the cilia, little hairlike structures that protrude from the inner surface of the bronchial tubes. If the cilia are destroyed or do not work, or if the pollution of inhaled air is more than the system can remove, this protection offered by cilia is lost.

Cigarette smoke first slows, then stops the action of the cilia. Eventually it destroys them, leaving delicate membranes exposed to injury from substances inhaled in cigarette smoke or from the polluted air in which the person lives or works. Special cells of the body, the **macrophages** (literally "big eaters"), also work to remove foreign particles from the respiratory tract by engulfing them. Cigarette smoking seems to make macrophages work less efficiently.

Although cigarette smoking can cause many respiratory disorders and diseases, the damage is not always permanent. Once a person stops smoking, he or she can usually look for steady improvement in overall respiratory function. Chronic coughing subsides, phlegm (mucus) production returns to normal, and breathing becomes easier. The likelihood of respiratory disease drops sharply. People of all ages, even those who have been smoking for decades, improve after they stop smoking. If given a chance, the human body has remarkable powers to restore itself.

Exploring Your Emotions

You are married and have children; you don't smoke, but your spouse does. How do you feel about his or her behavior? What will you do about it?

Other Health Hazards Cigarette smoking is associated with many other health hazards, and the list keeps getting longer. Many of these associations have only recently been discovered, however, so we are not sure if they are causally related or if they merely exist together. Further research may link cigarette smoking to still other disorders.

Premature skin wrinkling, premature baldness, gum disorders, and allergies have all been associated with cigarette smoking. Recent research also suggests that smoking may harm the immune system.

Smoking and Pregnancy Accumulated evidence indicates that smoking during pregnancy can seriously harm both the mother and the unborn baby. It is especially harmful for mothers who are very young or older, or who are poorly nourished, are anemic, or have other health

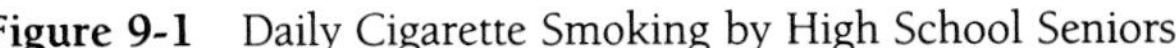

Figure 9-1 Daily Cigarette Smoking by High School Seniors

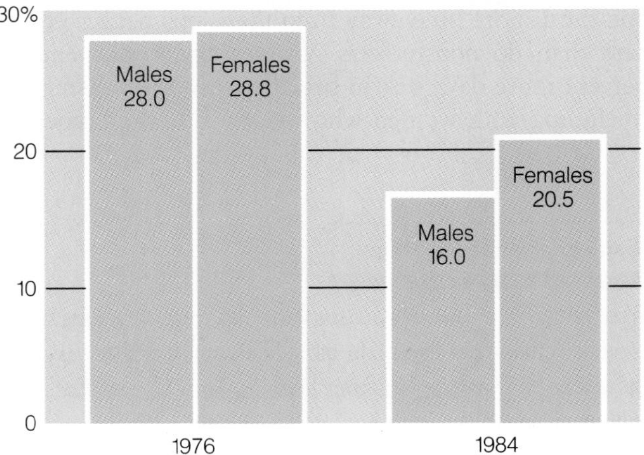

Sidestream smoke "Second-hand smoke" that comes from the burning end of a cigarette, cigar, or pipe.

Mainstream smoke Smoke that is inhaled by a smoker and then exhaled into the atmosphere.

Carboxyhemoglobin A compound formed when carbon monoxide displaces oxygen from red blood cells; it seriously limits the body's ability to use oxygen.

problems. These harmful effects include increased risk of spontaneous abortion, miscarriage, and stillbirths. If the baby is born alive, it runs an increased risk of congenital abnormalities and premature birth, and its birth weight is likely to be lower than otherwise. Lower birth weights are associated with increased mortality and a variety of diseases, especially infections.

In addition, other evidence suggests that infants born to smoking mothers are more likely to die from sudden infant death syndrome, or SIDS, also known as crib death, and are more likely to show long-term impairments in physical growth and intellectual development. Moreover, as if these problems were not enough, animal research evidence suggests that certain cancers are more common in animals that were exposed as fetuses to cigarette smoke.

Ulcers People who smoke cigarettes are more likely to have peptic ulcers than nonsmokers, and are more likely to die from them, especially ulcers of the stomach. People with ulcers should stop smoking immediately because smoking impairs the ability of the ulcer to heal.

Cumulative Effects Statistical data have shown the cumulative effects of smoking. These effects fall into the following two general categories.

Reduced Life Expectancy A boy who takes up smoking before age 15 and continues to smoke is only half as likely to live to age 75 as a boy who never smokes. If he inhales deeply, he risks losing one minute of life for every minute of smoking. Women who have similar smoking habits also have a reduced life expectancy.

Frequent Illness A national health survey begun in 1964 has produced some interesting findings. Smokers spend one-third more time away from their jobs because of illness than do nonsmokers. Women smokers spend 17 percent more days sick in bed than women nonsmokers (including both women who work inside the home and women who work outside). Lost workdays associated with cigarette smoking number in the millions.

Both men and women smokers show a greater rate of acute and chronic disease than those who have never smoked. The U.S. Public Health Service estimates that if all people had the same rate of disease as those who never smoked, there would be 1 million fewer cases of chronic bronchitis, 1.8 million fewer cases of sinusitis, and 1 million fewer cases of peptic ulcers in the country every year.

Exploring Your Emotions

You have been told to quit smoking, because you have severe smoker's cough. You quit, but your new boss spends hours in your office, smoking heavily. How do you feel about the problem, and how will you deal with it?

The Effects of Smoking on the Nonsmoker

The movement to protect people from tobacco smoke is gaining strength. As more nonsmokers become aware of the health hazards smokers are inflicting on them, they are insisting more on the right to breathe clean air.

Sidestream smoke (also referred to as "second-hand smoke") enters the atmosphere from the burning end of the cigarette, cigar, or pipe. Smoke that the smoker inhales and then exhales is referred to as **mainstream smoke.** Studies have shown that sidestream smoke has (1) twice as much tar and nicotine than in mainstream smoke; (2) three times as much benzopyrene, a cancer-causing agent; (3) almost three times as much carbon monoxide, which robs the blood of vital oxygen; and (4) three times as much ammonia. Nearly 85 percent of the smoke in a room where someone is smoking comes from sidestream smoke. Thus the nonsmoker is at risk both from the mainstream smoke exhaled by the smoker as well as from the sidestream smoke polluting the environment.

Carbon Monoxide and Other Harmful Agents Carbon monoxide is a poisonous, odorless gas commonly known as a pollutant from automobile exhausts. It is also one of the main ingredients of tobacco smoke. When inhaled, this gas displaces oxygen from red blood cells and forms **carboxyhemoglobin**, a dangerous compound that seriously limits the body's ability to use oxygen. Studies have shown that in rooms where people are smoking, levels of carbon monoxide can exceed those permitted by the Federal Air Quality Standards for outside air. Nonsmokers can still be affected by the harmful levels of sidestream smoke hours after they have left a smoky environment. Carbon monoxide still lingers in the bloodstream five hours later.

(continued on p. 210)

Why Do You Smoke?

Here are some statements made by people to describe what they get out of smoking cigarettes. How *often* do you feel this way when smoking them? Circle one number for each statement. For an accurate score, be sure you answer every question.

	ALWAYS	FREQUENTLY	OCCASIONALLY	SELDOM	NEVER
A. I smoke cigarettes in order to keep myself from slowing down	5	4	3	2	1
B. Handling a cigarette is part of the enjoyment of smoking it	5	4	3	2	1
C. Smoking cigarettes is pleasant and relaxing	5	4	3	2	1
D. I light up a cigarette when I feel angry about something	5	4	3	2	1
E. When I have run out of cigarettes I find it almost unbearable until I can get them	5	4	3	2	1
F. I smoke cigarettes automatically without even being aware of it	5	4	3	2	1
G. I smoke cigarettes to stimulate me, to perk myself up	5	4	3	2	1
H. Part of the enjoyment of smoking a cigarette comes from the steps I take to light up	5	4	3	2	1
I. I find cigarettes pleasurable	5	4	3	2	1
J. When I feel uncomfortable or upset about something, I light up a cigarette	5	4	3	2	1
K. I am very much aware of the fact when I am not smoking a cigarette	5	4	3	2	1
L. I light up a cigarette without realizing I still have one burning in the ashtray	5	4	3	2	1
M. I smoke cigarettes to give me a "lift"	5	4	3	2	1
N. When I smoke a cigarette, part of the enjoyment is watching the smoke as I exhale it	5	4	3	2	1
O. I want a cigarette most when I am comfortable and relaxed	5	4	3	2	1
P. When I feel "blue" or want to take my mind off cares and worries, I smoke cigarettes	5	4	3	2	1
Q. I get a real gnawing hunger for a cigarette when I haven't smoked for a while	5	4	3	2	1
R. I've found a cigarette in my mouth and didn't remember putting it there	5	4	3	2	1

How to Score

1. Enter the numbers you have circled to the smoking questions in the spaces below, putting the number you have circled to question A over line A, to question B over line B, and so on.

2. Total the 3 scores on each line to get your totals. For example, the sum of your scores over lines A, G, and M gives you your score on *Stimulation*—lines B, H, and N give the score on *Handling*, etc.

							TOTALS
____ A	+	____ G	+	____ M	=		____ STIMULATION
____ B	+	____ H	+	____ N	=		____ HANDLING
____ C	+	____ I	+	____ O	=		____ PLEASURABLE RELAXATION
____ D	+	____ J	+	____ P	=		____ CRUTCH: TENSION REDUCTION
____ E	+	____ K	+	____ Q	=		____ CRAVING: PSYCHOLOGICAL ADDICTION
____ F	+	____ L	+	____ R	=		____ HABIT

Why Do You Smoke? (*continued*)

Scores can vary from 3 to 15. Any score 11 and above is *high;* any score 7 and below is *low*.

What Your Scores Mean

What kind of smoker are you? What do you get out of smoking? What does it do for you? This test is designed to provide you with a score on each of six factors that describe many people's smoking. Your smoking may be well characterized by only one of these factors, or by a combination of factors. In any event, this test will help you identify what you use smoking for and what kind of satisfaction you think you get from smoking.

The six factors measured by this test describe one or another way of experiencing or managing certain kinds of feelings. Three of these feeling-states represent the *positive* feelings people get from smoking: (1) a sense of increased energy or *stimulation,* (2) the satisfaction of *handling* or manipulating things, and (3) the enhancing of *pleasurable feelings* accompanying a state of well being. The fourth is the *decreasing of negative feelings* by reducing a state of tension or feelings of anxiety, anger, shame, etc. The fifth is a complex pattern of increasing and decreasing "craving" for a cigarette, representing a psychological *addiction* to cigarettes. The sixth is *habit* smoking, which takes place in an absence of feeling and is purely automatic smoking.

A score of 11 or above on any factor indicates that this factor is an important source of satisfaction for you. The higher your score (15 is the highest), the more important a particular factor is in your smoking and the more useful the discussion of that factor can be in your attempt to quit.

A few words of warning: If you give up smoking, you may have to learn to get along without the satisfactions that smoking gives you. Either that or you will have to find some more acceptable way of getting this satisfaction. In either case, you need to know just what it is you get out of smoking before you can decide whether to forego the satisfactions it gives you or to find another way to achieve them.

Stimulation If you score high or fairly high on this factor, it means that you are one of those smokers who is stimulated by the cigarette —you feel that it helps wake you up, organize your energies, and keep you going. If you try to give up smoking, you may want a safe substitute, a *brisk walk* or moderate exercise, for example, whenever you feel the urge to smoke.

Handling Handling things can be satisfying, but there are many ways to keep your hands busy without lighting up or playing with a cigarette. Why not toy with a pen or pencil? Or try doodling. Or play with a coin, a piece of jewelry, or some other harmless object. There are plastic cigarettes to play with, or you might even use a real cigarette if you can trust yourself not to light it.

Accentuation of Pleasure—Pleasurable Relaxation It is not always easy to find out whether you use the cigarette to feel *good,* that is, get real, honest pleasure out of smoking or to keep from feeling so *bad*. About two-thirds of smokers score high or fairly high on *accentuation of pleasure,* and about half of those also score as high or higher on *reduction of negative feelings*.

Those who do get real pleasure out of smoking often find that an honest consideration of the harmful effects of their habit is enough to help them quit. They substitute eating, drinking, social activities, and physical activities—within reasonable bounds—and find they do not seriously miss their cigarettes.

Reduction of Negative Feelings, or "Crutch" Many smokers use the cigarette as a kind of crutch in moments of stress or discomfort, and on occasion it may work; the cigarette is sometimes used as a

The Smoky Work Environment Nonsmokers exposed to tobacco smoke at work for many years show decreased lung function. Some studies indicate that 50 percent of nonsmokers report problems working near a smoker. Another 36 percent said they were forced to move away from their work stations because of sidestream smoke.

A trend is gaining momentum to restrict smoking at work through state and city laws. The general approach of these laws is that although the preferences of nonsmokers and smokers are considered when possible, the rights of nonsmokers must be ensured first. This trend is also increasing among private companies as more and more of them adopt policies to protect the health of the nonsmoker.

tranquilizer. But the heavy smoker, the person who tries to handle severe personal problems by smoking many times a day, is apt to discover that cigarettes do not help him deal with his problems effectively.

When it comes to quitting, this kind of smoker may find it easy to stop when everything is going well, but may be tempted to start again in a time of crisis. Again, physical exertion, eating, drinking, or social activity—in moderation—may serve as useful substitutes for cigarettes, even in times of tension. The choice of a substitute depends on what will achieve the same effect without having any appreciable risk.

"Craving" or Psychological Addiction Quitting smoking is difficult for the person who scores high on this factor, that of *psychological addiction.* For him, the craving for the next cigarette begins to build up the moment he puts one out, so tapering off is not likely to work. He must go "cold turkey." It may be helpful for him to smoke more than usual for a day or two, so that the taste for cigarettes is spoiled, and then isolate himself completely from cigarettes until the craving is gone. Giving up cigarettes may be so difficult and cause so much discomfort that once he does quit, he will find it easy to resist the temptation to go back to smoking because he knows that some day he will have to go through the same agony again.

Habit This kind of smoker is no longer getting much satisfaction from his cigarettes. He just lights them frequently without even realizing he is doing so. He may find it easy to quit and stay off if he can break the habit patterns he has built up. Cutting down gradually may be quite effective if there is a change in the way the cigarettes are smoked and the conditions under which they are smoked. The key to success is becoming *aware* of each cigarette you smoke. This can be done by asking yourself, "Do I really want this cigarette?" You may be surprised at how many you do not want.

Summary

If you do not score high on any of the six factors, chances are that you do not smoke very much or have not been smoking for very many years. If so, giving up smoking—and staying off—should be easy. If you score high on several categories, you apparently get several kinds of satisfaction from smoking and will have to find several solutions. Certain combinations of scores may indicate that giving up smoking will be especially difficult. Those who score high on both *reduction of negative feelings* and *craving,* may have a particularly hard time in going off smoking and in staying off. However, there are ways to do it; many smokers represented by this combination have not been able to quit.

Others who score high on Factors 4 and 5 may find it useful to change their patterns of smoking and cut down at the same time. They can try to smoke fewer cigarettes, smoke them only half-way down, use low-tar-and-nicotine cigarettes, and inhale less often and less deeply. After several months of this temporary solution, they may find it easier to stop completely. You must make two important decisions: (1) whether to try to do without the satisfactions you get from smoking or find an appropriate, less hazardous substitute, and (2) whether to try to cut out cigarettes all at once or taper off. Your scores should guide you in making both of these decisions.

SOURCE: Daniel Horn and Associates, 1983 (October), *A Self-Test for Smokers* (Test 3), DHEW Publication No. (CDC) 75-8716 (Washington, D.C.: U.S. Public Health Service, Department of Health and Human Services).

Sidestream Smoke and Children As you may have noticed, young children and babies breathe faster than adults. And they therefore inhale more air as well as the pollutants in the air. Studies have shown that children inhale three times more pollutants per unit of body weight than do adults. This intake is particularly harmful because young lungs need clean air for optimal development.

Babies of parents who smoke at home suffer much more pneumonia and bronchitis than babies of nonsmoking parents. This is particularly true in their first year of life. Studies show that the mother's smoking has the most impact on the child's lung function, probably because the mother is usually the primary caretaker. And since women are smoking more, more children are affected.

Asthma, which can be a serious lung disease and is the most frequent cause of school absenteeism from a chronic condition, is aggravated by tobacco smoke. Many asthma deaths among children may be related to such exposure. And even among nonasthmatic children, researchers have found that respiratory illnesses twice as often hit children whose parents smoked at home, compared to those with nonsmoking parents.

One study divided 441 nonsmokers into those with a history of allergies and those without. Of both groups, 70 percent suffered from eye irritations caused by smoke. The allergic group suffered the most symptoms, from breathlessness to headaches, nasal congestion, and cough. Even among the nonallergic group, 30 percent developed headaches and nasal discomfort, while 25 percent developed coughs.

Sidestream Smoke and Lung Cancer Researchers have found an increased risk of lung cancer in nonsmoking wives married to men who smoke. This finding is not surprising, because we know that ingredients in tobacco smoke cause lung cancer at a high rate among smokers. There are probably no safe levels of tobacco smoke inhalation.

Tobacco Odors Have you ever gone to a party with smokers and noted, much later or even the next day, a strong odor of tobacco in your hair and clothes? The human body acts as a magnet to tobacco smoke. Burning tobacco smoke creates a high electrical potential, whereas the water-filled human body has a low one. The smoke in a room gravitates and clings to people in much the same way as iron filings are attracted to a magnet. Aldehydes and ketones (chemicals in tobacco smoke) produce the penetrating odor; the tars hold them to your skin and your clothes. The smoker may not be sensitive to the odor because smoke destroys the inner lining of the nose. Research has found that smoke contamination is so intense that demands on an air-conditioning system can increase to as much as 600 percent to control the smell.

What Can Be Done?

Nonsmokers have the right to breathe clean air, free from harmful and irritating tobacco smoke. This right supersedes the right to smoke when the two conflict. Nonsmokers have the right to express—firmly but politely—their adverse reactions to tobacco smoke. They have the right to voice their objections when smokers light up. Nonsmokers have the right to act through legislative channels, social pressures, or any other legitimate means—as individuals or in groups—to prevent or discourage smokers from polluting the environment and to seek the restrictions of smoking in public places. Here are a few things you can do

- Tell family, friends, co-workers, students, and strangers that you mind if they smoke.
- Put stickers and signs in your home, car, classroom, and office. Request seating in nonsmoking sections when you travel. Wear buttons.
- Ask your doctor and dentist or health professional to restrict smoking in their waiting rooms and to establish no-smoking regulations in all health care facilities, including hospitals.
- Contact the American Lung Association or the American Cancer Society to discuss ways to protect nonsmokers.

Exploring Your Emotions

You have just quit smoking, and you're still having a hard time with smoking urges. All your best friends smoke, and one of them (who knows you've quit) offers you a cigarette. How do you feel? How would you express your feelings?

Action at the Federal Level The Comprehensive Smoking Act was signed into law in 1984. One of the act's major provisions replaced the old health warning ("the U.S. Surgeon General has determined that cigarette smoking is dangerous to your health"). The new warnings read as follows:

- "Smoking causes lung cancer, heart disease, emphysema, and may complicate pregnancy."
- "Quitting smoking now greatly reduces serious risks to your health."
- "Smoking by pregnant women may result in fetal injury, premature birth, and low birth weight."
- "Cigarette smoke contains carbon monoxide."

The act also requires that cigarette companies disclose to the U.S. Department of Health and Human Services a complete list of all chemicals and other ingredients added to cigarettes during the manufacturing process.

There has been other action on the federal level. In 1986, Congress permanently extended the 16 cents excise tax on cigarettes, which was temporarily increased from 8 cents in 1982. Tax bills introduced in 1985 removed the tax deduction for cigarette advertising and promotion activities, such as sponsorship of sports events and music festivals. In addition, one federal court and three federal agencies have now held that sensitive nonsmokers are "handicapped persons" and can take legal action to require employers to provide a "reasonable accommodation" to the handicap.

Politics, Tobacco, and Tobacco Interests More and more restrictions are being placed on smoking in public buildings, on airliners, and in other public places. These efforts have been somewhat successful in reducing cigarette smoking in some age groups, but they are opposed by an impressive concentration of economic, social, and political power. Tobacco interests wield enough power to keep the U.S. government subsidizing them with $30 million cash each year despite the fact that government is paying for an aggressive antitobacco campaign.

Helping the Smoker to Quit Our national epidemic of tobacco-related disease and death will not be reversed until each individual takes responsibility for his or her own health and well-being. Studies have shown that most ex-smokers quit on their own without participating in a particular program. Yet some programs may be more helpful than others and may differ in their ability to help different kinds of people.

Most stop-smoking programs emphasize one of various pharmacological, psychological, or health education approaches. Some combine more than one approach. The health education programs often assume that if a person learns the facts about smoking he or she will make the rational decision to stop smoking. But human behavior is quite complex and not necessarily rational, and the failure rates of these programs tend to be quite high. For one reason, nicotine's powerful addicting qualities often overwhelm the smoker's conscious desire to stop smoking.

Most smoking programs treat quitting as an event and assume that when the program is over, the smoking problem will also be over. And, in fact, most programs can demonstrate a high quit rate initially, but after one year most people have started smoking again. These programs provide a social environment with psychological supports that no longer function for the smoker when the program ends. The behavioral reinforcers that maintained abstinence are no longer present. Learning theory suggests that when the reinforcers disappear, so does the behavior. Giving up smoking (or other drug dependencies) is a long-term, intricate process. Heavy smokers who just say they have stopped "cold turkey" are not showing the thinking

Exploring Your Emotions

How are these two advertisements intended to touch your feelings? Are they effective? Design a poster and a slogan to express your feelings about smoking.

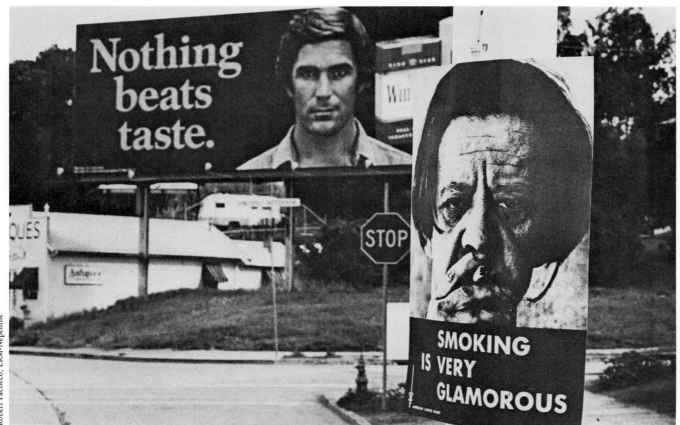

Robert Pacheco, EKM-Nepenthe

Nicotine Gum: New Hope for Smokers

Most smokers want to quit. They know that smoking cigarettes hurts their health, sets a bad example for children, annoys nonsmokers, and costs a lot of money. But breaking a long-standing habit can be tough.

A pack-a-day smoker inhales 75,000 puffs each year. Over the years, lighting up becomes linked to many events of everyday life, and habits are formed that can be psychologically difficult to give up. In addition, most smokers are physically addicted to nicotine and experience unpleasant withdrawal symptoms when they stop smoking.

Nicotine gum can be a valuable aid to smoking cessation under medical supervision. It is being marketed as a prescription product under the brand name Nicorette by Merrell Dow Pharmaceuticals, Inc., a subsidiary of the Dow Chemical Company. A 96-piece package of Nicorette costs about $20. Each piece of gum contains 2 mg of nicotine, which, when the gum is chewed slowly, is absorbed through the lining of the mouth over a 20- to 30-minute period. Chewing one piece of gum per hour produces blood nicotine levels comparable to those obtained with hourly cigarette smoking. Any nicotine that is swallowed has little effect on the body. The gum provides a substitute for oral activity and can prevent nicotine withdrawal symptoms, allowing the smoker to break the behavioral habits of smoking without suffering the discomforts of nicotine withdrawal.

Most users find that 8 to 10 pieces of gum a day are sufficient to control their craving for cigarettes. Side effects are common but mild. Most of them disappear by themselves within a week or can be controlled by chewing more slowly. After a few months, use of the gum is tapered off and stopped.

An FDA advisory committee that reviewed the evidence concluded that nicotine gum increases the likelihood of smoking cessation when used together with appropriate counseling. The product is most suitable for smokers in whom the addictive component is strongest—those who smoke 30 or more cigarettes per day or those who find that the most difficult cigarette to give up is the first one in the morning.

Nicotine gum is not a "miracle" drug and does not take the place of willpower. But it can be very helpful to those who have a strong desire to become nonsmokers for good. Recent studies involving hard-core smokers found that success rates using nicotine gum and counseling were three times as high as with counseling alone or with counseling and placebo gum containing nicotine in nonabsorbable form. Perhaps one day nicotine gum will also be approved for use as a temporary substitute for smoking in situations like airplane trips or meetings, so that smokers can maintain their nicotine levels without disturbing the people around them.

Merrell Dow supplies doctors with detailed information on how to select and prepare patients for using the gum. Users receive a 24-page booklet and, upon request, two newsletters about smoking cessation and nicotine gum treatment. Doctors are being urged to provide at least one follow-up visit per month over the treatment period (usually three to four months).

If you smoke, there is certainly good reason to stop. No matter how long one has smoked, it is still beneficial to quit. During the first day after quitting, the heart and lungs begin to repair the damage caused by cigarette smoke. Smokers cough usually disappears within a few weeks, energy and endurance may increase, and taste and smell may return for foods that haven't been enjoyed for years. After ten years, the risk of dying from heart and blood vessel disease goes down to the level of nonsmokers. The risk of lung cancer decreases, and so does the incidence of respiratory infections and lung tissue destruction, which are responsible for emphysema. A study of over 10 million ex-smokers found that the death rate ten years after quitting approached that of people who had never smoked.

SOURCE: Stephen Barrett, 1985 (May) Nicotine gum: New hope for smokers, *Healthline*.

and struggling and other mental processes that contributed to their final overt behavior.

Pharmacological programs usually substitute nicotine-containing substances such as chewing gum. Some of these programs are effective when combined with psychological and social reinforcement. However, success rates are usually lower than 25 percent after a one-year follow-up. Their major drawback is that the nicotine addiction remains untreated. When these nicotine-containing substitutes for cigarettes are discontinued, many people begin to smoke again. In addition, many people do not find these substitutes very satisfying and complain about side effects.

Bloom County □ Berke Breathed

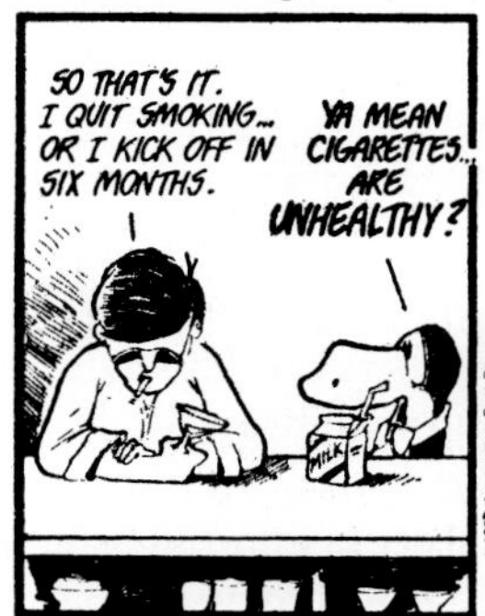
SO THAT'S IT. I QUIT SMOKING... OR I KICK OFF IN SIX MONTHS.
YA MEAN CIGARETTES... ARE UNHEALTHY?
MILK

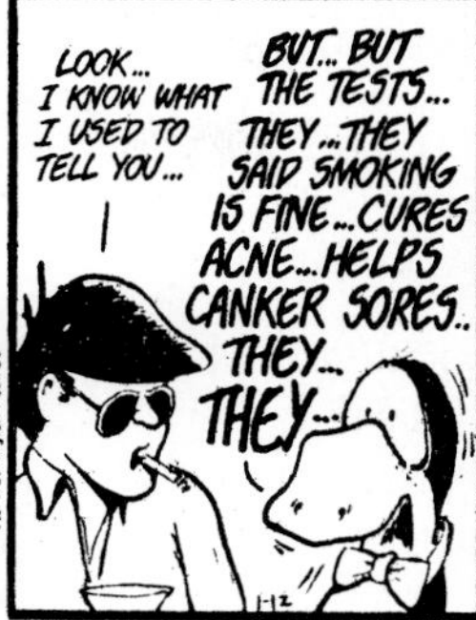

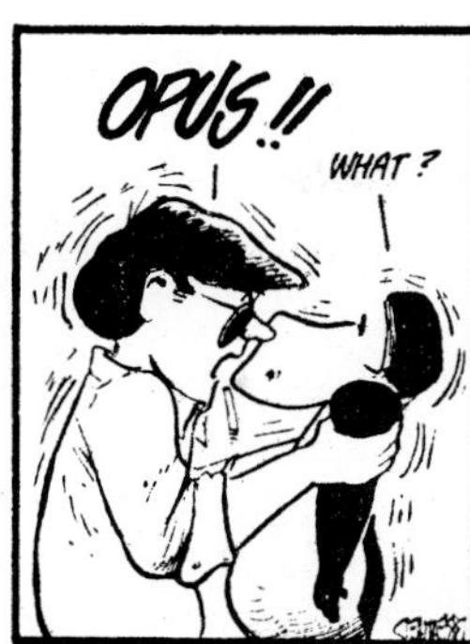
OPUS!!
WHAT?

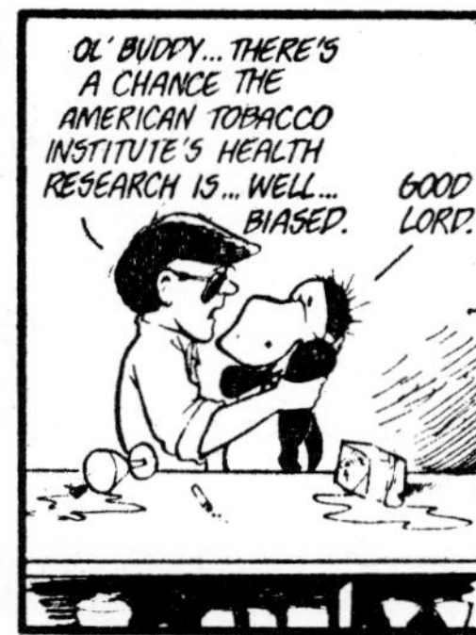
OL' BUDDY... THERE'S A CHANCE THE AMERICAN TOBACCO INSTITUTE'S HEALTH RESEARCH IS... WELL... BIASED.
GOOD LORD.

Giving up smoking is usually a lengthy process that is influenced by many factors. None, unfortunately, are highly predictive of success in quitting. Stop-smoking programs that combine several approaches have the most promise. These programs, which sometimes operate in industrial settings, may attract people who would not otherwise participate in a smoking clinic. They often alter the social environment by setting up demands and expectations against smoking. Peer support is often a powerful influence in behavior, as witnessed by the experience of Alcoholics Anonymous. The persistent encouragement of colleagues, family, and friends can be critical in giving up drug dependencies. Providing individual or group incentives is another intervention that can be combined with other techniques. Feedback on cardiac and respiratory status can be a compelling method to help some people stop smoking. And documenting improvement in vital functions after the person has quit smoking can continue to provide positive reinforcement.

Benefits from Quitting Studies have shown that when smokers stop, a number of changes start to occur. Food is absorbed more efficiently, appetite increases, and the senses of taste and smell improve. In some people, these changes lead to slight weight gain—but they are signs of health. Cardiovascular changes include improved circulation (in hands and feet especially), reduced heart rate, lowered blood pressure, and increased heart efficiency during rest and exercise. Many ex-smokers report more energy, increased alertness, and need for less sleep. Because of increased microcirculation in the skin, some people report improved facial complexion.

As one might expect, respiratory changes are often pronounced. An immediate improvement appears in the efficiency of oxygen exchange between the lungs and the circulatory system, maximal breath capacity increases, and breathing rate decreases. Gradually the "smoker's cough" declines and long-term respiratory conditions—such as bronchitis, emphysema, and asthma—improve.

The younger people are when they stop smoking, the more pronounced the health improvements. And these improvements gradually but invariably increase as the period of nonsmoking increases.

Take Action

Your answers to the Exploring Your Emotions questions in this chapter and your placement level on the Wellness Ladder will, we hope, encourage you to begin a process of self-exploration and self-discovery that you will continue. Reflect on the entire chapter's content and ask yourself how each point relates to your own life. Then take action:

1. In your notebook, list the positive behaviors that help you avoid smoking or a smoker's environment. Consider how you can strengthen those positive behaviors. Then list the behaviors that block your achieving wellness. Consider each behavior and decide which you can change. Begin with the easiest ones first. Reread Chapter 1 to review some general techniques for accomplishing these changes. Discuss them in class or with a close friend.

2. If you are a smoker, turn back to the personal contract for quitting smoking on page 11. Fill out and sign the contract and give it to a close friend. Ask him or her to return it to you after the target date on the contract.

3. If you are a smoker, go to the student health clinic and ask to take a lung function test. Take along a friend who doesn't smoke and ask that he or she be allowed to take the test, too. Compare the results. If you don't smoke, recruit a smoking friend.

4. Read the following Behavior Change Strategy, and take the appropriate action.

Behavior Change Strategy

Quitting Smoking

There are relatively few bright lights on the horizon of stop-smoking research. Many very intriguing, well-intentioned, and soundly based programs have failed to show any effectiveness. Most of the available research is based on people who have attended smoking cessation clinics, even though the vast majority of smokers try to quit without such "hands-on" assistance.

The following program has demonstrated relatively greater therapeutic benefits than alternative approaches. You are urged to approach quitting smoking as a significant problem-solving challenge.

No program, no matter how detailed, can possibly address all facets of the smoking habit in a way that will work for everyone. Yet some strategies and steps can improve personal chances—your probability of lasting success—if they are modified by feedback and experience.

There are three phases to quitting smoking: (1) preparation, (2) quitting, (3) and maintaining success. Each of these stages is discussed in order here.

Preparation for Quitting Preparation for quitting involves collecting personal smoking information in a detailed smoking diary. The format and a representative diary appear in Chapter 1. Notice that the diary enables the smoker to collect two major types of information—cigarettes smoked and smoking urges. Part of the job is to identify patterns of smoking that are connected with routine situations (for example, the coffee break smoke, the after-dinner cigarette, the tension reduction cigarette, and so on).

The second major task of this preparation phase is to learn how to use nonsmoking relaxation methods. Many smokers find that they use cigarettes to help them unwind in tense situations or to relax at other times. Because smoking performs this function, it will be difficult to eliminate unless you find effective substitutes. Since it takes time to become proficient at using progressive relaxation, initial practice of this procedure is recommended early in the process of preparation. Refer to the more detailed discussion of progressive relaxation found in Chapter 2.

Quitting Quitting smoking is the first goal most smokers want to reach, but staying off cigarettes is the ultimate objective. Quitting involves establishing a personal quit contract that specifies the day and time when you will stop smoking as well as possible rewards for quitting. In this regard, it might be useful to identify the amount of money that you will save by not smoking a pack or so of cigarettes a day. You might set this money aside as a nonsmoking "salary."

In regard to the personal contract, smokers are usually torn between quitting abruptly (the so-called cold turkey approach) or through gradual reduction (one step at a time). Research favors the abrupt approach but with enough time set aside to learn and practice effective quitting skills. One useful approach to quitting helps the smoker appreciate the natural unpleasantness of his or her smoking. The procedure that can help reawaken this unpleasant side of smoking is called *aversive smoking* or, as we will refer to it here, *focused smoking*.

In focused smoking, the smoker smokes only in unusual circumstances and in a manner that helps him or her concentrate only on the negative aspects of normal smoking. Here is a suggested schedule for this practice. Note that there are "yes" days and "no" days; these refer to whether smoking is permitted in the special smoking sessions. All normal smoking is automatically prohibited. (It is simply too hard to establish unpleasant associations if one continues normal smoking.)

Many people choose not to follow this focused smoking approach

Typical focused smoking schedule		Typical focused smoking session	
Monday:	YES	Step 1:	Smoke at regular pace with total concentration upon unpleasant aspects of the experience
Tuesday:	YES		
Wednesday:	YES		
Thursday:	No Smoking		
Friday:	YES	Step 2:	Five-minute rest period for reflection
Saturday:	No Smoking		
Sunday:	YES	Step 3:	Smoke one cigarette at normal pace with total concentration on the unpleasant features of that experience
Monday:	YES (Quit Day)		

SOURCE: Adapted from B. G. Danaher and E. Lichtenstein, 1978, *Become an Ex-Smoker*. Englewood Cliffs, N.J.: Prentice-Hall.

because they think that it is self-punishment. In fact, the procedure serves several useful functions in that it avoids the withdrawal problems that might be encountered if you quit smoking abruptly; it solidifies a personal commitment to change; and it can help revive vivid images of the unpleasant impact of smoking on your immediate physical sensations (burning eyes, throat, mouth, and so on).

Maintaining Nonsmoking Maintaining nonsmoking over time is the ultimate goal of any stop-smoking program, and it is the third phase of this program. The lingering smoking urges that remain once you have quit are the targets of work and planning because they will cause relapse if left unattended. Just as there are patterns to smoking, there are also patterns to lingering smoking urges that can be identified through the use of an urge diary that looks very much like the smoking diary that appears in Chapter 1. Patterns are often linked to situations in what seem like simple and innocuous ways. If you always used to sit the same way every evening to read the paper and watch the evening news—and have a cigarette—then even after you have quit smoking you may have smoking urges in that situation. By changing something in the situation—sitting in another chair or reading in another room—you may be able to break the strength of past associations. In the same way you will have to practice a new repertoire of nonsmoking skills if stress or boredom is a strong smoking-urge "signal" for you. It is very helpful to practice the relaxation procedures (which you should have been using since the preparation phase) to deal effectively with boredom or stress.

Cognitions, too, can be a source of considerable trouble during the maintenance phase of becoming an ex-smoker. Testing yourself ("I can prove that I'm strong; let me smoke just one to prove my personal strength") and remembering cigarettes as long-lost friends or part of a better time in your life ("the good old days") can erode your sense of resolve and your skills in resisting lingering smoking urges. Identifying and listing personal prosmoking self-statements can be very helpful in alerting you to how you can unwittingly undermine your own progress. Of course, it is essential to go beyond merely listing these thoughts; it is critical to *attack them* and *reduce their frequency*.

Finally, with the self-reward approach noted earlier (the nonsmoking "salary"), keep track of the emerging benefits that come from having quit smoking. Items that might appear on such a list include improved stamina, an increased sense of pride at having kicked a personally troublesome problem, improved sense of taste and smell, and so on.

There is no available cookbook of stop-smoking recipes that can be used word for word. This section has outlined some of the strategies that have helped others to quit smoking. Reread Chapter 1 to review the notion of personal problem solving, and adapt these suggestions.

Selected References

Cancer Facts and Figures 1987. 1986. New York: American Cancer Society.

The Health Consequences of Using Smokeless Tobacco. A Report of the Advisory Committee to the Surgeon General. 1986. Bethesda, Md.: U.S. Department of Human Services.

Heart Facts 1987. 1986. New York: American Heart Association.

Laurent, C. 1985 (January 16). Resolutions—Up in smoke? *Nursing Mirror* 160:30.

A Lifetime of Freedom from Smoking. 1986. New York: American Lung Association.

Miller, G. H., and D. R. Gerstein. 1985 (March 22). Smoking and longevity. *Science* 227:1412.

Overstreet, J. I. 1987 (January). How to help a friend quit smoking. *Healthline*.

The Pharmacologic Treatment of Tobacco Dependence: Proceedings of the World Congress. 1985. Cambridge, Mass.: Harvard University.

Smoking and Health. A Report of the Surgeon General. 1986. Bethesda, Md.: U.S. Department of Health and Human Services.

Troyer, Ronald J., and G. E. Markle. 1983. *Cigarettes: The Battle over Smoking*. New Brunswick, N.J.: Rutgers University Press.

Recommended Readings

The Health Consequences of Using Smokeless Tobacco, A Report of the Advisory Committee to the Surgeon General. 1986. Bethesda, Md.: U.S. Department of Human Services.
A comprehensive examination of the role of smokeless tobacco in the causation of cancer, noncancerous and precancerous oral diseases or conditions, addiction, and other adverse health effects.

Smoking and Health. A report of the Surgeon General. 1986. Bethesda, Md.: U.S. Department of Health and Human Services.
A careful examination of the evidence, showing that low levels of exposure to environmental tobacco smoke is harmful to the health of the nonsmoker.

Chapter 10

Contents

Rate Yourself

Your Alcohol Use and Attitudes Read the following statements carefully. Choose the one in each section that best describes you at this moment and circle its number. When you have chosen one statement for each section, add the numbers and record your total score. Find your position on the Wellness Ladder.

5 Rarely drinks alcohol
4 Rarely drinks alcohol except with meals
3 Has a drink at least once a day
2 Sometimes drinks in the morning
1 Usually drinks in the morning and evening

5 Drinks to be sociable
4 Drinks to reduce tension
3 Drinks to reduce inhibitions
2 Drinks because others are drinking
1 Drinks to avoid thinking about troubles

5 Never drives after having two or more drinks
4 Rarely drives after having two drinks
3 Often drives after having two drinks
2 Often drives after having more than two drinks
1 Drives regardless of amount of alcohol consumed

5 Is well informed about the effects of alcohol
4 Knows a good deal about the effects of alcohol
3 Knows something about the effects of alcohol
2 Knows little about the effects of alcohol
1 Is ignorant about the effects of alcohol

5 Avoids drinking on an empty stomach
4 Usually sips rather than gulps alcoholic beverages
3 Knows how much alcohol is enough
2 Gets intoxicated without realizing it
1 Drinks without regard to amount or effect

Total Score ______

Alcohol

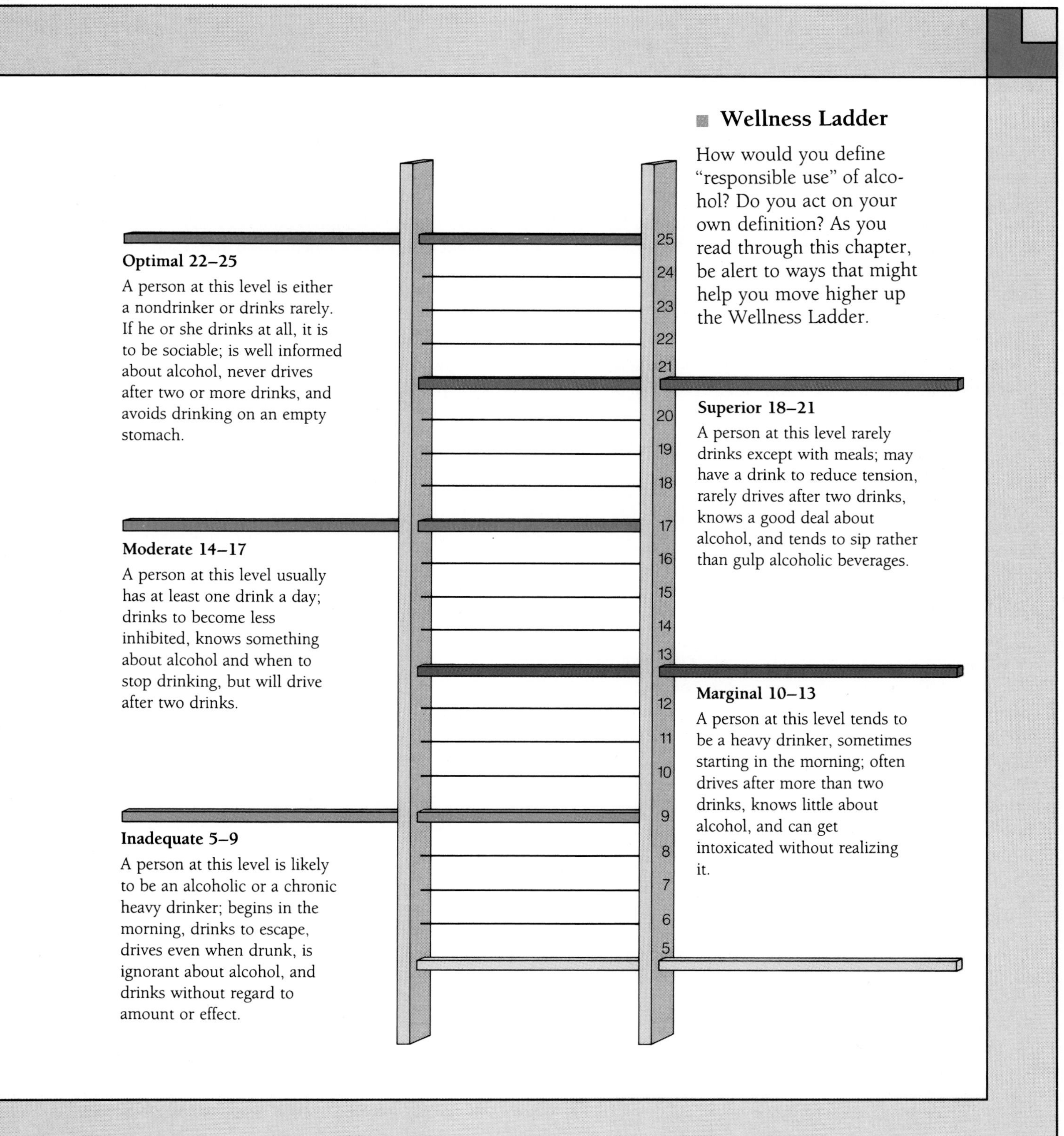

Optimal 22–25

A person at this level is either a nondrinker or drinks rarely. If he or she drinks at all, it is to be sociable; is well informed about alcohol, never drives after two or more drinks, and avoids drinking on an empty stomach.

Moderate 14–17

A person at this level usually has at least one drink a day; drinks to become less inhibited, knows something about alcohol and when to stop drinking, but will drive after two drinks.

Inadequate 5–9

A person at this level is likely to be an alcoholic or a chronic heavy drinker; begins in the morning, drinks to escape, drives even when drunk, is ignorant about alcohol, and drinks without regard to amount or effect.

Wellness Ladder

How would you define "responsible use" of alcohol? Do you act on your own definition? As you read through this chapter, be alert to ways that might help you move higher up the Wellness Ladder.

Superior 18–21

A person at this level rarely drinks except with meals; may have a drink to reduce tension, rarely drives after two drinks, knows a good deal about alcohol, and tends to sip rather than gulp alcoholic beverages.

Marginal 10–13

A person at this level tends to be a heavy drinker, sometimes starting in the morning; often drives after more than two drinks, knows little about alcohol, and can get intoxicated without realizing it.

Alcohol The intoxicating ingredient in fermented liquors. A colorless, pungent liquid.

Intoxication The state of being mentally affected by a chemical.

Fermented Describes a substance in which complex molecules have been broken down by the action of yeast or bacteria. Fermentation of certain substances produces alcohol.

Distillation The process of heating a mixture and recondensing the vapor. This process intensifies the mixture's properties and eliminates impurities. Distillation is used in manufacturing whiskey and brandy.

Psychoactive Affecting the mind; specifically said of drugs that affect the brain or nervous system.

Proof value Two times the percentage of alcohol.

Stimulant Something that increases nervous or muscular activity.

Inhibition The blocking of impulse or inclination.

Central nervous system depressant Any chemical that affects the brain or spinal cord and decreases nervous or muscular activity.

Stupor A state of dulled mind and senses in which an individual has little or no appreciation of his or her surroundings.

People long ago recognized the power of alcoholic beverages: The "spirit" changed feelings and behavior. Ever since, **alcohol** has had a somewhat contradictory role in human life. It has been associated with good times, cheerfulness, and conviviality, but it is also associated with escape, with blotting out the world, with inch-by-inch suicide, and with general self-destructiveness. Many of our slang expressions for **intoxication** reflect its less positive aspects—"blasted," "smashed," "bombed," "wasted."

Alcohol is probably the oldest drug in the world; we have evidence that beer and berry wine were used at least by 6400 B.C. and probably even earlier. Alcohol has been used in religious ceremonies, in feasts and celebrations, and as a medicine for thousands of years. Beer, a mild intoxicant brewed from a mixture of grains, usually contains from 3 to 6 percent of ethyl alcohol. Wines are made by **fermenting** the juices of grapes or other fruits.

Once the **distillation** process was developed (about A.D. 800), the spirit could be concentrated in a purer and more potent form. It was called *al-kuhl,* an Arabic word meaning "finely divided spirit." Throughout history alcohol has been more popular than any other drug, in spite of a great variety and number of prohibitions against it. In fact, forbidding the use of alcohol seems only to make it more popular. Even the newer **psychoactive** drugs have not diminished that popularity.

Ethyl alcohol, in various concentrations, is the common psychoactive ingredient in wine, beer, and what are called *hard liquors.* The concentration of alcohol in table wines is about 9 to 14 percent. Other wines such as sherry, port, and Madeira contain about 20 percent alcohol. These types are called *fortified wines* because distilled alcohol has been added to them. The stronger alcoholic beverages, such as gin, whiskey, brandy, and rum and liqueurs, are made by distilling brewed or fermented grains or other products. These beverages contain (usually) from 35 to 50 percent alcohol, a concentration about ten times that of beer.

Alcohol concentration in a beverage is indicated by the **proof value**, which is two times the percentage concentration. If a beverage is 100 proof, it contains 50 percent alcohol. Two ounces of 100-proof whiskey contain one ounce of pure alcohol. The proof value of the stronger alcoholic beverages can usually be found on the bottle labels. A convenient way of remembering alcohol concentrations is that the usual 12-ounce bottle of beer, 5-ounce glass of table wine, and cocktail with 1½ ounces of liquor all contain the same amount of alcohol—about 0.6 ounces.

Exploring Your Emotions

You have just come back from a football game and settled into a booth at a local tavern with some friends. Bill orders a ginger ale. What goes through your mind about Bill when you hear his order? Do you feel negative, neutral, or positive about him?

Immediate Effects of Alcohol

Alcohol acts as a depressant on the central nervous system. This fact is the overall reason for the changes that result from drinking. Physiologically, it first depresses a part of the brain that is involved in coordinating various parts of the nervous system. It also interferes with the processes that control inhibitions and depresses the function of nerves, muscles, including the heart muscle, and many other body tissues. We do not know precisely how alcohol exerts these effects.

Most people are familiar with the usual immediate effects of alcohol on behavior. These effects include anxiety reduction, mild euphoria, muscle incoordination, and slurring of speech.

When people drink in social settings, alcohol often seems to act as a **stimulant**, enhancing conviviality or assertiveness. This response probably occurs, however, because alcohol acts on people to make them lose their **inhibitions**, not because it stimulates the nervous system. Low doses of alcohol sometimes make people better able to perform simple tasks, but complex behavior, such as driving, is impaired. Moderate doses markedly interfere with coordination, intellectual functions, and verbal performance. At higher doses, the individual may be easily

Myths about Alcohol

Myth You can speed up the metabolism of alcohol by exercising, drinking coffee or taking other CNS stimulants, or by breathing fresh air.

Fact Once alcohol is absorbed, there are no ways of appreciably accelerating its breakdown.

Myth Alcoholics can "handle their alcohol" better than nonalcoholics.

Fact In later stages of alcoholism, tolerance to alcohol often decreases. In some severe alcoholics, tolerance fluctuates from day to day; on one day a liter of wine has little behavioral effect, on another day, he or she will be staggering after one glass of wine.

Myth When you are under the influence of alcohol, you are so relaxed you are less likely to get hurt in an accident.

Fact Alcohol slows protective reflexes and impairs coordination. People under the influence of alcohol are at much greater risk of injury (and death) from accidents.

Myth Most alcoholics are consciously aware of drinking too much.

Fact Denial—the unconscious psychological process that blocks awareness of reality—is an almost universal characteristic of alcoholics and other drug abusers. There is a clinical adage: "the two hallmarks of alcoholism are drinking too much and denying that you drink too much."

Myth Every alcoholic is unique.

Fact Although every alcoholic has some unique traits, the similarities among alcoholics usually are more pronounced than their differences.

Myth An alcoholic must want help before he or she will respond to it.

Fact Many alcoholics respond to coercive intervention—to save their relationships, their careers, or their driver license—even though they continue to deny their drinking problems.

Myth Only an alcoholic can understand and help another.

Fact Recovering alcoholics do have something unique to offer—a positive, encouraging example. But most of us have experienced and can empathize with the feelings associated with excessive drinking—anxiety, depression, loneliness, remorse.

Myth An alcoholic must "hit bottom" before he or she is ready to stop drinking.

Fact Alcoholics do not have to lose all before they are motivated to stop. People vary markedly in what induces them to change their behavior. For some, the first blackout or alcohol-related automobile accident fosters abstinence.

Myth The first step in the treatment of alcoholism is hospitalization.

Fact Most alcoholics can be treated on an outpatient basis. Those with medical complications such as delirium tremens or seizures may require hospital care.

Myth There is only one kind of effective treatment for alcoholism.

Fact Different treatments work for different people. Shopping is often required. Male alcoholics are more likely to respond to group therapy. Women often do better with individual or family therapy.

angered or given to crying. Drinkers who take very high doses risk pronounced depression of the **central nervous system**, with **stupor**, unconsciousness, even death.

Shakespeare accurately described the effects of alcohol on sexual performance. He said (in *Macbeth*) that "it stirs up desire, but it takes away the performance." Small doses may improve sexual performance for individuals who are especially anxious or self-conscious, but higher doses usually make it worse. Excessive alcohol use on either an acute or chronic basis can result in reduced erection response and reduced vaginal lubrication.

Alcohol causes blood vessels near the skin to dilate, and drinkers often feel warm; their skin flushes, and they may sweat more. Flushing and sweating contribute to loss of heat, and so the internal body temperature falls. High doses of alcohol may impair the body's ability to regulate temperature, causing it to drop sharply, especially if the surrounding temperature is low. Drinking alcoholic beverages to keep warm in cold weather does not work, and it can even be dangerous.

Alcohol, particularly in large amounts, definitely changes sleep patterns. Alcohol may facilitate falling asleep more quickly, but the sleep is often light, punctuated with awakenings, and unrefreshing. Even after the habitual drinker stops drinking, his or her sleep may be altered for weeks or months. Users of alcohol frequently awaken

Table 10-1 Drinking and Blood Alcohol Concentrations

Alcoholic Beverage Consumed in One Hour	Blood Alcohol Concentrations (mg/100 ml)					
	100 lb.		150 lb.		200 lb.	
	Female	Male	Female	Male	Female	Male
One can or bottle of beer (12 ounces of 5% beer) *or* One glass of wine (5 ounces of 12% table wine) *or* One cocktail or mixed drink (1½-ounce jigger or shot of 80-proof spirit)	0.05	0.04	0.03	0.027	0.024	0.020
Two cans/bottles of beer *or* Two glasses of wine *or* Two cocktails/mixed drinks	0.10	0.08	0.06	0.05	0.05	0.04
Four cans/bottles of beer *or* Four glasses of wine *or* Four cocktails/mixed drinks	0.20	0.16	0.12	0.10	0.09	0.08

SOURCE: Modified from California Department of Motor Vehicles, 1986.

with a "hangover"—headache, nausea, stomach distress, and generalized discomfort.

The Metabolism of Alcohol

Alcohol is absorbed into the bloodstream from the stomach and small intestine. How long absorption from the stomach takes depends on the amount, type, and proof of the beverage, the time taken to drink it, and whether or not there is food in the stomach. For example, a glass of champagne drunk quickly on an empty stomach will be absorbed at a more rapid rate (and could have greater immediate effects) than a larger amount of sherry sipped slowly after a large meal. Food in the stomach slows the absorption process by acting as a barrier between the alcohol and the stomach wall. Alcohol not absorbed in the stomach moves with any other undigested stomach contents into the small intestine. Here, absorption is rapid and complete because the walls of the small intestine have a large surface area and are highly permeable to alcohol. Neither the **blood alcohol concentration (BAC)** nor the presence of food affects absorption from the small intestine. Usually all alcohol is absorbed before it has the chance to reach the colon.

After alcohol is absorbed through the wall of the stomach or small intestine, it is distributed via the blood throughout the tissues of the body. In general, less alcohol becomes concentrated in fatty tissues. Since women usually have a higher percentage of fat at any given body weight than men do, women will have a higher BAC with the same amount of alcohol than will a man of the same weight (see Table 10-1). As the blood circulates through the liver, a certain amount of the alcohol passes into the liver cells, where it is transformed into energy and other products. The rate of this metabolic process stays about the same in each individual. A person who weighs 150 pounds and has normal liver function **metabolizes** on the average about 0.3 ounce of alcohol per hour.

About 2 to 10 percent of alcohol is not metabolized in the liver, but is excreted unchanged, mostly via the lungs and kidneys. This is the basis of breath and urine analyses for alcohol levels and the reason for the telltale smell of alcohol on a user's breath.

If an individual drinks slightly less alcohol each hour than the amount he or she can metabolize in an hour—about half a bottle of beer or half of an ordinary-size

Blood alcohol concentration (BAC) The amount of alcohol in the blood in terms of weight per unit volume. Also referred to as blood alcohol level (BAL).

Metabolize To chemically transform food and other substances in the body into energy and wastes.

Dose-response relationship The relationship between the amount of a drug taken and the intensity or type of drug effect.

Sedate To calm by the use of a drug that quiets the activity of the nerves.

drink—the BAC remains low. People can drink large amounts of alcohol this way over long periods of time without becoming noticeably intoxicated.

If this same individual drinks just a little bit more than he or she can metabolize, his or her BAC will steadily increase, and he or she will become more and more drunk (see Table 10-2). Despite popular myths, there is no way that people can significantly speed up their metabolism of alcohol. The rate of alcohol metabolism is the same whether the person is asleep or awake.

We do not know exactly how alcohol acts to influence individual behavior, but we can measure its effects according to relationships and factors that apply to most drugs. One important factor in the action of alcohol is the **dose-response relationship.** The influence of alcohol on behavior is likely to depend on how much the person takes in. The concentration of alcohol in the blood (BAC) is a major determinant of drug effects. Alcohol at low concentrations makes people feel relaxed, jovial, and euphoric, but at higher concentrations people are much more likely to feel angry, **sedated,** or sleepy. Subjects in experiments have been able to do simple motor tasks at low dose levels of alcohol better than when sober. They do worse in the same tasks when they have had moderate higher doses. Very high BACs can cause stupor and sometimes death.

The effects of alcohol are first recognized at BACs of about 0.03 to 0.05 percent. These effects may include light-headedness, relaxation, and release of inhibitions. When the BAC reaches 0.1 percent, a major reduction in most sensory and motor functioning occurs. At 0.2 percent, the drinker is totally unable to function, either physically or psychologically. Usually coma accompanies a BAC of 0.35 percent, and any higher level can kill a person. Figure 10-1 shows the results of a study of the relationship between drinking and driving. How much a person drinks (the dose) has an effect on how he or she drives (the response).

The estimated number of drinks is shown on the bottom axis of Figure 10-1. This representation is a rough guide in which one drink can be one cocktail, a 5-ounce glass of table wine, or one bottle of beer. The drinker is assumed to be a man of average weight (150 pounds), and the drinking takes place in one hour. It takes more drinks to achieve a given BAC if the person weighs more, if he or she has eaten recently, or if the drinking is done

Exploring Your Emotions

One of your friends often gets argumentative when he drinks. Lately, he seems to be getting even more angry while drinking, almost to the verge of hitting his girlfriend. Would you talk to him? What would you say?

Table 10-2 Physiological Effects of Alcohol

Blood Alcohol Concentrations (Percent)	Common Behavioral Effects	Hours Required for Alcohol to Be Metabolized
0.00–0.05	Slight change in feelings—usually relaxation and euphoria. Decreased alertness.	2–3
0.05–0.10	Emotional lability with exaggerated feelings and behavior. Reduced social inhibitions. Impairment of reaction time and fine motor coordination. Increasingly impaired during driving. Legally drunk at 0.08 in Utah and 0.10 in many other states.	4–6
0.10–0.15	Unsteadiness in standing and walking. Loss of peripheral vision. Driving is extremely dangerous. Legally drunk at 0.15 in all states.	6–10
0.15–0.30	Staggering gait. Slurred speech. Pain and other sensory perceptions greatly impaired.	10–24
More than 0.30	Stupor or unconsciousness. Anesthesia. Death possible at 0.35 and above.	More than 24

SOURCE: Modified from U.S. Department of Health and Human Services, 1986.

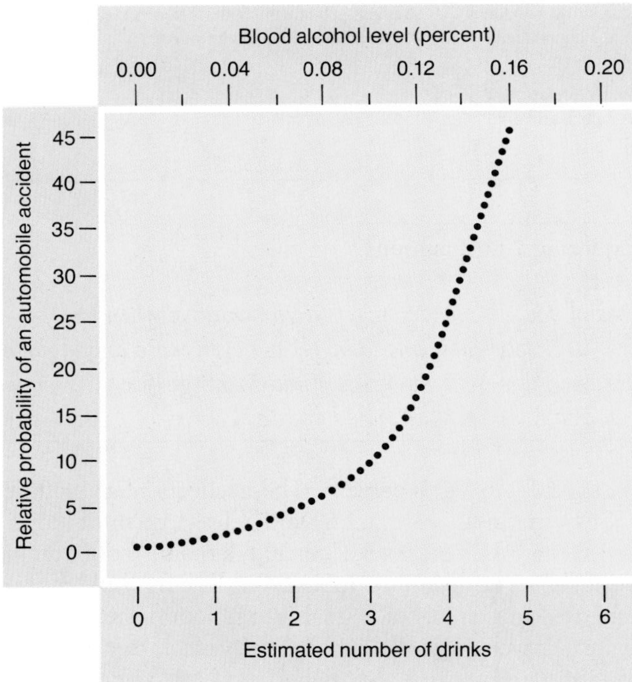

Figure 10-1 The dose-response relationship of alcohol levels and automobile accidents.

more slowly. The vertical axis represents how likely the drinker is to have an automobile accident compared to a sober driver. In other words, a man driving with a BAC of 0.10 (the legal limit in most states) is about ten times more likely to be involved in an accident than someone with no alcohol in his or her blood. Clearly, low doses of alcohol do not greatly increase risk, but as the dose increases, the risk of an automobile accident increases at a spectacular rate.

Exploring Your Emotions

Last Saturday you and three friends spent the evening drinking and dancing. When you drove home, you knew that alcohol was affecting your driving, but somehow you made it back without incident. The next day you don't remember precisely where you parked the car. In the morning paper you read of a drunk driver who lost control of his car, careened through a guard rail, and killed a pedestrian. You realize that accident could have been caused by you. How do you feel about the incident reported in the newspaper? How would you feel if the driver had been you?

Health Risks

Alcohol use has been linked to certain cancers of the upper digestive and respiratory tracts. It is difficult to get a clear picture of the relationship, however, because most heavy drinkers also smoke cigarettes, a practice that definitely increases the risk of several types of cancer. Alcohol may be the main factor in certain cancers. It may also increase the risk already present from tobacco use.

Recent studies of animals and humans indicate that alcohol ingested during pregnancy can harm the fetus. Women who drink, especially in excessive amounts, are at increased risk of giving birth to children who have a collection of birth defects known as the **fetal alcohol syndrome.** These children are small at birth, are likely to have heart defects, and often have abnormal anatomical features, including small, wide-set eyes. Even with the best of care, their physical and mental growth rate is slower during childhood than normal. In adolescence they sometimes catch up with their age mates in terms of physical size but not usually in mental abilities. Most remain mentally retarded, with IQs in the 40 to 80 range. Although researchers initially thought that fetal alcohol syndrome was caused by poor nutrition associated with the alcoholism of the mother, subsequent research indicates that it results directly from excessive alcohol intake. We should remember that alcohol is very soluble in water and blood is primarily water. Thus, any alcohol ingested rapidly enters the mother's blood and quickly crosses the placenta into the circulation of the fetus; when the mother has a blood alcohol concentration of 0.03, so does her fetus. There is no precise blood alcohol threshold level above which damage occurs and below which there is no danger. Instead the frequency and severity of defects progressively increase as the amount of drinking increases. As is the case with other drugs, the fetus seems especially vulnerable to alcohol during the first trimester of pregnancy. The safest course of action is abstinence.

Effects of Chronic Alcohol Use

Alcohol even in relatively small amounts can alter liver function. With continued use of alcohol, liver cells are damaged and then progressively destroyed. The destroyed cells are often replaced by fibrous scar tissue, a condition known as **cirrhosis of the liver.** As cirrhosis develops, the individual may progressively lose his or her capacity to tolerate alcohol, because there are fewer remaining liver cells to metabolize whatever alcohol is in the bloodstream. Alcohol can also irritate and inflame the pancreas, causing nausea, vomiting, abnormal digestion, and severe pains

Fetal alcohol syndrome Birth defects caused by excessive alcohol consumption by the mother.

Cirrhosis A disease of the liver caused by excessive and chronic drinking. Contrary to earlier medical belief, cirrhosis occurs even when nutrition is adequate.

Cardiac myopathy Weakening of the heart muscle through disease.

High-density lipoprotein (HDL) Waxy substance in the blood thought to protect against heart disease.

Alcohol abuse The use of alcohol to a degree that causes physical damage, impairs functioning, or results in behavior harmful to others.

Alcohol dependence Either pathological use of alcohol or impairment in functioning due to alcohol and tolerance or withdrawal; alcoholism.

Alcoholism Chronic psychological and nutritional disorder from excessive and compulsive drinking; alcohol dependence.

Exploring Your Emotions

Two close friends of yours who have been married for several years tell you they plan on starting a family. You know that the woman has several drinks every day, although you don't consider her an alcoholic. You also know that babies of mothers who drink are more likely to have birth deformities. What do you think about their plans? Should you tell them about fetal alcohol syndrome? Would you?

---

in the abdomen. It may harm the kidneys over longer periods of time, but such harm does not happen often.

Alcohol can affect the cardiovascular system. In many people, more than one or two drinks will elevate blood pressure, making strokes and heart attacks more likely. Some alcoholics show weakening of the heart muscle, a condition known as **cardiac myopathy.** Cardiac myopathy can be caused by the direct toxic effects of alcohol, or indirectly by the malnutrition and vitamin deficiencies that many alcoholics experience from their poor diets and gastrointestinal disturbances. Recent studies indicate that moderate amounts of alcohol increase blood levels of certain **high-density lipoproteins (HDLs).** However, the specific type of HDL that is increased with alcohol is not the kind that is thought to offer some protection against heart attacks. In summary, although the relationships between alcohol and cardiovascular disease are multiple and complex, the net result is clear—excessive drinking increases the risk of disease. These health risks progressively increase as the amount of excessive drinking increases.

Medical Uses of Alcohol

The value traditionally placed on alcohol "for medical purposes" is based more on imagination than fact. Alcohol sponges are commonly used to reduce fever because alcohol cools the skin by evaporation. In concentrations of 70 percent by weight, alcohol kills bacteria. It is used as an astringent and skin cleanser in treating skin disorders. Contrary to a popular myth, however, alcohol is not a good antiseptic for open wounds. It injures exposed tissues and may form a coagulant that protects rather than destroys bacteria. People who associate alcohol with dining pleasure may feel hungrier and digest their food better if they take a small amount of alcohol—a bottle of beer, a glass of wine—with their meals. Drinking alcohol has been thought by some to be useful in treating angina pectoris, a painful disorder in which the heart is unable to get enough oxygen. This remedy is doubtful. If the sufferer feels better, it is probably because he or she has been sedated rather than because his or her circulation is better.

Relationships between alcohol use and mortality rates are complex. As one would predict, both abstainers and moderate drinkers live longer than heavy drinkers. More surprisingly, some recent studies also suggest that people who regularly drink moderate amounts of alcohol—fewer than three drinks per day—live longer than those who abstain completely. However, these findings are controversial and may reflect unrepresentative sampling techniques. Claims that small amounts of alcohol are good for one's health express personal belief, not established scientific fact.

Alcohol Abuse and Alcoholism

Recent definitions make a distinction between alcohol abuse and alcohol dependence, or alcoholism. According to the third edition of the *Diagnostic and Statistical Manual of Mental Disorders* (1980) of the American Psychiatric Association, "The essential feature of **alcohol abuse** is a pattern of pathological use for at least a month that causes impairment in social or occupational functioning. The essential features of **alcohol dependence,** which is also called **alcoholism,** are either a pattern of pathological alcohol use or impairment in social or occupational functioning due to alcohol, and either tolerance or withdrawal."

Other authorities use different definitions to describe problems associated with drinking. The important point is that one does not have to be an alcoholic to have problems with alcohol. The person who only drinks once a month, perhaps on payday or after an exam, but then drives while intoxicated is an alcohol abuser.

People of all social and economic classes use alcohol excessively, not just people who are considered to be skid

Early Indications of Alcohol Abuse

1. Drinking alone or secretively.
2. Using alcohol deliberately and repeatedly to perform or get through difficult situations.
3. Feeling uncomfortable on certain occasions when alcohol is not available.
4. Escalating alcohol consumption beyond an already established drinking pattern.
5. Consuming alcohol heavily in risky situations; for example, before driving.
6. Getting "drunk" regularly or more frequently than in the past.
7. Drinking in the morning or at other unusual times.

row bums. Skid row bums account for only a small percentage of the total alcoholic population and usually represent the final stage of a drinking career that began years before. Among white American men, excessive drinking usually begins in the teens or twenties and gradually progresses through the thirties until the person is clearly identified as alcoholic by the time he is in his late thirties or early forties. It is relatively uncommon for alcoholism to begin in men after the age of 45 unless there are concomitant psychiatric problems such as depression. There are different patterns of alcohol abuse. Here are four common patterns:

1. *Regular daily intake of large amounts.* This continuous pattern is the most common adult pattern of excessive consumption in most countries.
2. *Regular heavy drinking limited to weekends.* This continuous pattern is commonly followed by teenagers.
3. *Long periods of sobriety interspersed with binges of daily heavy drinking lasting for weeks or months.* This episodic or "bender" pattern is common in the United States but quite uncommon in France, although the per capita consumption of alcohol is higher in France.
4. *Heavy drinking limited to periods of stress.* This "reactive" pattern is associated with periods of anxiety or depression; for example, examination or other performance fears, interpersonal difficulties, school or work pressures.

The "natural history" of alcoholism in women differs from that of men. Women tend to become alcoholic at a later age and with fewer years of heavy drinking. It is not unusual for women in their forties or fifties to become alcoholic after years of controlled drinking, whereas this pattern occurs infrequently in men. Women alcoholics also develop cirrhosis and other medical complications somewhat more often than men.

There are notable differences in patterns of alcoholic drinking among various racial and ethnic groups. For example, urban black males commonly start excessive drinking at a younger age than do urban white males, develop serious medical and neurological illnesses at an earlier age, and have a higher rate of alcoholism-related suicides. Excessive drinking among Native American Indians varies from tribe to tribe and does not follow a consistent pattern. There is a very low rate of alcoholism in Asia, and a high rate among the Irish.

Estimating the prevalence of alcoholism is complicated by disagreement about definition and other methodological problems. Although the figure of 9 or 10 million American alcoholics has often been cited, it is not based on scientific studies. More systematic studies of smaller geographic areas such as counties or states suggest that about 3 percent of all men are alcoholic and perhaps 0.1 to 1 percent of all women. It is somewhat easier to determine the quantity of drinking done by a given population. Studies show that about 20 percent of American men are heavy drinkers, meaning they drink daily and drink six or more drinks several times a month.

We do not know exactly what causes alcoholism. Probably a variety of factors are involved, all of which vary from individual to individual. Recent reliable studies have compared individuals who were adopted when they were young and individuals who lived with their biological parents. These studies showed that people are more likely to be alcoholics if their biological parents are alcoholics. Alcoholism in adopted parents, however, does not make individuals either more or less likely to become alcoholics. In other words, there apparently is a genetic contribution to susceptibility to alcoholism. Not all children of alcoholics become alcoholics, however, and it is clear that many other factors are involved. Personality disorders, being subjected as a child to destructive child-rearing practices, and imitating parents' and other important people's abuse of alcohol may all play a part. People who begin drinking excessively during their teenage years are especially prone to alcoholism later in life. Common psychological features of individuals who excessively use alcohol are denial ("I don't have a problem") and rationalization ("I drink because I need to socialize with my customers.")

Certain social factors have been linked with alcoholism. These include urbanization, disappearance of the extended family, and general loosening of kinship ties,

Alcohol-related Social Problems in the United States

1. Alcohol-precipitated cirrhosis is the sixth leading cause of death in the United States.

2. Alcohol abusers shorten their life spans by ten to twelve years.

3. One-half of all traffic fatalities are associated with alcohol use.

4. One-third of all homocides are associated with alcohol use.

5. One-third to one-half of all fatal accidents (other than traffic) are associated with alcohol use.

6. One-third to one-half of all crimes committed are associated with alcohol use.

7. One-third of all arrests are for public intoxication.

8. Alcohol abuse and alcoholism drain the economy of an estimated $15 billion per year. Of this total, $10 billion is attributable to lost work time; $2 billion is spent for health and welfare services provided to alcoholics and their families; and property damage, medical expenses, and other overhead costs account for another $3 billion.

9. One person in every five is closely related to someone who suffers from alcohol abuse.

Children of Alcoholics

One out of eight Americans—or about 30 million people—grow up in alcoholic households, according to the Children of Alcoholics Foundation. For these children and countless others like them, home is often a battlefield, and growing up a struggle to cope with constant stress and embarrassment. It's a time when needs are often ignored, and family life centers around the drinking parent.

The alcoholic household leaves emotional scars that can last a lifetime. The figures alone—for family violence, incest, and predisposition to self-abusive behavior—are staggering:

- 55 percent of all family violence occurs in alcoholic homes.
- Incest is twice as likely to be inflicted on daughters of alcoholics as on their peers.
- Children of alcoholics are three to four times more likely to become alcoholic than the general population;
- 50 percent of children of alcoholics marry an alcoholic; 70 percent develop a pattern of compulsive behavior as an adult, including alcoholism, drug abuse, and overeating.

And no statistic can measure the psychological pain and turmoil that children of alcoholics grow up with and often carry into adulthood.

Until recently, children of alcoholics were considered no different from other children with family difficulties and were largely ignored by treatment programs that tended to focus on the alcoholic parent. But all that is changing.

Today, professionals recognize the special problems and needs of children of alcoholics, and family-oriented therapy has become a major focus of alcoholism rehabilitation. And treating the problem—rebuilding shattered self-esteem and relearning how to talk and trust and love—must begin with identifying the problem.

What to Do if You're the Child of an Alcoholic . . .

Step 1. The first thing to do is to realize that you are not alone. Thousands of people across the country have been through the same problem, have felt the same fears, and have dreamed the same dreams that you have for a happy family life where drinking is not a problem. These people have been where you are and know what you're feeling, and they're on your side.

Step 2. The second thing to do about the problem is to tell someone about it. Maybe you have an interested teacher or a special friend or a favorite aunt or uncle. Talk with them about the problem and don't hold back. Even though it might seem easier and safer and less painful just to keep things a secret, the part that can really hurt you over the long term is keeping your pain and your problems all locked up inside you. Remember that other people understand and they can help.

Step 3. The third thing to do if you think you're the child of an alcoholic is to realize that it's not your fault. Your parents may love you, but your parents have a problem. The best way you can help them is to help yourself. Call one of the local Al-Anon or AlaTeen agencies listed in the phone book or call or write the Children of Alcoholics Foundation, 540 Madison Avenue, New York, NY 10022, (212) 980-5394.

SOURCE: Do It Now Foundation, 2050 East University Drive, Phoenix, AZ 85034.

Tolerance Lower sensitivity to a drug so that a given dose no longer exerts the usual effect and larger doses are needed.

Withdrawal symptoms Unpleasant physical and mental sensations experienced when abstaining from a drug to which one is addicted.

DTs (delirium tremens) A state of confusion brought on by reduction of alcohol intake in a person addicted to alcohol. Other symptoms are sweating, trembling, anxiety, and hallucinations.

Hallucinations False perceptions that do not correspond to external reality. A person who hears voices that are not there or who sees visions is having hallucinations.

Paranoia A mental disorder characterized by false beliefs that one is being persecuted, often beliefs of a grandiose and logically systematic nature. There are no hallucinations, and intelligence is not impaired.

---

increased mobility, and changing religious and philosophical values.

Complications of Alcoholism The consequences of alcoholism are well known. People definitely develop a **tolerance** to alcohol after repeated use. They require greater and greater amounts to produce the same psychological effect. Tolerance, however, develops at different rates to different effects of alcohol. For example, alcohol-induced depression of the respiratory system develops slowly and only to a small extent. Thus alcoholics are only slightly less susceptible to lethal respiratory depression from overdose than are moderate users. The same is true for users of barbiturates and most other sedating drugs.

When people continue to abuse alcohol for long periods of time, their tolerance may begin to decrease. Some chronic alcoholics have very little tolerance for alcohol, in part because their livers are so damaged that they no longer have adequate amounts of the enzymes necessary to metabolize alcohol.

When alcoholics stop drinking or cut their intake way down, they will have **withdrawal symptoms.** These can vary from merely unpleasant feelings to serious, even life-threatening, disorders. The jitters, or "shakes," are the most common withdrawal symptom and may last as long as two weeks. Seizures are less common, but they are more serious. Still less common is the severe withdrawal reaction known as the **DTs (delirium tremens)**, a dramatic state characterized by disorientation, confusion, and vivid **hallucinations**, often of vermin and small animals.

Since alcohol is water soluble and distributed throughout most of the body, it can harm many different organs and tissues. Damage to the liver in the form of cirrhosis is just one well-known example. Asthma, gout, diabetes, and recurrent infections are more common in heavy drinkers than in people who drink moderately or not at all. Inflammations of the stomach, intestines, kidneys, bronchi, and peripheral nerves also occur more frequently in alcohol abusers. Other medical and psychiatric complications are associated with excessive alcohol use. Some of these alcohol-related medical problems are made worse by nutritional deficiencies that often accompany alcohol abuse. Disorders of the liver, stomach, and intestine are especially common, as are diseases of the nervous system, but all vary among users. One individual may primarily have defects of the central nervous system, serious damage to the memory, and no liver or gastrointestinal damage. Another individual, with a similar drinking and nutrition history, may have advanced liver disease and no memory defects.

An alcoholic's medical and psychiatric problems often respond rapidly to hospitalization, tranquilizers, and the elimination of alcohol from the diet. These problems are likely to return, however, if the person starts drinking again. Some people have what is called **paranoid** personalities. If they use alcohol excessively, they may suffer delusions, jealousy, suspicion, and mistrust—so-called alcoholic paranoia.

Alcohol use causes more serious social problems than all other forms of drug abuse combined. The 1983 statistics of the National Council on Alcoholism concluded that 10 million Americans were alcoholic; for each of these, another three to four people were directly affected. In 1978, nearly one out of five people in a Gallup poll indicated that alcohol caused trouble in their family. An estimated 3.3 million 14- to 17-year-olds are showing signs of potential alcohol dependency. These numbers are far greater than those associated with cocaine, heroin, or marijuana use. Especially in young people, overdependence on alcohol not only increases chances of subsequent health problems, but also can stunt personality development.

Treatment It is important to realize that some alcoholics recover without professional help. It is unknown how often this occurs, but perhaps as many as 25 percent of alcoholics "spontaneously" stop drinking or reduce their drinking to the point where problems do not occur. In a 1981 study of "problem drinkers," 9 percent of American adults were currently experiencing drinking problems. Another 9 percent had had drinking problems in the past but no longer did. One of the great debates in the field is whether "true" alcoholics can become controlled or social drinkers. Studies indicate this may occur, but as the exception rather than the rule.

In any event, the majority of alcoholics do not stop their chronic excessive use of alcohol on their own. For these people, treatment is difficult. However, although we do not have satisfactory ways to treat all people who have alcohol problems, cautious optimism has replaced the widely held view of "nothing can be done" that prevailed a few years ago.

Many different kinds of treatment programs exist. Some,

such as Alcoholics Anonymous, emphasize group and "buddy" support as well as personal testimonies. By contrast, the Raleigh Hills system includes the use of aversion therapy in which the subject is conditioned to associate drinking alcohol with negative consequences such as medically produced nausea. The best treatment programs often involve a combination of a variety of techniques, such as Alcoholics Anonymous, psychotherapy (individual, group, and especially family or couple), and chemical therapies. None of these has been successful for all patients. As with the treatment of other drug dependencies, one major problem in treating alcoholics is predicting ahead of time which treatment will be most useful for a particular individual. Another major treatment problem has to do with long-term effectiveness. For example, one chemical treatment involves the use of disulfiram (trade name, Antabuse). Disulfiram causes patients to become violently ill whenever they drink. What usually happens is that after taking the drug for a while, the patient declares him- or herself to be "cured" and decides that he or she no longer needs the drug. The effect of the drug does not wear off for about four days, so the patient is able to avoid impulse drinking and may even gain enough momentum to stay "cured"—for a time. After weeks or perhaps months of not taking the drug, many patients start drinking again.

Prescribing chemical substitutes such as diazepam (Valium) or chlordiazepoxide (Librium) for alcohol is a controversial treatment. Proponents argue that at least the more toxic alcohol is being replaced by a less toxic drug and thus the health hazard is reduced. Others claim that one drug dependency is merely being exchanged for another and many of the behavioral problems associated with the chemical abuse are unchanged. Like many controversies in the field of alcoholism and drug abuse, this one is unlikely to be resolved, because value judgments are involved.

Exploring Your Emotions

You have just spent the evening enjoying a party you held at your home. In the early morning you are saying good-night to a group that is leaving. One person in the group is staggering drunk. You realize that he should not drive home. You suggest he leave his car and ride home with someone else. He shakes off your suggestion and weaves out to his car. How do you feel about this risk? If you feel responsible, what should you do? What would *you do?*

The Responsible Use of Alcohol

The responsible use of alcohol means drinking in such a way as to keep your blood alcohol level low so that your behavior is always under your control. Here are some tips.

1. *Drink slowly.* Learn to sip your drinks rather than gulp them. It helps to develop the habit of deliberately tasting and smelling the nuances of alcoholic beverages so that you can decide their similarities and differences. Learn to compare and contrast the different kinds of wines and beers.
2. *Space your drinks.* Learn to drink nonalcoholic drinks at parties—juices or tonic water without the alcohol, for example—or intersperse these with alcoholic drinks. Learn to refuse a round: "I've had enough for right now." Parties are easier for some people if they hold a glass of anything nonalcoholic that has ice and a twist of lime floating in it so that it looks as if they were drinking alcohol. Other people are comfortable in openly requesting "mocktails"—drinks like "virgin screwdrivers" that have all the ingredients of the cocktail except the alcoholic beverage. Such requests provide a healthy model for others.
3. *Eat before and while drinking.* Avoid drinking on an empty stomach. Food in your stomach will not prevent the alcohol from eventually being absorbed, but it will slow down the rate somewhat, and thus the peak blood alcohol level will usually be lower.
4. *Know your limits and your drinks.* Learn how different blood alcohol concentrations affect you. In a safe setting such as your home, with your parents or roommate, see how a set amount—say, two drinks an hour—affects you. A good test is walking heel to toe in a straight line with your eyes closed or standing with your feet crossed and trying to touch your finger to your nose with your eyes closed. However, be aware that in different settings your performance, and espe-

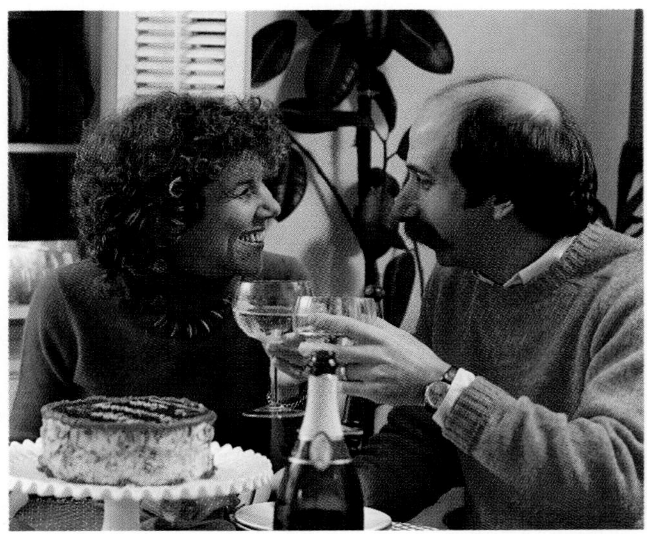

Richard Hutchings

The Designated Driver

What is a "designated driver?" The principle is simple: one individual refrains from drinking alcoholic beverages to assure the safe transportation home of the remaining guests. At the next party, another person volunteers and the responsibility is rotated. In Sweden and the United Kingdom, where the practice originated, designated drivers place their car keys in their empty beverage glasses so they are not served.

Social drinkers, as well as alcoholics, are a menace behind the wheel. Young drivers between the ages of 16 and 24 are involved in more than one-third of all alcohol-related traffic accidents. These "social drinkers" are unable to drive responsibly because judgment is impaired, reaction time is slowed, and coordination is reduced. No one can drive skillfully and safely after consuming alcoholic beverages.

How Can You Identify an Impaired Driver?

By learning to spot the following warning signs of an impaired driver, the chances of becoming involved in an alcohol-related motor vehicle accident are reduced:

- Unusually wide turns
- Straddling the center line or lane marker
- Driving with one's head out of the window or with the window down in cold weather
- Nearly striking an object or another vehicle
- Weaving or swerving
- Driving on other than the designated roadway
- Stopping with no apparent cause
- Following too closely
- Responding slowly to traffic signals
- Abrupt or illegal turns
- Rapid acceleration or deceleration
- Driving with headlights off at night

What Should You Do if You See an Impaired Driver?

- Maintain a safe following distance if the driver is ahead of you. Do not try to pass, because he or she may swerve into your vehicle.
- Turn right at the nearest intersection if the driver is behind you. Let him or her pass and then return to your route.
- Move to the shoulder and stop if the driver is approaching your vehicle. Avoid a head-on collision by sounding your horn or flashing your lights.
- Slow down and expect the unexpected when approaching an intersection.
- Fasten your safety belt. Place children in approved safety seats and keep all doors locked.
- Report suspected impaired drivers to the nearest law enforcement agency by phone or citizen's band radio. Give a description of the vehicle, license number, location, and direction the vehicle is headed.

If you are the "designated driver," get your passengers home safely. They will respect your act of caring.

Alcohol-related traffic accidents claim approximately 25,000 American lives, seriously injure 300,000 others and cost our society more than $10 billion annually. The National Safety Council asks you to help reduce these figures by adopting the "designated driver" concept and urging others to use it to avoid drinking and driving situations.

SOURCE: The designated driver: being a friend, 1986 (December), *Healthline*.

cially your ability to judge your behavior, may change. At a given blood alcohol concentration, you will perform less well when surrounded by activity and boisterous companions than you will in a quiet test setting with just one or two other people. This impairment results partially because alcohol reduces your ability to perform when your brain is bombarded by multiple stimuli. It is useful to discover the rate at which you can drink without increasing your BAC. Be able to calculate the approximate amount a given drink will increase your BAC.

5. *Determine your reasons for drinking.* How do they compare with those given by most college students (see Box)? In what other ways can you learn to fulfill your underlying needs? It is often helpful to keep a diary of your drinking. Include in the diary not only times, settings, and amounts, but what you were feeling and thinking before you started drinking.
6. *Cultivate and model responsible attitudes toward alcohol.* Our society teaches us attitudes toward drinking that increase the chances for alcohol-related problems, if not for ourselves, for others. Many of us have difficulty

Ten Most Common Reasons Given by College Students for Drinking Alcohol

1. "Increases my feelings of sociability."
2. "Relieves anxiety or tension."
3. "Makes me feel elated or euphoric."
4. "Makes me less inhibited in thinking, saying, or doing certain things."
5. "Enables me to go along with my friends."
6. "Enables me to experience a different state of consciousness."
7. "Makes me less inhibited sexually."
8. "Enables me to stop worrying."
9. "Alleviates depression."
10. "Makes me less self-conscious."

Mocktails

Healthier eating habits, an aging population, alcohol awareness, and crackdowns on drunk driving have greatly increased the market for nonalcoholic beverages. A recent Louis Harris poll for *Business Week* magazine found that 45 percent of those surveyed were consuming less alcohol than they did five years ago. Many beverage retailers are encouraging the use of nonalcoholic or low-alcoholic beverages as well as responsible drinking, designated driver programs, and the like.

Sparkling water sales have increased 600 percent in the last ten years, and sales of other "old-time" nonalcoholic drinks have been rising. Cider is being sold as sparkling cider. Ginger ale is being blended with orange juice and garnished with fresh flowers to make gingemosa. And "virgin" drinks (virgin mary, coherent colada, and mockarita) are becoming more popular.

Beverage manufacturers have been working at a furious pace to develop "mocktails" and mock beers that taste like their alcoholic counterparts. Seagram's spent over five years and $30 million to develop St. Regis, the first dealcoholized wine to be mass marketed in the United States. A nonalcoholic, low-calorie wine cooler was introduced to the Florida beverage market by Paradise Fruit Company. The alcohol was removed from a grape wine, and the residue was combined with fruit juices, NutraSweet, water, and carbonation to create an alcohol-free wine cooler with only 18 calories per 12-ounce bottle. More than thirty nonalcoholic versions of imported and domestic beers, labeled as "nonalcoholic malt beverages," are currently available.

In Hotels, Etc. . .

The hospitality industry is also involved. Holiday Inn has developed a mocktail program that has enjoyed an excellent response. Red Lobster has introduced "thirst-quencher nonalcoholic beverages" to its menu. And Chi Chi's cleverly markets margaritas and coladas as "nada" beverages. The trend is apparent: the U.S. consumer increasingly wants healthier beverages with fresh ingredients, attractive appearance, more flavor, and less or no alcohol.

At College. . .

Our experience at Purdue University makes it clear that the mocktail market for young adults is quite large. Last year, 102 participants filled out questionnaires while dining in the John Purdue Room, a student laboratory that offers formal dining. The survey found that 34 percent preferred mocktails over cocktails, but 60 percent would rather dine in a restaurant that offers both nonalcoholic and alcoholic drinks. And 81 percent said the price of a drink does not affect their choice between nonalcoholic and alcoholic drinks. The John Purdue Room began offering mocktails during the summer of 1985. According to its director, Jeffrey Graves, "the response has been excellent—80 to 90 percent of the guests enjoy a mocktail."

These figures should really not be surprising, because many peo-

(continued on next page)

Mocktails (*continued*)

ple drink in the presence of others for "social" reasons rather than a desire to ingest alcohol. Drinks provide something to do with one's hands, and a way to look busy when conversation lapses.

In a Health Care Setting. . .

The health care industry may also be affected by the increased attention to nonalcoholic beverages. Nonalcoholic specialty beverages have been available for patients for many years. For example, eggnogs and protein drinks provide nutrition for the gastrointestinally disabled. However, most such drinks have been bland, unpalatable, and unattractive. This need not be the case *in any food service setting* if imagination is used. Improvements can range from nutritious milkshakes for breakfast to sparkling nectar mocktails at afternoon social gatherings. Beverages can be made more appealing through creative use of glassware, garnishes, and service techniques.

Fruit and vegetable garnishes can add eye appeal and nutrients to any beverage. Garnishing ideas range from vegetable sticks and slices, to chunks of frozen fruit. Many ideas are available from ordinary cookbooks and pamphlets developed by major suppliers of the food service industry. LeGout's mocktail recipes use Equal (aspartame), nondairy creamer, and LeGout drink bases. Perrier suggests mocktail recipes for cooling drinks served the natural way. And V-8 Juice is a ready-to-serve mocktail enjoyed by today's light drinker. A 6-ounce portion has only 36 calories and is high in vitamins A and C.

The mocktail is not a new idea, but the expanding market for alternatives to alcoholic beverages *is* new. Party hosts, restaurateurs, bar owners, health professionals, and others involved in providing food or drink to others can capitalize on this trend by satisfying the growing number of people who want alcohol-free beverages.

Mock Beverages

Recipes

Chocolate Cinnamon Coffee (a LeGout mocktail)

Hot strong coffee	7 ounces
Nondairy creamer	1 ounce
Cinnamon powder	1/8 teaspoon
Unsweetened cocoa powder	1 teaspoon
Equal low-calorie sweetener	2 packets
Garnish:	
Cinnamon stick	1 stick
Whipped topping	1 dollop
Cinnamon powder	1 sprinkle

Directions: Combine all ingredients and stir well. Pour into a coffee mug, garnish, and serve.
Yield: One 8-ounce drink
Calories per serving: 54

Strawberry Squirt (from Perrier)

Fresh strawberries	6
Vanilla yogurt	1 cup
Chilled Perrier	6½ ounces

Directions: Blend berries and yogurt at high speed until smooth. Stir in chilled Perrier and garnish with a fresh strawberry and serve.

To make Strawberry Squirtsicles, pour the Strawberry Squirt drink into a 4-ounce paper cup. Insert a wooden stick in center and freeze. When frozen, peel off paper cup and eat as a frozen pop.
Yield: 2 servings.

Breakfast Shake (from Perrier)

Ripe bananas	2
Eggs	2
Papayas, peeled and seeded	2
Honey	2 tbsp.
Low-fat milk	1 cup
Chilled Perrier	6½ ounces
Nutmeg	Pinch

Directions: Place first five ingredients in blender and blend on high speed until smooth. Stir in Perrier until frothy and add nutmeg.
Yield: 2 servings.

New York Deli (from Campbell Soup, a prizewinning recipe by Marie Fattore of New York)

V-8 Juice	8 ounces
Dill pickle juice	1 tsp.
Coarse mustard	1 tsp.
Prepared horseradish	½ tsp.
Worcestershire sauce	Dash
Salt and pepper	To taste

Directions: Shake ingredients together and pour over crushed ice. Serve with a pickle spear.
Yield: 1 serving.

SOURCE: John R. Dienhart and G. Stewart Eidel, 1987 (January–February), Party drinks you can drive on, *Healthline*.

Students Against Driving Drunk (SADD)

Without question, drunk driving ranks today as one of the nation's most serious health and safety issues—accounting each year for an estimated 25,000 traffic fatalities, hundreds of thousands of injuries and billions of dollars in economic costs to society. Among no group is the problem more severe than teenagers and young adults.

Students Against Driving Drunk (SADD) was established in 1981 to improve young people's knowledge and attitudes about alcohol and drugs to help save their lives—and the lives of others. The program has three major components:

First, it provides a series of lesson plans to present the facts about drinking and driving, permitting students to make informed decisions.

Second, it mobilizes students to help one another through peer pressure to face up to the potential dangers of mixing driving with alcohol or drugs.

And third, it promotes a frank dialogue between teenagers and their parents through the SADD "Contract." Under this agreement both students and their parents pledge to contact each other should they ever find themselves in a potential DWI (driving while intoxicated) situation.

CONTRACT FOR LIFE

A Contract for Life
Between Parent and Teenager
The SADD Drinking-Driver Contract

Teenager I agree to call you for advice and/or transportation at any hour, from any place, if I am ever in a situation where I have been drinking or a friend or date who is driving me has been drinking.

Signature

Parent I agree to come and get you at any hour, any place, no questions asked and no argument at that time, or I will pay for a taxi to bring you home safely. I expect we would discuss this issue at a later time.

I agree to seek safe, sober transportation home if I am ever in a situation where I have had too much to drink or a friend who is driving me has had too much to drink.

Signature

Date

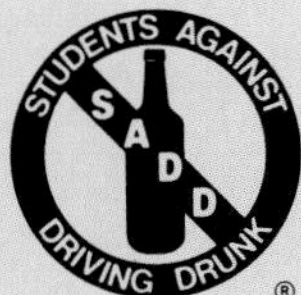

S.A.D.D. does not condone drinking by those below the legal drinking age. S.A.D.D. encourages all young people to obey the laws of their state, including laws relating to the legal drinking age.

Distributed by S.A.D.D., "Students Against Driving Drunk"

expressing disapproval to someone who has drunk too much. We are amused by the antics of the "funny" drunk. We tend to accept the alcohol industry's linking of drinking with virility or sexuality. And we treat abstainers as odd. These attitudes are not healthy.

7. *Learn to be a responsible host or hostess regarding alcohol.* In medieval England an important legal precedent, the dramskeeper's principle, was established. This principle put the responsibility for alcohol-related injuries or untoward results of the guest's drunken behavior on the innkeeper or tavern owner. Although the legal force of this principle has been muted over the centuries, it is a useful guide for our obligations to our guests. Acquire the habit of serving nonalcoholic beverages as well as alcohol and of not asking guests if you can get them another drink. Always serve food

along with alcohol. Be able to insist that a guest who had too much take a taxi, ride with someone else, or stay at your house rather than drive.

8. *Develop alternatives to alcohol.* There are many pleasant alternatives to drinking. For example, many people who have adopted programs of vigorous physical exercise—aerobic dancing, jogging, exercycling—find that their alcohol consumption correspondingly drops. Other people have learned to spend evenings and weekends without drinking by changing their usual routine and deliberately excluding alcohol—taking a walk before or after dinner instead of having drinks, for example.

Take Action

Your answers to the Exploring Your Emotions questions in this chapter and your placement level on the Wellness Ladder will, we hope, encourage you to begin a process of self-exploration and self-discovery that you will continue. Reflect on the entire chapter's content and ask yourself how each point relates to your own life. Then take action:

1. Attend an Alcoholics Anonymous meeting. What behavioral techniques are used to help people to stop drinking? How effective do you feel AA is?
2. Record or note advertisements for alcoholic beverages. What psychological techniques are used to sell the products? What are the hidden messages?
3. Drink a glass of wine at least one hour before dinner. Note both the physical effects and the behavioral effects. Do you feel warmer, cooler, dizzy, nauseated, excited, relaxed? Note the effects every 15 minutes for one hour.
4. List the positive behaviors that help you avoid alcohol entirely or keep your consumption to a minimum. Consider how you can strengthen your existing behavior. Also list the behaviors that block your achieving optimal health. Which ones can you change to improve your health?
5. Talk to your friends about alcohol. Ask about each other's drinking behavior. On what occasions does your drinking exceed moderate levels? When do you drive while under the influence? What can you do differently to avoid these situations? How can you influence each other toward more healthy drinking behavior?
6. Before leaving this chapter, review the Rate Yourself statements in this chapter. Have your feelings or values changed? Are you now better equipped to handle the complex and very human problems associated with alcohol consumption?

Selected References

Bean, Margaret. 1982 (April). Alcohol and adolescents. *Psychosomatics* 23(4):24–28.

Brown, Stephanie. 1985. *Treating the Alcoholic: A Developmental Model of Recovery*. New York: Wiley.

Dennison, D., T. Prevet, and M. Affleck. 1980. *Alcohol and Behavior: An Activated Education Approach*. St. Louis: Mosby.

Goodstadt, M. S., and A. Caleekal-John. 1984 (November). Alcohol education programs for university students: a review of their effectiveness. *International Journal of Addictions* 19(7):721–41.

Goodwin, Donald W. 1985 (February). Alcoholism and genetics. The sins of the father. *Archives of General Psychiatry* 42(2):171–74.

Kissin, Benjamin, and Henri Begleiter. 1983. *The Pathogenesis of Alcoholism: Biological Factors*. Vol. 7: *The Biology of Alcoholism*. New York: Plenum Press.

Kissin, Benjamin, and Henri Begleiter. 1983. *The Pathogenesis of Alcoholism: Psychosocial Factors*. Vol. 8: *The Biology of Alcoholism*. New York: Plenum Press.

Ludwig, A. M. 1985 (January). Cognitive processes associated with "spontaneous" recovery from alcoholism. *Journal of Studies on Alcoholism* 46(1):53–58.

Malfetti, J. L. 1985 (August). Public information and education sections of the Report of the Presidential Commission on Drunk Driving: A critique and a discussion of research implications. *Accident Analysis and Prevention* 17(4):347–53.

Mitchell, M. C. 1985 (July). Alcohol-induced impairment of central nervous system function: behavioral skills involved in driving. *Journal of Studies on Alcohol (Suppl)* 10:109–16.

Peele, S. 1986 (January). The implications and limitations of genetic models of alcoholism and other addictions. *Journal of Studies of Alcoholism* 47(1):63–73.

Russell, R. 1986. *What Should We Teach About Alcohol?* Piscataway, N.J.: Rutgers Center of Alcohol Studies.

Vogler, R. E., and W. R. Bartz. 1982. *The Better Way to Drink: The Alternative That Works*. New York: Simon & Schuster.

Recommended Readings

Goodwin, Donald. 1981. *Alcoholism: The Facts*. New York: Oxford University Press.
A scholarly, well-written book that critically reviews a great deal of research in alcoholism.

Jellinek, Elvin M. 1960. *The Disease Concept of Alcoholism*. New Haven, Conn.: Hillhouse Press.
A landmark book that helped make alcoholism a legitimate topic for scientific inquiry.

Kissin, Benjamin, and Henri Begleiter. 1976. *Social Aspects of Alcoholism*. New York: Plenum Press.
A classic reference text that summarizes social science studies in alcoholism.

Ray, Oakley, and Charles Ksir. 1987. *Drugs, Society, and Human Behavior*, 4th ed. St. Louis: Mosby.
An entertaining, popular college text that skillfully underscores societal factors that influence alcohol use.

Schuckit, Marc A. 1984. *Drug and Alcohol Abuse: A Clinical Guide to Diagnosis and Treatment*, 2nd ed. New York: Plenum Press.
A balanced, informative treatise that focuses on the clinical aspects of alcoholism.

Chapter 11

Contents

Rate Yourself

Your Psychoactive Drug Use and Attitudes Read the following statements carefully. Choose the one in each section that best describes you at this moment and circle its number. When you have chosen one statement for each section, add the numbers and record your total score. Find your position on the Wellness Ladder.

5 Avoids addictive drugs
4 Limits intake of caffeine
3 Drinks coffee or tea regularly
2 Uses marijuana
1 Uses cocaine

5 Believes drugs should be used to reduce pain
4 Believes drugs should be used routinely to relieve tension
3 Uses drugs to relieve depression
2 Uses stimulant drugs to feel elated
1 Uses drugs to enhance sexual sensations

5 Is well educated about the effects of drugs
4 Is knowledgeable about the effects of drugs
3 Knows something about the effects of drugs
2 Knows little about the effects of drugs
1 Is ignorant about the effects of drugs

5 Does not take any drug without fully knowing its effects
4 May experiment with medically prescribed drugs
3 May experiment with drug taking if advised by a close friend
2 May take a psychoactive drug to see what it is like
1 Might try LSD if it were available

5 Educates others about the effect on health of psychoactive drugs
4 Is aware of the health consequences of psychoactive drugs
3 Believes that only illegal drugs have serious health consequences
2 Believes that cocaine and marijuana are not addicting
1 Believes that cocaine and marijuana have no effect on health

Total Score ______

Other Psychoactive Drugs

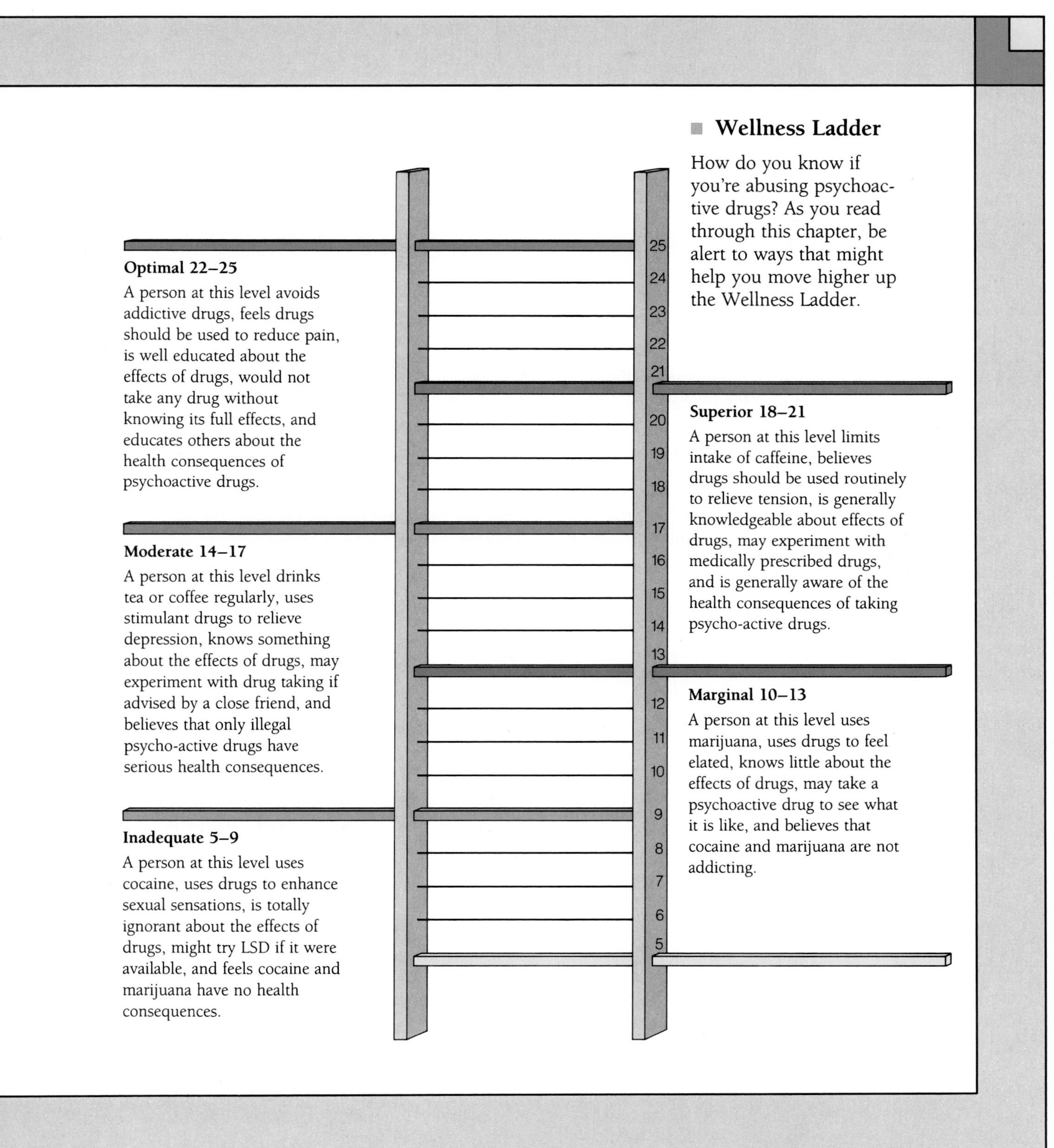

Optimal 22–25
A person at this level avoids addictive drugs, feels drugs should be used to reduce pain, is well educated about the effects of drugs, would not take any drug without knowing its full effects, and educates others about the health consequences of psychoactive drugs.
Superior 18–21
A person at this level limits intake of caffeine, believes drugs should be used routinely to relieve tension, is generally knowledgeable about effects of drugs, may experiment with medically prescribed drugs, and is generally aware of the health consequences of taking psycho-active drugs.
Moderate 14–17
A person at this level drinks tea or coffee regularly, uses stimulant drugs to relieve depression, knows something about the effects of drugs, may experiment with drug taking if advised by a close friend, and believes that only illegal psycho-active drugs have serious health consequences.
Marginal 10–13
A person at this level uses marijuana, uses drugs to feel elated, knows little about the effects of drugs, may take a psychoactive drug to see what it is like, and believes that cocaine and marijuana are not addicting.
Inadequate 5–9
A person at this level uses cocaine, uses drugs to enhance sexual sensations, is totally ignorant about the effects of drugs, might try LSD if it were available, and feels cocaine and marijuana have no health consequences.
25
24
23
22
21
20
19
18
17
16
15
14
13
12
11
10
9
8
7
6
5

Wellness Ladder

How do you know if you're abusing psychoactive drugs? As you read through this chapter, be alert to ways that might help you move higher up the Wellness Ladder.

Psychoactive drug Any substance that when taken into the body can alter the user's consciousness.

Drug abuse Taking drugs to a degree that causes physical damage, impairs functioning, or results in behavior harmful to others.

Pharmacological properties The overall effects of a drug on the individual's behavior, psychology, and chemistry. This term also refers to the amount of the drug required to exert various effects, the time course of these effects, and other characteristics of the drug such as its chemical composition.

Central nervous system (CNS) The brain and spinal cord.

Dose-response function The relationship between the amount of a drug taken and the intensity or type of drug effect.

Time-action function The relationship between the time elapsed since a drug was taken and the intensity of a drug effect.

Metabolize To chemically transform food and other substances into energy and waste.

In this chapter we define a **psychoactive drug** as any chemical that when taken into the body can alter a person's experience or consciousness—his or her sensations, feelings, thoughts, or the functions of the nervous system. We discuss psychoactive drugs from five arbitrarily defined categories: (1) opiates; (2) central nervous system depressants with barbiturate-like effects; (3) central nervous system stimulants such as cocaine, usually with amphetamine-like effects; (4) hallucinogens, including marijuana; and (5) inhalants. It should be remembered that alcohol, tobacco, prescription, and over-the-counter medications and caffeine are also drugs with psychoactive properties. They are discussed in other chapters.

Most of the drugs in the five categories discussed here are used, or have been used in the past, to treat pain or other symptoms. Sometimes the abuse of a drug came about unexpectedly as a by-product of its medical use. To distinguish between drug use and drug abuse, we define **drug abuse** as drug taking to the extent that it causes physical damage to the user, impairment of the user's ability to function in social situations or on the job, or behavior that is harmful to others.

Factors Influencing Drug Effects

As with alcohol and tobacco, the effects of the psychoactive drugs discussed in this chapter are extremely complex and highly variable. The same drug may affect different users differently or the same user in different ways under different circumstances. The effects of a single dose also do not stay the same. The effects change as the body absorbs and metabolizes the drug. For example, the initial effects of marijuana are usually stimulating; later, there is more CNS (central nervous system) depression. When the same drug has different effects, those differences must be due to factors not related to the drug itself—physical differences in individual users and psychological and social factors.

Drug Factors When different drugs or changes in dosage produce different effects, the differences are usually caused by drug factors—pharmacological properties of the drug, dose response, time-action function, cumulative effects, and method of use.

Pharmacological Properties In the last few years, a considerable amount has been learned about the effects of drugs on simpler nervous systems such as those of laboratory animals. These effects are usually quite complex and are usually affected by a host of variables. At a human level, it's useful to describe drugs in terms of their general **pharmacological properties.** For example, some drugs are classified according to which part of the body they affect. Drugs that stimulate the **central nervous system** are called **CNS** stimulants. Other drugs are classified by their chemical makeup; for example, opiates or cannabis products.

Dose-response Function Increasing the dose of a drug changes the way a drug affects people. This property is called the **dose-response function.** It is not true, however, that increasing the dose simply intensifies the first effect. A familiar example is the person who becomes friendly after one cocktail and belligerent and hostile after six.

Time-action Function The effects of a drug are greatest when tissue concentrations of the drug are changing the fastest, especially if they are increasing. This aspect of a drug is known as the **time-action function.** A constant drug level, even if it is high, is less likely to change the user's experience or behavior. We can use alcohol, one kind of drug, as an example. Immediately after a person takes a drink, the alcohol begins to be absorbed into the digestive tract, and the level of alcohol in the blood begins to rise rapidly. As the alcohol is **metabolized,** the blood alcohol level gradually falls (see Chapter 10). Intoxication is usually greater when the level is rising than when it is falling, even though there may actually be somewhat less alcohol in the blood.

Cumulative Effects Psychoactive drugs may over time cause physiological alterations in the body that change the effects of a drug. When habitual and occasional alcohol users take the same amount of alcohol, the habitual user is generally less affected.

Why People Use Drugs

In our society many people have come to expect that drugs will be a part of almost every aspect of daily living. Some believe that chemicals should be used to cure every discomfort and to enhance every pleasure. Through the powerful influence of peers, parents, and advertising, we are taught to seek solutions to many problems of living by using drugs rather than by other means. Common factors influencing drug use include

- Peer pressure and need to conform
- The desire to alter one's mood and physiological state
- The need to cope with difficulties
- Alienation and poor self-image
- Simple boredom
- Depression or anxiety
- Curiosity
- Ready availability of drugs
- The desire to enhance performance or obtain certain kinds of pleasure

Nonmedical Drug Use

Following are projected estimates of the numbers of people who report having used drugs nonmedically. The two categories are young adults and the total population over the age of 12. Estimates are developed from the *National Survey on Drug Abuse: 1979*, by the National Institute on Drug Abuse.

	18–25 years (pop. 31,985,000)				Total (pop. 179,358,000)			
	Ever Used[a]		Current User[b]		Ever Used		Current User	
	%	Number	%	Number	%	Number	%	Number
Marijuana and hashish	68	21,700,000	35	11,200,000	30	54,800,000	13	22,600,000
Inhalants	17	5,400,000	1	300,000	7	12,700,000	1	1,400,000
Hallucinogens	25	8,000,000	4	1,300,000	9	15,800,000	1	1,800,000
PCP	15	4,800,000	*	*	5	8,200,000	*	*
Cocaine	28	9,000,000	9	2,900,000	8	15,100,000	2	4,400,000
Heroin	4	1,300,000	—	—	1	2,600,000	—	—
Stimulants	18	5,800,000	4	1,300,000	6	13,900,000	1	2,100,000
Sedatives	17	5,400,000	3	1,000,000	6	13,900,000	1	2,100,000
Tranquilizers	16	5,100,000	2	600,000	5	9,800,000	—	—
Analgesics	12	3,800,000	1	300,000	5	8,200,000	—	—
Alcohol	95	30,400,000	76	24,300,000	90	160,800,000	61	108,600,000
Cigarettes	83	26,500,000	43	13,800,000	79	142,100,000	36	62,400,000

[a] one or more times in a person's life
[b] at least once in the 30 days prior to the survey
* not included in the survey
— amounts of less than .5% are not listed

Biochemical Describes the branch of chemistry that deals with the life processes of plants and animals.

Pharmacological factors The properties and reactions of drugs.

Setting The environment in which something is done.

Set A person's expectations or preconceptions in a given situation.

Placebo An inert or innocuous medication that is given in place of an active drug; it is often called a sugar pill.

"High" The subjectively pleasing effects of a drug, usually felt quite soon after the drug is taken.

Depressant Something that decreases nervous or muscular activity.

Stimulant Something that increases nervous or muscular activity.

Absorption The passage of substances through the skin, lungs, or gastrointestinal tract into the blood.

Exploring Your Emotions

How do you feel about people's using drugs that alter their consciousness? Most people feel strongly one way or the other about such habits. Why should passions be so strong regarding these psychoactive drugs? In what ways do people feel threatened by such patterns? Obviously, you would feel threatened if you were driving down the highway and knew that the approaching driver was high on cocaine. However, statistically, it is more likely than an approaching driver would be under the influence of alcohol or Valium. Many people either forget about or tolerate traditional drug abuses, but they feel threatened by newer psychoactive drugs. Why?

Method of Use When a drug is taken by a method that allows its rapid entry into the bloodstream and the brain, stronger effects are usually produced than when the method of use involves slower absorption. For example, injecting a drug generally produces stronger effects than swallowing the same drug. Drugs are usually injected one of three ways: intravenously (IV or mainlining), intramuscularly (IM), or subcutaneously (SQ or skin popping). Inhaling (smoking) marijuana produces about three times the effects of the same dose taken by mouth.

Physical Differences in Individual Users Even when the drug factors are the same, two individuals may respond quite differently. Weight can make a difference. For example, the effects of certain drugs on a 100-pound person will be twice as great as the effect of the same amount on a 200-pound person. Other causes of differing responses include general health and various subtle **biochemical** states. Interactions between drugs, including many prescription drugs and over-the-counter drugs, can also have unpredictable effects.

Psychological and Social Factors With large drug doses, **pharmacological factors**, the chemical properties of the drug itself, tend to have the strongest influence on the user's response. With small doses, psychological and social factors are often more important. These factors, or variables, are the setting. The **setting** is the physical and social environment surrounding drug use. If a person uses marijuana at home with trusted friends and pleasant music, the effects are likely to be different from the effects if the same dose is taken in an austere experimental laboratory with an impassive research technician. Similarly, the dose of alcohol that produces mild euphoria and stimulation at a noisy, active cocktail party might induce sleepiness and slight depression when taken at home while alone.

The term **set** refers to how the user expects to react. When people strongly believe that a given drug will psychologically affect them in a certain way, they are likely to experience those effects regardless of the drug's pharmacological properties. The **placebo effect**—when an individual receives an inert substance and yet responds as if it were an active drug—is an example of set.

Experiments have been conducted in which some subjects smoked small quantities of marijuana, while others (unknowingly) smoked a substance that smelled and tasted like marijuana but was not. The intensity of the **high** the subjects experienced was not related to whether or not they had actually smoked marijuana. Clearly, the setting and the set had greater effects on the smokers than the drug itself.

Major Psychoactive Drugs

We have classified psychoactive drugs into five groups—opiates, barbiturates, and other central nervous system **depressants**, central nervous system **stimulants**, hallucinogens, and inhalants. We have by no means included all psychoactive drugs in this classification; many drugs that we do not include also have great potency.

Opiates The opiates, also called narcotics, are natural or synthetic (laboratory-made) drugs that act as morphine does in the body. Opium, morphine, heroin, meperidine, methadone, and codeine are examples of drugs in this class. The various opiates have similar effects, but they do differ in dose-response and time-action characteristics. They are sometimes injected under the skin, into the muscles, or directly into the veins. They may also be taken into the body by **absorption** from the stomach and intestine, the membranes of the nose, and from the lungs. How

Endorphin A chemical produced naturally in the brain that has pain-killing effects.

Euphoria An exaggerated feeling of well-being.

Dependency syndrome A behavior pattern of compulsive drug users. The pattern is characterized by preoccupation with acquiring the drug and using it. This is also termed *addiction syndrome*.

Tolerance Lower sensitivity to a drug so that a given dose no longer exerts the usual effect and larger doses are needed.

Withdrawal The process of abstaining from a drug on which one has been dependent.

---

the drug is taken determines how quickly it enters body tissues. If it is injected, the tissue level will change rapidly, and behavioral changes will result. The same dose taken by mouth will be less effective immediately, but it may last longer. The reason for the more lasting effect is that the drug enters the tissues more slowly.

Recent studies have found that in humans there are naturally occurring opiates, called **endorphins.** The endorphins, which appear to control pain and regulate emotional states and sensory input, may be involved in the dependency process, and their specific role is currently the subject of much research activity.

Effects The opiates reduce pain and produce drowsiness, changes in mood, and mental clouding. Opiate users are unable to concentrate; they have trouble thinking; they feel apathetic and lethargic and cut down on physical activity; they cannot see as well; they feel less anxious; and they are less responsive to frustration, hunger, and sexual stimulation.

Opiates also induce **euphoria.** This property becomes important in the development of drug abuse, but many individuals at first feel vaguely uneasy and have muscular aches and other unpleasant sensations. It is not clear why some individuals go on to develop strong dependency on these drugs, but undoubtedly they do so because of a combination of psychological, social, and pharmacological factors.

All opiates in common use have a high potential for making people dependent on them; indeed, the chronic use of opiates is the usual example given of the classic **dependency (addiction) syndrome.**

A key feature of the classic dependency syndrome is **tolerance.** Users develop a tolerance for the drug and need larger and larger doses to achieve the same effect. Users often try to stay one step ahead in the game by using a technique called "chipping." (See Figure 11-1). They take only low doses and those not very often, in a usually futile attempt to avoid getting "hooked." But too often the time between doses shortens, the dose gets bigger, and tolerance develops. The usual starting dose of heroin is about 3 milligrams, but tolerance can lead within a few months to doses of 1,000 mg. Taking heroin can be a very expensive habit.

If the addict chooses to reduce the expense by giving up the habit or cutting way down on the dose, he or she faces yet another hazard of chemical dependency. He or she will have to endure **withdrawal** symptoms. If a certain level of the drug is not maintained in the blood, flu-like symptoms result. These include running nose and eyes, yawning, and sweating. These symptoms develop into worse ones as the level of the drug in the bloodstream continues to drop: weakness, nausea, vomiting, stomach pains, and diarrhea. The user may have goose pimples, and back muscles, bones, and limbs may ache severely. With heroin, these symptoms peak about 24 hours after the last dose and usually begin to fade in two to three days.

Many opiate users administer their drugs intravenously (IV). Nonmedical IV drug use has many health hazards,

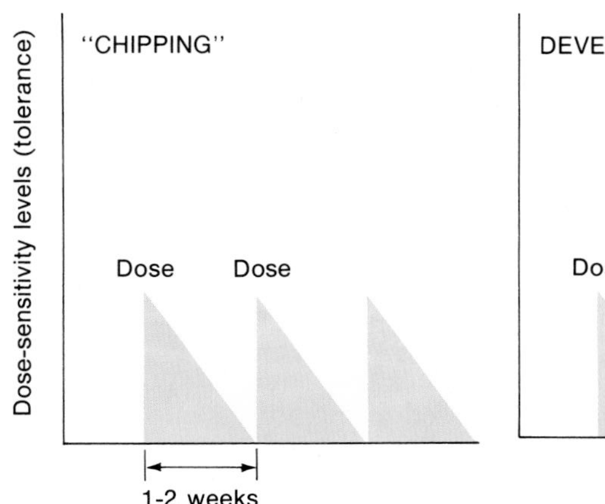

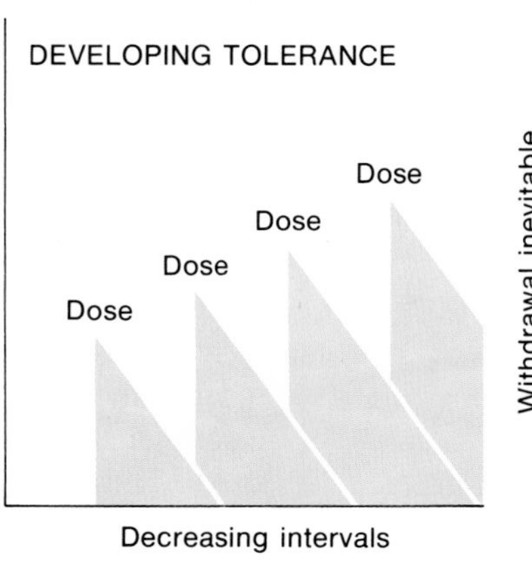

Figure 11-1 The key factor in avoiding developing a tolerance for a drug is to allow intervals between each dose.

Barbiturate A common sedative-hypnotic drug.

Sedative-hypnotics Another term for CNS depressants. These drugs cause drowsiness or sleep.

Anxiolytic A drug that can reduce tension and anxiety without putting the user to sleep; a tranquilizer.

especially from unsterile needles and impurities often contained in the drugs. AIDS (discussed further in Chapter 19), infectious hepatitis, systemic infections, and abcesses in the brain, heart, or lungs are the most lethal.

Treatment Most methods of treatment for opiate addiction have not worked very well. (See, e.g., Figure 11-2.) A fairly recent innovation is the substitution of methadone for heroin. Methadone maintenance reduces the possibility of a severe withdrawal reaction and decreases the craving for heroin without interfering with the individual's ability to function normally in personal, social, and vocational spheres. Methadone treatment clearly allows many former heroin addicts to live more useful lives.

Central Nervous System Depressants Central nervous system depressants slow down the overall activity of nerves, all muscles, including the heart, and many other body tissues. The result ranges from mild sedation to death, depending on which drug is used, how much is taken and in what way, the physical and emotional state of the user, and what his or her degree of tolerance is, if any.

The most common CNS depressants are alcohol (discussed in Chapter 10), **barbiturates,** and other various **sedative-hypnotics** that are not barbiturates but have similar effects. During the last twenty years, many new drugs have been marketed as "safe" and "nonaddicting" sedative-hypnotics, but most of these have turned out to have unwanted side effects and dangers, just as the barbiturates do.

Figure 11-2 Relapse rate over time for heroin, smoking, and alcohol.

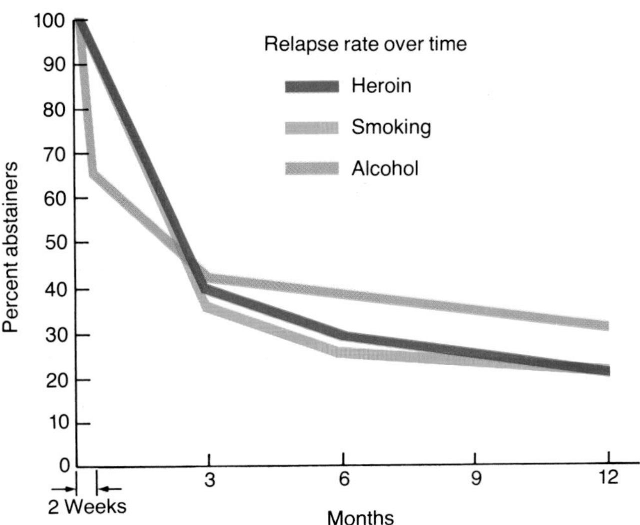

Methaqualone (Quaalude is the trade name of a common methaqualone compound) is an example of a sedative-hypnotic that was initially considered to be safe and to have little potential for abuse. Now, it is clear that methaqualone can have significant adverse effects and is often abused.

Anxiolytics, also termed **tranquilizers,** such as diazepam (Valium) can also be classified as CNS depressants. In low doses, the anxiolytics reduce anxiety without causing extreme drowsiness but in high doses sedation is inevitable.

In most countries a variety of barbiturates are available. They are all similar in chemical composition and action, but they do differ in how quickly they act and how long their action lasts. Drug users call barbiturates "downers" and refer to specific brands by names that describe the color and design of the capsules: "reds" or "red devils" for Seconal, "yellows" or "yellow jackets" for Nembutal, "blue heavens" for Amytal, and "rainbows" for Tuinal (a combination of secobarbital and amobarbital). People usually take barbiturates in capsules, but injecting them is also common.

Effects Barbiturates as well as many other sedative-hypnotics have much the same effects on behavior as alcohol. They reduce anxiety (although how much varies); they cause mood changes, muscular incoordination, slurring of speech, and drowsiness or sleep. Cognitive and motor functioning are also affected, but the degree varies from person to person and also depends on the kind of task the person is trying to do.

Most people become drowsy with small doses, although a few become more active. However, when people take these drugs deliberately to alter their awareness or for social reasons, they can overcome most of the sedative effects and remain awake even with large doses. It is particularly easy for the user to overcome drowsiness if the user has developed tolerance or if the environment is stimulating and exciting.

Medical Uses Barbiturates, methaqualone, and other sedative-hypnotics are widely used for treating people with insomnia, as daytime sedatives, and for control of seizures. They are also used to modify the effects of other drugs (for example, to reduce the excessive physical activity that often accompanies the use of CNS stimulants).

Co-dependency

A co-dependent is someone who is in a continuing relationship with a chemically dependent person, and whose actions help or enable that person to continue in his or her dependency. You may be a co-dependent if you have ever

1. Gotten into recurrent arguments with someone close to you because of his or her use of alcohol or other drugs.
2. Called his or her workplace (or other obligations) to make an excuse for someone who was hung over or otherwise debilitated from drug use.
3. Stayed up at night waiting for or gone out searching for someone who drinks or uses drugs.
4. Felt embarrassed, angry, betrayed, or hurt by someone close to you who uses alcohol or drugs.

The Valium Habit

Up to 2.4 million jittery Americans regularly take Valium or other tranquilizers of the benzodiazepine family. And while everyone knows that heavy use of such drugs can lead to serious addiction, the risk in taking ordinary prescribed doses has remained in doubt. Last week, however, a team of addiction experts announced a study that "unequivocally" shows that long-term "therapeutic" use of these antianxiety drugs can cause withdrawal—a sure sign of drug dependence.

Pharmacologist Usoa Busto and her colleagues at Toronto's Addiction Research Foundation carried out a controlled study: they selected 40 volunteers who had been taking antianxiety medication regularly and gave them either Valium or an inert placebo pill. Those unknowingly switched to the placebo exhibited such symptoms as headache, insomnia, sweating, difficulty in concentrating and feelings of anxiety. Such signs, the researchers noted, are also typical of withdrawal from heavy use of alcohol or barbiturates. The onset of withdrawal was immediate in those patients previously taking short-acting drugs, like lorazepam, that are quickly excreted by the body; symptoms appeared three to eight days later among those who had been taking Valium or other long-acting medication.

The results, says Busto, should make physicians more wary about prescribing benzodiazepine drugs in the first place. Doctors, she says, should "think twice now about whether the benefits . . . outweigh the risks of dependence." But to prevent withdrawal, the researchers note in last week's New England Journal of Medicine, all the doctor needs to do is gradually cut the dose and wean the patient off the drug.

SOURCE: The Valium habit, 1986 (October 13) *Newsweek*, p. 95.

Patterns of Abuse People who use CNS depressants for reasons other than medical ones use them in a variety of patterns. Some go on "sprees" from time to time; others take large doses every day for long periods. People usually have their first experience with barbiturates either by way of medical prescription or by way of friends in the drug subculture. Abuse for the medical patient may begin with repeated use for insomnia and progress to addiction through bigger and bigger doses at night coupled with a few capsules at stressful times during the day.

Most sedative-hypnotic drugs, including alcohol and the barbiturates, can lead to classical physical addiction, including pronounced tolerance and withdrawal symptoms. Tolerance, sometimes for up to 15 times the usual dose, can develop during a year or two of repeated use. Tolerance to the depression of the respiratory system caused by these drugs develops more slowly than tolerance to the behavioral effects of the dose. As with heroin and alcohol, the margin between a dose that does what the user wants and a lethal overdose narrows dangerously.

Withdrawal symptoms are more severe than those accompanying opiate addiction and are similar to the DTs of alcoholism. They begin as anxiety, shaking, and weakness but may turn into convulsions and possible cardiovascular collapse, which may result in death.

Addiction to CNS depressants and severe alcoholism are alike in many ways. While intoxicated, addicts cannot function very well. They are mentally confused and are frequently obstinate, irritable, and abusive. Both the alcoholic and the person addicted to CNS depressants commonly have poor general health, and both may suffer from (sometimes permanent) brain damage, with impaired ability to reason and make judgments. Furthermore, the incoordination caused by these drugs often results in injuries and accidents.

Barbiturates and other sedative-hypnotics are major agents of self-destruction. Barbiturate overdose is one of the most frequent methods of suicide among American women and accounts for over 3,000 known deaths each year in the United States. Many accidental deaths result when people use barbiturates and alcohol together. Even if a single dose of either would not have been fatal, combined depressant effects of both can halt breathing. Alcohol and barbiturates are not unique in this respect; combinations of many depressants can exert more deleterious effects than a single depressant used alone. Barbiturate addicts, like alcoholics and opiate addicts, often become preoccupied with having enough of the drug and sometimes resort to criminal activities to make sure they do. Violent behavior has also been linked with barbiturate addiction and with the use of methaqualone.

Central Nervous System Stimulants The most commonly used CNS stimulants are nicotine (discussed in Chapter 9), caffeine and related compounds, amphetamine and amphetamine-like drugs, and cocaine.

Table 11-1 Caffeine Content of Commonly Used Drugs

One Cup	Milligrams
Coffee (ordinary brewed or instant)	75–150
Coffee (decaffeinated)	2–5
Tea	25–150
Cocoa	10–50
One 12-ounce Can	
Cola drink	40–50
One tablet	
Caffedrine	250
No-Doz	100

Caffeine Caffeine is the main drug in coffee, tea, cocoa, and many cola drinks, and in some drugs sold over the counter for combating fatigue, such as No-Doz. In ordinary doses caffeine produces greater alertness and a sense of well-being. It also cuts down on feelings of fatigue or boredom, and using caffeine may enable a person to keep at physically exhausting or repetitive tasks longer. Such use is usually followed, however, by a sudden letdown. Caffeine does not noticeably influence a person's ability to perform complex intellectual tasks unless fatigue, boredom, alcohol, or other factors have already affected normal performance.

Caffeine mildly stimulates the heart and respiratory system, it increases muscular tremor, and it enhances gastric secretion. Higher doses may cause nervousness, irritability, headache, disturbed sleep, and gastric irritation or peptic ulcers. In women excessive caffeine consumption may cause development of breast cysts and may aggravate the symptoms associated with premenstrual syndrome.

Drinks containing caffeine are rarely harmful for most individuals, but some tolerance develops and withdrawal symptoms of irritability and headaches do occur. Excessive caffeine consumption causes excessive anxiety in many people. People with certain psychiatric problems often feel better when they decrease or eliminate their intake of caffeine. (See Table 11-1.) Recently, caffeine-free coffee and cola drinks have become popular; these are useful for people who are sensitive to the adverse effects of caffeine.

Amphetamines Amphetamines are a group of synthetic (laboratory-made) chemicals that are potent CNS stimulants. Some common amphetamines are dextroamphetamine (Dexedrine), *d-1*-amphetamine (trade name Benzedrine), and methamphetamine (trade name Methedrine). Popular names for these drugs change often and are different in different parts of the country. Some of the more common ones are "uppers" and "speed." The properties of amphetamines are also shared by another group of synthetic chemicals, which include methylphenidate (trade name Ritalin), phenmetrazine (trade name Preludin), and diethylpropion (trade names Tenuate and Apisate). These drugs are most commonly taken orally, although sometimes they are "mainlined' intravenously.

Small doses of amphetamines usually make people feel better, more alert and wide-awake, and less fatigued or bored. Small doses can produce some improvement in activities requiring extreme physical effort or endurance, such as certain athletic contests or military maneuvers. (See Chapter 14, "Exercise," for more information on the use of drugs and physical performance.) Amphetamines generally increase motor activity but do not measurably alter a normal, rested person's ability to perform tasks calling for complex motor skills or high-level thinking.

Psychosis A severe mental disorder in which there is a distortion of reality. Symptoms might include delusions or hallucinations.

Paranoid behavior Behavior caused by the false belief that one is being systematically persecuted.

Like caffeine, amphetamines do most to improve performance by counteracting fatigue and boredom.

Amphetamines in small doses also subdue the appetite, increase the heart rate and blood pressure, and change sleep patterns.

Amphetamine-like drugs, such as Ritalin, have been used to control the behavior of so-called hyperactive children. Instead of stimulating these children to an even higher level of excitement, for some reason, still not known, the drug calms them. The controversy surrounding such use of drugs is heated.

Amphetamines are sometimes used to curb appetite, but after a few weeks the user develops tolerance, and higher doses are necessary. Sometimes, too, when people stop taking the drug, their appetites rebound, and they gain back the weight they lost. One over-the-counter diet drug, propanolamine, has become popular. However, all these appetite-suppressant drugs have the intrinsic limitation of not permanently changing eating behavior. (See Chapter 13, "Weight Control," for more information on this topic.) Amphetamines have other medical uses, but many physicians doubt their usefulness and consider other approaches more worthwhile and not as risky.

Much amphetamine abuse begins as an attempt to cope with a passing situation. A student cramming for exams or an exhausted long-haul truck driver, executive, or soldier can go a little longer by "popping a benny," but the results can be disastrous. The likelihood of making bad judgments significantly increases. An additional danger is that the stimulating effects may wear off suddenly, and the user may precipitously feel exhausted or fall asleep ("crash").

Repeated use of amphetamines, even in moderate doses, often leads to tolerance and the need for larger and larger doses. The result can be severe disturbances in behavior, including paranoid **psychosis** with illusions, hostility, delusions of persecution, and unprovoked violence. These behaviors make up the "speed freak" syndrome. It is just like a nondrug psychosis except that it stops if the person stops taking the drug.

Some users inject large doses of amphetamines into their veins. Each injection immediately produces a feeling of intense pleasure, an orgasmic "flash," followed by sensations of vigor and euphoria that last for several hours. As these feelings wear off, they are replaced by feelings of irritability and vague uneasiness, along with physical aches. The discomfort strongly motivates the user to take another injection. The situation is somewhat similar to the injection of opiates. The result is a "run," a period of repeated injections of amphetamines. During a run, the individual often goes without sleep and without enough food or liquids. He or she is also likely to develop **paranoid behavior.**

A run ends when the user is too uncomfortable or too disorganized, or simply when the drug is all gone. The exhausted user will sleep for a day or two, then be lethargic or depressed. Injecting amphetamines instantly relieves the lethargy or depression, so the user is likely to begin another run.

Continued high-dose amphetamine use can develop into a dependency syndrome, with increasing tolerance and withdrawal symptoms (although these are less severe than with opiates). The individual is also likely to spend much of his or her time obsessively and compulsively seeking drugs.

People ending a run sometimes try to combat the stress and discomfort by using heroin or other CNS depressants. At least in this respect, amphetamines can be a steppingstone to other drugs.

There is no consistent evidence that certain personality traits make a person more likely to chose amphetamines or, for that matter, any one drug in preference to others. The main factors in choosing a drug are whether or not it is available and whether or not other people around are already using it.

Paranoia is only one of the hazards of amphetamine use. Others include malnutrition and loss of weight, damage to blood vessels, strokes, and other changes in the heart and blood vessels. As with opiates, the injection method brings an added danger, the risk of diseases caused by unsterile conditions.

Cocaine Cocaine, a potent CNS stimulant, can be made synthetically. It can also be obtained from the leaves of coca shrubs that grow high in the Andes Mountains in South America. For centuries natives of that region have chewed coca leaves both for pleasure and to increase their endurance. For a short time, Sigmund Freud was enthusiastic about the use of cocaine to cure morphine addiction and alcoholism. As is so often the case with new drug treatments, Freud's enthusiasm waned after he had more experience with the adverse side effects. At the beginning of the twentieth century, many patent medicines and nonalcoholic beverages such as Coca-Cola contained small amounts of cocaine. Commercial considerations such as cost cutting and later changes in drug control legislation ended this practice. Today, Coca-Cola (for example) uses the flavor from coca leaves, but all the cocaine has been extracted.

Cocaine produces a euphoria, which makes its illegal

The High Price of Abuse

HOW CRACK AFFECTS THE BODY
BRAIN
Causes euphoria, then depression, irritability, and craving for the drug. Long-term use can lead to psychological problems like paranoid psychosis resembling schizophrenia.
SKIN
Users can experience a sensation of bugs crawling over them.
LUNGS
Heavy use leads to lung damage similar to emphysema, and an acute overdose can cause respiratory arrest.
HEART
Heart rate and blood pressure increase, leading to risk of arrhythmia or even heart attack.
APPETITE
Suppresses desire for food, leading to weight loss, and in severe cases, malnutrition.

Crack is cocaine intensified. Its effects are cocaine's—but amplified, sharper, meaner, uglier. The assault on the body, brain and nervous system occurs in swifter, more profound fashion. "Crack, even more than plain cocaine, puts users at extremely high risk," says Dr. Nicholas Masi of the cocaine addiction treatment center in Plantation, Fla.

Crack's immediate effects are readily observable: chronic sore throats and hoarseness are common. Crack can leave a user gasping for breath and vulnerable to emphysema. But these complaints pale in comparison with the even more dangerous changes that crack triggers in the body. Crack, says Masi, "throws the entire cardiovascular system into turmoil. Your blood vessels rapidly constrict. You're a key candidate for respiratory failure." Dramatically increased blood pressure and heart rate can lead to coronary attacks, and the intense stimulation of the brain may trigger convulsions.

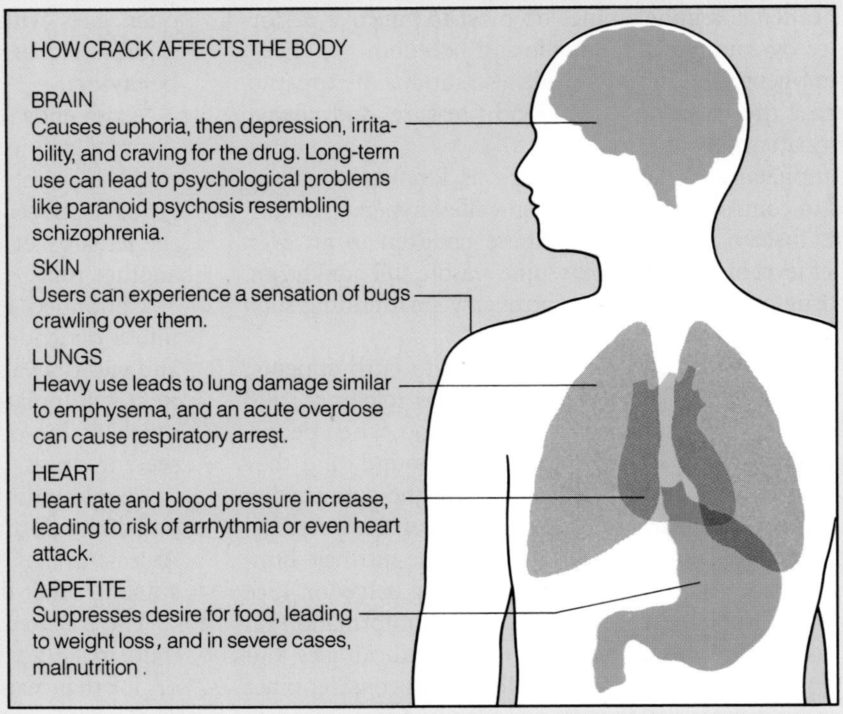

Far sneakier and subtler are the drug's invisible psychochemical changes. Dr. Ronald K. Siegel of UCLA outlines four stages to cocaine addiction. First comes euphoria, a feeling of stimulation and sexual excitement, soon followed by sadness and depression. Much later come irritability, sleeplessness and paranoia. The fourth stage, says Siegel, "is a schizophrenic-like psychosis, complete with delusions and hallucinations." One nightmare common to addicts is that bugs are crawling over their skin. Heavy crack smokers can go through all four stages in a single drug binge.

The stronger the craving for cocaine, the less a crack user cares for food. "You don't eat when you're smoking," says one California addict. Rats supplied with unlimited cocaine will use the drug until they die, ignoring food and water. Such intensely addictive behavior has helped change scientific opinion about cocaine's grip. Says Dr. Jeffrey Rosecan of New York City's Columbia-Presbyterian Medical Center: "If anyone had doubts as to whether cocaine is physically addicting, all he has to do is look at a couple of crack users."

Crack's addictive qualities affect the brain's biochemistry. The nerve cells of the brain communicate with one another with the help of chemicals called neurotransmitters. Crack triggers the brain to release these substances, chiefly dopamine, serotonin and norepinephrine, at once. This overstimulation, says Rosecan, "probably results in the euphoria experienced by the user."

But the effect is the same as overdrawing a bank account to go on a spending spree. Cocaine blocks the return of the neurotransmitters to the nerve cells for reuse. Eventually the brain is squeezed dry and craves stimulation. Addicts who try to recapture the high by smoking more crack only aggravate the neurochemical deficiency. Says Rosecan: "We think these physical changes correspond to the psychological changes of the crash—depression, irritability, paranoia and craving."

The higher someone soars on crack, the lower he falls. Says Dr. Arnold Washton of the National Cocaine Hotline: "It's impossible for the nonaddict to imagine the depth and viciousness of depression that an advanced cocaine addict suffers from." Users become anhedonic, all but incapable of pursuing or feeling normal pleasure. Addicts are prone to suicide, accidents and drug overdoses. Drawn by the prospect of a brief, inexpensive thrill, a user may find that he pays for crack with his life.

SOURCE: The high price of abuse, 1986, *Time* (June 2), p. 18.

Vasoconstriction A constriction of the blood vessels.

use very popular. In 1983, about 20 percent of all Americans aged 18–27 reported use of cocaine. However, it is very expensive, costing as much as $1,000 an ounce for high-quality supplies. As you would expect for anything so expensive, cheaper synthetic substitutes are now available. Vernacular names for cocaine are "coke" and "snow." As with other drugs, these names change over time and from place to place. Often the same name is used for both cocaine and substitutes.

Although cocaine can be swallowed and absorbed into the bloodstream from the stomach and intestine, it is usually snorted, sniffed, or injected intravenously since those methods of administration provide more rapid increases of cocaine concentrations in the blood and hence more intense effects. Another method of administration involves heating the cocaine with ether or other chemicals and then inhaling its alkaloid vapors. This is called "free-basing"; the user risks burns from sudden combustion, as in the well-publicized case of comedian Richard Pryor. A chemically similar method of processing cocaine involves baking soda and water. This yields an inexpensive, ready-to-smoke form of free-base cocaine, often called "crack." Crack is typically available as small beads or pellets smokable in glass pipes or sprinkled on tobacco or marijuana.

The effects of cocaine are like those of amphetamines, but they are more intense and do not last as long. When the cocaine is absorbed via the lungs, either by smoking or inhalation, it reaches the brain in 10 seconds or so and the effects are particularly intense. The effects from intravenous injections occur almost as quickly—20 seconds. Since the nasal mucosa briefly slows absorption, the onset of effects from snorting takes two or three minutes. Heavy users who want to maintain the effects inject cocaine intravenously every 10–20 minutes.

The larger the dose of cocaine and the more rapidly it is absorbed into the bloodstream, the greater the immediate, sometimes lethal acute effects. Acute fatalities from cocaine are most commonly caused by excessive CNS stimulation that induces convulsions and respiratory collapse, cardiac arrythmias (irregularities in heartbeat), damage to the heart muscle itself, or from brain damage, especially hemorrhage. These deaths can occur in young, athletic people who have no underlying health problems. Two days after being drafted as the top choice by the world champion Boston Celtics basketball team, Maryland University basketball star Len Bias died immediately after using cocaine. A few weeks later, Don Rogers, a star safety for the Cleveland Browns professional football team, died while using cocaine. Cocaine also contributed to the sudden death of standout University of Texas basketball player "Jeep" Jackson, who was playing in a charity game and headed for a promising professional career.

Exploring Your Emotions

You are invited to a school party where some well-known athletes are apparently using cocaine. What are your feelings? You know that small amounts of cocaine can trigger potentially lethal heart problems even in healthy young people. What do you do? Do you have responsibilities to the users? To the authorities?

Cocaine also constricts the blood vessels and acts as a local anesthetic. It is no longer used for anesthesia, however, because synthetic derivatives work better.

In the chronic cocaine snorter, repeated **vasoconstriction** produces a typical inflammation of the nasal mucosa, which may lead to a bloody nose and even to septal perforation of the septum between the nostrils. Weight loss is another common effect. Cocaine users, like amphetamine users, may develop paranoid and assaultive tenden-

DOONESBURY by Garry Trudeau

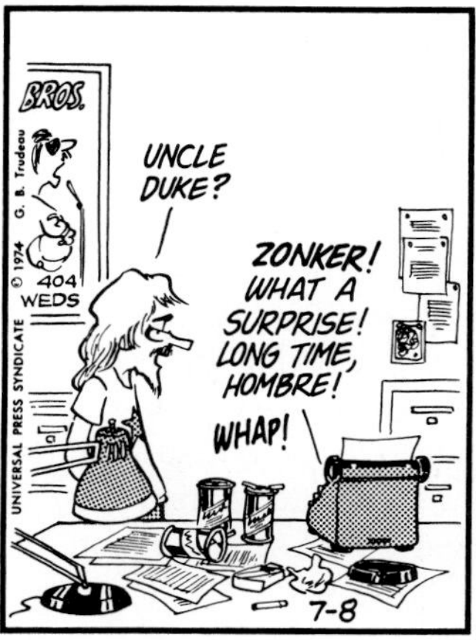
BROS.
UNCLE DUKE?
ZONKER! WHAT A SURPRISE! LONG TIME, HOMBRE!
WHAP!
404 WEDS
7-8

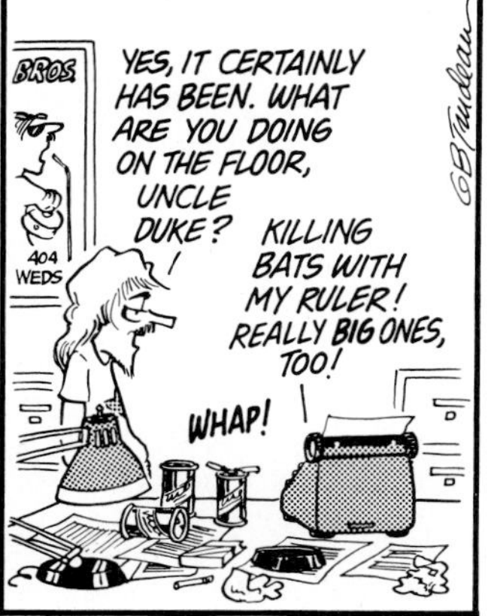
YES, IT CERTAINLY HAS BEEN. WHAT ARE YOU DOING ON THE FLOOR, UNCLE DUKE?
KILLING BATS WITH MY RULER! REALLY BIG ONES, TOO!
WHAP!

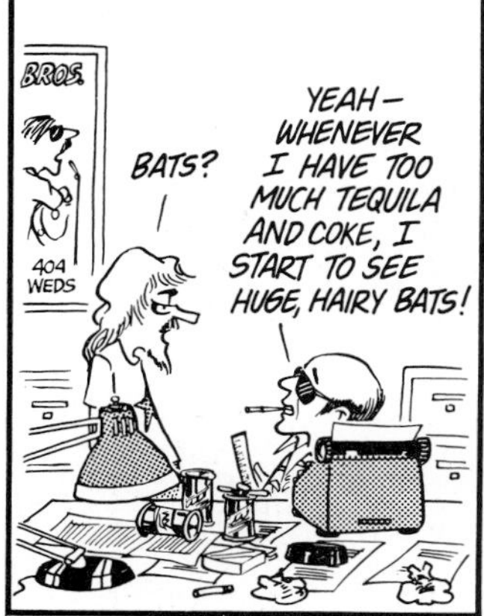
BATS?
YEAH—WHENEVER I HAVE TOO MUCH TEQUILA AND COKE, I START TO SEE HUGE, HAIRY BATS!

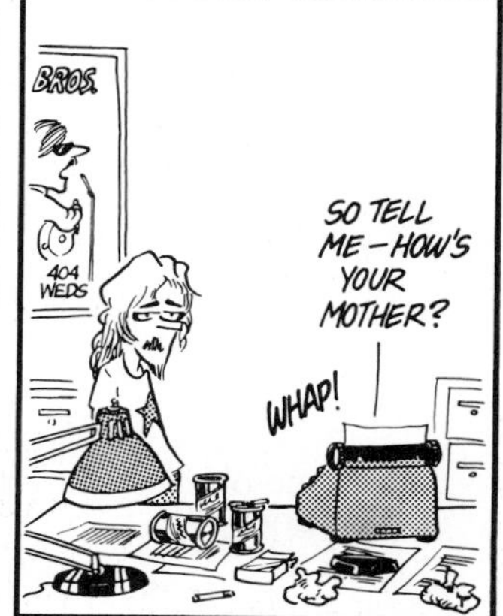
SO TELL ME—HOW'S YOUR MOTHER?
WHAP!

Synesthesia A condition in which a stimulus evokes not only the sensation appropriate to it but also another sensation of a different character. An example is when a color evokes a specific smell.

Depersonalization A state in which a person loses the sense of his or her own reality or perceives his or her own body as unreal.

Cross-tolerance The capacity of one drug to prevent withdrawal symptoms when another drug is abruptly discontinued.

Altered states of consciousness Profound changes in mood, thinking, and perception.

---

cies. The early stereotype of the crazed homicidal "dope fiend" was the cocaine user, not the heroin addict. However, even for the chronic cocaine user, the "dope fiend" stereotype seldom applies.

Cocaine users sometimes try to reduce paranoid feelings by using "speedball" mixtures, which combine cocaine and a depressant such as an opiate or barbiturate. However, the rapid changes thus imposed on the CNS are sometimes fatal. Comedian John Belushi died from a combination of intravenous cocaine and heroin.

Since cocaine (unlike the amphetamines) has a short time-action function, tolerance and pronounced withdrawal reactions require very frequent usage. Chronic use occurs anyway, probably because of psychological factors such as craving. Also, when a steady cocaine user stops taking the drug, he or she may feel pronounced depression and lethargy. The depression is transiently relieved by taking more cocaine, and thus continued use is perpetuated. In addition, some binge cocaine users go for weeks or months without using any cocaine and then compulsively and repetitively take large amounts. This pattern underscores the importance that psychological factors can play in chemical dependencies and refutes older conceptions of "addiction" that required physiological tolerance or withdrawal symptoms.

Hallucinogens The term hallucinogens refers to a group of drugs whose predominant pharmacological effect is to alter perception in the user. They are also called "psychedelics" for their alleged mind-expanding properties, or "psychomimetics" to focus on their psychosis-mimicking effects.

The hallucinogens include LSD (lysergic acid diethylamide), mescaline, psilocybin, STP (dimethoxy-methylamphetamine), DMT (dimethyl-tryptamine), PCP (phencyclidine), and many others. LSD is the most widely known of the hallucinogens, and we shall discuss it as an example of the entire group.

Marijuana, a cannabis product, can also be considered a hallucinogen and is discussed separately. MDMA (methylenedioxymethamphetamine), and other "designer" drugs are sometimes classified as hallucinogens, but in usual doses are more comparable to CNS stimulants. These drugs can be taken in a variety of ways, but are most commonly smoked or ingested.

LSD is one of the most powerful psychoactive drugs. A dose of 100 micrograms, an amount so small that it can hardly be perceived, will produce noticeable effects in most people. These effects include slight dizziness, weakness, nausea, and dilation of the pupils; disorders of vision, an improved sense of hearing, an altered sense of time, and a phenomenon known as **synesthesia**, rapid changes of mood, feelings of **depersonalization**, distortions in how people see their bodies, and alterations in the relationship between self and external reality.

Many hallucinogens induce biological tolerance so quickly that after a few days' use their effects are reduced greatly. The user must then stop taking the drug for several days before his or her system can be receptive to it again. These drugs cause little drug-seeking behavior and no physical dependence or withdrawal symptoms. Switching from one hallucinogenic drug to another does not also change the tolerance because many hallucinogenic drugs have **cross-tolerance.** An individual who is tolerant to one hallucinogenic drug is often tolerant to others.

In smaller doses especially, the immediate effects of the hallucinogens depend on psychological and social factors: the personality of the user and what he or she expects, recent events in his or her life, and the setting. Many effects of hallucinogens are hard to describe because they involve subjective and unfamiliar dimensions of awareness—the **altered states of consciousness** for which hallucinogens are famous.

Hallucinogens have acquired a certain aura not associated with other drugs. Some people have taken LSD in search of a religious or mystical experience, or in the hope of exploring new worlds, or as therapy, in an attempt to solve their problems. LSD has been acclaimed not only as a "mind blower" but also as an aid to creativity and personal growth.

Scientific research does not support these claims. People on LSD may make a greater number of original responses, but they are less able to synthesize them, to coordinate them into an appropriate pattern. Claims of increased sensitivity and powers of insight are also not supported by scientific evidence.

A severe panic reaction, which can be terrifying in the extreme, is more common with a large dose of LSD, but can sometimes happen even with a small dose. It is impossible to predict when a panic reaction will occur. Some LSD users report having hundreds of pleasurable and ecstatic experiences before an inexplicable "bad trip," or "bummer." If the user is already in a serene mood and

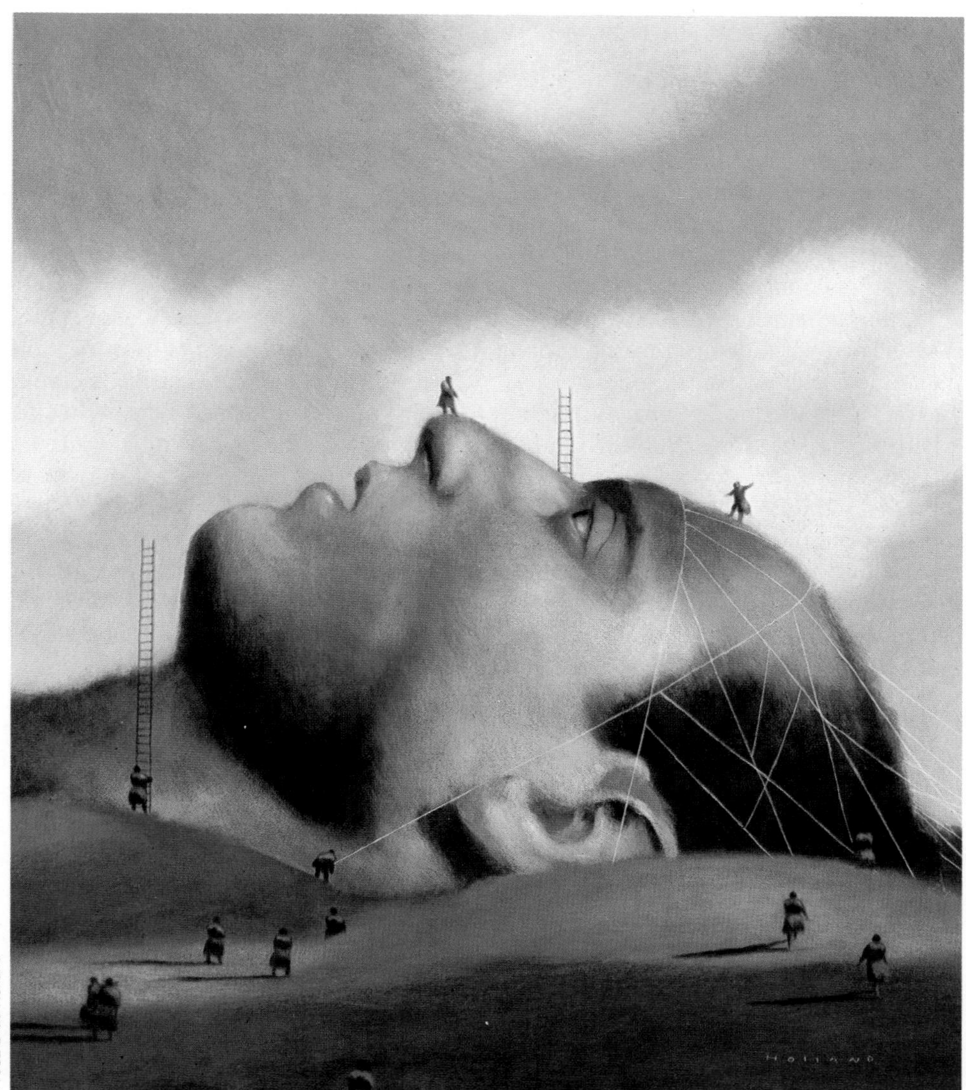

Exploring Your Emotions

How might feelings of depersonalization (as induced by drugs) give rise to feelings of "oneness with the universe"? To feelings of being lost and dispersed? What kinds of feelings might make a person seek depersonalization experiences, or conversely, avoid them?

feels no anger or hostility and if he or she is in secure surroundings with trusted campanions, a bad trip may be less likely, but a tranquil experience is not guaranteed.

Even after the drug's chemical effects have worn off, spontaneous flashbacks and other psychological disturbances can occur. Flashbacks, or **palinopia,** are perceptual distortions and bizarre thoughts that occur after the drug has been entirely eliminated from the body. Flashbacks are relatively rare phenomena, but they can be extremely distressing. They are often triggered by specific psychological cues associated with the drug-taking experience, such as certain mood states or even types of music.

Many of the bad trips attributed to LSD may actually be caused by impurities or other drugs and chemicals. The purity of LSD bought on the street varies widely, and it is a common practice to add other substances that purportedly heighten one or another of the drug's effects. Drug dealers often substitute less expensive psychoactive drugs (such as amphetamines or PCP) for more expensive ones (such as cocaine or LSD) so they can make more money.

Some researchers have claimed that LSD damages **chromosomes.** Evidence so far indicates that LSD in moderate doses does not damage chromosomes, at least not in laboratory settings; does not cause detectable genetic damage; and does not produce birth defects. Laboratory LSD is pure. Street LSD is not.

It can be risky for a pregnant woman to use any drugs, illegal or otherwise, especially during the first trimester when small chemical alterations in the mother's body can have a large effect on the developing embryo. Even later in pregnancy the fetus is usually more susceptible than the mother to adverse effects of any drug she takes.

Most other hallucinogens have the same general effects that LSD has, but there are some variations. As in LSD use, the effects of small doses depend largely on psychological and social factors, the set, and the setting. A DMT high does not last as long as a LSD high. An STP trip, in contrast, lasts longer than an LSD trip. Ditran and related compounds cause greater intellectual impairment and confusion than other hallucinogens.

Mescaline (peyote), the ceremonial drug of the Native North American Church, supposedly produces a "mellower" trip than LSD. Obtaining mescaline costs far more than making LSD, however, so most street mescaline is simply LSD that has been highly diluted. Hallucinogenic effects can be obtained from certain "magic" mushrooms (*Psilocybe mexicana*), certain morning glory seeds, nutmeg, jimsonweed, and other botanical products, but unpleasant side effects—nausea and dizziness—have limited the popularity of these products. Development and use of new psychedelics will probably continue, at least until they turn out to be less effective or to have more unpleasant side effects than older drugs. A few will probably have certain features that will make them useful for some purposes. Research on therapeutic applications of LSD practically stopped when LSD became illegal. Before then LSD was being tried with the terminally ill, with heroin addicts, in the treatment of alcoholism, and also under carefully controlled conditions, as an aid to psychotherapy. Many experts feel this research should be resumed since the therapeutic potential of hallucinogens has not been clearly determined.

Phencyclidine, also known as "angel dust," "PCP," "hog," and "peace pill," is a widely used synthetic hallucinogen. PCP reduces and distorts sensory input, especially **proprioception** (awareness of the position of arms and legs, joints, and so forth), and creates a state of sensory deprivation. This drug was initially used as a human anesthetic, but was unsatisfactory because of the postoperative agitation, confusion, and delirium its use caused. However, it is still used in veterinary medicine as an animal tranquilizer. Since the ingredients of PCP are readily obtainable and it can be easily made, it is often available on the illicit market and is sometimes used as a cheap adulterant for other psychoactive agents.

Following the faddish pattern of use of most psychedelics, PCP was extensively used in the mid-1960s. It declined in popularity when that generation became aware of the prevalence of adverse side effects including convulsions, memory impairments, coma, and occasionally death. In the mid 1970s PCP again became widely used and is currently a major drug problem. In some parts of the country, PCP is being replaced by a closely related drug, ketamine. Ketamine has most of the effects and associated risks of PCP.

Marijuana and Other Cannabis Products Marijuana is a crude preparation of various parts of the Indian hemp plant, *Cannabis sativa,* which grows in most parts of the world. THC (tetrahydrocannabinol) is the main active ingredient in marijuana. Concentrations of THC vary widely, depending on where the plant is grown and how it is cultivated, harvested, and cured. Hashish is a potent cannabis preparation derived mainly from the thick resinous materials of the flowering tops and upper leaves of the plant. It contains high concentrations of THC. THC can be synthesized, but it is a very expensive process. Because of the cost, pure THC is virtually never available on the illicit market. Drugs sold as THC are almost always something else, such as methamphetamine.

Marijuana is usually smoked, but can also be ingested. It is classified as a hallucinogen.

Effects of Marijuana As is true with most psychoactive drugs, what the user expects and what his or her previous experience with the drug has been strongly influence the effects of marijuana. At low doses, marijuana users typically experience euphoria, heightening of subjective sensory experiences, slowing down of the time sense, and a

Palinopia Condition of experiencing prolonged visual afterimages. One of the effects of hallucinogens.

Chromosome Microscopic bodies in the cell nucleus. The chromosomes carry the genes that convey hereditary characteristics.

Proprioception The sensory processes that identify the position and movement of muscles, tendons, and joints.

Psychotropic A general term referring to any chemical that can have effects on thinking, mood, or behavior.

relaxed laissez-faire attitude. These pleasant effects are the reason why this drug is so widely used. With moderate doses, these effects become stronger, and the user can also expect to have impaired memory function, disturbed thought patterns, lapses of attention, and subjective feelings of unfamiliarity.

The effects of marijuana with higher doses are determined mostly by the drug itself rather than by set and setting. Very high doses produce feelings of depersonalization in which the mind seems to be separated from the body, as well as marked sensory distortion and changes in the body image (such as a feeling that the body is very light). People who have not had much experience with marijuana sometimes think these sensations mean that they are going crazy and become anxious or even panicky. Such reactions resemble an LSD bad trip, but they happen much less often, are less severe, and do not last as long.

Physiologically, marijuana chiefly acts to cause increases in heart rate and dilatation of certain blood vessels in the eyes, which creates the characteristic bloodshot eyes. The user also feels less inclination for physical exertion.

Cannabis preparations were once medically prescribed for a variety of human illnesses, including insomnia, migraine, depression, and epilepsy. Now, however, none of these uses can be supported. Its medical use for sedative or euphoric effects is limited because of the perceptual and cognitive changes it brings about and also because individual reactions cannot be predicted. Somewhat more promising are current investigations into the use of THC to reduce nausea and improve appetite during cancer chemotherapy. In this situation, adverse side effects are less critical. THC and related compounds are also being studied for possible use in certain forms of glaucoma, the increased pressure within the eye sometimes leading to blindness.

We do not yet understand fully the long-term effects of cannabis use. We can predict, however, from experience with other drugs that the body systems and functions most affected in the beginning by marijuana are the ones most vulnerable to long-term injury. A small percentage of users will undoubtedly develop lung disorders. Some will perhaps show changes in brain functions. A persistent decrease in energy and drive has been described in a few chronic users but this so-called amotivational syndrome has not been conclusively established in scientific studies. It is unlikely that all chronic cannabis users will suffer harmful effects. Individuals vary greatly in how susceptible they are to both immediate and long-term effects of drugs. When we consider the long-term effects of marijuana (and of any other drugs), we should keep in mind the time-lag factor. A period of time must pass before long-term effects of a drug can be recognized. Tobacco, for example, was long thought to be a "harmless" drug.

Does marijuana cause dependence? Some tolerance can develop, but marijuana smoking irritates the throat and lungs. These unpleasant side effects make a steady increase in use of low-potency preparations unlikely. However, like all drugs that produce "good" feelings, marijuana can become the focus of the user's life to the exclusion of other activities. The chronic marijuana user will not necessarily limit his or her drug use to cannabis. Drug uses appear to be related, and the chronic marijuana user is more likely to be a heavy user of tobacco, alcohol, and other dangerous drugs.

Designer Drugs A relatively recent addition to the group of drugs that can be considered hallucinogens are the "designer drugs." The term designer drugs refers to new psychoactive compounds that are produced in laboratories by modifying the chemical structure of older, often naturally occurring drugs. For example, MDMA, also known as Ecstasy, is a derivative of oil of sassafras or oil of nutmeg. These designer drugs are often touted as having unique pharmacological properties and unique behavioral effects. Advocates of Ecstasy, for example, argue that it dissolves anxieties and permits you to think and talk about emotionally troubled issues that otherwise would be too frightening to face. However, proponents of Ecstasy and other designer drugs fail to acknowledge that the human brain has a limited repertory of chemical responses no matter what drug has been taken. Thus, effects of designer drugs fall in patterns that are very similar to traditional, better-known **psychotropics**; the few differ-

Exploring Your Emotions

You are at a party with college friends. Everyone is having a good time. Then someone in the group pulls out a bag of "grass" and begins rolling a joint. You are offered some. What do you do? What do you say? What changes would you expect in your relationships with your friends if you accepted or declined the offered joint?

Delirium A reversible state of mental confusion sometimes marked by emotional excitement.

Toxic psychosis A delirious state caused by brain dysfunction induced by a drug or by another agent such as fever.

Neuroleptics The group of powerful drugs useful in treating schizophrenia. These drugs are also called antipsychotics.

Psychoneurotic A term used to describe the mental disorders characterized by symptoms such as anxiety, depression, compulsion, obsessions, and phobias. Unlike psychosis, a psychoneurotic reaction is usually free of gross distortion of reality.

Depression A mild or severe emotional state characterized by dejection, low spirits, feelings of inadequacy, and inability to act.

Mania An emotional disorder characterized by excessive enthusiasm, unstable attention, and exaggerated activity.

Manic-depressive disorders A psychiatric disorder in which the patient's mood swings from mania to depression and back. This disturbance, which often runs in families, is also called bipolar disease.

ences are trivial, usually subjective, and most often related to dosage. Unwanted and in some instances dangerous side effects are inevitable in some people when higher doses are used. For example, the chemical name of Ecstasy is *3,4 methylenedioxymethamphetamine*. As one might expect from this name, the basic pharmacological effects are similar to amphetamine; with large-enough doses of MDMA, adverse effects virtually identical to amphetamine result.

"Designer heroin" or 3-methylfentanyl provides another example of a synthetic drug initially marketed as a "safe" opiate, which has subsequently been shown to have most of the negative effects of heroin. Underground chemists will undoubtedly continue to develop new drugs that will be "marketed" as uniquely safe and effective; however, they cannot expand the limited number of ways that the human body can respond to any psychoactive chemical.

Drugs and Delirium

Many drugs, and other substances not usually thought of as drugs, can bring on a form of abnormal behavior called **delirium**, or **toxic psychosis.** Delirium results from a temporary impairment of brain function. Different chemicals act on the brain in different ways, but the results are generally similar. They consist of changing levels of awareness to surrounding events, decreased ability to maintain attention to a task, and variable amounts of mental confusion. The person may also experience hallucinations, especially visual ones.

Some drugs, such as the belladonna alkaloid, datura, or jimsonweed, produce a delirium that is characterized by profound memory impairments. Delirium can be produced by inhaling certain chemicals such as some glues, gases in aerosols, kerosene, gasoline, amyl nitrite, and anesthetic agents such as laughing gas (nitrous oxide). Most inhaled chemicals interfere directly with brain function, but some do so indirectly by interfering with oxygen exchange in the lungs. Inhalants can be very dangerous to health; high concentrations of these substances in the blood can cause brain, liver, and kidney damage or even asphyxiation.

Exploring Your Emotions

Can you think of any legitimate recreational use of drugs? If so, where do you draw the line between legitimate and illegitimate use? Where do you place caffeine?

Psychiatric Use of Drugs

Certain classes of psychoactive drugs can be useful in treating psychiatric problems. The antipsychotic drugs, also called **neuroleptics** or major tranquilizers, are helpful in some individuals who have schizophrenia. We do not know exactly why they work the way they do, but there is no question that in psychotic individuals they reduce bizarre motor activity, decrease responsiveness to external and internal stimuli, and check hallucinations and delusions. In proper doses for the individual patient, the antipsychotic drugs accomplish these results without causing so much sedation that the individual cannot continue his or her daily activities.

A different class of drugs is the anxiolytic. Benzodiazepines such as Valium and Librium are examples of this group. They can reduce anxiety, relieve muscle tension, and cut down irritability in most people without causing extreme sedation. However, they can cause drowsiness, especially when combined with CNS depressants or when taken in tranquil, boring settings. Anxiolytic drugs are also used to treat other **psychoneurotic** reactions and many other conditions, but they are less effective in treating psychosis. They are extensively prescribed in contemporary medical practice. Patients demand them, and physicians often prescribe them for minor problems such as transient stresses that are an inevitable part of daily life. Virtually all such unpleasant stresses are better handled by learning appropriate psychological coping maneuvers. In addition, anxiolytic drugs can interfere with driving and do increase the effects of alcohol. All drugs, including anxiolytics, should be avoided during pregnancy, especially during the first three months. Because many women do not realize they are pregnant until the second month, obvious difficulties can occur.

As with other psychoactive drugs, distinctions between appropriate use of anxiolytic drugs and their abuse are often difficult to make. Most medical authorities would agree that ideally these drugs should be used primarily in time-limited situations where anxiety is so high the individual's usual coping abilities are completely overwhelmed. However, in our society these drugs are widely used where the situation is less clear-cut. Many people ingest anxiolytics on a frequent, often a daily, basis. The number of people who follow this pattern is far greater than the number of people who inject heroin, smoke opium, or inhale solvents. Is this pattern of consumption drug use or drug abuse? If we agree that any drug use resulting in impairment of functioning should be considered abuse, then the anxiolytics are commonly abused. When moderate or high doses are used daily or frequently, their anxiety-reducing effects tend to accumulate, alertness decreases, and various degrees of mental and behavioral impairment result.

In addition, some individuals clearly develop dependencies to the anxiolytics. These dependencies can involve pronounced craving, marked tolerance, and withdrawal reactions including seizures.

Recent research has produced many drugs for treating mood disorders. Some of these drugs, called antidepressants, are used to treat long-lasting severe **depression.** They are chemically very different from the stimulant drugs described earlier in this chapter. Results vary, but in some individuals antidepressants cause significant elevations in mood and increased activity and drive. As with most psychoactive drugs, it is not known precisely how they achieve these results. It is difficult for doctors to tell which individuals will benefit most from antidepressants, but studies show that these drugs work best with individuals who show "pure" severe depression with slowed body movements, reaction time, and speech pattern. The more a person's depressed behavior is combined with anxiety, hostility, or disorders in thinking, the less effective the antidepressants seem to be.

Among the newest drugs for treating severe mood disorders are the lithium salts. Lithium salts are effective in reducing **mania.** This condition is marked by exaggerated euphoria, inappropriate self-confidence, and poorly controlled overactivity. Lithium salts are also useful in treating **manic-depressive disorders,** in which the individual swings back and forth between mania and depression. As with the antidepressants, lithium salts appear to work best with people whose mood disorders are not combined with disturbances in thinking or perception. Despite the fears of many patients, lithium, antidepressants, and antipsychotic drugs do not produce dependence even when used chronically.

The study of the effects of drugs on the mind and behavior will undoubtedly see further development within the next few decades. We can especially expect to see refinements in people's abilities to predict which drug will be most useful for a given patient. New psychoactive drugs may present new possibilities for therapy or for social use. They also may present new possibilities for abuse. Making honest and unbiased information about drugs available to everyone, however, may cut down on their abuse. Lies about the dangers of drugs—"scare stories"—can lead some people to disbelieve *any* reports of drug dangers, no matter how soundly based and well documented they are.

Take Action

Your answers to the Exploring Your Emotions questions in this chapter and your placement level on the Wellness Ladder will, we hope, encourage you to begin a process of self-exploration and self-discovery that you will continue. Reflect on the entire chapter's content and ask yourself how each point relates to your own life. Then take action:

1. Find out what facilities are available in your community to handle chemical dependence. If none is available, what facilities are needed? Locate the public health agency that is responsible for your area and communicate these needs to them.

2. Survey three older adults and three young students about their attitudes toward legalizing marijuana. Are there any differences? If so, what would account for these differences?

3. Visit a chemical dependence treatment facility and interview the administrator about admission, treatment, and release procedures. Does this kind of firsthand observation affect your attitude about psychoactive drugs?

4. For one week, keep a daily log of all the psychoactive drugs that you use, the approximate dosage, the time of day, and what you think are the reasons for your taking each dose. Don't forget to include soft drinks and over-the-counter medications. What pharmacological categories do they fall into? Are there any patterns? Are there any signs of abuse?

5. Do you have any genetic susceptibility to drug abuse? Make a pedigree or family tree of your blood relatives. Have any of them had problems with alcohol or other drugs? You should remember that any biological vulnerability or resistance to drug problems is usually significantly modified by personal and environmental factors.

6. Before leaving this chapter, review the Rate Yourself statements in this chapter. Have your feelings or values changed? Are you now better equipped to handle the complex and very human problems associated with the use of psychoactive drugs?

Behavior Change Strategy

Lower Your Intake of Caffeine

One of the most frequently used drugs—caffeine—has almost no social constraints placed on it. And because it supports certain behaviors that are characteristic of our culture, such as sedentary, stressful, white-collar work, you may find yourself relying on coffee (or tea, chocolate, or colas) to get through a busy schedule. Such habits often begin in college. Fortunately, it's easier to break a habit before it becomes entrenched as a lifelong dependency.

Caffeine overdose can have some harmful effects on you (see text), and knowing what they are can help motivate you to reduce your intake. You may feel increased anxiety and irritability; some people may be especially sensitive to caffeine and may find such exaggerated states hard to manage. And women may develop breast cysts, as well as experience excess premenstrual tension, when they drink a lot of coffee.

When you are studying for exams, the forced physical inactivity and the need to concentrate even when fatigued may lead you to overuse caffeine preparations. But caffeine doesn't "help" unless you are already sleepy. And it does not relieve any underlying condition (you are just more tired when it wears off). So how can you change this pattern?

Diary Self-monitoring

Keep a log of how much caffeine you eat or drink. Use a standard measuring cup; heat-resistant ones are available. Using Table 11-1, convert the amounts you eat or drink into an estimate expressed in milligrams of caffeine. Be sure to include all forms, such as chocolate bars and pills, as well as caffeine candy, colas, cocoa or hot chocolate, chocolate cake, tea, and coffee.

A convenient way to keep a log is to tape a bracelet of paper onto your wrist, to record on as you go through a busy day. Don't be surprised if your intake falls sharply from this method alone—that's one benefit of paying attention to your habits. It's also a good conversation piece, which increases the attention you give to the behavior strategy.

Self-assessment

At the end of a week, add up your daily totals and divide by 7 to get your daily average in milligrams. How much is too much? At more than 250 mg. per day, you may well be experiencing some adverse symptoms. Are you experiencing at least five of the following? If so, you may want to cut down.

- Restlessness
- Nervousness
- Excitement
- Insomnia
- Flushed face
- Excessive sweating
- Gastrointestinal problems
- Muscle twitching
- Rambling flow of thought and speech
- Irregularities in rhythm of heartbeats
- Periods of inexhaustibility
- Excessive pacing or need to constantly move around

Set Limits

Can you restrict your caffeine intake to a daily total, and stick to this contract? If so, set a cutoff point, such as one cup of coffee. Pegging it to a specific time of day can be helpful, because then you don't confront a decision at any other point (and possibly fail). If you find you cannot stick to your limit, you may want to cut out caffeine altogether; abstinence can be easier than moderation for some people. Remember—tea, cocoa, and so on are not caffeine-free substitutes for coffee.

Find Other Ways to Keep Your Energy Up

If you are fatigued, it makes sense to get enough sleep or to exercise more rather than drowning the problem in coffee. Different individuals need different amounts of sleep; you may also need more sleep at different times, such as during a personal crisis or an illness. Also, exercise raises your metabolic rate for hours afterward—a handy fact to exploit when you want to feel more awake and want to avoid an irritable coffee jag. And if you've been compounding your fatigue by not eating properly, try chowing down on complex carbohydrates such as whole-grain bread and potatoes instead of candy bars.

Some Tips on Cutting Out Caffeine

Here are some more ways to decrease your consumption of caffeine:

1. Keep some noncaffeine drink on hand, perhaps hot water or bouillon, to give a warm feeling to your hands and mouth.
2. Alternate between hot and very cold liquids.
3. Drink decaffeinated coffee or herbal teas.
4. Fill your coffee cup only halfway.
5. Avoid the office or school lunchroom or cafeteria and the chocolate area of the grocery store. (Often people drink coffee or tea and eat chocolate simply because it is there.)

Selected References

Cohen, Sidney. 1985. *The Substance Abuse Problems*. Vol. 2: *New Issues for the 80s*. New York: Haworth Press.

Cregler, L. L., and H. Mark. 1986 (May 1). Cardiovascular dangers of cocaine abuse. *American Journal of Cardiology* 57:1185.

Drug Abuse Council. 1980. *The Facts about Drug Abuse*. New York: Free Press.

Duncan, D. F., and R. S. Gold. 1981. *Drugs and the Whole Person*. New York: Macmillan.

Fisher, Seymour, Allen Raskin, E. H. Uhlenhuth, eds. 1987. *Cocaine: Clinical and Biobehavioral Aspects*. New York: Oxford University Press.

Ray, Oakley, and Charles Ksir. 1987. *Drugs, Society, and Human Behavior*, 4th ed. St. Louis: Mosby.

Smith, D. E., H. B. Milkman, and S. G. Sunderwirth, eds. 1985. Addictive disease: Concepts and controversy. *The Addictions: Multidisciplinary Perspectives and Treatment*. Lexington, Mass.: Lexington Books.

Suggested Readings

Blum, R. H. et al. 1969. *Society and Drugs*. San Francisco: Jossey-Bass.
A well-written book that emphasizes the historical and social context of non-medical drug use.

Connell, P. H. 1958. *Amphetamine Psychosis*. New York: Oxford University Press.
The original treatise on adverse effects from amphetamine use.

Jones, R. T. 1983. Cannabis and health. *Annual Reviews of Medicine* 34:247–58.
A scholarly, balanced review of marijuana's effects on health.

Kaplan, J. 1970. *Marijuana—The New Prohibition*. New York: World Publishing Co.
The classic book on the politics of marijuana control in the United States.

Kaplan, J. 1983. *The Hardest Drug: Heroin and Public Policy*. Chicago: University of Chicago Press.
An excellent description of the scientific and political issues involving heroin.

Schuckit, M. A. 1984. *Drug and Alcohol Abuse: A Clinical Guide to Diagnosis and Treatment*, 2nd ed. New York: Plenum Press.
A balanced, informative text that focuses on the clinical aspects of drug use.

Chapter 12

Contents

Rate Yourself

Your Nutrition Behavior Read the following statements carefully. Choose the one in each section that best describes you at this moment and circle its number. When you have chosen one statement for each section, add the numbers and record your total score. Find your position on the Wellness Ladder.

5 Drinks only nonfat milk
4 Prefers nonfat milk
3 Prefers fat-containing milk
2 Consumes few dairy products
1 Avoids dairy products

5 Eats fruit twice daily
4 Eats fruit once daily
3 Eats fruit 3–4 times a week
2 Eats fruit once a week
1 Rarely eats fruit

5 Eats vegetables twice daily
4 Eats vegetables once daily
3 Eats vegetables 3–4 times a week
2 Eats vegetables once a week
1 Rarely eats vegetables

5 Maintains reasonable weight
4 About 5 pounds overweight
3 More than 10 pounds overweight
2 More than 20 pounds overweight
1 More than 30 pounds overweight

5 Has checked nutritional adequacy of diet
4 Eats a balanced and varied diet
3 Takes an occasional vitamin pill for "insurance"
2 Chooses foods with little variety
1 Takes "stress vitamins" or protein supplements

Total Score ______

Nutrition Facts and Fallacies

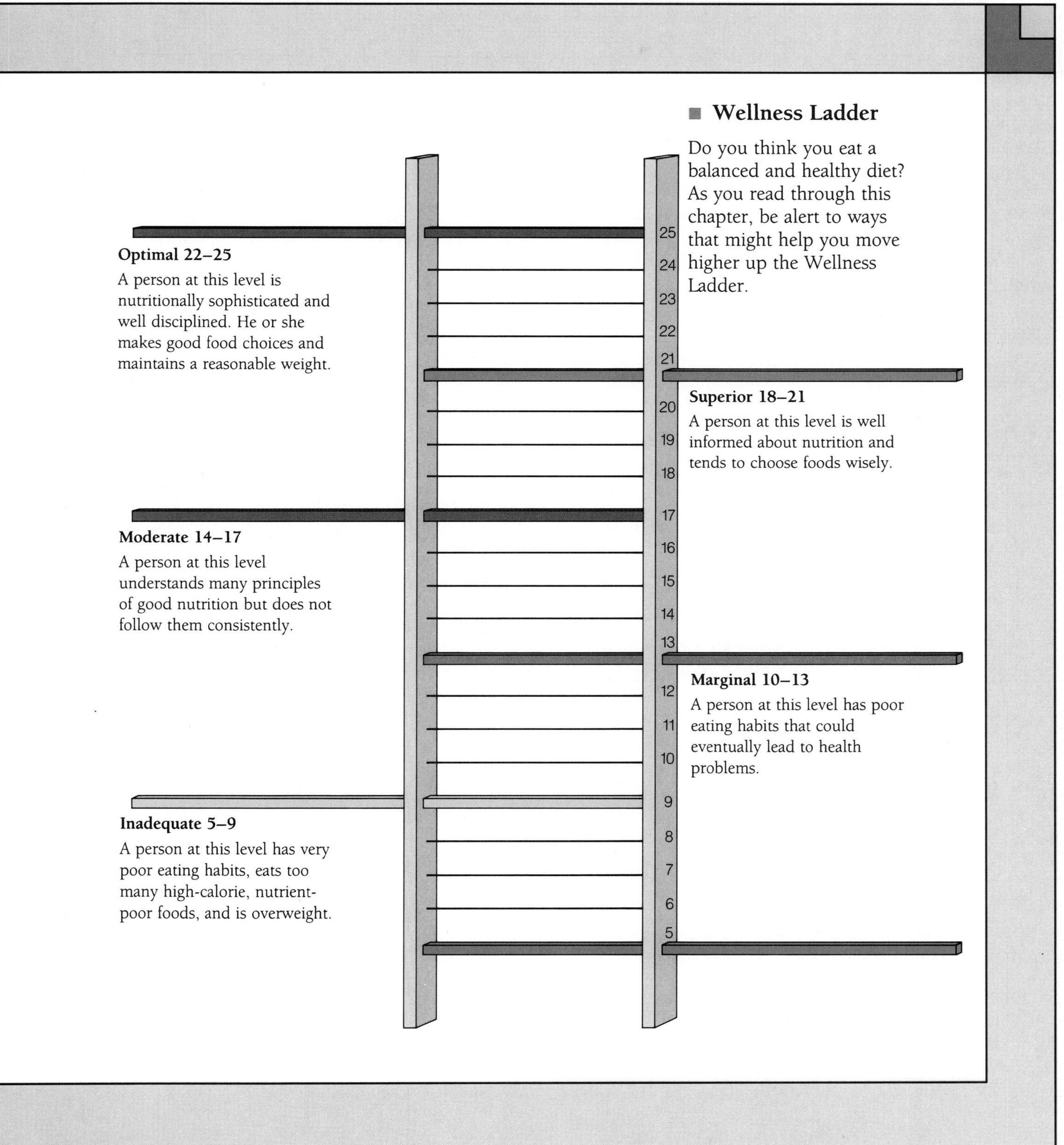

Wellness Ladder

Do you think you eat a balanced and healthy diet? As you read through this chapter, be alert to ways that might help you move higher up the Wellness Ladder.

Optimal 22–25
A person at this level is nutritionally sophisticated and well disciplined. He or she makes good food choices and maintains a reasonable weight.

Superior 18–21
A person at this level is well informed about nutrition and tends to choose foods wisely.

Moderate 14–17
A person at this level understands many principles of good nutrition but does not follow them consistently.

Marginal 10–13
A person at this level has poor eating habits that could eventually lead to health problems.

Inadequate 5–9
A person at this level has very poor eating habits, eats too many high-calorie, nutrient-poor foods, and is overweight.

Nutrition The science of food and how the body uses it in health and disease.

Caloric value The energy value of food. A calorie is the amount of energy, in the form of heat, required to raise the temperature of 1 kilogram of water 1 degree Celsius.

Essential nutrients Substances your body must get from foods because (with minor exceptions) it cannot manufacture them. They include vitamins, minerals, some amino acids, glucose, linoleic acid, and water.

Saturated fats Fats whose molecules are filled to capacity with hydrogen.

Amino acids The building blocks of proteins.

Monounsaturated fats Fats with room for two hydrogen atoms per molecule.

Polyunsaturated fats Fats with room for four or more hydrogen atoms per molecule.

Few of us escape childhood without at least a vague feeling that what tastes good must be bad for us and what's good for us should taste terrible. Then as adults we are exposed to an avalanche of conflicting nutrition advice from newspapers, magazines, books, and television programs. Many of us are left so confused about what makes up a nutritionally sound diet that we continue to eat what we like but worry that we may not be eating properly.

Exploring Your Emotions

Do you feel you eat properly? Do you feel guilty about anything you eat or don't eat? Or do you worry that some things you eat aren't good for you? Where do you feel you learned your eating habits?

This confusion should not be difficult to resolve. Although the science of nutrition is relatively young, scientists already know what nutrients are needed for an adequate diet and what foods provide them. Understanding just these basic facts can help you eat sensibly and protect yourself against nutrition fallacies.

Basic Food Components

Some basic **nutrition** concepts have existed since at least the fifth century B.C., when Hippocrates postulated that foods contain various amounts of a life-giving substance that is extracted by the body during digestion. In the eighteenth century (A.D.), a major step toward the science of nutrition was taken by the French chemist Antoine Lavoisier. He determined that metabolism of food in the body uses approximately the same amount of oxygen and produces about the same amount of heat as burning that amount of food in the laboratory. His experiments made clear that Hippocrates's "life-giving substance" was the **caloric value** or *energy value* of food.

Today we know that a diet adequate for human growth and development must contain vitamins, minerals, and other **essential nutrients**—about 50 in all. The word "essential" in this context means that we must get these substances from food, because, with few exceptions, our bodies cannot manufacture them.

Most plants use light energy from the sun to convert chemicals from air, water, and soil into all the complex chemicals they need. Animals, including we humans, must eat foods to get the nutrients needed for energy and to maintain body tissues and systems.

The nutrients in foods can be divided into six groups: proteins, fats, carbohydrates, vitamins, minerals, and water. Practically all foods contain mixtures of proteins, fats, and carbohydrates, although they are commonly classified according to the predominant one. Vitamins and minerals help regulate body functions and are needed in relatively small amounts. Water is actually the major component in both foods and the human body, which is about 60 percent water.

Proteins Proteins are the body's main *structural* component. The proteins in our food are too large to be absorbed through our intestines, so they are broken down during digestion into their component **amino acids.** These smaller components are then absorbed from the intestine and reassembled where needed into the large number of proteins needed to build and maintain the body's structure. Amino acids not used for this purpose are used for energy. Most Americans eat more protein than they need.

Of the twenty-two common amino acids, eight are *essential* for adults: isoleucine, leucine, lysine, methionine, phenylalanine, threonine, tryptophan, and valine. Protein sources are considered *complete* or of high quality if they supply all the essential amino acids in adequate amounts, and *incomplete* if they do not. Meat, fish, poultry, eggs, milk, cheese, and other foods from animal sources provide complete proteins. Incomplete proteins, which come from plant sources such as beans and peas, are good sources of most essential amino acids because they are usually low in only one or two of them. Vegetarians can get the essential amino acids they need by combining their foods properly.

Fats Fats are the most concentrated source of energy. Fatty deposits in your body not only store energy but also help insulate your body and support and cushion your organs. Fats also help your body absorb fat-soluble vitamins from your intestine.

Fats, also known as lipids, that are solid at room temperature are called *fats,* while those that are liquid at room temperature are called *oils.* The fats commonly found in food and in the body are composed of glycerol (an alco-

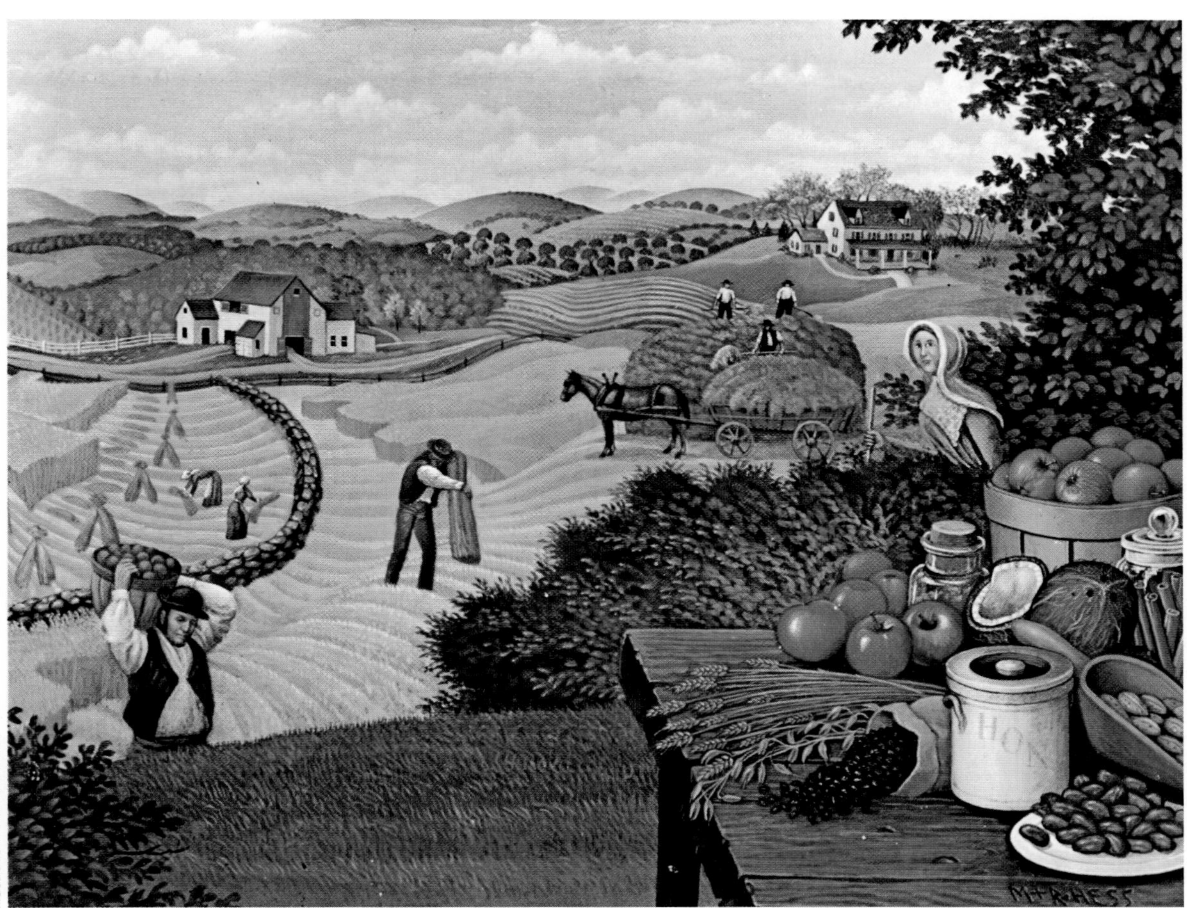

Illustration: Richard Hess

Exploring Your Emotions

How does this picture make you feel? How does tradition enter into your eating habits?

hol) plus three chainlike fatty acids. Fatty acids differ in the lengths of their chains and in the degree of saturation with hydrogen. Those filled to capacity with hydrogen are called **saturated;** those with room for two hydrogen atoms per molecule are called **monounsaturated;** and those with room for four or more are called **polyunsaturated.** Linoleic acid, which is polyunsaturated, is the only lipid nutrient recognized as essential for humans.

Food fats are mixtures of saturated and unsaturated fatty acids, but the dominant type determines their characteristics. Oils tend to be unsaturated. Olive and peanut oils contain mostly monounsaturated acids, while sunflower, corn, soybean, cottonseed, and safflower oils are mostly polyunsaturated. Most saturated fats are of animal origin, or are vegetable oils to which hydrogen has been added (*hydrogenation*). However, palm and coconut oils, which are used in cakes and nondairy creamers, are saturated.

The amount of saturated fat in the diet is an important factor that affects the level of blood *cholesterol,* a fatlike substance that, if elevated, is associated with increased risk of heart disease (see Chapter 17). Butter, shortening, and oil are obvious sources of fat in the diet, but well-marbled meats, poultry skin, whole milk, ice cream, nuts, seeds, salad dressings, and some baked products also provide considerable fat. Most experts believe that the American diet is too high in fat, particularly saturated fat.

Carbohydrates Carbohydrates can be divided into two groups: simple and complex. Sugars, such as table sugar, honey, and corn syrup, are simple carbohydrates and contain only one or two sugar molecules. Starches and most

Digestion Processes of breaking down foods in the gastrointestinal tract into compounds your body can absorb.

Glucose A simple sugar that is your body's basic fuel.

Metabolism The sum of the biochemical activities within your body. Substances changed by chemical reactions within your body are said to be *metabolized*.

types of dietary fiber are complex carbohydrates, which are chains of many sugar molecules. **Digestion** breaks down starches and sugars into single sugar molecules that are absorbed into your body. The links between the sugar molecules in dietary fiber cannot be broken down by human digestive enzymes, so fiber passes down your intestinal tract and provides bulk for stools (feces).

Within the body, **glucose** is the basic form of fuel. All foods must be digested or **metabolized** to glucose before the energy within them is accessible. Glucose circulates in your blood and is stored in the form of glycogen, mainly in your liver and muscles. However, when you eat more than your body needs, the excess is stored as fat, which is a more concentrated energy storage form than glycogen.

Carbohydrates are the best source of glucose and supply 35 to 50 percent of the calories in the average American diet. Carbohydrates are found in cereals, breads, fruits, and vegetables. When you don't have enough carbohydrates in your diet—which occurs during fasting or very low calorie diets—your body makes glucose from fats or proteins.

Most experts believe that Americans should increase their intake of carbohydrates—particularly complex carbohydrates—while lowering their intake of proteins and fats.

Dietary Fiber Dietary fiber (also called "bulk" or "roughage") includes a large number of plant substances that are difficult or impossible for us to digest. All foods of plant origin contain fiber in various quantities.

Fiber in the intestinal tract holds water, making feces bulkier and softer so they pass more quickly and easily through the intestines. Low-fiber diets can cause constipation. Research suggests that prolonged lack of dietary fiber is associated with such problems as diverticulitis (a painful condition in which abnormal pouches in the wall of the large intestine become inflamed), hemorrhoids (abnormally enlarged veins in the rectum), colon cancer, obesity, diabetes, and increased serum cholesterol levels (associated with increased risk of heart disease). Most scientists agree that fiber can be useful in treating constipation, hemorrhoids, and diverticulitis, but it is not yet clear how valuable it is in preventing other ailments. Nor is it known which components of fiber, if any, might be potentially most useful.

Although it is not yet clear exactly how much and what types of fiber would be ideal, most authorities believe that the average American would benefit from a *modest* increase in daily intake. But even fiber that occurs naturally in food should be eaten in moderation. A high-fiber diet can make you feel "stuffed" or "bloated," and can interfere with your absorption of essential minerals such as iron, copper, zinc, and calcium.

Although wood pulp fiber has been added to some foods as a selling point, it is not the same as dietary fiber. It has no nutritive value, and its long-term effect on health is unknown.

Vitamins Vitamins are organic (carbon-containing) substances required in tiny amounts to promote specific chemical reactions within living cells (see Table 12-1). Many vitamins are catalysts—substances that initiate or

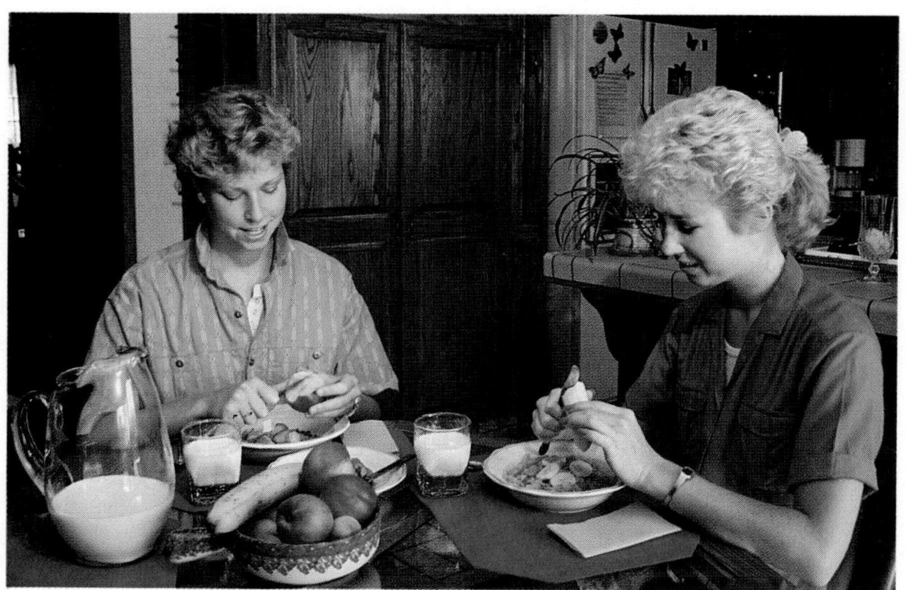
Myrleen Ferguson

Table 12-1 Functions and Food Sources of Vitamins

Vitamin	U.S. RDA[a]	Why Needed	Food Sources
Thiamin (B_1)	1.5 mg	Conversion of carbohydrates into energy	Yeast, rice husks, whole-grain and enriched breads and cereals, liver, pork, lean meats, poultry, eggs, meats, fish, many fruits and vegetables
Riboflavin (B_2)	1.7 mg	Energy release; maintenance of skin, mucous membranes, and nervous structures	Dairy products, liver, yeast, fruits, whole-grain and enriched breads and cereals, vegetables, lean meats, poultry
Niacin (B_3)	20 mg	Conversion of carbohydrates, fats, and protein into energy; essential for growth; synthesis of hormones	Liver, chicken, turkey, halibut, tuna, milk, eggs, grains, fruits and vegetables, enriched breads and cereals
B_6 (pyridoxine, pyridoxal, pyridoxamine)	2.0 mg	More than 60 enzyme reactions	Milk, liver, lean meats, whole-grain or enriched breads and cereals, vegetables
B_{12}	6 micrograms	Synthesis of red and white blood cells; many other metabolic reactions	Liver, meat, eggs, milk
Folic acid	0.4 mg	Blood cell production, maintenance of nervous system	Liver, many vegetables
Biotin	0.3 mg	Intermediary metabolism of fats, carbohydrates, and proteins	Widely distributed in foods
Pantothenic acid	10 mg	Metabolism of carbohydrates, fats, and proteins	Eggs, liver, kidneys, peanuts, whole grains, most vegetables, fish
A (retinol)	5,000 International Units	Maintenance of eyes, skin, linings of the nose, mouth, digestive and urinary tracts	Liver, whole milk, butter, cheese, fortified margarine, carrots, spinach, other vegetables
C (ascorbic acid)	60 mg	Maintenance and repair of connective tissues, bones, teeth, cartilage; promotes wound healing	Peppers, broccoli, Brussels sprouts, citrus fruits, tomatoes, potatoes, cabbage, other fruits and vegetables
D (cholecalciferol)	400 International Units	Regulation of calcium and phosphorus metabolism; promotion of calcium absorption; development and maintenance of bones and teeth	Fortified milk, fish liver oils; sunlight on skin produces vitamin D
E (tocopherol)	30 International Units	Protection and maintenance of cellular membranes	Vegetable oils, whole grains, leafy vegetables; smaller amounts widespread in foods
K	—	Production of prothrombin (essential for blood clotting)	Green leafy vegetables, soybeans, beef liver; widespread in other foods

[a]For adults and children age 4 or older

Vitamin A carbon-containing substance whose lack causes a specific deficiency disease curable by that substance.

Scurvy A disease caused by lack of vitamin C in which the gums bleed and teeth are loosened.

Recommended Dietary Allowances (RDAs) Amounts of certain nutrients considered adequate to meet the needs of most healthy people.

Basic Four Food Group system A method of grouping foods according to nutrient content.

Dietary Guidelines for Americans Seven general principles of good nutrition intended to help prevent certain diet-related diseases.

---

speed up chemical reactions but remain unchanged while performing their tasks repeatedly. Unlike foods, vitamins provide no significant amount of energy for your body but are needed in other ways, for example, to help release the energy in carbohydrates, fats, and proteins. A substance is considered a **vitamin** if lack of it causes a specific deficiency disease that is cured when the substance is resupplied. Probably the best-known deficiency disease is **scurvy**, which killed many sailors on long ocean voyages until people realized in the eighteenth century that oranges and lemons could prevent it. Today we know that the victims of this disease lacked vitamin C in their diets.

Humans need thirteen known vitamins. Four are fat soluble (A, D, E, and K), and nine are water soluble (C and the eight "B-complex" vitamins: thiamin (B_1), riboflavin (B_2), niacin (B_3), B_6, B_{12}, folic acid, biotin, and pantothenic acid). Since patients can survive for many years without becoming ill on intravenous feedings fortified with these substances, it appears that no vitamins remain to be discovered.

Most vitamins must be obtained from food because the human body cannot manufacture them, but a few are also made within the body. (Vitamin D is made in your skin when you are exposed to sunlight, and biotin and vitamin K are made by intestinal bacteria.) Vitamin deficiency diseases are rare in the United States because vitamins are readily obtainable from our food supply.

Minerals Minerals are inorganic (not carbon-containing) compounds you need in relatively small amounts to help regulate body functions, aid in growth and maintenance of body tissues, and act as catalysts for the release of energy (see Table 12-2). We know of seventeen essential minerals. The major minerals are present in the body in amounts exceeding five grams: calcium, phosphorus, magnesium, sulfur, sodium, potassium, and chloride. The essential trace minerals (which you need in tiny amounts) are chromium, cobalt, copper, fluoride, iodide, iron, manganese, molybdenum, selenium, and zinc.

Table 12-2 Functions and Food Sources of Selected Minerals

Mineral	U.S. RDA[a]	Why Needed	Food Sources
Calcium	1,000 mg[b]	Maintenance of bones and teeth; blood clotting; maintenance of cell membranes; control of nerve impulses	Milk and milk products
Phosphorus	1,000 mg	Bone growth and maintenance (teams with calcium); energy transfer in cells	Present in nearly all foods
Magnesium	400 mg	Transmission of nerve impulses; energy transfer; composition of many enzyme systems	Widespread in foods and water (except soft water)
Iron	18 mg	Component of hemoglobin (carries oxygen to tissues) and myoglobin (in muscle fibers), and enzymes	Liver, lean meats, legumes, enriched flour; absorption enhanced by presence of vitamin C
Iodine	150 micrograms	As essential part of thyroid hormones, regulation of body metabolism	Iodized salt, seafood
Zinc	15 mg	More than 70 enzyme reactions including synthesis of proteins, RNA, and DNA	Meat, eggs, liver, and seafood (especially oysters), milk, whole grains
Copper	2 mg	Iron metabolism and red blood cell formation	Liver, shellfish, nuts, dried beans

[a]For adults and children age 4 or older.
[b]For women, most authorities now recommend 1,000–1,200 mg daily before menopause and 1,500 mg after menopause.

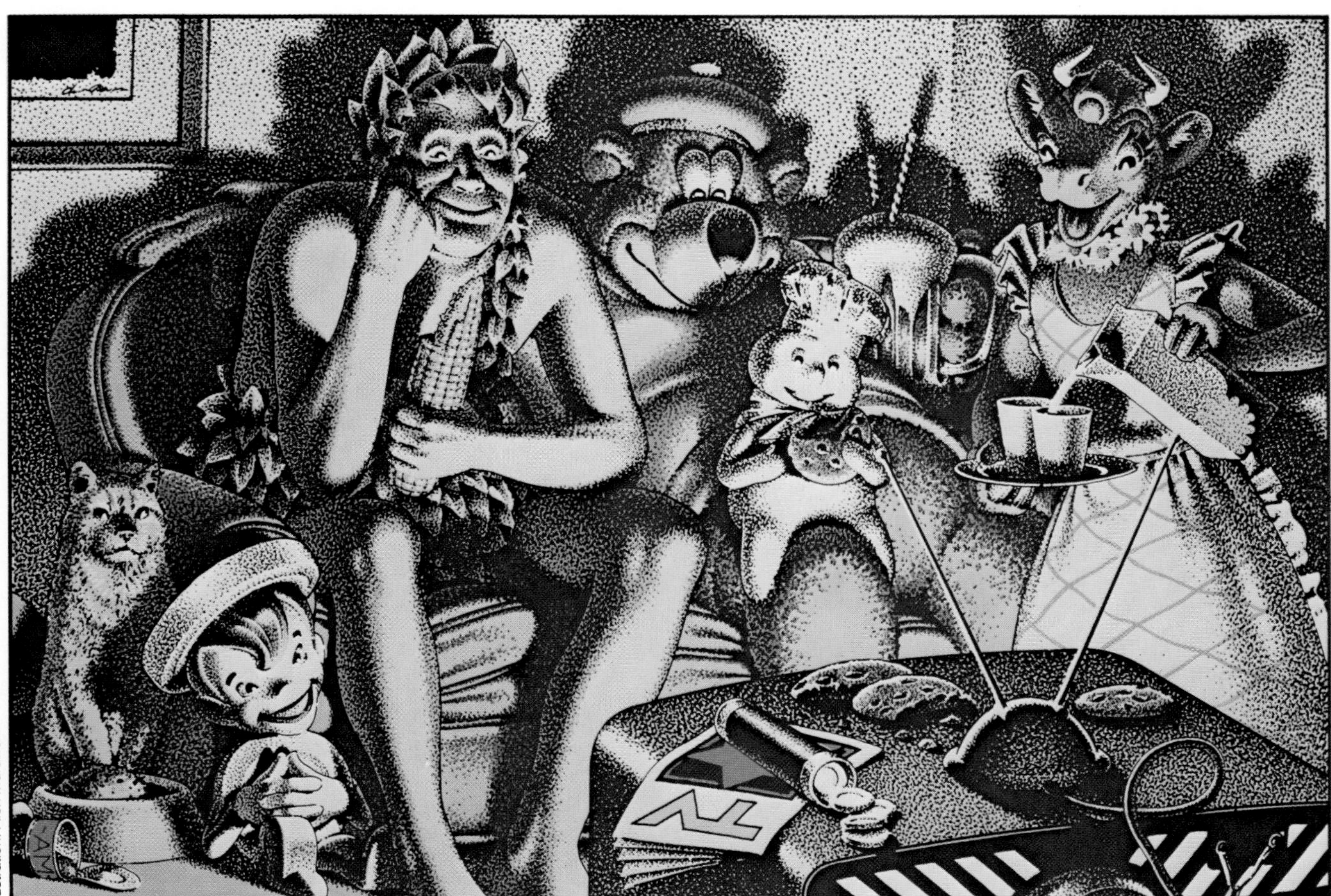

Illustration: Alex Murawski

Exploring Your Emotions

To what extent is your diet affected by television commercials? How many of these characters can you identify?

Choosing a Daily Diet

Three sets of well-publicized guidelines are available to help you make dietary choices. The **Recommended Dietary Allowances** (RDAs) are standards for preventing nutrient deficiencies. The **Basic Four Food Group system** is a method of food classification to help ensure a balanced diet of the essential nutrients. The **Dietary Guidelines for Americans** are intended to help prevent certain diet-related diseases.

Recommended Dietary Allowances Since 1943, the Food and Nutrition Board of the National Research Council/National Academy of Sciences has been publishing nutrient guidelines known as the Recommended Dietary Allowances (RDAs). These amounts are defined as "the levels of intake of essential nutrients considered adequate to meet the known nutritional needs of practically all healthy persons." The RDA for each vitamin is usually derived by estimating the range of normal human needs, selecting the number at the high end of that range, and adding a safety factor high enough to allow for body storage but not too high to cause trouble.

RDAs have been established for ten vitamins and six minerals. "Estimated safe and adequate intakes" have also been established for twelve additional vitamins and minerals for which fewer data are available. These values are revised periodically to take new research findings into account. Usually the revisions are minor.

It is important to understand that RDAs are not "requirements" or minimums, but are recommended daily *averages*. They were developed to guide food service personnel who feed large groups and are deliberately set higher

U.S. Recommended Daily Allowances A simplified version of the RDAs used in food products labels.

than most people need in order to cover the range of individual variations. Intakes equivalent to two-thirds of the RDAs are usually adequate, and higher than RDA amounts are seldom advisable.

RDA values vary somewhat according to age and sex, and are higher for pregnant and breastfeeding women. Because tables constructed from these values are relatively cumbersome for public use, the U.S. Food and Drug Administration (FDA) has devised a simpler table called the **U.S. Recommended Daily Allowances (U.S. RDAs).** These are the largest values for each age-and-sex category of the RDA values set in 1968. Tables 12-1 and 12-2 show the amounts and food sources of the vitamins and minerals for which U.S. RDAs have been established. Percentages of U.S. RDAs per portion are listed on cereal boxes and the labels of many other food products. They are also required by law on the packaging of all vitamin and mineral products.

Basic Four Food Groups Nearly all people in the United States can have a nourishing diet without having to eat foods they don't like or entirely give up foods they especially do like. This statement doesn't mean that your food choice doesn't matter; it means that each person can meet nutritional needs in many different ways. The fundamental principles of healthy eating are *moderation, variety,* and *balance.* A diet is balanced if it contains appropriate amounts of each nutrient.

The most practical guidelines for simplifying food selection comprise the Basic Four Food Groups system devised in 1955 by scientists at Harvard University's Department of Nutrition. This system groups foods according to similarity in nutrient content and designates the size and number of servings needed daily from each group to provide nutritional adequacy. The system lets you select foods from groups rather than having to calculate the amount of each nutrient in each individual portion of food. The key to using the Basic Four is to eat a variety of foods within each food group and to use moderation in choosing portion sizes.

The U.S. Department of Agriculture and many nutritionists use a fifth group—"fats, sweets, and alcohol"—composed of foods that provide calories but few, if any, vitamins. You should limit these "extras" so that you can meet your basic needs with nutrient-rich foods from the Basic Four Food Groups.

Dietary Guidelines for Americans Although the Basic Four system provides practical guidelines for avoiding nutrient deficiencies, it doesn't directly address the prevention of other diet-related health problems. To deal with this matter, the U.S. Department of Agriculture and the Department of Health and Human Services have published *Dietary Guidelines for Americans* for those who want to decrease their chances of developing certain chronic diseases. The guidelines are recommended especially for people who have risk factors such as a family history of obesity, diabetes, high blood pressure, high blood cholesterol, or heart disease early in life.

Although specific individuals at risk might benefit from quantitative advice about diet (how much of this or that to eat), the advisory committee that developed the guidelines decided that data are not extensive or clear-cut enough to make quantitative recommendations for the general public. Rather than recommending specific quantities of food or nutrients as ideal or optimal, the advisory committee suggested seven general guidelines:

1. *Eat a variety of foods.* To assure variety and a well-balanced diet, choose foods each day from five food groups: fruits; vegetables; cereals and other foods made from grains; dairy products; and meats, fish, poultry, eggs, and dry beans and peas. (These groups are identical to the traditional "Basic Four" except that fruits and vegetables are categorized separately.) Vitamin or mineral supplements are rarely needed except by some women who menstruate, are pregnant, or are breastfeeding. For babies, the guidelines suggest breastfeeding unless there are special problems, delaying solid foods until the age of 4–6 months, and not adding salt or sugar to baby foods.
2. *Maintain desirable weight.* Because obesity is associated with many serious illnesses, the guidelines suggest that the weight of adults should usually be not much more than it was at about 25 years of age (assuming it was normal at that time). For those who are overweight, the recommended loss of 1 or 2 pounds a week should be accomplished by increasing physical activity and eating low-calorie, nutrient-rich foods—more fruits, vegetables and grains, less fat and fatty foods, less sugar and sweets, and less alcoholic beverages. Diets below 800 calories per day can be hazardous and should be followed only under medical supervision.
3. *Avoid too much fat, saturated fat, and cholesterol.* Acknowledging that controversy exists, the guidelines state that "for the U.S. population as a whole, it is sensible to reduce daily consumption of fat. This suggestion is especially appropriate for individuals who have other cardiovascular risk factors such as cigarette smoking, high blood pressure, diabetes, or a family

Basic Four Food Groups

You can get all essential nutrients by eating a balanced variety of foods each day from the food groups listed here. Eat a variety of foods in each food group, and adjust serving sizes appropriately to reach and maintain your optimal weight.

Basic Food Group	Recommended Number of Servings Daily	Serving Size	Food Sources
Fruit and vegetable	4 or more	½ cup juice, or ½ cup cooked, 1 cup raw	Fruit or juice, including citrus daily Dark green leafy or bright yellow vegetables 3–4 times weekly
Grain and cereal	4 or more	1 slice	*Breads:* whole-grain and enriched, muffins, rolls, tortillas
		½–¾ cup	*Cereals:* cooked, dry, whole-grain, rice, grits, barley, flours, buckwheat, millet
		½ cup	*Pasta:* macaroni, noodles, spaghetti
			Starchy vegetables: corn, lima beans, peas, potato, pumpkin, winter squash
Milk and cheese	2 (adult)	1 cup	Milk, yogurt
	3 (child)	1½ oz.	Cheese (calcium content greater in harder varieties)
	4 (teen)		
		1–1¾ cup	Milk-containing foods
Meat and alternates	2	2–3 oz. cooked	Meat, poultry, fish
		2	Eggs
		2 tbsp.	Peanut butter, nuts
		½ cup	Cottage cheese
		1 cup	Dried beans and peas

SOURCE: From Stare, F. J., and Aronson, V. 1983. *Your Basic Guide to Nutrition*. Philadelphia: Stickley. Reprinted with permission.

history of premature heart disease." The guidelines recommend choosing lean meat, fish, poultry and dry beans and peas as protein sources; using nonfat or low-fat milk and milk products; limiting your intake of fats and oils, especially those high in saturated fat; trimming fat off meats; broiling, baking, or boiling instead of frying; and moderate use of fat-containing foods such as breaded or deep-fried foods.

4. *Eat foods with adequate starch and fiber*. Because foods differ in the kinds of fiber they contain, include a variety of fiber-rich foods such as grains, breads, cereals, fruits, and vegetables. Adding fiber to foods that do not normally contain it is not recommended.
5. *Avoid too much sugar*. The major health concern with excess sugar consumption is tooth decay. But the risk does not depend simply on how much sugar and sugar-containing foods you consume but on how often and whether you eat them between meals and stick to the teeth. Brush after eating sugary foods, take in enough fluoride, and use fluoridated toothpaste. Contrary to popular belief, too much sugar in the diet does not cause diabetes.
6. *Avoid too much sodium*. Noting that high sodium intake is sometimes a factor in high blood pressure, the guidelines suggest that you consider reducing sodium intake. You can do so by learning to enjoy the flavors of unsalted foods; adding little or no salt during cooking or at the table; flavoring foods with herbs, spices, or lemon juice; and limiting your intake of foods that are obviously salty or contain significant amounts of hidden salt.
7. *If you drink alcoholic beverages, do so in moderation*. Since many alcoholic beverages are high in calories and almost all are low in other nutrients, even moderate drinkers will need to drink less if they are overweight and wish to reduce. Because the level of con-

The Vegetarian Diet—Advantages and Disadvantages

Variety and balance in the diet are as important to the vegetarian as to anyone else. Although vegetarians usually consume far more of some nutrients than other people do–namely, those nutrients present in plant foods, such as folic acid, vitamin A, and vitamin C—other vitamins and minerals are of particular concern.

Protein

A common concern of many vegetarians is whether they consume adequate protein. By including milk and/or eggs in their diets along with a variety of plant proteins, ovolactovegetarians can easily meet the U.S. Recommended Daily Allowance (RDA) for protein, although if they rely too heavily on dairy products they risk consuming excess fat. Since children, proportional to body weight, have a greater need for protein than do adults, it is especially important to give them a variety of protein-rich foods each day.

Current research indicates that eating complementary proteins to ensure adequate intake of essential amino acids may not be as critical to vegans as previously believed. Although consumption of essential amino acids is certainly important, as long as vegetarians consume enough varied plant protein each day (about 60 grams), they will maintain nitrogen balance. An advantage of vegetarian protein foods is that they are often higher in fiber than meats, richer in certain vitamins and minerals, and lower in fat.

Vitamin B_{12}

Plant foods do not contain vitamin B_{12}. It is found only in foods of animal origin and in special nutrient supplements such as vitamin B_{12}-enriched food. The ovolactovegetarian has no problem getting enough vitamin B_{12}, but the vegan needs a reliable source, such as vitamin B_{12}-fortified soy milk or yeast.

It takes a long time for vitamin B_{12} deficiency to develop after someone has given up animal foods, because the body can store up to four years' worth.

When the deficiency does occur, it can damage the brain and nerves irreversibly. A pregnant or lactating vegan should be aware that her infant can develop a vitamin B_{12} deficiency even if she remains healthy. This deficiency is extraordinarily damaging to developing infants; all vegan mothers must consume vitamin B_{12}-fortified products or take the appropriate supplements.

Vitamin D

Although the milk drinker is protected from deficiency as long as the milk is vitamin D-fortified, there is no practical source of vitamin D in plant foods. Regular exposure to sun will prevent a deficiency, but the homebound or vegans living in a northern climate or a smoggy city probably should take vitamin D supplements or drink soy milk fortified with vitamin D. Supplements should not exceed the RDA of 5 micrograms: excesses are toxic.

Riboflavin

Again, the milk-drinking vegetarian is protected from this deficiency, but the vegan must take special care to frequently include ample servings of dark greens to ensure that riboflavin needs are met. Nutritional yeast is another rich source of riboflavin for the vegan.

Calcium

It is next to impossible for the vegan to meet calcium needs without drinking two to three cups of calcium-fortified soy milk each day. Also recommended are ample and regular servings of self-rising flour and cornmeal, almonds and filberts, tofu, sesame seeds, and blackstrap molasses. Vegan children should receive calcium-fortified soy milk daily. If not, then calcium supplements must be taken daily, along with the other food sources just mentioned.

Iron

Vegetarians should pay special attention to their iron intake because the best iron sources are meats. Good sources include legumes, whole-grain breads and cereals, dark-green leafy vegetables, and dried fruits. But though iron absorption is three times higher from meat, vitamin C in fruits and vegetables can triple absorption from other iron-containing foods eaten at the same meal.

Overall Health

Compared to their meat-eating peers, informed vegetarians are more likely to be at their ideal weight and to have lower blood cholesterol levels, lower rates of certain kinds of cancer, and better digestive function. However, one must consider nondietary factors as well. For example, vegetarians often abstain from smoking and drinking. It is therefore hard to know whether their dietary practices alone account for their improved health, though they clearly contribute to it.

Cost

Because grains and other plant foods often cost less than meats, provide larger servings of food per ounce, and contain a greater variety of vitamins and minerals, vegetarians receive more nutrients for their food dollars. They also receive more nutrients for their calories, because most fruits and vegetables are nutrient-dense.

Environment

The consumption of plant proteins, such as legumes and grains, permits a much more economical use of land than the consumption of animal proteins. A million calories in wheat can be produced on less than an acre of land; a million calories in beef require 17 acres. We may soon find that we cannot afford the luxury of using seventeen times as much land to produce the same amount of food energy.

Social Aspects

One social advantage the vegetarian has is a unique opportunity to introduce meat-eating friends to a new and different way of eating. A vegetarian meal prepared with several familiar and some not-so-familiar, but delicious, foods can be a real treat for the person whose meal is usually centered around meat. Not only does such a meal generate conversation and interest, but it can also inspire new ways to select, prepare, and eat foods.

One social disadvantage is that the vegetarian's meat-eating friends may be hesitant to extend dinner invitations. They simply don't know what to prepare. One can easily overcome this hesitation by assuring them that they need not prepare a tofu and lentil bean casserole, because a simple meal such as macaroni and cheese, steamed vegetables, and a fruit salad is quite satisfying to anyone. Another social disadvantage is that many restaurants offer limited vegetarian choices. One must be creative and skillful in selecting menu items if one excludes meat or seafood. Chinese, Mexican, and Italian restaurants often have good vegetarian selections.

SOURCE: Linda K. DeBruyne, M.S., R.D., 1985 (August), *Healthline*.

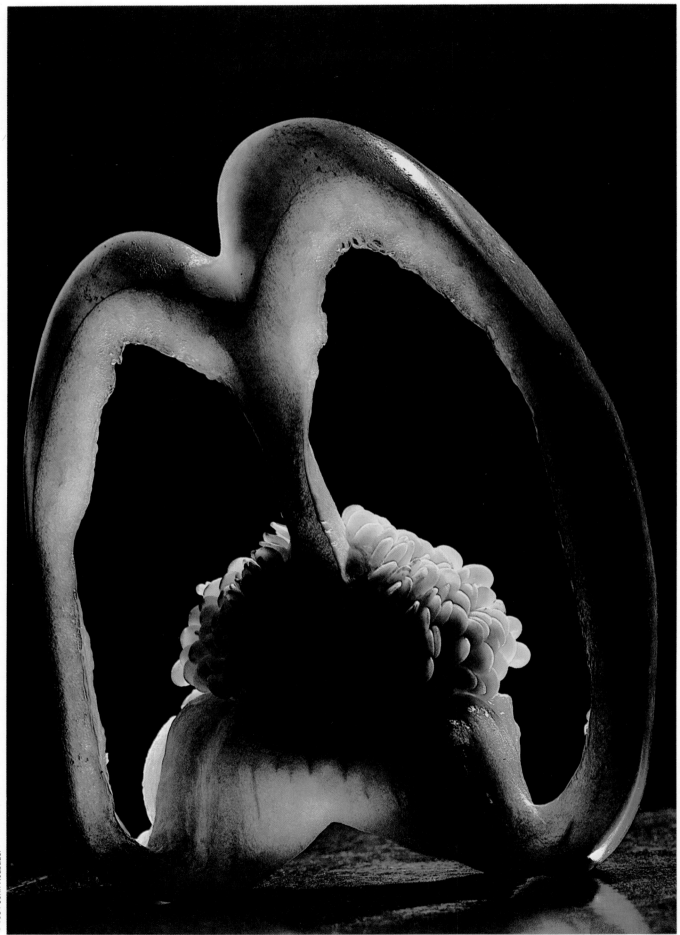

Vegans Vegetarians who eat no animal products at all.

Lactovegetarians Vegetarians who include milk and cheese products in their diet.

Lactovovegetarians Vegetarians who eat no meat, poultry, or fish, but do eat eggs and milk products.

Legumes Vegetables such as peas and beans.

Tofu A custardlike food made from soybeans.

sumption at which there is risk of birth defects to unborn children has not been established, pregnant women are advised to abstain completely from alcohol.

Vegetarian Eating Several million Americans restrict or eliminate foods of animal origin (meat, poultry, fish, eggs, milk) from their diet. Most do so because they think foods of plant origin are healthier, more natural, and take less energy to produce. Some do so for religious reasons. Vegetarians may be classified into three main categories: strict vegetarians (**vegans**), who eat no animal products at all; **lactovegetarians,** who eat milk and cheese products in addition to vegetables; and **lactovovegetarians,** who eat no meat, poultry, or fish but do include eggs and milk products.

A vegetarian diet can provide all the nutrients needed for proper growth and health. However, you must select foods carefully to ensure that your diet contains an adequate supply of protein, iron, calcium, zinc, and vitamin B_{12}. (The more foods you avoid, the more careful your selection should be.) Strict vegetarianism is undesirable for children under 5 years old because it is difficult for vegans to meet children's high requirements for protein and several other nutrients. Growing adolescents may have difficulty getting adequate caloric and nutrient intake from a vegan diet. Nor is strict vegetarianism a good idea for pregnant or lactating women. Since B_{12} is present only in animal foods and a limited number of specially fortified foods, vegans should probably take B_{12} supplements.

Proteins from some legumes—particularly soybeans and garbanzo beans (ceci beans, or chickpeas)—are close in nutritional quality to those from animal sources. Combining a small amount of animal protein with plant foods helps improve the overall protein quality of the diet. You can also get high-quality protein by combining plant foods that have complementary amino acids—that is, the amino acids that are insufficient in one food are provided by the complementing food. Legumes are complementary to grains and also to nuts and seeds. **Legumes** include blackeyed peas, peanuts, split peas, garbanzos, **tofu** (soybean curd), lentils, and many other types of beans and peas.

Labeling Foods Under current regulations, food labels must contain the following information if a nutrient has been added or a nutrition claim is made about the food: serving size and number of servings per container; calorie, protein, carbohydrate, fat, and sodium content; and percentage of U.S. RDAs of vitamin A, vitamin C, thiamin, riboflavin, niacin, calcium, and iron.

Exploring Your Emotions

Are you worried about additives and other chemicals in your food? Research one of your concerns, and write a "letter to the editor" of your student paper.

An optional listing may include the fat content by degree of saturation, the amount of cholesterol, the amount of potassium, and the percentage of U.S. RDAs of vitamins D, E, B_6, and B_{12}, folic acid, phosphorus, iodine, magnesium, zinc, copper, biotin, and pantothenic acid.

For most food products, ingredients must also be listed. The ingredient used in the largest amount by weight must be listed first, followed by others in descending order. However, the actual amounts do not have to be stated.

Vitamin and Mineral Supplementation

Many vitamin promoters suggest that everyone should take supplements to be sure that they get enough nutrients. They say, for example, that "eating on the run" and "overprocessing" of foods make the typical American in danger of deficiency. Some also claim that "soil depletion," snack-

(*Text continues on p. 272*)

Exploring Your Emotions

Are your tastes in food "your own," or do they derive from your childhood family customs? When you entered college, how did your eating habits change? Do you feel more comfortable with your current habits, or less? Why?

How to Keep the Natural Goodness in Food

- To preserve water-soluble vitamins, avoid prolonged soaking of fresh vegetables. Don't wash rice before cooking; you'll wash B vitamins down the drain.
- Prepare salads just before serving. Also delay cutting up and cooking vegetables until the last minute to reduce the loss of vitamin C. (The most nutritious way to eat fruits and vegetables is raw.)
- Boil vegetables until just tender in a minimum amount of water, using a pot with a tight-fitting lid to prevent vitamin loss. Do not thaw or wash frozen vegetables before cooking.
- Pressure cooking is the least damaging to vitamins. Steaming is second best, boiling less desirable. Frying leads to some vitamin loss, but a more serious disadvantage is that it adds fat and significantly increases the ratio of calories to nutrients.
- Broiling, frying, and roasting retain more B vitamins in meats than do braising and stewing. But in braised meats and stews, you can recapture lost vitamins by consuming the broth. Meats cooked rare retain more heat-sensitive thiamin than well-done meats.
- Potatoes boiled or baked whole in the skin retain nearly all their vitamins. In general, the smaller the pieces into which you cut vegetables before cooking, the greater the vitamin loss.
- Foods that are cooked ahead and later reheated can lose significant amounts of vitamins, especially C. This is not of major significance, however, as long as you have other sources of vitamin C in your diet.
- Cooking in copper pots can destroy vitamins C and E and folacin, unless the pots are well lined. Pots made of iron, brass, or monel (a nickel alloy) also destroy some of the vitamin C. But glass, stainless steel, aluminum, and enamel cookware do not affect nutrients.
- Use the cooking water from vegetables and the drippings from meats (after skimming off the fat) in soups and gravy. That way you recapture many of the lost vitamins. You can also use the vitamin-rich liquid from canned fruits to prepare gelatin desserts or fruit-flavored beverages.

Jane E. Brody, *Jane Brody's Nutrition Book*

Food Additives

Additives make up less than 1 percent of our food. The most widely used are sugar, salt, and corn syrup. These three, plus citric acid (found naturally in oranges and lemons), baking soda, vegetable colors, mustard, and pepper, account for 98 percent by weight of all food additives used in the United States.

By broadest definition, a food additive is any substance that becomes part of a food product when added directly or indirectly. Today some 2,800 substances are intentionally added to foods for one or more of the following reasons:

- *To maintain or improve nutritional quality*. Vitamins and minerals can be added to enrich (replace those lost in processing) or fortify (add nutrients lacking in the diet). Breads and cereals are enriched with B vitamins lost or destroyed during milling and processing of grains. Common examples of fortification include the addition of vitamin D to milk, vitamin A to margarine, vitamin C to fruit drinks, and iodine to table salt. These measures have helped eradicate such once-prevalent deficiency diseases as rickets, scurvy, pellagra, and goiter.
- *To maintain freshness*. Foods last as long as they do on the shelf or in the refrigerator because of additives that retard spoilage, preserve natural color and flavor, and keep fats and oils from turning rancid. Nitrates and nitrites, for example, protect meats from contamination with the toxin responsible for botulism, a deadly form of food poisoning. Antioxidants such as butylated hydroxyanisole (BHA) or butylated hydroxytoluene (BHT) help prevent changes in color, flavor, or texture that occur when foods are exposed to air. And vitamin C keeps

Food Additives (*continued*)

uncooked peaches from turning brown. The use of sulfites for maintaining the freshness of foods in salad bars was recently banned because some people developed severe allergic reactions after eating foods thus treated.

- *To help in processing or preparation.* Many products give body and texture to foods, blend food components, improve baking qualities, control acidity or alkalinity, retain moisture, and prevent caking or lumping. For example, emulsifiers give peanut butter a smooth flavor and texture and prevent it from separating into an oily layer at the top of the jar and a solid layer at the bottom. Thickeners create smoothness and prevent ice crystals from forming in frozen foods such as ice cream. Leavening agents such as yeasts and baking powder make baked goods rise by releasing carbon dioxide during the cooking process.
- *To alter taste or appearance.* Products to improve flavor or looks include coloring agents, natural and synthetic flavors, flavor enhancers such as monosodium glutamate (MSG), and sweeteners. More than 30 coloring agents are currently permitted for use in food. About half are vegetable extracts, and the rest are laboratory creations not found in nature. About 1,700 natural and synthetic substances are used to flavor foods. Some artificial flavors (such as vanillin, the chemical that gives vanilla its taste) are chemically identical to their natural counterparts, while others (such as saccharin) are not. However, the general concept of using artificial colors and flavors has been controversial, with proponents saying they are needed to enhance consumer enjoyment and critics saying that they present unnecessary risks. A few artificial colors have been banned by the Food and Drug Administration (FDA) because they were suspected of causing cancer.

"Natural food" advocates suggest that too many chemicals are being added to our foods. However, the important issue is not the number of chemicals, but whether they are safe and serve useful purposes. It is illogical to condemn additives with sweeping generalizations; the only proper way to evaluate them is to do so individually. This evaluation is the responsibility of the FDA, which has been paying a great deal of attention to this matter. Food additives, particularly those introduced in the past twenty years, have survived rigid testing procedures and scientific review not applied to the great majority of natural products. To remain on the market, additives must be judged both safe and significantly useful.

Food irradiation is regulated by the FDA under the terms of the 1958 Food Additives Amendment to the Federal Food, Drug, and Cosmetic Act, which specifies that irradiation must be regarded as an additive. Although irradiation is a process, Congress wanted to ensure that it would have to meet the stringent safety standards of food additives.

Irradiation can cause minor changes in the taste of foods similar to those caused by cooking, canning, or freezing, but it does not significantly affect nutritional contents. Unlike chemical pesticides, radiation leaves no residue in food; nor does it expose those who eat the foods to radiation. Foods processed with irradiation do not become radioactive, just as people do not become radioactive from a chest X-ray.

Low-dose irradiation was approved more than twenty years ago to inhibit sprouting of potatoes and to kill insects in wheat and wheat flour, but it has not been used for these purposes commercially. Recently, low-dose radiation was approved to inhibit ripening and spoilage of harvested fruits and vegetables and to kill the parasite in pork that causes trichinosis. High-dose irradiation is now permitted to kill micro-organisms in herbs and spices. Irradiated foods must be identified by the words "Treated with radiation" and the international logo shown here:

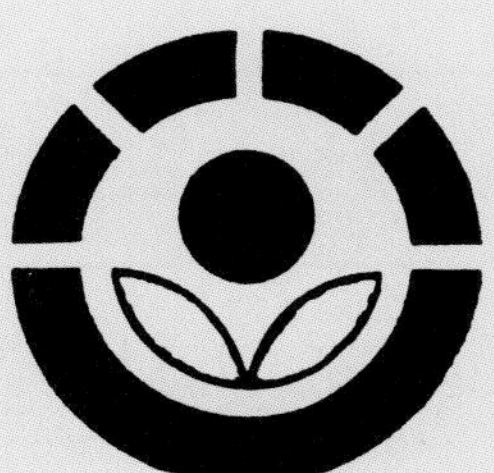

Problem Additives

Two additives remaining on the market can cause adverse reactions in susceptible individuals: sulfites and monosodium glutamate (MSG).

(continued on next page)

Food Additives (*continued*)

Sulfites are used to control micro-organisms in wine and to delay spoilage in many foods and drugs. As already mentioned, they have also been used to keep vegetables looking fresh in salad bars. Recently, however, it was determined that some people can experience asthmatic attacks, hives, diarrhea, or other symptoms when exposed to sulfites. Most reactions have been mild, but a few deaths from anaphylactic shock have been reported. The FDA has therefore banned use of sulfites on raw fruits and vegetables and requires warning labels on all packaged foods that contain detectable amounts of sulfites.

MSG is the sodium salt of glutamic acid, an amino acid abundant in both plant and animal proteins. MSG is used as a flavor enhancer, but most of the MSG we ingest is naturally present in our foods, not added. Most people have no trouble with MSG, but some experience unpleasant effects such as dizziness, weakness, headaches, chest pain, palpitations, nausea, and vomiting. This problem is referred to as the "Chinese restaurant syndrome" because MSG is commonly added to Chinese foods. Individuals sensitive to MSG can limit their intake by checking food labels, particularly of commercial soups, broths, soy sauce, gravies, spice blends, sausages, and salad dressings. They may also have to avoid restaurants where MSG is used in cooking. (Some Chinese restaurants will omit it if asked to do so.)

The Feingold Diet

In 1973, Benjamin Feingold, M.D., a pediatric allergist from California, proposed that salicylates, artificial colors, and artificial flavors were causes of hyperactivity in children. To relieve this problem, he suggested a diet free of these additives. He recommended further that the hyperactive child be included in the preparation of special foods and encouraged the family to participate in the dietary program.

Many parents who have followed Feingold's recommendations have reported improvement in their children's behavior, and many have joined Feingold Societies to promote the dietary program. However, carefully designed experiments have failed to support the idea that additives cause hyperactivity. Improvement, if any, appears related to changes in family dynamics such as paying more attention to the children. Because the Feingold diet appears to do no physical harm, it might seem sensible to try. However, the potential benefits must be weighed against the potential harm of falsely communicating to a child that behavior is determined by what he or she eats rather than by what he or she feels.

There's No Such Thing as "Junk Food" But There Are Junk *Diets*

During the past fifteen years, the term "junk food" has become part of America's everyday vocabulary. But as a nutritionist, I contend that this term is meaningless and should be discarded. In my opinion, there is no totally worthless food any more than there is a perfect food that meets *all* our nutritional needs.

Obviously, some foods contribute greater amounts of nutrients than others do. But most foods have *some* redeeming value under the right circumstances. The problem arises when foods that contribute more calories than nutrients crowd out foods of higher nutritional value in our diet. It is equally possible to make an unbalanced selection of nutritious foods and wind up with a diet overabundant in some nutrients yet deficient in others. In other cases, the result is a junk *diet*.

Some foods have little nutritional virtue by themselves. For example, in some cakes and cookies, most of the calories come from ingredients such as fat and sugar, and relatively few come from milk, flour, and eggs. However, if eating a cookie means that a child also drinks milk or fruit juice, we should look at cookie-and-milk or cookie-and-juice as a unit and judge them together rather than condemn one and applaud the other. For an 8-year-old, milk and

There's No Such Thing as "Junk Food" But There Are Junk *Diets* (*continued*)

one or two cookies make a nutritious combination. Milk and five cookies, though, may create an imbalance between calories and nutrients—and thus be considered lower in nutrition.

Potato chips are another example of a food that can be valuable in the right context. Eaten alone, potato chips add vitamin C, vitamin B_6, and copper to our diet. Eaten with a sandwich, potato chips become part of a balanced meal. But if we stuff ourselves with so many potato chips that we're too full to eat dinner, we are misusing them. "And what about the salt?" you may ask. One ounce of potato chips provides about 0.25 gram of sodium—less than sodium in sandwich bread and considerably less than in two slices of bread spread with salted butter. Just because you see and taste the salt doesn't mean that potato chips contain too much.

For another example, consider pizza. Some people see it as a junk food because it is high in calories, cholesterol, and fat. But pizza has nutritional merits comparable to a meat-and-cheese sandwich served with tomato.

How about the classically "healthful" foods like milk, eggs, orange juice, and oatmeal? Are they always desirable? Surprisingly, no. Milk, especially nonfat milk, has one of the most impressive nutrient profiles of any food. But it isn't perfect. While high in calcium, protein, and riboflavin, it is low in iron and vitamin C. In contrast, oranges are high in iron and vitamin C, but low in calcium, protein, and riboflavin.

What does this have to do with junk food? When a food doesn't meet an immediate nutritional need, its nutritional value is limited. After an adult has had two or three glasses of milk (which meet many nutritional needs), additional milk becomes less and less useful. If milk (which does not provide vitamin C) displaces fruit juice that does, it becomes worthless except as a source of calories. In this context, the extra milk would be a "junk" food. The key point to remember is that food should not be judged in isolation but in relation to your total diet and your individual needs.

If all your daily nutrient needs are met except for calories, you can obtain the rest of your calorie requirements from any food. Of course, moderation is a virtue. And so is avoiding excess amounts of saturated fats, sodium, calories, and cholesterol. Getting a maximum of 10 to 15 percent of your total daily calories from foods of limited nutritional value is a reasonable limit. Frequent eating of sticky sweets, especially between meals, should also be questioned because of its possible contribution to tooth decay.

In choosing nutritious foods, we might also consider the cost per nutrient. Many parents feel good about giving their children buttered toast and honey for breakfast but feel guilty if they serve a doughnut. Since both bread and doughnuts are made with enriched flour—and often with whole-wheat flour—there is no appreciable difference in their vitamin content. Considering cost, however, the doughnut is not as good a buy. Similar considerations hold for french-fried and baked potatoes. Nutritionally, a serving of french fries cooked in oil compares favorably with a baked potato served with a fat such as sour cream or butter. However, the cost per nutrient of commercially prepared french fries can be considerably higher than that of home-prepared baked potatoes.

People should eat the right amounts and combinations of nutrients to promote health, but they should eat in a rational way, without feeling guilty about including a favorite food merely for the pleasure it provides. Special medical considerations aside, a healthful diet can include at least small amounts of any food you enjoy—as long as your overall diet is moderate in calories and properly balanced.

SOURCE: Helen A. Guthrie, Ph.D., R.D., 1986, *Healthline*.

Anemia A deficiency in the oxygen-carrying material in the red blood cells.

Osteoporosis A condition, mostly affecting women, in which the bones become extremely thin and brittle.

ing, and dieting are additional reasons people need supplements; however, such claims are misleading.

Vitamin deficiency is rare unless a person's diet is extremely unbalanced. Eating large quantities of fast foods can result in an excessive intake of fats, calories, and sodium, but rarely results in vitamin deficiency. Nor will dieting cause vitamin deficiency unless it is prolonged or highly unbalanced. Although some types of food processing remove nutrients, other types add them. Some vitamins are lost in cooking, but such losses are usually only partial and are taken into account in the Basic Four system's recommendation to include uncooked fruits and vegetables in the daily diet. The idea that "depleted soils" rob the American diet of nutrients is also incorrect. The vitamin content of plants is determined by their heredity, not the soil they're grown in. Although the mineral content of plants *is* influenced by soil composition, crop rotation and fertilizers ensure that plants get adequate amounts of minerals.

Exploring Your Emotions

Onions are a main vegetable in human diets all over the world. Do you like them? Why or why not? Do some research to find out which nutrition claims are scientific and which are based on folk myths.

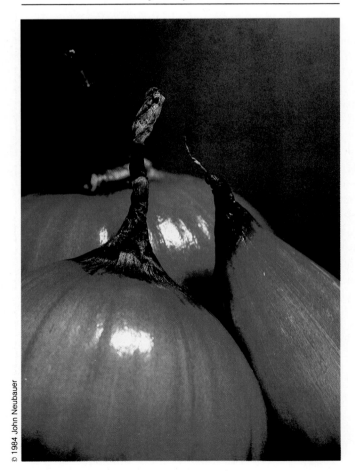

Although mineral deficiencies are not difficult to prevent, special attention should be paid to the minerals iron, calcium, and fluoride. You need iron to form red blood cells, and lack of it produces **anemia**. Because women who menstruate or are pregnant need ample amounts of iron, they should be careful to include iron-rich foods such as liver, veal, other meats, fish, and soybeans in their diet. However, self-medication with supplementary iron is unwise unless iron deficiency anemia is medically diagnosed through a blood test.

Women should also pay close attention to their calcium intake. Adequate calcium intake is one factor that can help prevent **osteoporosis**, a condition where bones become thinner and weaken later in life. Women who don't consume several portions of dairy products daily should consult their doctors about taking calcium supplements.

Fluoride, needed to build decay-resistant teeth during their formative years, cannot be obtained in adequate amounts from food. The best way to obtain it is from fluoridated water. Children raised in nonfluoridated communities should be given supplements from birth through age 12 as recommended by their physician or dentist.

The best way to get vitamins is from foods in a balanced diet, and balancing one's diet is not difficult. Vitamin supplementation may be appropriate for children up to 2 years old or who have poor eating habits, for some persons on prolonged weight reduction programs, for pregnant women (who may need folic acid), and for strict vegetarians (who may need B_{12} supplements). But the decision to supplement or not should be made on a logical basis. *Consumer Reports* magazine suggests,

> Rather than taking vitamins for "insurance," evaluate your diet to determine whether you are eating a variety of foods from the Basic Four groups. If you have trouble figuring that out by yourself, record what you eat for a week and ask a registered dietitian or physician whether you are missing anything. If you are, the best course of action will probably be to improve your eating habits. As a rule, don't take more than RDA amounts except on medical advice. And avoid doctors or nutrition consultants who recommend vitamins as cure-alls.

CSPI's Fast Food Eating Guide

For better or for worse, fast foods are here to stay. If you choose carefully, however, it's possible to get a fast food meal that isn't overburdened with fat, sodium, sugar, and calories. When you evaluate different foods, first consider their calorie, fat, sodium, and sugar content. Keep in mind that the average adult should consume no more than about 10–15 teaspoons of fat and 1,100 to 3,300 milligrams of sodium per day.

Fish

	Calories	Fat (tsp)	Sodium (mg)
Chilled shrimp, 1 piece *(L. J. Silver)*	**6**	0	19
Battered shrimp, 1 piece *(L. J. Silver)*	**47**	1	154
Baked fish w/sauce *(L. J. Silver)*	**151**	0	361
Catfish, one ¾ ounce piece *(Church's)*	**67**	1	151
Trout w/lemon-garlic butter *(Carl's Jr.)*	**200**	3	190
Fish *(Treacher's)*	**355**	5	450
¼-pound fish filet sandwich *(D'Lites)*	**390**	5	520
Fisherman's filet *(Hardee's)*	**469**	5	1013
Whaler sandwich *(Burger King)*	**540**	5	745
Moby Jack *(Jack-Box)*	**444**	6	820
Filet-o-Fish *(McDonald's)*	**435**	6	799
Filet of fish sandwich *(Carl's Jr.)*	**570**	6	790
Shrimp *(Treacher's)*	**381**	6	538
Whaler sandwich w/cheese *(Burger King)*	**590**	6	885
Fish sandwich *(Treacher's)*	**440**	5	836

Potatoes

Baked & Others	Calories	Fat (tsp)	Sodium (mg)
Baked potato *(several)*	**215**	0	10
Mashed potatoes *(Ky. Fd. Chkn.)*	**64**	0	268
Potato skins, per skin *(D'Lites)*	**90**	1	174
Potato w/margarine *(Roy Rogers)*	**274**	2	161
Mexiskins, per skin *(D'Lites)*	**99**	2	227
Hash brown potatoes *(McDonald's)*	**125**	2	325
Wedge cut potatoes *(Carl's Jr.)*	**252**	3	8
Potato cakes (2) *(Arby's)*	**201**	3	476
Potato w/chicken a la king *(Wendy's)*	**350**	1	820
Hash rounds *(Hardee's)*	**200**	3	310
Potato w/broccoli & cheddar *(D'Lites)*	**410**	4	820
Potato w/chili & cheese *(Wendy's)*	**510**	5	610
Potato w/sour cream & chives *(Wendy's)*	**460**	5	230
Mexican potato *(D'Lites)*	**510**	4	1000
Broccoli & cheddar potato *(Arby's)*	**541**	5	475
Mushroom & cheese potato *(Arby's)*	**510**	5	640
Potato w/taco beef & cheese *(Roy Rogers)*	**463**	5	726
Potato w/stroganoff & sour cream *(Wendy's)*	**490**	5	910
Home fries *(Wendy's)*	**360**	5	745
Taco potato *(Arby's)*	**620**	6	1060
Potato w/cheese *(Wendy's)*	**590**	8	450
Potato w/bacon & cheese *(Wendy's)*	**570**	7	1180
Deluxe potato *(Arby's)*	**650**	9	480

Fries	Calories	Fat (tsp)	Sodium (mg)
Kentucky fries *(Ky. Fd. Chkn.)*	**184**	2	174
Fries, regular *(McDonald's)*	**220**	3	109
Fryes, bigger better *(L. J. Silver)*	**247**	3	6

(continued on next page)

CSPI's Fast Food Eating Guide (*continued*)

Fries	Calories	Fat (tsp)	Sodium (mg)
French fries, regular (*D'Lites*)	**260**	3	100
French fries, small (*Hardee's*)	**239**	3	121
French fries, regular (*Burger King*)	**210**	3	230
French fries (*Arby's*)	**211**	2	39
French fries, regular (*Wendy's*)	**280**	3	95
Chips (*Treacher's*)	**276**	3	393
French fries, large (*Hardee's*)	**381**	5	192

Chicken

	Calories	Fat (tsp)	Sodium (mg)
Original Recipe drumstick (*Ky. Fd. Chkn.*)	**117**	1	207
Chicken breasts (2) (*Carl's Jr.*)	**200**	1	600
Litely breaded chicken (*D'Lites*)	**170**	2	430
Original Recipe wing (*Ky. Fd. Chkn.*)	**136**	2	302
Fried chicken leg (*Church's*)	**147**	2	286
Chicken sandwich, multi-grain bun (*Wendy's*)	**320**	2	500
Roasted chicken breast (*Arby's*)	**254**	2	930
Original Recipe breast (*Ky. Fd. Chkn.*)	**199**	3	558
Chicken filet sandwich (*D'Lites*)	**280**	3	760
Original Recipe thigh (*Ky. Fd. Chkn.*)	**257**	4	566
Chicken breast (*Roy Rogers*)	**324**	4	601
Fried breast (*Church's*)	**278**	4	560
Kentucky Nuggets (6) (*Ky. Fd. Chkn.*)	**282**	4	810
Chicken McNuggets (6) (*McDonald's*)	**323**	5	512
Fried wing (*Church's*)	**303**	4	583
Charbroiler chicken sandwich (*Carl's Jr.*)	**450**	3	1380
Fried thigh (*Church's*)	**305**	5	448
Chicken filet sandwich (*Hardee's*)	**510**	6	360
Extra Crispy thigh (*Ky. Fd. Chkn.*)	**343**	5	549
Chicken sandwich (*Treacher's*)	**413**	4	708
Turkey club sandwich (*Hardee's*)	**426**	5	1185
Chicken breast filet sand. (*Ky. Fd. Chkn.*)	**436**	5	1093
Chicken breast & wing (*Roy Rogers*)	**466**	6	867
Chicken salad croissant (*Arby's*)	**460**	8	725
Chicken club sandwich (*Arby's*)	**620**	7	1300
Chicken Supreme (*Jack-Box*)	**601**	8	1582
Specialty chicken sandwich (*Burger King*)	**690**	10	775

Burgers, Roast Beef, Steak, Ham

Burgers	Calories	Fat (tsp)	Sodium (mg)
Jr. D'Lite (*D'Lites*)	**200**	2	210
Hamburger, kid's meal (*Wendy's*)	**200**	2	265
Hamburger (*McDonald's*)	**263**	3	506
Hamburger (*Burger King*)	**310**	3	560
Hamburger (*Hardee's*)	**305**	3	682
Happy Star hamburger (*Carl's Jr.*)	**330**	3	670
Hamburger, multi-grain bun (*Wendy's*)	**340**	4	290
Cheeseburger (*McDonald's*)	**318**	4	743
Cheeseburger (*Burger King*)	**360**	4	705
Bacon cheeseburger (*D'Lites*)	**370**	4	730
Whopper Jr. (*Burger King*)	**370**	4	545
Double D'Lite (*D'Lites*)	**450**	5	290
Cheeseburger (*Hardee's*)	**335**	4	789
Double hamburger (*Burger King*)	**430**	5	585
Whopper Jr. w/cheese (*Burger King*)	**410**	5	685

Burgers	Calories	Fat (tsp)	Sodium (mg)
Quarter-Pounder *(McDonald's)*	**427**	5	718
Hamburger *(Roy Rogers)*	**456**	6	495
Jumbo Jack *(Jack-Box)*	**485**	6	905
Mushroom 'n' Swiss burger *(Hardee's)*	**512**	5	1051
Big Deluxe *(Hardee's)*	**546**	6	1083
Bacon cheeseburger, white bun *(Wendy's)*	**460**	6	860
Famous Star hamburger *(Carl's Jr.)*	**530**	7	705
Quarter-Pounder w/cheese *(McDonald's)*	**525**	7	1220
Big Mac *(McDonald's)*	**570**	8	979
Bacon double-cheeseburger *(Burger King)*	**600**	8	985
Whopper *(Burger King)*	**670**	9	975
Cheeseburger *(Roy Rogers)*	**463**	8	1404
Western bacon cheeseburger *(Carl's Jr.)*	**670**	9	1330
McD-L-T *(McDonald's)*	**680**	10	1030
RR-Bar Burger *(Roy Rogers)*	**611**	9	1826
Whopper w/cheese *(Burger King)*	**760**	10	1260
Bacon Cheeseburger Supreme *(Jack-Box)*	**724**	10	1307
Super Star hamburger *(Carl's Jr.)*	**780**	11	785
Double-beef Whopper *(Burger King)*	**890**	12	1015
Double-beef Whopper w/cheese *(Burger King)*	**980**	14	1295
Triple cheeseburger *(Wendy's)*	**1040**	15	1848

Roast Beef Sandwiches	Calories	Fat (tsp)	Sodium (mg)
California roast beef *(Carl's Jr.)*	**300**	2	505
Junior roast beef *(Arby's)*	**220**	2	530
Roast beef sandwich *(Roy Rogers)*	**317**	2	785
Regular roast beef *(Arby's)*	**350**	3	880
Roast beef sandwich *(Hardee's)*	**377**	4	1030
Roast beef sand w/cheese *(Roy Rogers)*	**424**	4	1694
Large roast beef w/cheese *(Roy Rogers)*	**467**	5	1953
Super roast beef *(Arby's)*	**620**	6	1420
Bac'n cheddar deluxe *(Arby's)*	**561**	8	1375

Steak	Calories	Fat (tsp)	Sodium (mg)
Top sirloin steak *(Carl's Jr.)*	**210**	2	85
Steak biscuit *(Hardee's)*	**419**	5	804
Charbroiler steak sandwich *(Carl's Jr.)*	**630**	8	700

Ham Sandwiches	Calories	Fat (tsp)	Sodium (mg)
Hot ham 'n cheese *(D'Lites)*	**280**	2	1160
Hot ham 'n cheese *(Hardee's)*	**376**	3	1067
Hot ham 'n cheese sandwich *(Arby's)*	**353**	3	1655
Ham biscuit *(Hardee's)*	**349**	4	1415
Specialty ham & cheese *(Burger King)*	**550**	7	1550

Desserts

	Calories	Fat (tsp)	Sodium (mg)	Sugar (tsp)
Chocolate D'Lite *(D'Lites)*	**203**	1	70	5
Soft serve with cone *(McDonald's)*	**185**	1	109	4
Strawberry sundae *(McDonald's)*	**320**	2	90	9
Caramel sundae *(McDonald's)*	**361**	2	145	10
Lemon meringue pie *(L. J. Silver)*	**200**	1	254	5
Brownie *(Roy Rogers)*	**264**	3	150	5
McDonaldland cookies *(McDonald's)*	**308**	2	358	6

(continued on next page)

CSPI's Fast Food Eating Guide (*continued*)

	Calories	Fat (tsp)	Sodium (mg)	Sugar (tsp)
Hot fudge sundae (*Roy Rogers*)	**337**	3	186	9
Lemon Luv fried pie (*Treacher's*)	**276**	3	314	3
Frosty dairy dessert, 12 oz. (*Wendy's*)	**400**	3	220	10
Apple turnover (*Hardee's*)	**282**	3	310	5
Big cookie (*Hardee's*)	**278**	3	258	5
Apple pie (*Burger King*)	**330**	3	385	4
Cherry pie (*McDonald's*)	**260**	3	427	4
Chocolaty chip cookies (*McDonald's*)	**342**	4	313	5
Danish (*Wendy's*)	**360**	4	340	2
Carrot cake (*Carl's Jr.*)	**350**	4	375	4
Blueberry turnover (*Arby's*)	**340**	5	255	6
Strawberry shortcake (*Roy Rogers*)	**447**	4	674	7
Pecan pie (*L. J. Silver*)	**446**	5	435	10
Apple turnover (*Jack-Box*)	**410**	5	350	7

Shakes, Milk

	Calories	Fat (tsp)	Sodium (mg)	Sugar (tsp)
Milk, 2.0% butterfat (*McDonald's*)	**86**	1	125	0
Whole milk (*several*)	**150**	2	125	0
Milk shake, average (*Jack-Box*)	**323**	2	147	9
Milk shake (*Hardee's*)	**391**	2	74	11
Milk shake, average (*McDonald's*)	**367**	2	236	10
Shakes, regular size (*Carl's Jr.*)	**490**	2	350	14
Milk shake, average (*Roy Rogers*)	**326**	2	278	9
Milk shake, average (*Arby's*)	**368**	2	275	10
Milk shake, average (*Burger King*)	**340**	2	300	9

Breakfast Items

	Calories	Fat (tsp)	Sodium (mg)
Grapefruit or orange juice, 6 oz.	**80**	0	2
English muffin w/butter (*McDonald's*)	**186**	1	310
Arby's butter croissant (*Arby's*)	**220**	2	225
Scrambled eggs (*McDonald's*)	**180**	3	205
Omelet w/mush., onion, green pepper (*Wendy's*)	**210**	3	200
Biscuit (*Roy Rogers*)	**231**	3	575
Breakfast Jack (*Jack-Box*)	**307**	3	871
Egg McMuffin (*McDonald's*)	**340**	4	885
Mushroom & swiss croissant (*Arby's*)	**340**	5	630
Crescent roll (*Roy Rogers*)	**287**	5	547
Omelet-ham, cheese & mushroom (*Wendy's*)	**290**	5	570
Hot cakes w/syrup & butter (*Carl's Jr.*)	**480**	3	530
French toast, 2 slices (*Wendy's*)	**400**	4	850
Biscuit w/egg (*Hardee's*)	**383**	5	819
Bacon & egg croissant (*Arby's*)	**420**	6	550
Bacon 'n cheese omelette (*Carl's Jr.*)	**290**	6	660
Pancake platter w/ham (*Roy Rogers*)	**506**	4	1264
Breakfast crescent sandwich (*Roy Rogers*)	**401**	6	867
Sausage biscuit (*Hardee's*)	**413**	6	864
Sausage McMuffin (*McDonald's*)	**427**	6	942
Steak & egg biscuit (*Hardee's*)	**527**	7	973

	Calories	Fat (tsp)	Sodium (mg)
Ham & egg biscuit *(Hardee's)*	**458**	6	1585
Sausage & egg croissant *(Arby's)*	**530**	10	745
Sausage McMuffin w/egg *(McDonald's)*	**517**	7	1044
Biscuit with sausage *(McDonald's)*	**467**	7	1147
Sausage & egg biscuit *(Hardee's)*	**521**	8	1033
Pancake platter w/sausage *(Roy Rogers)*	**608**	7	1167
Biscuit w/bacon, egg, cheese *(McDonald's)*	**483**	7	1269
Sunrise sandwich w/bacon *(Carl's Jr.)*	**410**	5	780
Egg & biscuit platter w/sausage *(Roy Rogers)*	**550**	9	1059
Sausage crescent *(Jack-Box)*	**584**	10	1012
Biscuit w/sausage and egg *(McDonald's)*	**585**	9	1301
Brkfst crescent sandwich w/ham *(Roy Rogers)*	**557**	9	1192
Scrambled eggs breakfast *(Jack-Box)*	**720**	10	1110

Miscellaneous

	Calories	Fat (tsp)	Sodium (mg)
Reduced cal. Italian dressing (1 Tbsp.) *(Wendy's)*	**25**	0	180
Cole slaw *(Ky. Fd. Chkn.)*	**121**	2	225
Thousand island dressing (1 Tbsp.) *(Wendy's)*	**70**	1	115
Pick-up window side salad *(Wendy's)*	**110**	1	540
12″ cheese pizza, 2 slices *(Domino's)*	**340**	1	660
Potato salad *(Roy Rogers)*	**107**	1	696
Regular taco *(Jack-Box)*	**191**	2	406

	Calories	Fat (tsp)	Sodium (mg)
Club Pita *(Jack-Box)*	**284**	2	953
Chili, 8 oz. *(Wendy's)*	**260**	2	1070
Macaroni *(Roy Rogers)*	**186**	2	603
Vegetarian D'Lite *(D'Lites)*	**270**	3	610
Chef salad *(Hardee's)*	**277**	4	517
16″ pepperoni pizza, 2 slices *(Domino's)*	**440**	3	1080
Onion rings *(Burger King)*	**270**	4	450
Taco salad *(Wendy's)*	**390**	4	1100
Hot dog *(Hardee's)*	**346**	5	744
Veal parmigiana *(Burger King)*	**580**	6	805
Pasta seafood salad *(Jack-Box)*	**394**	5	1570
Shrimp salad *(Hardee's)*	**362**	7	941
Seafood salad *(L. J. Silver)*	**471**	7	993
Crispirito *(Carl's Jr.)*	**670**	9	1050

SOURCE: Copyright © 1986: Center for Science in Public Interest, 1501 16th St., NW, Washington, DC. 20036. First Printing 1986.

Calcium for Bones: Second Thoughts

Conventional wisdom says that dietary calcium can prevent, or at least delay, the onset of osteoporosis. But conventional wisdom may be wrong, a number of researchers are reporting.

Not only is there no evidence that those who consume the most calcium build the densest bones, but now two careful studies show that the amount of calcium women consume may have nothing to do with the rate at which they lose bone with age.

One unchallenged fact is that osteoporosis is a serious problem. A consensus panel convened by the National Institutes of Health in 1984 reported that this degenerative bone disease afflicts as many as half of all elderly women and nearly a quarter of all older men in the United States.

Women aged 55 to 75 with osteoporosis tend to repeatedly fracture the vertebrae of their spines, which leads to severe back pain and the dowager's hump that is characteristic of the disease. Older men and women tend to fracture their hips.

The consensus panel's recommendations were that women take estrogen supplements after menopause to prevent the accelerated bone loss that occurs when the body stops making estrogen and that all but postmenopausal women consume 1,000 milligrams a day of calcium.

Postmenopausal women, the panel said, should consume 1,500 mg of calcium a day. A glass of milk, one of the best sources of calcium, contains 275 mg of calcium.

The evidence that people might require large amounts of calcium come from studies done by Dr. Robert Heaney of Creighton University in Omaha. Heaney performed calcium balance studies, which are extremely difficult metabolic studies meant to determine how much calcium individuals must consume to take in exactly as much as they excrete. His figures were 1,000 mg a day for all but menopausal women, who require 1,500 mg a day.

Yet others, doing similar studies, have come up with strikingly different figures, as low as 550 mg a day. It is unclear how much calcium is required to stay in metabolic balance, according to Dr. B. Lawrence Riggs of the Mayo Clinic in Rochester, Minn.

But what is clear, says Dr. Richard Mazess of the University of Wisconsin, is that numerous studies, including studies of thousands of people in the United States, the Netherlands, Switzerland, and other places, consistently fail to find any relationship between dietary calcium and bone density.

At a recent meeting of the American Society for Bone and Mineral Research, Riggs and Dr. C. Christiansen of Golstrup Hospital in Denmark independently reported results that cast even more doubt on the calcium hypothesis. Riggs studied 107 women living in Rochester between ages 23 and 88. He followed the women for an average of 4.3 years, carefully noting their daily calcium consumption and regularly measuring their bone density.

The women consumed anywhere from 269 to 2,000 mg a day of calcium, but each woman's calcium consumption tended to be fairly constant throughout the study period. Yet, Riggs says, "we found no correlation at all between

Where to Get Reliable Advice

If you have a question about nutrition, the most convenient person to ask is probably your physician, a local dietitian, or a home economist. If your doctor is unable to provide what you need, he or she can refer you to someone who will—usually a registered dietitian (R.D.).

Registered dietitians are specially trained to translate nutrition requirements into healthful, tasty diets. The "R.D." certification is usually sought by bachelor's- and master's-level nutrition graduates. To qualify, they must have additional professional experience and pass a comprehensive test on nutrition and food service management. They must also participate regularly in educational programs approved by the American Dietetic Association. Nutritionists with a doctoral degree (M.D. or Ph.D.) may also seek certification by the American Board of Nutrition.

Most conditions for which detailed nutrition advice is needed require medical diagnosis first. These include high blood cholesterol, diabetes, severe food allergy or sensitivity, high blood pressure, certain digestive problems, osteoporosis, severe kidney disease, cancer, and obesity. Consultation with an expert can also be worthwhile for pregnant and lactating women, competitive athletes, and people who just feel confused about nutrition.

Since the titles "nutritionist" and "nutrition consultant" are unregulated in most states, they have been adopted by many people who lack recognized credentials. In addition, a small percentage of licensed practitioners are engaged calcium intake and bone loss, not even a trend."

Riggs tried breaking down the data, looking for an effect of calcium. He took into account age, menopausal status, and serum estrogen levels. Still nothing. Then he compared the women in the upper quarter of calcium consumption—those who consumed more than 1,400 mg a day—to women in the bottom quarter—those who consumed less than 500 mg a day. Once again, there was no relationship between calcium consumption and bone loss.

Christiansen looked specifically at forty-three women who had just gone through menopause and were, therefore, rapidly losing bone. He divided the women into three groups, giving one group 2,000 mg a day of calcium, one group an estrogen supplement, and one group a placebo. Only the estrogen, he found, significantly slowed bone loss.

Given these findings, should anyone take calcium supplements? Citing the results of Riggs and Christiansen, some osteoporosis researchers are saying no.

"I don't advise anyone to take calcium," says Dr. Michael Parfitt of Henry Ford Hospital in Detroit. Riggs tells his patients not to take supplements but, to be on the safe side, they should try to get 1,000 mg a day from foods such as milk, cheese and yogurt. "Osteoporosis is a serious disease, and the nutritional value in dairy products goes beyond calcium," he said.

Calling calcium "the laetrile of osteoporosis," the University of Wisconsin's Mazess said he strongly opposes calcium supplements because no one has ever proved they help and no one has determined whether they are even safe to take. Susceptible people may get kidney stones if they take calcium supplements, and excess calcium cuts off vitamin D, which is necessary for strong bones, he notes.

In fact, he said, what elderly people may be lacking is not calcium but vitamin D.

Riggs and Mazess stress, however, that their remarks apply to adults only. Dietary calcium does seem to be linked to bone density in children and adolescents.

The only proven way to slow bone loss and prevent osteoporosis, the researchers say, is with estrogen therapy, and that applies exclusively to postmenopausal women. For everyone else, Riggs remarks, the best advice is to avoid smoking—which doubles the risk of osteoporosis—and to drink only very moderately. As few as two alcoholic drinks a day double a person's chances of getting the disease.

In addition, weight-bearing exercise seems to increase bone density. Some studies indicate that exercise—such as running and walking, but not swimming—does slow bone loss and prevent osteoporosis, says Riggs, who added that more research needs to be done.

But calcium, as an osteoporosis panacea, may be on its way out. Riggs says he considers the calcium question to be open and notes that it remains possible that the mineral has an effect. Yet, for now, that effect has proved elusive, if it exists at all.

SOURCE: Gina Kolata, 1986 (August 6), *Washington Post Health,* p. 10.

in unscientific nutrition practices. Experts on quackery suggest that consumers steer clear of

- Anyone who says that *everyone* needs vitamin supplements to be sure of getting enough. As noted earlier, most people can get all the vitamins they need by eating a varied and balanced diet.
- Anyone who suggests that most diseases are caused by faulty nutrition.
- Anyone who suggests that large doses of vitamins are effective against many diseases and conditions.
- Anyone who suggests hair analysis as a basis for determining the body's nutritional state or for recommending vitamins and minerals. Hair analysis is not reliable for this purpose.
- Anyone who uses a computer-scored "nutrient deficiency test" as the basis for prescribing vitamins. Computers used for such tests are programmed to recommend them for everyone.
- Any practitioner—licensed or not—who sells vitamins in his or her office. Scientific nutritionists do not sell vitamins. Unscientific practitioners often do—at two to three times their cost.

Future Nutrition Research

Although it is clear that diet is related to the development of a number of serious diseases, including heart disease and cancer (discussed in Chapters 17 and 18), much research of this type is still needed. Research needs to determine whether there is an optimal diet for everyone, or whether dietary strategy should differ according to heredity, biochemical traits, environmental factors, exercise patterns, or other factors. And it should also determine whether specific foods or food components cause trouble or can provide special benefit.

Take Action

We hope that your answers to the Exploring Your Emotions questions in this chapter and your placement level on the Wellness Ladder will encourage you to begin and maintain a process of self-exploration and self-discovery. Reflect on the entire chapter's contents and ask yourself how each point relates to your own life. Then take action:

1. In your Take Action notebook, keep track of everything you eat and drink for three or four days. Then see how well your average daily intake meets the Basic Four Food Group guidelines.
2. Read the lists of ingredients for three or four canned or packaged foods that you enjoy eating. If any ingredients are unfamiliar to you, find out what they are and why they have been used.
3. Find five advertisements or labels that use the word *natural* to describe a food product. Why do you think the word is used? Does the product have any advantages or disadvantages over competing products?
4. Read the following Behavior Change Strategy, and take the appropriate action.

Behavior Change Strategy

Nutrition

It is not at all unusual to hear people announcing the fact that they are trying to eat more "natural foods" or telling their friends that they are going to a particular restaurant because it serves "healthful food." At one time the content of our food was considered important primarily in terms of its calorie content. Even the term *diet* has come to mean a weight-loss program instead of its more complete definition: the food we eat. But there is a growing trend in our society toward a concern about the preparation, preservation, and derivation of our food. References to "natural" and "health" foods have become so commonplace that today these terms are used almost indiscriminately.

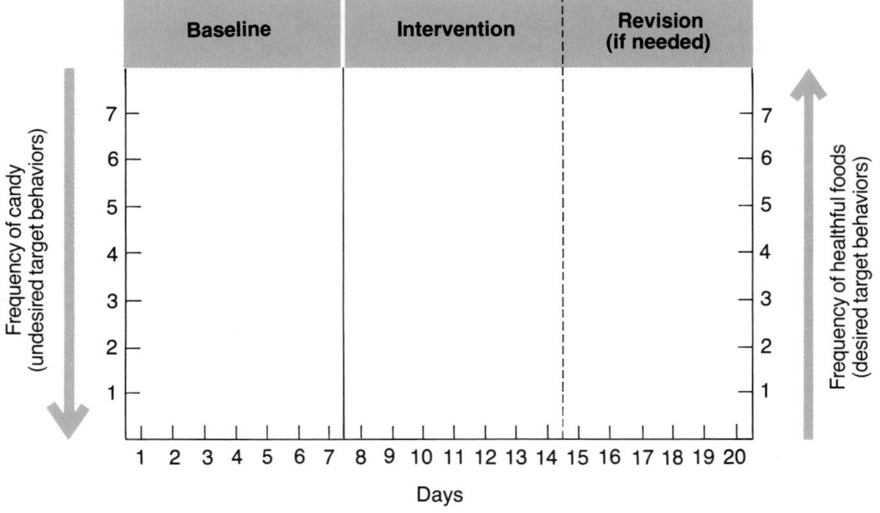

Establishing Baseline Levels If you want to alter your diet, some of the major health behavior change strategies we have already examined can help you. For example, you can keep track of your target behavior or set of behaviors by means of a diary (see Chapter 1). Let's say that you want to do two things to your diet: (1) you want to cut out all candy while walking between classes or while on errands in town, and (2) you want to eat more fresh fruits and raw vegetables.

Begin by keeping track of your candy consumption. In a diary jot down the time of day and what occurred before and after the eating event. On a chart such as the one shown here, keep track of the number of eating events. Because you also want to add more fruits and vegetables to your diet, you will want to keep notes on the kinds of foods you have been eating at meals. You can include this information on the same chart that you are already using (only on the right-hand vertical axis) or you can simply keep two graphs.

Intervention Once you have established your "baseline" levels, begin to make some changes in those routines that seem to precede your eating candy. For example, you might find that you have been eating candy from a vending machine that you walk by every day after class. If this is the case, try another route that allows you to avoid the machine. You might also find that you usually are hungry at one particular time of day and that you rarely have lunch or a healthful snack with you. If this is the case, try to keep a healthful snack on hand so that you will not be caught off guard and then be pushed toward eating candy (which always seems to be available). You can use the same sort of strategy to increase the number of fruits and vegetables in your diet: specifically, you will need to shop for these food items *in advance* and prepare them *ahead of time* so that they are readily available.

Revision (If Needed) You may discover that your initial plan works perfectly or that it works well for three weeks but then loses its effectiveness. You will have to watch out for programs that become stale and lose their strength, and, of course, you will want to revise an ineffective program entirely once you have given it a real try. The critical data from your diary can help you to decide how to revise your program. Plotting the data on a prominently displayed chart can encourage your progress.

Social Eating Events Avoiding an attractive (seductive) candy vending machine may be a lot easier than cutting back on late-night pizza binges; the former involves only you while the latter involves you and your friends. It is harder to make adjustments in social eating patterns, but there are some strategies that you can try. First, tell your friends that you would prefer to try something new to eat instead of pizza (popcorn, etc.). Being assertive in such matters can be very helpful; you may discover some allies who share your views about the type of food you want to eat. Second, try to cut down somewhat on these group activities without eliminating them entirely. Of course, you can try to change or limit the kinds of food you eat at these times, but it is generally very difficult to refrain from joining in once you are actually in the social situation.

Systematic Changes in Other Habits Many people take up sports activities or begin to increase their routine activity levels (walks after meals, etc.) at the same time that they try to adjust their diet. While it is not a good idea to try to make too many significant changes at one time, you may want to personally experiment with other changes while you make adjustments in what you are eating.

Selected References

Gibney, M. J. 1986. *Nutrition, diet and health*. New York: Cambridge University Press.

Lehmann, P. 1979 (April, May, June). More than you ever thought you would know about food additives. *FDA Consumer* 13(3):12–19, 13(4):18–23, 13(5):10–16.

Meister, K. A. 1985. Update on Food Irradiation. Philadelphia: Stickley. *Nutrition Forum*, Vol. 2, pp. 25–27.

Nutrition and Your Health: Dietary Guidelines for Americans. 1985. USDA/HHS (U.S. Department of Agriculture/Health and Human Services) Home and Garden Bulletin No. 232.

Sheridan, M. J., and K. M. Meister. 1982. *Food Additives and Hyperactivity*. New York: American Council on Science and Health.

Stare, F. J., and V. Aronson. 1983. *Your Basic Guide to Nutrition*. Philadelphia: Stickley.

The vitamin pushers. 1986 (March). *Consumer Reports* 51:170–75.

Recommended Readings

Hartbarger, J. C., and N. J. Hartbarger. 1981. *Eating for the Eighties*. Philadelphia: Saunders Press, Stickley.
A comprehensive guide to vegetarian nutrition.

Herbert, V., and S. Barrett. 1981. *Vitamins and "Health" Foods: The Great American Hustle*. Philadelphia: Stickley.
A comprehensive investigative report on nutrition quackery.

Marshall, C. W. *Vitamins and Minerals: Help or Harm?* 1985. Philadelphia: Stickley.
Tells what nutrients do, how much we need, and how to obtain them. Also covers megavitamin controversies.

Yetiv, J. 1986. *Popular Nutrition Practices: A Scientific Appraisal*. Toledo, Ohio: Popular Medicine Press.
A thorough, referenced analysis of more than 100 topics of contemporary interest.

Chapter 13

Contents

Rate Yourself

Your Weight Control Behavior Read the following statements carefully. Choose the one in each section that best describes you at this moment and circle its number. When you have chosen one statement for each section, add the numbers and record your total score. Find your position on the Wellness Ladder.

5 Slender
4 Close to ideal weight
3 Slightly above ideal weight
2 Overweight
1 Obese

5 Maintains regular eating schedule
4 Eats three times a day
3 Has irregular eating habits
2 Usually snacks between meals
1 Eats frequently during the day

5 Eats a balanced diet
4 Emphasizes vegetables in diet
3 Prefers meat and potatoes
2 Eats high-fat foods
1 Enjoys desserts with every meal

5 Vigorously active
4 Relatively active
3 Moderately active
2 Minimally active
1 Inactive

5 Believes weight is mostly affected by diet and exercise
4 Believes weight is mostly affected by diet
3 Believes exercise weight loss is offset by increased appetite
2 Believes weight is mostly affected by genetics
1 Believes weight is least affected by diet

Total Score ______

Weight Control

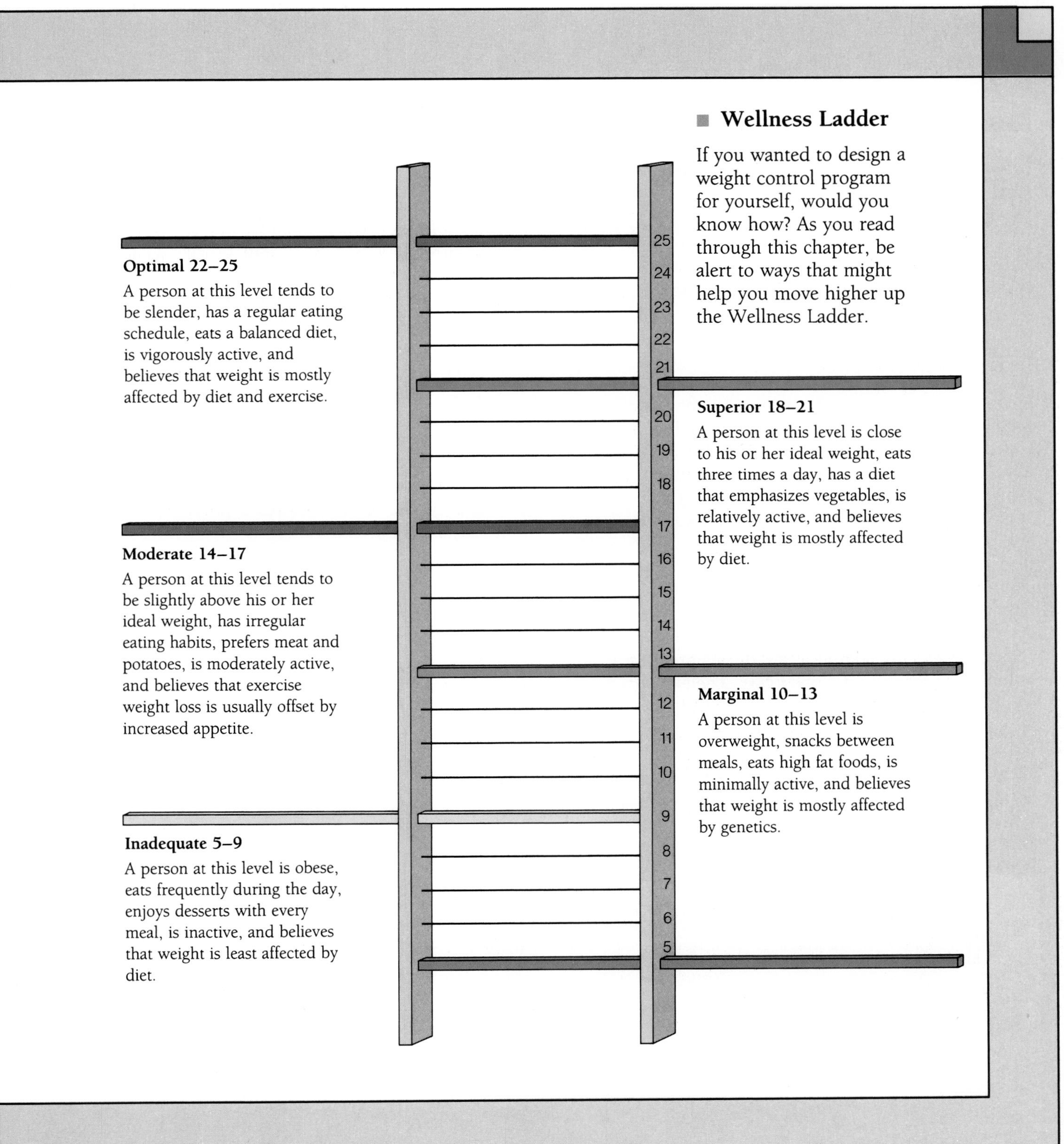

Wellness Ladder
If you wanted to design a weight control program for yourself, would you know how? As you read through this chapter, be alert to ways that might help you move higher up the Wellness Ladder.
Optimal 22–25
A person at this level tends to be slender, has a regular eating schedule, eats a balanced diet, is vigorously active, and believes that weight is mostly affected by diet and exercise.
Superior 18–21
A person at this level is close to his or her ideal weight, eats three times a day, has a diet that emphasizes vegetables, is relatively active, and believes that weight is mostly affected by diet.
Moderate 14–17
A person at this level tends to be slightly above his or her ideal weight, has irregular eating habits, prefers meat and potatoes, is moderately active, and believes that exercise weight loss is usually offset by increased appetite.
Marginal 10–13
A person at this level is overweight, snacks between meals, eats high fat foods, is minimally active, and believes that weight is mostly affected by genetics.
Inadequate 5–9
A person at this level is obese, eats frequently during the day, enjoys desserts with every meal, is inactive, and believes that weight is least affected by diet.
25
24
23
22
21
20
19
18
17
16
15
14
13
12
11
10
9
8
7
6
5

Overweight A condition in which a person weighs between more than the upper limit of what is considered "normal" or average and 20 percent above that limit for people of the same height and sex. (Note that average weight is increasing in the United States.)

Anorexia nervosa A diet-related disorder characterized by loss of appetite and severe weight loss.

Bulimia A diet-related disorder in which the person binges on food and then purges by means of self-induced vomiting, laxatives, or diuretics.

Overfat A condition in which a person has more body fat (adipose tissue) than is normal or healthy for people of the same height and sex. (For example, in males over 25 percent of total weight is body fat; in females, over 30 percent.)

Exploring Your Emotions

How do you feel about obese people? What kinds of personal judgments do you make about them? Do you feel similarly about extremely thin people?

Although "slimness as an ideal" has dominated American culture in recent years, it is very clear that most Americans are slowly gaining more and more weight, particularly with age. Indeed, some evidence shows that Americans are the heaviest people in the world, gaining an average of one or two pounds a year after the age of 20. (See Figure 13-1.) From 30 to 50 million Americans are **overweight.** One can, of course, be "overmuscled" in the sense of weighing more because one has a lot more muscle tissue than most people of the same age. But almost all overweight people have an excess of body fat.

Seriously overweight people risk their physical and emotional health. They have a significantly higher risk than normal-weight people for many diseases and disorders, including high blood pressure, high blood fats (hyperlipidemia), diabetes, heart disease, cerebrovascular diseases (strokes), diseases of the blood vessels, kidney and lung problems, complications during pregnancy, and serious risks for any kind of surgery. The National Institutes of Health recently declared excessive body fat to be a *serious* disease. Extreme body weight, or morbid obesity, may be especially dangerous for younger people, because it has been found to be a strong predictor of premature death in people under 35. Some experts also consider the social and personal problems of being seriously overweight to be as serious as the medical hazards. Many studies, for example, have shown that people rate others who are seriously overweight as less likeable and less popular. Many overweight people also report feeling more critical and less positive about themselves. Excess body fat is clearly hazardous to physical, social, *and* emotional health.

Figure 13-1 Degree of overweight in people aged 40–49 in population samples of seven countries.

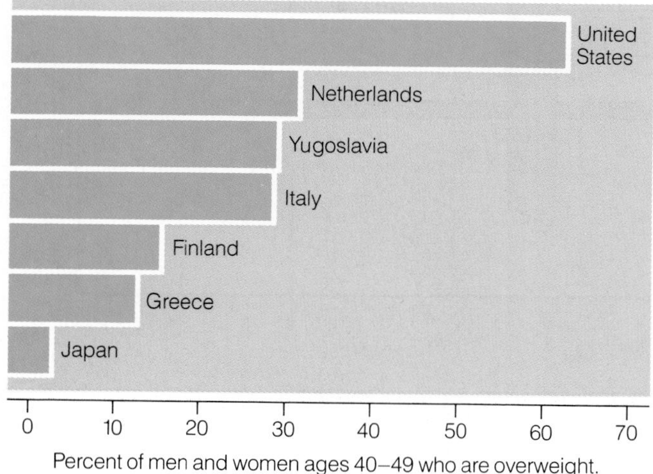

Problems of body weight and weight control, however, are not limited to excessive body fat. A growing number of people, especially teenagers and young adults, experience what are called "eating disorders," problems associated with food and eating. The most common disorders involve not eating enough food to maintain a reasonable body weight (that is, more than 25 percent below normal weight). Such people maintain themselves on starvation diets, and often combine eating very little with being very physically active. Called **anorexia nervosa,** this eating and body weight problem affects between 1 and 3 million Americans, mostly women. Perhaps the key characteristic of people suffering from anorexia is their intense fear of becoming fat and their view of themselves as "feeling fat" and looking heavy. The other major eating disorder is called **bulimia.** This problem shares a great deal with anorexia, with one important difference: someone who is bulimic is not seriously underweight. Bulimia typically involves trying to stay on a strict low-calorie diet, interrupted by going on a food-eating binge or eating more than intended and then deliberately forcing oneself to vomit before the food is digested. Often, the problems of anorexia and bulimia merge: the anorexic person also binges on food and then purges by inducing vomiting or using laxatives.

Serious problems in controlling body weight involve the extremes: weighing too much or too little. Two major points about body weight are becoming very clear: (1) many Americans of all ages weigh too much, and (2) some younger Americans are much too fearful and concerned about weighing too much.

What Should You Weigh?

Most weight tables list the average weight for Americans in terms of body build, age, and sex. However, because many people tend to weigh more, such tables can be misleading. For example, when the most commonly used

Obesity A complex disorder characterized by excessive body fat. Obesity may refer to weight 20 percent or more above a person's upper limit for weight, adjusted for sex and height. Also refers to what percent of total body weight is body fat. For males, over 25 percent body fat, and for females over 30 percent body fat, is clearly obese.

weight tables (1959 Metropolitan Life Insurance Company tables) were revised in 1983, after almost twenty-five years, the average weight of Americans clearly showed substantial increases. Because this increase represents gains in body fat, the Metropolitan tables are no longer called "tables of desirable weight." Instead, they are labeled as "average weights of Americans."

Any determination of ideal weight should consider such things as muscle size, body structure, and tendency to retain water. Ideal weight must reflect not only total weight but also the body's proportion of fat to lean tissue (such as muscle and bone). Generally, for women 20 to 24 percent of body weight as fat tissue is considered desirable, while for men the range is from 12 to 15 percent (Table 13-1).

Use Table 13-2 to see approximately how much you should weigh. This table uses the earlier, more conservative 1959 Metropolitan tables because of the higher body weights found in the newer 1983 tables. Table 13-2 suggests a range from minimum to maximum desirable weight (weights in parentheses), plus the ideal weight (the single number). Thus, for a woman 5 feet 6 inches in shoes with a medium frame, her ideal weight would be 128 pounds, with a desirable range between 120 to 135 pounds. (If in doubt about your body frame, use the medium category.) If you weigh 10 pounds or more above the upper limit for your category, you might want to lose some body fat. How much you should lose depends on several things. Unless you are obviously **overfat**—well beyond the 10 extra pounds for your desirable upper limit—how much you should lose depends on how *you* feel and what *you* think about your weight. You should be careful not to overreact to a few extra pounds beyond the upper or lower limit. Staying as you are or changing your weight is a personal choice, not a health problem. If you feel well and comfortable and are not gradually losing or gaining weight beyond the limit, then you may wish to stay as you are.

What Is Obesity?

Obesity is a physical condition characterized by excessive body fat. Usually a person is considered obese if his or her body weight is 20 percent above the upper limit weight given in Table 13-2. A person is morbidly obese if body weight is more than 50 percent above the upper limit.

Table 13-1 Percent Components of Body Weight in Normal Weight Adult Males

Water	60%
Protein	17
Fat	17
Minerals, glycogen, other	6

NOTE: For women, fat is about 25%, with less protein and minerals, etc., accordingly.
SOURCE: Adapted from J. S. Garrow, 1981, Treat Obesity Seriously (Edinburgh: Churchill Livingstone).

Exploring Your Emotions

How do you feel about your own body weight? Do you have strong feelings about the ideal body weight or shape of a sexual partner? Where do you think you learned these ideals?

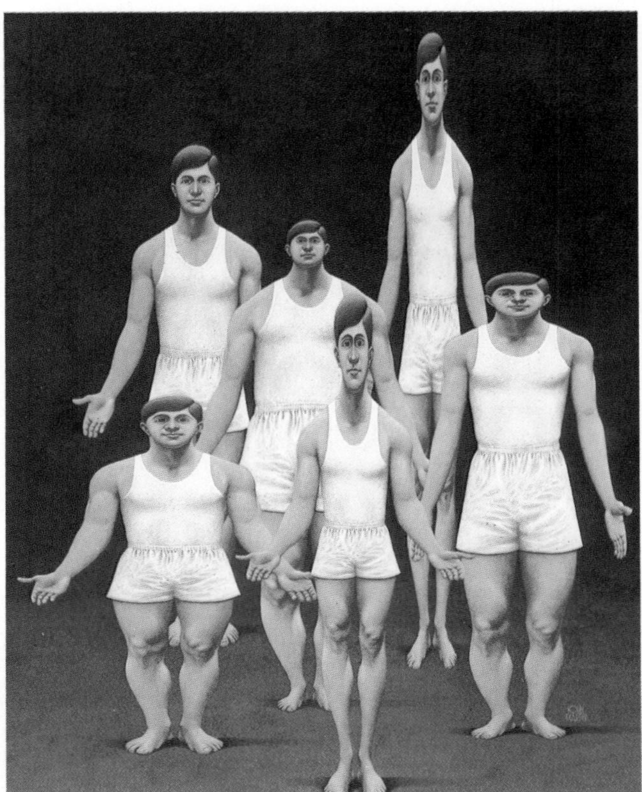

Illustration by John Martin

Table 13-2 Ideal Weight (Pounds) and Range[a]

Men				Women			
Height[b]	Small frame	Medium frame	Large frame	Height[b]	Small frame	Medium frame	Large frame
5′2″	116 (112–120)	124 (118–129)	134 (126–141)	4′10″	95 (92–98)	102 (96–107)	112 (104–119)
5′3″	119 (115–123)	127 (121–133)	137 (129–144)	4′11″	98 (94–101)	104 (98–110)	114 (106–122)
5′4″	122 (118–126)	130 (124–136)	140 (132–148)	5′0″	101 (96–104)	107 (101–113)	117 (109–125)
5′5″	125 (121–129)	133 (127–139)	144 (135–152)	5′1″	103 (99–107)	110 (104–116)	120 (112–128)
5′6″	129 (124–133)	137 (130–143)	147 (138–156)	5′2″	106 (102–110)	113 (107–119)	123 (115–131)
5′7″	133 (128–137)	141 (134–147)	152 (142–161)	5′3″	109 (105–113)	116 (110–122)	126 (118–134)
5′8″	137 (132–141)	145 (138–152)	157 (147–166)	5′4″	112 (108–116)	120 (113–126)	130 (121–138)
5′9″	141 (136–145)	149 (142–156)	161 (151–170)	5′5″	115 (111–119)	123 (116–130)	134 (125–142)
5′10″	145 (140–150)	153 (146–160)	165 (155–174)	5′6″	119 (114–123)	128 (120–135)	138 (129–146)
5′11″	149 (144–154)	158 (150–165)	169 (159–179)	5′7″	123 (118–127)	132 (124–139)	142 (133–150)
6′0″	153 (148–158)	162 (154–170)	174 (164–184)	5′8″	127 (122–131)	136 (128–143)	146 (137–154)
6′1″	157 (152–162)	167 (158–175)	179 (168–189)	5′9″	131 (126–135)	140 (132–147)	150 (141–158)
6′2″	162 (156–167)	171 (162–180)	184 (173–194)	5′10″	135 (130–140)	144 (136–151)	154 (145–163)
6′3″	166 (160–171)	176 (167–185)	189 (189–199)	5′11″	139 (134–144)	148 (140–155)	159 (149–168)
6′4″	170 (164–175)	181 (172–190)	193 (182–204)	6′0″	143 (138–148)	152 (144–159)	163 (153–173)

NOTE: The numbers in parentheses are reproduced with permission from the Metropolitan Life Insurance Company's Desirable Weight Table (1959). The ideal weight is based on the Fogarty Table of Desirable Weights (Bray, 1986).
[a]For adults aged 18 and above, in light clothes.
[b]Height in shoes—assume 1-inch heel for men and 2-inch heel for women.
SOURCE: Peter Wood, 1983, *The California Diet and Exercise Program* (Mountain View, Calif.: Anderson World Books). Reprinted by permission of Anderson World Books, Inc.

Other ways to define obesity include 25 percent or more total weight as body fat for men and 30 percent for women. How many people are obese, using the criteria of more than 20 percent above the upper limit for a particular height? Estimates vary between 30 to 40 million Americans. Roughly, 1 in 7 people are obese in the United States.

Currently, the best *simple* measure of body weight takes height and total weight into account. It is called the **Body Mass Index (BMI).** To compute BMI, total body weight is divided by height squared (weight/height^2). Table 13-3 presents the BMI values for men and women. The BMI for a 5-foot 8-inch woman would be about 21.5. (Note that BMI uses the metric system so that pounds are changed to kilograms and inches to centimeters). By placing a ruler or straight edge between your height in inches and weight in pounds, you can see if your BMI is in the "acceptable," "overweight," or "obese" range. The biggest advantage in using the BMI method over height-weight tables and total weight is that it comes closest to estimating how much of the total body weight is body fat.

Body mass index (BMI) A measure of relative body weight that divides total body weight (in kilograms) by the square of a person's height (in centimeters). A BMI above 25 indicates overweight and above 30, obesity.

Calorie A measure of the energy your body gets from food and uses in exercise. Technically, energy used to raise 1 kilogram of water 1° C.

What Causes Obesity? Most people believe that excessive body weight is simply caused by eating too much. This is not entirely true. Obesity is tied to a number of factors besides how much is eaten. Genetics, family and culture, body chemistry, eating and exercise habits, and psychological factors all play important roles. Scientists do not yet understand how these factors and others contribute to excessive body weight. The most popular and simple theory is often referred to as the "energy balance problem"; that is, people gain weight, mostly body fat, if the amount of energy (**calories**) used each day is less than the calories consumed each day. Generally speaking, to increase body weight more calories must be eaten than are used. However, several other factors are involved in

Table 13-3 Body Mass Index (BMI)

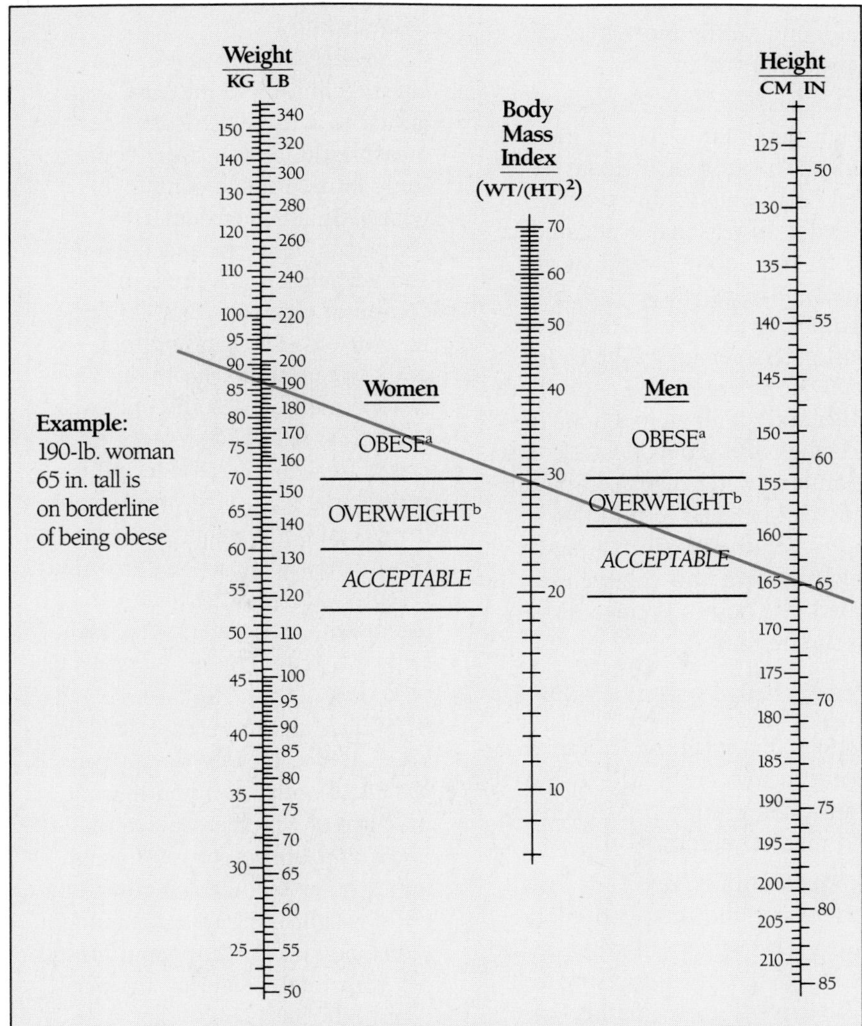

Note: To determine BMI, place a ruler or other straight edge between the body weight column on the left and the height column on the right and read the BMI from the point where it crosses the center. In the example, a 190 pound woman, 65 inches tall (5 foot, 5 inches) would be on the borderline between overweight and obese, with a BMI of 29.5.

[a]*Obesity:* BMI above 30 kg/m^2.

[b]*Overweight:* Body mass index (BMI) of 25 to 30 kg/m^2.

SOURCE: Reprinted with permission from G. A. Bray, 1978, Definitions, measurements and classification of the syndrome of obesity, *International Journal of Obesity* 2:99–112.

How Fat Are You?

You can use several methods to find out what percentage of your total body weight is fat, compared to water, muscle, skin tissue, bones, and so on:

1. *The Eyeball (or Mirror) Test.* Stand naked in front of a full-length mirror. If you readily see a lot of bulges, ripples, and soft, flabby tissue, then you are probably too fat. Note that a pregnant woman would of course look fat.

2. *The Ruler Test* (especially for males). Lie flat on your back on the floor and place a 12-inch ruler along midline of your stomach from lower rib cage to pelvic area (in direction from head to feet). If ruler lies flat, each end touching rib and pelvic area at the same time, you probably do not have excessive body fat in the abdominal area (no fair holding in your stomach!). This test often is not valid for females, who store most excessive fat below the waist.

3. *The Pinch (Skin fold) Test.* Because you may not readily see the more obvious signs (flabby, loose, ripples of tissue) of being overfat, the pinch test can be used. Certain locations on the body tend to store fat tissue, such as the back side of the upper arm (triceps area) and the back area just below the shoulder blade (subscapular area). You can check the triceps area by yourself (the back test requires another person). With your elbow bent and your arm relaxed (don't flex or tense your muscles), use the thumb and forefinger of your other hand. Gently lift the soft tissue away from the muscle. If you can lift between your thumb and forefinger more than ½ inch of "flab," then you may have more body fat than you need. If you can pinch clearly more than 1 inch, then you definitely are overfat.

4. *Skin Calipers Test.* For a more precise measure of body fat, use constant-tension **skin calipers** to "pinch" the soft fat tissue stored in the underarm and subscapular areas. One definition of being obese is a combined skin fold (triceps plus subscapular areas) of a little more than 1¾ inches for males and a little more than 2¾ inches for females.

5. *Underwater Test.* Fat tissue weighs less than water, protein, or bones. The ratio of body fat to total body weight can be determined with reasonable accuracy if all "fat-free" body weight (water, bones, muscles, and so on) is assumed to average 1.10 g/cubic centimeters versus 0.90 g/cc for fat. By submerging the entire body underwater with as much air in the lungs released as possible, the amount of water displaced by the body can be used to find the body's volume. With total body weight known and volume estimated, the body's average density (*d*) can be found:

$$\text{Percent body fat} = \frac{495}{d} - 450$$

Underwater weighing is often available in health clubs, YMCA programs, community health centers and medical clinics.

6. *Radioactive Isotope Tests* (total body water and total body potassium). The percent of body fat can also be determined by using a radioactive isotope (marker) of hydrogen or oxygen. Generally, fat-free tissue contains 73 percent water. If total body water is known, the amount of fat-free body tissue can be determined and, by subtraction from total body weight, the amount of body fat. The person is given a known dose of water with the isotope of hydrogen or oxygen marked (radioactively). After three to four hours, a blood sample is taken and total body water is calculated. Fat content of the body is then calculated. A similar procedure using radioactive isotopes of potassium can also be used, since the amount of potassium in fat-free tissue is known.

7. *Bioelectrical Impedence.* The latest technique to measure body fat uses a weak electrical current to measure the body's water content (only fat-free tissue contains water). Small electrodes are clipped to the wrist and the ankles and a briefcase-size programmed computer estimates total fat-free weight from determining total body water (similar to the radio isotope method described above). With total lean body weight estimated, total body fat is found by subtracting lean or fat-free weight from total body weight. Inaccurate results may occur if the person has recently eaten a large meal (increases body water) or if the person is retaining too much water or is dehydrated.

8. *Pounds and Percentage Body Fat.* You can also easily estimate your *pounds* of body fat if you have a measure of your percentage of body fat, from underwater weighing or other methods. If your total body weight is 120 pounds and your body fat is 30 percent, multiply your total weight by the percent body fat (120 × .30 = 36 pounds). Your lean (nonfat) body weight is 120 − 36 = 84 pounds. One researcher argues that females should not exceed 22 percent body fat and males should be no more than 15 percent body fat, *regardless* of their height and frame.

Skin calipers An instrument used to measure thickness of skin folds (fat tissue) in various parts of the body, such as triceps and mid-back.

Set point theory A theory that tries to explain why the body seems to maintain body weight around a certain level, making it more difficult at first to lose or gain weight.

this energy balance, including the body's tendency to resist weight change, the influence of foods and physical activities on how much energy the body uses when at rest (resting metabolic rate), the role of emotions and moods, as well as important family, sociocultural, and other environmental factors.

Changing Food and Activity Patterns At the turn of the century in 1900, most Americans consumed diets primarily composed of complex carbohydrates, especially bread, potatoes, pasta, rice, along with beans and legumes, fresh vegetables, and other whole grains. Small amounts of fats, especially animal fats, and simple or refined carbohydrates (sugars) were eaten. Since then Americans have dramatically increased how much fat of all kinds they eat (up by 31 percent) and refined sugars (up 50 percent) while eating much less complex carbohydrates (down 43 percent). Furthermore, Americans today are actually consuming somewhat *fewer* calories overall (down about 3 percent) compared to those in 1900—eating less and gaining more.

What has changed dramatically is the lifestyle of Americans. Despite the exercise and jogging craze of recent years, most people are much less physically active today than in 1900. Many work at white-collar office jobs that involve sitting for long periods of time, plus a lot of stress. This combination of stressful work conditions, much less vigorous physical activities in part due to career choices, combined with eating much more fats and refined carbohydrates (sugars), especially snacking on candy, ice cream, cookies, pastries—over 50 percent of all calories today are from fats and sugars compared to less than 25 percent in 1900—has greatly contributed to what is now called the epidemic of obesity and overweight in the United States.

A study by Dr. Peter Wood at Stanford University illustrates the connections among eating, weight change, and physical activity. In this study eighty-one men (between ages 35 and 55), selected because they were very physically sedentary, volunteered for a year-long study. Of these men forty-eight were assigned randomly to an exercise program of jogging regularly three times a week. The remaining thirty-three served as a control group. These men were asked to maintain their usual sedentary habits and routines. None was encouraged to change his diet. Careful records were kept of the number of miles run each week by those in the exercise group, along with changes in their body fat. After one year the men who jogged (they averaged 8 miles a week) not only had lost more weight than those in the control group but they actually were eating more food than the men who continued to be physically sedentary. Furthermore, the weight lost by the physically active men was mostly body fat, not lean weight, such as muscle tissue.

Genetic Factors Obesity can be produced in animals through selective breeding. That is, some animals are born with a greater tendency to gain body weight. We must assume, therefore, that heredity plays an influence in human obesity. (Unfortunately, many studies with humans confuse genetic and early environmental influences.) We do not understand how genetics influences body weight, especially obesity. Obesity clearly runs in families, but separating out genetic from social influences has proved difficult. We do know that obese infants are two to three times more likely to become obese as adults compared to normal weight infants. Obese teenagers are six times more likely to be obese adults. Furthermore, if both parents are obese, their children are two to three times more likely to be obese. And well over 50 percent of children with obese parents are destined to become obese as adults. By contrast, if parents are normal weight, fewer than one in five obese children will be obese as adults. Family size makes a difference. An only child is two to three times more likely to become an obese adult than a child with three or more siblings.

Set Point Researchers have found a great variability in body weights between humans but a remarkable consistency of body weight for the same person over time. Such findings suggest that each person may have his or her own biological weight—often referred to as **set point**—and that some people may have a point that is "set" far above what a particular culture considers normal or healthy. According to this theory, set point acts much like a room thermostat that tries to keep the room temperature at a certain level, such as 68° F. Researchers have long known that laboratory animals will adjust food intake and physical activity to compensate for either too little food or forced feeding of a great deal of food. With little food, the animals are less physically active, and with too much they are much more active. Theoretically the same kind of set point regulation may occur in humans.

Set point theory may help explain why some people have great difficulty in trying to lose or gain weight. Thus, initial efforts to lose or gain are resisted by the body's attempt to maintain weight around a certain level. If one is seriously overweight, then early efforts to lose weight would prove very difficult. However, if efforts persist,

Resting metabolic rate (RMR) The rate at which the body uses energy, as measured in calories, to stay alive while at rest: for example, while sitting quietly or sleeping. Over 70 percent of calories used by the body are used during rest.

Adipocyte A fat cell.

Triglycerides A type of fatty compound that circulates in the blood and is stored inside adipocytes (fat cells).

Thyroid A gland in the neck that influences the rate of body metabolism.

---

body weight will in time change. Critics of set point theory argue that while the body may strive at first to maintain weight, the influences of how much food is eaten and physical activity level are much stronger factors in explaining changes in body weight. Also, in controlled studies not everyone shows evidence of a set point working to resist weight changes.

Resting Metabolic Rate Your biggest single spender of energy (calories) is your body's **resting metabolic rate (RMR).** The RMR represents the number of calories used to stay alive while at complete rest (breathing, circulating blood, maintaining body temperature). The typical RMR is about 1 calorie per minute or 1,440 calories per day (60 × 24). About 74 percent of all calories used each day goes for RMR. Factors that influence RMR may be very important in controlling body weight. Several studies found that RMR changed when eating patterns changed. Confronted with a starvation-type diet, many people showed a sharp RMR reduction. In one study, RMR fell 20 percent. By contrast, if people substantially increased their number of calories, the RMR tended to increase. Such changes are sometimes cited as evidence for set point theory; the body may attempt to stay at a certain weight by altering its RMR.

Vigorous, consistent physical activity can raise RMR. Indeed, one current major approach to reducing body fat combines an improved diet (fruits, vegetables, whole grains, nonfat milk products, beans and legumes) with increasing physical activities on a regular basis. One major effect of more activity is to increase the body's RMR. Peter Wood points out that a 20 percent increase in RMR (for example, from 1 to 1.2 calories per minute) can lead to a loss of 25 to 30 pounds over a year. Note that much of this weight loss occurs while the person is resting.

Another metabolic-related problem that influences body weight has been called diet-induced obesity or the consequences of "yo-yo" dieting; that is, losing, gaining, losing, gaining. . . . Researchers such as Dr. Kelly Brownell at the University of Pennsylvania have repeatedly found in animal studies that when weight is lost, and then regained, the body becomes more resistant to losing weight the next time food intake is reduced (going on a diet). Apparently what happens is that the body becomes more energy conscious, using up fewer calories. Thus, after a few cycles of losing and regaining weight, it takes two to three times longer to lose the same amount of weight on the same diet compared to those who have not repeatedly lost and then regained weight. This "yo-yo" or down-and-up effect also has been found to trigger more overeating and to increase the number of fat cells. Thus, going on severe diets where weight is lost and then going off these diets with a regaining of the lost pounds *contributes* to obesity.

Sex Differences Differences exist between males and females as to *where* excessive fat tissue is stored. For women it is "below the belt," especially in the hips and buttocks. For men it is above the waist, especially in the abdominal ("pot belly") area. Researchers have found dramatically higher risk for heart disease in abdominal obesity. (For men the increased coronary risk was ten times greater over 20 years!) Women also ran greater coronary risk from excess weight held primarily above the waist (when the waist is larger than the hip circumference).

Developmental Factors Childhood obesity is a major problem that is becoming more prevalent. Approximately 25 percent of all American children are overweight, and parents who hope an obese child will "grow out of it" are waiting for something that is unlikely to happen. Indeed, most obese children become obese adolescents, and most obese adolescents become obese adults. It has been estimated, for example, that if an obese eighth-grader does not reduce body weight to a reasonably normal level by the end of adolescence, the odds are strongly against becoming normal weight later in life. Fourteen percent of obese infants in the United States later are obese as adults. The parallel figures for obese 7-year-olds and obese 10- to 13-year-olds are 41 and 70 percent, respectively. Furthermore, the contribution of obese parents to the weight status of the child, as already noted, is quite substantial. In effect, obese parents breed obese children who later become obese adults and parents. Thus, a vicious and

Exploring Your Emotions

Were you or someone you know fat as a child? How might someone be affected by being fat in childhood? In adolescence? How do you feel parents should help such children?

Where to Find Your Calories

If you eat like most Americans do, 40 percent of your energy (calories) comes from eating fats—saturated, monounsaturated, and polyunsaturated. That is altogether too much fat—because it raises your risk of obesity, cardiovascular disease, and some cancers. A whopping 17 percent typically comes from saturated fat—the kind of fat you can least afford to eat because it contributes most to heart disease.

Real		Ideal
17%	Saturated fats	6%
17	Monounsaturated fats	17
6	Polyunsaturated fats	10
45	Carbohydrate	55
15	Protein	11

Experts recommend other proportions for your calories sources. Begin by cutting total fats to about one-third of all calories and saturated fats to less than 10 percent of all calories. The proportion of monounsaturated fats should remain the same, while your polyunsaturated fat intake can be increased slightly.

You can reduce your protein slightly and expand the proportion of complex carbohydrates (vegetables, grains, and legumes) to 55 percent of your total calories.

hazardous cycle is established—one that fortunately can be altered with careful and consistent efforts.

The persistence of childhood obesity may be explained by studies showing that body weight is a function of the size and the number of fat cells. Weight gain can take place in two ways: by increasing the number of fat cells (which commonly occurs in childhood), or by enlarging the size of existing cells (typically what goes on with adults).

What increases the size and the number of **adipocytes** or fat cells? At a simple level, the answer is overeating. That is, when the body faces more energy than it is using, energy in the form of **triglycerides**, a type of fatty compound, is stored inside the fat cells. At first the fat cell stretches as it stores more and more triglycerides, but as the cells reach their maximum size, new fat cells are formed.

Major differences exist between people of the same sex and age in terms of the size and the number of fat cells at different regions of the body. Also, men have *larger* fat cells in the abdominal area than women; by contrast, women have *more* fat cells in the hip and buttock regions.

Some researchers believe that a larger number of fat cells may prompt greater appetite and more eating behavior. They also suspect that the body tends to keep fat cells full. Thus if overweight people try to lose weight, these fat-depleted cells help stimulate more eating and weight gain.

Combinations of weight loss methods can work for those with a larger number of fat cells. Such people may, however, have to work harder to maintain fat cells at a smaller size, and they may not become as slim as others.

Metabolic Factors Some cases of obesity can be due to severe metabolic problems, such as **thyroid** disturbances that lower resting metabolic rate level, or *Cushing's syndrome* (a disorder of the adrenal cortex). Recent evidence suggests that resting metabolic rate plays a major role in maintaining excessive body weight. (Note: taking thyroid pills to change metabolic rate is seldom effective, nor is it a safe way to reduce body weight.)

Metabolic factors, such as the person's resting metabolic rate, are related to genetic and biological differences. For example, obesity among identical twins is significantly greater than among fraternal twins. Furthermore, adopted children are much more likely to weigh the same as their biological parents compared to their adoptive parents. We do not yet fully understand what the specific mechanisms are. We do know, however, that metabolic differences between people do exist and these differences are related to the chances of becoming and remaining overweight. As already discussed, differences in the resting metabolic rate (RMR) play a major role in how many calories the body uses minute by minute under resting and relaxed conditions (sleeping, sitting quietly). We also know that the RMR changes in response to major changes in food intake—RMR drops if food is restricted and goes up if food intake is decreased. We also are beginning to understand how regular vigorous physical activity can increase RMR. And some drugs, such as d-fenfluramine which influences appetite level, can alter metabolic processes, reducing eating of high-calorie foods. Furthermore some evidence suggests that higher insulin sensitiv-

Fat Calories Are Getting Fatter

The conventional wisdom used to be that if you burn as many calories as you eat, you will maintain your weight. But not *all* calories are created equal; some turn out to be "heavier" than others. Several studies, such as those of Dr. Mark Hegsted at Harvard, have recently demonstrated that 1 gram of fat used within the body is worth 11 calories, not 9. While burning 1 gram of fat in the laboratory yields 9 calories of energy (and 1 gram of protein or carbohydrate yields 4 calories), the body's use of fat differs. This caloric gain for fat has to do with the body's use of carbohydrates and fats. Carbohydrates are designed primarily to be "burned" immediately by the body, or stored in the liver or muscles as glycogen until needed for energy. The body also uses considerably more calories to make fat from carbohydrates than when it is made from dietary fat.

By contrast, fat in the diet is directly stored as fat tissue and seldom used for energy. In addition, when the body converts dietary fat into fat cells it uses about 3 percent of the calories to make the change. However, the caloric cost of converting carbohydrates into body fat amounts to 23 percent of the calories eaten.

The upshot of this recent research is to raise very serious questions about the wisdom of "calorie counting," as if every calorie of food eaten was equal in its effect on body weight (and body fat). The new wisdom suggests that the same number of calories from dietary fat are more fattening than from carbohydrates. This may help explain why some people have difficulty losing weight on a fairly low-calorie diet. If most of those calories come from fats, then the weight loss will be more difficult. The kind of food you eat—some would say its quality—can make a difference. Maybe it's time to say no to foods high in fats.

ity levels may encourage better weight control. Obese people often suffer from lowered insulin sensitivity in response to increased blood glucose. This lowered sensitivity is related to impaired metabolic processes that can contribute to weight gain. Because metabolic as well as other physiological and genetic factors are involved, rather than just overeating, obesity is not considered an "eating disorder."

Physical Factors In terms of controlling weight and reducing body fat, physical activity (1) uses calories, (2) counteracts ill effects of obesity, (3) suppresses appetite, (4) increases resting metabolic rate (RMR) and possibly overcomes set point effects, and (5) minimizes loss of lean body tissue when losing weight. Note that losing weight through dieting alone, particularly through "starvation" diets of 300 to 600 calories per day, can result in a loss of as much as 50 percent in lean tissue, particularly muscle tissue. However, in a combination of dieting *and* physical activity, lean body tissue lost is only about 5 percent. This difference is very crucial since the goal is losing body fat, not muscle, organ, and other lean body tissue.

Exercise has commonly been ignored as a major factor in obesity because so many calories of physical activity must be spent to lose one pound. For example, in Scandinavia a traditional 49-mile cross-country ski race, which lasts about 10 hours, uses the energy equal to about two pounds of fat tissue. Another way of looking at the relationship of exercise to expending calories is to ask how many minutes of activity are required to use up 100 calories (keep in mind that the energy provided by a medium-sized piece of apple pie is about 350 calories). When running or jogging on the flat, you can take about 10 minutes to burn 100 calories. The same applies to sawing wood, playing racquetball, and swimming. Aerobic dancing may take 15 minutes of activity to burn 100 calories, as might roller skating and playing soccer; playing volleyball, cleaning windows, washing the car, or raking leaves each requires 20 minutes. The energy used (measured in calories) for 10 minutes of various activities based on people who weigh 125, 175, or 250 pounds is presented in Table 13-4. Note that *more* calories are used by heavier people—roughly twice as much by someone weighing 250 pounds as by someone weighing 125 pounds.

Such figures might seem discouraging to a person who is considering physical activity as a direct means of losing weight. Yet a crucial fact is commonly overlooked. Exercise works slowly yet continuously in influencing body weight. The typical American gains from one to two pounds a year between the ages of 20 and 50. All together this gain amounts to about 45 extra pounds by the age of 50. An average weight gain of 1½ pounds a year roughly equals 5,250 calories spread over 365 days. On a daily basis, this equals slightly more than 14.4 calories per day. Thus, just a slight yet consistent and steady increase in

Table 13-4 Calories Used in Ten Minutes of Various Activities

	Body Weight		
	125 Pounds	175 Pounds	250 Pounds
Personal Necessities			
Sleeping	10	14	20
Sitting (watching TV)	10	14	18
Sitting (talking)	15	21	30
Dressing or washing	26	37	53
Standing	12	16	24
Locomotion			
Walking downstairs	56	78	111
Walking upstairs	146	202	288
Walking at 2 mph	29	40	58
Walking at 4 mph	52	72	102
Running at 5.5 mph	90	125	178
Running at 7 mph	118	164	232
Running at 12 mph	164	228	326
Cycling at 5.5 mph	42	58	83
Cycling at 13 mph	89	124	178
Housework			
Making beds	32	46	65
Washing floors	38	53	75
Washing windows	35	48	69
Dusting	22	31	44
Preparing a meal	32	46	65
Shoveling snow	65	89	130
Light gardening	30	42	59
Weeding garden	49	68	98
Mowing grass (power)	34	47	67
Mowing grass (manual)	38	52	74
Sedentary Occupation			
Sitting writing	15	21	30
Light office work	25	34	50
Standing, light activity	20	28	40
Typing (electric)	19	27	39

	Body Weight		
	125 Pounds	175 Pounds	250 Pounds
Light Work			
Assembly line	20	28	40
Auto repair	35	48	69
Carpentry	32	44	64
Bricklaying	28	40	57
Farming chores	32	44	64
House painting	29	40	58
Heavy Work			
Pick and shovel work	56	78	110
Chopping wood	60	84	121
Dragging logs	158	220	315
Drilling coal	79	111	159
Recreation			
Badminton	43	65	94
Volleyball	43	65	94
Baseball	39	54	78
Basketball	58	82	117
Bowling (nonstop)	56	78	111
Canoeing (4 mph)	90	128	182
Dancing (moderate)	35	48	69
Dancing (vigorous)	48	66	94
Football	69	96	137
Golfing	33	48	68
Horseback riding	56	78	112
Ping-Pong	32	45	64
Racquetball	75	104	144
Skiing (downhill)	80	112	160
Skiing (water)	60	88	130
Skiing (cross country)	98	138	194
Squash	75	104	144
Swimming (backstroke)	32	45	64
Swimming (crawl)	40	56	80
Tennis	56	80	115

NOTE: Heavier people use *more* calories than lighter people, because more energy is needed for the extra weight. This table is for *continuous* activity (not for the minutes of resting during an activity). Energy used varies greatly with the *intensity* of doing the activity.
SOURCE: Reprinted with permission from K. D. Brownell, 1987, *The LEARN Program of Weight Control* (Philadelphia: University of Pennsylvania), pp. 64–65.

physical activity over the months and years can literally make the difference between maintaining ideal weight and becoming seriously overfat.

Social, Emotional, and Cultural Factors Eating, as with other human activities, is closely tied not only to how the person is feeling and thinking but also to social relationships and cultural values. We may know, for example, that a person consistently skips breakfast, seldom eats lunch, and chronically eats heavy meals at night. This pattern of eating may be closely tied to family patterns concerning food, sleep, and socializing at dinner. It may also be modeled by other people at school or work. Other examples come readily to mind. The intimate, relaxed dinner may have a special significance for lovers, as does the "working lunch" for business associates or political leaders and the birthday celebration. Food is often invested with religious significance and/or positive family feeling, as in the traditional American Thanksgiving dinner and in the Jewish seder.

Social and emotional meanings are also attached to patterns of eating. Thus, being obese can have an intimate significance for the person, but the nature of that significance depends on both personal and cultural factors.

While looking very slim and trim may be highly valued, especially for women in today's dominant American culture, many other cultures of the world view the round and plump image as very attractive. The growing American obsession with a superslim profile is closely tied to a number of physical, medical, and eating disorders, especially problems of weighing too little.

For young people it is particularly important to start planning a lifestyle that will allow for a reasonable balance of eating healthy foods and getting regular physical activities. With the increasing pressures of time and the growing tendency to eat "convenience" foods that are often very high in fats, salt, and calories plus the lack of vigorous physical activity in most jobs, the young person of today needs to consider ways to eat a balanced nutritious diet and get regular physical activities that together will control body weight.

Exploring Your Emotions

Do you sometimes overeat? If so, what do you feel motivates you? What kinds of food do you tend to overeat, and in what situations?

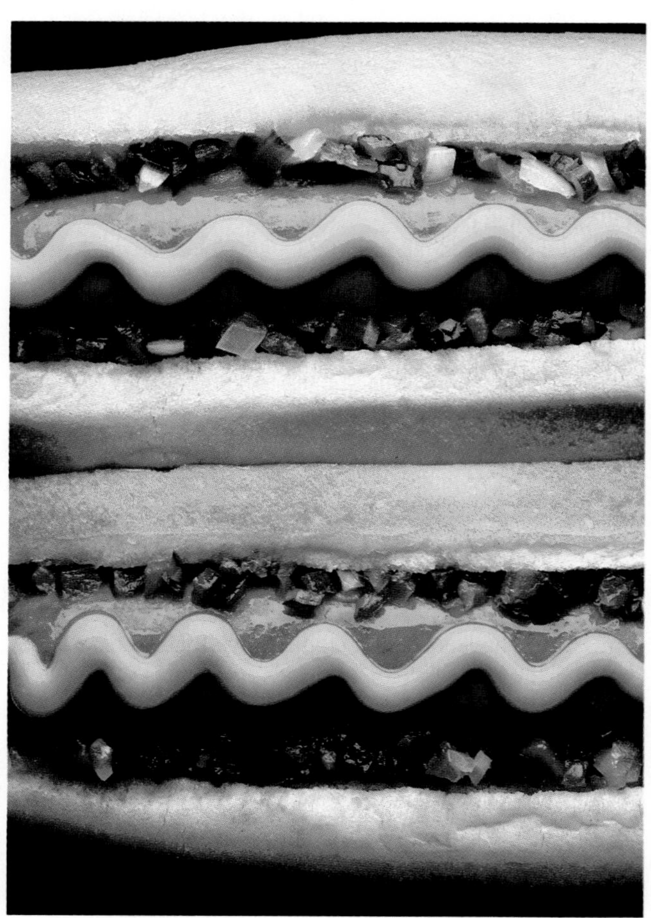
John Katz, photographer

Exploring Your Emotions

Given the higher rates of illness and mortality associated with obesity, how do you feel about the risks of obesity in regard to your chosen career? How do you feel about planning now to take action to reduce such risks?

Failure to Perceive Internal Cues If you need rest you become sleepy, and as soon as you give in to the feeling you fall asleep. When you need food, you feel hunger pangs in your stomach and increased taste sensitivity in your mouth. The sleepy feeling and the hunger pangs are examples of internal cues—sensations in your body that seek a specific response. But people often learn to ignore these cues, sometimes replacing them with external ones. For example, a clever fast food television commercial can make you feel hungry, even without any internal cues. External cues often reflect social and economic demands, but once you have "internalized" them, they seem to be coming from inside you. The internal cue "Eat something now!" is crowded out of consciousness by the external cue "It isn't lunchtime yet." The internal cue "Stop eating!" is often overridden by the external cue "Clean your plate."

Some people are clearly more externally stimulated or cued to eat than others. Learning to become more aware of how external cues influence your eating and other weight-related behaviors can be very helpful in altering unnecessary or compulsive eating as well as changing your choices of what to eat in various situations (for example, party, restaurant, week-end snacks).

Socioeconomic Factors Socioeconomic status (SES) and other socioeconomic factors are involved in obesity as well as eating disorders. Researcher Albert Stunkard notes a very strong relationship between SES level and obesity, especially for women: the prevalence of obesity goes down as SES level goes up. One major study found that the rate of obesity in women was 30 percent for the lower SES group, 16 percent for the middle group, and only 5 percent for the higher SES women. Obesity and SES level are also gender related. More women are obese at lower SES levels than men, but men are somewhat more obese at the higher SES levels than women. These differences may reflect the greater sensitivity and concern for a slim physical appearance among upper SES women. Another social factor in obesity is the number of family generations that have lived in the United States. Among first-generation Americans, 24 percent are obese, as compared to only 5 percent of fourth-generation Americans. These differences are independent of SES level.

Exploring Your Emotions

What cultural and socioeconomic patterns seem to influence the rate of obesity and overweight in your community? What causes for such overweight do you recognize and perhaps identify with to some extent?

Exploring Your Emotions

Have you ever been tempted to engage in self-starvation and/or purging? What kinds of pressures made you feel this way? How do you feel about the fact that most anorexics and bulimics are women?

Why is obesity linked to SES level? Several reasons exist. First, for thousands of years most people have lived at the edge of survival, with famines often occurring. Few people were overweight, and obesity was the mark of affluence and success. To be overweight was direct evidence of being powerful. Fat also served as a protection against future famines brought on by droughts or wars. "Feast or famine" was a regular event. One had to build up a reservoir of available energy now to survive future shortages of food. In more recent times, immigrants to the United States have often come from lands where the basic necessities of life were scarce. These new Americans often have viewed excessive body weight as positive evidence of success and perhaps as a protection against possible hard times in the future.

The role of cultural and ethnic factors was demonstrated in a recent study of Hispanics and Anglo adults in a Texas town. Hispanics of all SES levels were somewhat heavier than Anglos. However, Hispanic and Anglo women weighed more than men at lower SES levels yet considerably less than men at higher SES levels. This study demonstrates that social and economic factors may play a powerful role in determining body weight.

Age Obesity by the age of 50 is three times more prevalent than at the age of 20 and then declines, possibly because of the premature deaths of obese men from cardiovascular problems. In one study morbidly obese males (more than 50 percent over upper weight limit) between the ages of 25 and 54 were twelve times more likely to die than normal weight men of the same age. In general, if young adults (between ages 20 and 40) gain considerable weight, the risk of heart disease and stroke is notably higher. Somewhat more women are obese than men, and the prevalence of obesity for the female population persists beyond age 50 more so than for men. However the health problems of obese women are much *less* than obese men of the same age. This advantage of obese women in having fewer health problems is important to note. Significant biological and genetic factors may allow or even encourage women to gain and to maintain more body weight at less physical health risk than men. Thus the preoccupation and worry of many younger women, especially of higher SES levels, with weighing "a few extra pounds" seems unfounded from a physical health perspective.

Eating Disorders

As discussed earlier, two major eating disorders deserve note: anorexia nervosa and bulimia. Both these disorders have to do with social and psychological problems associated with eating and body weight as well as serious physiological disruptions and disorders. Anorexia is life threatening, leading to death between 15 and 20 percent of the time.

Anorexia In 1694 Dr. Richard Morton, a British physician, described a medical disorder called *anorexia* (from the Greek meaning "loss of appetite"). These people suffered from being on a starvation diet. Morton described them "like a skeleton only clad in skin." They also suffered from other physical and psychological problems associated with starving. Recently the dramatic increase (for example, over 300 percent between the 1950s to 1970s) in anorexia among young women has prompted a great deal of scientific research in what is now considered a serious psychological and medical disorder. Note that about 95 percent of anorexics are women.

What are the major characteristics of anorexia? The diagnostic criteria established by the American Psychiatric Association in 1980 (*DSM III*) include:

1. Intense fear of becoming obese that does not diminish as weight loss progresses
2. Disturbance of body image (such as claiming to "feel fat" or see oneself as fat, even though emaciated)
3. Weight loss of at least 25 percent of original normal body weight (if under 18, projected weight gain from growth charts for age is also considered)
4. Refusal to maintain body weight at minimal normal weight for age and height
5. No known physical illness or biologic factor that could explain extreme weight loss

There are different *types* of anorexics: (1) "restricting" type, who rigidly stick to a starvation-like diet; and (2) the "bulimic" type, who swing between overeating ("binge" eating), purging, often through self-induced vomiting, and back to restrained eating. Both types also commonly use vigorous and prolonged physical activities to reduce body weight. Second, the personalities of anorexics tend to differ from women who are of normal weight or who suffer from other problems, such as depression or anxiety. Researchers describe the anorexic as (1) somewhat obsessive, (2) usually introverted, (3) emotionally reserved and socially insecure, (4) very self-critical, (5) self-denying and deferential to others, and (6) overly rigid and stereotyped in their thinking. The two types commonly differ in personality, the bulimic type being more socially outgoing, more labile (up and down) in emotional state, and more socially deviant (for example, more likely to smoke, abuse alcohol and other drugs).

The physical complications of anorexia are considerable. Essentially, the person is starving, and death may occur if the condition is not reversed. The problems include serious metabolic problems, such as irregular cholesterol levels, liver dysfunction, low blood glucose levels (prolonged hypoglycemia), heart problems, including disruptions in the electrical control of the heart (arrhythmias), and serious endocrine (hormonal) abnormalities, such as low estrogen and growth hormone levels and elevated cortisol levels (cortisol is a hormone associated with negative emotional arousal). One of the most common symptoms, almost always present, is amenorrhea (stopping of menstrual cycle). Constipation, low blood pressure, skin discoloration (yellowing) and dryness, and hypothermia (low body temperature) are also common.

The causes of anorexia remain unclear, although most researchers believe social and family problems (especially with parents) are major causes, plus tremendous social and peer pressures to look very slim and trim. No evidence suggests any major genetic causes. Clearly, much of the problem stems from how the young woman thinks and feels about herself in relation to others, especially during early adolescence. Some theorists consider anorexia as a weight or fat phobia, an intense fear of being overweight. Thus, anorexia seems closely tied to a variety of social maturational problems as the person moves toward adulthood. How prevalent is anorexia? Estimates generally range between 1 to 2½ million Americans.

Treatment programs often share much in common with comprehensive programs focused on obesity. The first phase involves immediate help, often using reward techniques for eating, and sometimes requiring the person to be hospitalized. The primary goal is to increase body weight to a less dangerous level (for example, from 47 pounds to 70 pounds). The second phase is a counseling program to help the person continue to gain weight and begin to solve the various social and psychological problems that have contributed to the extreme fear of weighing too much as well as the other social and psychological characteristics (for example, feeling very self-critical and socially insecure). With considerable patience and persistence, plus social support and a behaviorally oriented program, the anorexic may become a normal weight person who is less obsessed with the shape and size of her body and is less fearful of "feeling fat" and looking heavy.

Bulimia This eating disorder commonly involves normal weight women (and a few men) in their late teens and twenties who adhere to strict dieting and restrained eating, then engage in binging; that is, rapid eating of large amounts of food within a two-hour period. Binge eating is then followed by a purging, usually by self-induced vomiting or taking large amounts of laxatives. The criteria used to identify bulimia are as follows:

1. Recurrent episodes of binge eating
2. At least three of the following:
   a. Eating high-calorie, easily digested food (for example, cookies, cakes, candy)
   b. Eating alone or inconspicuously
   c. Stopping eating when abdominal pain, sleep, social interruption, or self-induced vomiting occur
   d. Repeated attempts to lose weight by severely restricted diets, self-induced vomiting, diuretics, or laxatives
   e. Frequent weight fluctuations greater than 10 pounds due to binges and fasts
3. Awareness that the eating pattern is abnormal and fear of not being able to stop voluntarily
4. Depressed mood and self-critical thoughts after food binges
5. Lack of any known physical disorder

Understanding of bulimia, sometimes called *bulimia nervosa* or the "dietary chaos syndrome," is limited, because research started less than a decade ago. Bulimics and anorexics share many personality characteristics and much behavioral style. Both share a preoccupation with body shape and size as well as with food; both adhere to very strict or highly limited diets, often feel depressed, have low self-esteem, and have rigid beliefs about the need to diet and lose weight. Furthermore, roughly 40 to 50 percent of anorexics engage in binging and purging (the bulimic type), and many bulimics have been anorexic or shift back and forth from anorexia to bulimia.

The major difference is that the bulimic is not abnormal in body weight. The causes of bulimia are unclear, although some researchers believe causes involve a combination of behavior, emotions, and physiology. As with anorexia, little evidence suggests that bulimia is caused by genetic or biological factors.

Dehydration A potentially dangerous condition in which a person has less than a normal amount of body water.

What contributes to this cycle of strict dieting, binging, and purging? One view is that the person is under considerable pressure to comply with a severely restricting diet and experiences a lapse (gives in to the hunger and anticipated pleasure of high-calorie food). Once engaged in eating a small amount of so-called forbidden food, the person becomes upset about eating. This upset in turn interferes with the person's self-control, and the person gives in to intense hunger ("I've blown it, so what's the use of trying"). Binging then triggers purging as a way of trying to solve the problem of having eaten too much.

Unfortunately, vomiting as a solution to the binge eating creates a number of problems. First, it can intensify hunger and contribute to starting the cycle again. It also reinforces the very hungry person sometimes to yield to strong urges to overeat, because vomiting does eliminate weight gaining as a consequence of overeating. Furthermore, vomiting—sometimes two to three times a day—can create serious medical and physiological problems. These may include potassium deficiency, dehydration, gastrointestinal problems, liver disease, abnormal brainwave patterns (EEG), and endocrine (hormonal) problems.

The prevalence of bulimia among young women in the United States has not been carefully studied. Estimates range from 1 to 15 percent of American women. Among high school women, the estimate is 5 percent while it may be as high as 10 to 15 percent among college women. Controlled studies to help bulimics have only recently been conducted. As with anorexia, the most promising programs combine procedures to help the bulimic alter lifestyle, especially eating and purging behavior, as well as feelings and thoughts about self- and body image.

How Can Weight Be Controlled?

Controlling weight depends on several factors:

1. Degree of overfat
2. Past experience in controlling weight, including eating habits and physical activities
3. Age and gender
4. Social, cultural, and ethnic factors
5. Genetics, metabolic processes, and family history

Dieting alone is a very poor long-term solution for taking off fat and keeping it off. Diets that offer simple solutions to the complex problems of being overweight may actually be bad for you—especially by not supplying the full range of nutrients you need and, even more importantly, by possibly setting you up for long-term failure.

Knowing what kinds of food are eaten and how much is important. But you also need to realize that the weight control game involves many players and requires a variety of game strategies, including teamwork. As we have seen, the causes of being overfat involve a variety of factors. It is not just eating too much. Although they may seem very complex and confusing, some strategies for losing body fat and keeping it lost turn out to be straightforward and successful when people are patient yet persistent in their efforts.

The average number of pounds lost in controlled weight loss studies in 1984 was 15.4 pounds, up from an 8.4-pound average in 1974. The improvement was due to longer treatment programs (about three months in length compared to two months) and to a greater variety of treatment methods. Using behavioral methods—such as monitoring and recording calories and physical activity, establishing short-term goals about how much to eat and exercise each day, and providing self-rewards for progress—commonly leads to losses of 0.5 to 2 pounds per week, losses that are mostly body fat and not lean tissue. Furthermore, discouraging long-term results are mostly due to going on diets without also trying other procedures. When controlled eating (but not crash or rash diets) is *combined* with regular physical activities and attention to improving social relationships and support plus reducing self-defeating attitudes (cognitive processes), the results are much more encouraging.

Dieting Most low-calorie diets cause a rapid loss of body water at first. The weight loss shows up on scales, and many beginning dieters think that they are losing body fat. It soon becomes obvious to all but the most blindly optimistic dieters that they cannot keep on losing weight so quickly. If they somehow manage to persist, they can suffer serious **dehydration.** Rapid weight loss stemming from loss of body water is usually followed by an equally rapid weight gain.

Eating the right foods is very important (see Chapters 12 and 14). Nonfat or low-fat dairy products and complex carbohydrates—that is, fresh fruit and vegetables high in water and fiber—are best. Some examples of complex carbohydrates include potatoes (not fried), broccoli, tomatoes, pasta (spaghetti, macaroni), oatmeal, multigrain breads, and beans. Foods high in fats are loaded with calories and tend to add to weight problems, especially for inactive people. Balance in the diet is crucial. Most experts agree that you should eat some food in the

Myths about Crash Diets

Myth "Crash" or very low-calorie diets will lead to a permanent loss of body weight, and to a swift loss of body fat in a short time ('Lose 10 pounds in 10 days!').

Fact Actually, what is mostly lost rapidly in the first several days of dieting is body water, not fat. Going "on a strict diet" is usually followed by going "off a diet," and a return of the lost weight, sometimes even more weight than before.

Myth Very restricted dieting (for example, only eating fresh fruits or milk products) can be safe and effective in losing weight rapidly.

Fact Such diets are very unsafe because the body needs a complete balance of four basic food types (beans, grains, and nuts; fruits and vegetables; milk products; and poultry, fish, eggs) to ensure sufficient intake of complex carbohydrates, proteins, and fats as well as vitamins, minerals, and electrolytes daily.

Myth Fasting is the most powerful strategy to use in taking off excessive weight rapidly.

Fact Complete fasting can be very dangerous for several reasons. First, the body can lose almost as much lean body mass (from 30 to 50 percent), such as muscle tissue, as fat tissue. This protein malnutrition can seriously disrupt liver, kidney, and lung functioning as well as the nervous system. Also, fasting can reduce the body's level of antibodies that are essential in fighting disease. Fasting also reduces the storage of glucogen (glucose) in the body's muscles. Reduced glucogen can lower physical activity levels and may encourage diabetes. Finally, fasting stimulates the liver to release more poor-quality cholesterol into the bloodstream (low-density lipoprotein, or LDL) and reduces availability of the better-quality cholesterol (high-density lipoprotein, or HDL cholesterol).

Myth Obesity is caused by overeating, and strict dieting by itself can cure obesity.

Fact Seems logical, but it's not true. Excessive storage of body energy (mainly fat) is caused by several factors, not just how much food is eaten. Saying that people get fat only because they overeat is like saying that the sun comes up because it's morning. Total body weight depends on the body's "set point," the resting metabolic rate (RMR), the heat producing ("thermic") effects of food, and the amount of energy used in various physical activities. Thus, dieting by itself to lose and maintain weight loss, especially fat loss, is seldom successful and, more importantly, can be harmful to future efforts to lose body fat. The "yo-yo" effect of losing and then regaining body fat several times builds more and more resistance to future weight loss by dieting. Researchers have recently called this problem "diet-induced obesity."

Myth Skipping meals helps lose weight.

Fact Actually, skipping meals, such as breakfast, commonly leads to overeating at the next meal, *and, more importantly,* contributes to energy and mood changes that make it more difficult to lose weight. Eating *more* often, such as minimeals four to six times a day ("grazing"), and avoiding fats and refined sugars encourage weight loss by controlling appetite and increasing energy levels so that vigorous aerobic-type physical activities can be performed.

four major food groups: dairy products, fruits and vegetables, breads and cereals, and fish, poultry, and meats. Experts disagree about how much of each group is needed. Some argue that meats high in animal fat and cholesterol (for example, beef, sausage, pork) should be avoided along with eggs and dairy products, also because of fat and cholesterol. (Nonfat dairy products are the exception.) From a weight loss perspective, you should definitely cut down eating most meats, whole-milk dairy products, and "sweets" because they are high in fat.

Three balanced meals a day are important, especially breakfast. Skipping breakfast to save time and calories is a bad strategy in the weight control game. Snacks planned ahead of time also help reduce impulsive eating of foods high in fat and sodium. Watch out especially for foods high in fats. Remember that 1 gram of fat has 9 calories while 1 gram of carbohydrate or protein has only 4 calories. Table 13-5 provides a contrast of high- and low-fat foods. Any diet should minimize high-fat foods. By following these suggestions and by increasing physical activity, many overweight people can gradually achieve and maintain a healthy weight that reduces their excess body fat.

The goal in treating obesity is twofold. The person's

first aim should be to reach ideal weight; the second should be to maintain that weight for the rest of his or her life. Speed is not what counts, and is physiologically impossible, yet most popular diets promise just that. Consider, for example, a diet that promises a 220-pound man that he will lose 22 pounds in 10 days. Even if he eats nothing, his calorie deficit will only be about 3,500 calories a day, or 35,000 calories in 10 days. At the rate of 1 pound of fat lost per 3,500-calorie deficit, he will lose only about 9 pounds in those 10 days. And remember, this loss is what would occur if he ate absolutely nothing. Also remember that about 3 to 5 of those pounds will not be lost fat but lost muscle and other lean body tissue. (That is why starvation-type diets can be very dangerous.) If he did indeed lose 22 pounds, much of it would be lost body water, which would replenish itself once he started eating again.

Why is the "quick and fast" approach to weight loss so appealing? Probably because some people want immediate results, so they can feel good about making progress in losing weight. That's why so many advertisements in magazines and on television focus on losing weight quickly. What those ads fail to tell you is that most of the loss is body water, not fat. Trying to lose weight and keep it off involves saying no to eating rich and often fatty foods that taste good. Also involved is doing more physical activities and that requires time and effort. Thus, the attraction of going on a quick diet and quickly shedding many pounds is very appealing. While there is much to be said for the encouragement of feeling successful, it should be based on real success. In reducing body fat, the result of quick success is often fast failure.

Table 13-5 Foods and Their Fat

Percent Fat	Foods
90–100%	Fats, lard, salad and cooking oils
80–90	Butter, margarine
70–80	Mayonnaise, macadamia nuts, pecans
50–70	Almonds, walnuts, dried unsweetened coconut, bacon, baking chocolate
30–50	Steaks, spareribs, pork chops, goose, cheddar and cream cheeses, potato chips, French dressing, chocolate candy
20–30	Pot roast, lamb chop, frankfurters, ground beef, chocolate chip cookies
10–20	Round steak, veal chop, turkey, eggs, avocado, olives, chocolate cake and icing, french fries, ice cream, apple pie
1–10	Pork and beans, most fish, broiled chicken, crab, cottage cheese, liver, milk, creamed soups, sherbet, most cereals
Less than 1	Potatoes, most vegetables and fruits, egg whites, chicken, consommé

SOURCE: Reprinted with permission from K. D. Brownell, 1987, *The LEARN Program of Weight Control* (Philadelphia: University of Pennsylvania), p. 105.

Altering the amount and the type or quality of food eaten is very important. But it is far from the whole story. *Moderation* in quantity and variety in types of food eaten are crucial qualities of a healthy diet. A sensible weight loss strategy should strive for reducing body fat gradually by no more than 1 to 2 pounds per week. The key to successful dieting, as with other effective strategies needed to stay at your ideal low fat weight, lies in *permanently* altering your eating habits—what you eat, how much you eat, and how often you eat. Above all, the nutritional quality of what goes in is key to whether the fat goes on. By reducing fats in your diet, you will be reducing fats in your body.

Physical Activity Walking one mile every day for two years will expend about 73,000 calories, the equivalent of 18.2 pounds of body fat. (See Table 13-4.) Probably the most common myth about exercise is that it increases appetite and eating. Studies with experimental animals have shown this belief to be false. When normally sedentary animals were required to perform a moderate amount of exercise regularly, their consumption of food *decreased* and so did their weight. Only strenuous regular exercise causes people to eat more, and in such instances this increase is appropriate to the increased energy expenditure. The additional food intake does not result in a weight gain; it often does not even make up weight that is lost because of the energy used in being active.

Vigorous aerobic activities typically *reduce* food intake for a few hours and sometimes for the whole day of the activity. Obese people often experience less appetite after exercising vigorously, and they also use more calories in such activities because of their greater weight (see Table 13-4).

Exercising once in a while, however, is no more effective than eating balanced meals once in a while. A good physical program for weight loss does not produce spectacular results overnight (nor does a good diet), but if the program is followed faithfully over a long period of time, the total amount of weight lost will be reasonably large. Anyone beginning an activity program should start slowly

(continued on p. 302)

25 Tips from the Diet Center

By now, everyone knows about the Diet Center, but just in case . . . it is the world's largest weight-loss organization, with 1,758 offices across the country and a common-sense approach to diet that works so well, members lose a million pounds a month. Diet Center counselors gave us this batch of tried-and-true suggestions, practically guaranteed to keep you slim.

1. When you feel the urge to overeat, head for the nearest mirror and take a good, long look at yourself. (Do you still crave those extra calories?)

2. Parties needn't sabotage a diet: Call your hostess in advance and ask if you may bring one of your special (low-cal) dishes, beautifully prepared, to share with the guests.

3. If boredom is your downfall—if you tend to eat because there's nothing else to do—realize it's not food you want, but something to fill the void. Write letters, clean a closet, take a walk—anything to keep your mind and body occupied.

4. Midafternoon is the toughest time for many dieters. Be prepared for the four o'clock slump with an appropriate snack, such as any one of these items, each less than 100 calories: small baked potato; sliver of angelfood cake; twenty-eight chocolate chips; "Danish" made with thin-sliced bread topped with 1 tablespoon cottage cheese, 1 teaspoon sugar, cinnamon; popcorn flavored with Parmesan cheese; mug of hot chicken bouillon. (Keep snacks handy in a desk drawer if you work.)

5. Avoid the temptation to finish what the kids leave on their plates by having them, or your spouse, remove the plates and then wrap or dispose of leftovers as soon as the children have gotten up from the table.

6. Start thinking of food as fuel for your body's engine and eating as simply a way to keep your motor humming.

7. Make a "dream-come-true" bulletin board and hang it in a prominent place. Pin up pictures of how you want to look, slinky clothes you'd love to wear, things you'd like to do when you're thinner.

8. Be firm with people who "love you" with food. If your mother makes lasagna each time you visit, explain that losing weight is your top priority and she can *really* show she cares by broiling a piece of chicken for you.

9. Don't be discouraged if you're not losing pounds as fast as you think you should. When you hit a plateau, get out the tape measure and check for inch loss. Often the tape will show what the scales do not.

10. Read labels carefully when you shop for food. Bear in mind that any ingredient ending in "-ose" (dextrose, sucrose, fructose, maltose, for example) is a sugar.

11. Avoid wearing clothes you can hide in. Big, shapeless dresses and skirts with elastic waistbands disguise excess poundage, but offer little incentive to lose. Neatly fitted clothes with zippers, buttons and belts keep you and others aware of your progress.

12. Use modified "aversion conditioning" techniques to help you deal with temptation: When faced with a plate of cookies, french fries, anything you love, try to visualize the food soaking wet, covered with sand or ashes, stale or moldy.

13. Eat elegantly, even though you're counting calories. Smaller portions seem much more satisfying when arranged artfully, dressed up with colorful garnishes, served on best china and glassware.

14. Keep the fridge stocked with appropriate food so you'll never be caught with nothing but no-nos to eat. Boil a dozen eggs, cook up lots of fish and chicken breasts at once, cut up and store huge quantities of salad vegetables, etc.

15. When stress threatens to wear down your willpower, get away from the source of the tension if possible. Most important, ask yourself, "How would overeating help me in this situation?"

16. Shopping for a party? Don't store chips, cookies or other goodies where they might tempt you. Keep them out of sight and out of mind until the big day . . . locked in the trunk of your car if need be.

17. Get started on an exercise routine to burn off additional calories and tone muscles. Program your workout into the same time slot daily; don't allow anything but an emergency to interfere.

18. Shop for a really sensational dress or suit in the size that you want to be. Use the store's layaway plan and pay something on the outfit each time you lose five pounds. By the time you finally reach your weight goal, your new clothes will be paid for and ready to wear.

19. Plan meals carefully so that there will be little if any food left over for snacking later. (When

25 Tips from the Diet Center (*continued*)

entertaining, send leftovers home with guests.)

20. Hang a calendar near the bathroom scale and record your weight weekly. Take a moment or two at weigh-in time to give yourself a pep talk and plan your day's diet.

21. Eat an apple or munch on a carrot or celery sticks if preparing the evening meal makes you ravenous. Something to nibble on while fixing dinner helps you break the destructive taste-as-you-cook habit.

22. Cooperate with a dieting friend if you're both having trouble finding the time to shop and prepare special low-cal meals. One week, you shop for the two of you; she cooks. The next week, she shops; you cook.

23. Carry a "fat" picture of yourself in your wallet. (The more unflattering the photo, the better.) Take a peek at it whenever you feel your resolve beginning to waver.

24. If you need extra help getting from Friday P.M. to Monday A.M. without bingeing, map out a weekend diet strategy, listing in detail exactly what you will eat and when. Prepare food ahead and follow your plan exactly. It's when you *don't* have a plan that problems arise.

25. Get out of the mind set that uses food as a reward. Make a list of nonfood treats for when you need a psychic lift—a new lipstick, a paperback book, a long-distance call to your best friend, a movie. And of course, promise yourself something extra special when you reach your long-term goal.

Ladies' Home Journal (February 1984), pp 93, 122.

Evaluating a Fad Diet

We cannot possibly examine all the diets and reducing aids that promise quick, easy results, but we can use several criteria to evaluate a weight reduction program:

1. *Does it have any real advantages over existing or conventional diets?* Most fad diets have a gimmick, such as eating grapefruit or using liquid protein supplements. Do these gimmicks work, or are they only a means of attracting attention to the diet?

2. *Is the diet easy to follow?* Fasting, for instance, produces a weight loss, but it requires a great deal of willpower. Most people cannot keep it up for very long.

3. *Does the diet provide any long-term modification of eating habits that will allow the weight loss to be maintained after the diet is over?* Many diets, such as liquid protein diets and fasting, and diet aids, such as drugs, can produce a weight loss. However, because eating behavior is not changed, the person usually regains the weight.

4. *Does the diet present any hazard to health?* Very restrictive diets may lead to malnutrition; others, such as liquid protein diets, have caused injury and even death.

5. *How much does it cost?* Often the dieter is enticed into buying expensive equipment or overpriced "special" foods. Seldom are these items of any value.

6. *Does the diet promise quick results in return for little effort on the part of the dieter?* This is one of the hallmarks of a fad diet. Many of these claims simply are not true. Rapid weight losses observed on some diets, such as the low-carbohydrate diet, are caused by water loss.

7. *Are there any inconsistencies with established knowledge?* Examples include the assertion that carbohydrates rather than excess kilocalories are fattening and that grapefruit possesses some magical weight-reducing property.

William L. Scheider
Nutrition: Basic Concepts and Applications

Diuretic An agent that increases excretion of water by the kidneys, thus reducing water in the body.

and increase demands over time. The weight lost through exercise is primarily body fat (over 90 percent). Regular exercise produces a trimmer and healthier-looking body and will not deplete lean muscle tissue. Increasing exercise is easier if you approach it gradually. For example, increase your daily activities by walking up stairs instead of using elevators, by walking or cycling to school or work, or by parking far enough away from your destination to allow yourself to walk some distance. The benefits of weight loss via frequent planned physical activities are also extremely positive because the body's RMR often increases. Thus, over time the person will continually use more energy at all times, even while sleeping!

People who have lost considerable weight (over 50 pounds) and who have *kept* it off have continued to exercise vigorously, often increasing their physical activity levels after the initial weight loss. The most successful weight losers have been those who have combined a lower-calorie, lower-fat yet balanced diet with regular vigorous activity. In addition, some evidence suggests that increased activity coupled with reduced caloric intake may help the body to "reset" its weight point at a lower level. Thus, the weight loss from physical play and exercise is gradual yet much more likely to be permanent. Sustaining a well-balanced routine of physical activities, especially play activities that one enjoys, is just as important as a well-balanced diet.

Medical and Psychological Approaches A variety of medical and psychological methods have been used in weight control. Treatment with drugs involves the use of amphetamines and similar drugs to suppress appetite. In combination with a diet and under medical supervision, drugs have very limited usefulness. Furthermore, they have a serious potential for abuse that far outweighs their effectiveness. No scientific data support the use of drugs to suppress the appetite. And their side effects may include insomnia, marked irritability, dry mouth, and addiction. Recently, a Food and Drug Administration (FDA) investigation disclosed several deaths of obese people from using various combinations of drugs to lose weight. A particularly lethal combination involved amphetamines (stimulants) to suppress appetite, another drug that combines stimulants and depressants to control appetite, and a diuretic drug to reduce body fluids.

Some drugs act on the kidneys to promote loss of water from the body. These **diuretics** are also often advocated for the treatment of obesity. However, uncontrolled use of diuretics risks severe dehydration. Besides, obesity is a problem of too much fat, and diuretics have no effect on reducing body fat. The attraction of diuretics is the rapid weight loss from water that occurs. Standing on the scale will show a loss, but with the next glass of water (or any liquid) this weight is regained.

"Starch blockers," tablets containing the protein phaseolamin extracted from kidney beans, are another so-called solution to weight loss. No scientific evidence exists that weight loss occurs or is maintained by starch blockers; furthermore, they may cause cramps, nausea, and diarrhea. And eating complex carbohydrate (starchy) foods (fruits and vegetables, including beans and legumes as well as whole grains such as wheat, oats, rice, barley) helps greatly in curbing appetite, adds bulk and fiber, and reduces the excessively high amounts of fat and protein foods that most Americans eat.

Fasting as a method for losing weight is no longer widely favored. In the first place, total starvation leads to substantial loss of body constituents other than fat—notably, proteins and lean body tissue. Second, this approach can be dangerous. To be safe, the program must be carried out under strict medical supervision, an expense that most people cannot meet. Finally, people have suffered significant complications as a result of total starvation. These include acute attacks of gout (painful swelling of the feet), severe anemia, sudden drops in blood pressure, and in a few cases severe metabolic disturbances.

More importantly, total fasting does little, if anything, to change eating habits and to encourage regular vigorous physical activities. Indeed, fasting weakens people, discouraging them from being more active. Almost all people who have lost weight under starvation conditions have gained it back rapidly, especially if they lost it under unusual conditions such as in a hospital or at a fashionable "fat farm." When they return home, they resume their poor eating and exercise habits and rapidly regain the lost weight.

Are there any advantages to fasting, or to a near fasting or very low-calorie approach? Some medical authorities have argued for a very low-calorie (VLC), high-protein diet (between 200–800 calories per day) carefully supplemented with vitamins, minerals, and electrolytes. (Electrolyte balance helps maintain proper fluid levels and prevent dehydration and excessively low blood pressure.) Recent results of using VLC diets under strict medical supervision supplemented with vitamins and minerals have not been encouraging. Some studies report losses averaging 65 pounds over six months. But follow-up studies indicate that the dieters regain most of the lost weight. For example, one study followed people for two years. Although most had lost over 40 pounds on a supple-

Play Plans for Exercise and Weight Loss

Peter Wood has developed a variety of ways in which people can reduce weight and avoid unpleasant dieting. One strategy concerns using so many calories each day in play activities—doing things that are fun and interesting. If a person gets into the habit of expending a few more calories each day, then in time he or she can lose many pounds. Here are three plans, each designed to use up a different number of calories. Plan A is a minimum plan, while Plans E and J are more vigorous.

Play Plan A (25 calories per day)

Choose *one* playful act *each* day from the accompanying list. These are *extra* play calories to *add* to your usual routine.

Walk a quarter mile (3 blocks).

Cycle a mile, slowly.

Swim for 3 minutes.

Dance (aerobic) for 5 minutes.

Clean windows for 6 minutes.

Rake leaves for 6 minutes.

Scrub floor for 6 minutes.

Feel free to try different activities on different days.

Playful Hints . . .

- Get off to a good start—don't overdo!
- Find a playful friend!
- Don't forget—keep your play record.
- Yes—it's easy to start with, but there's lots more fun to come!

Play Plan E (150 calories per day)

Choose *one* activity every day.

Walk at moderate speed for 30 minutes.

Cycle for 25 minutes.

Swim for 15 minutes.

Dance (aerobic) for 25 minutes.

Dance (disco) for 30 minutes.

Play volleyball for 30 minutes.

Play table tennis for 30 minutes.

Clean windows to music for 30 minutes.

Scrub floors to music for 30 minutes.

Playful Hints . . .

- Do you have a companion to play with? Whom do you know who would like to lose weight with you?
- Make some of your play useful: clean windows or scrub floors to music! The exercise is burning fat.
- Think "play" whenever you have to go somewhere: Can you walk over, not ride? Is the bike handy? Why not walk to and from the restaurant? Go on, even jog a little on the way!
- If you don't drive, you won't have a parking problem (or a parking ticket).

Play Plan J (500 calories per day)

Choose *one* activity each day:

- Walk five miles in 75 to 90 minutes.
- Run for 45 minutes.
- Cycle for 60 minutes.
- Play racquetball for 60 minutes.
- Dance (aerobic) for 60 minutes.
- Play soccer for 60 minutes.
- Roller skate for 65 minutes.
- Mow the lawn for 60 minutes.
- Saw wood for 50 minutes.

This high level of fitness should be approached slowly. It involves playing vigorously for about an hour a day, or 4 percent of our 24-hour day. The player is very fit, eats a lot, and has banished weight problems!

Playful Hints . . .

- Major league stuff!
- Remember, drink more water than you feel you need when it's hot.
- To avoid injuries, do your stretching exercises and vary your plan.
- You are now twenty times more playful than you were at month 1.
- You have played away 4½ pounds of fat this month!
- This level of play will keep you slim and fit forever!

Peter Wood, 1983, *The California Diet and Exercise Program* (Mountain View, Calif.: Anderson World Books).

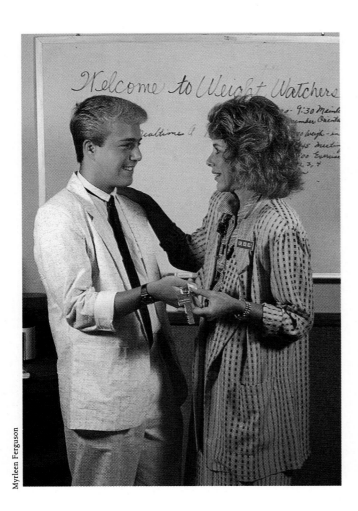

Myrleen Ferguson

mented fast during the first year, over 30 pounds were regained after the second year.

Group treatment of obesity is available through self-help organizations such as TOPS (Take Off Pounds Sensibly) and commercial organizations such as Weight Watchers (which has a membership of several million). Many obese people are apparently more inclined to use the services of Weight Watchers than to seek medical or self-help group assistance. The effectiveness of Weight Watchers, however, is somewhat difficult to evaluate, because few controlled studies have been conducted. Furthermore, commercial (for profit) organizations typically do not release information about their results.

Individual psychotherapy can also be a treatment for obesity. Over half the people seeing a professional (for example, psychiatrist) for obesity treatment report emotional disturbances, including anxiety and depression, associated with fasting or restricted-calorie diets. It is unclear if the obesity precedes or follows anxiety and depression. However, no evidence exists that exploring the historical causes of overeating can reduce overeating or body fat in any substantial fashion.

Cognitive-Behavioral Treatment A real breakthrough in treating obesity was reported in 1967 when Richard Stuart described a very successful treatment using behavior modification. Eighty percent of his subjects lost more than 20 pounds and some lost 30 to 40 pounds over one year. Many other studies have demonstrated successful use of behavior modification to treat mild to moderate obesity.

Since Stuart's initial results, other behavioral programs have been tried, but few matched these impressive results until recently. Currently, due to expanded time and methods, most behavioral programs now yield weight losses of 15 pounds over three months, with some programs showing losses of 20 pounds maintained after twelve months. Some of the advantages of behavioral programs, compared to other approaches, include (1) few emotional symptoms arise during treatments, (2) the dropout rates are fairly low, and (3) overall positive psychological functioning tends to increase.

Behavioral approaches vary widely but often focus on changing behavior associated with poor eating and physical activity habits. Such programs teach people specific ways to change maladaptive eating habits. Most programs include recording of food intake and weight (see Figure 13-2); the setting of reasonable weight loss goals (usually from 1 to 1½ pounds per week); rewards for success in changing habits; nutritional counseling; social rewards (achieved by teaching family and friends to praise, not criticize); cognitive strategies for directing appropriate behavior and countering self-defeating thoughts; and stimulus-control procedures that reduce the presence and availability of calorie-rich foods. Several major factors are associated with successful weight control programs: (1) behavioral focus on the person's "lifestyle"; (2) increasing physical activities, especially aerobic type; (3) changes in "cognitive" area, such as certain attitudes, beliefs, and self-talk; (4) increasing social support and improving interpersonal relationships; and (5) increasing accurate knowledge and understanding of nutrition and diet. Within these five areas, the nature of complex cycles and chains of events—interlocking events—is important to understand. Figure 13-3 presents two simple chains, illustrating how what a person thinks and feels influences eating and how a particular setting (such as sitting in front of the television set) also influences actions. Also important in successful weight and fat reduction programs are frequent and "intensive" sessions that continue beyond a few weeks. The strong temptations to slip back into old habits and attitudes require patient and persistent help from others. Keeping "on task" is hard work, and discouragement comes easy. Knowing that you will be often "checking in" with others about your weight, eating habits, physical activities, and emotional state goes a long way in providing the motivation to keep at it.

FOOD (KIND & AMOUNT)	TIME	FEELINGS	ACTIVITY	CALORIES
BREAKFAST				
Coffee 8oz.	7:30	Tired	Paper	0
Scram eggs, 2				222
Orange juice, 1 cup				122
			Total	344
LUNCH				
Roast beef sandwich	12:30	Hurried	Officework	241
Ritz crackers, 6				90
Hot cocoa, 1 cup				175
			Total	506
DINNER				
Chicken pot pie	7:00	Relaxed	T.V.	545
Carrot-raisin salad				310
Cauliflower, 1 cup				28
Skim milk, 1 cup				88
			Total	971
SNACKS				
Candy bar, 1½ oz.	2:45	Content	Reading report	210
Coke, 12oz.	3:15	Angry	Phone	144
Saltines, 5	9:15	Bored	T.V.	75
Peanut butter, 2 tbs.	"	"	"	188
			Total	617
DAILY CALORIE TOTAL 2,438				

Figure 13-2 Food Diary

Is Sugar Addictive?

A member of the board of Overeaters Anonymous, who calls herself a "recovered sucroholic," says she is convinced that refined sugar can be as addictive as alcohol:

> Many of us use sugar like a drug. It is our lover, friend, comforter, and when stress comes into our lives we reach for it automatically. Giving it up is terribly difficult; many people go through withdrawal and get the shakes. For some of us, complete abstinence is the only way out. We cannot be social sugar eaters just the way other people cannot be social drinkers.[1]

Another person who calls himself an "addict" is William Dufty, the author of the bestseller *Sugar Blues*.[2] Dufty describes how he kicked the sugar habit:

> I threw out everything that had sugar in it, cereals and canned fruit, soups and bread. . . . In about forty-eight hours, I was in total agony, overcome with nausea, with a crashing migraine. . . . I had it very rough for about twenty-four hours, but the morning after was a revelation. I went to sleep with exhaustion, sweating and tremors. I woke up feeling reborn.[3]

According to *Sugar Blues,* if you allow yourself to get "hooked" on sugar, your addiction can lead to physical and mental ruin. The front cover describes sugar as "the killer in your diet," while the back cover states, "Like opium, morphine and heroin, sugar is an addictive, destructive drug."

Is sugar an addictive drug? Can it lead to total destruction? Can it kill? Some intricate reasoning from experiments with animals sheds some needed light on the question. The outcome of the experiments was that animals can appear addicted to sugar under certain artificial circumstances; but when allowed access to normal food, they will not eat too much sugar. On a poor (low-protein) diet, however, their reliance on sugar becomes excessive. *Addiction,* then, is too strong a term to use for their relationship to sugar, but they certainly could be said to indulge in sugar *abuse.*

Can the same be said of people? Are they sugar abusers, or are they addicts? We should tell you right away that we have no final answer to this question, but can perhaps shed a little light on it. People's behavior seems more complex than animals' behavior, partly because people are conscious of what they do. They not only respond to stimuli (such as a sweet taste); they know they are responding. They think about it—and what they think may influence how they respond the next time.

You may have noticed the intensity of the feelings expressed by the two people quoted here. They shared a belief system; they *knew* they were addicted. Question: which comes first—the behavior or the belief? Some think the belief causes the behavior, and an interesting experiment provides evidence that supports the idea. The subjects were people who thought they were addicted to sugar, and who were therefore abstaining from its use. They believed that if they were to allow themselves to indulge at all, they would begin eating out of control; they would go on a binge. When made to believe they had overindulged, they did indeed proceed to overindulge some more; it was not what they actually ate, but what they believed they had eaten, that determined their subsequent behavior.[4]

This finding suggests that addiction may be a characteristic of the person, rather than of the substance. Some researchers who subscribe to this view have defined addiction . . . largely in psychological terms. They state that loss of control is a feature of all addictive behaviors and that "low self-regard is a crucial factor." Addictive people may differ biochemically from others, but the changes are self-induced.[5]

That addictive behavior may be a characteristic of the person, rather than of the substance, is supported by abundant additional research. People who tend to overeat compulsively resemble alcohol addicts on psychological tests—even if they don't drink alcohol.[6] In fact, people with all sorts of addictions—to alcohol, tobacco, heroin, other drugs, and food—have much in common.[7]

Notes

1. J. Pekkanen and M. Falco, Sweet and sour, *Atlantic Monthly,* July 1975, as quoted in *The Great American Nutrition Hassle* (Palo Alto, Calif.: Mayfield, 1978), pp. 252–259.
2. W. Dufty, *Sugar Blues* (New York: Warner Books, 1975).
3. Dufty, 1975, pp. 22–23.
4. J. Wardle and H. Beinart, Binge eating: A theoretical review, *British Journal of Clinical Psychology* 20 (1983): 97–109.
5. H. Milkman and S. Sunderwirth, The chemistry of craving, *Psychology Today,* October 1983, pp. 36–44.
6. J. B. Lauer and coauthors, Psychosocial aspects of extremely obese women joining a diet group, *International Journal of Obesity* 3 (1979): 153–167.
7. P. K. Levison, D. R. Gerstein, and D. R. Maloff, eds., *Commonalities in Substance Abuse and Habitual Behavior* (Lexington, Mass.: Lexington Books, 1983); abstract 83-1409 cited in *Alcohol Awareness Service* (National Institute on Alcohol Abuse and Alcoholism), December 1983, p. 28.

Source: E. N. Whitney, C. B. Cataldo, *Nutrition,* pp. 84–87.

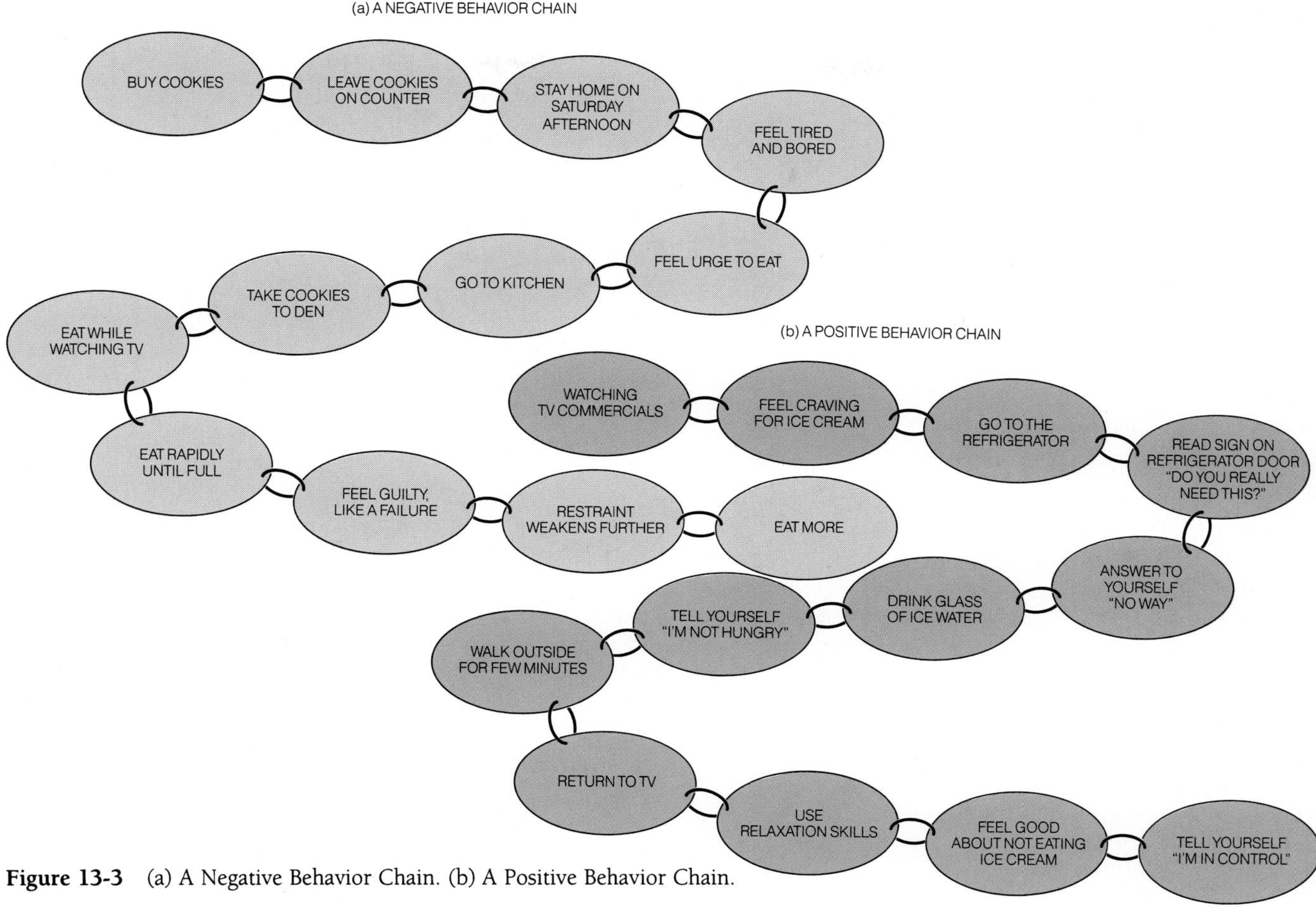

Figure 13-3 (a) A Negative Behavior Chain. (b) A Positive Behavior Chain.

Take Action

Your answers to the Exploring Your Emotions in this chapter and your placement level on the Wellness Ladder will, we hope, encourage you to begin a process of self-exploration and self-discovery that you will continue. Reflect on the entire chapter's content and ask yourself how each point relates to your own life. Then take action:

1. Read at least three currently popular diet plans. (Your library probably has copies of several diet programs.) Evaluate each plan in terms of the seven criteria given in the "Evaluating a Fad Diet" box. Which plan appears to be the best? Why? Would you consider going on any of the three diets? Would you recommend any of them to an overweight friend?

2. In your Take Action notebook keep track of your eating behavior for four or five days. Note the time, setting, amount of food, your mood, and what activities preceded your eating. What are the relationships between your eating and any of these elements? For instance, do you eat more food or certain kinds of foods when you are happy as opposed to upset?

3. List the positive behaviors that help you control your weight. Consider how you can strengthen these behaviors. Don't forget to congratulate yourself for these positive aspects of your life. Now list the behaviors that tend to block your maintaining optimal weight. Consider each of these behaviors and decide which ones you can change to improve your health and lifestyle.

4. Read the following Behavior Change Strategy, and take the appropriate action.

Behavior Change Strategy

Weight Control

Two central goals of any weight control program are (1) reduce the quantity and calories of food eaten, and (2) increase physical activities that use up calories. The strategies included to accomplish these goals follow the self-management format described in more detail in Chapter 1 of this book. Dietary and nutritional counseling is often included in many of these weight control programs. However, this section focuses only on cognitive behavioral strategies.

Self-monitoring

Keeping a chart or diary of body weight is a basic behavioral strategy. In addition to weight, a variety of additional data often is collected. For example, you can record the quantity, type, and caloric content of food consumed, as well as where your eating occurred, who was present at the time, and a description of hunger and other feelings associated with the eating episode. You can also include a physical activity record: type and duration of activity, estimated calories expended, where the exercise occurred, who was present, and your associated feelings.

Some people find such recording too burdensome. Adapt the process in ways that will help you do it. Remember, you need to know what you are doing. You can easily forget or distort things.

Stimulus Control

Eating and even internal feelings about being hungry are linked to certain situations. One way to lose weight is to limit the number of situations (times and places) in which food is permitted. Re-establishing—and narrowing—stimulus control over eating plays a major role in behavioral programs. Other stimulus controls involve getting rid of high-calorie foods or putting them out of sight in the refrigerator or on shelves, and instead displaying low-calorie foods. It can also help to use smaller plates (gives appearance of more food), to eat more slowly, and not to eat something just to clean your plate and avoid throwing food out.

Relaxation Methods

Eating that is linked to feelings—so-called emotional eating—can be a big contributor to overweight. The emotions can include tension, anxiety, boredom, depression, and anger. Most programs include instruction and practice in deep mental and muscular relaxation. Relaxing can really help you control your overeating. Managing your anger and/or depression may require some extra help.

Thoughts and Self-statements

Weight control programs should also emphasize the role of thoughts and self-statements in sticking to a personal program or contract. Some people find it helpful to keep a diary of self-statements that relate to losing weight. The following illustrates what such a diary might look like:

Time	Thoughts
7:30	"I'd really like a doughnut, but I'm not going to blow my day."
8:15	"It's not fair; I'm really trying and I haven't lost anything."
9:10	"Wish I had a doughnut or something; I'm hungry."
10:00	"It's not fair; it's snack time and all I get is water."
11:30	"Nothing tastes as good when I know there's no dessert."
12:10	"Look at them; they stuff themselves with sweets and stay skinny."
1:15	"Maybe I could have just a couple of cookies after school. I've earned them."
2:30	"Look at them—running off to their afternoon snacks. It's not fair."
3:15	"I don't care if I'm fat; I'll never lose anyway. It's not worth it."
4:30	"I might as well eat and enjoy it. I'll never be thin, no matter what I do."
5:45	"You pig. Now you feel stuffed and you've ruined your day."
7:30	"What a failure I am. I don't deserve to be thin."
9:00	"I'll never learn, will I? It's no use."
10:30	"I feel hopeless. I've tried everything and I always blow it."

SOURCE: M. J. and K. Mahoney, 1976, *Permanent Weight Control* (New York: Norton), p. 65.

Notice the number of discouraging and self-critical thoughts. These can be the biggest barrier to losing fat and changing eating habits. Such self-statements can set the stage for binge eating and purging. Counterstatements can reduce the influence of such negative "self-talk."

Self-contracts and Rewards

Contracts can also play a major role in your weight control program. Set a schedule for doing behavioral tasks, such as exercising as well as weight loss goals. Setting up positive consequences is also crucial.

Many people forget how important it is to reward themselves for making progress, often because they don't think they deserve it. Rewarding yourself for progress is very important.

Selected References

Brody, J. 1985, 1987. *Jane Brody's Good Food Book.* New York: Norton.

Brownell, K. D., and J. P. Foreyt, eds. 1986. *Handbook of Eating Disorders.* New York: Basic Books.

Jacobson, M. 1986. *The Fast-Food Guide.* New York: Workman Publishing.

Jeffrey, D. B., and R. C. Katz. 1977. *Take It Off and Keep It Off.* Englewood Cliffs, N.J.: Prentice-Hall.

Kolata, G. 1985. Obesity declared a disease. *Science* 227:1019–20.

Price, R. A. 1987. Genetics of human obesity. *Annals of Behavioral Medicine* 9:9–14.

Wurtman, J. J. 1983. *The Carbohydrate Craver's Diet.* Boston: Houghton Mifflin.

Recommended Readings

Bailey, C. 1984. *The Fit or Fat Target Diet.* Boston: Houghton Mifflin.
Provides sensible suggestions for dieting to lose excess body fat.

Brownell, K. D. 1985. *The LEARN Program for Weight Control.* Philadelphia: Department of Psychiatry, University of Pennsylvania.
Covers changes in lifestyle, exercise, attitudes, social relationships, and nutrition in losing and then maintaining weight.

Brownell, K. D., and J. P. Foreyt, eds. 1986. *Handbook of Eating Disorders.* New York: Basic Books.
Scholarly reviews by leading researchers of obesity, anorexia nervosa, and bulimia, including various theories and treatments.

Wood, P. 1983. *California Diet and Exercise Program.* Mountain View, Calif.: Anderson World Books.
Combines moderate dieting with progressively active programs of "play" or exercise.

Chapter 14

Contents

Rate Yourself

Your Fitness Behavior Read the following statements carefully. Choose the one in each section that best describes you at this moment and circle its number. When you have chosen one statement for each section, add the numbers and record your total score. Find your position on the Wellness Ladder.

5 Maintains a regular exercise program
4 Often engages in physical activity
3 Occasionally exercises
2 Rarely exercises
1 Is sedentary

5 Trim, highly toned body
4 Firm, toned body
3 Firm, poorly toned body
2 Slack body
1 Flabby body

5 Vigorous
4 Energetic
3 Active
2 Excessive sleep pattern
1 Awakes tired

5 Feels exhilarated after vigorous exercise
4 Recovers rapidly after vigorous exercise
3 Is tired after vigorous exercise
2 Overweight
1 Sluggish

5 Excellent stamina
4 Good stamina
3 Limited endurance
2 Easily tired
1 Easily exhausted

Total Score ______

Exercise for Health and Performance

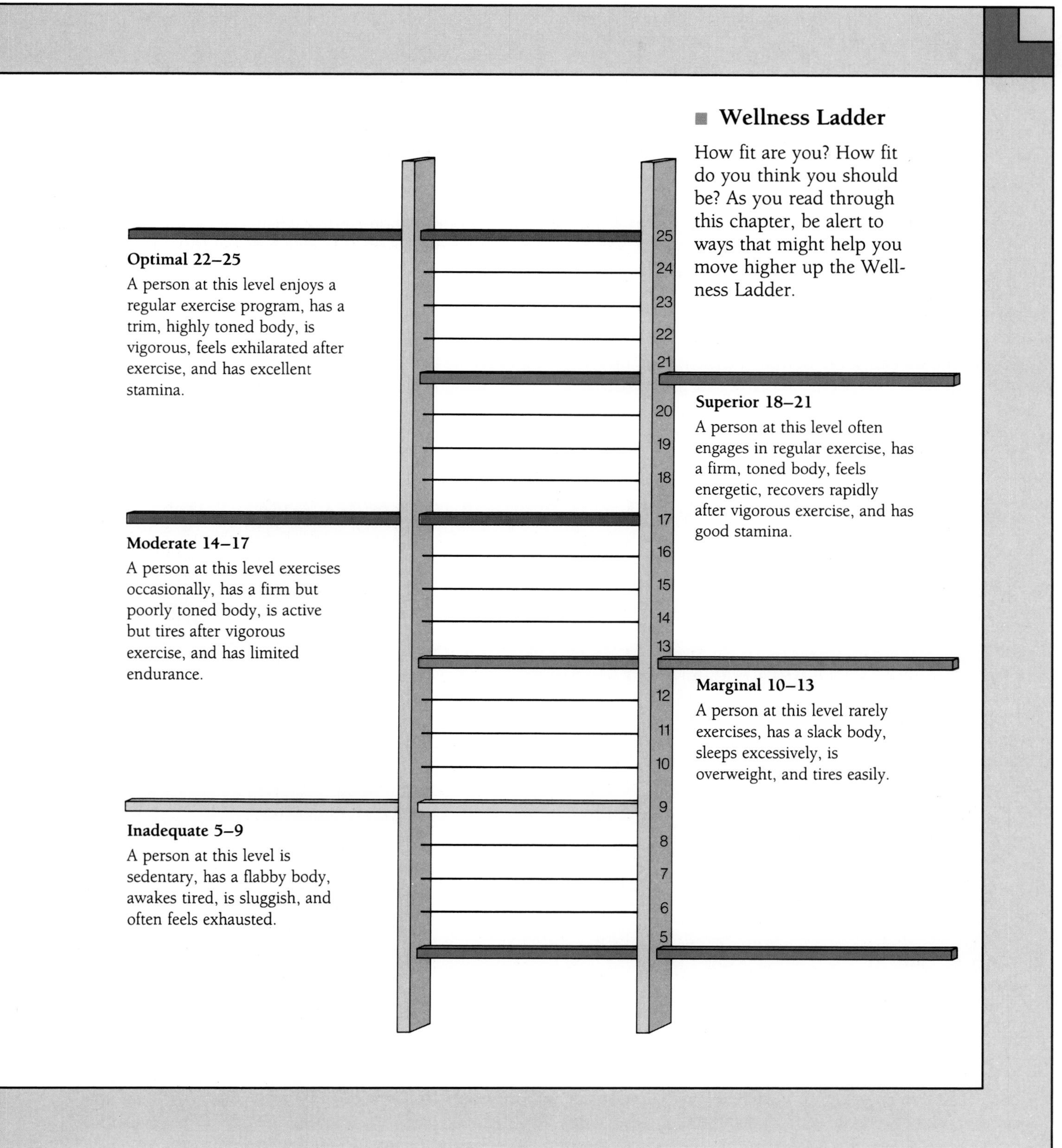

25
24
23
22
21
20
19
18
17
16
15
14
13
12
11
10
9
8
7
6
5
Optimal 22–25
A person at this level enjoys a regular exercise program, has a trim, highly toned body, is vigorous, feels exhilarated after exercise, and has excellent stamina.
Superior 18–21
A person at this level often engages in regular exercise, has a firm, toned body, feels energetic, recovers rapidly after vigorous exercise, and has good stamina.
Moderate 14–17
A person at this level exercises occasionally, has a firm but poorly toned body, is active but tires after vigorous exercise, and has limited endurance.
Marginal 10–13
A person at this level rarely exercises, has a slack body, sleeps excessively, is overweight, and tires easily.
Inadequate 5–9
A person at this level is sedentary, has a flabby body, awakes tired, is sluggish, and often feels exhausted.

Wellness Ladder

How fit are you? How fit do you think you should be? As you read through this chapter, be alert to ways that might help you move higher up the Wellness Ladder.

Exercise is in. Nowadays, if you don't backpack, jog, play tennis, or lift weights, people think there must be something wrong with you. Clearly, more and more people believe that regular exercise is good for them and can be an enjoyable way to spend their leisure time. Even big business is getting into the act; many companies have established recreational and fitness facilities for their employees because they believe it improves productivity and decreases health care costs.

Unfortunately, the "fitness boom" creates some problems for many exercise enthusiasts. Some people start in a wave of eagerness only to quit a few months later because the programs are boring. "Weekend warriors" suffer any number of overuse injuries. And athletic injuries strike down many novice exercisers. In sports such as tennis and jogging, over 50 percent of the participants can expect to experience injuries serious enough to interrupt their activities. These interruptions, in turn, often frustrate and discourage injured exercisers.

Most such difficulties stem from a basic lack of understanding of what exercise is. Many people participate in inappropriate activities or do too much too soon. Approached correctly, exercise and sports can contribute to health and well-being and can provide a continuing source of pleasure. With a little knowledge and planning, you can formulate a good program that is fun and takes little time.

What Is Physical Fitness?

Physical fitness is the ability to adapt to the demands and stresses of physical effort. It has a number of components, such as cardiorespiratory endurance, muscular strength and power, flexibility, body composition, speed, agility, coordination, and skill. Although some may overlap, each component is largely independent and requires specific types of exercise. Your body has the ability to adapt to physical stress and improve its function. Likewise, in the absence of such positive stress, its function deteriorates. For the most part, your physical capacity reflects the amount and intensity of your physical activity.

Your body's ability to adapt to levels of physical activity has profound effects on your biological well-being. If you are chronically inactive, then your body reflects the inac-

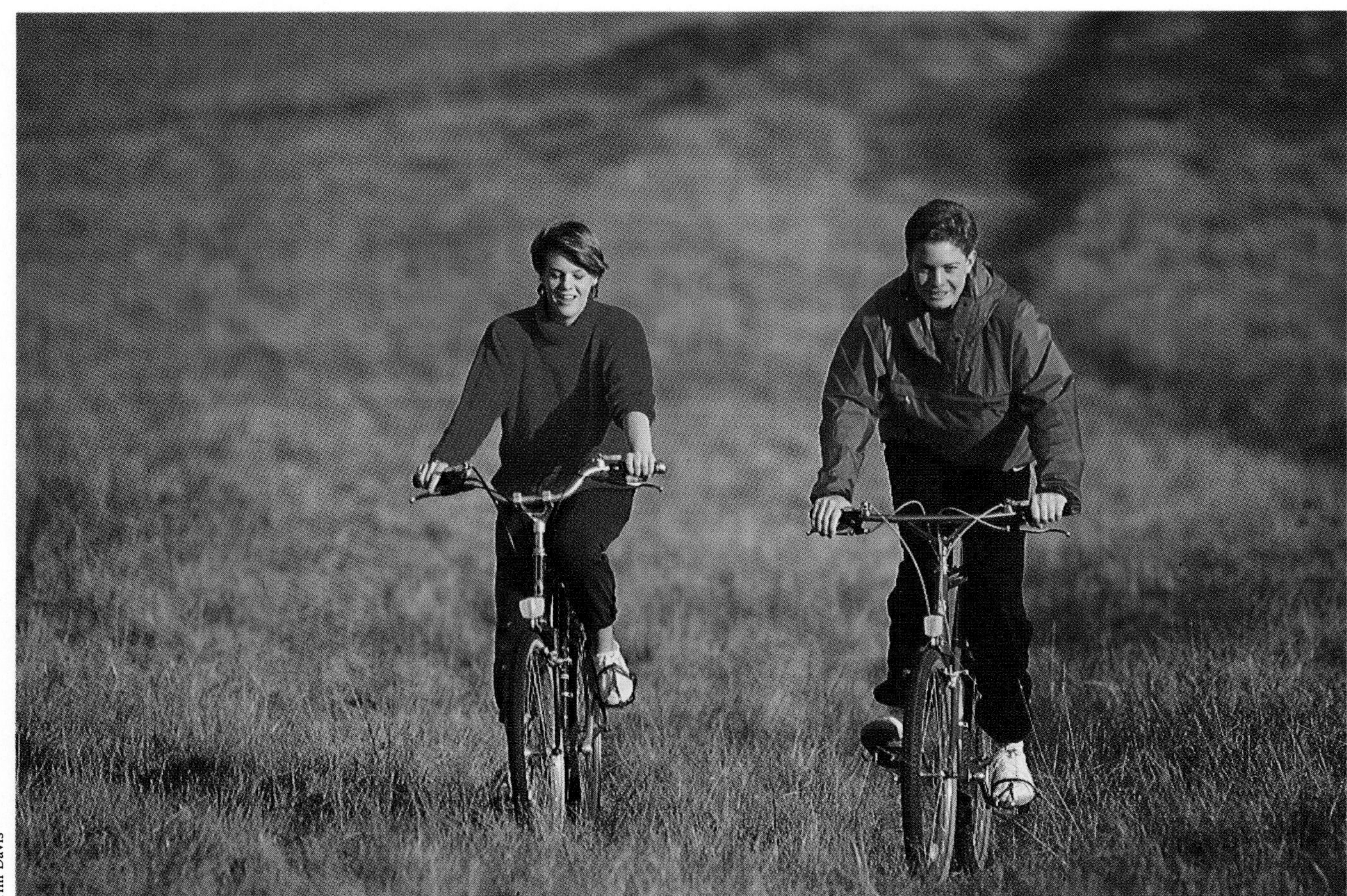

Tim Davis

Physical fitness The extent to which the body can respond to the demands of physical effort.

Sedentary Sitting much of the time; engaged in little physical activity.

Endurance exercise Rhythmical, large-muscle exercise for a prolonged period of time. Partially dependent on the ability of the cardiovascular system to deliver oxygen to tissues. Also known as aerobic or cardiorespiratory endurance exercise.

Aerobics Exercise that emphasizes increased use of oxygen.

Cardiorespiratory endurance The extent to which the heart and lungs can respond to physical exercise.

---

tivity: your heart and lungs have a lower capacity; your muscles, bones, and joints are weaker; and your body chemistry is impaired. Research studies show that an unfit person runs a higher risk of many health hazards such as heart disease, obesity, high blood pressure, backache, and difficulty in coping with emotional stress. Likewise, a consistently active person improves physiological function and tends to become healthier.

Why Get into Shape?

People have a variety of reasons for exercising and participating in sports. Some want to improve their health and well-being, while others feel that performance is also an integral part of an active and exciting lifestyle. For convenience, we will discuss health and performance separately.

Exercise and Health

Advances in public health and medicine have wiped out many diseases that have plagued human beings for centuries. Now we face an array of perplexing degenerative diseases that demand significant changes in personal lifestyle, rather than diseases that require traditional medical crisis intervention. Diseases and disabilities such as heart disease, stroke, obesity, cancer, diabetes, hypertension (high blood pressure), and backache can all be seriously affected by lifestyle factors such as diet, smoking, and exercise. Growing evidence points to the prime importance of regular physical activity in reducing the risk of these health problems.

Many technological advances have aimed at increasing convenience and reducing effort. Driving automobiles is more convenient than walking, a gasoline lawn mower is easier to use than a push mower, and an escalator can replace stairs. And more and more jobs require people to sit at a desk all day. We have to make a special effort to be physically active.

Our **sedentary** lifestyles mean that many of us have sedentary bodies, ripe for a number of degenerative diseases. Over the last forty years, researchers have established relationships between low levels of physical activity and the increased risk of heart disease and other diseases. Typically, the studies compared people working in sedentary occupations with those in active ones, or the leisure activities of workers in the same kinds of jobs. The findings: physically active people have up to 50 percent fewer health problems than sedentary people. A study of almost 17,000 male Harvard alumni found that the death rate from heart disease, respiratory disease, cancers, suicide, and all causes of death combined was significantly higher in sedentary men compared to active men. Still other studies, such as one by aerobics expert Kenneth Cooper and his co-workers, showed that the physical fitness level is critical in lowering the risk of health problems, such as heart disease.

Exercise is important because it improves body function and reduces the risk of degenerative diseases. The risk factors reduced include obesity, high blood sugar, high blood pressure, high cholesterol, and tissue weakness. Two basic kinds of exercise that are considered important for good health: endurance and musculoskeletal exercise.

Exploring Your Emotions

Let's say you have two hours per day free from job work or schoolwork. How will you spend it? What percentage of it do you feel good about using in physical activity?

Benefits of Endurance Exercise **Endurance exercise,** also known as **aerobic** or **cardiorespiratory endurance** exercise, is most important for health. As Cooper remarked, "You can live without big muscles or a nice figure, but you can't live without a healthy heart." Table 14-1 describes some of the ways regular endurance exercise can reduce the risk of severity of heart disease. Exercise helps your body become a more efficient "machine" that can cope better with challenges. Two major adaptations occur: (1) improved ability to transport oxygen, and (2) more efficient metabolism (body chemistry). In addition, people almost always become more interested in establishing healthful living habits.

Improved Cardiovascular System Perhaps the most important benefit of endurance exercise is the improved

Exercise and Calories

A preliminary study at Stanford University has shown that exercise alone was more successful in reducing weight than dieting alone. However, the combination of diet and exercise has been shown to have more permanent results.

Here's a sample of common exercises and the number of calories you can expend.

How Many Calories a Minute?

Activity	Calories/Minute			
Dancing, rock	3.3	3.8	4.4	4.9
Golf, hand cart	3.3	3.8	4.4	4.9
Lawn mowing, power	3.5	4.0	4.8	5.2
Baseball, fielder	3.7	4.4	4.9	5.4
Walking, 3 mph	3.9	4.5	5.3	5.8
Hiking, 20 lb. pack, 2 mph	3.9	4.5	5.3	5.8
Rowing machine	3.9	4.5	5.3	5.8
Sexual intercourse, active partner	3.9	4.5	5.3	5.8
Swimming, crawl, 20 yds./min.	3.9	4.5	5.3	5.8
Badminton, singles	4.6	5.2	6.2	6.8
Skating, leisure	4.6	5.2	6.2	6.8
Calisthenics	3.9	4.5	7.3	7.9
Gardening, weeding, digging	5.1	5.8	6.8	7.5
Sawing wood, hand	5.1	5.8	6.8	7.6
Bicycling, 10 mph	5.4	6.2	7.3	7.9
Dancing, square	5.5	6.3	7.4	8.0
Tennis, doubles	5.6	6.3	7.5	8.3
Aerobic dancing	5.8	6.6	7.8	8.6
Stair climbing, normal	5.9	6.7	7.9	8.8
Basketball, half-court	7.3	8.3	9.8	10.8
Handball	7.8	8.9	10.5	11.6
Volleyball	7.8	8.9	10.5	11.6
Snow shoveling, light	7.9	9.1	10.8	11.8
Jogging, 5.5 mph	8.6	9.8	11.5	12.7
Running, 6.5 mph	8.9	10.2	12.0	13.2
Skiing, cross-country, 5 mph	9.2	10.4	12.3	13.3
Trampolining	10.3	11.8	13.9	15.3
Bicycling, stationary, 20 mph	11.7	13.3	15.6	17.2
Weight (lbs.):	**105–115**	**127–137**	**160–170**	**182–192**

SOURCE: Adapted from Dr. Charles T. Kuntzleman, 1981, *Diet Free* (Rodale Press).

ability of your heart, lungs, and circulatory system to carry oxygen to your body's tissues. Your heart pumps more blood per beat, resting heart rate slows, the number of red blood cells increases, blood supply to the tissues improves, and resting blood pressure decreases. A fit cardiorespiratory system doesn't have to work as hard at rest and at low levels of exercise, because it functions more efficiently. A trained heart can better withstand the stresses and strains of daily life and meet the occasional emergencies that make extraordinary demands on your body's cardiorespiratory resources.

More Efficient Metabolism Your body survives by converting chemical or food energy into mechanical or work energy. This complicated process involves hormones, oxygen, fuels, and enzymes. A physically fit body adapts to facilitate these chemical reactions. The fit person shows an improved ability to generate useful energy, to use fats as fuel, and to regulate hormones.

Better Control of Blood Fats Blood lipids, or fatlike substances, such as cholesterol and triglycerides, are involved in the formation of plaques on the inner lining of the

Lipoproteins *(low-density lipoproteins, LDL; very low-density lipoproteins, VLDL; high- density lipoproteins, HDL)* Substances in blood, classified according to size, density, and chemical composition, that transport fats.

Lipid balance The levels of fats in the blood.

Preventive medicine A medical philosophy that stresses prevention of disease.

Table 14-1 Endurance Exercise and the Risk of Coronary Heart Disease

Endurance exercise tends to increase	Endurance exercise tends to decrease
1. Efficiency of the heart	1. Blood levels of triglycerides, total cholesterol, and low-density lipoprotein cholesterol
2. Size of blood vessels	2. Glucose intolerance
3. Blood supply to the heart	3. Obesity and body fat
4. Efficiency of distribution of blood to the tissues	4. Platelet stickiness (overadhesiveness in this type of blood cell has been implicated in the development of coronary artery disease)
5. Return of blood to the heart	5. Arterial blood pressure
6. Enzymes in the tissues that help supply energy	6. Heart rate
7. Efficiency of blood coagulation factors	7. Vulnerability to dysrhythmias of electrical conduction in the heart
8. High-density lipoprotein (HDL) cholesterol	8. Overreaction by "stress" hormones
9. Blood volume and number of red blood cells	9. Strain associated with psychic stress
10. Efficiency of the thyroid gland	
11. Growth hormone production, which increases the use of fats	
12. Tolerance to stress	
13. Prudent living habits	
14. The joy of living	

SOURCE: Modified from W. L. Haskell, 1984, Cardiovascular benefits and risks of exercise: the scientific evidence, in R. H. Strauss, ed., *Sports Medicine* (Philadelphia: Saunders), p. 65.

coronary arteries. Cholesterol is carried in the blood by **lipoproteins,** which are classified according to size and density. Three such lipoproteins are *low-density lipoprotein (LDL), very low-density lipoproteins (VLDL),* and *high-density lipoproteins (HDL).* Excess LDL cholesterol sticks to the walls of the coronary arteries, while HDLs pick up excess cholesterol in the bloodstream and carry it back to the liver for excretion from the body. Therefore, we can speak of "good cholesterol" (HDL) and "bad cholesterol" (LDL). Some researchers say that the relative amounts of HDL and LDL may be the most important factor involved in developing coronary heart disease. Endurance exercise has a marked positive effect on the **lipid balance** (Figure 14-1).

Easier to Control Body Fat Endurance exercise also influences body chemistry in regulating energy balance. We need nutritious food to supply vitamins and minerals as well as energy. However, a diet high in the right nutrients can be relatively high in calories. Regular exercise enables a person to eat a good diet without getting fat. Research indicates that without exercise it is extremely difficult to eat a nutritious diet and maintain an ideal body weight. Sedentary people may gain weight on a good diet simply because they are taking in more calories than they are using.

Promotes a Healthy Lifestyle In addition to allowing for a balanced diet, physical activity tends to promote prudent living habits—a "halo effect." People seem to become more aware of their bodies when they exercise, so they tend to live more healthful lifestyles. Their sense of well-being and physical capacity increases if they get enough sleep, do not smoke, and are not overweight. Getting regular endurance exercise is emphasized in **preventive medicine** (medical prevention of disease) because it improves so many health factors.

Figure 14-1 HDL Blood Levels for Runners and Sitters

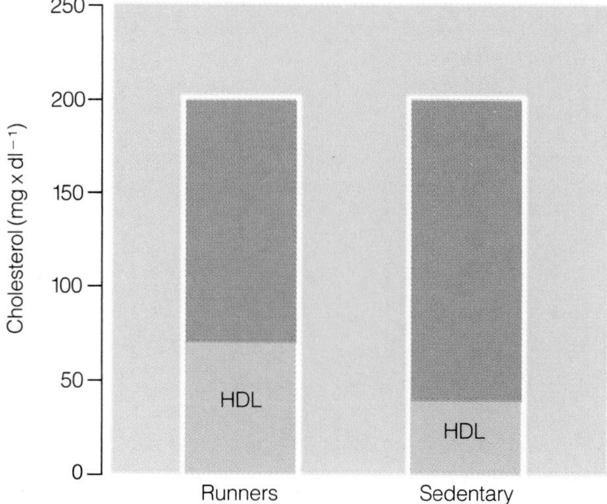

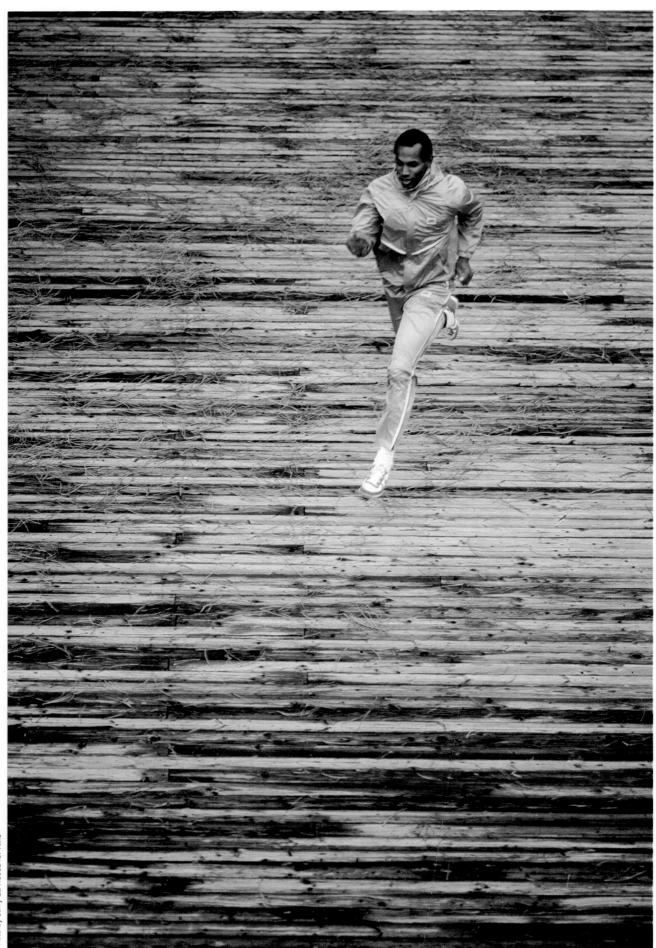

Photo by Jerry La Rocca for Nike

Epinephrine A hormone secreted principally by the adrenal medulla with a wide variety of functions, such as stimulating the heart, making carbohydrates available in the liver and muscles, and releasing fat from fat cells.

Norepinephrine A hormone released from the adrenal medulla and nerve endings of the autonomic nervous system. Has many of the same effects as epinephrine.

Endorphins Substances resembling opium that are secreted by the brain. They seem to be involved in modulating pain.

Exploring Your Emotions

The mind-body split has dominated thought and feeling about individual functioning for centuries. How do you feel about the results of that split? Do you feel that people who are physically active give up some of their claim to mental activity? Or the reverse?

Improves Mental Health and Neural Function Not only do exercise and sports enhance health and well-being, but most committed participants also point out the emotional benefits. The joys of a well-hit cross-court backhand, the euphoria of a run alone in the park, or the rush of a downhill schuss through deep snow powder provide pleasures that transcend possible health benefits. Physical activity can offer harmonious interaction or invigorating competition with other people. It can be an arena in which we strive to win or to perform better than we now do. Competent performance of a physical skill assures us that we control ourselves well.

Exploring Your Emotions

Has physical activity ever made you very happy? What kind of activity? How long did the pleasure last, and do you seek it out often?

Physically fit people have plenty of energy. They are productive and ready for whatever opportunities and activities present themselves. Their lifestyles are interesting and varied. Sedentary people, however, miss many pleasures that life has to offer. Often they don't have the stamina to enjoy many of the options open to them. A walk in the mountains, a game of volleyball, a dream vacation in Europe, or a game of frisbee on the beach can be exhausting or impossible. Even the activities of daily life can sap the energy of inactive people.

Many studies have shown that excessive stress and anxiety are often associated with poor health. Psychological stress prompts increased secretion of **epinephrine** and **norepinephrine** (the so-called fight-or-flight hormones), which are thought to speed the development of atherosclerosis (hardening of the arteries). In addition, excessive stress is thought to depress the immune system (which helps the body fight disease). Type A behavior—a personality type characterized by hostility, aggressiveness, and extreme competitiveness—is also associated with an increased risk of heart disease. Exercise training reduces anxiety and depression and decreases hormone secretion triggered by emotional stress.

Researchers have recently identified a group of substances resembling morphine, called **endorphins,** that are secreted by the brain. These substances seem to have many functions: they play a role in decreasing pain, in producing euphoria, and in suppressing fatigue. Some researchers credit endorphins with the "runner's high" that some people claim to experience during exercise. There may in fact be a physiological basis for what many exercise advocates previously attributed to a state of mind but controversy remains.

The Benefits of Strength, Flexibility, and Postural Exercises In addition to cardiorespiratory endurance, exercises that develop muscular strength, muscular endurance, joint flexibility, and posture are also critical to well-being. Backaches, for example, plague nearly 85 percent of the population. In most cases they can be directly traced to weak abdominal and spinal muscles with poor muscular endurance; poor flexibility in the spine, hips, and legs; and chronically poor posture. If the affected people could spend even five minutes a day working on these problems, their back trouble would be significantly eased. Any good book on athletic injuries (see Selected References) contains exercises to prevent back pain.

A basic principle of human functioning is "Use it or lose it!" Joint stiffness in the shoulders, neck, knees, and

Exploring Your Emotions

How does this picture make you feel? Are your feelings about it mainly positive or negative? (If you feel ambivalent, what divides your feelings?)

Exercises for Flexibility

- Perform stretching exercises statically. Stretch and hold the position 10 to 30 seconds (as long as 60 seconds if your muscles are tight). *Never bounce.*
- To develop more flexibility, practice stretching after exercise because your muscles are warmer then and can be stretched farther.
- You should feel a mild stretch rather than pain while performing these exercises. Emphasize relaxation.
- Avoid positions that increase the risk of low back injury. For example, if you are performing straight leg toe-touching exercises, bend your knees slightly when returning to a standing position.
- As with other forms of physical conditioning, develop flexibility gradually over time.
- There are large individual differences in joint flexibility. Do not feel you have to compete with others during stretching workouts.
- Practice flexibility exercises at least five days per week. Set aside a special time to develop this type of fitness.

For best results, do the exercises in the following numerical sequence. The body parts affected by each exercise are noted in parentheses.

SOURCE: I. Kusinitz and M. Fine, 1987, *Your Guide to Getting Fit* (Mountain View, Calif.: Mayfield).

1. Shoulder blade scratch (shoulders, arms)
Reach back with one arm as if to scratch your shoulder blade. Use your other hand to extend the stretch. Alternate arms.

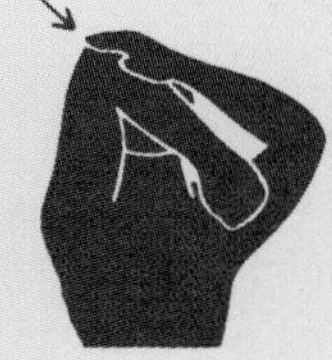

2. Towel stretch (triceps, shoulders, chest)
Grasp a rolled towel at both ends and slowly bring it back over your head as far down as possible. Keep your arms straight. (The closer your hands are, the greater the stretch.)

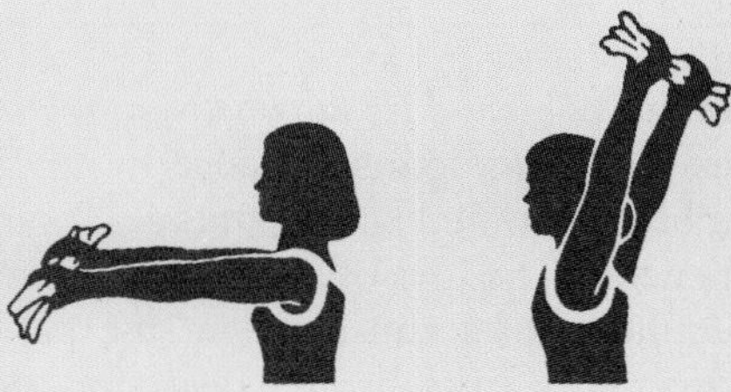

3. Alternate knee-to-chest (lower back)
Bring one knee up to your chest. Curl your head toward your knee. Keep the other leg on the floor.

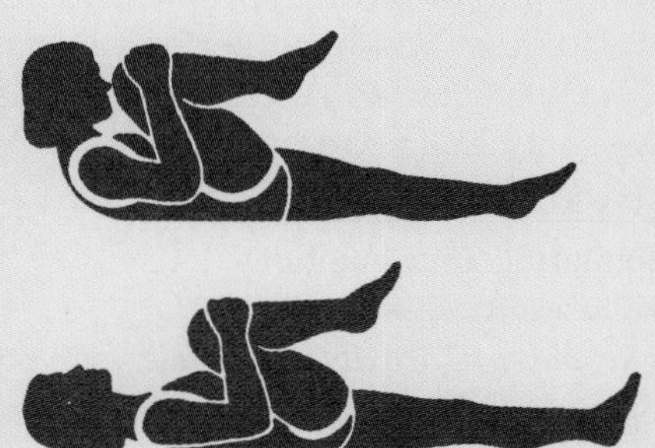

4. Double knee-to-chest (lower back)
Same as alternate knee-to-chest (3), except bring both knees up to your chest.

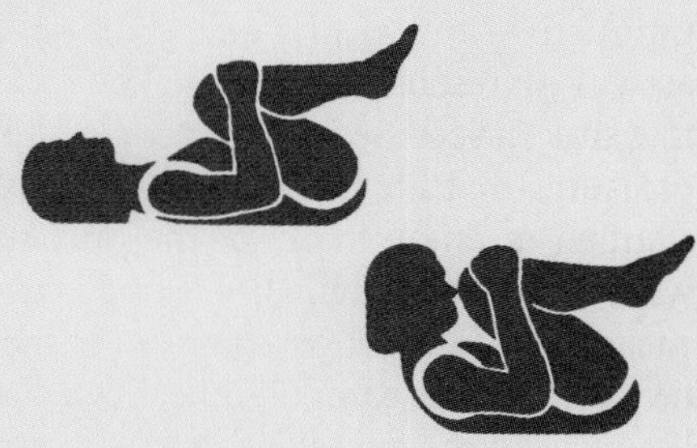

5. Sole stretch (groin)
With the soles of your feet pressed together, pull your feet toward you while pressing your knees down with your elbows.

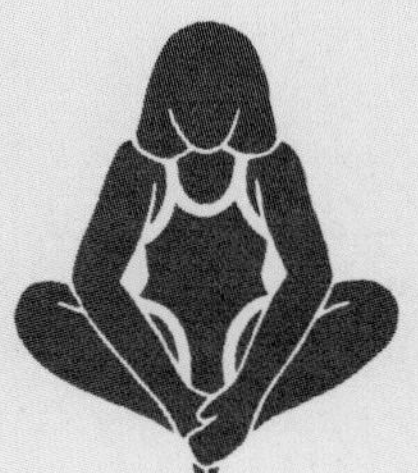

6. Seated toe touch (hamstrings)
Sit with your legs straight. Fold one leg in front and gradually reach for the toes of your other foot. Eventually you will be able to grasp your feet at the instep. Keep your head down. Alternate legs.

7. Seated foot-over-knee twist (hips)
Seated as depicted, turn at the hips to face the rear. Hold your ankle to keep your foot on the floor. Alternate legs.

8. Prone knee flexion (quadriceps)
Lying on your side with one arm tucked behind your head, use the other arm to slowly pull one foot up toward your buttocks. Flex the leg up until you feel the stretch in your quadriceps.

9. Wall lean (lower legs)
Lean against the wall with one leg bent and the other straight. Keep your back straight and your heels on the floor. Bend the knee of the straight leg—this changes the stretch from the calf muscle to the Achilles tendon. Alternate legs.

10. Stride stretch (hips, hamstring)
Assume the racer's starting position and stretch one leg backward. Keep your head down. Alternate legs.

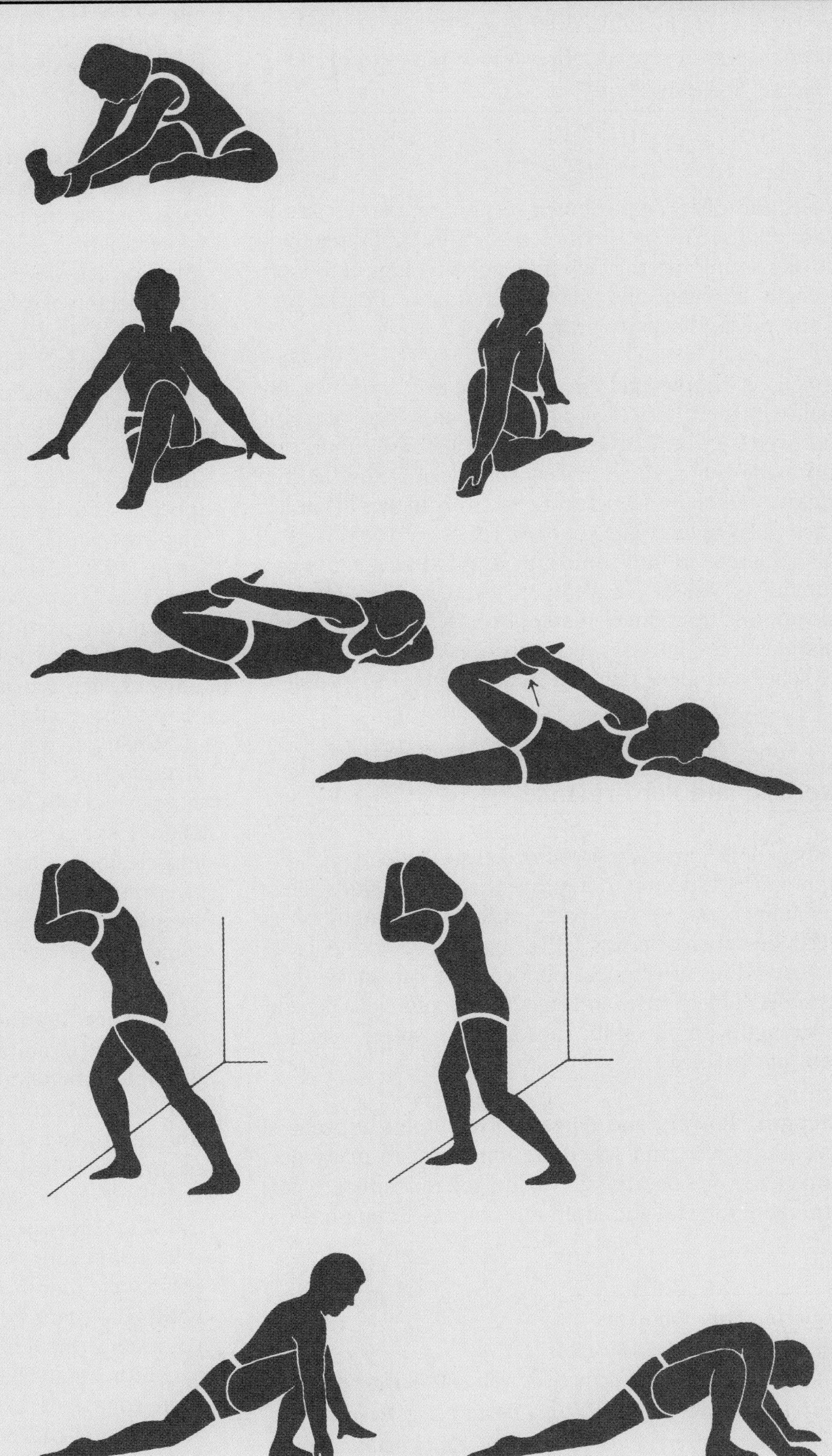

Exploring Your Emotions

Look ahead in your life; how will you be feeling about your present level of physical activity at age 30? 45? 60? 90? What changes in your lifestyle might be suggested by the principle "use it or lose it?"

ankles can often be attributed to nonuse, particularly in older adults. You can reduce such stiffness by regularly moving your joints through their normal range of motion. Strength, flexibility, and muscular endurance are vital parts of any physical activity program.

Aging As people age, exercise obviously improves the quality of their lives. Roy Shephard, an expert on aging and exercise from the University of Toronto, notes that improving the cardiovascular capacity of a middle-aged or older person by 15 percent effectively makes his or her functional age ten years younger. He says, "You'd have to go a long way to find something as good as exercise as a fountain of youth." In addition, exercise helps prevent calcium loss from bones (**osteoporosis**). And it improves musculoskeletal fitness, which enhances mobility and eases the aches and pains that can so debilitate older people.

Exercise and Performance

Many people, particularly young college students, actively enjoy sports and want to improve their sports skills. They play tennis, ski, or backpack with little thought of its effects on atherosclerosis, HDL, or endorphins. A basic understanding of physical performance can make their workouts more effective and enjoyable. Sports skills depend on strength, power, skill, coordination, speed, reaction time, and balance.

Strength, Power, and Speed The fitness aspects of strength, power, and speed are important in many performance sports because they allow the individual to perform more forceful and rapid movements. Strength is the ability to exert force, and power is the ability to apply force rapidly. Strength is largely improved by increasing muscle size through overload exercises; power is increased by improving both strength and skill.

When your nervous system calls on a muscle group to initiate a movement, it recruits specific muscle fibers according to the force required. Muscle fibers are subdivided into fast- or slow-twitch fibers. These fibers are classified according to their size, biochemistry, preferential fuels, nerve size, strength, endurance, and blood supply. In general, fast-twitch fibers are stronger and more powerful than slow-twitch fibers but fatigue more rapidly. Slow-twitch fibers have much more endurance, but are considerably weaker and slower.

Muscle fibers are recruited or used according to the requirements of the muscle contraction and the muscle's basic fiber characteristics. Slow-twitch muscle fibers are recruited when a muscle must perform low-intensity or repeated contractions. For example, slow-twitch muscle fibers are called on to maintain your body in the upright posture or to perform low-intensity exercise such as walking. Fast-twitch muscle fibers are recruited for high-intensity contractions such as heavy weight lifting or sprinting. Successful power athletes, such as sprinters, baseball players, and discus throwers, have a greater percentage of fast-twitch fibers in their active muscles, while elite endurance athletes, such as marathon runners and cross-country skiers, tend to have more slow-twitch fibers.

When you are building strength and power for a particular sport or type of exercise, you need to train the fibers you will use in the activity. The training program should specifically reflect the desired adaptation. The muscle fibers used in maximal strength speed sports, such as sprinting, are trained by high-intensity exercises. Low-intensity, prolonged exercise such as endurance swimming requires more prolonged muscle contractions.

Skill, Coordination, Balance, and Reaction Time The complexity of animal movements is mind-boggling. For example, when you want to hit a tennis ball, your brain must translate complex input from sight, sound, and various receptors in your muscles, joints, skin, and inner ear in order to initiate complex movements in your musculoskeletal system. Movement begins in a part of your brain called the **motor cortex**, which sends commands to nerve cells within your spinal cord that control specific muscles. Meanwhile, another part of your brain called the **cerebellum** constantly compares the intended movement with your actual movement so that each movement sequence is coordinated. The functioning of the motor cortex has been compared to running a computer program. This concept was called the **memory drum theory** and was formulated by F. M. Henry of the University of California, Berkeley. According to this theory, muscle fibers are pro-

Exploring Your Emotions

What kinds of physical activity do you enjoy? How does competition make you feel? What about being observed? What kinds of exercise do you feel you could maintain in a regular program?

Osteoporosis A bone disease characterized by the loss of bone mineral. It is particularly prevalent in postmenopausal women.

Motor cortex A portion of the brain responsible for movement.

Cerebellum A portion of the brain responsible for movement and balance.

Memory drum theory A theory that states that motor movements are imprinted in the motor cortex, then "replayed" by reflex when a person wishes to repeat the movement.

Electrocardiogram (EKG or ECG) A recording of the changes in electrical activity of the heart.

Triathlon An athletic contest involving three different sports events, usually swimming, running, and cycling.

Exploring Your Emotions

Would you like to be more fit? What do you feel keeps you from becoming more fit? Would it be easy or hard to overcome those barriers?

grammed to contract in an incredibly precise order that is regulated in terms of time, intensity, and duration. The skill sequence is somehow "imprinted" on the motor cortex in a manner analogous to the magnetic imprint on a computer floppy disk. The purpose of practicing a skill is to imprint a precise movement sequence in the brain. Repeated practice of the correct movement will eventually result in an almost reflex performance of the skill.

How to Get into Shape

Exercise can be a real pleasure in your life rather than a chore. Your individual program should promote good health and be fun at the same time. A little planning and reflection will go a long way in helping you achieve these goals.

Most young people probably don't need a medical examination before beginning an exercise program unless they have health problems. Diabetes, asthma, heart disease, or extreme obesity require a modified program. However, because your body experiences profound changes in capacity and function as a result of exercise, baseline medical measurements can help you assess the effects of exercise on your health.

If you are over 35 years old or have an increased risk of heart disease because of smoking, high blood pressure, or obesity, be sure to have an exercise **electrocardiogram (ECG)** before beginning a program. This checkup can help ensure that your program is a benefit to your health instead of a potential hazard.

Choosing the Appropriate Activities Although good health is an important *reason* to exercise, it is a poor *motivator* for consistent adherence to an exercise program. If you don't enjoy your program, you won't continue it for very long. It is easy to say, "Missing this workout isn't going to kill me." Unfortunately, that missed workout can stretch into several weeks or months. However, if you select a physical activity that you like and look forward to, you will be much more faithful.

Personality should have a great deal to do with your choices. If you like competitive sports and dread the idea of running around a track, you might choose activities like racquetball, basketball, and squash. If you are the solitary type, you might consider a sport like cross-country skiing, **triathlon**, or road running. If you don't have a favorite sport or exercise, try some new activities. Take a physical education class, join a health club, go on a sports vacation. You can find an activity that's both enjoyable and good for you.

Try to choose activities that contribute to your general health and well-being. Improved physiological function is a major benefit of exercise. However, some activities don't do very much in this regard. Endurance exercises such as walking, jogging, swimming, and cycling produce a cardiovascular training effect, while bowling, archery, and weight lifting do not (see Table 14-2). Although a variety of activities is desirable in a well-rounded program, cardiorespiratory endurance exercises should play a central role in your routine.

Be realistic. Consider the constraints that some sports present. Factors such as accessibility, expense, and time can make many activities impossible. For example, if you live in a warm climate, snow skiing isn't something you're likely to do on a regular basis. Some sports, like tennis, require a lot of time to achieve a reasonable skill level; you may be better off walking to get a good workout. Similarly, if you don't have four-hour blocks of time available, you will have difficulty squeezing in eighteen holes of golf. Examine your own situation and develop a reasonable plan.

Variety is also important to an enjoyable exercise program. If you are interested in a particular sport, supplement it with conditioning activities. For example, if you are a tennis player, support your playing with strength, flexibility, and endurance exercises. Participate in new activities and try to improve in old ones. The more variety, the less boredom.

Structuring Your Program To develop cardiorespiratory endurance, strength, power, speed, flexibility, or skill, you must work on specific exercises. Lifting weights will not develop the heart and lungs, and running contributes little to strength and power. As discussed, cardiovascular endurance exercise is the most important component of

Maximal oxygen consumption (MOC) The body's maximum ability to transport and use oxygen.

---

your program, but you should supplement it with other forms of exercise.

Cardiovascular Endurance (Aerobic) Exercises The best exercises for developing cardiorespiratory endurance are those that stress a large portion of the body's muscle mass for a prolonged period of time and include running and jogging, walking and hiking, swimming, and bicycling. Games such as racquetball, tennis, basketball, and soccer are also good if the skill level and intensity of the game are sufficient to provide a vigorous workout.

Table 14-2 Examples of Endurance Exercises

Activity	Exertion Level
Backpacking	M–H
Badminton	M
Basketball	M–H
Bicycling	M–H
Calisthenics	M
Canoeing	L–M
Dancing	M
Fencing	M
Fishing	L
Football (touch)	M
Golf (walking)	M
Handball	M–H
Hiking	L–M
Horseback riding	L–M
Hunting	L–M
Mountain climbing	M–H
Racketball	M–H
Rope jumping	M–H
Running	M–H
Scuba diving	L–M
Skating (ice and roller)	M
Skiing (cross country)	M–H
Skiing (downhill)	M
Skiing (water)	M
Snowshoeing	M–H
Soccer	M–H
Squash	M–H
Swimming	L–M
Tennis	L–H
Volleyball	L–M
Walking	L–M
Weight training (circuit)	M

Note: L, light exercise, activity increases metabolism less than 5 times above rest; M, moderate exercise, activity increases metabolism 5–10 times above rest; H, heavy exercise, activity increases metabolism more than 10 times above rest.

Cardiorespiratory endurance exercise should play the prominent part in any physical activity program. The American College of Sports Medicine has made recommendations based on scientific research for the quantity and quality of training required for developing and maintaining cardiorespiratory fitness in healthy adults (see Table 14-3).

Frequency of Training The optimal workout schedule for endurance training is three to five days per week. Beginners should start with three and work up to five days. Training more than five days a week often leads to injury for recreational athletes. Training less than three days a week provides little health benefit, and you risk injury because your body never gets a chance to fully adapt to regular exercise training.

Intensity of Training The most misunderstood aspect of conditioning, even among experienced athletes, is training intensity. Problems are caused by doing too little or too much. Many recreational swimmers, for example, get very little benefit from their exercise because they don't work hard enough—their activity is closer to bathing than swimming. Yet working too hard will result in injury.

A primary purpose of endurance training is to increase **maximal oxygen consumption (MOC).** MOC represents the maximum ability of the cells to use oxygen and is considered the best measure of cardiovascular capacity. Intensity is the crucial factor in attaining a training effect and improving MOC. Although several methods for cal-

Table 14-3 Recommended Quantity and Quality of Exercise for Developing and Maintaining Fitness in Healthy Adults

Mode of activity

Aerobic or endurance exercises, such as running-jogging, walking-hiking, swimming, skating, bicycling, rowing, cross-country skiing, rope skipping, and various game activities.

Frequency of training

3 to 5 days per week

Intensity of training

60 percent of capability range plus resting pulse rate, or 50 percent to 85 percent of maximum oxygen uptake

Duration of training

15 to 60 minutes of continuous aerobic activity. Duration depends on the intensity of the activity.

SOURCE: American College of Sports Medicine, 1978, *Sports Medicine Bulletin* 13:1–4.

Walk Your Way to Fitness

If you are one of those many people for whom jogging holds no attraction, and if you have never learned to ski, can't play tennis, don't own a bicycle, and dislike swimming, there is no need to give up all hope of ever becoming more physically fit. Regardless of real or imagined limitations due to age, sex, body weight, or lack of athletic prowess, you can still get into great shape. You can walk your way to fitness!

Often Overlooked

Unfortunately, the physical conditioning value of walking often goes unrecognized—partly because it is such a simple, natural, everyday part of living. Also, with so many people running marathons, playing racquet sports, and taking up vigorous outdoor activities such as downhill and cross-country skiing, it's understandable that many might think walking is just not physically demanding enough to qualify as a worthwhile fitness developer.

In reality, however, walking—if it is done briskly enough and long enough—can be just as good as jogging, or any other endurance exercise, for developing a high level of cardiorespiratory fitness. And for those who are exceptionally overweight, or have been extremely sedentary for a long period of time, have limiting medical or orthopedic problems, or are of advanced years, it is the preferred route to fitness!

Walking Can Work Wonders

Properly organized, a walking program can provide three of the most important benefits to be gained from exercise—cardiovascular endurance, weight control, and reduction of emotional stress. It promotes increased lung action, stimulates the circulation, activates many large muscle groups and can burn up a significant number of calories. Research has also shown it to be helpful in lowering elevated blood pressures.

Walking for Fitness

A leisurely stroll is relaxing, aids circulation, and burns up some calories, but for cardiorespiratory conditioning, a more vigorous pace is essential. It must be fast enough to adequately tax your heart and lungs.

For fitness improvement, three exercise factors—intensity, duration, frequency—must be properly balanced. The formula calls for walking briskly enough to bring your exercise heart rate into the "target zone" for your age group, continuing for 30–60 minutes, and doing this at least three to four times per week.

Numerous Advantages

Walking, as a form of regular exercise, offers a great many advantages. It requires no special clothing or equipment, other than a suitable pair of shoes, and it is the easiest of all exercise activities to fit into your normal daily living pattern. You can walk all or part of the way to work, walk at the noon hour, walk home again after work, incorporate a walking workout into a shopping trip, walk those errands to the corner store, and you can easily combine brisk walking with other recreational pursuits such as picnic outings, visits to the museum, or just general sightseeing, all without changing clothes or raising your neighbors' eyebrows. It's also the easiest fitness activity to take with you wherever you go, even on vacation, because it can be done almost anywhere and anytime.

Highly Adaptable Walking is an almost universally acceptable fitness activity because it is so easily adaptable to people of every age and level of physical condition, and requires no special athletic skills whatsoever. It is also considerably less stressful on muscles and joints than faster-paced, more jarring activities such as jogging, tennis, squash, or racquetball. And in addition to being simple and safe, it can be used for many different purposes—for cardiorespiratory fitness, weight control, relaxation, or for strengthening and conditioning the legs.

Socially Rewarding Another special advantage associated with walking is its social aspect. It lends itself ideally to sharing with a friend or loved one, and its benefits are multiplied when it's enjoyed amid the wonders of nature. Nothing is so exhilarating and yet so relaxing as a brisk walk in the countryside, especially on a crisp autumn day.

Walking can be an excellent preliminary to a program of more vigorous activities, but it's also an exceptionally effective fitness program in its own right and one that can be safely followed all the years of your life.

To make sure you are walking fast enough, you can check your exercise heart rate by carefully counting your pulse at the wrist or at the side of your throat. If necessary, stop your walking long enough to do this (count the pulses for 10 seconds and multiply by 6) then resume your walking.

(continued on next page)

Walk Your Way to Fitness (*continued*)

Adjust your pace as required to keep your heart rate high enough, looking for hills to walk, or carry some extra weight in a knapsack.

If you are exercising in the upper half of your "target zone," 30–40 minutes will be sufficient. At lower levels of effort, however, you should continue for at least 60 minutes. Done three to five times per week, this kind of program can be highly effective, as well as enjoyable, and those who use it will soon realize why that sage physician, Hippocrates, once said, "Walking is man's best medicine."

Source: Walk your way to fitness, 1985 (February), *Healthline*.

culating this effect have been devised, one of the easiest involves heart rate. It is not necessary to exercise at the maximum heart rate in order to improve MOC. Beneficial effects occur at lower heart rates with a much lower risk of injury. The maximum heart rate is the fastest rate possible before exhaustion sets in.

To determine the rate at which you should exercise—your target heart rate—first find out what your heart rate is after ten minutes of complete rest. Then subtract your resting heart rate from your maximum heart rate. The most reliable way of calculating this maximum rate is by means of a **treadmill test,** which is administered in physicians' offices, hospitals, and sports medicine laboratories. Maximum heart rate can also be estimated by subtracting your age from 220, or it can be taken from Table 14-4. Although these last two methods are usually fairly accurate, they can be grossly inadequate for some people. For example, a 20-year-old college student may have a maximum heart rate as low as 180 beats per minute or as high as 215 beats per minute.

The difference between your resting and maximum pulse rates is your **capability range (CR)** or **heart rate reserve.**

Table 14-4 Maximum and Target Heart Rates Predicted from Age

Age	Predicted Maximum Heart Rate	Target Heart Rate 60%	80%
20–24 years	200	149	174
25–29	200	149	174
30–34	194	145	170
35–39	188	142	165
40–44	182	138	160
45–49	176	134	155
50–54	171	131	151
55–59	165	128	146
60–64	159	124	142
60+	153	121	137

SOURCE: Derived from Metropolitan Life Insurance Company charts and Karvonen formula (target heart rate = 0.6 or 0.8 $[HR_{max} - HR_{rest}] + HR_{rest}$).

For example,

Maximum heart rate	200
Resting heart rate	− 70
Capability range	130 beats

The training effect occurs when the heart rate is higher than the resting heart rate by an amount that is 60–80 percent of the capability range plus the resting heart rate. For example,

Capability range	130
Minimum intensity	× .6
60% CR	78
Resting heart rate	+ 70
Target heart rate	148 beats per minute

Measure your heart rate either at the wrist or at one of the carotid arteries, located on each side of your Adam's apple. Begin counting immediately after you have finished exercising. The pulse rate usually drops rapidly after exercise, so the most accurate procedure is to count beats for 15 seconds and then multiply the number by 6. To build fitness, the heart rate must be maintained at the target for a minimum of 15–20 minutes.

The more fit you become, the harder you will have to work to improve. By monitoring your heart rate, you will always know if you are working hard enough to improve or if you are overdoing it. You can maintain fitness by exercising at the same intensity approximately three times per week. For most people, a fitness program involves attaining an acceptable level of fitness and then maintaining that level. There is no need to keep working indefinitely to improve; doing so only increases the chance of injury.

A relatively new technique that is practiced by some athletes is **periodization of training** (cycle training). With this technique, the intensity of the workout varies from one training session to another. The benefit of cycle training is that you are rested on a day that calls for a heavy workout. For example, the intensity sequence of a week-long series of workouts might be (1) hard, (2) easy, (3) moderate, (4) easy, (5) moderate, (6) rest, and (7) rest. A

Treadmill test A controlled exercise test to measure exercise capacity.

Capability range (CR) The capacity of the heart to increase its heart rate above a resting level.

Heart rate reserve The capacity of the heart to increase its heart rate above a resting level. Same as capability range.

Periodization of training A training technique that systematically varies the volume and intensity of the workouts.

Resistive exercise Exercise that forces muscles to contract against increased resistance; for example, weight training.

Isometric exercise Application of force without movement. Also called *static* exercise.

Isotonic exercise Application of force with movement.

Isokinetic exercise Application of force at constant speed. A form of isotonic exercise.

hard workout might be practiced at 80 percent of the heart rate reserve, a moderate workout at 70 percent, and an easy workout at 60 percent (see Table 14-4). This method helps you to work hard when you have a lot of energy and lets you rest when you are tired.

Duration of Training The length of time you should spend on a workout depends on its intensity. If you are walking, swimming slowly, or playing a stop-and-start game like tennis, you should participate for 45 to 60 minutes. High-intensity exercises such as running can be practiced for a shorter period of time (such as 20 minutes). The recreational athlete should start off with less vigorous activities and only gradually increase intensity. For most people, continuous endurance exercise should last from 15 to 60 minutes.

Other Forms of Exercise Exercise that will develop muscular strength and muscular endurance should also be included in any program designed to promote health. Your ability to maintain correct posture and to move efficiently depends in part on adequate muscle fitness. Good muscle tone is also important for appearance. After all, if you are physically fit, you want to look physically fit.

Muscular strength and endurance can be developed in many ways, from weight training to calisthenics. Common exercises such as sit-ups, push-ups, pull-ups, and wall-sitting (leaning against a wall in a seated position and supporting yourself with your leg muscles) satisfy the strength needs of most people if they practice a few exercises for the major muscle groups three to five days a week.

Resistive exercise—exercises that require muscles to exert force against a significant resistance—is necessary to increase strength. Modes of resistance include weights, exercise machines, or your own body weight. In general, you must train at least twice a week for an hour to experience significant results. Using heavy resistance with few repetitions (one to ten) builds strength and muscle size, while employing more repetitions improves muscular strength endurance (the ability to exert force over a longer period of time). Strength training improves performance in most sports and has become a prominent part of the training program of many athletes.

There are three categories of strength exercises. **Isometric exercise** is applying force without movement; **isotonic exercise** is applying force with movement; and **isokinetic exercise** is exerting force at a constant speed. Isotonic exercise seems to be most valuable for developing strength that can be transferred to other forms of physical activity.

Flexibility is perhaps the most neglected part of fitness, even though it is extremely important. You lose flexibility when you do not move your joints through their normal range of motion. Some exercises, such as running, actually decrease flexibility because they require only a partial range of motion. It is therefore important to do exercises that maintain mobility in the major joints. At least once a day, do some stretching or mobility exercises for the hamstrings, hips, lower spine, neck, and shoulders. (See "Exercises for Flexibility" box.) If you get into the habit of doing these exercises regularly, you can prevent many of the muscle and joint pains that plague most people.

Developing Skill in Physical Activity The ability to learn a skill and the rate at which it is learned are specific and therefore unrelated to other activities. In other words, if you want to learn a particular skill, you have to practice that skill and not something else.

Many people do not exercise, or dislike exercise, because they feel silly or self-conscious. They feel ridiculous hitting tennis balls over the fence instead of over the net; they are embarrassed by running a 12-minute mile or trying to touch their toes and barely getting past their kneecaps. Such people do not give themselves a chance. They try an activity once or twice and then give it up in despair. If they would take the time and effort to acquire some competence, they would begin to enjoy physical activity.

The first step in learning a skill is to get help. If you want to acquire competence in tennis, golf, or sailing, it is best to receive instruction. Most sports require a mastery of certain skill, so instruction from a qualified teacher can save you hours of frustration, and it can increase your enjoyment of the sport. Take a physical education class, sign up for lessons at the recreation department, or get private instruction.

Skill is also important in conditioning activities such as jogging, swimming, and cycling. Know your own capacity, and be able to gauge the intensity of exercise

Anabolic Steroids: How Do They Work?

Anabolic steroids are drugs that resemble male hormones such as testosterone and are widely used by athletes in such sports as track and field, weight lifting, and football. Athletes take them in the hope of gaining weight, strength, power, speed, endurance, and aggressiveness. Although research findings are divided, most experts feel that they are effective in improving some types of athletic performance. They have dangerous side effects. A recent, alarming trend is young nonathletes taking these drugs to improve appearance and sex appeal.

Male hormones, principally testosterone, are partially responsible for the tremendous developmental changes that occur in boys during puberty and adolescence. Male hormones have both androgenic and anabolic effects. **Androgenic effects** are characterized by changes in primary and secondary sexual characteristics such as enlargement of the penis and testes; changes in the voice; hair growth on the face, armpit, and genital areas; and increased aggressiveness. The **anabolic effects** of androgens include accelerated growth of muscle, bone, and red blood cells, and enhanced neural conduction. Anabolic steroids have been manufactured to enhance the anabolic properties (tissue building) of the androgens and to minimize the androgenic (sex-linked) properties. However, no steroid has completely eliminated the androgenic effects.

Anabolic steroids can have dangerous side effects. Although they improve athletic performance, the benefits are not worth the health risks. The principal side effects of anabolic steroids can be subdivided into (1) normal physiological actions of male hormones that are inappropriate in the recipient, and (2) toxic effects caused mainly by oral forms.

The *physiological side effects* include reduced testosterone production, testicular function, and sperm cell production. Libido (sex drive) may increase or decrease. Anabolic steroids increase fluid retention. Steroid use by women and immature children may induce masculinizing hair growth on face and body, deepening of the voice, oily skin, increased sweat gland activity, acne, and baldness. In women, some of these changes are irreversible. Women may also experience clitoral enlargement and menstrual irregularity. Children initially experience accelerated maturation followed by premature closure of growth centers in the long bones.

Anabolic steroids can result in testicular atrophy and decreased sperm production. These changes may also reverse themselves after usage stops, but prolonged use may permanently disturb the delicate hormone regulatory system.

Anabolic steroids may also harm the immune system. These drugs are thought to block the action of hormones called corticosteroids involved in breakdown and repair after a heavy workout. In reaction, the body increases production of corticosteroids and their receptors. Corticosteroids suppress the immune system, which fights off diseases. Athletes often get colds or flu when going off steroids because of the increased corticosteroids.

Oral anabolic steroids, such as methandrostenolone (Dianabol), present the greatest risk of toxicity, particularly to the liver, because their structure has been altered to make them more biologically active. Such steroids concentrate in the liver much earlier and in greater quantity than the injectable varieties. Prolonged use has been linked to severe liver disorders such as blood-filled cysts, liver cancer, and bile duct obstruction.

Several factors in steroid use are linked to increased risk of coronary heart disease: high levels of cholesterol and triglycerides, high blood pressure, and low levels of high-density lipoproteins (HDLs). Many weight-trained athletes use steroids from ten to more than twenty years, risking premature death from atherosclerosis. Hypertension (high blood pressure) is also common, probably due to fluid retention.

A variety of other side effects have been reported including muscle cramps, gastrointestinal distress, headache, dizziness, sore nipples, and abnormal thyroid function. Some of these side effects even show up in people who have only taken low doses for short periods of time.

Anabolic steroids Synthetic male hormones used to increase muscle size and strength.

Androgenic effects Effects of anabolic steroids that cause changes in secondary sexual characteristics, such as hair growth, aggressiveness, and deepening of the voice.

Anabolic effects Effects of anabolic steroids that tend to build tissues such as muscle.

that will result in improvement without injury. Some instruction on technique from a coach or fellow participant can often help you to move and train more efficiently.

Managing Your Program After you have chosen the nature of your program and determined its basic structure, a few basic considerations will make your program run more smoothly. Adhering to these principles will help you to improve at the fastest rate, have more fun, and minimize the risk of injury.

Buy Good-quality Equipment When you are sure of your activities, buy the best equipment you can afford. Good equipment will enhance your enjoyment and decrease your risk of injury. Along with the recent growth in physical activity has come a wave of new equipment and clothing. Some of it is truly revolutionary: the new skis allow you to go faster with better control, new tennis rackets make it easier to hit the ball over the net, and new materials make sports clothing more comfortable and fashionable. Unfortunately, some new products are either overpriced or of poor quality. A flashy but overweight tennis racket can produce an elbow injury, while a shoe that can't absorb shock can cause leg pains. Before you invest in a new piece of equipment, investigate it. Is it worth the money? Does it produce the results it is supposed to? Ask the

Exploring Your Emotions

What would you be thinking about if you were the person in this picture?

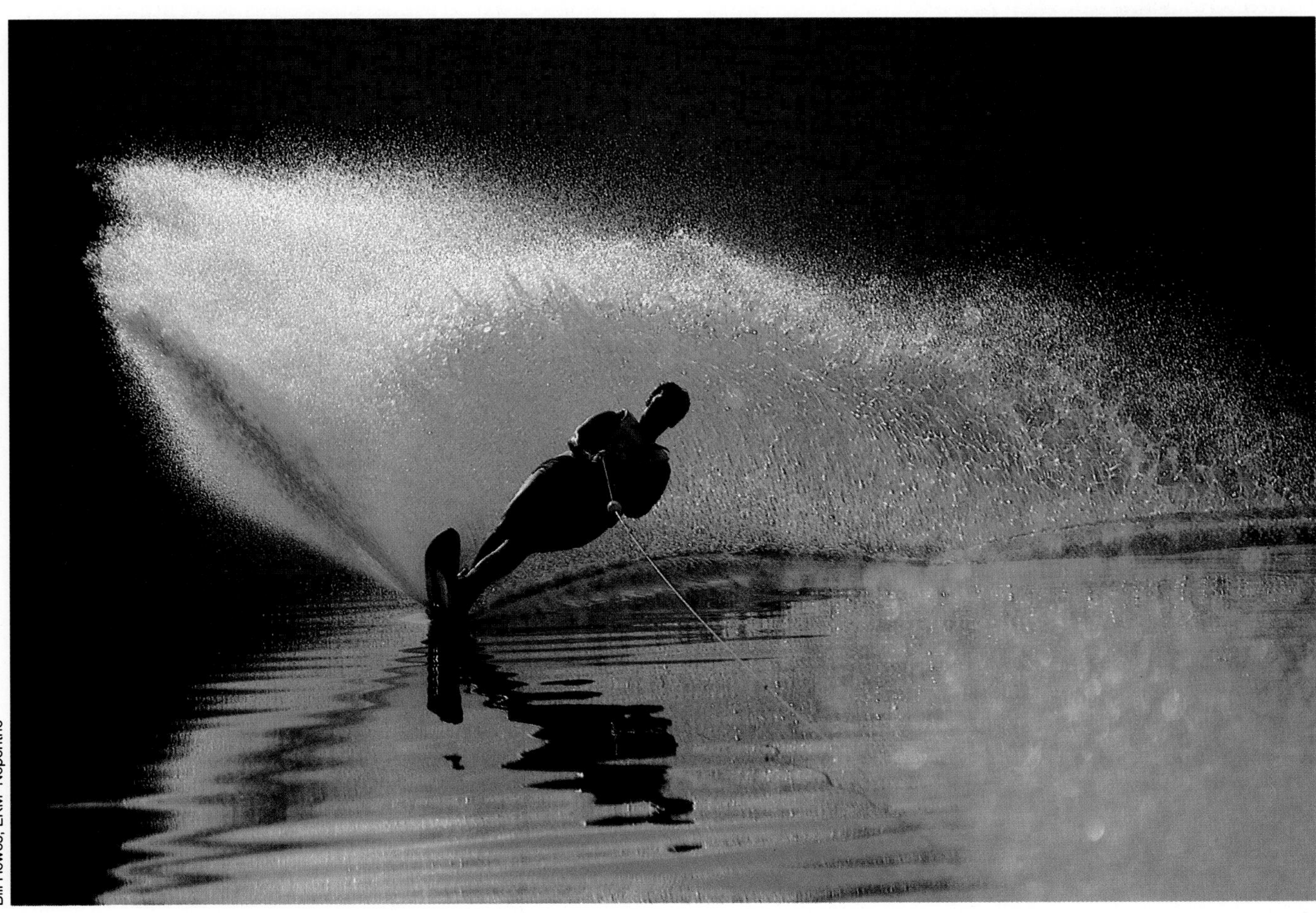

Bill Hewes, EKM–Nepenthe

Synovial fluid Fluid found within many joints that provides lubrication and nutrition to the cells of the joint surface.

Glycogen A complex carbohydrate, found largely in the liver and skeletal muscle, that serves as a carbohydrate storage depot.

Overload Subjecting the body to more stress than it is accustomed.

experts (coaches, physical educators, and sports instructors) for their opinion. Better yet, educate yourself. Every sport, from running to volleyball, has magazines devoted to every aspect of it. A little effort to educate yourself will be well rewarded.

Footwear is perhaps the most important item of equipment for almost any sport. Buy shoes that are appropriate for the activity. Don't jog in shoes designed for tennis or basketball, and vice versa. Make sure the shoes fit; a shoe's five-star rating doesn't make any difference if your feet hurt. (Figure 14-2 shows the characteristics of an ideal running shoe.)

Warm Up and Cool Down Warming up before exercising enhances your performance and decreases your chances of injury. Your muscles work better when their temperature is slightly above resting level. Warming up helps your body's physiology gradually progress from rest to exercise. Blood needs to be redirected to active muscles, and this takes time. Your heart needs time to adapt to the increased demands of exercise. Warm up helps spread **synovial fluid** throughout joints, which helps protect surfaces. (This is like an automobile: warming up a car spreads oil through the engine parts before you shift into gear.)

A warm-up session should include low-intensity movements similar to those in the activity that will follow. Low-intensity movements include hitting forehands and backhands before a tennis match, skiing down an easy run before tackling a more difficult one, and running a 12-minute mile before progressing to an 8-minute one. Some experts also recommend warm-up stretching (flexibility) exercises.

Figure 14-2 What to look for in a running shoe

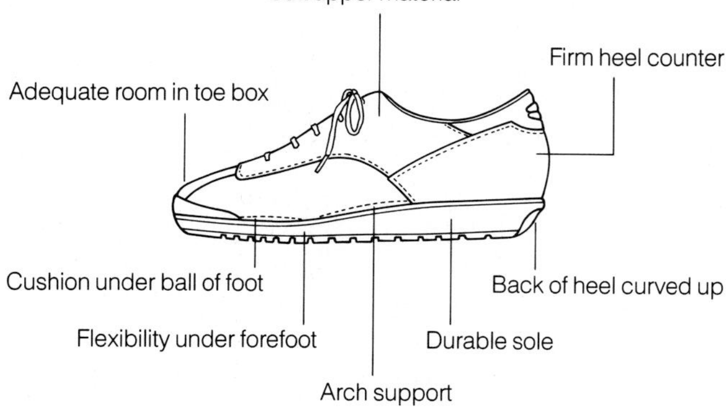

Cooling down after exercise is also important, to protect the heart and prevent fainting. At rest, a relatively small percent of your total blood volume is directed to muscles. However, during exercise as much as 85 percent of the heart's output is directed to them. During recovery from exercise, it is important to continue exercising at low level (cool down) in order to provide a smooth transition to the resting state. Cooling down helps maintain the return of blood to your heart during recovery and thus facilitates the delivery of oxygen to the heart.

Maintain Proper Diet and Fluid Intake The relationship between diet and exercise is widely misunderstood. Many athletes and other physically active people waste millions of dollars on vitamins, minerals, and protein supplements. For most people, a nutritionally balanced diet (see Chapter 12) contains all the energy and nutrients needed to sustain an exercise program.

Long-distance runners as well as other athletes benefit from diets that are higher than average in carbohydrates because carbohydrates increase the amount of glycogen in the muscles and liver. **Glycogen**, a carbohydrate stored in muscles and the liver, is vitally important for sustaining physical activity over long periods of time. When levels of this substance are low, the athlete feels sluggish, weak, and tired.

Your body depends on water to maintain a healthy body chemistry. Water is important for many chemical reactions and for maintaining correct body temperature. Because sweating reduces water level, it is important to drink fluids during exercise sessions. As a rule of thumb, try to drink about half a pint of water for every 30 minutes of heavy exercise. Increase this amount in hot weather. Water—preferably cold—or diluted carbohydrate drinks are the best fluid replacements. You do not need to replace electrolytes, such as sodium and potassium, during exercise because the body is very efficient at sparing them.

The best way to detect water loss after exercise is by weighing yourself in the nude (sweaty clothes can weigh a lot). An average endurance workout uses about 200 calories, while a pound of fat contains 3,500 calories. The majority of weight loss after physical activity obviously is due to water loss. Relying on thirst alone, you can take 24 hours or more to replace this fluid loss. Ideally, you should restore your body fluids before exercising vigorously again.

Dealing with Athletic Injuries

Injuries can happen even to the most careful physically active person. Although annoying, most are neither serious nor permanent. However, an injury that isn't cared for properly can escalate into a chronic problem, sometimes serious enough to permanently curtail the activity.

"When should I call a doctor?"

Consult a doctor for head and eye injuries, possible ligament injuries, broken bones, and internal disorders such as chest pain, fainting, and intolerance to heat. Also seek medical attention for apparently minor injuries that do not get better within a reasonable amount of time.

"How should I manage minor athletic injuries when they occur?"

For minor cuts and scrapes, stop the bleeding and clean the wound. Treat soft tissue injuries (muscles and joints) immediately with ice packs. Elevate the affected part of the body, and compress it with an elastic bandage to minimize swelling. Use ice for 48 hours after the injury or until all swelling is gone. Some experts recommend taking over-the-counter medication that decreases inflammation, such as aspirin or ibuprofen, to treat soft tissue injuries.

"How do I rehabilitate my body after a minor athletic injury?"

Several rehabilitation procedures can be used for most types of athletic injuries: (1) reduce the initial inflammation, (2) restore normal joint motion, (3) restore normal strength and endurance, and (4) restore functional capacity. This fourth step involves gradually reintroducing the stress of the activity until you are capable of returning to full intensity.

"When can I return to full participation after an athletic injury?"

Before returning to full exercise participation, you should meet the following criteria: (1) full range of motion in the joints, (2) normal strength and balance among muscles, (3) normal coordinated patterns of movement, with no injury compensation movements, such as limping, and (4) little or no pain.

How to Maintain Fitness

Your ultimate level of fitness depends on your goals, the intensity of your program, and your natural ability. It is important to recognize when your fitness is adequate.

The Training Effect: Stress versus Distress When your body is subjected to a physical stress that it can tolerate, it adapts and improves its function. However, if the stress is too high, your body breaks down and becomes distressed or injured. This is the cornerstone of exercise training.

You won't improve unless you push yourself. For example, to improve flexibility you have to push your joints past their normal ranges of motion. Improved fitness is an adaptation to **overload** (an exercise stress that is more severe than the body is used to). If there is no stress, there is no improvement. You have to overload your body consistently over a long period of time.

Overdoing exercise is just as bad as not exercising hard enough, however. No one can become fit overnight. Your body needs time to adapt to increasingly higher levels of stress. The process of training involves a countless number of stresses and adaptations. If you feel sore and tired the day after exercising, then you have worked too hard. Injury will slow you down just as much as a missed workout.

Consistency is the key to fitness improvement and freedom from injury. A training diary, or record of your workouts, can help you apply the stresses of exercise more scientifically. All you need are a pencil and notebook to write down the details of your program. This record keeping will help you evaluate your progress and plan your exercise intelligently.

Commercial Health Clubs

There are exceptions to all generalizations: some health clubs do an outstanding job and others are frauds or near-frauds. The range can be found among national chains as well as among one-person operations. It is extremely difficult to make blanket statements, but *Consumers Guide®* can at least set down some guidelines.

High-pressure Selling

When you enter a health club, you can expect a tour followed by a high-pressure sales pitch. Be ready for it. Instructors and managers are well schooled in making an effective representation. They want your business.

Consumers Guide® sees nothing wrong with the health club manager's making a strong case emphasizing the value of exercise. But that's it. Under no circumstances should you feel badgered, embarrassed, belittled, threatened, detained, or mocked. If you feel any excessive amount of pressure, leave or at least ask for more time. If you are told this is a once-in-a-lifetime deal or that the rates go up tomorrow, etc., forget it. It's a high-pressure outfit interested in the dollar figure, not yours.

The Contract

Read the contract carefully. If you want more time, take it. If you feel you should read it at home or want to discuss it with other members of your family or anyone else, do so. If the health club won't permit you to take the contract home, steer clear of that organization. Make sure the contract commits you to no more than two years; one year is preferable. All contracts should provide for a minimum three-day cooling-off period; look for a "use of facility" clause permitting you to use the club during those three days.

Key Considerations

During the tour, explanation of facilities, and closing, you should be aware of the following:

1. Is there a discussion of your individual problems? This should take place prior to signing the contract. Is there a discussion of your physical limitations, risk factors, and the possibility of stress tests? Do they recommend that you talk to your doctor before you embark on an exercise program?

2. Is the person conducting the tour an instructor, a manager, or what? Does he or she seem to be well trained and not just well built? Ask if he or she is a physical education or physical therapy graduate with additional training in fitness. If not, does the club have an in-service training program emphasizing cardiovascular fitness? Do you sense that the person has a genuine interest in you? Is he or she able to explain how the machines operate, their value and limitations?

3. Does the spa manager or instructor emphasize cardiovascular fitness, or is the focus on muscle strength and muscle endurance? If the emphasis is on muscle strength and endurance, you can eliminate that club. Be careful—even the official statement of the Association of Physical Fitness Centers notes that "the modern health spa . . . offers programs of physical fitness incorporating concepts of progressive resistance exercise for both sexes. . . ." Progressive resistance exercise is the development of muscle endurance and strength. Remember, the primary focus should be on cardiovascular fitness.

4. Visit the club *at a time of day when you plan to use it.* This is crucial. Every club has a peak usage time. Waiting in line to run on the treadmill, ride a bicycle, or lift weights can be a serious inconvenience. Consider time and use of facilities as important factors.

5. Before signing anything, talk to several of the people who are exercising (or who have just finished, if you don't want to interrupt their work.) If the manager doesn't permit you to do this, cross the club off your list. Ask what they think of the program, what the emphasis is, and whether personal attention is given. Try to find out what the dropout rate is. European Health Spas claim that nearly three-fourths of their new members are referrals from other members. If the three-fourths figure is correct—and there is no way to check on it—it would indicate that this chain must be doing something right.

6. Find out how long the club has been in your area. The longer the better, and if under the same management, that's another plus. Approach a new club with caution—especially "pre-opening" sales. There have been cases where con artists have held pre-opening sales for clubs that never opened.

7. Find out if the club belongs to the Association of Physical Fitness Centers. This trade association for full-service health spas is dedicated to upgrading the industry. The Association has established a code of ethics that covers programs, facilities, employees, and consumers' rights.

8. The spa needs you more than you need the spa. Don't forget that. A club is an extra. It can provide you with some social contacts, motivation, and a special place to exercise—if you need these things.

SOURCE: Charles T. Kuntzleman, 1978, *Rating the Exercises, pp. 300–301.*

Table 14-5 Standards for the 1.5-Mile Run/Walk (Min:Sec)

	High	Good	Fair	Poor
Males				
20–29	9:45	12:00	13:00	15:00
30–39	10:00	12:15	13:30	16:00
40–49	10:30	12:30	14:00	16:30
50–59	11:00	13:30	15:00	18:30
60+	11:15	14:30	16:30	19:00
Females				
20–29	11:00	13:15	14:15	16:15
30–39	11:15	13:30	14:45	17:15
40–49	11:45	13:45	15:15	17:45
50–59	12:15	14:45	16:15	19:45
60+	12:30	15:45	17:45	20:15

Note: This test should not be attempted without at least six weeks of conditioning. Check with your doctor if you are over 35.

How to Know When You Are in Shape You are in shape when your body has reached your desired degree of adaptation. A 4-minute miler may be out of shape if he or she is running a mile in 4 minutes and 20 seconds, while the average person may be in adequate shape if he or she can comfortably run 2 miles in 18 minutes.

The best way to assess your fitness is in a modern sports medicine laboratory. Such laboratories are widely available and can be found in university physical education departments or medical centers. Here you will receive an accurate profile of your capacity to exercise. Typically, your endurance will be measured on a treadmill or bicycle, your body fat will be estimated, and your strength and flexibility will be tested. This evaluation will reveal whether you are in shape and suggest an exercise program that's appropriate for your level of fitness.

Testing your own fitness is more difficult because endurance, strength, coordination, and agility are specific to an activity or task. It is meaningless to compare the number of pull-ups or push-ups you can do with the strength requirements of, for example, tennis, skiing, or jogging.

To get a rough estimate of your cardiorespiratory fitness, check your speed in the 1.5-mile run or walk. Keep in mind, however, that this test may be totally inadequate for activities such as swimming and cycling. Nevertheless, it can provide an estimate of whether your fitness is consistent with good health. Table 14-5 provides standards for both men and women.

Staying Fit You can only maintain fitness by exercising on a regular basis at a consistent intensity. Three days per week seems to be the minimum number of days to maintain most types of fitness. You must work at the intensity that brought you to your desired fitness level. If you don't, your body will become less fit because less is expected of it. In general, if you exercise at the same intensity over a long period, your fitness will level out and can be maintained easily.

Psychologically, people seem to be able to do this only if they have a goal. The goal can be anything from fitting into a dress bought last year to skiing down a new slope. The important thing to remember is that you can have goals without striving to improve your fitness.

Varying a program is another good way to maintain interest. For example, you might consider competitive sports (swimming, running, racquetball, volleyball, golf, and so on) at the recreational level. Exposing yourself to new experiences can add zest to any program.

Take Action

Your answers to the Exploring Your Emotions in this chapter and your placement level on the Wellness Ladder will, we hope, encourage you to begin a process of self-exploration and self-discovery that you will continue. Reflect on the entire chapter's content and ask yourself how each point relates to your own life. Then take action:

1. On the left side of a page in your Take Action notebook, list the positive behaviors that help you avoid a sedentary lifestyle and keep you fit. How can you strengthen these behaviors? On the right side of the page, list the behaviors that block a physically active lifestyle. Consider which ones would be easiest to change and start to change them.

2. Track and monitor your physical activity during the next two weeks by doing the following: Indicate in your Take Action notebook the activity and the time, date, and duration of the activity. After you have accumulated this information, draw a graph that looks like the one here, adding your own appropriate dots. At the end of the two weeks,

connect the dots with a solid line. This line is called a *trend line*. Is your trend line generally up, down, or horizontal?

3. Look in your closet and take out the shoes you use for your most frequent physical activity. Consider whether they are appropriate for the activity. Find an expert (coach, physical educator, or sports instructor) and ask his or her opinion.

4. Read the following Behavior Change Strategy, and take the appropriate action.

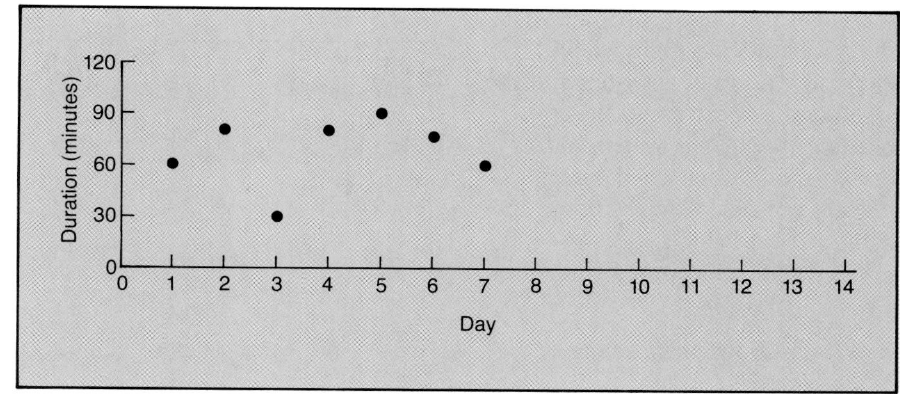

Behavior Change Strategy

Exercise

Perhaps more than any other topic area in health promotion, exercise has caught the spirit of the 1980s. Books on running and other forms of exercise appear almost daily. Exercise spas and special sports centers have become a major business enterprise in many parts of the country. With all this development and apparent popular interest, it may be a surprise that there has been relatively little behavioral research to provide tested guidelines for following personal exercise programs. The research published has focused, instead, on the physiological changes and benefits associated with training. Moreover, most of this limited research has reflected the training experiences of subjects such as athletes, armed forces personnel, students in physical education classes, and people recovering from seriously debilitating events such as heart attacks.

What, then, can be recommended to individuals who do not have the incentives or motivation of these special groups? The best recommendations are drawn from behavior self-management approaches.

Diary (Self-monitoring) As with the other behavior change strategies suggested throughout this book, the best first step involves collecting detailed information, in this case about beginning or "baseline" activity levels. There are a number of ways to go about measuring your personal exercise activity. For example, you can measure the number of times per week (*frequency*) you participate in a certain type of exercise. You can also measure the *duration* of your activity (for example, how much time you spend walking or swimming laps). By combining frequency and duration, you begin to assess the *intensity* of your usual exercise. This approach is satisfactory if you are trying to increase only one or possibly two types of exercise, but it grows more complicated if you want to increase your general level of activity, including a range of different types of behavior, such as walking, running, climbing stairs, swimming, and lifting weights.

Dr. Kenneth Cooper has devised an aerobic point system to handle specifically the complexity that comes with increasing different types of physical activity. The term *aerobic* refers to the amount of oxygen the body can process per unit of time, and it reflects on the conditioning of the lungs, heart, and vascular system. In essence, Cooper has assessed the relative fitness benefits from different activities in terms of the amount of oxygen the activity requires at different levels of training. By awarding points to various forms of activity, Cooper's system allows for a varied "menu" of activities while linking practice to physiological indices of fitness. Cooper also uses a standardized fitness self-test that permits classification into fitness levels. More specifically, in a special running exam, the participant merely measures the distance he or she can cover in 12 minutes. If we know that distance, we can determine his or her level of fitness (excellent, very poor, or somewhere in between). With a gradually increasing range of activities and the associated aerobic points accumulated per week, this system builds on self-monitoring to encourage significant personal changes in exercise habits.

Cooper offers four key guidelines:

1. Progress slowly.
2. Warm up properly before exercising.
3. Exercise within your personal tolerance.
4. Cool down slowly following exercise.

Aerobic Points

Activity	Distance or Time	Min.:Sec.	Points
Walking, running	1 mile	19:59–14:30	1
		14:29–12:00	2
		11:59–10:00	3
		9:59–8:00	4
		7:59–6:31	5
		6:30–5:45	6
		under 5:45	7
Cycling	2 miles	12:00 or longer	0
		11:59–8:00	1
		7:59–6:00	2
		under 6:00	3
Swimming	200 yards	6:40 or longer	0
		6:39–5:00	1
		4:59–3:20	1.5
		under 3:20	2.5
Handball	10 minutes		1.5

SOURCE: Adapted from K. H. Cooper, 1970, *The New Aerobics* (New York: Bantam).

Stimulus Control You can change your personal environment in a number of ways that will encourage you to follow through with an exercise program. For example, you might put your jogging shoes in an obvious place where you cannot miss them (in the hallway or by the bedroom door). This compels you to think about jogging. Although *thinking about* jogging is not the same thing as jogging (thoughts do not merit aerobic points), it is part of the chain of events that leads to that behavioral goal. This use of stimulus control is similar to the way in which we use alarm clocks—setting up the environment to help us later.

Another example of stimulus control is posting your diary of practice on the bedroom door or some other highly visible place. This will serve as a *reminder* and provide you with additional incentive to increase your activity. You can even set up special study areas, or "dedicated activity zones," to make other work more efficient so that you have enough time in your daily schedule to participate in physical activities.

Cognition (Self-statements) Thoughts can play a critical role in a personal exercise program. Rationalizations can discourage your efforts. ("The more I play tennis, the more uncoordinated I become." Or, "I'm just making a fool out of myself!") Thoughts don't need to be so personal, however, to undermine your enthusiasm. ("It's too cold outside to run right now." Or, "I just don't want to take too many showers in one day—I'll just wait until tomorrow to do x, y, and z.") As in all behavioral programs, it is wise to begin by keeping a list and identifying such thought patterns and *then* to directly attack negative thoughts in order to reduce their frequency.

Self-contracts and Reward Systems Personal contracts can provide an important and added incentive to your exercise program. A typical contract specifies in detail the target behaviors of concern: the kinds of exercise activities you want to increase and by how much. It identifies the day and time of practice and usually includes your signature. Of course, some benefits come directly from improving your personal fitness level—in terms of both psychological and physical improvements—but these benefits are often delayed. A reward system can provide more immediate positive consequences and can even be related to your target behavior (for example, paying yourself a certain amount of money for each day you follow your program and with the money you "earn" buying new jogging shoes or a subscription to a jogging or running magazine).

Exercising with other people often offers the incentives of both structure and companionship. However, this happens only if the other person or members of the group maintain a thorough and regular exercise schedule. In any case, you must be prepared to exercise independently should the group break apart or become less conscientious.

The problem-solving approach described more fully in Chapter 1 of this book, combined with the specific strategies outlined in this section, can improve your chances of becoming more physically fit.

Selected References

American College of Sports Medicine. 1986. *Guidelines for Graded Exercise Testing and Exercise Prescription.* Philadelphia: Lea & Febiger.

Brooks, G. A., and T. D. Fahey. 1984. *Exercise Physiology: Human Bioenergetics and Its Applications.* New York: Macmillan.

Brooks, G. A., and T. D. Fahey. 1987. *Fundamentals of Human Performance.* New York: Macmillan.

Fahey, T. D., ed. 1986. *Athletic Training: Principles and Practice.* Mountain View, Calif.: Mayfield.

Kramsch, D. M., A. J. Aspen, B. M. Abramowitz, T. Kreimendahl, and W. B. Hood. 1981. Reduction of coronary atherosclerosis by moderate conditioning exercise in monkeys on an atherogenic diet. *New England Journal of Medicine* 305:1483–89.

Nieman, D. C. 1986. *The Sports Medicine Fitness Course.* Palo Alto, Calif.: Bull Publishing.

Noakes, T. 1984. *The Lore of Running.* Cape Town, South Africa: Oxford University Press.

Paffenbarger, R. S., R. T. Hyde, A. L. Wing, and C. H. Steinmetz. 1984. A natural history of athleticism and cardiovascular health. *Journal of the American Medical Association* 252:491–95.

Pollock, M. L., J. H. Wilmore, and S. M. Fox. 1978. *Health and Fitness Through Physical Activity.* New York: Macmillan.

Recommended Readings

Brooks, G. A., and T. D. Fahey. 1987. *Fundamentals of Human Performance.* New York: Macmillan.
A general overview of the physiology of exercise.

Kusinitz, I., and M. Fine. 1987. *Your Guide to Getting Fit.* Mountain View, Calif.: Mayfield.
The latest fitness applications from the field of exercise physiology.

Chapter 15

Contents

Rate Yourself

Your Self-care Behavior Read the following statements carefully. Choose the one in each section that best describes you at this moment and circle its number. When you have chosen one statement for each section, add the numbers and record your total score. Find your position on the Wellness Ladder.

5 Well educated about when to see the doctor
4 Reads reference materials before visiting the doctor
3 Schedules an annual physical exam
2 Prefers asking the doctor before buying medicines
1 Sees the doctor for minor complaints such as colds and sore throats

5 Keeps medicine chest up-to-date
4 Throws away old medications
3 Occasionally throws away old medications
2 Prefers to keep old medications
1 Uses old medications, even after expiration date

5 Knows blood pressure and cholesterol levels
4 Knows blood pressure level
3 Vaguely knows that blood pressure is normal
2 Thinks that blood pressure or cholesterol level is high
1 Has no idea what constitutes high blood pressure or cholesterol levels

5 Well educated about home medical tests
4 Familiar with home medical tests
3 Vaguely familiar with home medical tests
2 Unfamiliar with home medical tests
1 Would not consider using a home medical test

5 Reads medical self-care reference materials regularly
4 Reads medical self-care reference materials when sick
3 Occasionally reads self-care reference materials when sick
2 Rarely reads self-care reference materials
1 Never reads self-care reference materials

Total Score ______

Medical Self-care: Skills for the Health Care Consumer

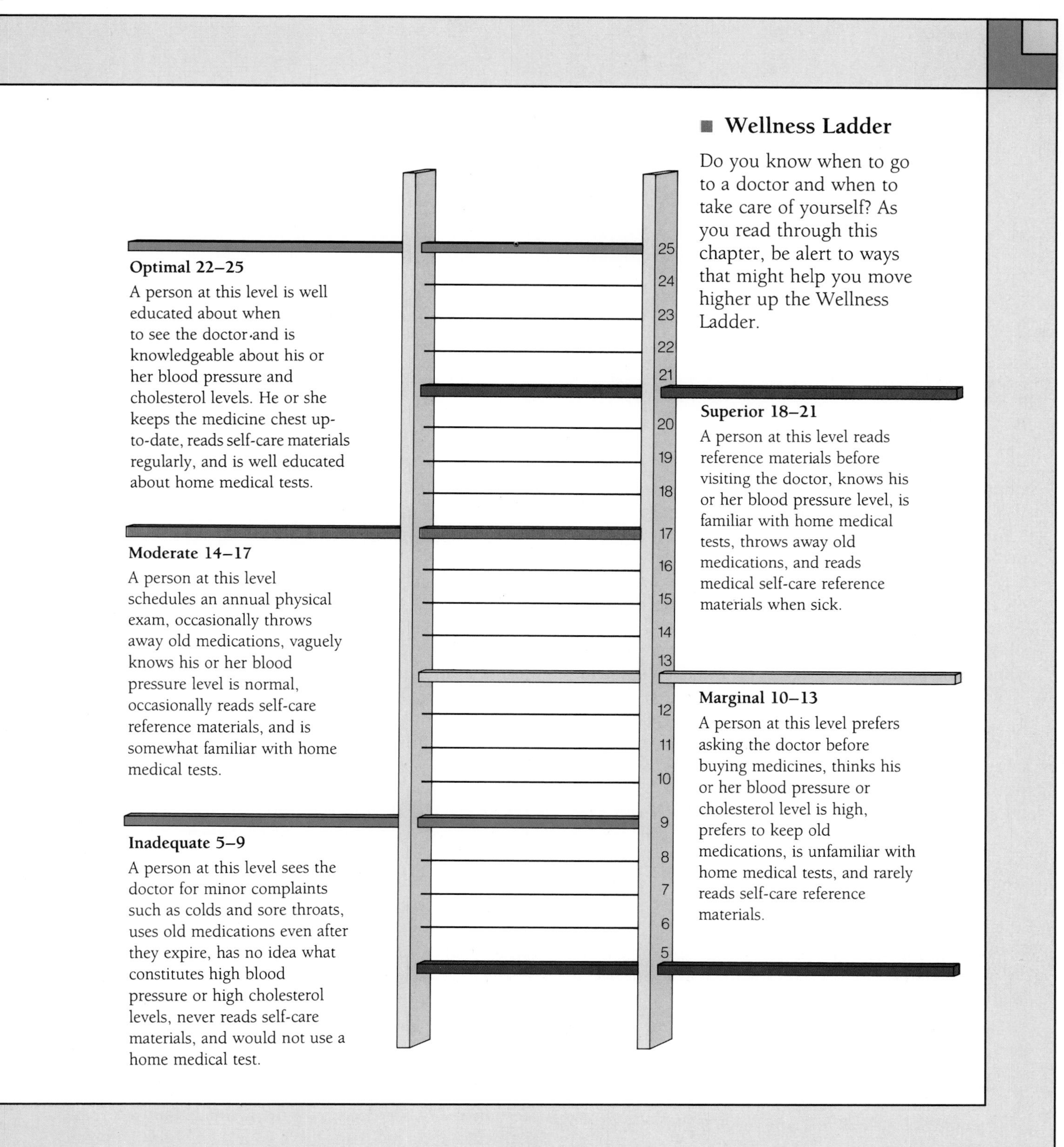

Wellness Ladder
Do you know when to go to a doctor and when to take care of yourself? As you read through this chapter, be alert to ways that might help you move higher up the Wellness Ladder.
Optimal 22–25
A person at this level is well educated about when to see the doctor and is knowledgeable about his or her blood pressure and cholesterol levels. He or she keeps the medicine chest up-to-date, reads self-care materials regularly, and is well educated about home medical tests.
Superior 18–21
A person at this level reads reference materials before visiting the doctor, knows his or her blood pressure level, is familiar with home medical tests, throws away old medications, and reads medical self-care reference materials when sick.
Moderate 14–17
A person at this level schedules an annual physical exam, occasionally throws away old medications, vaguely knows his or her blood pressure level is normal, occasionally reads self-care reference materials, and is somewhat familiar with home medical tests.
Marginal 10–13
A person at this level prefers asking the doctor before buying medicines, thinks his or her blood pressure or cholesterol level is high, prefers to keep old medications, is unfamiliar with home medical tests, and rarely reads self-care reference materials.
Inadequate 5–9
A person at this level sees the doctor for minor complaints such as colds and sore throats, uses old medications even after they expire, has no idea what constitutes high blood pressure or high cholesterol levels, never reads self-care materials, and would not use a home medical test.
25
24
23
22
21
20
19
18
17
16
15
14
13
12
11
10
9
8
7
6
5

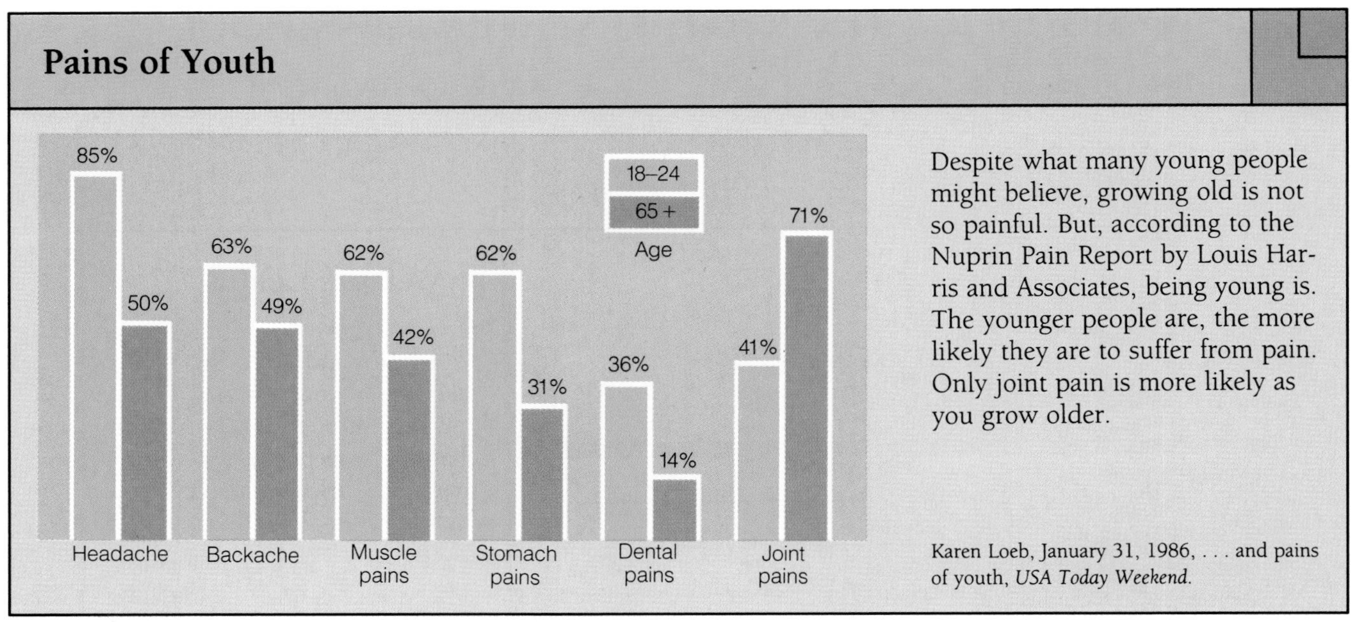

Pains of Youth

Despite what many young people might believe, growing old is not so painful. But, according to the Nuprin Pain Report by Louis Harris and Associates, being young is. The younger people are, the more likely they are to suffer from pain. Only joint pain is more likely as you grow older.

Karen Loeb, January 31, 1986, . . . and pains of youth, *USA Today Weekend.*

Over the past month, how many medical problems or symptoms did you have? Colds, backaches, stomachaches, rashes, fatigue, headache, minor eye irritations, and so on? For how many of those symptoms did you see a doctor or seek medical advice?

Studies show that the average person has about four new symptoms each *month* yet only consults or visits a doctor four times per *year*. At least 80 percent of all medical symptoms are self-diagnosed and self-treated. Yet this profile is not the traditional view of the health care system.

When we think of health care resources, we tend to think of doctors, nurses, clinics, and hospitals. Professional health care, however, is in reality just the tip of the iceberg. Below the surface is a massive *hidden* health care system, people taking care of themselves, their families, and their friends. This vast nonprofessional health care system dwarfs the professional system in size and function (see Figure 15-1).

The professional medical care system depends on the functioning of nonprofessional care. If people were to stop practicing self-care and seek professional care for even a small percentage of the complaints they usually manage by themselves, the professional health care system would be swamped. Moreover, if the competence of people to manage their own health problems could be increased by just a small amount, the demand for costly professional services would decrease dramatically.

This critical role of people as the *primary* providers of health care for themselves and their families has gone largely unnoticed. People's confidence in managing their own health problems has been undermined, and the knowledge of when to self-treat and when to seek professional care has not been widely shared.

A shift is occurring in health care toward informed self-care. People are beginning to reclaim their power, and the doctor-patient relationship is changing. Many patients are asking more questions of their doctors, considering a wider range of options, and educating themselves about the determinants of their health.

Central to this transition is the recognition that people manage their own health and health care. Managers, whether tending a home or a business, don't do everything themselves. They use others, including consultants, to get the job done. The role of the manager is to take responsibility for decisions and to make sure they are carried out. As self-manager of your own health, you will need to seek information from a wide variety of sources:

Exploring Your Emotions

You wake up in the morning with a stuffy nose and a mildly sore throat. By the next day you feel chilled and achy all over and have a dry cough. You decide to go to the doctor. After a brief exam, the doctor tells you that you have a cold and that there is no cure for the common cold. He or she tells you to go home, rest, and drink plenty of fluids. How would you feel about your encounter with the medical care system? What did you expect to happen?

friends, family members, books, magazines, and self-help groups. At times you may even hire a consultant or team of consultants, including physicians and other health professionals. Once they have given you their best advice, it is up to you to make choices and to follow through.

The essence of self-care and self-management is an attitude. This attitude centers around a sense of confidence and competence to manage your own health, with help when necessary. It involves accepting personal responsibility for your health and participating more actively in every phase of your health care. It involves recognizing that the everyday choices that you make with regard to health habits and personal relationships are critical determinants of your health. Self-care also means working to change physical, social, and economic forces that undermine health into forces that support the full development of your health potential.

You can develop this self-care attitude by learning skills to manage medical problems and to make the health care system work effectively for you.

Managing Medical Problems

Effectively managing medical problems involves developing several skills. First, you need to learn how to be a good observer of your own body and assess your symptoms. Second, you need to be able to decide when to seek professional advice and when you can safely deal with the problem on your own. Third, you need to know how to safely and effectively self-treat common medical problems.

Self-assessment Self-care begins with careful observation of your own body. We are constantly observing our bodies, scanning for unusual sensations, aches, or pains. Symptoms are signals from our bodies. They alert us that something may be wrong.

Symptoms are often an expression of the body's attempt to heal itself. For example, the pain and swelling that occur after an ankle injury immobilize the injured joint, to allow healing to take place. A fever may be an attempt to make the body less hospitable to infectious agents (pathogens). A cough can help clear the airways and protect the lungs. Understanding what a symptom means and what is going on in your body helps reduce anxiety about symptoms and allows you to practice safe self-care that supports your body's own healing mechanisms.

Carefully observing symptoms also helps you identify those signals that suggest you need professional assistance to help your body heal. You should begin by noting when the symptom began, how often and when it occurs, what makes it worse, what makes it better, and if you have any associated symptoms. You can also monitor your body's "vital signs" such as temperature and pulse rate (see Appendix I, "Home Medical Tests"). These signs may give important clues as to how your body is managing an illness.

Not too long ago, the thermometer was the only tool available to evaluate medical problems at home. Now a new generation of medical self-tests are available: screening tests for colon cancer, home blood pressure machines, home blood glucose tests for diabetics, pregnancy tests, self-tests for urinary tract infections, and over a dozen other do-it-yourself kits and devices. All these tools are designed to help you make a more informed decision about when to seek medical help and when to self-treat.

Home medical tests offer several advantages: cost savings, convenience, privacy, an increased sense of control, and sometimes more comprehensive information. Blood pressure measurements taken at home can give a more complete picture of what your blood pressure is like throughout the day, not just during visits to the doctor. Many people suffer from "white-coat hypertension"—their blood pressure may go up during the stress of a visit to the doctor. Home blood pressure checks can also help hypertensives under medical supervision try nondrug

Exploring Your Emotions

A friend tells you she has noticed a lump in her breast but is afraid to see a physician and would rather risk cancer than face its possible confirmation. How do you counsel her? Remember that she is unlikely to respond to your merely saying, "See a doctor."

Figure 15-1 The hidden health care system

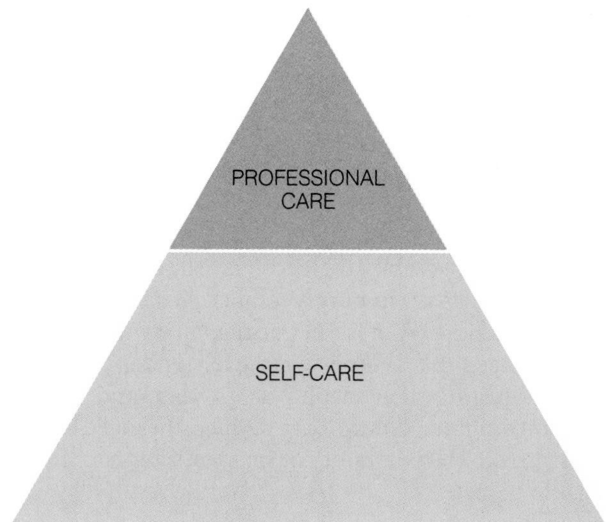

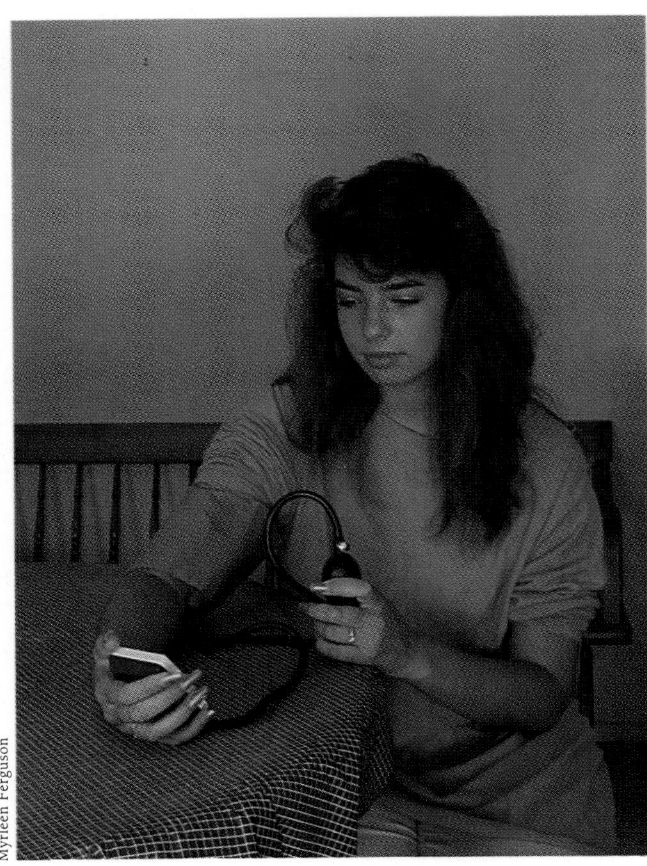
Myrleen Ferguson

treatments such as diet, exercise, or relaxation. One study even suggests that home blood pressure monitoring *itself* may lower blood pressure. Why? One theory is that checking your own blood pressure may be a form of biofeedback—as you become aware of pressure changes you can voluntarily control them. It may be that over time you experience less anxiety while checking your pressure. Or you may begin, unconsciously, to change your diet and other factors that affect blood pressure.

Home blood glucose monitoring can be a more efficient, less expensive way to check blood glucose levels, because it allows frequent, rapid measurements without interrupting normal daily activities to go to a laboratory. Before home blood glucose monitoring was available, diabetics had to rely on urine tests, which may lag behind blood levels and therefore may give misleading information about very low blood glucose levels **(hypoglycemia)** or very high levels **(hyperglycemia).** With home monitoring, diabetics can work in partnership with their physicians to keep their blood sugar levels under better control by adjusting their insulin doses, diet, and exercise. Sometimes tighter control can reduce the need for frequent visits to the laboratory or hospitalization to manage unstable diabetes.

Privacy is also an important factor in the growth of home medical tests. A self-test for pregnancy lets a woman find out for herself whether she is pregnant. Another new test allows people to check stool specimens at home for small amounts of blood. This test for "hidden" blood is recommended annually for people over age 50 as a screening test for colon cancer. If blood is found, then further tests are necessary to determine whether the bleeding is from a colon cancer or some other source.

Although home medical tests have many benefits, they are not foolproof. Just like laboratory tests, some may show abnormal results even though you are quite healthy (a **false positive** result), while others may fail to detect abnormalities (a **false negative**). Careful reading of the instructions with the test kits, including when *not* to test, as well as coaching from your doctor, will minimize these problems. If you do find an abnormal test result, repeat the test. If it is still abnormal, if you are at all doubtful about the test results, or if your symptoms persist even if the tests are normal, consult your physician.

Careful self-observation and selective use of self-tests may help provide you with the type of information you need to make informed self-care decisions and participate more actively in your care.

Decision Making: Knowing When to Go to the Doctor To self-treat or not self-treat, that is the question. When confronted with a symptom, a person must ask a series of questions: "What's going on in my body?" "Is this dangerous?" "Have I or anyone else I know had something like this before?" Some of the answers you can make to these questions are conscious and rational; others are more unconscious, emotional responses. The goal of your deliberations is to decide whether to ignore the symptom, self-treat, or seek professional care.

People often make two kinds of mistakes in deciding what to do when faced with symptoms. They may rush to the doctor too often or too quickly for minor complaints they could easily and effectively manage on their own. Or they may ignore symptoms and self-treat when they should be seeking professional assistance.

For example, suppose you develop diarrhea and some mild abdominal cramping. If you immediately rush off to the doctor, you are likely to waste your time and the doctor's. However, if you knew what key signs to look for (such as blood in the stool, high fever, and dehydration) and how to practice effective self-care for the symptoms (clear liquid diet, and so on), you would be in a position to make a more informed choice.

At the other extreme, people too often ignore symptoms that *should* trigger a visit to the doctor. For example, any breast lump should be medically evaluated. Although 80–90 percent of breast lumps turn out to be noncan-

Hypoglycemia Abnormally low levels of glucose (sugar) in the blood. Usually occurs when a diabetic takes too much insulin.

Hyperglycemia Abnormally high levels of glucose (sugar) in the blood. Usually found in diabetes.

False positive An inaccurate test result that indicates an abnormality in a person who is actually healthy.

False negative An inaccurate test result that indicates that a person is normal when he or she is actually diseased.

Triage A screening and sorting out of people who are sick or injured so that the most seriously ill can be treated first or so that the patient is directed to the most appropriate type of medical practitioner.

---

cerous, early treatment of the few that are cancerous can save lives. Informed self-care involves knowing how to evaluate symptoms so that you don't go to the doctor either too early *or* too late.

Your decision to seek professional assistance for a symptom is generally guided by your previous history of medical problems and the nature of the symptom you are experiencing. In general, you should check with a physician for symptoms that are

1. *Severe.* If the symptom is very severe or intense, medical assistance is advised. Examples include severe pains, major injuries, and other emergencies.
2. *Unusual.* If the symptom is very peculiar and unfamiliar, it is wise to check it out with your doctor. Examples include unexplained lumps, changes in a skin blemish or mole, problems with vision, difficulty swallowing, numbness, weakness, unexplained weight loss, and blood in sputum, urine, or bowel movement.
3. *Persistent.* If the symptom lasts longer than expected, seek medical advice. Examples include fever for more than five days, a cough lasting longer than three weeks, a sore that doesn't heal within a month, and hoarseness lasting longer than four weeks.
4. *Recurrent.* If a symptom tends to return again and again, medical evaluation is advised. Examples include recurrent headaches, stomach pains, and backache.

Sometimes a single symptom is not a cause for concern, but when the symptom is accompanied by other symptoms the combination may suggest a more serious problem. For example, a fever with a stiff neck suggests meningitis. A cough with green sputum and a high fever might mean pneumonia.

If you evaluate your symptoms and think that you need professional assistance, then you must decide how urgent the problem is. If it is a true emergency, then you should go (or be taken) to the nearest emergency room. Emergencies would include such things as

- Major trauma or injury such as head injury, suspected broken bone, deep wound, severe burn, eye injury, or animal bite
- Uncontrollable bleeding
- Intolerable and uncontrollable pain
- Severe chest pain
- Severe shortness of breath
- Poisoning or drug overdose
- Loss of consciousness or seizure
- Stupor, drowsiness, or disorientation that cannot be explained
- Severe or worsening reaction to an insect bite or sting, or to a medication, especially if breathing is difficult

Unfortunately, most visits to an emergency room (ER) are not emergencies. One study by the Indiana Hospital Association reviewed 13,523 emergency room visits. Over 50 percent were judged not to be true emergencies. In fact, even 25 percent of those patients arriving by ambulance were not emergencies.

There are many reasons not to go to a hospital emergency room if it is not a true emergency. Emergency rooms do not operate on a first come, first served basis. Patients are **triaged**, a screening process in which those patients with the most urgent needs are treated first. So if your problem is not a true emergency, you may have to wait hours while more critically ill patients are seen before you. Your past medical records are usually not available in the emergency room, and it is harder to get appropriate follow-up care. Also, many insurance policies do not cover nonemergency visits to emergency rooms, so if you go to an ER with a sore throat, cough, rash, or other mild symptom, you could end up paying the bill. And emergency room medical bills are much higher than office or urgent care center visits.

If your problem is not an emergency, but still requires medical attention, consider a call to your doctor's office. Often you can be given medical advice over the phone without the inconvenience of a visit. If you do require a visit, it can often be arranged at the most convenient and appropriate time and place. Nearly 16 percent of all outpatient medical advice and 30 percent of pediatrics advice is now dispensed by telephone.

To help you make wise medical decisions, a "Self-care Guide for Common Medical Problems" is provided in Appendix II. This guide includes some specific guidelines on when to call the doctor for certain medical problems and on when and how to self-treat.

Self-treatment When confronted with a new symptom, many people try to find some pill or potion that will relieve or cure it. However, other self-treatment options are available. In most cases, your body can itself relieve

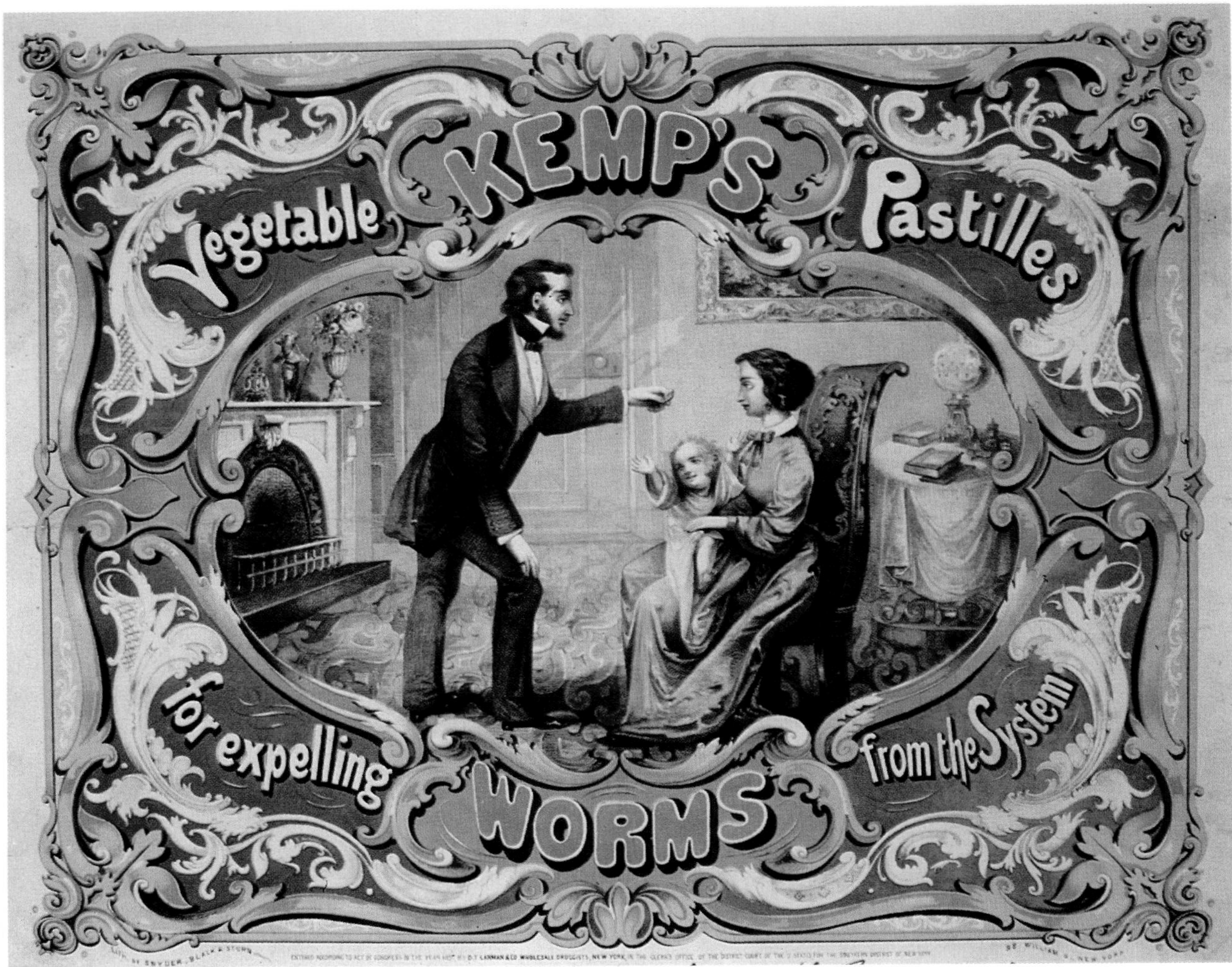

The Bettmann Archive

Exploring Your Emotions

In early America all medications were available without a doctor's prescription. Today many drugs from antibiotics to pain medications require a prescription. How do you feel about this? How should it be determined which medications should be available only with prescriptions and which without?

your symptoms and heal the disorder. The prescriptions filled by your body's internal pharmacy are frequently the safest and most effective treatment. So patience and careful self-observation are often the best choices in self-treatment. Nondrug treatments are also sometimes highly effective. For example, massage, ice packs, and neck exercises may be, at times, more helpful than drugs in relieving headaches and other aches and pains. For a variety of disorders either caused or aggravated by stress, relaxation and stress management strategies may be the treatment of choice (see Chapter 2). So before reaching for medications, consider *all* your options for self-treatment.

Self-medication Self-treatment with nonprescription medications is an important and valuable part of our health care system. Within every two-week period, nearly 70 percent of people self-medicate with one or more drugs. If even a small percentage of people stopped using such **over-the-counter (OTC)** drugs and began making appointments with doctors for their colds, sore throats, backaches, and headaches, doctors could not possibly handle the load. Many OTC drugs are highly effective, not only in relieving symptoms but also in curing conditions. Doctors themselves may recommend OTC products when they can be helpful. But if you do self-medicate,

OTC (over-the-counter) Medications and products that can be purchased by the consumer without a prescription.

Generic drug Non-brand name drug that is not registered or protected by a trademark.

you should know what you are taking, why you are taking it, how it works, and how to use medications wisely.

More than 200,000 nonprescription drug products are offered for sale to the U.S. public, representing only about 500 active ingredients. An estimated $8 billion is spent each year on such products. Nearly 75 percent of the public receives its education on OTC drugs solely from TV, radio, newspaper, and magazine advertising. Unfortunately, many claims for drugs are either untrue or subtly misleading.

You need to be aware of the barrage of drug advertising aimed at you. The implicit message of such advertising is that every symptom, every ache and pain, every problem, can be solved by a product. Many of the OTC products *are* effective; but many simply waste your money and divert your attention from better ways of coping.

In 1972 the Food and Drug Administration (FDA) initiated a massive review of the safety, effectiveness, and labeling of OTC products. The study identified many ingredients in OTC products that are either ineffective or of questionable safety. In addition, the review panels recommended that some drugs, formerly available only by doctor's prescription, be shifted to nonprescription status. The law actually states that a prescription should not be required for any drug if the instructions for its safe use can be understood by the patient without the intervention of a doctor. The result is that many more effective medications, such as hydrocortisone cream and antifungal agents, have become available to consumers without a prescription. Increased consumer choice brings increased responsibility to use these medications wisely.

It is important to remember that any drug, whether bought in the supermarket or prescribed by a doctor, may have side effects. However, following some simple guidelines will improve your chances of safely and effectively self-medicating:

1. Always read drug labels and follow directions carefully. A surprising number of people do not read medication labels before taking the contents. The label must by law include the names and quantities of the active ingredients, precautions, and adequate directions for safe use. Carefully reading the label, and reviewing the individual ingredients, may help prevent you from taking medications that have caused problems for you in the past. If you don't understand the information on the label, ask a pharmacist or doctor before using it.
2. Do not exceed the recommended dosage or length of treatment unless you discuss this change with your doctor.
3. Use caution if you are taking other medications. OTC and prescription drugs can interact, either canceling or enhancing the effects of the medications. If you have questions about drug interactions, ask your doctor or pharmacist before you mix medicines.
4. Try to select medications with single active ingredients rather than combination ("all-in-one") products. A product with multiple ingredients is likely to include drugs for symptoms you don't even have, so why risk the side effects of medications you don't need? Using single-ingredient products also allows you to adjust the dosage of each medication separately for optimal symptom relief with minimal side effects.
5. When choosing medications, learn the ingredient names and try to buy generic products. **Generics** contain the same active ingredient as the brand name product but generally at a much lower cost.
6. Never take or give a drug from an unlabeled container or in the dark when you can't read what the label says.
7. If you are pregnant, nursing, or have a chronic disease such as kidney disease, consult your doctor before self-medicating.
8. Many medications have an expiration date of about two to three years. Dispose of all expired medications.
9. Store your medications in a safe place away from the reach of children. Poisoning with medications is a common and preventable problem. The usual bathroom medicine chest is usually not a particularly secure or dry place to store medications. Consider a lockable tool chest or fishing box.

The Home Pharmacy If you were to survey home medicine chests, what would you find? On average, there would be twenty-two medications, including seventeen OTC products. You would probably find an oversupply of expired medications, leftover prescription drugs, and useless medications. At the same time, certain essential medications and equipment would be absent. Most people wait until a crisis arises. They then search frantically through a poorly stocked medicine chest and often have to make an inconvenient midnight dash to a pharmacy, if they can find one open.

There are only a few essential supplies; the rest varies depending upon the particular health problems you or your family are likely to face. Since many of the medications deteriorate, buy small quantities of infrequently used medications and replace them about every three years.

Your Home Self-care Kit

Medications:

- **Anesthetic throat lozenges, spray, or gargle**
  Sore throat
- **Antacids (aluminum hydroxide/magnesium hydroxide)**
  Indigestion and heartburn
- **Antibacterial ointment cream**
  Minor skin wounds
- **Antifungal creams/powders**
  Fungal infections (e.g., athlete's foot, ringworm)
- **Antihistamines**
  Allergies
- **Antimotion sickness medication**
  Motion sickness
- **Aspirin/acetaminophen/ibuprofen**
  Fever, headache, minor pain
- **Burow's solution**
  Minor skin irritations/rashes
- **Decongestant tablets, nose sprays, drops**
  Nasal congestion
- **Ear wax dissolver**
  Ear wax
- **Expectorant/cough suppressant (dextromethorphan)**
  Coughs
- **Eye drops and artificial tears**
  Minor eye irritations
- **Hemorrhoid preparations**
  Hemorrhoids
- **Hydrocortisone cream (0.5%)**
  Minor skin irritations/rashes
- **Hydrogen peroxide**
  Wound cleansing
- **Kaolin/pectin or attapulgite preparations**
  Diarrhea
- **Milk of magnesia or bulk laxative**
  Constipation
- **Sodium bicarbonate (baking soda)**
  Wounds, rashes, insect bites
- **Sunscreen agents**
  Prevention of sunburn
- **Syrup of ipecac**
  Poison ingestion

Supplies and Tools

- **Adhesive tape**
  Minor injuries
- **Adhesive bandages**
  Minor wounds
- **Elastic bandages**
  Strains and sprains
- **Eye cup**
  Washing out foreign bodies
- **Heating pad/hot water bottle**
  Minor pains and strains
- **Ice pack**
  Minor injuries and pain
- **Needle-nosed tweezers**
  Splinters
- **Thermometer**
  Fever

Getting the Most Out of Your Medical Care

Self-care involves more than self-diagnosis and self-treatment. It includes knowing when to seek professional care and how to get the most out of your medical care. The key to making the health care system work for you lies in good communication with your physician and with the other members of the health care team. Unfortunately, many people are intimidated by their doctors and afraid to communicate freely. Medical jargon can be very confusing. One study revealed that 20–30 percent of college-educated people had significant misunderstandings about the meaning of such common medical terms as *hypertension, virus, herpes, tumor, Pap smear, strep throat,* and *uterus.* Yet patients tend not to ask their doctors what such medical jargon means, because they fear appearing stupid. Others are afraid to ask why a test or treatment is needed for fear of appearing to challenge the authority of the physician. Patients often conceal personal concerns about sexuality, drug abuse, emotional problems, and cancer. All these fears and others block open communication with the physician.

Physicians share the responsibility for poor communication. They may feel too busy or important to take the time to talk with patients. They may ignore questions, use incomprehensible medical jargon, and respond in an unsupportive way to your attempts to assert yourself.

Exploring Your Emotions

You have been having recurrent stomach pain so you decide to go to the doctor. The doctor does a brief physical examination and tells you that you probably have a hiatal hernia with reflux esophagitis. He or she wants you to have an upper GI series X-ray examination, hands you a prescription for medication, and walks out of the room. How would you feel about this encounter? What would you do?

Medispeak

Ever wonder why doctors say "clavicle" instead of "collarbone," and "diaphoresis" instead of "sweat"?

When you walk out of your doctor's office, can you honestly say that you understood everything he or she told you? If you don't, you're not alone. Call it *medicalese* or *medispeak,* it comes out the same—confusing.

According to two language specialists, jargon has proved convenient to politicians, bureaucrats, lawyers, educators, physicians and others because it conceals fuzzy thinking while projecting an illusion of wisdom.

"Mysterious-sounding words are often so intimidating they ward off any challenges from listeners," says Lois DeBakey and Selma DeBakey, professors of scientific communication at Baylor College of Medicine in Houston.

Doctors who use unnecessary jargon "rely on the uncritical acceptance of their words by their audiences. Few people are courageous enough to ask a doctor to translate ominous scientific terms into plain English," say the DeBakeys.

Yet incomprehensible language ill serves the user. It "drives a wedge between the medical community and the rest of the public."

More important, they add, "It perverts the purpose of language—communication—by creating confusion and misinterpretation. If patients misunderstand the physician's explanation, they may become apprehensive or depressed; if they misinterpret instructions, they will be unable to cooperate in their treatment."

You can avoid these problems by becoming fluent in medicalese yourself. Begin by taking this medical quiz, selecting the word or phrase that best describes each term.

Questions

1. *Adipose*
   a. Fatty
   b. Additional X-rays
   c. Totaling the bill
2. *Ambulatory*
   a. Transported by ambulance
   b. Able to walk
   c. Unable to walk
3. *Analgesic*
   a. Painkiller
   b. Rectal medicine
   c. Antibiotic
4. *Antipyretic*
   a. Bleeding gums
   b. Antacid
   c. Fever reducer
5. *Atrophy*
   a. Prize for best patient
   b. Weight loss
   c. Shrinkage (of muscle or other tissue)
6. *Benign*
   a. Noncancerous
   b. Fast-growing
   c. Cancerous
7. *Congenital*
   a. Friendly disposition
   b. A disorder of the genitals
   c. Condition present at birth
8. *Contraindicated*
   a. Recommended
   b. To be avoided
   c. Makes no difference
9. *Dermatitis*
   a. Tight skin
   b. Inflammation of the skin
   c. Numbness of the skin
10. *Edema*
    a. Swelling
    b. Pertaining to an enema
    c. Bruising
11. *Etiology*
    a. The study of eating
    b. The study of nutrition
    c. Pertaining to the causes of disease
12. *Febrile*
    a. High in fibre
    b. Feverish
    c. Weak
13. *Hematoma*
    a. Bruise
    b. Broken toe
    c. Iron deficiency
14. *Hemorrhage*
    a. Bleeding
    b. Pertaining to hemorrhoids
    c. Old blood
15. *Idiopathic*
    a. Of lower intelligence
    b. Not able to walk a straight line
    c. Of unknown cause
16. *Lesion*
    a. Any sore or wound
    b. A group of health practitioners
    c. Relief from stress
17. *Negative test result*
    a. The patient has a disorder
    b. The patient doesn't have the disorder
    c. The patient died
18. *Parenteral*
    a. Disease inherited from parents
    b. Medicine given by parents
    c. Medicine given by injection
19. *Prognosis*
    a. Disease of the nose
    b. A chronic condition
    c. Expected outcome of a disease
20. *Pruritis*
    a. Infection producing pus
    b. Itching
    c. Of highest purity

(continued on next page)

Medispeak (*continued*)

21. *Psychogenic*
   a. Of unsound mind
   b. Having an emotional origin
   c. Having a genetic origin
22. *Q.I.D.*
   a. Take four times a day
   b. Take for four days
   c. "Quit if disagreeable"
23. *Sepsis*
   a. Infection
   b. Cleanliness
   c. Waste removal
24. *Sequela*
   a. After-effect of a disease
   b. Quiet atmosphere
   c. Food poisoning
25. *Subclinical*
   a. The basement of the hospital
   b. A poorly equipped hospital
   c. Having no visible symptoms
26. *Subcutaneous*
   a. Not very pretty
   b. Beneath the skin
   c. Underfed
27. *Syndrome*
   a. Infected sinus
   b. A recurring infection
   c. A specific collection of symptoms
28. *Systemic*
   a. Affecting the whole body
   b. Methodical
   c. Cyst-forming
29. *Topical*
   a. Overheated
   b. On the surface
   c. Pertinent discussion
30. *Urticaria*
   a. Hives
   b. Burping
   c. Standing upright

Answers

1. *Adipose:* a. It refers to the layer of connective tissue beneath the skin that contains many fat cells.

2. *Ambulatory:* b. Being ambulatory is actually good.

3. *Analgesic:* a.

4. *Antipyretic:* c.

5. *Atrophy:* c. This wasting away of tissue usually occurs with lack of use.

6. *Benign:* a. This is good news.

7. *Cogenital:* c. This is something that developed before you were even born.

8. *Contraindicated:* b. If your doctor says that estrogen replacement therapy is contraindicated for someone with a family history of cancer, he or she means don't take it.

9. *Dermatitis:* b. A catchall phrase for any skin irritation in which there is redness, itching, and rash.

10. *Edema:* a. This is a condition in which the tissues contain an excessive amount of fluid.

11. *Etiology:* c. Simply a sophisticated way of discussing the cause of an illness.

12. *Febrile:* b. If your doctor says you are in a febrile state, he or she means that you also have the symptoms that accompany a rise in temperature.

13. *Hematoma:* a. Here's a fancy way to say you've got a black-and-blue mark.

14. *Hemorrhage:* a. You may think that hemorrhage always refers to an enormous flow of blood, but in fact even minor bleeding can be called a hemorrhage.

15. *Idiopathic:* c. Any time a doctor uses this word to preface the name of a disease, he or she is simply telling you that they don't know what causes it.

16. *Lesion:* a. Here's another catchall word that covers everything from skin sores associated with eczema, to the lung damage in tuberculosis.

17. *Negative test result:* b. A negative test result indicates normal.

18. *Parenteral:* c. This just means "not by mouth." So when a medicine is given parenterally, it means by injection.

19. *Prognosis:* c. If your doctor says "the prognosis is good," he or she expects you to recover.

20. *Pruritis:* b. Why can't they just say itching?

21. *Psychogenic:* b. Some headaches may be psychogenic disorders if they are caused by emotional upset or stress.

22. *Q.I.D.:* a. Now you know what those letters on your prescription mean. Actually they stand for the Latin *"quarter in die."*

23. *Sepsis:* a. This kind of infection refers to the presence in your system of bacteria or their poisons.

24. *Sequela:* a. Think of sequel and you've got the answer. In medicine, when a second disorder develops as a result of the first, it's called a *sequela.*

25. *Subclinical:* c. Refers to the period before the appearance of typical symptoms of a disease. In other words, when you're only a little bit sick, the doctor may say you have a subclinical case of the disease.

26. *Subcutaneous:* b. You're most likely to hear this word when your doctor is ordering an injection of medicine. He or she means that the drug should be administered just below the skin.

27. *Syndrome:* c. The grouping of symptoms always indicates a particular disease or abnormal condition.

Medispeak (*continued*)

28. *Systemic:* a. If your doctor says he or she is giving you a systemic remedy, he or she means it's a drug that will work on the whole body.

29. *Topical:* b. A medicine applied topically simply means that it is to be spread (as in an ointment) to a specific area of the skin surface.

30. *Urticaria:* a. Usually from an allergic reaction to foods, drugs, emotional stress, or insect bites.

Scoring

Give yourself one point for each correct answer. If you scored:

24–30: You're already well versed in medispeak, and because of that you rarely misunderstand your doctor's explanations or instructions.

12–23: You're on your way to fluency, but you still need some assistance. That's why you often ask your doctor to explain the words you are unfamiliar with, even though it sometimes makes you feel uncomfortable.

0–11: You need to invest in a medical dictionary for laypeople—and use it. Only then will you be able to change your feelings of intimidation to those of self-confidence.

SOURCE: *San Jose Mercury News,* November 22, 1983.

The doctor-patient relationship is undergoing an important transformation. The image of the physician as a God-like, all-knowing authority and the patient as a passive supplicant is slowly fading. What is emerging is more of a doctor-patient *partnership,* in which the doctor acts more like a consultant and the patient participates more actively. The necessary ingredients in a successful doctor-patient partnership are a sympathetic, caring physician and a prepared, assertive patient. As physician Marvin Belsky commented "It is not enough for the doctor to stop playing God. You've got to get off your knees."

You should try to remember that physicians are human, they have off days, they make mistakes like everyone else. You don't have to "love" your doctor as a best friend, but you should expect someone who is attentive, caring, able to listen, and able to clearly explain things to you. You also have to do your part. You need to be assertive in a kindly but not aggressive manner. You need to express your feelings and concerns, ask questions, and, if necessary, be persistent. If your physician is unable to communicate clearly with you in spite of your best efforts, then you probably need to change physicians. Remember, the physician works for you.

Here are several tips that can help ensure good communication before, during, and after your visit to the doctor:

Preparing for the Visit

- Before visiting your physician, make a written list of questions or concerns that you have. Also include notes about your symptoms (when it started, how long it lasts, what makes it worse or better, and so on). This list prepares you to clearly state your major concerns as well as concisely answer the questions your physician is likely to ask. Have you ever thought to yourself after you walked out of the office, "Why didn't I ask about . . ."? Making a list beforehand helps ensure that your concerns get addressed.
- Bring a list of all medications (prescription and nonprescription) you are taking, or bring all these medications with you to the office so that your physician can review them. Also, if you have previous medical records or test results that might be relevant to your problems, bring them along.

During the Visit

- Take notes during the visit, or consider bringing along someone else to act as a second listener. Another set of eyes and ears may help you later recall some of the details of the visit or instructions.
- Try to be as open as you can in sharing your thoughts, feelings, and fears. Remember, your physician is not a mindreader. If you are worried, try to explain why: "I am worried that what I have is contagious, my father had similar symptoms before he died," and so on.
- Don't be afraid to ask what you may consider a "stupid" question. These questions can often indicate an important concern or misunderstanding.
- If you don't understand or remember something the physician said, admit that you need to go over it again.

Exploring Your Emotions

Your appointment with the doctor is for 3 P.M. At 4 P.M. a nurse ushers you into a dressing room, and you wait there, shivering in a plastic sheet, for half an hour. How do you feel when the doctor walks in briskly and asks, "Well, how do you feel today?"

For example, "I'm pretty sure you told me some of this before, but I don't recall what the answer was."

- Give your physician feedback. If you don't like the way you have been treated by the physician or someone else on the health care team, let your physician know. If you have been unable to follow the physician's advice or had problems with a treatment, tell your physician so adjustments can be made. Also, most physicians very much appreciate compliments and positive feedback, but patients are often hesitant to praise their doctors. So, if you are very pleased, let your physician know.
- When appropriate, ask your physician to write down instructions or recommend reading material for more information on a particular subject.

After the Visit

- At the end of the appointment, briefly repeat back—in your own words—what you understood the physician to say about the nature of the problem and what you are supposed to do. This repetition helps check your understanding, to ensure the best care.
- Make sure you understand what the next steps are. Should you return for a visit and, if so, when and why? Should you phone for test results? Are there any danger signs you should watch for and report back to your physician?

In addition to developing effective communication skills, understanding something about how a diagnosis is made, what treatment options are available, and what questions you should ask will help equip you to take a more active role in your own health care.

The Diagnostic Process Solving a medical problem is sometimes like solving a mystery. The problem is presented, clues are discovered, evidence is sought, possibilities are tracked down, and finally (and hopefully) a correct diagnosis is made.

There are three main sources of clues and information on which to base a diagnosis. The first is the medical history, which is the patient's own description of what has happened. The second is the physical examination of the patient. The third is the results from various diagnostic tests and procedures. All this information is then combined to reach a diagnosis that names and explains the problem and guides treatment.

The Medical History: Telling It Like It Is The most important part of medical diagnosis is the medical history. This is the description that you give the physician of your problem, concerns, and background. In well over 70 percent of cases, a careful history alone can lead to a correct diagnosis. Your ability to clearly, concisely, and accurately describe your illness is an essential first step in the diagnostic process. Understanding how the physician elicits your medical history can help you tell the story. Most physicians use a standard procedure to elicit the medical history. A complete medical history usually consists of five parts: the chief complaint, the present illness, the past medical history, review of systems, and social history. Depending on the nature of the problem, you may be asked about some or all of these areas.

THE CHIEF COMPLAINT The first step is to record the chief complaint, preferably in your own words. The physician may ask you a question such as "What brings you here today?" "What kind of problem have you been having?" or "What problem concerns you the most?" This is your opportunity to express what's uppermost in your mind. If you have more than one concern, say so: "I am most bothered by a cough, but I also have been experiencing pain in my shoulder and a fever." Briefly and concisely list your concerns. Now is not the time for lengthy descriptions. A study of medical interviews found that physicians generally let the patient talk about 18 seconds before interrupting with questions. So take advantage of this time to state your agenda for the visit. Try to be direct and honest. If you are concerned about a sexual problem or a possible cancer, don't disguise your concerns or wait until the end of the visit to bring them up.

THE PRESENT ILLNESS During this part of the history, the physician will try to learn more about your chief complaint. You will be asked a series of questions that will clarify the nature, character, and time course of your major symptom. You may be asked, "When did it begin? Is it constant or episodic? How long does it last? Where is it located? How does it feel? (sharp? dull? aching? intense? mild?) What brings it on or makes it worse? What makes it better? Are there any associated symptoms? What do you think has caused the problem?" Try to be concise and specific in answering these questions. If your doctor asks when the symptom started and you reply "a while ago," this is not very helpful. Was it a few minutes ago, hours, days, years—decades? The more specific you can be, without embellishing your description with irrelevant details, the clearer a picture the doctor will have of your needs and the less time you will waste.

THE PAST MEDICAL HISTORY Next you may be asked about your health in general and your medical history, including previous illnesses, hospitalizations, operations, immunizations, allergies, and medications. Such information may provide important clues in solving your current problems. For example, if you have had an appendectomy, then something other than appendicitis must be causing your abdominal pain. If you are taking certain medications, their side effects might explain your current symptoms.

Be careful to report to your physician *all* the medications that you are taking, including birth control pills, vitamins, and nonprescription medications such as aspi-

Palpation The act of feeling some organ or part of the body in order to make a diagnosis.

Auscultation The act of listening to sounds made by the body in order to make a diagnosis.

Ophthalmoscope A lighted instrument used to view the interior of the eye.

Otoscope A lighted instrument used to view inside the ear.

Murmur An abnormal sound heard over a blood vessel or the heart due to some blockage of blood flow.

rin, antacids, and laxatives. Knowing about these medications may be important in diagnosing and treating your problem. It is important to know the names and dosages of all the medications you are taking; it is a good idea to carry an up-to-date list with you. Saying that you are taking "the little green pills" usually doesn't help identify the medication.

When asked about allergies to medications, describe which medication you had taken and the exact type of symptoms it caused. A rash, fever, or wheezing developing after taking a medication is often a true allergic reaction while nausea, ringing in the ears, lightheadedness, agitation, and so on are likely to be side effects rather than true drug allergies.

REVIEW OF SYSTEMS Your physician may next review symptoms you may be experiencing in all your different body organs and physiological systems. You may be asked questions about your gastrointestinal, urinary, nervous, cardiovascular, and respiratory systems. For example, a review of your cardiovascular system will include questions about such symptoms as chest pains, shortness of breath, difficulty in breathing while lying down, and swelling in your feet. Although such questions may not seem to be related to your chief complaint, your responses may reveal vital information to managing your present illness or detecting unrecognized problems.

SOCIAL HISTORY Finally you may be asked about your job, living conditions, travel experiences, family, life stresses, and health habits such as smoking and alcohol use. Exposure to chemicals and toxic materials at work might help explain certain symptoms. A recent trip to a foreign country might account for diarrhea and stomach pain. Some diseases are inherited, or tendencies to develop them may be inherited. Clotting disorders, diabetes, and heart disease are examples. Other diseases, such as infections of the lungs, intestines, or skin, are contagious and easily spread within a family.

Giving an accurate and concise medical history is critical to good medical care. You are the expert about how you feel and how you experience symptoms. Through the medical history, you can share your expertise with the physician.

The Anatomy of a Physical Examination The physician then proceeds to examine you. Depending upon your chief complaint this examination may be a complete, head-to-toes exam or may be directed to certain areas or physiological systems.

Traditionally, the physical examination consists of inspection (looking), **palpation** (feeling), and **auscultation** (listening). A physical examination might include

VITAL SIGNS Pulse rate, breathing rate, temperature, and blood pressure may be measured.

HEAD, EARS, EYES, NOSE, AND THROAT The physician may look at the ear canal and ear drum with a lighted instrument (**otoscope**) for signs of infection or blockage. Your hearing may be tested by whispering, a ticking watch, a tuning fork, or an electronic device. The doctor may inspect the external parts of the eye; redness may indicate an infection, paleness may suggest anemia. The pupil of the eye normally constricts when light shines in. The blood vessels, retina, and optic nerve at the back of the eye can be seen with a special lighted instrument called an **ophthalmoscope**. The physician may check the mucous membranes of your nose, and tapping over the sinus cavities that elicits tenderness may suggest infection. He or she may check your tongue, gums, mouth, and throat for abnormalities.

NECK The physician may feel your neck for the presence of swollen lymph nodes during an infection, or for irregularities in the thyroid gland, which lies just below the Adam's apple. A stethoscope can detect abnormal sounds called **murmurs** in the arteries of the neck, which may signal atherosclerotic blockage and risk of stroke.

CHEST The physician may tap on your chest with his or her fingers to detect possible fluid accumulation or pneumonia. You will be asked to take deep breaths in and out through your mouth as your physician listens with a stethoscope. The stethoscope can also be used to detect irregularities in heart rhythm or abnormal clicks and murmurs as the heart valves open and close. Women's breasts are checked for lumps as a possible sign of breast cancer.

ABDOMEN The physician will use his or her fingers to probe your belly, checking your liver in the upper right side, your spleen in the upper left, your stomach in the upper middle, and intestines throughout. Any tenderness or masses will be noted. Your physician may also listen with a stethoscope to the sounds your intestines make.

RECTUM The physician may insert a gloved finger into your rectum to check for abnormal growths. In men, the prostate gland can be checked through the rectum for lumps, enlargement, or tenderness.

GENITALS In men, the penis and testicles will be checked for sores, tenderness, or growths. The physician may press a finger against the scrotal sac and lower abdomen to feel for a weakness in the abdominal wall. A bulge in the abdominal contents when you cough is a sign of a hernia. In women, a pelvic examination includes inspection, palpation, and a Pap smear, which is a test that checks for cancer in cells gently scraped off the cervix.

EXTREMITIES The doctor may check your legs and feet for swelling, redness, or tenderness of the joints suggesting arthritis. Painless but swollen ankles and feet may be a sign of heart, liver, or kidney disease. The pulses in your feet and wrists may be checked for adequate blood flow through the arteries. Your calves may be squeezed to check for blood clots in the veins.

SKIN Your skin will be checked for sores, moles, lumps, and rashes. Paleness may suggest anemia; a yellow color (jaundice) may suggest a liver abnormality such as hepatitis.

NEUROLOGICAL Depending on your symptoms, the physician might check your nervous system. This check might include testing your muscle strength, balance, coordination, reflexes, and sensation. For example, tapping the tendon below your kneecap normally elicits a reflex contraction of a thigh muscle. This knee-reflex action brings many parts of the nervous system into play, and a malfunction can indicate problems in the nervous system and/or quadraceps muscle in the thigh.

If you notice any pain or unusual sensations during the examination, let your physician know. Your response may provide important information. Also, if you are curious about what is being done during the exam or why, ask your physician. (But not when your doctor has the stethoscope in his or her ears!)

Medical Testing In addition to the medical history and physical examination, diagnostic testing now provides a wealth of new information to help solve medical problems. Gone are the days when medical tests meant only a microscope and a drop of blood or urine. High-tech and high-cost medical testing is now a burgeoning industry, accounting for nearly a third of our national health bill. No body fluid, orifice, or cavity is beyond the reach of a medical probe: blood and urine tests, X-rays, biopsies, taps, scans, electronic monitors, and a bewildering array of **endoscopies** (bronchoscopy, arthroscopy, sigmoidoscopy, and so on), the scoping procedures that peer into nearly every part of the body.

More than 10 billion medical tests are done in the United States each year—over 40 tests per person—at a staggering cost of $140 billion, or $600 for each of us. Patients can no longer afford to take a passive role in this important phase of their medical care.

Valid reasons for doing a medical test are to help your doctor diagnose symptoms accurately, to monitor the progress of a known disease, or to screen for a hidden disease. However, many unnecessary tests are performed for other reasons. Many doctors order tests simply to protect themselves from malpractice. An American Medical Association survey found that at least three out of every four doctors admitted having ordered tests for the sole purpose of having a better defense should a patient bring a suit against them.

Medically unnecessary tests may also be ordered because they are profitable. Many physicians can earn more by ordering tests and doing diagnostic procedures than by taking the same amount of time to question, examine, counsel, or think about a patient's problem.

However, patients are not helpless in the face of overtesting. You may be surprised to learn that except for life-threatening emergencies, doctors cannot order medical tests (or for that matter, surgical procedures or treatments) without your permission. Although most doctors make certain to get written consent for tests with significant risks—those requiring general anesthesia or the insertion of tubes or catheters—other tests are usually "ordered" without much explanation. Data from several studies suggest that at least 25 percent of all medical tests contribute little to patient care, but a lot to patient bills. For example, when researchers at the University of California, San Francisco, studied 2,000 patients hospitalized for surgery, they found that 60 percent of the blood tests routinely ordered were unnecessary. In fact, of these *unindicated* tests only one in about 400 revealed abnormalities that could have changed preoperative management. Further, in those rare cases where abnormalities were detected, the results were ignored, presumably because they either were not noticed or were dismissed as not significant. The researchers conclude that if a thorough history turns up no hint of a medical problem, routine testing on hospital admissions is a waste.

Many patients feel that more tests automatically mean better care. People often say, "My doctor is so thorough—he did nearly every test available!" Although tests can provide a measure of reassurance, a diagnosis can be made

Exploring Your Emotions

You have been seeing a doctor about a funny-looking growth on your shoulder. Now she says she is sending you to the laboratory to get a biopsy. You have two days to wait before you see the doctor again. How do you deal with your feelings?

Endoscopy A medical procedure in which a viewing instrument is inserted into body cavities or openings. The specific procedures are named for the area viewed: inside joints (arthroscopy), inside airways (bronchoscopy), inside the abdominal cavity (laparoscopy), and inside the lower portion of the digestive tract, called the *sigmoid colon* (sigmoidoscopy).

80 to 90 percent of the time with only a thorough history and physical exam. Also, the tests ordered may be the wrong ones.

Consider Anne Garber, a 23-year-old woman complaining of a mild burning discomfort in her upper abdomen for about two weeks. Her doctor asked her several brief questions, examined her abdomen, and ordered "a few tests": a urinalysis, a twelve-test blood panel, a complete blood count, and an upper GI series (X-rays that outline the esophagus and stomach).

All these studies added an extra $150 to her bill but did little to change her suspected diagnosis of esophagitis—an inflamed esophagus caused by stomach acid backup. Nor did the tests affect her treatment—antacids. The most likely diagnosis and treatment could have been determined from her history without a lot of testing. In this respect, Anne Garber was overtested. But she was also undertested. In the previous five years, she hadn't had a Pap smear and pelvic exam, both cancer-screening tests generally recommended for women her age.

When you visit a doctor, you can help assure that medical tests are not "just what the doctor ordered" but what you really *need*. Ask the following questions, particularly when your physician recommends any expensive, uncomfortable or potentially risky test:

"WHY DO I NEED THE TEST?" Start by asking how the test will help diagnose your problem or change your treatment. "Because you need it" or "because we usually do it in this situation" are not satisfactory answers. Here's an example of a better explanation: "I'm recommending a barium enema because you've been passing blood in your stool. A previous test shows the blood isn't due to hemorrhoids, so we need to find the source of the bleeding. It may be quite harmless, but it could be a serious problem such as a bowel cancer that needs prompt treatment."

Ask about alternatives. For example, if you have already had the proposed test, can those earlier results be used? To this end, it is wise to keep a record of all your medical tests—when and where they were done and the results.

Then ask your physician about the risk of waiting and not testing. Sometimes the best test is the test of time. Monitoring the symptoms under a doctor's supervision for a specific period of time may provide the necessary diagnostic clue, or the symptoms may simply resolve on their own.

"WHAT ARE THE RISKS?" No test entirely lacks risks. Begin by weighing the balance between potential benefits and risks. To start with, the test itself may be wrong. An inaccurate result can lead to a wrong diagnosis, or delayed or inappropriate treatment. A false positive, an abnormal finding when you're actually healthy, may label you as "sick," provoking needless anxiety and sometimes job or insurance difficulties.

There can also be direct physical risks. Any time your body is penetrated by a needle, tube, or viewing instrument, you risk infection, bleeding, or damage to vital structures. The hazards of radiation exposure, though modest, must also be considered. Reactions to anesthetics, drugs, or dye contrast materials used in certain imaging techniques may also produce complications. Physical risks vary depending on the nature of the test, your age, past medical history, general state of health and ability to cooperate, and the skill and experience of your physician.

"HOW DO I PREPARE FOR THE TEST?" For some tests, preparation is very important. Be sure to remind your physician about any allergies, especially to medications, anesthetics, or X-ray contrast materials. Mention medications you may be taking (including nonprescription drugs like aspirin), bleeding problems, or whether you might be pregnant. Ask whether you should do anything special before the test, such as fasting or discontinuing medications. For example, eating breakfast may interfere with a "fasting" blood sugar test for diabetes.

"WHAT WILL THE TEST BE LIKE?" For many tests, knowing how the test is done and how it will feel can decrease your anxiety and discomfort before and during a test. You may want to ask, "Will it hurt? How long will it take? How will I feel afterward? How is the test done? Who will do it?"

When you ask if a certain test will hurt, doctors often say, "Not at all" or "It only lasts a few minutes." Many doctors simply don't know how the procedure feels. Others downplay the discomfort to avoid alarming you or discouraging you from undergoing a needed test.

Health professionals tend to significantly underestimate the physical and mental impact of tests on patients. Patients, however, tend to overestimate the discomfort before a test. Discomfort may vary considerably with the skill, sensitivity, and gentleness of the professional doing the test.

With certain tests, such as a pelvic exam, sigmoidoscopy (to check the rectum), or a barium enema, the discomfort may be due more to embarrassment than pain.

(text continues on p. 355)

Medical Tests for Healthy People

Each year patients faithfully flock to their physicians for their annual physical exam and testing. They are questioned, tapped, probed, bled, and X-rayed—all in the name of health. But is all this testing really necessary? If you are generally healthy without symptoms, should you undergo medical testing, and, if so, which tests should you have? In order to answer such questions you need to understand the uses and limits of medical tests.

At first glance, it may seem like a great idea to undergo batteries of screening tests on a periodic basis. Then diseases can be detected even before symptoms develop and you can be treated at an earlier, more curable stage in the disease. On this basis doctors and patients alike tend to assume that if a few tests are good, more must be better. Unfortunately, very few screening tests have been shown to be of benefit. To carefully select only those screening tests that might be useful to you, consider asking the following questions:

1. "Is the disease or condition being tested for an important health problem?"

It doesn't make much sense to screen for a trivial health problem. You should be more interested in tests that detect conditions significantly influencing the quality and quantity of your life. So a screening test for pitch appreciation is unlikely to be of much benefit (unless you are a musician), while one for cancer or heart disease is more promising.

2. "Am I at significant risk for the disease or condition detected by the test?"

Many diseases occur primarily in men or women, in certain ethnic groups, or at certain ages. For example, colon cancer tends to occur in people over the age of 45 or 50, so in younger people there is little reason to screen for the disease unless special risk factors (such as family history of polyps or colon cancer) make the disease more likely. If you are not at increased risk due to your age, sex, or medical history, then the proposed test is unlikely to benefit you.

3. "Can the proposed screening test detect the disease or condition before symptoms alert me that something is wrong?"

Most diseases signal their presence with characteristic symptoms that, when evaluated, can lead to a diagnosis. For some diseases, however, waiting for symptoms to develop can mean that the disease will spread and perhaps become incurable. For example, early diagnosis of cervical cancer is very desirable, because a Pap smear can detect the cancer before symptoms appear, when it is most easily cured. But you don't really need a screening test for appendicitis, since the condition is usually announced promptly by abdominal pain.

4. "Do early diagnosis and treatment favorably alter the progress of the disease?"

It makes little sense to screen for a disease for which there is no effective treatment. However, even if an effective treatment is available and acceptable, it must be shown to be more effective when applied in the stage before symptoms develop. For example, if an *incurable* lung cancer is discovered six months before symptoms would have signaled its presence, the person doesn't actually survive any longer as a result of early diagnosis and treatment. The test merely informs the person of the cancer six months earlier. The result is that the person lives six months longer knowing that he or she has an incurable disease, but actual survival is not enhanced by the screening effort. Similarly, the laboratory diagnosis of arthritis before symptoms develop is not useful, because available treatments are not any more effective when started in the early stages of the disease. Fortunately, for a few diseases such as high blood pressure, breast cancer, and colon cancer, early diagnosis and treatment do make a difference.

5. "Is the proposed screening test reasonably accurate, acceptable, and inexpensive?"

One of the greatest stumbling blocks to effective screening programs is test inaccuracy. If a test is not sensitive enough to identify people who have the disease in question, then many diseased people will be missed (false negatives).

But if the test is positive in many healthy people (false positives), mistaken diagnoses may occur and further testing is usually required to sort this out. Unfortunately, no test is 100 percent accurate, so we must choose the best available.

The proposed test must also be acceptably comfortable and safe. For example, examining the colon with a long, flexible viewing instrument (colonoscope) may be the most effective way to detect early colon cancer. But it is unlikely that this procedure will be acceptable as a routine screening test for healthy people because of the discomfort, risk, and expense.

Because screening tests are usually performed on large numbers of people, the expense of even low-cost tests can mount rapidly. The expense of a screening program also includes the cost of follow-up investigations of people who showed positive screening results. Since medical resources are limited, it is generally agreed that screening tests should be shown to offer significant savings in terms of prolonged life or decreased suffering to justify the effort. Otherwise, health resources would be better spent elsewhere.

In summary, for a screening test to be worthwhile, it must reliably detect a significant disease before symptoms develop, the treatment must be more effective when begun before symptoms arise, and the detection and treatment must be accomplished at an acceptable risk and cost. Very few tests currently meet these requirements.

So back to the original question: which tests should a generally healthy person have and how often should he or she have them? Nearly everything you read and every doctor you ask will give you a different opinion. Some say, "Have electrocardiograms (EKGs)"; others disagree. Some argue for many blood tests, others shun them. While many experts might agree on the value of a certain test, they may disagree on who should have it or how often. In truth, we often lack the kind of controlled scientific data that would allow us to know with much certainty which tests should be performed.

Despite these limitations, some rough guidelines can be offered to help you select which medical tests to have and approximately how often they should be performed. These recommendations are intended for generally healthy adults. They are based for the most part on several large studies and reviews by panels of medical experts. You will notice that instead of recommending the same tests for everyone, there is an attempt to individualize the tests to some degree depending on age and sex. Some of the recommended tests have not been shown definitively to meet the most stringent requirements for effective screening tests, and yet are included because it seems likely that their benefits outweigh their risks.

These guidelines represent the minimum tests recommended for people *without symptoms*. If you have symptoms or are at increased risk for certain conditions, due to your medical or family history, additional tests may be advised. Use these guidelines as a starting point, and discuss your particular needs with your doctor.

And remember, if you have a normal test result, still keep on the alert for signs or symptoms that may suggest disease. While carefully selected screening tests can help you protect your health, remember that the most important factors that determine your health do not show up on medical tests at all. In truth, choosing not to smoke, drinking alcohol moderately or not at all, wearing seat belts, exercising regularly, eating wisely, managing stress effectively, and so on, will do more to protect and promote your health than all the tests in the world.

SOURCE: Adapted from David S. Sobel and Tom Ferguson, 1985, *The People's Book of Medical Tests* (New York: Summit Books).

Medical Tests for Healthy People (*continued*)

Recommended Medical Tests for Healthy People

Test and Condition	Age 18–39	Age 40–49	Age 50–59
History and physical exam for various disorders and risks	Every 5–10 years	Every 3–5 years	Every 2–3 years
Blood pressure measurement for hypertension	Every 2–3 years	Every 2–3 years	Every 2–3 years
Vision test for vision problems	Every 5 years Every 2–3 years if corrective lenses worn	Every 5 years Every 2–3 years if corrective lenses worn	Every 5 years Every 2–3 years if corrective lenses worn
Tuberculin skin test (PPD) for tuberculosis	Every 5 years until age 35 or every 1–2 years if high risk		
Urinalysis for kidney and urinary tract disease, liver disease, diabetes, metabolic disorders	Every 10 years	Every 5–10 years	Every 5–10 years
Hematocrit for anemia	Every 3–5 years (women) Every 10 years (men)	Every 3–5 years (women) Every 5–10 years (men)	Every 5–10 years
Blood glucose for diabetes	Every 10 years	Every 5–10 years	Every 5–10 years
Cholesterol for heart disease risk	Every 5–10 years	Every 5–10 years	Every 5–10 years
Glaucoma test (Tonometry) for glaucoma		Every 3 years	Every 3 years
Hearing test for hearing impairment			Every 3–5 years
Test for hidden blood in the stool for bowel cancer			Every year
Sigmoidoscopy for bowel cancer			Every 5 years
For men add: Testicular self-exam for testicular cancer	Monthly until age 40		
For women add: Pap smear for cervical cancer	Every 3 years after 2 normal yearly exams	Every 3 years after 2 normal yearly exams	Every 3 years
Breast self-exam for breast cancer	Monthly	Monthly	Monthly
Breast exam by doctor for breast cancer	Every 2–3 years	Every 1–2 years	Every 1–2 years
Mammography for breast cancer	Once between the ages of 35–39	Every 1–2 years	Every 1–2 years
Rubella antibody titer for immunity to German Measles	Once		

Age 60–69	Age 70+
Every 2–3 years	Every 2–3 years
Every 2–3 years	Every 2–3 years
Every 5 years Every 2–3 years if corrective lenses worn	Every 5 years Every 2–3 years if corrective lenses worn
Every 5–10 years	Every 5 years
Every 5–10 years	Every 5 years
Every 5–10 years	Every 5 years
Every 5–10 years	
Every 3 years	Every 3 years
Every 3–5 years	Every 3–5 years
Every year	Every year
Every 5 years	Every 5 years
Every 3 years	Every 3 years
Monthly	Monthly
Every 1–2 years	Every 1–2 years
Every 1–2 years	Every 1–2 years

It helps to remember that the physician and staff understand. If you are particularly anxious, try talking it out beforehand.

During and after the test, it is important to let the doctor or assistants know what you are feeling. If you're uncomfortable, something can usually be done. But if you don't speak up or signal your doctor, there's no way to help you. Besides, your sensations may provide the first clue to averting a developing complication.

"WHAT DO THE RESULTS MEAN?" No test is 100 percent accurate. When faced with an abnormal result, the natural tendency is to assume that you are sick. However, as noted earlier, it may be a false positive—an abnormal result even though you are healthy.

A false positive can be caused by a statistical fluke in the way normal values are set. For example, the "normal," or reference, values for many blood and urine tests are often established by testing young, white, healthy volunteers—often lab technicians or medical students. The normal range is then constructed to include *only* 95 percent of those healthy people. Thus 5 percent of all healthy patients will automatically show abnormal or borderline results on any lab test. Statistically, if you have twelve separate tests done, you run a 50 percent chance of having one "abnormal" result, even though you are healthy. Are you older, overweight, nonwhite? If you differ significantly from the reference group, the normal range may not be appropriate for you.

Other test inaccuracies stem from certain medications, exercise, stress, eating, or time of day. Even in the best labs, 2 to 5 percent of results may be wrong because of variation in test reagents or errors in handling or labeling test specimens. Repeating the test may cure the "disease."

Conversely, normal results do not necessarily indicate health. A certain percentage of tests are false negatives—normal results even though the person is sick. Many smokers, for example, are falsely reassured by a negative (normal) chest X-ray. Yet a chest film does not necessarily show early lung cancer or emphysema.

Also, normal usually means average—that is, you will be compared with average values characteristic for the population. However, normal in this sense does not necessarily mean optimal, healthy, or desirable. For example, you might have a "normal" (average) blood pressure or cholesterol level but lower levels may actually be healthier. As one observer commented, "It is 'normal' to die of heart disease in the United States."

Medical tests often give the impression of objectivity and precision. Yet some tests, such as X-rays, electrocardiograms (EKGs), and scoping procedures, require subjective interpretation and may miss important abnormalities. A study of chest X-ray interpretation, for example, found that more than 70 percent of the reports contained disagreements among experienced radiologists; in 25 per-

Antibiotic A drug that has the ability to destroy bacteria.

Steroid A drug of hormone origin. Certain of these medications can decrease inflammation.

cent of the reports, the doctors missed important findings. Therefore, getting an experienced second opinion on diagnosis may be important, particularly when ominous symptoms are present or when risky therapies or procedures are prescribed on the basis of an abnormal test.

Above all, remember that medical tests are only part of the diagnostic puzzle. Such clues must always be viewed in the context of other information about you: medical history, family, age, habits, medications, symptoms, and physical examination. Good physicians treat patients, not test results.

Medical and Surgical Treatments Once a diagnosis is made, the treatment options can be considered. The treatments offered for diseases should reflect the wide variety of physical, chemical, and psychosocial factors that cause or aggravate the disease condition. Although some diseases can be cured or ameliorated by medical or surgical treatment, other diseases require no treatment at all or may be aggravated by attempts at therapy. Therefore, whenever a treatment is recommended, whether medications or an operation, it is important that you understand the reasons for treatments, options, risks, and expected benefits. Asking the following key questions may help ensure that you are getting the best possible care for yourself.

"WHAT ARE MY CHOICES IN TREATMENTS?" Many conditions can be treated in a variety of ways, and your physician should be able to explain the alternative choices to you. In some cases, management with medications is a viable alternative to surgery. In other cases, lifestyle changes including exercise, diet, and stress management should be considered alongside medications or surgery before making a choice. When any treatment is recommended, also ask what the consequences are likely to be if you postpone treatment.

"WHAT ARE THE RISKS, COSTS, AND EXPECTED BENEFITS OF EACH TREATMENT OPTION?" To make an informed choice about any treatment, you need to know what each of the options would cost you. This cost includes how likely possible complications such as drug reactions, bleeding, infection, injury, or death might be. To understand a proposed treatment, you should also ask about costs both personal (such as time loss from work) or financial (whether your insurance will pay for part or all of the proposed treatments). You also need to understand how likely it is that the proposed treatment will benefit you in terms of prolonging your life, relieving your symptoms, or improving your ability to function. No one can tell you which choice is right for you. However, to make an informed choice you need information about the treatment options. Informed *choice,* not merely informed *consent,* is an essential ingredient in quality medical care.

Prescription Medications Each year Americans swallow nearly 40 billion doses of medication. Over a lifetime, that amounts to an average of nearly 76,000 pills per person. Each year an average of seven prescriptions are written for each person. We live in a society that believes in "better living through chemistry," and so for every ailment we tend to seek a pill. And medications *can* be miraculous. Thousands of lives are saved each year by antibiotics, heart medications, insulin, and scores of other drugs. Pain medications and anesthetics make the unbearable bearable. Arthritis medications help preserve function for thousands of people. The list goes on.

We also pay a price for having such powerful tools. Of all admissions to hospitals, nearly 5 percent are due primarily to drug reactions and 20 percent of these patients are likely to have a second drug reaction during their hospital stay. And adverse drug reactions contribute significantly to deaths during hospitalization.

Part of the problem lies with physicians who overprescribe or misprescribe drugs. Mishaps also occur because patients do not receive adequate information about medications and often don't understand how to take them or fail to follow instructions given to them. Consumers must ask the following questions about their medications.

"DO I REALLY NEED THIS MEDICATION?" Many physicians often prescribe medications not because they are really necessary, but because they think that patients want and expect drugs. Physicians often feel pressured to do "something" for the patient, so they reach for the prescription pad. As Abraham Maslow observed, "When the only tool you have is a hammer, you tend to treat everything as if it were a nail." So ask about nondrug alternatives. Sometimes the best medication of all is no medication.

Even useful medications sometimes have contraindications. So remember to mention the names of the prescription and OTC medications you are now taking, the drugs to which you may be allergic, whether you are or think you might be pregnant, or whether you are breastfeeding or have any chronic diseases like heart or kidney disease that could complicate the use of medications.

"WHAT IS THE NAME OF THE MEDICATION, AND WHAT IS IT SUPPOSED TO DO?" Your doctor should tell you why the medication is being prescribed and how the prescription might be expected to help you. For example, antibiotics for a

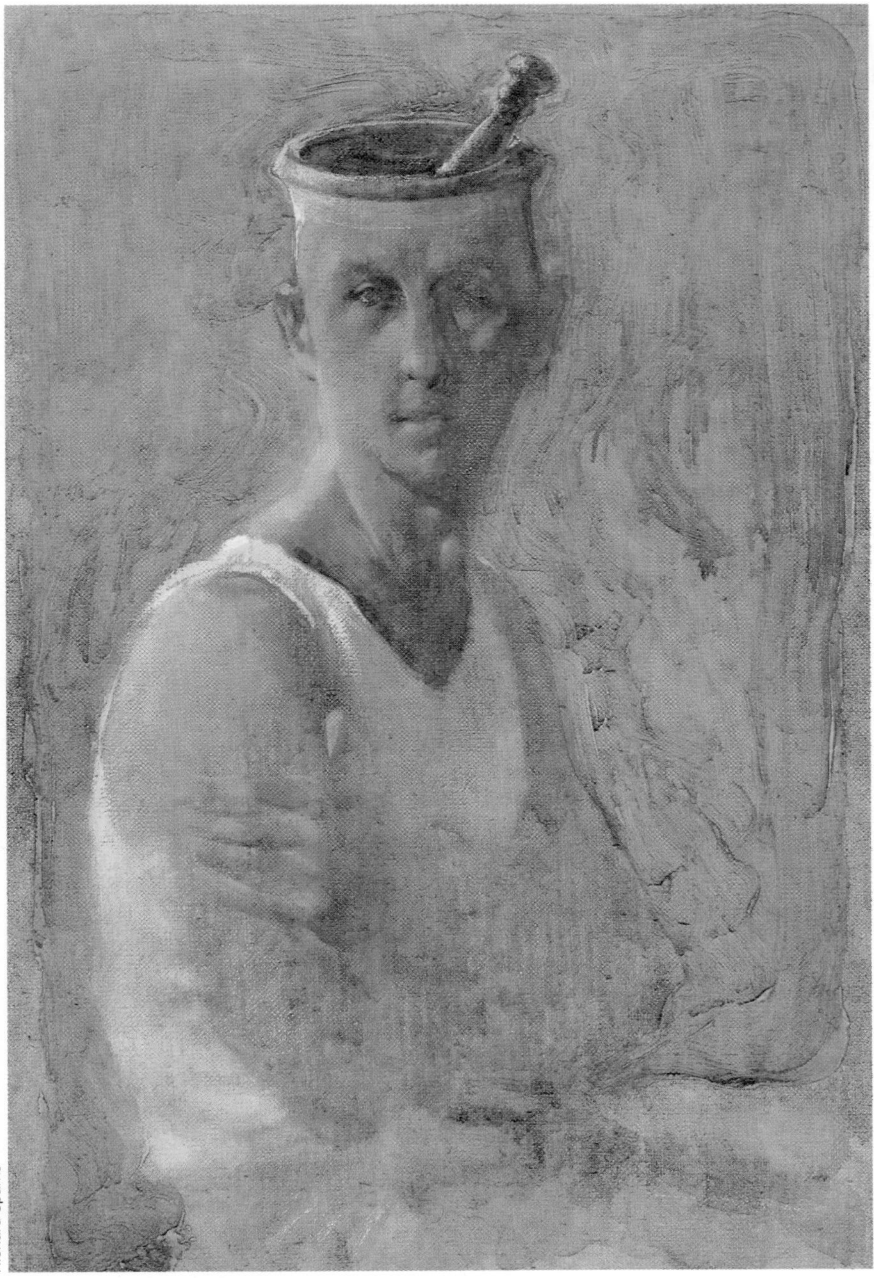
Richard Sparks

Exploring Your Emotions

Suggest a caption for this picture, to express your feelings about it. What "message" might the author be trying to convey?

strep throat infection are given primarily to prevent later complications (rheumatic fever and heart disease) rather than to stop the sore throat pain. An anesthetic solution to gargle is intended to ease sore throat pain. You should also know how soon you should expect results. For instance, drugs may take one to two days to reduce infections or inflammation, while antidepressant medications may not show effects for a week or more.

"HOW AND WHEN DO I TAKE THE MEDICATION, AND FOR HOW LONG?" Understanding how much of the medication to take and how often to take it is often critical to the safe, effective use of medications. Does "every six hours" mean "every six hours while awake?" Should the medication be taken before meals, with meals, or between meals? What should you do if you accidentally miss a dose? Should you skip it, take a double dose next time, or take it as soon as you remember? Should you continue taking the medication until the symptoms subside or until the medication is finished? The answers to such questions are important. For example, if you are taking an **antibiotic** for a bacterial infection, you may feel better within a few days but you should still take the medication as prescribed for a week or two to prevent a recurrence. Or if you stop taking **steroid** medications used to treat poison oak or poison ivy when the rash subsides rather than

Preventing Surgery

Life is better without surgery. Not only is there some inevitable operative risk and some anesthesia risk, the whole experience of having an operation and recovering from it is expensive, painful, cumbersome, and often unnecessary. Much emphasis on avoiding unnecessary surgery has come along with recommendations for "second opinions." These may help somewhat, but they are by far the lesser of measures available to you. You can prevent the need for surgery. The basic principle is to eliminate the risk factors that lead to the common surgical operations. Surprisingly, the strong relationship of elective surgery to risk factors has not been emphasized in medical writing, but there are very strong risk factors that are related to the most common elective surgical procedures.

Inguinal hernia repair: Hernias result from coughing from cigarettes, overweight, poor general fitness, specific weakness of the abdominal muscles, a tendency toward bursts of activity, or bad techniques in lifting. Avoidance of these risk factors greatly reduces the possibility that you will need this operation.

Hemorrhoidectomy: Hemorrhoids or "piles" occur most commonly in the inactive, those with low-fiber diets, and those who are not physically fit. Most hemorrhoidectomies can be avoided by lifestyle modifications.

Varicose veins: These result usually from overweight, inactivity, use of constricting garters, or failure to use support stockings when standing for long periods of time. Take care of the risk factors and avoid the operation.

Appendectomy: The frequency of appendectomy operations is going down rapidly, for reasons that are not fully understood. It appears that prompt treatment of abdominal pain (often with antibiotics), reduction in the frequency of pinworms, and a gradual increase in dietary fiber are important. Again, the dietary risk factors that influence development of other bowel diseases affect the likelihood of this operation.

Hysterectomy: This is an operation for which you should seek a second opinion. The indications for hysterectomy are somewhat controversial, and the decision is a personal one. Many physicians believe that the operation should be done seldom just for irregular or heavy periods and not very often for fibroid tumors.

Gall bladder surgery: Gall bladder problems are most frequently found in individuals with at least moderate obesity, high-fat diets, personal inactivity, and low fluid intake. Most gall bladder operations are necessary when recommended, but many could have been prevented by appropriate attention to these risk factors.

Gastric resection: Abdominal operations because of intestinal hemorrhage, ulcer, or bowel obstruction are related to stress, often to medications, and even more frequently to alcohol intake. Healthy lifestyles greatly decrease the likelihood that the need for these operations will appear.

Hiatal hernia repair: A hiatus hernia is a herniation of part of the stomach upward through the diaphragm. It occurs in people who are overweight, who are in poor physical condition, and who cough a lot. Medical measures, instead of surgery, can

taking the full course of treatment, the rash can erupt again. Taking the medication properly is vital. Yet when patients are surveyed, 40 percent report that their physicians did not say how to take the medication or how much to take. If you are not told how to use the medication, be sure to ask or consult the prescription bottle.

"WHAT FOODS, DRINKS, OTHER MEDICATIONS, OR ACTIVITIES SHOULD I AVOID WHILE TAKING THIS MEDICATION?" The presence of food in the stomach may help protect the stomach from some medications, but it can render other drugs ineffective. Milk products or antacids block absorption of the antibiotic tetracycline, so this drug is best taken on an empty stomach. Other drugs you may be taking, even over-the-counter drugs and alcohol, can either amplify or inhibit the effects of the prescribed medication. Taking aspirin along with an anticoagulant medication can thin your blood and possibly result in hemorrhage. The more medications you are taking, the greater the chance of an undesirable drug interaction.

"WHAT ARE THE SIDE EFFECTS, AND WHAT DO I DO IF THEY OCCUR?" All medications have side effects. Some may be tolerable, minor annoyances while others may be life-also relieve symptoms. A second opinion can be useful in avoiding operation for this condition.

Tonsillectomy and adenoidectomy: There are almost no indications for these operations. They are generally performed out of ignorance. The tonsillar and adenoid tissue will gradually reduce by itself as the subject grows older, and it becomes almost undetectable by age 30 even without surgery. In fact, the tonsillar tissues are useful and help to fight early life infections. If a tonsillectomy and adenoidectomy are suggested, a second opinion is indicated. Perhaps even a third or fourth.

Caesarean section: The frequency of Caesarean section has greatly increased in recent years in the United States, with some benefits in treating fetal distress syndromes. But almost all authorities agree that, in some hospitals and in some areas of the country, C-sections are performed far too frequently. Seek a hospital and an obstetrician that has a low percentage of C-sections among deliveries (anything over one-third of all deliveries by C-section should be considered high); ask your doctor directly. It used to be felt that once a C-section had been performed, all subsequent deliveries would have to be by C-section. However, many doctors now accept that a vaginal delivery is often possible even though there has been a previous C-section.

Coronary artery bypass graft: These operations, or equivalent procedures that dilate the coronary arteries, are precipitated by symptoms that come from coronary atherosclerosis, which is highly related to the cardiac risk factors of inadequate exercise, obesity, smoking, hypertension, high fat intake, and stress. The problem can be prevented. Even after symptoms develop, there should be attempts to control these symptoms by medicine and by improvements in lifestyle. Only a small percentage of bypass operations actually improve life expectancy. Improvement in survival is possible only when the major obstruction is in the left main coronary artery and, to a lesser extent, when all three major coronary arteries are involved. Because these operations are major procedures and because there may be other nonsurgical approaches that have not been tried, we believe that second opinions should be sought and that your family physician should agree with the need for these procedures.

Operations that are generally clearly indicated: In contrast, there are some operations for which the need is usually obvious and in which good results may be anticipated with some confidence. These include total hip replacement operations, total knee replacement operations, extraction of cataracts, and transplantation of the cornea of the eye.

SOURCE: From Donald M. Vickery and James F. Fries, 1986, *Take Care of Yourself: The Consumer's Guide to Medical Care,* 3rd ed. (Reading, Mass.: Addison-Wesley), pp. 12–13.

threatening allergic reactions. You need to know what symptoms to look out for and what action to take should they develop. Should you seek immediate medical care, discontinue the medication, or call your doctor? Unfortunately, a recent survey showed that 70 percent of patients starting a new medication did not recall being told by their physicians or pharmacists about precautions and possible side effects. It is your responsibility to ask.

"CAN YOU PRESCRIBE AN ALTERNATIVE OR GENERIC MEDICATION THAT IS LESS EXPENSIVE?" Every drug has three names—a chemical name, a generic name, and a brand name. The chemical name refers to the chemical structure. The generic name, which may be the same as the chemical name, is the usual scientific name used to refer to the medication. The brand name is a company's unique name for the drug. When a drug company develops a new drug in the United States, it is granted exclusive rights to produce that drug for seventeen years. After this seventeen-year period has expired, other companies may market chemical equivalents of that drug (sometimes formulated with different fillers, in different strengths, and so on). These generic medications are generally considered as safe and effective as the original brand name drug, but often cost half as

The Dangers of Drug Interaction

Who needs to be concerned about drug interactions? You do, if you answer yes to some of the following questions.

- Do you have more than one doctor, or do you patronize more than one pharmacy for prescription and over-the-counter (OTC) drugs?
- Do you currently take several different medicines a day?
- Do you drink coffee or alcoholic beverages?
- Do you smoke?
- Do you use sedatives and oral contraceptives?
- Do you take vitamins, antacids, pain relievers, laxatives, or other OTC medicines?
- Do you take medicine for a chronic disorder such as diabetes, high blood pressure, allergies, epilepsy, or asthma? Literally hundreds of different drug interactions have been reported. They vary in severity and clinical importance. Such things as vitamin deficiencies, treatment failures, and even sudden death may result from a drug interaction, although many are harmless.

Drugs interact not only with other drugs, but with foods, environmental agents, and diagnostic laboratory tests as well. Some interactions warrant cautionary statements on package labels, but others get little or no notice.

The next time you have an OTC cold remedy in your hand, for example, read the label. If it contains a decongestant drug and an antihistamine, the label will warn you not to take the remedy if you are taking a monoamine oxidase inhibitor, and to avoid taking alcohol and the remedy at the same time.

Monoamine oxidase inhibitors (such as Nardil, Marplan and Parnate) are prescription drugs used for the treatment of mental depression. If you take one of these drugs with a decongestant drug (such as phenylpropanolamine, phenylephrine, or pseudoephedrine), the interaction between the two may precipitously elevate blood pressure, causing severe headaches and increasing risk of a heart attack or stroke.

The warning about alcohol is there to prevent another kind of interaction. Antihistamines cause sedation. So does alcohol. Together, the sedative effects of both drugs are additive and likely to make you drowsy. This interaction is potentially dangerous for people who drive motor vehicles or operate mechanized machinery.

A similar, but much more dangerous interaction occurs between alcohol and other sedative drugs such as Valium, Librium, Xanax, phenobarbital, and Nembutal. The sedation caused by the combined effects of alcohol and any of these drugs may be enough to make you stop breathing as you sleep.

Other less common drug interactions may not be mentioned on the labels of OTC remedies. Aspirin, for example, may enhance the "blood-thinning" action of anticoagulant drugs (such as Coumadin and Dicoumarol) and cause bleeding. Vitamin B-6 (pyridoxine) may interfere with the action of levodopa (Dopar, Larodopa), which is used to treat Parkinsonism. Remedies for diarrhea (such as Kaopectate and Pepto-Bismol) may prevent the absorption of many drugs.

Interactions between food and drugs are common. Most often, food delays or prevents drug absorption simply by getting in the way, but specific interactions also occur.

One of the most dangerous of these involves monoamine oxidase inhibitors and such foods as aged cheddar cheese, yogurt, chicken liver, and Chianti wine, which contain large amounts of a chemical called *tyramine*. When we eat such foods, the tyramine is rapidly inactivated and produces no noticeable effects. However, monoamine oxidase inhibitors prevent the inactivation of the tyramine, which, when it accumulates in the blood, may elevate blood pressure enough to precipitate a heart attack or stroke.

Environmental agents such as insecticides and tobacco smoke may influence the action of certain drugs by altering the rate at which the body eliminates them.

Interactions between drugs and diagnostic laboratory tests can delay proper treatment or lead to an improper diagnosis and unnecessary treatment, hospitalization, or, perhaps, surgery. Literally scores of such tests can be affected by drugs. Always tell your doctor or nurse about the medicines you take whenever a diagnostic test is conducted.

L. R. Willis, *Healthline*

Elective surgery A nonemergency operation that the patient can choose to schedule.

Mortality rate The number of deaths occurring in the population being studied.

Morbidity rate The number of illnesses or injuries occurring in the population being studied.

much. In some cases, your physician may have a good reason for preferring a particular brand.

"Is there any written information about the medication?" Even if your physician takes the time to carefully answer all your questions about medications, you will probably find it difficult to remember all this information. Fortunately, there are now many sources of information, from package inserts to pamphlets and books where you can read more about the medications you are taking (see Appendix III, "Resources for Self-care").

Surgery Americans are the most operated-on people in the world. Each year over 20 million operations are performed. About 20 percent of these operations are in response to an emergency such as a severe injury while 80 percent are **elective** surgeries, meaning the patient can generally choose when and where to have the operation if at all. The number of operations performed varies widely from country to country, city to city, and even surgeon to surgeon. The most important factor predicting rates of surgery in a given community is the number of surgeons, not the amount of disease. The more surgeons, the more surgery. All this suggests that you would do well to ask some questions when surgery is recommended for you or a family member to help ensure the operation is really necessary.

"Why do I need surgery at this time?" Although operations have become commonplace in our society, we should not take them lightly. Operations can save lives, but they can also take lives and cause injury. Many experts estimate that about one in five operations is unnecessary and that many more could be prevented if we would change our lifestyles.

Your physician should be able to explain to you the reason for the surgery, alternatives to surgery, and what is likely to happen if you don't have the operation. You should also ask about how the surgery is likely to benefit you.

With most surgery, getting a *second opinion* is advised, and many health insurance plans now require a second opinion before all or certain elective operations. Studies show that when second opinions are required on elective surgical procedures, in 27 percent of cases the second surgeon does not agree that the recommended operation is necessary. Failure to confirm the need for surgery is most common with recommendations for operations of the uterus, tonsils, varicose veins, back, knee, nose, and prostate gland. A second opinion should be an independent opinion. Therefore, consult another physician who is not a partner or associate of the physician who recommended the surgery. Getting a second opinion is not the same as changing physicians. The second physician should not be sought as another possible surgeon, for example. Instead, he or she is only to give a disinterested opinion, in the sense that there will be no personal financial gain in recommending surgery. Consulting a nonsurgeon may also be helpful in exploring alternatives to surgery. For more information about how to get a second opinion, you can call the Second Surgical Opinion Hot Line, sponsored by the U.S. government, at 800-638-6833 (or 800-492-6603 in Maryland).

If your second opinion agrees with the recommendation for surgery, then you can feel more confident in proceeding. If the second opinion conflicts with the first, you may wish to have the doctors confer with each other to clarify the recommendations or you may want to get a third opinion. Disagreements among doctors are usually honest differences of opinion in gray areas of medical knowledge where an expert consensus has not yet been reached. In all cases, you yourself must weigh the opinions carefully, and make the final decision about your treatment.

Although second opinions are most commonly sought for elective surgical procedures, you should also consider getting one for any treatment or diagnostic procedure with significant risk or cost.

"What are the risks and complications of the surgery?" All surgical procedures carry some risk. The average risk of death from surgery is about thirteen deaths for every 1,000 operations. Of course, this overall risk will vary depending on the type of operation performed, the surgeon, and your general state of health. You should ask about the **mortality rate** (risk of death) and **morbidity rate** (risk of nonlethal complications). You should also ask how often the surgeon has performed the operation and what his or her personal experience has been with the procedure. Studies show that surgical teams with more experience with an operation tend to have lower rates of complications.

Sometimes an operation can be performed in several different ways using different incisions, techniques, and anesthetics. Discuss these options with your surgeon so that you can better understand what choices you have.

Some of the risk from a surgical procedure is due to the use of an anesthetic. There are two basic types of anesthesia—general and local. General anesthesia affects your entire body and blocks pain by making you unconscious. Local anesthesia involves injecting a medication that numbs only one area of the body so you remain awake during the operation. There are advantages and

Autologous donation A process in which a person can receive a transfusion of his or her blood that was previously withdrawn and stored.

Outpatient A person receiving medical attention without being admitted to the hospital.

Vasectomy Surgical cutting of the tube that transports sperm (vas deferens), performed as a method of birth control.

Dilation and curettage (D&C) Scraping of the interior of the uterus, usually performed to diagnose cancer or stop bleeding.

Tonsillectomy Surgical procedure to remove the lymph tissue (tonsils) at the back of the throat.

---

disadvantages to each type of anesthesia. Many patients prefer being asleep during the operation so they choose general anesthesia. However, general anesthesia carries a greater risk of heart irregularities and collapse of the cardiovascular system. The risk of death from general anesthesia is estimated somewhere between one in 3,000 to one in 10,000. Local anesthesia is much safer and is now replacing general anesthesia in many types of operations. Be sure to discuss your options in anesthesia with your surgeon.

Blood transfusions may be required during some operations. If you need a transfusion, blood banks have adopted techniques to screen donor blood to generally assure its safety. Nevertheless, if an elective operation is planned, ask if you can donate and store some of your own blood in the months preceding the surgery. Then if you need blood during surgery you can receive a transfusion of your own blood. This technique, known as **autologous donation**, reduces the risk even further of developing a transfusion reaction or contracting an infection such as viral hepatitis or AIDS from infected donor blood.

"CAN THE OPERATION BE PERFORMED ON AN OUTPATIENT BASIS?" More than 30 percent of all operations can now be safely performed on an **outpatient** (ambulatory) basis without requiring an overnight stay in the hospital. You generally enter the hospital or ambulatory care facility in the morning. The procedure is performed, and then you are observed for a period of time and sent home the same day unless serious complications develop. Ambulatory operative procedures are generally less complex and require less postoperative monitoring. Among the 200 different operations that can now be performed on an ambulatory basis are **vasectomies**, hysterotomies, laparectomies, tubal ligations, some hernia repairs, breast biopsies, **dilation and curettage (D&C), tonsillectomies**, cataract surgery, some types of plastic surgery and orthopedic procedures, and scores of other minor surgical procedures.

Outpatient surgery offers many advantages. In most cases, it is nearly one-half the cost of comparable in-hospital operations. It prevents some of the family disruption and psychological trauma that often accompany hospitalization. And it decreases the opportunities for the patient to develop a hospital-acquired medical complication such as infection.

"WHAT CAN I EXPECT BEFORE, DURING, AND AFTER SURGERY?" Knowing what to expect before, during, and after surgery can help you prepare psychologically and physically for the operation. Preparation also appears to decrease postoperative discomfort and need for pain medications, and to shorten postoperative hospital stays.

Proper preparation can also make the operation safer. For example, for some operations you will be asked not to eat for eight to twelve hours before the procedure. This reduces the chances of nausea, vomiting, and inhaling food into the lungs.

You should also ask about how long it should take you to recover and what you can do to speed recovery. You should also be informed about what to expect after surgery in terms of symptoms and which symptoms might signal a complication and should be reported to your doctor.

You are an important part of the health care system; not only as a *consumer* of medical care but as a primary health care *provider*. Managing common medical problems; knowing when and how to self-treat and when to seek professional care; communicating clearly and concisely with your physician; asking questions about medical tests, medications, and surgery; and knowing how to get more information on health topics are some of the essential skills for a health-wise consumer. Developing these skills will not only result in better health care but will also help you develop a real sense of competence and confidence about managing your health.

Take Action

Your answers to the Exploring Your Emotions questions in this chapter and your placement level on the Wellness Ladder will, we hope, encourage you to begin a process of self-exploration and self-discovery that you will continue. Reflect on the entire chapter's content and ask yourself how each point relates to your own life. Then take action:

1. Consider the following medical problem: You bend over to lift a box of books and feel a sharp pain in the right side of your lower back. You can barely move without feeling

pain. You think that you have just "pulled a muscle," but you're not certain. What signs and symptoms might indicate a more serious injury? What symptoms might prompt you to visit a doctor? What self-care strategies could you use to manage a back strain? How could you prevent a similar injury in the future? Compare your responses with the advice given in Appendix II.

2. Review all the medications in your medicine cabinet. Discard any expired or unlabeled medications. Ask your doctor or pharmacist whether you should keep any medications you are uncertain about. Compare the contents of your medicine chest to those listed in the box, "Your Home Self-care Kit," and expand your supplies if you need to.

3. Before your next visit to a doctor, make a *written* list of your concerns. Be prepared to ask questions. After the visit, review how it went. Were your concerns satisfactorily addressed? Were you better able to communicate your needs and answer questions? Did you feel more involved and in control? What aspects would you like to handle more easily?

4. Read the following Behavior Change Strategy and take appropriate action.

Behavior Change Strategy

Following Through with Suggestions: Compliance and Adherence

Many of the chapters in this book describe steps that you can take to accomplish health goals. Personal responsibility for change makes obvious good sense when we look at topics like quitting smoking, losing weight, managing stress, and so on. But when people seek and receive medical care they tend to give away their personal responsibility—to resign their fate to "omniscient, modern medicine." But following medical advice still requires you to manage your behavior. For example, in outpatient or ambulatory situations, the patient is often asked to attend meetings in regular fashion, told to take medications according to a certain schedule, asked to engage in special exercise or stretching movements, and asked to make modifications in the selection and/or preparation of foods.

Medicine recognizes the important role of self-management in health care and supports research in the area of *patient adherence* or *compliance*. The kinds of strategies that have been tested and found to be helpful include the following:

1. Using reminders placed in one's personal environment (home, car, workplace) that improve follow-through in taking medication and keeping scheduled appointments
2. Using diary systems and other forms of self-monitoring to keep a detailed account of a wide variety of health behaviors such as diet, pill taking, exercise practice, and so on
3. Using self-reward systems so that practice of certain self-change programs is encouraged by access to desired activities or items (emphasizing the extrinsic short-term incentives to complement the important but often too distant long-term intrinsic benefits for change)
4. Using self-monitoring and self-rewards to encourage small changes at first followed by larger ones (beginning with only one pill per day, for example, in the first week followed by the needed two-pill-per-day regimen in the second week)

Communication is one of the key requirements of improved adherence. The patient must fully understand what needs to be done, and the physician (or physician staff member) must listen to the scheduling and personal concerns about the regimen from the patient's perspective. A sharing of information contributes to a sense of shared responsibility for following through with the medical regimen. Successful medical care necessarily involves more than following doctor's orders. What is needed from a medical care perspective must accommodate a person's individual schedule and habits. Although changes in packaging and recommendations from medicine are easing this process (for example, availability of pills that can be taken fewer times and still have the same pharmacological benefits), the patient must recapture the sense of responsibility for self-management that characterizes so much health behavior.

Appendix I Home Medical Tests

Taking Your Temperature

Breathing, digesting, moving, even thinking, all generate body heat. Your body temperature reflects your overall body metabolism and muscular activity. Warm-blooded animals have evolved a remarkable mechanism to keep body temperature within a narrow, safe range in spite of considerable variations in environmental temperatures.

Why Performed It is a good idea to measure your temperature a few times when you are feeling well, to establish your normal baseline. Be sure to include both morning and evening readings, because body temperature is typically 0.5 to 1 degree Fahrenheit higher in the evening than in the morning. Then if you develop symptoms such as a cough, earache, diarrhea, or skin rash, check your temperature. It can provide a clue as to the cause or severity of the symptoms.

Equipment The most common and least expensive (about $1–2) thermometer is the glass thermometer filled with mercury or a red liquid. There are two types: oral (with a thinner bulb tip) and rectal (with a thicker tip). Plastic fever strips are also available (about $3) containing heat-sensitive liquid crystal that changes color to indicate the temperature. Finally, new electronic thermometers (about $12) show temperature on an easy-to-read digital display.

Procedure Oral temperatures should not be measured for at least ten minutes after smoking, eating, or drinking a hot or cold liquid. When using a glass thermometer, first clean it with rubbing alcohol or cool (hot water may break it) soapy water. Then grip the end opposite the bulb and shake vigorously as though trying to shake drops of water off the tip. Shake it down until it reads 95°F or lower. Place the oral thermometer under the tongue and keep your mouth tightly closed around it. Leave the thermometer in place for a *full three minutes*. If you leave it in for only two minutes, nearly one-third of temperature readings will be off by at least a half a degree.

To read the glass thermometer, grip it at the end opposite the bulb and hold it in good light with the numbers facing you. Roll the thermometer slowly back and forth between your fingers until you see the silver or red reflection of the column. Note where the column ends, and compare it with the degrees marked in lines on the thermometer. Each long line is a full degree, and each short line counts for 0.2 (two-tenths) of a degree. Most thermometers have a special mark, usually an arrow, indicating a "normal" temperature of 98.6°F. Most thermometers for home use are calibrated in degrees Fahrenheit (F), but some may have the alternative scale of degrees Celsius (C).

Results "Normal" temperature varies from person to person, so it is important to know what is normal for you. Your normal temperature will also vary throughout the day, lowest in the early morning and rising by as much as a degree in the early evening. If you exercise or if it is a hot day, your temperature may normally rise. Also, in women body temperature typically varies by a degree or more through the menstrual cycle, peaking around the time of ovulation. Rectal temperatures normally run about 0.5 to 1 degree higher than oral temperatures. If your recorded temperature is more than 1.0–1.5 degrees above your "normal" baseline temperature, you have a fever. Most often fevers are due to an infection, but fevers may also be caused by drug reactions, inflammation, arthritis, hormone abnormalities, cancer, or severe injuries.

Home Ear Exam

Ear infections are a common problem, especially among young children. Nearly any parent may want to learn how to examine ears. The infection may involve only the external ear canal (external otitis) or the middle ear behind the ear drum (otitis media). With the aid of an instrument called an *otoscope,* you can learn to examine someone else's ear canal and ear drum at home.

Why Performed Home ear exams can be useful in the initial evaluation of earaches, ear fullness, or hearing loss. It may also be useful in monitoring the progress of treatment.

Equipment An otoscope is a hand-held instrument with a built-in light source, a magnifying lens, and a cone-shaped viewing end that is inserted into the ear canal. Home otoscopes are available for about $20.

Procedure Gently insert the instrument in the opening of the ear canal and view the canal and ear drum. Ask your pediatrician, family physician, or nurse practitioner to show you the proper way to do the exam. Practice on healthy adults and children so that you develop an understanding of what a normal ear looks like.

Results You may be able to identify wax in the ear canal or a swollen, red canal, which suggests an infection. If the ear drum looks red or bulging, it may mean a middle ear infection. Discuss any abnormal findings with your physician. Even if the ear exam appears normal, consult a doctor if there is severe ear pain, fever, hearing loss, dizziness, ringing in the ears, or ear discharge.

Self-exam for Dental Plaque

Dental disease is the most common chronic disease; nearly 95 percent of all Americans suffer from tooth decay (dental caries) and/or gum disease (periodontal disease). The major culprit in both of these preventable diseases is dental plaque, a sticky substance composed of millions of bacteria that accumulates around and between teeth. If not removed by proper daily brushing and flossing, plaque can cause tooth decay, gum infection, and tooth loss.

Why Performed Plaque is nearly invisible, so how can you know if you are brushing and flossing adequately? Regular dental checkups will help, but you can also test for plaque at home.

Equipment Disclosing tablets are available in most pharmacies for $2 for 30 tablets. The disclosing tablets contain a harmless red vegetable dye that stains food debris and dental plaque so that you can spot areas not thoroughly cleaned.

Procedure After brushing and flossing, chew one of the tablets thoroughly, swishing the mixture of saliva and dye over your teeth and gums for about 30 seconds. Then gently rinse your mouth and examine your teeth in the mirror.

Results Areas of plaque will stain bright red. The stained areas, usually along the gum margins and between teeth, indicate places you missed while brushing and flossing. Don't be discouraged if you "fail" your first few plaque tests with glowing colors. With this feedback, your brushing and flossing techniques will improve until you no longer leave areas of harmful plaque.

Home Blood Pressure Monitoring

Blood pressure is the force exerted against the walls of blood vessels as your heart pumps blood through your body. Your blood pressure changes from day to day, even minute to minute, depending on activity, diet, drugs, and emotions. Even talking has been shown to raise blood pressure. About one in five Americans has high blood pressure (hypertension). If not controlled, it increases a person's risk of stroke, heart failure, kidney failure, and heart attack. High blood pressure is often referred to as the "silent killer" because most of us cannot accurately sense, without measuring it, if our own blood pressure is increased.

Why Performed Everyone should have their blood pressure checked, or check it themselves, at least every two to three years. If it is normal, more frequent testing is not necessary. If it is elevated, you should check with your doctor to plan appropriate home blood pressure monitoring and, if necessary, treatment. Self-recording of blood pressure is most useful for people with hypertension or borderline high blood pressure. It can offer a more complete and accurate picture of what your blood pressure is like throughout the day and in different environments, not just the doctor's office. It can let you monitor the effects of diet, exercise, weight loss, and medications on your blood pressure. Many people find that home blood pressure monitoring is sufficient to help them lower their blood pressure to safer levels without medications or with a minimum of medication.

Equipment There are several types of blood pressure devices: cuffs with a stethoscope, electronic cuffs with built-in microphone, and the newest electronic "mikeless" cuffs. The cost is generally $40–50, up to $200 for models that inflate automatically and give a printed record. Almost all these devices come with a standard-size cuff that fits, at most, an arm that's 13 inches (33 centimeters) in diameter at its widest point. If your arm is thicker than that, the standard-size cuff will be too small for you and may give falsely elevated readings. Larger cuffs can be ordered from some companies, but ask before buying a device.

Procedure The instructions on how to take your blood pressure will vary depending on the type of blood pressure device you use. The basic principles are similar. Wrap the inflatable bag (cuff) firmly around your upper arm. As the cuff is inflated, blood flow to your arm is temporarily blocked. Then, as the cuff is slowly deflated, blood first begins to flow in the arteries when the pressure produced by your heart contracting is high enough to overcome the pressure in the cuff. This higher measurement is called *systolic* and reflects the maximum pressure produced when the heart is contracting. As the cuff continues to deflate, at some point the blood flow through the artery is no longer restricted at all. This pressure is called the *diastolic* pressure and reflects the lowest pressure in the system that occurs when the heart is relaxing. These two pressures are recorded as systolic/diastolic. For example, if your systolic pressure is 122 and your diastolic pressure is 78, your blood pressure would be recorded as 122 /78, which is read as "122 over 80." All pressures are expressed in terms of millimeters of mercury (mm Hg) because the original blood pressure devices measured pressure using a column of mercury.

Results There is no "magic number" for normal blood pressure, but there are some rough guidelines. A systolic pressure below 140 and a diastolic below 90 are considered "normal" even though lower pressures are actually healthier. If you get repeated readings higher than these, you should consult your physician. Also, test the accuracy of your blood pressure device by occasionally bringing it with you to your doctor's office. Measure your pressure on your machine and then on the doctor's. The readings should match fairly closely. Have a health professional observe and check your technique. Remember, a single measurement of elevated blood pressure does not constitute hypertension. Repeat the procedure if elevated readings are obtained, and check with your physician. Do not adjust your blood pressure medications based on home blood pressure readings without first discussing this more with your physician.

Home Pregnancy Tests

The new home pregnancy test kits are similar to the ones used in doctors' offices and laboratories. They are designed to test for the presence of a hormone in the urine. This hormone, called *human chorionic gonadotropin (HCG),* is produced by the developing placenta and excreted in the urine in increasing amounts during the first weeks of pregnancy. If the hormone is detected in the urine test, it is a sign of pregnancy.

Why Performed When a menstrual period is late, a home pregnancy test can sometimes provide confirmation and reassurance without having to visit a doctor or laboratory. Early confirmation of pregnancy can be very useful. It may allow you to start proper prenatal care right away, during the first month of pregnancy when the risk to the fetus is greatest. Such care includes changes in nutrition and avoidance of cigarettes, drugs, alcohol, and X-ray exposure. Or if you so decide, an abortion can be arranged early on, when the procedure is simpler and safer.

Equipment Home pregnancy tests are now available without a doctor's prescription in most drugstores and supermarkets. They cost about $10.

Procedure Manufacturers claim that the tests are sensitive enough to detect the pregnancy hormone as early as one day after a missed menstrual period. However, by waiting at least until your period is a week late you improve the accuracy of the test and save money on unnecessary testing. The tests involve collecting a first-of-the-morning urine specimen; this is the most concentrated urine and more likely to contain the pregnancy hormone. The instructions for the various kits need to be followed exactly: mix the various chemicals together and wait the prescribed amount of time.

Results Results are available in anywhere from 30 minutes to an hour or two. Positive and negative results are indicated in different ways depending on the test kit used; a solution may change color, a ring-shaped deposit may form in the bottom of a tube, a dipstick may turn blue, and so on. These tests are not foolproof. They're better at telling you that you are pregnant than in making sure that you are not. A positive test on these tests is 99 to 100 percent accurate, but if the test is negative, there's still a 10 to 20 percent chance that you really are pregnant. So, if your period still hasn't come a week after a negative test, repeat the test. If the problem continues or if you are having lower abdominal pain, see your doctor.

SOURCE: Adapted from David S. Sobel and Tom Ferguson, 1985, *The People's Book of Medical Tests* (New York: Summit).

Appendix II Self-care Guide for Common Medical Problems

The following self-care guide will help you manage a dozen of the most common symptoms:

- Fever
- Sore throat
- Cough
- Nasal congestion
- Ear problems
- Nausea, vomiting, or diarrhea
- Headache
- Low back pain
- Strains and sprains
- Cuts and scrapes

Each symptom is described here in terms of what's going on in your body. Particular emphasis is given to the fact that most symptoms are part of the body's natural healing response and reflect your body's wisdom in attempting to correct disease. Self-care advice is also given, along with some guidelines as to when to seek professional advice. In most cases, the symptoms are self-limiting; that is, they will resolve on their own with time and simple self-care strategies.

No medical advice is perfect. You will always have to make the decision as to whether to self-treat or get professional help. This guide is intended to provide you with more information so that you can make better, more informed decisions. If the advice here differs from that of your doctor, discuss the differences. In most instances, your doctor will be best able to customize the advice to your individual medical situation.

The guidelines given here apply to *generally healthy adults*. If you are pregnant, nursing, or have some chronic disease, particularly one that requires medication, check with your doctor for special self-care advice appropriate for you. For example, if you have a condition such as inflammatory bowel disease (colitis), your doctor should give you specific advice on how to manage diarrhea and when to call for help. Also, if you have an allergy or suspected allergy to any recommended medication, please check with your doctor before using it. For guidelines appropriate for children, see *Taking Care of Your Child: A Parent's Guide to Medical Care,* 1984, by Robert H. Pantell, M.D., James F. Fries, M.D., and Donald M. Vickery, M.D. (Reading, Mass.: Addison-Wesley).

If you have several symptoms, read about your main symptom first and then proceed to the lesser symptoms. Above all, use your common sense. If you are particularly concerned about a symptom or confused about how to manage it, call your doctor to get more information.

Fever

A fever is an abnormally high body temperature, usually over 100°F. It is most commonly a sign that your body is fighting an infection. Fever may also be due to inflammation, an injury, or a drug reaction. Chemicals released into your bloodstream during an infection reset the thermostat in the hypothalamus of your brain. The message goes out to your body, "Quick, turn up the heat!" The blood vessels in your skin constrict, you curl up, and throw on extra blankets to reduce heat loss. Meanwhile, your muscles begin to shiver to generate enormous additional body heat. The result is a fever.

Later when your brain senses that the temperature is too high, the signal goes out to increase sweating. As the sweat evaporates, it carries heat away from the body surface.

A fever may not be all bad; it may even help us fight infections by making the body less hospitable to bacteria and viruses. A high body temperature appears to bolster the immune system and may inhibit the growth of infectious micro-organisms.

Most generally healthy people can tolerate a fever as high as 103–104°F without problems. Therefore, if you are generally in good health there is little need to reduce a fever unless you are very uncomfortable. The elderly and those with chronic health problems such as heart disease may not tolerate the increased metabolic demand of a high fever, and fever reduction may be advised.

Most problems with fevers are due to the excessive loss of fluids from evaporation and sweating, which may cause dehydration.

Self-assessment

1. Take your temperature several times throughout the day.
2. Look for signs of dehydration (excessive thirst; very dry mouth; infrequent urination with dark, concentrated urine; and lightheadedness).

Self-care

1. Drink plenty of fluids to prevent dehydration; at least 8 ounces of water, juice, or broth every two hours.
2. Sponge baths using lukewarm water will increase evaporation and help reduce body temperature naturally.
3. Don't bundle up. This decreases the body's ability to lose excess heat.
4. Take aspirin or aspirin substitute (acetaminophen). For adults, two standard-size tablets every 4 to 6 hours can be used to reduce the fever and the associated headache and achiness. Do not use aspirin if you have a history of allergy to aspirin, ulcers, or bleeding problems. In addition, most pediatricians recommend using an aspirin substitute, not aspirin, for fever in children. This is because of the finding that some children with chicken pox or influenza when treated with aspirin have developed a life-threatening complication, Reye's syndrome.

When to Call the Doctor

1. Fever over 103°F (102°F if over 60 years old)
2. Fever lasting more than five days
3. Recurrent unexplained fevers
4. Fever accompanied by rash, stiff neck, severe headache, cough with brown/green sputum, severe pain in flank or abdomen, painful urination, convulsions, or mental confusion
5. Fever with signs of dehydration
6. Fever after starting a new medication

Sore Throat

A sore throat is caused by inflammation of the throat lining due to an infection, allergy, or irritation (especially from cigarette smoke). With an infection, you may also notice some hoarseness from swelling of the vocal cords and "swollen glands," which are enlarged lymph nodes that produce white blood cells to help you fight the infection. The lymph nodes, part of your body's defense system, may remain swollen for weeks after the infection subsides.

Most throat infections are caused by viruses. Your body knows how to fight virus infections, and antibiotics are not necessary or helpful with virus infections. However, about 20–30 percent of throat infections are due to streptoccocal bacteria. This type of bacteria can cause complications such as rheumatic fever and rheumatic heart disease and therefore should be treated with antibiotics. Strep throat is usually characterized by very sore throat, high fever, swollen lymph nodes, a whitish discharge at the back of the throat, and the absence of other cold symptoms such as a cough and runny nose (which suggest a virus infection). Allergy-related sore throats are usually accompanied by running nose and watery, itchy eyes.

Self-assessment

1. Take your temperature.
2. Look in a mirror at the back of your throat. Is there a whitish, puslike discharge on the tonsils or back of the throat?
3. Feel the front and back of your neck. Do you feel enlarged, tender lymph nodes?

Self-care

1. Stop smoking to avoid further irritation of your throat.
2. Drink plenty of liquids to soothe your inflamed throat.
3. Gargle warm salt water (¼ tsp. salt in 4 oz. water) every one to two hours to help reduce swelling and discomfort.
4. Suck on throat lozenges, cough drops, or hard candies to keep your throat moist.
5. Use throat lozenges, sprays, or gargles that contain an anesthetic, to temporarily numb your throat and make swallowing less painful.
6. Try aspirin or aspirin substitute to ease throat pain.
7. For an allergy-related sore throat, try an antihistamine such as chlorpheniramine.

When to Call the Doctor

1. Great difficulty swallowing saliva or breathing.
2. Sore throat with fever over 101°F, especially if you do not have other cold symptoms such as nasal congestion or cough.
3. Sore throat with a skin rash.
4. Sore throat with whitish pus on the tonsils.
5. Sore throat and recent contact with a person who has had a positive throat culture for strep.
6. Enlargement of lymph nodes lasting longer than three weeks.
7. Hoarseness persisting longer than three weeks.

Cough

A cough is a protective mechanism of the body to help keep the airways clear. There are two types of cough: a dry cough (without mucus) and a productive cough (with mucus). Common causes of cough include infection (viral or bacterial), allergies, and irritation from smoking and pollutants. If you have a cold, the cough may be the last symptom to improve, because the airways may remain irritated for several weeks after the infection has resolved.

Your airways are lined with hairlike projections called *cilia,* which move back and forth to help clear the airways of mucus, germs, and dust. Infections and cigarette smoking paralyze and damage this vital defense mechanism.

Self-assessment

1. Take your temperature.
2. Observe your mucus. A thick green, brown, or bloody mucus suggests a bacterial infection.

Self-care

1. Stop smoking. Smoking irritates the airways and undermines your body's defense mechanisms, leading to more serious infections and longer lasting symptoms. Most people do not feel like smoking when they have a cold with a cough. If you want to quit, a cold may provide an excellent opportunity to do so.
2. Drink plenty of fluids (at least six 8-oz. glasses a day) to help thin mucus and loosen chest congestion.
3. Breathe steam through a vaporizer or in a hot shower to help loosen chest congestion.
4. Suck on cough drops, throat lozenges, or hard candy to keep your throat moist and help relieve a dry, tickling cough.
5. If you have a dry, nonproductive cough or the cough keeps you from sleeping, you can use a cough syrup or lozenge that contains the over-the-counter cough suppressant dextromethorphan. Since a cough that produces mucus is protective, it is generally not advised to suppress a productive cough.

When to Call the Doctor

1. Cough with thick green, brown, or bloody sputum.
2. Cough with high fever (above 102°F) and shaking chills.
3. Severe chest pains, wheezing, or shortness of breath.
4. Cough that lasts longer than two weeks.

Nasal Congestion

Nasal congestion is most commonly caused by infection or allergies. With infection, the nasal passages become congested due to increased blood flow and mucus production. This congestion is actually part of the body's defense to fight the infection. The increased blood flow raises the temperature of the nasal passages, making them less hospitable to germs. The nasal secretions are rich in white blood cells and antibodies to help fight and neutralize the invading organisms and flush them away. Nasal congestion associated with sore throat, cough, and fever usually indicates a virus infection.

Nasal congestion caused by allergies is often accompanied by a thin, watery discharge, sneezing, itchy eyes, and sometimes a seasonal pattern. In an allergic reaction, the offending allergen (pollen, dusts, molds, dander, and so forth) trigger the release of histamine and other chemicals from the cells lining the nose, throat, and eyes. These chemicals cause swelling, discharge, and itching. Antihistamine drugs block the release of these irritating chemicals.

Self-assessment

1. Take your temperature.
2. Observe the color and consistency of your nasal secretions. A thick green, brown, or bloody discharge suggests a bacterial sinus infection.
3. Tap with your fingers over the sinus cavities above and below the eyes. If this causes increased pain, a bacterial sinus infection may be present.

Self-care

1. Stop smoking to prevent continuing irritation of the nasal passages.
2. Use moist heat from a hot shower or vaporizer to help liquify congested mucus.
3. Use a decongestant nasal spray or drops to temporarily relieve congestion. However, if these decongestants are used for more than three days they can cause "rebound congestion" that actually creates more nasal congestion. As an alternative, use salt water nose drops (¼ tsp. salt in ½ cup of boiled water).
4. Try an oral decongestant such as pseudoephedrine 60 mg every six hours to help shrink swollen mucous membranes and open nasal passages. In some people, these medications can cause nervousness, sleeplessness, or heart palpitations. If you have uncontrolled high blood pressure, heart disease, or diabetes, check with your doctor before using decongestants.
5. To help relieve nasal discharge and sneezing, try an antihistamine such as chlorpheniramine, 4 to 8 mg every eight hours. These medications can cause drowsiness, dry mouth, and excessive drying of the nose and air passages. If you have asthma, glaucoma, or difficulty urinating due to an enlarged prostate gland, check with your doctor before using these medications.

When to Call the Doctor

1. Nasal congestion with severe pain and tenderness in the forehead, cheeks, or upper teeth and a high fever (above 102°F).
2. Thick green, brown, or bloody nasal discharge.
3. Nasal congestion and discharge unresponsive to self-care treatment and lasting longer than three weeks.

Ear Problems

Ear symptoms include earache, discharge, itching, stuffiness, and hearing loss. They may be caused by problems in the external ear canal, ear drum, middle ear, or Eustachian tube (the passageway that connects the middle ear space to the back of the throat). The ear canal can become blocked by excess wax, producing a sense of the ear being plugged and hearing loss. An infection of the external ear canal due to excessive moisture and trauma is often referred to as "swimmer's ear." It can cause pain, fullness, discharge, and itching. Congestion and blockage of the Eustachian tube by a cold or allergy can result in pain, fullness, and hearing loss. A middle ear infection often produces severe pain, hearing loss, and fever.

Self-assessment

1. Take your temperature. A fever may be a sign of infection.
2. Have someone look into the ear canal with a flashlight or otoscope. Look for wax blockage or a red, swollen canal indicating an external ear infection.
3. Wiggle the outer part of the ear. If this increases the pain, an infection or inflammation of the external canal is the likely cause.

Self-care

1. If blockage of the ear canal with wax is the problem, first try a hot shower to liquify the wax and use a wash cloth to wipe out the ear canal. You can also use a few drops of an over-the-counter wax softener and then flush the canal gently with warm water and a bulb syringe. Do not use sharp objects or cotton swabs; they can scratch the canal or push the wax in deeper.
2. To treat mild infections of the external ear canal, you must thoroughly dry the ear canal. A few drops of a drying agent (Burow's solution) on a piece of cotton gently inserted into the canal can act as a wick to dry the canal.
3. To relieve congestion and blockage of the Eustachian tube, try a decongestant like pseudoephedrine, a nasal spray (but no longer than three days), or an antihistamine. Hot showers or a vaporizer may help loosen secretions, and yawning or swallowing may help open your Eustachian tube. For a mild plugging sensation without fever or pain, pinch your nostrils and blow gently to force air up the Eustachian tube and "pop" your ears.

When to Call the Doctor

1. Severe earache with fever.
2. Puslike or bloody discharge from the ear
3. Sudden hearing loss, especially if accompanied by ear pain or recent trauma to the ear
4. Ringing in the ears or dizziness
5. Any ear symptom lasting longer than two weeks

Nausea, Vomiting, or Diarrhea

Nausea, vomiting, and diarrhea usually are defensive reactions of your body to rapidly clear your digestive tract of irritants. These symptoms are most commonly caused by the "stomach flu," a virus infection, but may also be caused by food poisoning, medications, or other types of infection. Vomiting dramatically ejects irritants from your stomach, and nausea discourages eating to allow the stomach to rest. In diarrhea, overstimulated intestines flush out the offending irritants.

The major complications of vomiting and diarrhea are dehydration from fluid losses and decreased intake and the risk of bleeding from irritation of the digestive tract.

Self-assessment

1. Take your temperature. A fever is often a clue that an infection is causing the symptoms.
2. Observe the color and frequency of vomiting and diarrhea. This helps estimate severity of fluid losses and checks for bleeding (red, black, or "coffee grounds" material in stool or vomit).
3. Look for signs of dehydration: very dry mouth, marked thirst, infrequent urination with dark, concentrated urine, and lightheadedness.
4. Look for signs of hepatitis, an infection of the liver that produces a yellow color in the skin and white parts of the eyes.

Self-care

1. To replace fluids, take frequent, small sips of clear liquids such as water, non-citrus juice, broths, flat ginger ale, or ice chips.
2. When the vomiting and diarrhea have subsided, you can try nonirritating, constipating foods like the BRAT diet: Bananas, Rice, Applesauce, and Toast.
3. For several days avoid alcohol, milk products, fatty foods, aspirin, and other medications that might irritate the stomach. Do not stop taking regularly prescribed medications without discussing this change with your doctor.
4. Medications are not usually advised for vomiting. For diarrhea, over-the-counter medications containing kaolin, pectin, or attapulgite may help thicken the stool. Medications containing paregoric may help decrease painful intestinal spasms.

When to Call the Doctor

1. Inability to retain any fluids for twelve hours, or signs of dehydration
2. Severe abdominal pains not relieved by the vomiting or diarrhea
3. Blood in the vomit (red or "coffee grounds-like" material) or in the stool (red or black, tarlike material)
4. Vomiting or diarrhea with a high fever (above 102°F)
5. Yellow color in skin or whites of eyes
6. Vomiting with severe headache and history of recent head injury
7. Vomiting or diarrhea that lasts three days without improvement
8. Recurrent vomiting and/or diarrhea
9. If you are pregnant or have diabetes

Headache

Headache is one of the most common symptoms. There are three major types of headache: muscle tension (the most common type), vascular (related to the blood vessels), and sinus (involves blocked sinus cavities). Muscle tension headaches are often due to emotional stress or physical stress such as poor posture. The muscles in the neck, scalp, and jaws tighten, producing a dull, aching sensation or band of tension around the head. Vascular headaches, which include the common migraine, are due to a constriction and then dilation of blood vessels in the head. Vascular headaches are usually severe, one-sided, throbbing headaches often associated with nausea, vomiting, and visual disturbances (flashing lights or stars). Sinus headaches are caused by blockage of the sinus cavities with resulting pressure and pain in the cheeks, forehead, and upper teeth. These headaches are often associated with nasal congestion. Sometimes a combination of these types of headaches will occur. Headache caused by elevated blood pressure is very uncommon and occurs only with very high pressures.

Self-assessment

1. Take your temperature. The presence of fever may indicate a sinus infection. Fever, severe headache, and very stiff neck suggest meningitis, a rare, but serious infection around the brain and spinal cord.
2. Tap with your fingers over the sinus cavities in your cheeks and forehead. If this causes increased pain, it may indicate a sinus infection.
3. For recurrent headaches, keep a headache diary. Record how often and when your headaches occur, associated symptoms, preceding activities, food and beverage intake.

Self-care

1. Try ice packs or heat on your neck and head.
2. Gently massage the muscles of your neck and scalp.
3. Try deep relaxation or breathing exercises.
4. Take aspirin or aspirin substitute for pain relief.
5. If pain is associated with nasal congestion, try a decongestant medication like pseudoephedrine.
6. Try to avoid emotional stressors and physical stressors (like poor posture and eye strain)
7. Try avoiding certain foods that may trigger headaches. These often include aged cheeses, chocolate, nuts, red wine, alcohol, avocados, figs, raisins, and any fermented or pickled foods.

When to Call the Doctor

1. Unusually severe headache
2. Headache accompanied by fever and very stiff neck
3. Headache with sinus pain and tenderness and a fever
4. Severe headache following recent head injury
5. Headache associated with slurred speech, visual disturbance, numbness or weakness in face, arms, or legs
6. Headache persisting longer than three days
7. Recurrent unexplained headaches
8. Increasing severity or frequency of headaches

Low Back Pain

Pain in the lower back is a very common condition that results in large part from our upright posture, which puts tremendous strain on our lower backs. The pain is most often due to a strain of the muscles and ligaments along the spine, which may or may not be triggered by bending, lifting, or other activity. Low back pain can also be due to bone growths (spurs) irritating the nerves as they leave the spine or to pressure from ruptured or protruding discs, the "shock absorbers" between the vertebrae. In addition to back pain, nerve irritation can produce lower leg pain, numbness, tingling, weakness, and loss of bowel or bladder control. Sometimes back pain is actually caused by an infection or stone in the kidney. Fortunately, however, simpler muscular strain is the most common cause of low back pain and can usually be effectively self-treated.

Self-assessment

1. Take your temperature. Back pain with high fever may indicate a kidney or other infection.
2. Check for blood in your urine or frequent, painful urination, which may also indicate a kidney problem.
3. Observe for tingling or pain traveling down one or both legs below the knee with bending, coughing, or sneezing. These symptoms suggest a disc problem.

Self-care

1. Lie on your back or in any comfortable position on the floor or on a firm mattress with knees slightly bent and supported by a pillow. Rest for twenty-four hours or longer if the pain persists.
2. Use ice packs on the painful area for the first twenty-four hours, then apply ice or heat.
3. Take aspirin or aspirin substitute for pain relief as needed.
4. After the acute pain has subsided, begin gentle back and stomach exercises. Practice good posture and lifting techniques to protect your back. To learn more about proper back exercises and use of your back, consult a physical therapist or your doctor.

When to Call the Doctor

1. Back pain following a severe injury such as an accident or fall
2. Back pain radiating down the leg below the knee on one or both sides
3. Persistent numbness, tingling, or weakness in the legs or feet
4. Loss of bladder or bowel control
5. Back pain associated with high fever (above 101°F),

frequent or painful urination, blood in the urine, or severe abdominal pain
6. Back pain that does not improve after one week of self-care

Strains and Sprains

Missteps, slips, falls, accidents, and athletic misadventures result in a variety of strains, sprains, and fractures. A strain occurs when you overstretch a muscle or a tendon (the connective tissue that attaches muscle to bone). Sprains are caused by overstretching or tearing of ligaments (the tough fibrous bands that connect bone to bone). Depending on the severity and location, a sprain may actually be more serious than a fracture because bones generally heal very strongly while ligaments may remain stretched and lax after healing. A sprain may take six weeks for the ligament to heal.

After most injuries, you can expect pain and swelling. This is the body's way of immobilizing and protecting the injured part so that healing can take place. The goal of self-assessment is to determine whether you have a minor injury that you can safely self-treat or a more serious injury to an artery, nerve, or bone that should be treated by your doctor.

Self-assessment

1. Observe for coldness, blue color, or numbness to the limb beyond the injury. These may be signs of damage to artery or nerve.
2. Look for signs of a possible fracture, which would include misshapen limb, reduced length of the limb on the injured side compared to the uninjured side, inability to move or bear weight, grating sound with movement of injured area, extreme tenderness at one point along the injured bone as you press with your fingers, or a sensation of snapping at time of the injury.
3. Gently move the injured area through its full range of motion. Immobility or instability suggest a more serious injury.

Self-care

1. Immediately immobilize, protect, and rest the injured area until you can bear weight on it or move it without pain. Remember, if it hurts, don't do it.
2. To decrease pain and swelling, immediately apply ice (cold pack or ice wrapped in a cloth) for 15 minutes every hour for the first twenty-four to forty-eight hours. Then apply ice or heat as needed for comfort.
3. Immediately elevate the injured limb above the level of your heart for the first twenty-four hours to decrease swelling.
4. Immobilize and support the injured area with an elastic wrap or splint. Be careful not to wrap so tightly as to cause blueness, coldness, or numbness.
5. Take aspirin or aspirin substitute for pain as needed.

When to Call the Doctor

1. An injury that occurred with great force such as a high fall or motor vehicle accident
2. Hearing or feeling a snap at the time of the injury
3. A limb that is blue, cold, or numb
4. A limb that is bent, twisted, or crooked
5. Tenderness at specific points along a bone
6. Inability to move injured area
7. Wobbly, unstable joint
8. Marked swelling of the injured area
9. Inability to bear weight after twenty-four hours
10. Pain that increases or lasts longer than four days

Cuts and Scrapes

Cuts and scrapes are common disruptions of your body's skin. Fortunately, the vast majority of these wounds are minor and don't require stitches, antibiotics, or a doctor's care. An abrasion involves a scraping away of the superficial layers of skin. Abrasions, though less serious, are often more painful than cuts because they disrupt more skin nerves. Cuts come in two varieties: lacerations (narrow slices of the skin) and puncture wounds (stabs into deeper tissues).

Normal healing of a cut or abrasion is a wondrous process. After the bleeding stops, small amounts of serum, a clear yellowish fluid, may leak from your wound. This fluid is rich in antibodies to help prevent an infection. Redness and swelling may normally occur as more blood is shunted to the area, bringing white blood cells and nutrients to speed healing. There may also be some swelling of nearby lymph nodes, which are another part of your body's defense against infection. Finally, a scab forms. This is "nature's Band-Aid," which protects the area while it heals.

The main concerns about cuts are the possibilities of damage to deeper tissues and the risk of infection. Damage to underlying blood vessels may lead to severe bleeding as well as blueness and coldness to areas beyond the wound. Injured nerves may produce numbness and loss of ability to move parts of the body beyond the injured area. Damaged muscles, tendons, and ligaments can also result in inability to move areas beyond the cut.

Wound infection usually does not take place until twenty-four to forty-eight hours after an injury. Signs of infection include increasing redness, swelling, pain, pus, and fever. One of the most serious, though fortunately uncommon, complications of cuts is tetanus ("lockjaw"). This bacterial infection thrives in areas not exposed to oxygen, so it is more likely to develop in deep puncture wounds or dirty wounds. Tetanus is very unlikely to develop in minor cuts or wounds caused by clean objects like knives. You need a tetanus shot following a cut

- If you have never had the basic series of three tetanus immunization injections
- If you have a dirty or contaminated wound and it has been longer than five years since your last injection
- If you have a clean, minor wound and it has been longer than ten years since your last injection

Self-assessment

1. Look for warning signs of complications: persistent bleeding, numbness, inability to move injured area, or the later development of pus, increasing redness, and fever.
2. Measure the size of the cut. If your cut is shallow, less than an inch long, not in a high-stress area (such as a joint, which bends), and you can easily hold the edges of the wound closed, it probably won't need stitches.

Self-care

1. Apply direct pressure over the wound until bleeding is stopped. The only exception is puncture wounds, which should be encouraged to bleed freely (unless spurting a large amount of blood) for a few minutes to flush out bacteria and debris.
2. Try to remove any dirt, glass, or foreign material from the wound with tweezers or by scrubbing.
3. Wash the wound vigorously with soap and water, followed by an application of hydrogen peroxide solution as an antiseptic.
4. If it is an abrasion, cover the area with a Band-Aid until a scab forms. For minor lacerations, close the cut with a butterfly bandage or a sterile adhesive tape (Steristrips), drawing the edges close together but not overlapping. If there is an extra flap of clean skin, leave it in place for extra protection. Do not attempt to close puncture wounds. Instead soak puncture wounds in warm water for 15 minutes several times a day for several days. Soaking helps keep the wound open and thus prevents infection.

When to Call the Doctor

1. Bleeding that can't be controlled with direct pressure
2. Numbness, weakness, or inability to move injured area
3. Any large, deep wound
4. A laceration in an area that bends and the edges of the cut cannot be easily held together
5. Cuts on the hands or face unless clean and shallow
6. Contaminated wound in which you cannot remove the foreign material
7. Any human or animal bite
8. If you need a tetanus immunization (see indications noted earlier)
9. Development of increasing redness, swelling, pain, pus, or fever twenty-four hours or more after the injury
10. If the wound is not healing well in three weeks

Appendix III Resources for Self-care

Books

Brody, Jane E. 1982. *Jane Brody's Guide to Personal Health.* New York: Times Books.
A compilation of highly readable newspaper columns on common medical problems and concerns.

Graedon, Joe, and Teresa Graedon. 1980, 1984, 1986. *The People's Pharmacy.* Vols. 1–3. New York: Avon.
Three lively and highly informative books discussing the pharmacology, profits and politics that affect the drugs we use.

Griffith, H. Winter. 1985. *Complete Guide to Symptoms, Illness, and Surgery.* Tucson, Ariz.: Body Press.
A mammoth book discussing over 700 symptoms, 500 illnesses, and 160 surgeries.

Griffith, H. Winter. 1986. *Complete Guide to Prescription & Nonprescription Drugs.* Tucson, Ariz.: Body Press.
A comprehensive guide to side effects, warnings, and precautions for safe use for over 4,000 brand name and generic drugs.

Inlander, Charles B., and Ed Weiner. 1985. *Take This Book to the Hospital with You.* Emmaus, Pa.: Rodale Press.
The lively and informative guide from The People's Medical Society on how to survive a hospital stay.

Kemper, Donald W., Kathleen E. McIntosh, and Toni M. Roberts. 1986. *Healthwise Handbook: The Practical Guide to Family-based Care.* Boise, Idaho: Healthwise, Inc.
Practical, straightforward guidelines on the best home care for a variety of common medical problems in adults and children.

Kunz, Jeffrey R.M. (Ed.). 1982. *The American Medical Association Family Medicine Guide.* New York: Random House.

A mammoth volume discussing more than 650 diseases. Contains ninety-nine question-and-answer charts to help evaluate common medical symptoms and decide when to see the doctor.

Pantel, Robert H., James F. Fries, and Donald M. Vickery. 1984. *Taking Care of Your Child: A Parent's Guide to Medical Care.* Reading, Mass.: Addison-Wesley.

An indispensable guide for common health problems of children, containing over ninety-five easy-to-use decision charts to help parents decide when to call the doctor and when to treat at home.

Sehnert, Keith W. and Howard Eisenberg. 1985. *How to Be Your Own Doctor (Sometimes).* New York: Putnam.

The first modern self-care guide offering advice for self-management of the thirty-eight most common illnesses and accidents.

Sobel, David S., and Tom Ferguson. 1985. *The People's Book of Medical Tests.* New York: Summit Books.

A consumer's guide that answers questions about 200 medical and home diagnostic tests.

Vickery, Donald M. 1986. *Taking Part: The Survivor's Guide to the Hospital.* Reston, Va.: Center for Corporate Health Promotion.

Using decision-making charts, this book offers a second opinion to help the patient decide whether hospitalization and surgery are necessary for the treatment of twenty common medical problems.

Vickery, Donald M., and James F. Fries. 1986. *Take Care of Yourself: The Consumer's Guide to Medical Care.* Reading, Mass.: Addison-Wesley.

Over 3 million copies are in print of this excellent self-care guide, which includes over 100 easy-to-follow decision charts outlining when to see the doctor and how to apply safe and effective home treatment.

Wurman, Richard Saul. 1985. *Medical Access.* Los Angeles: Access Press.

A travel guide to medical care containing descriptions of medical tests, surgical procedures, and the most commonly asked consumer health questions.

Zimmerman, David R. 1983. *The Essential Guide to Nonprescription Drugs.* New York: Harper & Row.

The most comprehensive and authoritative review of the safety and effectiveness of over-the-counter products.

Newsletters and Magazines

American Health (80 Fifth Avenue, New York, NY 10011)

Harvard Medical School Health Letter (79 Garden Street, Cambridge, MA 02138)

Health Facts (Center for Medical Consumers, 237 Thompson St., New York, NY 10012)

Healthline (1149 Chestnut St., #10, Menlo Park, CA 94025)

Health Information Centers

Boston Women's Health Collective (445 Mt. Auburn Street, Watertown, MA 02172, 617-924-0271)

Center for Medical Consumers (237 Thompson St., New York, NY 10012, 212-674-7105)

Consumer Information Center (Pueblo, CO 81009 or 18th and E Streets, N.W., Washington, DC 20405, 202-566-1794)

Planetree Health Resource Center (2040 Webster Street, San Francisco, CA 94115, 415-923-3680)

Self-help and Mutual Aid Groups

In the United States alone, an estimated over 500,000 self-help groups and chapters of self-help organizations provide information and peer support for nearly every conceivable medical condition or problem. There are groups for diabetes, cancer, stroke, heart surgery, Alzheimer's disease, child abuse, drug abuse, infertility, asthma, cystic fibrosis, nursing mothers, blindness, epilepsy, DES (diethylstilbestrol) exposure, eating disorders, colitis, mental retardation, phobias, sleep disorders, sexual problems, women's health, and hundreds of others. You can look in the white pages of the telephone book for your local chapter or contact one of the following self-help clearinghouses for the names of self-help groups in your community.

- National Self-help Clearinghouse (City University of New York, 33 West 42nd St., New York, NY 10036, 212-840-1258)
- The Self-help Center (Center for Urban Affairs, Northwestern University, 2040 Sheridan Road, Evanston, IL 60201, 312-328-0470)
- Self-help Resource Center (UCLA Psychology Department, 405 Hilgard Avenue, Los Angeles, CA 90024, 213-825-1799 or in California 800-222-5465).

Telephone Hotlines

While you can't be cured by a telephone, you can often get medical information—often free—by calling a hotline number. These services are set up to help people learn about various diseases and conditions, keep up to date on the latest research, and find out how to get further assistance. In many communities throughout the country, you can call a free service called Tel-Med and request to hear one of several hundred brief taped health information messages. Check your white pages of the telephone book for the local access number.

- Acne: Acne Help Line, sponsored by the Acne Research Institute, in Newport Beach, CA, 800-235-ACNE (in California, 800-225-ACNE).
- Acquired Immune Deficiency Syndrome (AIDS): AIDS Hot Line, 800-342-AIDS (in Hawaii and Alaska, 404-329-3534 collect).
- Agoraphobia (fear of open spaces): The Agoraphobia and Anxiety Program of Temple University, Philadelphia, 215-667-6490.

- Alcohol: National Clearinghouse for Alcohol Information, 301-468-2600.
- Alzheimer's disease: Alzheimer's Disease and Related Disorders Association, 800-621-0379 (in Illinois, 800-572-6037), 24 hours.
- Anorexia and bulimia: National Association of Anorexia Nervosa and Associated Disorders, 312-831-3438.
- Blindness: American Council of the Blind, 800-424-8666.
- Blindness and physical handicaps, available programs: The National Library Service for the Blind (part of the Library of Congress), 800-424-8567 (in Washington, DC, 202-287-5100).
- Cancer: Cancer Information Service, part of the National Cancer Institute, 800-4-CANCER (in Washington, DC, 202-636-5700).
- Cocaine: Cocaine Abuse Hot Line, 800-COCAINE, 7 days, 24 hours.
- Diabetes: Juvenile Diabetes Foundation, 800-223-1138 (in New York State, 212-889-7575).
- Digestive disorders (from heartburn to ulcers): Gutline, sponsored by the American Digestive Disease Society, 301-652-9293, Tuesdays between 7:30 and 9:00 P.M. Eastern time.
- Drugs, drug interactions, drug side effects: Food and Drug Administration (FDA) Center for Drugs and Biologics Office of Consumer and Professional Affairs, Rockville, MD, 301-443-1016.
- Food and cosmetics safety: The Consumer Inquiries Section of the Office of Consumer Affairs of the FDA, 301-443-3170.
- Hearing problems: Dial-a-Hearing Screening Test, part of Occupational Hearing Services, 800-222-EARS (in Pennsylvania, 215-565-6114).
- Heart disease: Heart Line, sponsored by the Association of Heart Patients, 800-241-6993.
- Infertility: Resolve National Phone Counseling Line, 617-484-2424.
- Kidney disease: American Kidney Fund, 800-638-8299 (in Maryland, 800-492-8361; in Washington DC, 301-986-1444).
- Lung disease, respiratory disorders, allergies: Lung Line, sponsored by the National Jewish Center for Immunology and Respiratory Medicine in Denver, CO, 800-222-LUNG.
- Lupus: Lupus Foundation of America, Inc., 800-558-0121.
- Nutrition for infants and pregnant women: BeechNut Nutrition, 800-523-6633 (in Pennsylvania, 800-492-2384).
- Spina bifida: Spina Bifida Association, 800-621-3141 (in Illinois, 312-663-1562).
- Sports and sports injuries: Women's Sports Foundation, 800-227-3988 (in Hawaii, Alaska, and California, 415-563-6266).
- Sudden Infant Death Syndrome (SIDS): American Sudden Infant Death Syndrome Institute, 800-232-SIDS (in Georgia, 800-847-SIDS).
- Surgery: Second Opinion Hot Line, sponsored by the U.S. government's Department of Health and Human Services, 800-638-6833 (in Maryland, 800-492-6603).

Selected References

Gartner, Alan, and Frank Riessman, 1977. *Self-help in the Human Services*. San Francisco, Calif.: Jossey-Bass.

Greenfield, Sheldon, Sherrie Kaplan, and John E. Ware. 1985. Expanding patient involvement in care: Effect on patient outcomes. *Annals of Internal Medicine* 102:520–28.

Herman, P. G., D. E. Gerson, S. J. Hessel, and others. 1975. Disagreements in chest roentgen interpretation. *Chest* 68:278–82.

Kaplan, Eric B., Lewis B. Sheiner, and others. 1985. The usefulness of preoperative laboratory screening. *Journal of the American Medical Association* 253:3576–81.

Levin, Lowell S., and Ellen L. Idler. 1981. *The Hidden Health Care System*. Cambridge, Mass.: Ballinger.

Louis Harris and Associates. 1983 (March). *Patient Information and Prescription Drugs: Parallel Surveys of Physicians and Pharmacists*. Washington, D.C.: U.S. Food and Drug Administration.

Medical Practices Committee, American College of Physicians. 1981. Periodic health examination: A guide for designing individualized preventive health care in the asymptomatic patient. *Annals of Internal Medicine* 95:729–32.

Runkle, Cecilia, and Catherine Regan. 1985. The role of self-care in medical care. In Wendy Squyres, ed., *Patient Education and Health Promotion in Medical Care*. Palo Alto, Calif.: Mayfield.

Self-medication: The New Era . . . A Symposium (condensation of papers and discussions). 1980 (March 31). Washington, D.C.: The Proprietary Association.

Vickery, Donald M., Howard Kalmer, Debra Lowry, Muriel Constantine, Elizabeth Wright, and Wendy Loren. 1983. Effect of a self-care education program on medical visits. *Journal of the American Medical Association* 250:2952–56.

Williamson, John D., and Kate Kanaher. 1978. *Self-care in Health*. London: Croom Helm.

Recommended Readings

See Appendix III of this chapter for annotated readings.

Chapter 16

Contents

Rate Yourself

Your Attitudes about Health Care Professionals Read the following statements carefully. Choose the one in each section that best describes you at this moment and circle its number. When you have chosen one statement for each section, add the number and record your total score. Find your position on the Awareness Ladder.

5 Has family doctor (M.D. or D.O.)
4 Prefers M.D. or D. O. for medical problems
3 Relies on chiropractors for medical advice
2 Uses unorthodox medical care, such as acupuncture
1 Prefers faith healers to orthodox medicine

5 Is well informed about prescription and over-the-counter drugs
4 Seeks expert advice before buying medicines
3 Reads label before taking medicine
2 Takes medicine without reading label
1 Likes whatever cure-all fad comes along

5 Is skeptical of advertising about health products
4 Cannot be persuaded by advertising alone to purchase health products
3 Is occasionally influenced by advertising to buy health products
2 Believes ads must be true or they wouldn't be published
1 Keeps buying health products by mail despite being dissatisfied

5 Selects comprehensive health insurance after careful review
4 Selects health insurance on the recommendations of friends
3 Has health insurance but doesn't know what it covers
2 Believes having health insurance is a waste of money for young adults
1 Doesn't believe in having health insurance

5 Knows how to file complaints with consumer protection agencies
4 Is familiar with consumer protection agencies
3 Is vaguely familiar with consumer protection agencies
2 Would resist complaining to a consumer protection agency
1 Is unfamiliar with consumer protection agencies

Total Score ______

Choosing Health Care Services and Insurance

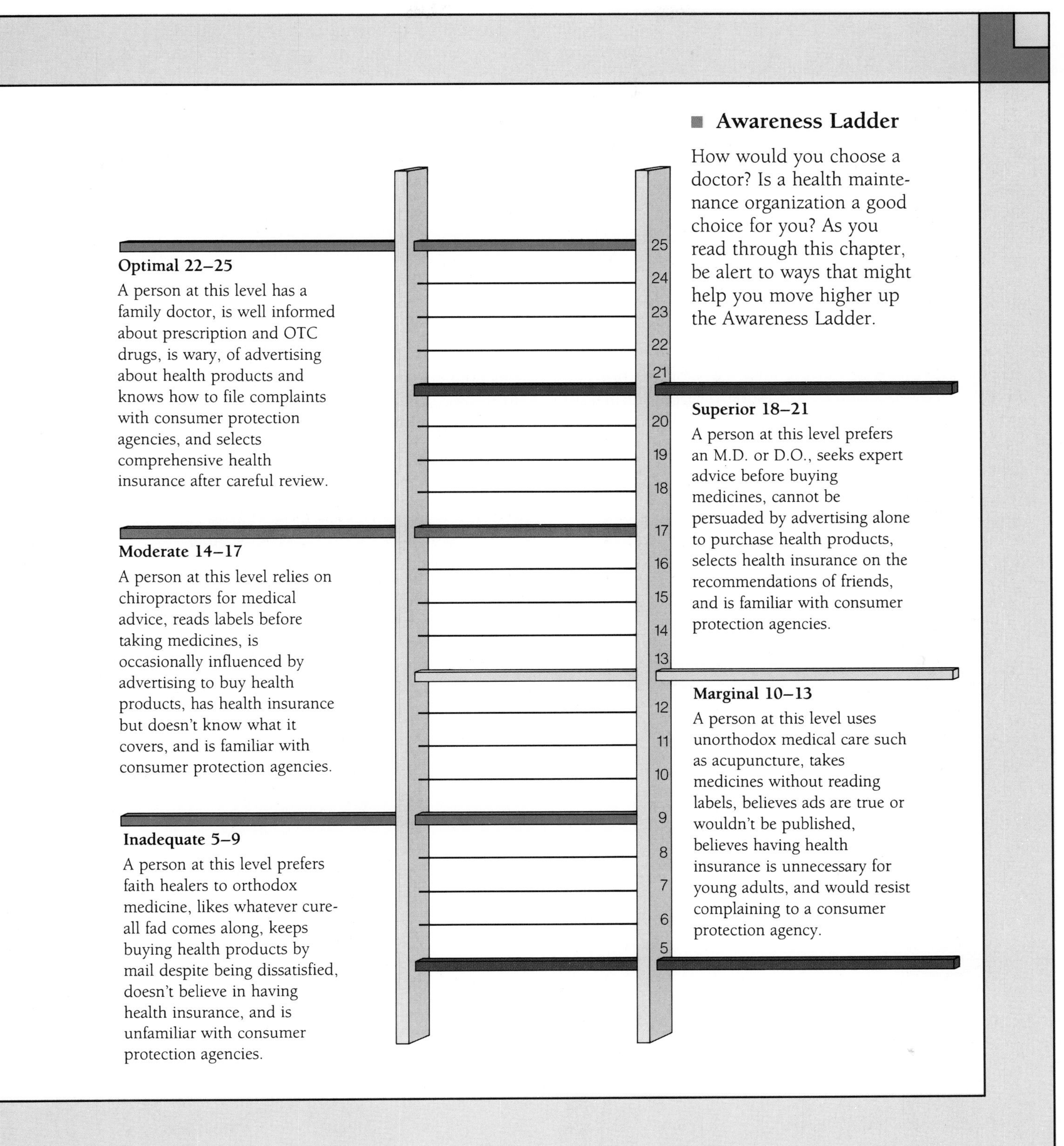

Awareness Ladder
How would you choose a doctor? Is a health maintenance organization a good choice for you? As you read through this chapter, be alert to ways that might help you move higher up the Awareness Ladder.
25
24
23
22
21
20
19
18
17
16
15
14
13
12
11
10
9
8
7
6
5
Optimal 22–25
A person at this level has a family doctor, is well informed about prescription and OTC drugs, is wary, of advertising about health products and knows how to file complaints with consumer protection agencies, and selects comprehensive health insurance after careful review.
Superior 18–21
A person at this level prefers an M.D. or D.O., seeks expert advice before buying medicines, cannot be persuaded by advertising alone to purchase health products, selects health insurance on the recommendations of friends, and is familiar with consumer protection agencies.
Moderate 14–17
A person at this level relies on chiropractors for medical advice, reads labels before taking medicines, is occasionally influenced by advertising to buy health products, has health insurance but doesn't know what it covers, and is familiar with consumer protection agencies.
Marginal 10–13
A person at this level uses unorthodox medical care such as acupuncture, takes medicines without reading labels, believes ads are true or wouldn't be published, believes having health insurance is unnecessary for young adults, and would resist complaining to a consumer protection agency.
Inadequate 5–9
A person at this level prefers faith healers to orthodox medicine, likes whatever cure-all fad comes along, keeps buying health products by mail despite being dissatisfied, doesn't believe in having health insurance, and is unfamiliar with consumer protection agencies.

When you seek medical care, how should you go about it? Should you go to a general practitioner? A specialist? A hospital emergency room? An emergicenter? Whom should you see? Of course, the best time to look for a doctor is before you are ill.

Most experts believe it is best to have a primary physician who gets to know you and can treat you or coordinate referrals to specialists when needed. Doctors who are board certified in family practice (for adults and children), internal medicine (for adults only), or pediatrics (for children only) are likely to be good choices because they have extensive training in the diagnosis and treatment of general medical problems.

Staff affiliation with a hospital connected with a medical school indicates that a physician is working with up-to-date colleagues and is apt to have up-to-date skills and information. Affiliation with a hospital that trains residents is also favorable. Less certain is affiliation with only privately owned hospitals—especially small ones—unless they are the only ones in the area. Lack of any hospital affiliation may be a sign of substandard care. Information on a doctor's credentials may be obtainable from the doctor's office, the local medical society, a local hospital, or a directory available at a medical or public library.

When choosing an outpatient facility, you should consider such factors as quality of care, cost, convenience, and whether follow-up care is available. Table 16-1 lists the advantages and disadvantages of various sources of medical care.

Orthodox Practitioners

Health professionals are regulated by state licensing laws. To become licensed, they must graduate from an accredited professional school, have additional clinical experience, and pass a licensing examination given by a state or national board.

Medical Doctors Medical doctors are independent practitioners who hold an M.D. (doctor of medicine) degree from an accredited medical school. Once licensed, they are legally authorized to administer any type of medical

Table 16-1 Outpatient Health Care Facilities

Facility	Advantages	Disadvantages
Medical office	Maximum personal attention. Low cost per visit.	Limited hours.
Multispecialty group practice	Low cost per visit. Consultations may be more readily available.	Same physician may not always be seen (varies with setup of group). May have less choice of consultants.
Student health service	Convenient location. Minimal cost.	Hours and scope of practice may be limited.
Emergicenter	Costs less than hospital emergency room. Open long hours. Convenient appointment times.	Costs more than private office. May not be ideal setup for follow-up care. When care is episodic, doctor does not get to know the patient as an individual.
Hospital emergency room	Open 24 hours a day. Able to handle serious emergencies. Sophisticated equipment available.	Highest cost. Nonemergency cases may not receive much attention. Follow-up care may be minimal. Care is episodic and less personal.
Hospital outpatient clinic	Fees may be reduced for individuals who cannot afford private care.	Patients may have to wait a long time to be seen. Tend to have high staff turnover so different doctors may be seen.
Ambulatory surgical facilities	Surgery costs less than it would in a hospital.	Unsuitable for major surgery.

Recognized Medical Specialties and Subspecialties

Administrative medicine Operation and management of organizations and institutions such as health departments, hospitals, clinics, and health care plans

Aerospace medicine Subspecialty of preventive medicine dealing with problems of aviation and space flight

Allergy and immunology Subspecialty of internal medicine

Anesthesiology Administration of drugs to prevent pain or to induce unconsciousness during surgical operations or diagnostic procedures

Cardiovascular disease (cardiology) Subspecialty of internal medicine that deals with the heart and blood vessels

Child psychiatry Subspecialty of psychiatry that deals with nervous and emotional problems of children

Colon and rectal surgery (proctology) Diagnosis and treatment of disorders of the lower digestive tract

Dermatology Diagnosis and treatment of skin diseases

Emergency medicine Diagnosis and treatment of emergencies

Endocrinology and metabolism Subspecialty of internal medicine that deals with glandular and metabolic disorders

Family practice General medical services for patients and their families

Forensic pathology Subspecialty of pathology that deals with medicine and the law

Gastroenterology Subspecialty of internal medicine that deals with disorders of the digestive tract

General surgery Surgery of parts of the body that are not in the domain of specific surgical specialties (some overlapping areas)

Head and neck (otolaryngology) Care of diseases of the head and neck except for those of the eyes or brain

Infectious disease Subspecialty of internal medicine

Internal medicine Diagnosis and nonsurgical treatment of internal organs of the body of adults

Neonatal-perinatal medicine Subspecialty of pediatrics that deals with disorders of newborn infants, including premature infants

Neurological surgery (neurosurgery) Diagnosis and surgical treatment of diseases of the brain, spinal cord, and nerves

Neurology Diagnosis and nonsurgical treatment of diseases of the brain, spinal cord, and nerves

Nuclear medicine Use of radioactive substances for diagnosis and treatment

Obstetrics and gynecology (ob/gyn) Care of pregnant women and treatment of disorders of the female reproductive system

Occupational medicine Subspecialty of preventive medicine that deals with the special physical and psychological risks in industry

Ophthalmology Medical and surgical care of the eyes, including the prescription of glasses

Orthopedic surgery (orthopedics) Care of diseases of the muscles and diseases, fractures, and deformities of the bones and joints

Pathology Examination and diagnosis of organs, tissues, body fluids, and excrement

Pediatrics Care of children from birth through adolescence

Pediatric allergy Subspecialty of pediatrics

Pediatric cardiology Subspecialty of pediatrics that deals with diseases of the heart

Pediatric hematology-oncology Subspecialty of pediatrics concerned with the treatment of blood disorders and cancers

Pediatric nephrology Subspecialty of pediatrics that deals with kidney disorders

Pediatric surgery Subspecialty of pediatrics

Physical medicine and rehabilitation (physiatry) Treatment of convalescent and physically handicapped patients

Plastic surgery Surgery to correct or repair deformed or mutilated parts of the body, or to improve facial or body features

Preventive medicine Prevention of disease through immunization, good health practice, and concern with environmental factors

Psychiatry Treatment of mental and emotional problems

Public health Subspecialty of preventive medicine that deals with promoting the general health of the community

Pulmonary disease Subspecialty of internal medicine that deals with diseases of the lungs

Radiology Use of radiation for the diagnosis and treatment of disease

Rheumatology Subspecialty of internal medicine that deals with arthritis and related disorders

Thoracic surgery Surgical treatment of the lungs, heart, and large blood vessels within the chest cavity

Urology Treatment of male sex organs and urinary tract and treatment of female urinary tract

SOURCE: *Consumer Health*, 1985.

Osteopaths Medical practitioners who have graduated from an osteopathic medical school. Osteopathy incorporates the theories and practices of scientific medicine but tends to focus on musculoskeletal problems.

Podiatrists Nonmedical practitioners whose practice is limited to the feet and legs.

Optometrists Nonmedical practitioners who primarily examine the eyes to detect vision problems and prescribe corrective lenses.

Chiropractic A system of health care based on the premise that misalignments of the vertebrae contribute to most diseases and ailments.

---

or surgical treatment. What they actually do depends on their training, their inclinations, and the available facilities. Because the scope of medicine is so vast, most physicians take additional training after graduation. Those choosing to become specialists take three or more years of hospital-based specialty training, after which they can become "board certified" by taking a stringent specialty examination. A few specialty boards require periodic recertification, to ensure updated skills and knowledge. To work in a hospital, doctors must apply for staff privileges, which are based on training and experience and are reviewed annually.

Exploring Your Emotions

Your knee has been bothering you for several weeks, possibly as a result of jogging. You have seen your family doctor, who recommended surgery. You want to get a second opinion, but are hesitant to alienate this old friend of your father's. How will you handle your feelings?

Osteopaths **Osteopaths** are independent practitioners who have received a D.O. (doctor of osteopathy) degree. Osteopathy was founded, more than a hundred years ago, on a belief that the main cause of disease was mechanical interference with nerve and blood supply, correctable by spinal manipulation. As medical science developed, osteopathy gradually incorporated all of its theories and practices. Today, osteopathic practice is virtually identical to medical practice except that osteopaths tend to have greater interest in musculoskeletal problems and manipulative therapy.

Exploring Your Emotions

Your small daughter has had repeated ear infections, and you have tried everything your pediatrician suggests, with no success in reducing their frequency. A friend shows you an advertisement for megavitamin therapy for childhood illnesses. You try it, and your daughter is now hospitalized from the toxic effects of excess Vitamin A. Who is responsible? What feelings do you have about the situation?

Podiatrists **Podiatrists** are independent practitioners whose care is limited to problems of feet and legs. They are not medical doctors but hold a D.P.M. (doctor of podiatric medicine) degree. The length of their training is similar to that of physicians but emphasizes problems of the feet and legs. Podiatrists can prescribe drugs and do minor surgery in their offices. Those who wish to do major foot surgery must secure hospital privileges.

Optometrists **Optometrists** are independent practitioners who are trained to examine the eyes and related structures to detect vision problems, eye diseases, and other problems. They are not physicians but hold an O.D. (doctor of optometry) degree. Most states allow them to use drugs for diagnostic purposes. If they detect eye disease, they are expected to refer the patient to an appropriate physician. However, a few states permit them to treat minor ailments.

Dentists Dentists form another group of practitioners who can practice without medical supervision. They hold either a D.D.S. (doctor of dental surgery) or D.M.D. (doctor of medical dentistry) degree. Those who wish to become specialists complete two or more years of specialty training after graduation from dental school. Dentists are permitted to perform certain types of surgery and to prescribe a limited number of drugs within the scope of their training.

Alternative Health Care

This section discusses seven systems of diagnosis and treatment that are based on theories not accepted by the scientific community: chiropractic, applied kinesiology, homeopathy, iridology, acupuncture, reflexology, and naturopathy. Chiropractic is unique among these approaches because its practitioners are licensed in all fifty states and most of its schools are accredited by a recognized agency. A few states license naturopaths and nonmedical acupuncturists. Three states have separate boards for licensing physicians as homeopaths. In most states, unlicensed individuals who use the methods described in this section could be convicted of practicing medicine without a license. But few are ever prosecuted.

The fact that an approach is based on unorthodox ideas does not mean that its practitioners never help people. People whose symptoms are stress related often lose these

How to Spot a Quack

The many published lists of tips on how to spot a quack all seem to include these seven factors:

1. *Secrecy.* The machine or product has been developed by a special formula. Purchasers of the Drown radiotherapeutic device had to promise to have their machines repaired only at the Drown offices. The actual circuit was so simple that a junior high school science student would have recognized its simplicity.

2. *Cure.* While orthodox medicine uses the term *cure* guardedly, the quack sometimes guarantees a cure for many or all diseases.

3. *Spurious degrees.* The quack's offices are covered with degrees that the unsuspecting victim believes are legitimate indications of special skills in medicine.

4. *Scare tactics.* The quack speaks of horrible medical consequences if treatment is delayed for as much as an hour. Be wary of signing any contracts for a specified number of treatments. Such contracts are a sure sign of quackery. Any time speed is emphasized, the patient should become immediately suspicious.

5. *Testimonials.* "Case histories" depicting a long line of successes appear as advertisements, as planted stories in newspapers, or on television talk shows. Talk show hosts like to interview quacks because they tend to "liven" things up. This gives the quack instant exposure to millions of people. There is little incentive for giving equal time to scientists to refute the quack's claims because the scientist must be more cautious in his or her statements and is therefore a less entertaining figure.

6. *Medical conspiracy.* Quacks are quick to claim that they are being persecuted by the medical community because their cures will cut into the incomes doctors make "by keeping people sick." They are also quick to state publicly that they are willing to make their substances, machines, or other products available for testing, but the material is rarely delivered.

7. *Law suits.* Many quacks are legally belligerent and travel with an entourage of lawyers. Whenever someone challenges the quack's claims, he or she threatens to sue.

symptoms following treatment by an unorthodox health provider. Moreover, many of the practitioners described here persuade patients to develop healthier living habits. Also, some refer patients who need it for appropriate medical care. However, reliance on unorthodox methods can delay effective care. Further, there may be financial exploitation.

Some of the health providers described in this section refer to themselves as "holistic" (or "wholistic"), meaning that they treat the whole patient, giving attention to emotions and lifestyle as well as physical problems. The best medical doctors have always practiced in this manner. The holistic label is used by a few scientific practitioners who operate wellness clinics. But most holistic practitioners use a wide variety of unscientific methods of diagnosis and treatment, including high doses of vitamins.

Chiropractic **Chiropractic** is based on the beliefs of Daniel David Palmer, who concluded in 1895 that the main cause of disease is misplaced spinal bones. He theorized that subluxations (partial dislocations) of spinal vertebrae cause disease by interfering with the flow of nerve energy from the brain to the rest of the body, and that spinal adjustments can restore the vertebrae to their proper places, enabling the body to heal itself.

Chiropractors today can be classified into two main groups, "mixers" and "straights." Mixers, the larger group, acknowledge that germs, hormones, and other factors play a role in disease but regard mechanical disturbances of the spine as the major underlying cause. In addition to manipulation, mixers use physical therapy methods and may prescribe food supplements. Straights still cling to Palmer's original doctrines and tend to confine themselves to manual manipulation of the spine. Chiropractors are not licensed to prescribe drugs or perform surgery. A

Exploring Your Emotions

Because of arthritis pain your grandfather has been wearing a copper bracelet for about six months and has stopped his medication. How do you feel about this and how will you handle your feelings?

small number of chiropractors completely reject Palmer's theories and limit their practice to musculoskeletal disorders that have been medically diagnosed.

Applied Kinesiology **Applied kinesiology** is based on the premise that every organ dysfunction is accompanied by a specific weak muscle. Its proponents also believe that nutritional deficiencies, allergies, and other adverse reactions to food substances can be detected by placing substances in the mouth so that the patient salivates. "Good" substances will lead to increased strength in specific muscles, whereas "bad" substances will cause specific weaknesses. Treatment of muscles diagnosed as "weak" may include special diets, food supplements, acupressure, and/or spinal manipulation. These concepts do not conform to accepted scientific beliefs about the nature of health and disease, and critics believe that any apparent beneficial results are the result of patient suggestibility.

Homeopathy **Homeopathy** is based on the theories of Samuel Hahnemann (1755–1843), a German physician. Hahnemann was justifiably alarmed about bloodletting, leeching, purging, and other medical procedures of his day that did far more harm than good. He was also critical of medications such as calomel (mercurous chloride), which was given in doses that caused mercury poisoning. Instead, he proposed his "law of similars"—that the symptoms of disease can be cured by substances that produce similar symptoms in healthy people. The word *homeopathy* is derived from the Greek words *homeo* ("similar") and *pathos* ("suffering" or "disease").

Hahnemann believed that diseases represent a disturbance in the body's ability to heal itself and that only a small stimulus is needed to foster the healing process. After experimenting on himself and others, he concluded that the smaller the dose, the more powerful the effect—just the opposite of what pharmacologists believe today.

As scientific drug use developed, homeopathy declined sharply, particularly in America, where its schools either closed or converted to modern methods. But a few hundred modern-trained physicians have kept the practice alive in this country by taking courses here or abroad or by training with a practicing homeopath.

Homeopathic remedies were recognized as drugs by the 1938 amendment to the Federal Food, Drug and Cosmetic Act. They can be obtained from practitioners and are also available without a prescription from health food stores, pharmacies, and manufacturers. These products appeal primarily to people who are afraid of doctors or of taking more potent drugs.

Iridology **Iridology** was devised more than a hundred years ago by Ignatz von Peczely, a Hungarian physician. It is based on the belief that each area of the body is represented by a corresponding area in the iris of the eye (the colored area surrounding the pupil). It is claimed that states of health and disease can be diagnosed from the color, texture, and location of various pigment flecks in the eye. According to a leading proponent, "Nature has provided us with a miniature television screen showing the most remote portions of the body by way of nerve reflex responses." Practitioners claim to diagnose imbalances that can be treated with vitamins, minerals, herbs, and similar products.

Iridologists use elaborate charts that indicate where various organs are represented in the eye. As the American Medical Association Council on Scientific Affairs has noted, these charts are similar in concept to those used years ago in phrenology, the pseudoscience that related protuberances of the skull to the mental faculties and character of the individual. Regarding iridology's appeal, the council remarked, "Iridology does offer the dual attraction of simplicity and mystery without the inconvenience, and sometimes positive discomfort, that often accompanies diagnostic medical procedures; nevertheless, iridology has not yet been established as having any merit as a diagnostic technique." Of course, medical doctors can diagnose a few conditions by examining the interior of the eye with an opthalmoscope, but that is not what iridologists do.

Acupuncture **Acupuncture** is a technique that began in Stone Age China. It consists of the insertion of needles into the skin, or muscles or tendons beneath, as one or more "acupuncture points." These points, said to represent various internal organs, are generally located along meridians on the surface of the body. Good health is said to be produced by a harmonious mixture of yin and yang, the fundamental activities characteristic of the universe, which combine to form the life force (*Ch'i*). Illness is said to occur when the flow of *Ch'i* is imbalanced. Proponents claim that stimulation of acupuncture points can balance yin and yang so that internal organs can return to normal function. Similar claims are made for **acupressure (Shiatsu)** where no needles are used.

Acupuncture defines the body according to systems that have no relation to established facts about body physiology. The systems are said to be affected by color, weather, emotion, and other factors. Meridians and acupuncture points on the surface of the body cannot actually be seen or measured. They are part of the mystical ancient Chinese way of looking at the body, health, disease, and nature.

Acupuncture works by suggestion, somewhat like hypnosis, and can also trigger release of the body's own morphine-like drugs (endorphins). Either of these mechanisms may produce temporary pain relief, but there is no evidence that acupuncture can affect the course of any physical illness. The American Medical Association Council on Scientific Affairs recommends that acupuncture for

Applied kinesiology A treatment method based on the theory that organ dysfunction is accompanied by muscle weakness that may be correctable by nutritional methods.

Homeopathy A treatment method based on the theory that tiny doses of certain substances can exert powerful effects within the body.

Iridology A diagnostic method based on the theory that each area of the body is represented by a corresponding area in the eye.

Acupuncture A technique based on the theory that insertion of needles into points on the skin can restore health.

Acupressure (Shiatsu) A technique based on the theory that pressing on various body parts can restore health.

Reflexology A treatment method based on the theory that pressing on certain areas of the hands or feet can help relieve pain and remove the underlying cause of disease in other parts of the body.

Naturopathy A treatment approach based on the belief that the basic cause of disease is violation of nature's laws.

---

pain relief be regarded as experimental and performed only in medical research settings.

Reflexology **Reflexology**, also known as "zone therapy," is based on the theory that pressing on certain areas of the hands or feet can help relieve pain and remove the underlying cause of disease in other parts of the body. Proponents claim that (1) the body is divided into ten zones that begin or end in the hands and feet; (2) each organ or part of the body is represented by an area on the hands and feet; (3) the practitioner can diagnose abnormalities by feeling the feet; (4) massaging or pressing each area can stimulate the flow of energy, blood, nutrients, and nerve impulses to the corresponding body zone; and (5) reflexology has been effective against anemia, arthritis, asthma, cataracts, deafness, diabetes, heart disease, high blood pressure, kidney disease, and many other health problems.

Naturopathy **Naturopathy** is a treatment approach based on the belief that the cause of disease is the violation of nature's laws. Naturopaths believe that diseases are the body's effort to purify itself, and that cures result from increasing the patient's vital force by ridding the body of toxins. Naturopathic treatment can include "natural food" diets, vitamins, herbs, tissue minerals, cell salts, manipulation, massage, remedial exercise, diathermy, colonic enemas, acupuncture, reflexology, hypnotherapy, and homeopathy. Radiation may be used for diagnosis but not for treatment. Drugs are forbidden except for compounds that are components of body tissues. Naturopaths, like many chiropractors, believe that virtually all diseases are within the scope of their practice.

Faith Healing Beliefs that prayer and other rituals can heal have existed since ancient times. Moreover, the idea accepted by ancient practitioners that demons cause disease is prevalent today among segments of the American public. In the United States, several religions include faith healing as part of their dogma, and many evangelistic healers have attracted large followings.

Few scientific attempts have been made to evaluate faith healing. Although testimonials abound, it is difficult and time consuming to investigate such claims. Some cures attributed to faith healing are undoubtedly cases of spontaneous remission (including some in which the original diagnosis was wrong).

Probably the most extensive study of faith healing was made by William A. Nolen, M.D., a Litchfield, Minnesota, surgeon who spent two years investigating various practitioners and evaluating their results. Among other things, Dr. Nolen was able to record the names of twenty-five people who were "miraculously healed" by Kathryn Kuhlman at a service in Minneapolis. When he followed up on these cases, he found that not one had been helped.

During the past two years, several prominent faith healers have been exposed as outright frauds by magician James Randi and associates. In several instances, people capable of walking had been placed in wheelchairs before the performance so that the healer could help "cripples" walk. In another case, the investigators found that the healer was not getting information about the ailments of members of his audiences from God, as he claimed, but from radio transmissions from his wife backstage.

Health Insurance

Health insurance enables people to budget in advance for health care costs that may otherwise be unpredictable and ruinously high. Hospital care costs hundreds of dollars a day, and surgical fees can cost thousands. So health insurance is important for almost everyone.

Types of Policies There are three basic types of health insurance coverage: basic, major medical, and comprehensive.

Exploring Your Emotions

You have decided to get married the day after you graduate from college. Your in-laws say that they will pay your health insurance premiums for one year after the marriage, or until both of you have insurance through your job(s). How do you feel about this wedding gift?

Basic protection includes expenses for hospital, surgical, and medical care. Hospital benefits may provide payment of a specific amount for a specified number of days. Or full charges may be paid for daily room, board, routine nursing services, and intensive care up to a maximum number of days. Coverage may also be provided for various inpatient and outpatient services such as laboratory tests, X-ray films, medications, and physical therapy. Visits to doctors' offices are not usually covered.

Major medical insurance (also called "extended benefit" or "catastrophic coverage") is designed to help protect against medical expenses resulting from prolonged illness or serious injury. These contracts generally include a deductible clause, a co-insurance provision, high maximum limits, and coverage of a broad spectrum of services not included under basic coverage. Typically they pay 80 percent of covered services after a $100 deductible. Psychiatric benefits are usually more limited than others.

Comprehensive major medical insurance policies integrate basic and major medical insurance into one program.

Health insurance policies may be sold to groups or individuals. Group policies generally offer more coverage and cost less than individual policies. Most people are insured through a group policy obtained through their place of employment. Because the extent and type of covered services vary widely from contract to contract, policies should be read carefully to understand what protection they provide.

Government Programs In many states, certain categories of indigent people (people who have no money) are eligible for **Medicaid**, a state-run, federally subsidized program that covers a broad spectrum of health care services.

Individuals who are chronically disabled or have reached age 65 are eligible for **Medicare**, a federal program comprising two parts. Part A provides hospital insurance financed through Social Security taxes. Part B helps pay for medical services and is financed through monthly premiums paid by those who wish to subscribe. Private insurance companies also sell "medigap" policies to supplement Medicare coverage.

Under Medicare, a doctor who "accepts assignment" may not bill the patient for the difference between the usual fee and the amount the patient pays (except for amounts that involve deductibles and co-insurance).

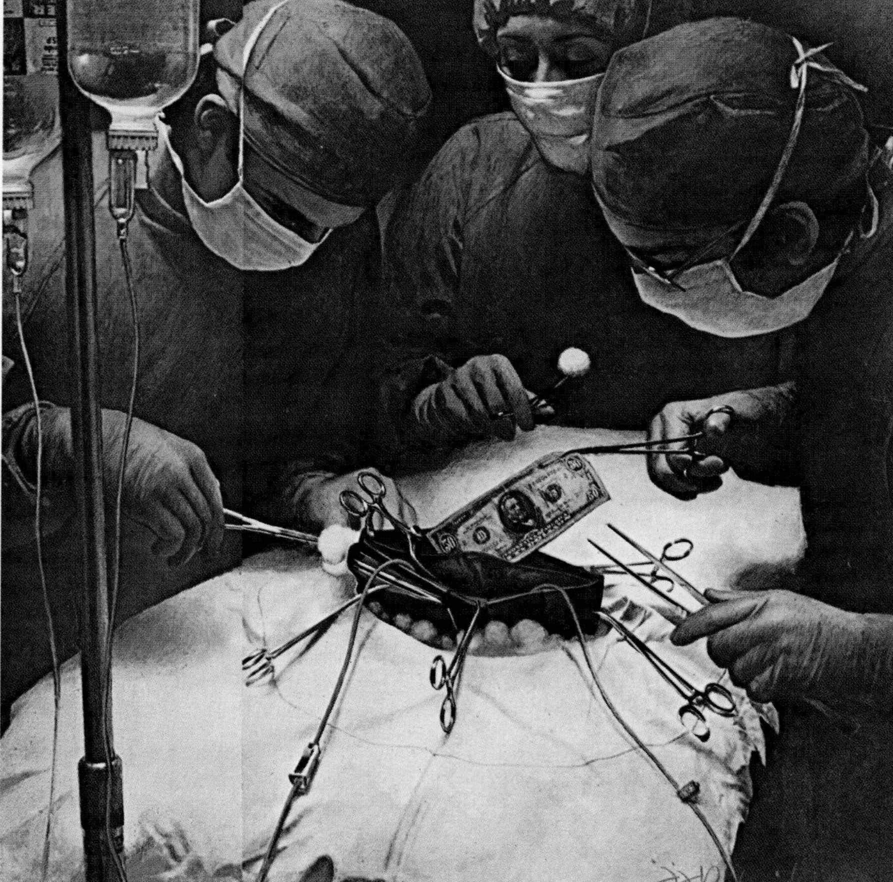

Exploring Your Emotions

How do you feel about the financial aspects of health care? Do you feel doctors are paid too much? Do you feel surgery is often done for financial gain rather than patient gain? How do you express your feelings?

Glossary of Health Insurance Terms

Because health insurance policies are legal contracts, they use precise legal language. Some of these terms appear in all policies, while others appear just in some. Understanding them will help you figure out how a policy works and what it actually covers.

Assignment of benefits By signing a form (usually the insurance claim form), you authorize the insurance company to pay the doctor directly. Otherwise payment must be made directly to you. Most doctors will ask you to sign the form if you don't want to pay your bill before the insurance company pays its share. Under Medicare, a doctor who "accepts assignment" may not bill the patient for the difference between the usual fee and the amount the patient pays (except for amounts that involve deductibles and co-insurance).

Basic protection Insurance that includes hospital, surgical, and medical care.

Capitation Payment to health providers according to number of patients they agree to serve rather than amount of service rendered.

Co-insurance This is an arrangement whereby you and the insurance company share costs. Typically, the insurer pays 75 to 85 percent of covered costs and you pay the rest. Some policies set an upper limit to co-insurance expense, after which the company pays all additional charges.

Comprehensive major medical insurance Policies that integrate basic and major medical insurance into one program.

Conversion privilege A provision that enables those insured by group contracts to obtain an individual policy under various circumstances, such as leaving the job that provided the group coverage.

Coordination of benefits A term that prohibits you from collecting identical benefits from two or more policies, thereby profiting when you are ill. After the primary company pays, other companies will calculate their coverage of the remainder. All group policies contain a coordination clause, but most individual policies do not.

Deductible The amount you must pay before the insurance company starts paying.

Endorsement or rider An attachment to the basic insurance policy that changes its coverage.

Exclusions Specified conditions or circumstances for which the policy does not provide benefits.

Grace period The number of days that you may delay payment of your premium without losing your insurance.

Guaranteed renewability A policy where the company agrees to continue insuring you up to a certain age (or for life) as long as you pay the premium. Under this provision, the premium structure cannot be raised unless it is raised for all members of a group or class of insured, such as all people living in your state with the same kind of policy.

Health maintenance organization (HMO) A prepaid health plan in which patients receive health care from designated providers.

Inpatient services Services received while hospitalized.

Major medical insurance Insurance designed to help protect against medical expenses resulting from prolonged illness or serious injury.

Medicaid Federally subsidized, state-run plan of health care for indigent people.

Medicare Federal health insurance program for people 65 or older and for certain disabled younger people.

Notice of claim Written notice the company must receive when a claim exists. Typically it must be received within twenty days or as soon thereafter as reasonably possible.

Outpatient services Services obtained at a hospital by people who are not confined to the hospital.

Participating physician A physician who agrees to abide by the rules of a plan in return for direct payment by the insurance company. The agreement includes acceptance of a fixed fee schedule, a monthly fee per eligible patient, or other fee limitation.

Pre-existing condition A health problem you had before becoming insured. Some policies exclude these conditions, while others do not.

Preferred provider organization (PPO) A prepaid insurance plan in which providers agree to deliver services for discounted fees. Patients can go to any provider, but using nonparticipating providers results in higher cost to the patient.

Provider Any source of health care services, such as a hospital, doctor, pharmacist, or laboratory.

Reasonable charge The amount a company will pay for a given service based on what most providers charge for it.

Waiting period A specified time between issuance of a policy and coverage of certain conditions. Typically there are waiting periods for pre-existing conditions and maternity benefits.

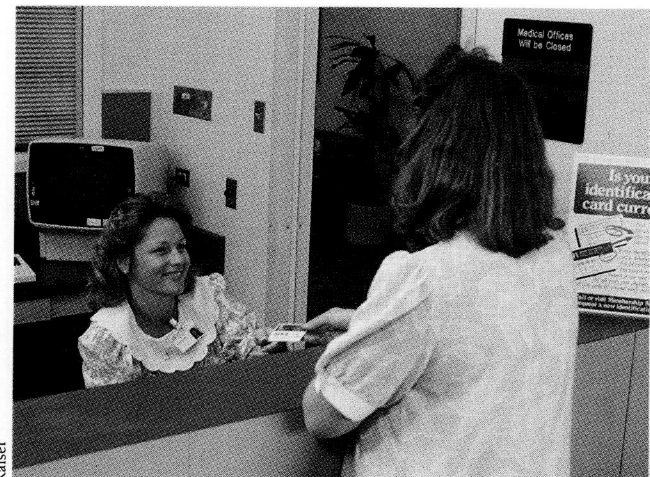

Kaiser

Prepaid Group Plans Most insurance companies permit the policyholder complete freedom to decide where to obtain treatment. Because health care costs have been rising, insurance companies, hospitals, and private groups have been marketing plans aimed at controlling these costs. The doctors in these plans must agree to certain cost controls, and the patients are restricted in their choice of doctors.

Health maintenance organizations (HMOs) are comprehensive programs in which doctors agree to accept a monthly fee (**capitation**) per patient or to charge for actual services rendered according to a fee schedule. Usually the agreed fees are lower than the doctor's standard fee. Then, if the plan has made a profit, a portion of the profit will be shared with the participating doctors. This type of plan is designed to encourage doctors to avoid unnecessary services. The doctors belonging to the HMO may be located in their own offices or at a central facility where the doctors are salaried. Under HMO programs, patients can choose their primary physician from a list of participating doctors, and need a referral by the primary physician for services by specialists to be covered.

Preferred provider organizations (PPOs) are programs in which participating doctors and hospitals agree to accept fixed fees that are usually 15 to 20 percent less than their usual fees. Patients can go to any provider, but using nonparticipating providers results in considerably higher cost to the patient.

Choosing a Policy Choosing health insurance can be complicated because there are many types of plans and contracts can vary greatly from company to company and even within the same company. Probably the best first step in choosing a suitable plan is to see whether you can get group coverage through work or membership in an organization. If you work for a large company, several plans may be available. If no group coverage is available, contact Blue Cross/Blue Shield and agents for several other insurance companies. After discussing your needs with them, get a copy of each policy that sounds suitable, read them carefully, and be sure you understand what they say. If you want both basic and major medical coverage, it is often best to get both from the same company to avoid gaps in coverage. However, your aim should be to insure mainly against the most serious types of losses. In the long run, it is more economical to absorb the cost of minor medical expenses as part of your overall budget. "Dread disease" policies that cover only one disease, such as cancer, are inadvisable, and other types of overlapping policies should also be avoided. Mail-order policies that pay a daily amount generally have low limits and a waiting period, which make them unsuitable for basic coverage.

Asking the following questions may help you evaluate prospective policies:

- What services are covered?
  - Inpatient hospital costs
  - Surgical costs, including anesthesia
  - Inpatient medical services
  - Doctors' office visits
  - X-ray examinations
  - Outpatient diagnostic tests
  - Medications
  - Psychiatric treatment
  - Physical therapy
  - Maternity fees
  - Private-duty nursing
  - Skilled nursing home care
- Which of these services am I most likely to need?
- Are there exclusions for any pre-existing conditions I have?
- How do the various policies compare in cost?
- Are the deductible and co-insurance provisions suitable for me?
- Are the maximum limits high enough?
- Will I be able to see the doctors I prefer?
- Does my present doctor participate?

Consumer Protection Agencies

Legal protection against health frauds and quackery is based on a framework of federal and state laws. Professional and voluntary agencies can sometimes apply pressure to wrongdoers. Educational information is available from many sources.

Federal Agencies The U.S. Food and Drug Administration (FDA) has jurisdiction over advertising of prescription drug products and labeling of nonprescription products and health devices. It is illegal to market a product without FDA approval (which usually means that the agency considers it safe and effective). When the FDA learns that a product is being marketed with unapproved claims, it can issue a warning letter, seize the product, or obtain an injunction. Criminal prosecution is also possible, but it is rarely done.

The FDA has a very active public educational program. Its magazine, *FDA Consumer,* provides excellent coverage of health, nutrition, and safety issues. Its Office of Consumer Affairs distributes pamphlets, sponsors talks and conferences, and answers individual inquiries. Its field offices, located in major cities throughout the country, distribute educational materials, answer inquiries, and provide speakers.

The Federal Trade Commission (FTC) has jurisdiction over interstate advertising of all health products and services except for prescription drugs. However, it rarely takes action against licensed health practitioners because they are subject to supervision by state licensing boards. When the FTC becomes aware of wrongdoing, it can obtain a cease-and-desist order, which, if violated, can trigger penalties up to $10,000 a day for each violation.

The U.S. Postal Service has jurisdiction over the sale of products or services by mail. When misleading mail-order promotions are detected, the agency can seek voluntary discontinuation or obtain administrative permission to intercept orders and return them to the senders. After a scheme has been stopped, a promoter who resumes similar activity can be fined up to $10,000 per day.

Although actions by federal agencies can be extremely

Exploring Your Emotions

What conflicting feelings are suggested by the term "sterile environment"? How would you feel if you were a "bubble child," a child permanently encased in a sterile suit to ward off infection that might overpower a defective immune system?

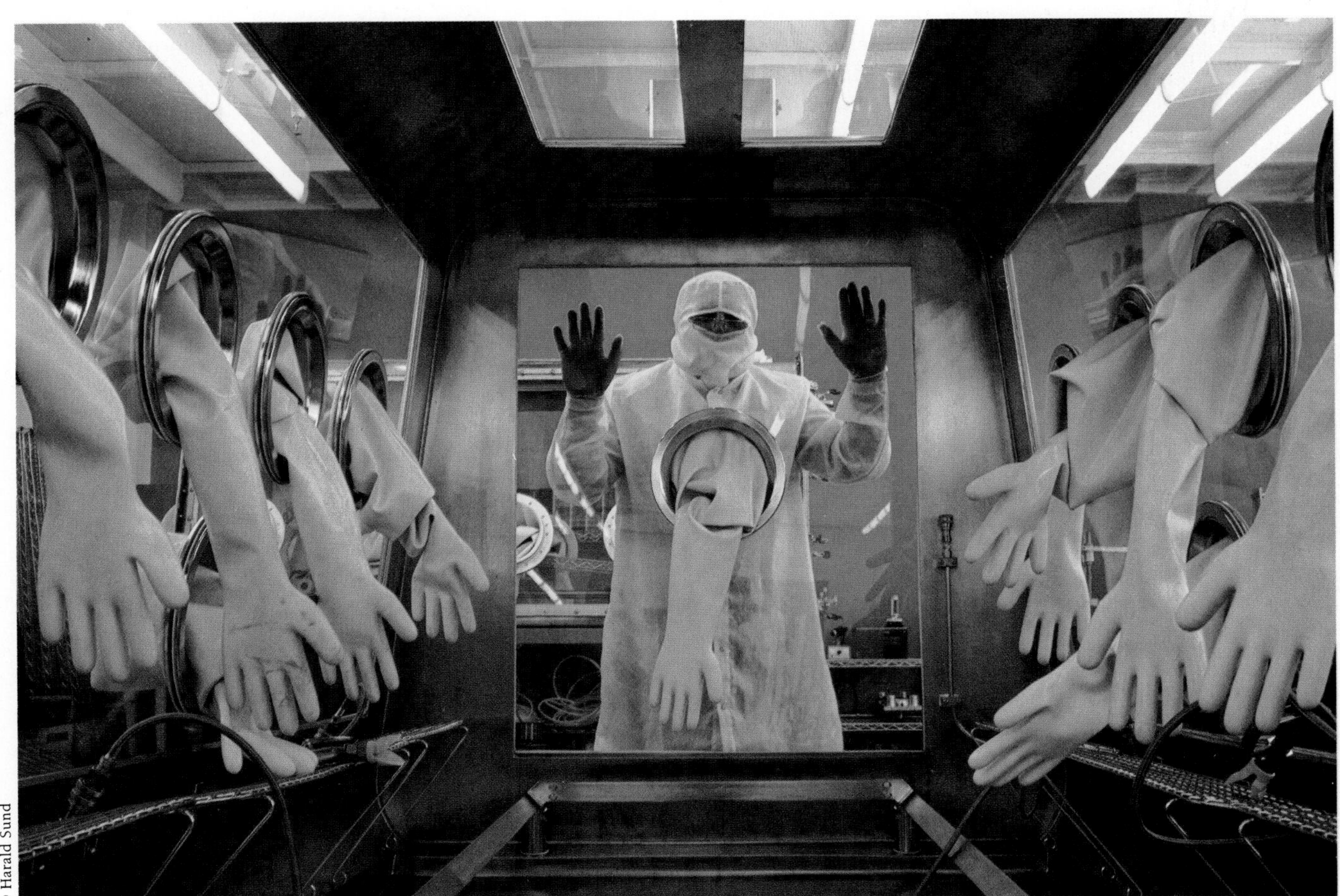

Patient's Bill of Rights

The American Hospital Association presents a Patient's Bill of Rights with the expectation that observance of these rights will contribute to more effective patient care and greater satisfaction for the patient, the physician, and the hospital organization. Further, the Association presents these rights in the expectation that they will be supported by the hospital on behalf of its patients, as an integral part of the healing process. It is recognized that a personal relationship between the physician and the patient is essential for the provision of proper medical care. The traditional physician-patient relationship takes on a new dimension when care is rendered within an organizational structure. Legal precedent has established that the institution itself also has a responsibility to the patient. It is in recognition of these factors that these rights are affirmed.

1. The patient has the right to considerate and respectful care.

2. The patient has the right to obtain from his [or her] physician complete current information concerning his diagnosis, treatment, and prognosis in terms the patient can be reasonably expected to understand. When it is not medically advisable to give such information to the patient, the information should be made available to an appropriate person in his behalf. He has the right to know by name the physician responsible for coordinating his care.

3. The patient has the right to receive from his physician information necessary to give informed consent prior to the start of any procedure and/or treatment. Except in emergencies, such information for informed consent should include but not necessarily be limited to the specific procedure and/or treatment, the medically significant risks involved, and the probable duration of incapacitation. Where medically significant alternatives for care or treatment exist, or when the patient requests information concerning the medical alternatives, the patient has the right to such information. The patient also has the right to know the name of the person responsible for the procedures and/or treatment.

4. The patient has the right to refuse treatment to the extent permitted by law, and to be informed of the medical consequences of his action.

5. The patient has the right to every consideration of his privacy concerning his own medical care program. Case discussion, consultation, examination, and treatment are confidential and should be conducted discreetly. Those not directly involved in his care must have the permission of the patient to be present.

powerful and put illegal operators out of business, federal enforcement has serious limitations. Some illegal schemes are never detected, while others are detected long after their promoter has done considerable harm. In some cases, offenders can remain in business for years by appealing to federal courts. Most important, the number of illegal schemes is so great that federal agencies do not have sufficient resources to act against all they detect.

State and Local Agencies Licensed practitioners are regulated by state boards that can conduct investigations into alleged wrongdoing. When an offense takes place, the practitioner can be ordered to take corrective action and can be placed on probation or have his or her license suspended or revoked.

State attorneys general have jurisdiction over illegal health activities such as illegal representations by unlicensed practitioners, marketing of unapproved drugs, and false advertising. In cases involving individual victims, local district attorneys may have primary jurisdiction.

The extent to which individual states protect their residents from quackery and health fraud depends on the strength of their laws and the resources allotted to the problem. While some states conduct extensive investigations and prosecute many promoters of quackery, others do virtually nothing.

Professional and Voluntary Organizations Professional groups such as state and local medical societies can often help individuals check the reputation of practitioners or products. These groups can also investigate

6. The patient has the right to expect that all communications and records pertaining to his care should be treated as confidential.

7. The patient has the right to expect that within its capacity a hospital must make reasonable response to the request of a patient for services. The hospital must provide evaluation, service, and/or referral as indicated by the urgency of the case. When medically permissible, a patient may be transferred to another facility only after he has received complete information and explanation concerning the needs for and alternatives to such a transfer. The institution to which the patient is to be transferred must first have accepted the patient for transfer.

8. The patient has the right to obtain information as to any relationship of his hospital to other health care and educational institutions insofar as his care is concerned. The patient has the right to obtain information as to the existence of any professional relationships among individuals, by name, who are treating him.

9. The patient has the right to be advised if the hospital proposes to engage in or perform human experimentation affecting his care or treatment. The patient has the right to refuse to participate in such research projects.

10. The patient has the right to expect reasonable continuity of care. He has the right to know in advance what appointment times and physicians are available and where. The patient has the right to expect that the hospital will provide a mechanism whereby he is informed by his physician or a delegate of the physician of the patient's continuing health care requirements following discharge.

11. The patient has the right to examine and receive an explanation of his bill regardless of the source of payment.

12. The patient has the right to know what hospital rules and regulations apply to his conduct as a patient.

No catalogue of rights can guarantee for the patient the kind of treatment he has a right to expect. A hospital has many functions to perform, including the prevention and treatment of disease, the education of both health professionals and patients, and the conduct of clinical research. All these activities must be conducted with an overriding concern for the patient, and, above all, the recognition of his dignity as a human being. Success in achieving this recognition assures success in the defense of the rights of the patient.

American Hospital Association

accusations of unethical and unprofessional conduct and can sometimes persuade wrongdoers to take corrective action. Professional societies can reprimand or expel members. Hospital officials can reduce, suspend, or revoke a practitioner's privileges at their particular hospital. But practitioners who neither belong to a professional group nor work in a hospital are unlikely to be affected by the disciplinary efforts of these organizations.

Local Better Business Bureaus (BBB's) investigate unethical business practices but rarely get involved in disputes involving licensed practitioners. The National Council of Better Business Bureaus investigates and publishes occasional reports about quack products and their promotion. BBB's National Advertising Division investigates questionable product advertising and can sometimes persuade offending advertisers to stop.

The National Council Against Health Fraud, P.O. Box 1276, Loma Linda, CA 92354, is a membership organization of more than 2,000 persons concerned about quackery and health frauds. It sponsors meetings, publishes a newsletter and position papers, distributes other publications, and operates an information clearinghouse for individuals, government agencies and media representatives. Information and advice are also available from many local, state, and national professional and voluntary organizations.

Table 16-2 summarizes where to obtain information or complain about questionable health matters. Remember that people who make appropriate complaints may not only help themselves, but may also help to protect others.

Table 16-2 Where to Complain or Seek Help

Problem	Agencies to Contact
False advertising	Bureau of Consumer Protection, Federal Trade Commission, Washington, DC 20580 National Advertising Division, National Council of Better Business Bureaus, 845 Third Avenue, New York, NY 10022 Editor or station manager of media outlet where ad appeared
Product marketed with false or exaggerated claims	Health Fraud Branch, Food and Drug Administration, 5600 Fishers Lane, Rockville, MD 20857 Regional FDA office State health department Congressional representatives
Phony mail-order promotion	Chief Postal Inspector, U.S. Postal Service, Washington, DC 20260 Editor or station manager of media outlet where ad appeared
Improper treatment by licensed practitioner	Local medical society (if member) Local hospital (if staff member) State licensing board
Improper treatment by unlicensed individual	Local district attorney State attorney general Local newspaper or TV station
Advice needed about questionable product or service	National Council Against Health Fraud, Inc., P.O. Box 1276, Loma Linda, CA 92354 Local, state, or national professional groups

Take Action

We hope that your answers to the Exploring Your Emotions in this chapter and your placement level on the Awareness Ladder will encourage you to begin and maintain a process of self-exploration and self-discovery. Reflect on the entire chapter's contents and ask yourself how each point relates to your own life. Then take action:

1. Visit the student health center or other health care facility, and write a brief evaluation of the quality and kinds of services available. Consider such things as hours, waiting time, health literature, scope of services, availability of specialists, and so forth. Give your evaluation to the manager or other appropriate official, or to the student newspaper.

2. Talk to a hospital official to get some idea of hospital care costs in your community. Then find out what health insurance programs are available for college students. Which one(s) would you recommend? Which one(s) would you not recommend?

3. Talk to one or more "alternative" practitioners about their work. Ask what training they have, what conditions they treat most often, how they make diagnoses, what treatments they give, and whether they have any pamphlets you can inspect. List the questions you have about these practices, and discuss the questions in class. Where would you go to find answers that satisfy you?

Selected References

AMA Council on Scientific Affairs. 1982. *Reports of the Council 1981*. Chicago: American Medical Association.

Barrett, S., ed. 1980. *The Health Robbers—How to Protect Your Money and Your Life,* 2nd ed. Philadelphia: Stickley.

Nolen, W. A. 1974. *Healing: A Doctor in Search of a Miracle*. New York: Random House.

Stalker, D., and C. Glymour, eds. 1985. *Examining Holistic Medicine*. Buffalo, N.Y.: Prometheus Books.

Recommended Readings

Brody, J. 1982. *Jane Brody's Guide to Personal Health*. New York: Times Books.
A guide to health strategy based on the author's newspaper columns.

Butler, K., and L. Rayner. 1985. *The Best Medicine: The Complete Health and Preventive Medicine Handbook*. San Francisco: Harper & Row.
A comprehensive discussion of disease prevention and treatment plus tips on avoiding quackery.

Cornacchia, H., and S. Barrett. 1985. *Consumer Health—A Guide to Intelligent Decisions*. St. Louis: Times Mirror/Mosby.
A comprehensive guide to the health marketplace.

Inglis, B., and R. West. 1983. *The Alternative Health Guide*. New York: Knopf.
Seventy "alternative" therapies from the viewpoint of two proponents.

Jarvis, W. T. *Quackery and You*. 1985. Washington, D.C.: Review and Herald Publishing Association.
A 32-page booklet of basic facts about quackery.

Chapter 17

Contents

Rate Yourself

Your Cardiovascular Health Behavior Read the following statements carefully. Choose the one in each section that best describes you at this moment and circle its number. When you have chosen one statement for each section, add the numbers and record your total score. Find your position on the Wellness Ladder.

5 Keeps blood pressure and cholesterol level normal
4 Has had blood pressure and cholesterol level checked within the last year
3 Does not know blood pressure or cholesterol level
2 Has elevated or unknown blood pressure or cholesterol level
1 Has clearly elevated blood pressure and cholesterol level

5 Avoids smoking and, in many ways, discourages others' smoking
4 Avoids smoking, no ashtrays in house
3 Avoids smoking
2 Smokes occasionally and is indifferent to others' smoking
1 Smokes regularly and offers cigarettes to others

5 Eats little or no red meat, very moderate on other higher-fat foods
4 Eats little ice cream, french fries, chocolate, rich cakes
3 Eats few eggs, some fatty foods almost daily
2 Eats eggs and fat-rich foods almost daily
1 Eats eggs, red meats, fat-rich desserts daily

5 Often feels relaxed, very seldom feels angry, seldom feels time urgent and competitive
4 Feels somewhat relaxed, occasionally angry, seldom hurried
3 Occasionally feels relaxed, sometimes angry, and time urgent
2 Often angry, feels competitive, in a hurry
1 Gets angry almost daily, extremely competitive, time urgent

5 Does aerobic exercise three to four times a week, keeps body weight normal with low body fat
4 Exercises once a week, keeps normal body weight
3 Exercises two to three times a month, body weight normal
2 Seldom exercises, has body weight clearly above normal
1 Does little or no aerobic exercise and is definitely overweight or obese.

Total Score ______

Cardiovascular Health

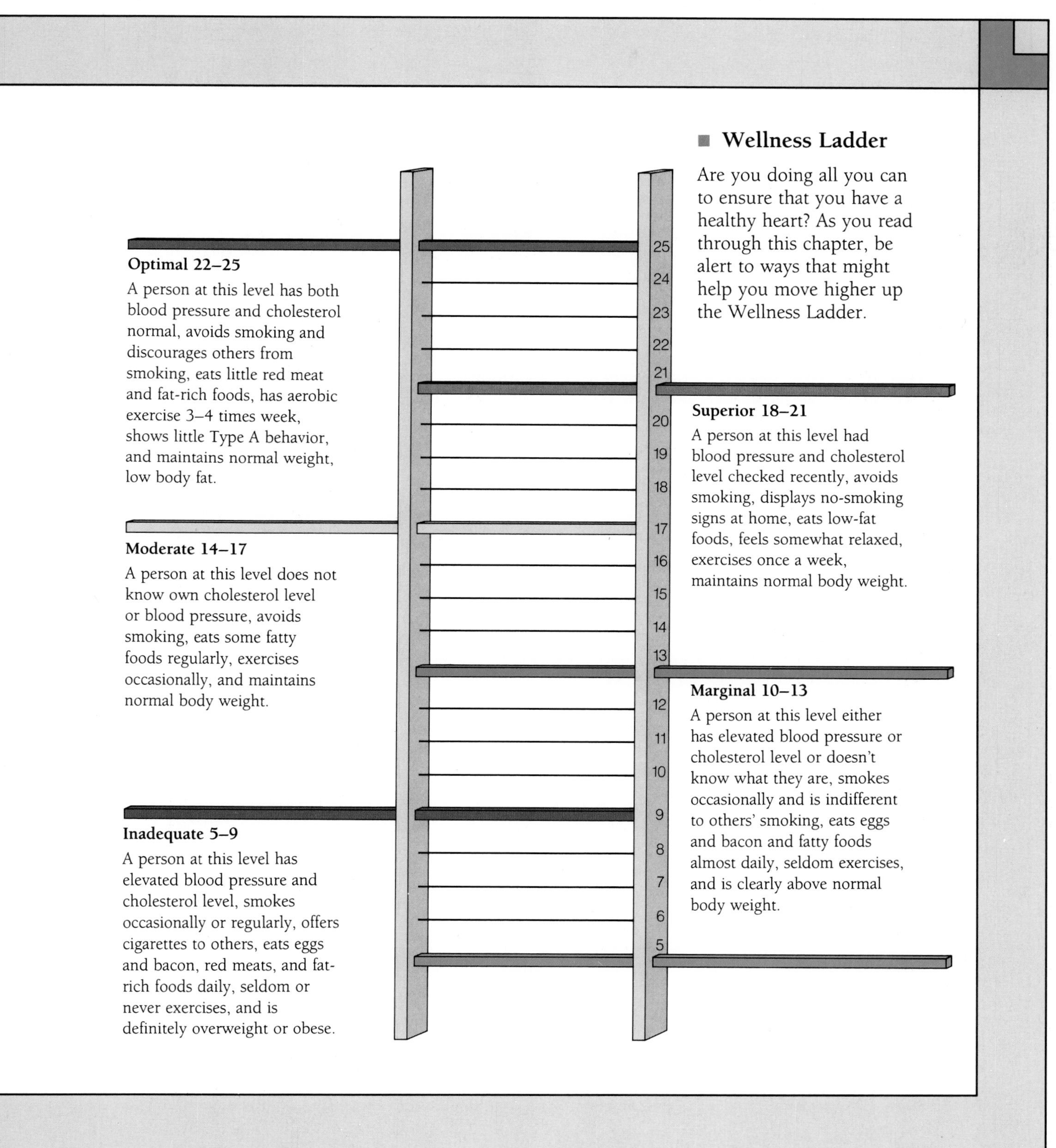

Wellness Ladder
Are you doing all you can to ensure that you have a healthy heart? As you read through this chapter, be alert to ways that might help you move higher up the Wellness Ladder.
Optimal 22–25
A person at this level has both blood pressure and cholesterol normal, avoids smoking and discourages others from smoking, eats little red meat and fat-rich foods, has aerobic exercise 3–4 times week, shows little Type A behavior, and maintains normal weight, low body fat.
Superior 18–21
A person at this level had blood pressure and cholesterol level checked recently, avoids smoking, displays no-smoking signs at home, eats low-fat foods, feels somewhat relaxed, exercises once a week, maintains normal body weight.
Moderate 14–17
A person at this level does not know own cholesterol level or blood pressure, avoids smoking, eats some fatty foods regularly, exercises occasionally, and maintains normal body weight.
Marginal 10–13
A person at this level either has elevated blood pressure or cholesterol level or doesn't know what they are, smokes occasionally and is indifferent to others' smoking, eats eggs and bacon and fatty foods almost daily, seldom exercises, and is clearly above normal body weight.
Inadequate 5–9
A person at this level has elevated blood pressure and cholesterol level, smokes occasionally or regularly, offers cigarettes to others, eats eggs and bacon, red meats, and fat-rich foods daily, seldom or never exercises, and is definitely overweight or obese.
25
24
23
22
21
20
19
18
17
16
15
14
13
12
11
10
9
8
7
6
5

Risko: Your Chances of Developing Heart Disease

0–4	You have one of the lowest risks of heart disease for your age and sex.
5–9	You have a low to moderate risk of heart disease for your age and sex but there is room for improvement.
10–14	You have a moderate to high risk of heart disease for your age and sex with considerable room for improvement on some factors.
15–19	You have a high risk of developing heart disease for your age and sex with a great deal of room for improvement on all factors.
20 & over	You have a very high risk of developing heart disease for your age and sex and should take immediate action on all risk factors.

Warning

- If you have diabetes, gout, or a family history of heart disease, your actual risk will be greater than indicated by this appraisal.
- If you do not know your current blood pressure or blood cholesterol level, you should visit your physician or health center to have them measured. Then figure your score again for a more accurate determination of your risk.
- If you are overweight, have high blood pressure or high blood cholesterol, or smoke cigarettes, your long-term risk of heart disease is increased even if your risk in the next several years is low.

Men

Find the column for your age group. Everyone starts with a score of 10 points. Work down the page *adding* points to your score or *subtracting* points from your score.

	54 or Younger	55 or Older
	Starting Score 10	Starting Score 10
1. Weight Locate your weight category in the following table. If you are in . . .		
☐ Weight category A	Subtract 2	Subtract 2
☐ Weight category B	Subtract 1	Add 0
☐ Weight category C	Add 1	Add 1
☐ Weight category D	Add 2	Add 3
	Equals ☐	**Equals** ☐
2. Systolic blood pressure Use the "first" or "higher" number from your most recent blood pressure measurement. If you do not know your blood pressure, estimate it by using the letter for your weight category. If your blood pressure is . . .		
A 119 or less	Subtract 1	Subtract 5
B Between 120 and 139	Add 0	Subtract 2
C Between 140 and 159	Add 0	Add 1
D 160 or greater	Add 1	Add 4
	Equals ☐	**Equals** ☐
3. Blood cholesterol level Use the number from your most recent blood cholesterol test. If you do not know your blood cholesterol, estimate it by using the letter for your weight category. If your blood cholesterol is . . .		
A 199 or less	Subtract 2	Subtract 1
B Between 200 and 224	Subtract 1	Subtract 1
C Between 225 and 249	Add 0	Add 0
D 250 or higher	Add 1	Add 0
	Equals ☐	**Equals** ☐

4. Cigarette smoking If you . . .
(If you smoke a pipe, but not cigarettes, use the same score adjustment as those cigarette smokers who smoke less than a pack a day.)

☐ Do not smoke	Subtract 1	Subtract 2
☐ Smoke less than a pack a day	Add 0	Subtract 1
☐ Smoke a pack a day	Add 1	Add 0
☐ Smoke more than a pack a day	Add 2	Add 3
	Final Score Equals ☐	**Final Score Equals** ☐

Weight Table for Men

Look for your height (without shoes) in the far left column and then read across to find the category into which your weight (in indoor clothing) would fall.

Your height ft. in.	Weight category (lbs.) A	B	C	D
5 1	up to 123	124–148	149–173	174 plus
5 2	up to 126	127–152	153–178	179 plus
5 3	up to 129	130–156	157–182	183 plus
5 4	up to 132	133–160	161–186	187 plus
5 5	up to 135	136–163	164–190	191 plus
5 6	up to 139	140–168	169–196	197 plus
5 7	up to 144	145–174	175–203	204 plus
5 8	up to 148	149–179	180–209	210 plus
5 9	up to 152	153–184	185–214	215 plus
5 10	up to 157	158–190	191–221	222 plus
5 11	up to 161	162–194	195–227	228 plus
6 0	up to 165	166–199	200–232	233 plus
6 1	up to 170	171–205	206–239	240 plus
6 2	up to 175	176–211	212–246	247 plus
6 3	up to 180	181–217	218–253	254 plus
6 4	up to 185	186–223	224–260	261 plus
6 5	up to 190	191–229	230–267	268 plus
6 6	up to 195	196–235	236–274	275 plus
Estimate of systolic blood pressure	119 or less	120 to 139	140 to 159	160 or more
Estimate of blood cholesterol	199 or less	200 to 224	225 to 249	250 or more

Because both blood pressure and blood cholesterol are related to weight, an estimate of these risk factors for each weight category is printed at the bottom of the table.

Risko: Your Chances of Developing Heart Disease (*continued*)

Women

Find the column for your age group. Everyone starts with a score of 10 points. Work down the page *adding* points to your score or *subtracting* points from your score.

1. Weight Locate your weight category in the following table. If you are in . . .

	54 or Younger	55 or Older
	Starting Score 10	Starting Score 10
☐ Weight category A	Subtract 2	Subtract 2
☐ Weight category B	Subtract 1	Subtract 1
☐ Weight category C	Add 1	Add 0
☐ Weight category D	Add 2	Add 1
	Equals ☐	Equals ☐

2. Systolic blood pressure Use the "first" or "higher" number from your most recent blood pressure measurement. If you do not know your blood pressure, estimate it by using the letter for your weight category. If your blood pressure is . . .

	54 or Younger	55 or Older
A 119 or less	Subtract 2	Subtract 3
B Between 120 and 139	Subtract 1	Add 0
C Between 140 and 159	Add 0	Add 3
D 160 or greater	Add 1	Add 6
	Equals ☐	Equals ☐

3. Blood cholesterol level Use the number from your most recent blood cholesterol test. If you do not know your blood cholesterol, estimate it by using the letter for your weight category. If your blood cholesterol is . . .

	54 or Younger	55 or Older
A 199 or less	Subtract 1	Subtract 3
B Between 200 and 224	Add 0	Subtract 1
C Between 225 and 249	Add 0	Add 1
D 250 or higher	Add 1	Add 3
	Equals ☐	Equals ☐

4. Cigarette smoking If you . . .

	54 or Younger	55 or Older
☐ Do not smoke	Subtract 1	Subtract 2
☐ Smoke less than a pack of day	Add 0	Subtract 1
☐ Smoke a pack a day	Add 1	Add 1
☐ Smoke more than a pack a day	Add 2	Add 4
	Equals ☐	Equals ☐

5. Estrogen use Birth control pills and hormone drugs contain estrogen. A few examples are:
*Premarin *Ogan *Menstranol *Provera *Evex
*Menest *Estinyl *Meurium
*Have you ever taken estrogen for five or more years in a row?
*Are you age 35 years or older and are now taking estrogen?

☐ No to both questions	Add 0	Add 0
☐ Yes to one or both questions	Add 1	Add 3
	Final Score Equals ☐	**Final Score Equals** ☐

Weight Table for Women

Look for your height (without shoes) in the far left column and then read across to find the category into which your weight (in indoor clothing) would fall.

Your height	Weight Category (lbs.)			
ft. in.	A	B	C	D
4 8	up to 101	102–122	123–143	144 plus
4 9	up to 103	104–125	126–146	147 plus
4 10	up to 106	107–128	129–150	151 plus
4 11	up to 109	110–132	133–154	155 plus
5 0	up to 112	113–136	137–158	159 plus
5 1	up to 115	116–139	140–162	163 plus
5 2	up to 119	120–144	145–168	169 plus
5 3	up to 122	123–148	149–172	173 plus
5 4	up to 127	128–154	155–179	180 plus
5 5	up to 131	132–158	159–185	186 plus
5 6	up to 135	136–163	164–190	191 plus
5 7	up to 139	140–168	169–196	197 plus
5 8	up to 143	144–173	174–202	203 plus
5 9	up to 147	148–178	179–207	208 plus
5 10	up to 151	152–182	183–213	214 plus
5 11	up to 155	156–187	188–218	219 plus
6 0	up to 159	160–191	192–224	225 plus
6 1	up to 163	164–196	197–229	230 plus
Estimate of systolic blood pressure	119 or less	120 to 139	140 to 159	160 or more
Estimate of blood cholesterol	199 or less	200 to 224	225 to 249	250 or more

Because both blood pressure and blood cholesterol are related to weight, an estimate of these risk factors for each weight category is printed at the bottom of the table.

SOURCE: American Heart Association.

Atria The two upper chambers of the heart in which blood collects before passing to the ventricles; also called auricles.

Ventricles The two lower chambers of the heart from which blood flows through arteries to the lungs and other parts of the body.

Endocardium A membrane lining the cavities of the heart.

Myocardium The muscular wall of the heart.

Epicardium A membrane covering the heart.

Vena cava Large vein through which blood is returned to the right atrium of the heart.

Cardiovascular system The heart and blood vessels.

Aorta The large artery that receives blood from the left ventricle and distributes it to the body.

Arterioles The smallest arteries that end in capillaries.

Capillaries Very small blood vessels that distribute blood to all parts of the body.

Venules Small veins.

Coronary Bypass Surgery Surgery in which a vein is grafted from a point above to a point below an obstruction in a coronary artery, improving the blood supply to the heart.

Transluminal angioplasty A technique in which a catheter with a balloon on the tip is inserted into an artery; the balloon is then inflated at the point of obstruction in the artery, pressing the plaque against the artery wall to improve blood supply.

Carotid artery The major blood vessel carrying blood to the brain.

Cardiovascular disease (CVD) Diseases of the heart and blood vessels: hardening of the arteries, high blood pressure, and heart attacks.

Most of us are familiar with the stereotype of the future heart attack victim: the harried, frenzied, superambitious executive. We nod and say, "He's working on a coronary." He knows the stereotype, too, and may acknowledge it with a wry grin before hurrying on to his coronary. But that stereotype is only part of the truth. The other part may be closer to home for all too many of us—the overweight and underactive person sprawled in front of the television set after too much dinner, with a cigarette in one hand and a potato chip in the other. This person is also working on a coronary. Until more of us make changes in our living habits and begin to move toward a healthier lifestyle, cardiovascular disease will continue to be the Number One Killer in America.

The Cardiovascular System

The heart is a four-chambered muscle, about the size of your fist, shaped roughly like a cone. Its two upper chambers are usually called the **atria** (plural of *atrium*) but are sometimes called *auricles*. Oxygen-poor blood enters the right atrium through the vena cava. It then passes through the right **ventricle** and is pumped into the lung through the pulmonary artery. In the lung, the blood absorbs oxygen from inhaled air. The now oxygen-rich blood flows back through the pulmonary vein into the left atrium, then the left ventricle, and finally out the aorta to the rest of the body. The wall of the heart has three layers. The interior layer, called the **endocardium**, is a membrane lining the chambers of the heart. The middle layer, the "muscle," is called the **myocardium**. The third layer, a membrane called the **epicardium**, covers the heart. The heart and the blood vessels (veins, arteries, and capillaries) together make up the **cardiovascular system**. See Figure 17-1.

The heart pumps blood through the blood vessels. When blood flows into the ventricles from the atria, the heart muscle contracts, squeezing blood out into the pulmonary artery and the largest artery, the aorta. Valves prevent the blood from flowing in the wrong direction.

Blood vessels are classified by size and function. Veins carry blood *to* the heart; arteries carry it *away* from the

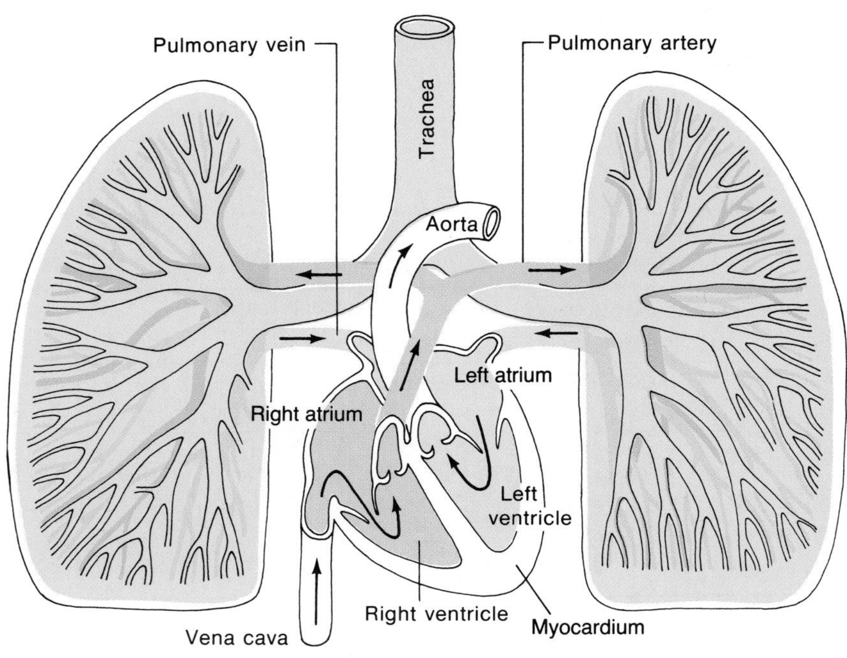

Figure 17-1 Cross section of the heart and lungs showing paths of blood flow.

Bypassing Heart Surgery

More than 200,000 Americans undergo **coronary bypass surgery** each year, at a total cost of over $4 billion. Despite the fact that it is a major operation, such surgery has become almost routine in many medical centers throughout the country.

A healthy blood vessel, usually a vein from one of the patient's own legs, is inserted between the aorta and the blocked coronary arteries. During the operation, a heart-lung machine maintains circulation. Coronary bypass patients usually spend two to three days in an intensive recovery unit after the operation and then another week in the hospital. The costs of this procedure can range from $15,000 to $30,000 depending on which part of the country you're in and what services are requested.

The operation carries a certain amount of risk. About 1 to 3 percent of bypass patients do not survive the operation or die soon after it. The risk is highest for the elderly, women, and people who have other medical conditions.

Studies have recently indicated that for at least 20 percent of these patients, surgery may not be necessary. One study, conducted at fifteen medical centers in the United States and Canada, involved patients without pain who had suffered one heart attack. These patients also showed significant blockages in one or more coronary arteries. The results of the study indicated that bypass surgery was not superior to medications in preventing further heart attacks. Patients who have severe angina pectoris, a disabling pain felt behind the breastbone, are often candidates for bypass surgery. However, even among these patients it is unclear that a medical regimen including daily aspirin does not achieve similar or even better results than major surgery.

Why doesn't bypass surgery help more people avoid future heart attacks, including death? Cardiologist Eugene Passamani suggests, "Bypass surgery only fixes the plumbing. It does nothing to stem the progression of the underlying disease." In many cases—some studies suggest 50 percent—three to five years later the newly implanted blood vessel becomes clogged again and the patient is faced with major surgery. Another 30 percent of bypass surgery patients have other arteries that become seriously blocked.

Angioplasty

One new technique increasingly used in the United States with great success is **transluminal angioplasty**. It is being used to treat severely blocked coronary arteries as well as blocked arteries in other parts of the body.

The technique involves threading a catheter with an inflatable balloon tip through the artery until it reaches the area of blockage. The balloon is then inflated, flattening the fatty plaque and widening the arterial opening. The procedure has several advantages: it is done under a local anesthesia and does not involve surgery or the use of a heart-lung machine. The cost is only a fraction of that for bypass surgery, nor does it usually involve more than one or two days of hospitalization.

Unfortunately, it is not appropriate for all types of coronary artery disease. Some patients who undergo an unsuccessful angioplasty may still require bypass surgery. In about 25 percent, the blockages reform and a repeat angioplasty may be required.

Angioplasty is also being used to treat blockages in the arteries of the legs and the **carotid artery**, the major vessel carrying blood to the brain.

heart. The main trunk of the arterial system, the **aorta**, branches into smaller arteries, which in turn branch into even smaller arteries. The smallest arteries, called **arterioles**, branch still further into the smallest blood vessels, the **capillaries**.

By way of the capillaries, blood from arterioles is transferred to small veins called **venules**, then to larger veins, which return it to the heart. Two important blood vessels supply blood to the heart itself, directly to the myocardium. These blood vessels, branching from the aorta, are the coronary arteries.

Major Forms of Adult Cardiovascular Disease

The diseases that affect the heart and blood vessels are called collectively **cardiovascular diseases CVD**. Chief among them are atherosclerosis, hypertension (high blood pressure), stroke, congestive heart failure, rheumatic heart disease, and congenital heart disease. Cardiovascular disease was once considered a disease of old age. This is no longer the case, since many men in their forties die from cardiovascular disease. Although often hereditary, these

Atherosclerosis An early form of arteriosclerosis in which the inner layers of artery walls are made thick and irregular by deposits of a fatty substance. The internal channel of arteries become narrowed, and blood supply is reduced.

Arteriosclerosis Hardening of the arteries.

Plaque A deposit of fatty (and other) substances on the inner wall of the arteries.

Coronary thrombosis A clot in a coronary artery, often causing sudden death.

Cerebral thrombosis A clot in a vessel that supplies blood to the brain.

Cholesterol A fatty compound in the blood that is also found in deposits on the walls of arteries.

Platelets Microscopic disk-shaped cell fragments in the blood. These disintegrate on contact with foreign objects and release chemicals that are necessary for the formation of blood clots.

Blood plasma The fluid portion of the blood.

Antibodies Proteins in the blood that are generated in reaction to foreign proteins. Antibodies neutralize the foreign proteins, producing immunity from them.

Omega-3 fatty acids A group of fatty acids found in marine life that reduce the tendency of blood clots.

Hypercholesterolemia An excess amount of cholesterol in the blood.

---

early deaths can also be traced to self-indulgent lifestyles and common misconceptions of what "the good life" is. Many early deaths could be prevented if people changed their patterns of daily living, especially their smoking habits, exercise programs, diets, and control over such problems as hypertension and diabetes.

Atherosclerosis The most common form of hardening of the arteries, or **arteriosclerosis**, is **atherosclerosis**, a slow progressive process that begins early in life, sometimes before puberty. In this disease arteries become narrowed by deposits of fat, cholesterol, and other substances. As these deposits, called **plaques**, accumulate on the walls of the arteries, the arteries lose their elasticity and are unable to expand and contract. The flow of blood through the narrowed arteries is restricted. A clot (thrombus) may form, blocking the artery and depriving the heart, brain, or other organ of the vital oxygen carried by the blood. When a coronary artery is blocked, the result is a **coronary thrombosis**, which is one kind of heart attack. When an artery leading to the brain is blocked, the result is a **cerebral thrombosis**, a kind of stroke.

Several factors have been linked to the development of atherosclerosis in susceptible individuals. These include high concentration of blood lipids (fats and fatlike substances), of which **cholesterol** is one, genetic disorders, cigarette smoking, diets high in animal fats, and hypertension. The interaction of these factors is not yet fully understood.

The Growth of Arterial Plaques One theory advanced to explain the growth of arterial plaques is called the "response to injury" theory. Apparently, the narrowing of an artery is not caused solely by the accumulation of substances forming the blockage. Studies with animals suggest that arterial blockages can begin with repeated or chronic injury to the endothelium, a thin layer of cells lining the inner surface of the artery. The injury to the inner surface allows the smooth muscle cells of the middle wall to come into contact with the blood. The muscle cells then multiply, forming a plaque.

Arterial plaques resembling but not identical to those occurring in people have been brought on in animals by injuring their arteries in several ways, among them (1) mechanically, by inserting catheters (tubes); and (2) by increasing the amount of the blood lipids carrying cholesterol.

The direct cause of atherosclerosis may not, however, be the injury itself. It may instead be the presence of some substance in the blood that causes the smooth muscle cells to multiply.

When the endothelium is injured, **platelets** (particles in the blood that are involved in the clotting mechanism) cluster around the exposed smooth muscle cells and release chemicals into the **blood plasma**. One group of investigators has shown that one protein released by the platelets can cause smooth muscle cells to divide and that when this protein is absent the muscle cells do not divide. This research was done in tissue cultures, however, not in live animals.

Other investigators have shown (in rabbits) that when the platelets are destroyed by **antibodies**, injury to the endothelium no longer causes plaques to form. Evidence implicating platelets in the formation of plaques in people is less direct and still inconclusive. Data on humans are more difficult to obtain because experiments must not produce atherosclerosis or injure the subject in any way.

Another substance implicated in the multiplying of smooth muscle cells is cholesterol. One of its functions is as a building block for cell membranes. Cholesterol has been found to be a major component of plaques. People suffering from the genetically transmitted disease **hypercholesterolemia** have abnormally high concentrations of cholesterol in their blood plasma and frequently die of atherosclerosis as young adults.

Exploring Your Emotions

You are eating your favorite Sunday breakfast, steak and eggs, and your daughter says to you, "My science teacher says steak and eggs are not good for your heart." How do you respond to this, knowing that parents are important models for their children's behavior?

Fishing for Cardiovascular Health

When you were a child, your folks probably told you that fish and codliver oil were good for you. And, unlike some other things you may have been told (such as "finish *everything* on your plate"), the fish recommendation may have some basis in fact.

Recently, Dutch researchers reported that fish eaters had half the mortality from heart disease as fish noneaters! And the really remarkable fact was that the fish eaters had to eat only 1 ounce of fish per day to achieve this protective effect.

Another report in the same journal suggested a possible reason for the improved longevity—fish lowered the cholesterol levels. In this study, two groups of 10 patients each were studied. Both groups had very high levels of both cholesterol (CHOL) and fat (triglyceride, or TG), although the specific type of abnormality differed. The patients were fed three diets, varying primarily in the amount and type of fat. The decreases in both CHOL and TG with the fish-rich diet were extraordinary. In fact, they were greater than could be expected even with the best prescription drugs currently available:

Group	Cholesterol Level Control Diet	Cholesterol Level Fish Diet	Triglyceride Level Control Diet	Triglyceride Level Fish Diet
Abnormality Type IIb	324	236	334	118
Abnormality Type V	373	207	1353	281

Although these two studies are the best publicized, they certainly do not stand alone. Many other articles support the improved mortality experience of fish eaters, although some studies do not show such a relationship. Also, many studies demonstrate the CHOL- and TG-lowering effects of fish and fish oils.

Why the sudden interest in fish and fish oil? Well, scientists sought an explanation for the observation that Greenland Eskimos have a very low rate of heart disease, even though their diet is very high in fat. This seeming paradox may be due to the fact that much of their fat intake comes from marine sources (fish, whale, seal, walrus). Marine fat is especially rich in a group of fatty acids called **omega-3 fatty acids**. These acids tend to decrease the "stickiness" of platelets, the blood cells that are responsible for blood clotting. Excessively "sticky" platelets are believed to play a major role in blocking arteries. Sudden arterial blockage, of course, causes many strokes and heart attacks.

Omega-3 fats seem to have two potentially beneficial effects: (1) they lower blood CHOL and TG, and (2) they decrease the tendency of platelets to "clump" together. Preliminary evidence suggests that these two beneficial effects of the fish fats probably occur at two different dose levels. Probably only high doses of fish (or fish oil supplements) affect CHOL levels. High doses are in the range of ½ to 1 pound of marine foods per day (the amount that Greenland Eskimos eat!), or about thirty 1-gram fish oil supplement pills per day! A much lower dose, (probably in the range of two to three 4-ounce fish servings per week, or one to two supplement pills per day), may decrease platelet stickiness.

This assessment is strictly an educated guess, and that much more data must be gathered before scientific recommendations may be made. For instance, the Danish study quoted earlier found that men who ate lean fish containing about 1.5 percent omega-3 fatty acids had as low a mortality as the men who ate the fattier fishes (which contain 5 to 10 percent omega-3 fats). This finding suggests that *something else in fish—not necessarily the omega-3 content—may be beneficial to the heart.* This is one reason why some researchers recommend eating the fish themselves, rather than taking supplements.

But supposing you absolutely refuse to eat fish. Is taking a fish oil supplement reasonable? You might consider several factors in answering this question:

First, children, adolescents, pregnant women, individuals on anticoagulants (blood thinners), or those with bleeding or bruising problems should not take any sort of fish oil supplement. Little is known about fish oil use in the first three groups of patients, and some fish oils may have large amounts of vitamin A, an excess of which can cause birth defects. The last two groups are usually in a precarious balance, and adding substances that increase bleeding tendency may lead to a serious, or perhaps even fatal, episode of bleeding.

Second, patients under a doctor's care for a serious medical disorder should discuss any plans for fish

(continued on next page)

Fishing for Cardiovascular Health (*continued*)

oil supplementation with their physician. If he or she is not receptive to even discussing the issue, they may wish to search for a *bona fide* fish oil researcher in their geographic area. Finding such an individual may take some effort—but a literature search in the local medical library may turn up a local researcher. Alternatively, the chief dietitian at a local hospital may be able to direct the patient to an appropriate research facility. *Your local health food store does not qualify as a bona fide research facility.*

Third, patients with very high CHOL levels (over 300–350) and/or very high TG levels (over 500) are very reasonably treated with fish oils, *under medical supervision.* None of the drugs currently used to treat such high CHOL and TG levels are very satisfactory, and although current experience with fish oil supplements is limited, sufficient evidence allows at least a trial of fish oil supplementation. This trial would have to be considered experimental at the present time. Other experts in this field may legitimately disagree with this view, and may appropriately prefer to use agents with which they are more familiar. And of course these suggestions are subject to modification as further research accumulates.

Fourth, it seems reasonable to increase fish intake to the levels noted to be beneficial in the Danish study—two or three fish dishes per week.

To prepare the fish, emphasize broiling, baking, and poaching (unfortunately, some researchers have implicated barbecuing as a source of carcinogens). Breading and deep frying the fish partially defeat the healthy effects of eating fish. Fatty fishes, such as mackerel, salmon, and tuna, may add calories, but may also be more useful. Finally, shellfish, which have been traditionally off limits to cholesterol-restricted individuals, have been shown to have little deleterious effect on serum cholesterol, and may in fact be beneficial. Thus, intake of lobster and shrimp has been liberalized, and should be discussed with one's physician and/or registered dietitian or qualified nutritionist.

SOURCE: Jack C. Yetiv, 1987 (March), Fishing for cardiovascular health, *Healthline.*

Two kinds of cholesterol have been identified as having opposite effects on the development of atherosclerosis: **low-density lipoprotein (LDL)** and **high-density lipoprotein (HDL)**. LDL causes arteries to thicken by accumulating on artery walls. HDL helps keep LDL in solution, or in a watery state returning excess amounts of cholesterol to the liver for recycling, so that blood can pass freely through the arteries to the heart. Carefully conducted medical surveys have indicated that high concentrations of LDL in the blood plasma are a serious risk factor for atherosclerosis. See Figure 17-2.

Cigarette Smoking Studies have firmly established that cigarette smoking is a risk factor for atherosclerosis. One

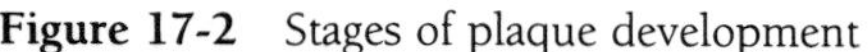

Figure 17-2 Stages of plaque development

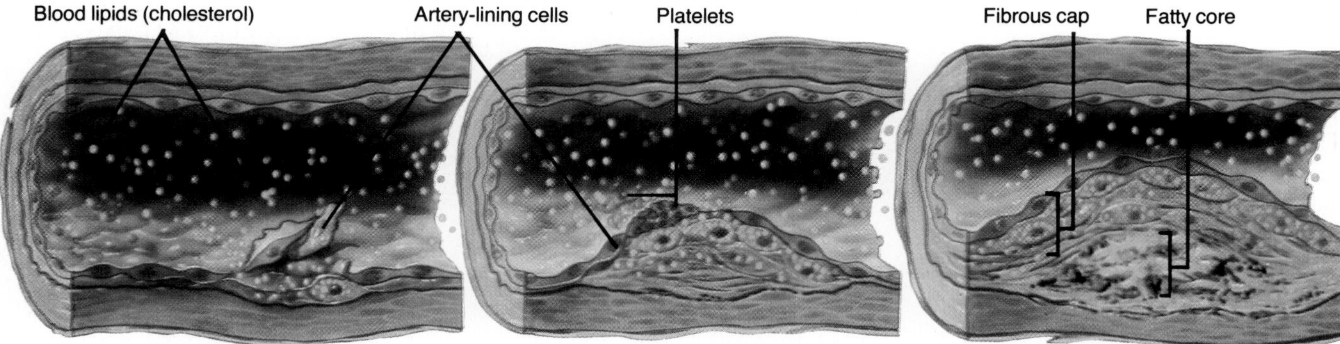

1 Plaque buildup begins when excess fat particles, called *lipids,* collect beneath cells lining the artery that have been damaged by smoking, high blood pressure, or other causes.

2 Platelets, one of the body's protective mechanisms, collect at the damaged area and cause a cap of cells to form, isolating the plaque within the artery wall.

3 The narrowed artery is now vulnerable to blockage by clots that can form if the cap breaks and the fatty core of the lesion combines with the clot-producing factors in the blood.

Low-density lipoproteins (LDLs) Blood fats that result in cholesterol acumulating on artery walls, which eventually block the flow of blood to the heart and brain.

High-density lipoproteins (HDLs) Blood fats that help transport cholesterol out of the arteries and thus protect against heart diseases.

Lipoprotein A protein and lipid connected as one chemical.

Heparin A natural substance in the body that prolongs clotting time.

Hypertension Sustained abnormally high blood pressure.

mechanism by which smoking may increase the incidence of the disease has been suggested by Edwin Bierman of the University of Washington Medical School: plaques that are associated with atherosclerosis contain smooth muscle cells with very high concentrations of **lipoproteins**. Normally, the lipoproteins that deliver cholesterol to the cells are broken down by the cell. Bierman discovered that the breakdown process slows when the concentration of oxygen is lowered. Cigarette smoking produces carbon monoxide, which enters the blood and tends to replace oxygen, thus lowering its concentration. Thus, cigarette smoking may promote the accumulation of lipoproteins in the cells and facilitate the formation of plaques. Cigarette smoke also appears to destroy **heparin**, the body's natural anticoagulant (blood thinner)—thus making blood cells more prone to clotting. In addition, passive smoke (smoke generated by others) has been strongly implicated in the development of atherosclerosis as well as of lung cancer. Consequently, just being around smokers for long periods of time may in itself be a risk factor for heart disease.

Diet Does lowering the concentrations of blood lipids or cholesterol prevent or reverse plaque formation? In one controlled study with monkeys, a low-cholesterol diet retarded progression of atherosclerosis. In a study of men who had already suffered one heart attack, the use of drugs that lowered blood cholesterol levels did not lessen the likelihood of a second attack. However, in a recent 10-year study of 3,800 middle-aged men with abnormally high cholesterol levels, it was conclusively demonstrated that for every 1 percent reduction in cholesterol, there was a 2 percent drop in heart attacks. Although the study used a cholesterol-lowering drug to achieve its results, the researchers concluded that their findings should apply to the general population with elevated cholesterol levels.

Hypertension The medical term for persistent or sustained high blood pressure is **hypertension**. Hypertension is in itself the primary cause of more than 60,000 deaths each year in the United States. It also contributes to 1.5 million heart attacks and strokes each year. See Figure 17-3.

Hypertension is called a "silent killer," because it presents no symptoms. Victims thus have no way of knowing without testing that they have the disease. Recent studies have shown that more people have become aware of their hypertension and are being treated for it. Control of high blood pressure is thought to have significantly contributed to the recent decline in heart attacks.

Hypertension cannot be cured, but it can be treated and controlled. Lack of treatment can result in serious damage to vital organs, particularly the heart, brain, and kidneys. Blood vessels in the kidneys, for example, may rupture from constant high blood pressure, making it difficult if not impossible for them to clear waste material from the bloodstream. In the eyes, pressure on the cap-

Exploring Your Emotions

Your parent suffers from persistent high blood pressure (hypertension), for which the doctor has prescribed drugs and regular exercise. However, your parent is somewhat sedentary, doesn't believe much in taking medicine, and tends to neglect the problem. How does such apparently irrational behavior make you feel? How can you help him or her understand the seriousness of the disease and the necessity for taking the medication without alienating him or her?

Figure 17-3 Estimated prevalence of the major cardiovascular diseases in the United States, 1987.

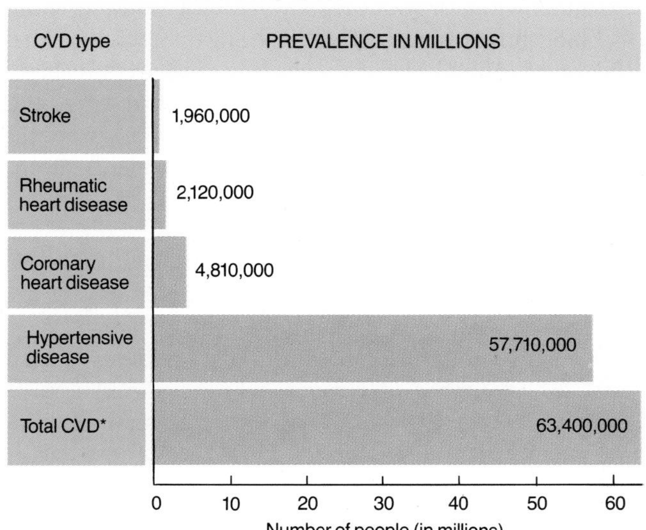

*The sum of the individual estimates exceeds 63,400,000, since many people have more than one cardiovascular disorder.
Source: American Heart Association.

Diastole Relaxation of the heart.

Systole Contraction of the heart.

Sphygmomanometer An instrument for measuring blood pressure.

Essential hypertension Persistent elevated blood pressure without known or specific cause.

Secondary hypertension High blood pressure caused by disease such as kidney dysfunctioning or tumor.

Renin An enzyme found in the kidney.

Angiotensin A naturally occurring substance that constricts blood vessels.

Viscosity The quality in the blood of "syrupiness."

---

illaries in the retina may cause swelling and tiny hemorrhages and may eventually result in blindness. Hypertension may also cause arteries to lose their elasticity from being constantly stretched.

Blood Pressure Defined Blood pressure is the force per area exerted by blood against the walls of the arteries. This force is created by the pumping action of the heart. Every time the heart contracts, or beats (called **systole**), blood pressure increases. When the heart relaxes between beats (**diastole**), the pressure decreases. Blood pressure is highest in the arteries, which transport blood away from the heart, and lowest in the veins, which return blood to the heart.

Measuring Blood Pressure Blood pressure is measured with a stethoscope and an instrument called a **sphygmomanometer**. A sphygmomanometer consists of an airbag or cuff and a column of mercury marked off in millimeters. The cuff is wrapped around the upper arm and inflated by squeezing an attached rubber bulb. The inflated cuff depresses the branchial artery in the arm, stopping the flow of blood. Air pressure supports the column of mercury. As air is slowly released from the cuff, the column of mercury falls. When the cuff is no longer tight enough to prevent the passage of blood through the artery, the examiner will hear with the stethoscope a thudding sound as blood flow resumes. The height of the mercury when the sound is first heard is the reading of the systolic blood pressure, the pressure when the heart is contracting. After noting the systolic blood pressure, the examiner continues to release air until the sound can no longer be heard. The pressure at this point is diastolic blood pressure, the blood pressure when the heart is relaxed. Blood pressure is expressed as two numbers—for example, 120/80. The first and larger number is the systolic blood pressure, and the second number is the diastolic blood pressure.

A single blood pressure reading is not necessarily accurate, for a number of reasons, including measurement error, anxiety, excitement, and so on. Several readings, preferably taken over a period of time, are a more reliable indication of a person's "real" blood pressure.

Physicians have long regarded a blood pressure reading of 160/95 as the level at which treatment is required. Several recent studies, however, including a study of 8,000 patients sponsored by the National Institutes of Health and called the Hypertension Detection and Follow-up Program, have indicated that substantial reductions in deaths from heart attacks and strokes can be achieved by treating people whose blood pressure is in the 140/90 range.

The Causes of Hypertension Hypertension is a complex disease that has various causes, many of which are unknown. Hypertension for which no specific cause has been found is called **essential hypertension**. Hypertension that can be ascribed to particular organic defects, such as kidney disease, is called **secondary hypertension**.

Atherosclerotic plaques increase friction within arteries, elevating the blood pressure. The higher pressure is thought to increase the incidence of injury to the endothelium, thereby promoting further plaque growth. All risk factors relating to atherosclerosis must be regarded as risk factors of hypertension.

The kidneys release the enzyme **renin**, which promotes the formation of **angiotensin** proteins. These in turn cause the blood vessels to constrict. The release of renin is inhibited by high pressure in the kidney arteries. If these arteries have been narrowed by atherosclerosis or by some other cause, their pressure will be low, so renin will continue to be secreted, proteins will continue to be produced, and all arteries will continue to be constricted. Hypertension is the result. Damage to the kidneys by wound, infection, or tumor can also cause an excess of renin. Removal of the kidney or repair of the kidney arteries sometimes produces a cure.

Hypertension in patients who have no evident damage to either kidneys or kidney arteries is classified as essential. Some such patients have higher than normal levels of renin. For them, high blood pressure may be caused primarily by constriction of arteries. Under these conditions, the kidneys tend to excrete water, lowering blood volume, increasing blood **viscosity** ("syrupiness"), and placing great stress on the blood vessels. People with high renin levels have an increased incidence of heart attacks, strokes, and kidney failure.

Some individuals with essential hypertension have lower than normal renin levels. For them, hypertension may be caused primarily by increased blood volume. Either decreased sodium excretion by the kidneys or increased secretion of the hormone aldosterone (a hormone produced by the adrenal glands that causes the kidneys to

Lowering Cholesterol to Prevent Heart Attacks

Cholesterol is a waxy substance found only in animal products. It is often confused with saturated fats, which are only rarely found in vegetable sources. Coconut oil is an example. Although fats do not contain cholesterol, they do enhance absorption of cholesterol from the intestine into the bloodstream. Saturated fats especially enhance this absorption. Dairy products—which are animal products—are sources of both cholesterol and saturated fat. Studies have shown that if you eat foods rich in cholesterol (such as egg yolks) but you do not consume saturated fats, your blood cholesterol level may not rise much.

Three kinds of cholesterol are commonly described: total cholesterol (CHOL), high-density lipoproteins (HDL), and low-density lipoproteins (LDL). HDL is regarded as the "good" cholesterol, while LDL is considered "bad."

What Are the Facts?

Much evidence links elevated blood cholesterol to coronary heart disease. In fact, lowering elevated blood cholesterol (specifically LDL cholesterol) will reduce the risk of heart attacks due to coronary heart disease. This reduction has been demonstrated conclusively in men who have elevated blood cholesterol levels: evidence strongly suggests that women with elevated levels can achieve similar protection.

Cholesterol is carried in the bloodstream in several protein-lipid combinations, called *lipoproteins*. Some cholesterol is carried by the high-density lipoproteins (HDL), but most blood cholesterol in humans is carried by specific low-density lipoproteins (LDL). The LDL cholesterol, when present in excess form a major part of that buildup in the artery wall that is called *atherosclerosis*. Atherosclerosis narrows the coronary arteries, which furnish most of the blood supply to the heart.

Remarkably, although LDL cholesterol appears to promote disease, HDL cholesterol appears to protect against the disease process. The relative distribution of cholesterol into the two types, HDL and LDL, has shown to be a better gauge of coronary risk than is the total blood cholesterol level.

What Are the Risks?

Blood cholesterol levels of most Americans are too high, largely because we eat too many calories, and too much saturated fat and cholesterol. According to a panel of experts convened by the National Institutes of Health, the following total cholesterol levels carry either moderate or high risk of heart disease.

Age	Moderate Risk	High Risk
2–19	170–185 mg	Above 185 mg
20–29	201–220	Above 220
30–39	221–240	Above 240
40 +	240–260	Above 260

These numbers are only rough estimates of risk; however, it is possible to substantially increase the accuracy of predicting risk by including HDL cholesterol values and forming a "risk ratio." This ratio is produced by dividing the total cholesterol value by the HDL value. Ratios above 4 are considered undesirable. So it is important to find out the HDL value as well as the total cholesterol value. In some instances a person with a total value of 210 may be at greater risk than a person with a total value of 240. If, for example, Person A with 210 milligrams of total cholesterol had an HDL value of 35 milligrams, he or she would have a risk ratio of 6 (210/35 = 6). Person B, with a total value of 240 and an HDL of 60 has a risk ratio of 4 (240/60 = 4). The higher the ratio, the greater the risk.

The level of HDL cholesterol alone is a good measure of risk of heart disease. The higher the level, the lower the risk.

It has been demonstrated that women, nonsmokers, lean people, people who exercise regularly, and people who drink moderately have higher HDL levels than men, smokers, obese people, sedentary people, and nondrinkers.

Another important risk factor is an inherited tendency toward elevated levels of LDL (the bad cholesterol). Such people may be "cholesterol sensitive." That is, they are affected much more by eating saturated fats and cholesterol than are people who are not particularly sensitive. Thus a person with a family history of elevated LDL or total cholesterol may have to work twice as hard to bring HDL up and/or LDL down.

What You Can Do

Many foods and nutrients, as well as behaviors such as smoking and exercise, have been studied to see whether or not they raise or lower cholesterol. The single most important dietary factor in raising

(continued on next page)

Lowering Cholesterol to Prevent Heart Attacks (*continued*)

LDL and/or total cholesterol is saturated fat. Cholesterol itself, as found in foods such as eggs and shellfish, does not appear to have a great effect on blood cholesterol—with the possible exception of especially susceptible individuals. Aerobic exercise has been shown so far to be the single most powerful effective way to raise HDL. Giving up the smoking habit runs a close second. The following checklists contain recommendations that can help people lower LDL and/or total cholesterol (TC) and raise HDL cholesterol.

To Lower LDL/CHOL

- Reduce saturated fat (eat less pork, beef, lamb).
- Increase monounsaturated fats (eat more olive and peanut oil).
- Increase polyunsaturated fats (eat more corn, safflower, sesame oils).
- Take calcium supplements.
- Take niacin (a B vitamin).
- Eat fatty fish (salmon, mackerel, sardines, herring).
- Eat oat bran (for example, in cereal, muffins, or cookies).
- Eat legumes (beans, chick peas).
- Use more garlic.
- Eat more pectin (apples, grapes, berries, grapefruit).
- Consume more vegetable fiber (carrots, broccoli, cabbage).

To Raise HDL

- Engage in regular aerobic exercise.
- Stop smoking.
- If overweight, lose weight.
- Eat fish oil.

SOURCE: Paul Insel, 1986 (March), Lowering cholesterol to prevent heart attacks, *Healthline.*

What You Should Know about Heart Attack

An estimated 4,810,000 people have coronary heart disease. An estimated 540,000 died of heart attack in 1984—350,000 before they reached the hospital. Many thousands of these might have been saved if the victims had heeded the signals.

Delay spells danger. When you suffer a heart attack, minutes—especially the first few minutes—count.

Know the Signals

The signals of heart attack are

- Uncomfortable pressure, fullness, squeezing, or pain in the center of the chest lasting two minutes or more.
- Pain may spread to shoulders, neck, or arms.
- Severe pain, dizziness, fainting, sweating, nausea, or shortness of breath may also occur. Sharp, stabbing twinges of pain are usually not signals of a heart attack.

Emergency Action

If you are having typical chest discomfort that lasts for two minutes or more, call the local emergency rescue service immediately. If you can get to a hospital faster by car, have someone drive you. Find out which hospitals have 24-hour emergency cardiac care and discuss with your doctor the possible choices. Plan in advance the route that's best from where you live and work. Keep a list of emergency rescue service numbers next to your telephone and in a prominent place in your pocket, wallet, or purse.

Be a Heart Saver

If you are with someone who is having the "signals," and if they last for two minutes or longer, act at once.

Expect a "denial." It is normal to deny the possibility of anything as serious as a heart attack—but insist on taking prompt action.

1. *Call* the emergency rescue service, or

2. *Get* to the nearest hospital emergency room that offers 24-hour emergency cardiac care, and

3. *Give* mouth-to-mouth breathing and chest compression **(CPR)** if it is necessary and if you are properly trained.

SOURCE: American Heart Association.

Cardiopulmonary resuscitation (CPR) A technique involving mouth-to-mouth breathing and chest compression to keep oxygen flowing to the brain.

Antihypertensive drugs Prescribed drugs that lower blood pressure.

Diuretics Drugs that increase the flow of urine.

Prostaglandins Hormones that act on the kidneys.

Coronary occlusion Partial or total obstruction of a coronary artery, as by a clot; usually resulting in myocardial infarction.

Myocardial infarction A heart attack in which the heart muscle is damaged through lack of blood supply.

Collateral circulation The movement of blood by a system of smaller blood vessels when a main vessel is blocked.

---

retain water) could produce such an effect. The ultimate causes remain elusive.

About half the patients with essential hypertension have normal levels of renin in their blood. Many researchers have tried without success to discover subtle defects in the kidneys of such patients. They *have* found, however, that the angiotensins act on the sympathetic and central nervous systems as well as on the blood vessels, so the search for causes has broadened.

Hypertension appears to have a strong genetic component. But Harvard University researchers have found in young children an environmental influence on blood pressure as well. Whatever is responsible for essential hypertension may be acquired in childhood, but separating genetic from environmental factors has been traditionally a knotty problem in human biology. The National Heart, Lung, and Blood Institute is now researching high blood pressure in children and adolescents, investigating the effects of diet, psychological factors, lifestyles, genetic factors, and physical activity.

Treatment of Hypertension Treatment of hypertension often consists of **antihypertensive drugs** and changes in diet. Recent studies have shown that regular exercise also lowers blood pressure.

One group of antihypertensive drugs is the **diuretics**, which increase fluid excretion by the kidneys. Use of diuretics is recommended for low-renin patients, whose hypertension is thought to be due primarily to increased blood volume.

Another group of antihypertensive drugs blocks the action of angiotensin proteins. This treatment is appropriate for patients with higher than normal renin levels. Other drugs under study as possibly having an effect on hypertension are **prostaglandins** and kinins, protein fragments that seem to cause dilation (widening) of blood vessels.

Mild hypertension can frequently be treated by changes in diet alone, such as restricted salt intake in salt-sensitive people, caloric intake, or both. Not everyone's blood pressure is affected by eating salt. However, some people's blood pressure will go up as soon as they eat salt. These salt-sensitive people have to restrict their salt intake to control their blood pressure. Overweight people are more susceptible to hypertension because added weight places greater demands on the cardiovascular system. Adipose (fatty) tissue, such as organ and muscle tissue, requires blood to nourish it. In overweight people, the heart must pump more blood through a more extensive system of blood vessels. Restricting salt intake tends to curb fluid retention, thus reducing blood volume.

"Heart Attack" A "heart attack" is the end result of a long-term disease process. It does not just happen, although the attack itself may come without warning. The most common form of heart disease is coronary artery disease caused by atherosclerosis. When the coronary arteries cannot supply oxygenated blood to the heart muscle, because of a blood clot, a heart attack results. A heart attack caused by a clot is called a *coronary thrombosis*, a **coronary occlusion**, or a **myocardial infarction**. In myocardial infarction, part of the heart muscle (myocardium) may suffocate from lack of oxygen. If the heart attack is not fatal—that is, if enough of the muscle is undamaged to permit life to continue—the muscle begins to repair itself. It does so through a process called **collateral circulation**, in which small blood vessels open to take over the functions of the blocked artery and to move more blood through the damaged area. As healing takes place, scar tissue replaces part of the injured muscle. Collateral circulation can be developed even before a heart attack takes place. Aerobic exercise (discussed in Chapter 13) increases collateral circulation and may delay or prevent heart attacks due to blocked coronary arteries.

Exploring Your Emotions

There is a history of cardiovascular disease in your family. Your grandfather had a heart attack when he was 42, your father had a heart attack when he was 50, and your uncle had a stroke when he was 53. Although you are much younger, you are worried. Because you are much younger, however, you are not taking any preventive action. How do you feel about putting off the consequences of your lifestyle, which will inevitably affect your heart's health? At what age will you take action? Why haven't you started?

Angina pectoris A condition in which the heart muscle does not receive enough blood, causing severe pain in the chest and often in the left arm and shoulder.

Stroke An impeded blood supply to some part of the brain resulting in the destruction of brain cells (also called *cerebrovascular accident*).

Cerebral embolism Blockage of a blood vessel in the brain, caused by blood clots or other material carried in the blood from other parts of the body.

Cerebral hemorrhage Bleeding in or near the brain.

Aneurysm A sac formed by a distension or dilation of the artery wall.

Congestive heart failure A condition resulting from the heart's inability to pump out all the blood that returns to it. Blood backs up in the veins leading to the heart, causing an accumulation of fluid in various parts of the body.

Pulmonary edema Accumulation of water in the lungs.

Electrocardiogram (ECG) A test to detect abnormalities by measuring the electrical activity in the heart.

Electroencephalogram (EEG) A test that measures nerve cell activity in the brain.

Computerized tomography (CT) scan A test using computerized X-ray images to detect brain damage.

Arteries narrowed by disease may still be open enough to deliver blood to the heart. However, at times—chiefly during emotional excitement, stress, or physical exertion—the heart requires more oxygen than narrowed arteries can accommodate. When the need for oxygen outstrips the supply, the heart's electrical system may be disrupted, also causing a heart attack. Chest pain, called **angina pectoris**, is a signal that the heart is not getting enough blood to supply the oxygen it needs. Angina pain is felt as an extreme tightness in the chest and heavy pressure behind the breastbone or in the shoulder, neck, arm, hand, or back. This pain, although not actually a heart attack, is a warning that the load on the heart must be reduced. Angina may be controlled in a number of ways (with diet and drugs), but its course is unpredictable.

Stroke For brain cells to function as they should, they must have a continuous and ample supply of oxygen-rich blood. If brain cells are deprived of blood for more than a few minutes, they die. A **stroke**, also called a "cerebrovascular accident," occurs when the blood supply to the brain is cut off. Stroke can be particularly serious because injured brain cells, unlike those of other organs, cannot regenerate themselves.

A common cause of stroke is the buildup of a blood clot in one of the cerebral arteries of the brain. This condition, called *cerebral thrombosis*, is likely to occur when the cerebral arteries become damaged by atherosclerosis. Deposits formed on the artery walls encourage the formation of clots. The risk of stroke is much higher among hypertensives than among those with normal blood pressure. If an artery to the brain is clogged from atherosclerotic deposits, the high blood pressure accelerates the disease.

Occasionally a wandering blood clot, called an *embolus*, is carried in the bloodstream and becomes wedged in one of the cerebral arteries. This result is called a **cerebral embolism**. Another type of stroke, called *cerebrovascular occlusion*, occurs when a clot plugs up a cerebral artery.

Sometimes a diseased artery bursts in the brain. Blood pours into the surrounding tissue, and cells normally nourished by the artery are deprived of blood and cannot function. This event is called a **cerebral hemorrhage**. Patients who suffer from both atherosclerosis and high blood pressure are more likely to suffer cerebral hemorrhage than those who have only one condition or neither.

Bleeding of an artery in the brain may also be caused by a head injury or by the bursting of an aneurysm. An **aneurysm** is a blood-filled pocket that bulges out from a weak spot in an artery wall. Aneurysms in the brain may remain stable and never break, but when they do, the result is a stroke.

An interruption of the blood supply to any area of the brain prevents the nerve cells there from functioning. Nerve cells control sensation and most of our bodily movements. Which parts of the body are affected by the stroke depends on the area of the brain affected. A stroke may impair speech, cause walking disability, or cause loss of memory. The severity of a stroke and its long-term effects depend on which brain cells have been injured, how widespread the damage is, how effectively the body can restore the blood supply, and how rapidly other areas of brain tissue can take over the work of damaged cells.

Congestive Heart Failure A number of conditions, including high blood pressure, heart attack, atherosclerosis, rheumatic fever, and birth defects, can cut down on the heart's pumping efficiency. When the heart cannot maintain its regular pumping rate and force, fluids begin to back up and collect in the lungs and other parts of the body. When this extra, collected blood seeps through capillary walls, edema (swelling) results. Blood accumulating in the lungs causes swelling there, and this condition is called **pulmonary edema**. Pulmonary edema, in turn, causes shortness of breath. The entire process is **congestive heart failure**.

When people with impaired heart function stand or sit upright for long periods of time, the effect of gravity causes excess blood to accumulate in the legs. But in the prone position that people usually assume while resting, gravity no longer keeps the extra blood in the legs, and it goes into the lungs. There it interferes with breathing, which becomes extremely labored. If the heart weakens further, congestion in the lungs may be present all the time.

Congestive heart failure can be controlled. Treatment includes reducing the workload on the heart, modifying

Stroke: Prevention and Treatment

Stroke can often be prevented today. In fact, the death rate from stroke has fallen as much as 45 percent since 1970. This decline in deaths has come about, in part, because of new diagnostic tests and treatments. In addition, many Americans are adopting sensible health habits that lower the risk for stroke.

Yet stroke remains a leading cause of death among the elderly and is responsible for a large number of nursing home admissions.

What Is a Stroke?

Stroke is a sudden disruption in the flow of blood to an area of the brain. Deprived of blood, the affected brain cells either become damaged or die. While cell damage can often be repaired and the lost function regained, the death of brain cells is permanent and results in disability. There are three major types of stroke:

The *thrombotic* stroke is most common. Fatty deposits (plaques) build up in the arteries (blood vessels) that supply blood to the brain. This severely reduces the blood flow until, eventually, a clot or lump (called a *thrombus*) in an artery entirely blocks the path of blood.

An *embolic* stroke results when a blood clot forms somewhere else in the body, usually in arteries of the heart or neck, and the clot (embolus) travels through the circulatory system to the brain.

A *hemorrhagic* stroke is the most severe type of stroke. It occurs when a blood vessel in the brain bursts, allowing blood to pour into the brain outside of normal channels.

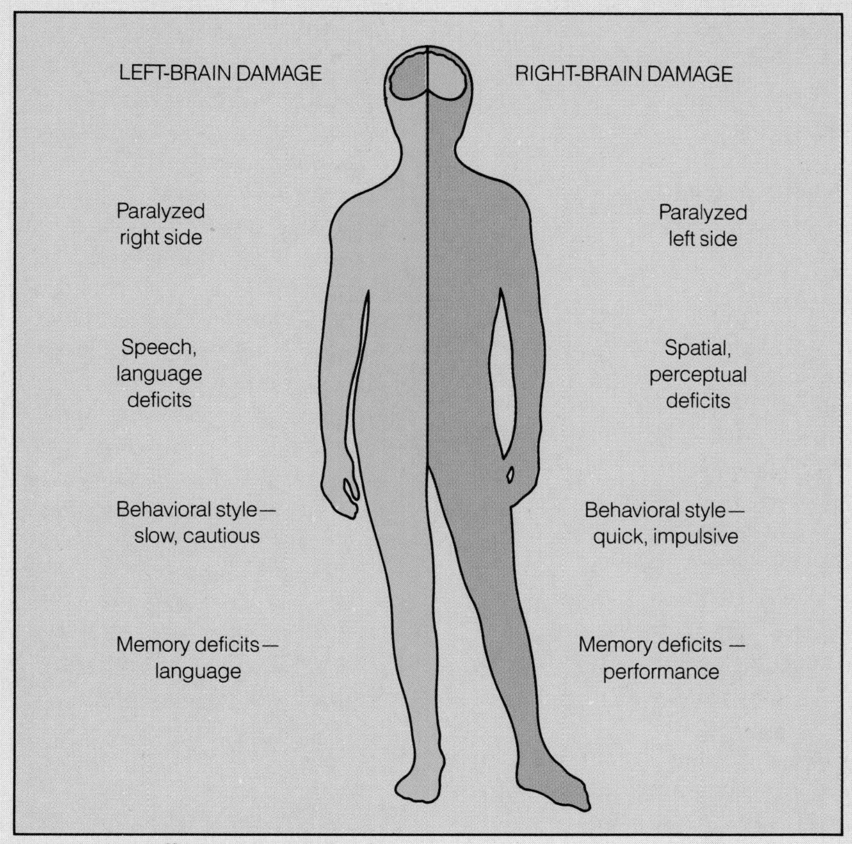

Brain damage affects opposite side of body.

Diagnosis and Treatment

A stroke is a medical condition that requires immediate care. Patients may be treated by the family physician or internist, or may be referred to a neurologist, a doctor who specializes in diagnosing and treating disorders of the brain. The neurologist first evaluates the patient to determine if a stroke in progress has been completed. The entire episode can last from minutes to hours and sometimes (although rarely) days.

An early diagnosis is made by evaluating symptoms, reviewing the patient's medical history, and performing routine tests. Tests that may be given include an **electrocardiogram** (a test that measures the electrical activity of the heart), and **electroencephalogram** (a test that measures nerve cell activity in the brain), and a **computerized tomography (CT)** scan (a painless technique that can assess brain damage). The CT scan uses a computer to construct black-and-white pictures of the brain from X-rays beamed through the head.

Treatment begins as soon as the stroke is diagnosed, to ensure that no further damage to brain cells occurs. Strong drugs, called *anticoagulants,* may be prescribed to prevent blood clots from becoming

(continued on next page)

Stroke: Prevention and Treatment (*continued*)

larger; or, in the case of a hemorrhagic stroke, drugs may be prescribed to lower the blood pressure, which is usually high.

What You Can Do to Prevent Stroke

Stroke was once viewed as a single devastating attack, but we now know it develops over a period of many years. The risk factors or conditions that lead to stroke include high blood pressure, atherosclerosis, heart disease, diabetes, smoking, and being overweight.

You can prevent stroke by taking these steps:

- Control your blood pressure. Have your blood pressure checked regularly, and, if it is high, follow your doctor's advice on how to lower it.
- Stop smoking.
- Eat a healthy diet that includes protein sources low in cholesterol (such as chicken, turkey, fish, and beans), skimmed milk, fruits, and vegetables.
- Exercise regularly. There is evidence that exercise strengthens the heart and improves circulation. It will also help in weight control; being overweight increases the chance of developing high blood pressure, heart disease, and atherosclerosis. Check with your doctor about what is an appropriate weight for your height and age.
- Control diabetes. If untreated, diabetes can cause destructive changes in the blood vessels throughout the body.
- Promptly report warning signs to your doctor. **Transient ischemic attacks (TIAs)** are the clearest warning that a stroke may occur; they produce temporary strokelike symptoms, such as numbness or weakness in an arm or leg, difficulty with speech, unexplained headaches, dizziness, momentary blindness, and impaired judgment.

Rehabilitation

Rehabilitation should begin as soon as possible after the patient's condition is stable. It consists of various types of therapy: *physical therapy* helps strengthen muscles and improves balance and coordination (patients may learn to use mechanical aids such as a walker, crutches, a cane, or braces); *speech and language therapy* helps those whose speech has been damaged; *occupational therapy* helps improve eye-hand coordination and strengthens skills needed to wash and dress, use tools, or prepare food.

Rehabilitation usually begins while the patient is still in the hospital and, for most, continues at home. Health care experts (physicians, physical and occupational therapists, nurses, social workers, and speech and language specialists) work together as a team to coordinate activities that will help the patient as well as the patient's family.

Progress in rehabilitation varies from person to person. For some, recovery is completed within weeks following a stroke; for others, it may take many months or years.

SOURCE: U.S. Department of Health and Human Services, 1986 (July–August), Stroke: Prevention and treatment, *Healthline*.

salt intake, and using drugs that help the body eliminate excess fluid. Heart stimulants taken orally, particularly digitalis, will improve the heart's efficiency.

Cardiovascular Disease, Personality, and Lifestyle

Historian Arnold Toynbee comments, "At the earliest moment at which we catch our first glimpse of man on Earth, we find him not only on the move but already moving at an accelerated pace. This crescendo of acceleration is continuing today. In our generation it is perhaps the most difficult and dangerous of all current problems of the human race." And Harvard nutritionist Jean Mayer says, "We are again in the age of the great pandemics. Our plague is cardiovascular." We are social animals. We respond to the world with our hearts, our arteries, and our internal juices. Even while we lie in bed, a random thought can make our heart race and our blood pressure rise. No wonder many of us will eventually become disabled or die from cardiovascular disease.

The increased occurrence of cardiovascular disease has essentially been restricted to populations that are industrially and socially advanced. Perhaps the most widely publicized research linking cardiovascular disease with lifestyle comes from cardiologists Meyer Friedman and

Transient ischemic attack (TIA) A small stroke; usually a temporary interruption of blood supply to the brain causing numbness or difficulty with speech.

Congenital heart disease Disease present at birth due to malformation of the heart or its major blood vessels.

Patent ductus arteriosus A congenital defect in which the opening between a branch of the aorta and a branch of the pulmonary artery fails to close after birth.

Coarctation of the aorta A congenital defect in which the aorta is narrowed or constricted.

Blue baby A baby with a blue coloration of the skin due to insufficient oxygen in the blood.

Ray Rosenman, who wrote *Type A Behavior and Your Heart* (1974). After extensive studies of thousands of working men, they concluded that men vulnerable to cardiovascular disease have much in common. They tend to be people who are extremely punctual and greatly annoyed if kept waiting. They are individuals with few hobbies; they find routine jobs at home bothersome because they feel the time could be spent more profitably. They walk rapidly, eat quickly, and attempt to do several things at one time. They are impatient, often anticipating what others will say, frequently interrupting before questions or replies are fully completed. These coronary-prone individuals (Friedman and Rosenman call them Type A's) seem to aspire to some vague, ill-defined achievements in their social environments. Add to this portrait a sedentary life, with little or no exercise, a tobacco-smoking habit, and one deadline after another, and you have the perfect candidate for a heart attack or stroke. In contrast, Type B's are more relaxed, and competition does not dominate their lives. They have more patience and more time for recreational activities. (See Chapter 2 to find out if you are Type A or B).

In a sense, some of us choose our diseases by the way we live. If we see no options, we can choose only one road. A competitive society that values status and material wealth is likely to foster only certain kinds of behaviors. Within such a society, few of us can resist these important influences. If we can see that we have a choice and are able to exercise it, however, our road will fork. Figure 17-4 shows only the economic costs of cardiovascular disease.

Heart Diseases in Children

Congenital Heart Disease Out of every 125 children born in the United States, one has a defect or malformation of the heart or major blood vessels. These conditions are referred to collectively as **congenital heart disease**. The development of the heart can go astray at any point, but in most cases medical scientists do not know why. Rubella, commonly called German measles contracted by the mother during the first three months of pregnancy is believed to be a prime cause of abnormal fetal development. Other viral diseases may also contribute. There may be a genetic component, too, although rarely is more than one child in a family affected.

The most common congenital defects are holes in the wall dividing the lower chambers of the heart. Holes may also occur in the wall between the upper chambers. With these defects, the heart produces a distinctive sound, making diagnosis relatively simple.

Other defects cannot be diagnosed without elaborate tests. One such defect is **patent ductus arteriosus**, a condition in which the prenatal channel between a branch of the aorta (a main artery delivering blood to the body) and a branch of the pulmonary artery (an artery delivering blood to the lungs) fails to close as it should. Another defect, **coarctation of the aorta**, is a narrowing, or constriction, of the largest artery of the body. Heart failure may result unless the constricted area is repaired by surgery. Another common defect results when the arteries delivering the blood to the body and lungs are transposed and attached to the wrong ventricles. The red, oxygen-rich blood that should be going to the body is returned to the lungs. The blue, oxygen-poor blood going to the body fails to supply enough oxygen for essential cell functions.

Most of the common congenital defects, including those causing **"blue baby"** conditions, can now be accurately

Figure 17-4 Estimated economic costs, in billions of dollars, of cardiovascular diseases by type of expenditure, United States, 1987.

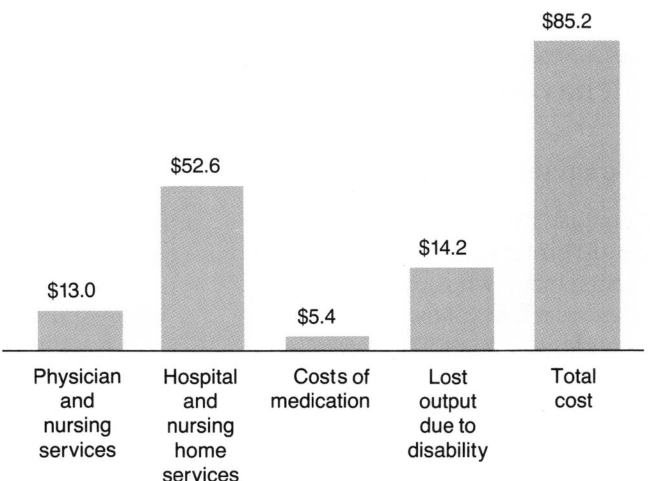

Rheumatic fever A disease, mainly of children, characterized by fever, inflammation, and pain in the joints; often damages the heart muscle.

Trachea Tube through which air passes to and from the lungs; the windpipe.

Biofeedback A method of controlling physiological responses once considered involuntary, such as blood pressure.

diagnosed. Important in saving lives is the early recognition that the newborn infant who shows blue appearance, respiratory difficulty, or failure to thrive may be suffering from congenital heart disease. Surgery to correct defects is also possible. Although such operations are hazardous, they give many children the chance for a normal life that would otherwise be denied them.

Rheumatic Heart Disease Ninety percent of heart trouble in children can be attributed to **rheumatic fever**, a disease associated with the hemolytic streptococcus bacterium (commonly called strep throat). The symptoms of rheumatic fever are generally vague, making diagnosis rather difficult. Among the symptoms observed in children are loss of weight or failure to gain weight; a low but persistent fever; poor appetite; repeated nosebleeds without apparent cause; jerky body movements; pain in the arms, legs, or abdomen; fatigue; and weakness. Antibiotics can usually prevent rheumatic fever. One attack of rheumatic fever will not prevent another and, in fact, often predisposes the child to later attacks. A child who has had an attack will usually have to take a daily dose of antibiotics for several years.

Rheumatic heart disease sometimes develops as a secondary response to rheumatic fever. This disease cripples the heart by scarring the muscle or damaging the heart valves. Treatment of rheumatic heart diseases often consists of surgery to restore the efficiency of damaged valves.

Take Action

Your answers to the Exploring Your Emotions questions in this chapter and your placement level on the Wellness Ladder will, we hope, encourage you to begin a process of self-exploration and self-discovery that you will continue. Reflect on the entire chapter's content and ask yourself how each point relates to your own life. Then take action:

1. Blood pressure is extremely variable. Have your blood pressure measured four times on four different occasions. Average the measurements to get an accurate picture of your blood pressure level. For information on home blood pressure monitoring, see Appendix I in Chapter 15.
2. Call the American Red Cross and sign up for a brief course in cardiopulmonary resuscitation (CPR).
3. Find out the route to the nearest hospital or clinic that has a coronary care unit. Educate family members and friends about the hospital and the route.
4. Read the following Behavior Change Strategy and take the appropriate action.

Behavior Change Strategy

Behavioral Management of High Blood Pressure

Because high blood pressure apparently produces few noticeable symptoms, many who suffer from it never seek or follow medical advice. In addition, high blood pressure is an ongoing, chronic problem that requires a course of treatment of long—possibly, lifelong—duration. Furthermore, the recommended medical treatment often calls for the use of antihypertensive medications that sometimes produce side effects. When all these factors are considered, it is clear that treatment may be difficult for people who must manage their blood pressure.

A considerable and still-growing body of behavioral research concerns ways to help people manage blood pressure. Results have not been consistent, and considerable controversy exists for any specific behavioral recommendations. Nevertheless, current behavioral strategies seem to assume at least one of three roles: (1) they may *substitute* for drug treatment for people who cannot (or will not) tolerate drug side effects, (2) they may be used as *adjuncts* to medication in that they may help to reduce the dosage needed to effectively manage blood pressure, or (3) they may play a *preventive* role in work with "at risk" groups such as children with elevated blood pressure readings and the relatives of patients already diagnosed as having hypertension.

Some of the strategies currently being used include the reduction of salt (sodium) intake, weight reduction, increased physical exercise, and relaxation techniques. By far the greatest amount of research on methods of blood pressure management has been in the areas of relaxation and biofeedback.

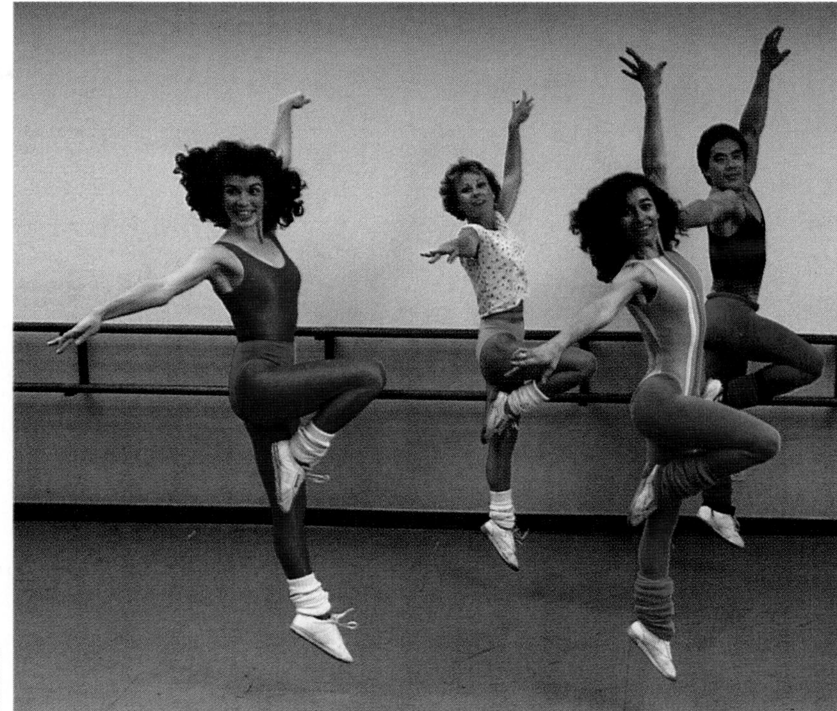

Tim Davis

Biofeedback and Relaxation Training

Biofeedback experiences can be used in conjunction with relaxation training or alone.

By means of biofeedback training, certain people are apparently able to reduce their intake of medications. It is extremely important to note, however, that antihypertensive medication should not be discontinued during biofeedback or relaxation training without close medical supervision.

Is biofeedback better than relaxation training? An incisive review of the available literature concluded that there was "no consistent advantage for one form of treatment over the other" but that relaxation was somewhat more convenient to use and decidedly less expensive. Furthermore, they found that relaxation was probably the more fundamental approach (the "final common pathway") in the sense that it produces a more general decrease in heart rate, blood pressure, and muscle activity, which are attacked separately and narrowly by specialized biofeedback training.

Selected References

Heart Facts. 1987. The American Heart Association.

Kromhout, D. et al. 1985. The inverse relation between fish consumption and 20-year mortality from coronary heart disease. *New England Journal of Medicine* 312:1205.

National Institute of Health. NIH Consensus Development Conference Statement: Lowering blood cholesterol to prevent heart disease. *Journal of the American Medical Association* 253:2080.

Rahimtoola, S. H. 1985. Cholesterol and coronary heart disease: A perspective. *Journal of the American Medical Association* 253:2094.

Walker, W. J. 1983. Changing United States' lifestyle and declining vascular mortality: Cause or coincidence? *New England Journal of Medicine* 308:649.

Recommended Readings

Richards, N. 1987. *Heart to Heart*. New York: Atheneum.
The author discusses what technology combined with human skills can do to combat heart disease.

Sobel, D., and Ferguson, T. 1985. *The People's Book of Medical Tests*. New York: Summit Books.
A consumer's guide that answers questions about 200 medical and home diagnostic tests.

Yetiv, J. Z. 1986. *Popular Nutritional Practices: A Scientific Appraisal*. Toledo: Popular Medicine Press.
A thorough, referenced analysis of more than 100 topics of contemporary interest.

Chapter 18

Contents

Rate Yourself

Your Cancer Risk Behavior Read the following statements carefully. Choose the one in each section that best describes you at this moment and circle its number. When you have chosen one statement for each section, add the numbers and record your total score. Find your position on the Wellness Ladder.

5 Knows the risk factors in cancer
4 Knows that lifestyle is implicated in cancer
3 Knows that 90 percent of lung cancer is caused by smoking
2 Defends cancer risk behaviors such as smoking
1 Denies that cancer can be prevented by lifestyle

5 Knows the recommendations for early detection of cancer
4 Checks breasts or testicles regularly
3 Knows cancer's warning signals
2 Avoids thinking about cancer detection
1 Resists cancer prevention

5 Avoids excessive sun exposure
4 Uses sunscreens when exposed to the sun
3 Sunbathes occasionally without protection
2 Sunbathes regularly without protection
1 Sunbathes frequently without protection

5 Avoids carcinogens
4 Limits X-rays
3 Limits intake of foods with preservatives
2 Prefers cured meats such as ham or bacon
1 Eats burnt food

5 Lives in an area with little smog
4 Has a job without exposure to carcinogens
3 Has a job with exposure to carcinogens but is protected
2 Lives in an area with heavy smog
1 Has a job with exposure to carcinogens and is not protected

Total Score ______

Cancer

Wellness Ladder

What can you do to help lower your risk of cancer? As you read through this chapter, be alert to ways that might help you move higher up the Wellness Ladder.

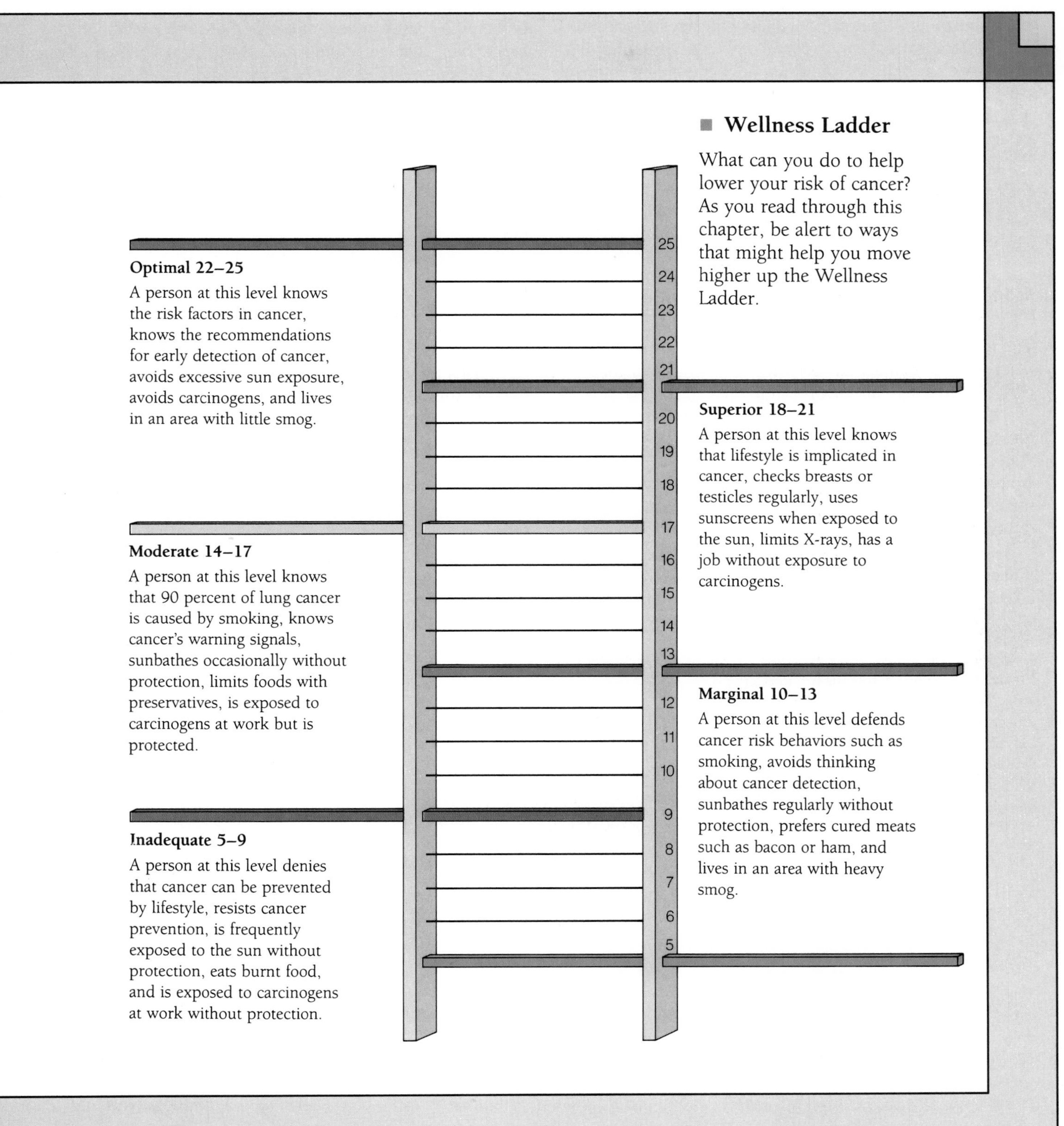

Optimal 22–25

A person at this level knows the risk factors in cancer, knows the recommendations for early detection of cancer, avoids excessive sun exposure, avoids carcinogens, and lives in an area with little smog.

Superior 18–21

A person at this level knows that lifestyle is implicated in cancer, checks breasts or testicles regularly, uses sunscreens when exposed to the sun, limits X-rays, has a job without exposure to carcinogens.

Moderate 14–17

A person at this level knows that 90 percent of lung cancer is caused by smoking, knows cancer's warning signals, sunbathes occasionally without protection, limits foods with preservatives, is exposed to carcinogens at work but is protected.

Marginal 10–13

A person at this level defends cancer risk behaviors such as smoking, avoids thinking about cancer detection, sunbathes regularly without protection, prefers cured meats such as bacon or ham, and lives in an area with heavy smog.

Inadequate 5–9

A person at this level denies that cancer can be prevented by lifestyle, resists cancer prevention, is frequently exposed to the sun without protection, eats burnt food, and is exposed to carcinogens at work without protection.

Cancer is both frightening and fascinating. Frightening because of many myths and misconceptions combined with feelings of hopelessness. And fascinating because it is mysterious, challenging, and capable of being conquered. About 50 percent of cancer patients survive it to lead normal lives. This survival rate has been rapidly increasing since the 1930s, when only 20 percent of cancer patients survived more than five years. Despite the real gains made in treating cancer, the total number of cancer deaths is on the increase. The reason for this is the increase in lung cancer—the leading cancer killer among men and women. This dramatic rise in cancer deaths can be attributed almost entirely to cigarette smoking (see Chapter 9).

What Is Cancer?

The term *cancer* refers to disorders of cell growth. These disorders, sometimes called **malignant tumors** or malignant **neoplasms,** all involve unregulated unrestrained growth of the body's cells. Normally (in adults), cells divide and grow at a rate sufficient to replace dying cells. When you cut your finger, for example, the cells around the wound divide more rapidly to heal the wound. When the wound is healed, the rate of cell growth and division returns to normal.

The cancer growth process is controlled by DNA in the nucleus of the cell. If nuclei lose their ability to regulate, cells divide at random, resulting in growths called *tumors.*

Tumors serve no physiological purpose. Some are made up of cells similar to the surrounding cells and are enclosed in a membrane that prevents them from penetrating other tissues. Such tumors, called **benign tumors,** are dangerous only if their physical presence interferes with bodily functions. A benign tumor, for example, can cause death if it blocks the blood supply to the brain.

Cancers are malignant tumors. They kill by invading normal tissues, eventually destroying normal cells. The nuclei of cancer cells are larger than those of normal cells. They also have a greater number of **chromosomes.** Some researchers have suggested that an increase in the number of chromosomes produced may be the first detectable sign of cancer.

Cancer cells do not stick as closely together as normal cells or as tightly to their original site, called the *primary tumor.* They break away easily, which enables them to invade nearby tissue directly or spread to other parts of the body, where they establish new colonies of cancer cells. This traveling process is called **metastasizing,** and the new tumors are called *secondary tumors,* or *metastases.* Traveling cancer cells can follow two courses. They can produce secondary tumors in the lymph nodes and be carried through the lymph system to form secondary sites elsewhere, or they can invade blood vessels and circulate through the vessels to colonize other organs (see Figure 18-1).

This ability of cancer cells to metastasize makes early cancer detection critical. To control the cancer and prevent death, every cancerous cell must be removed. Once

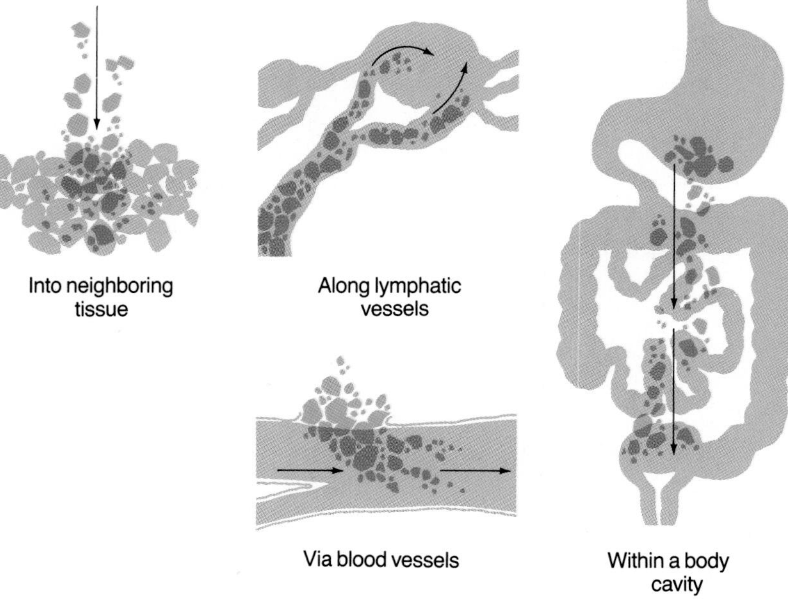

Figure 18-1 Cancer spreads in three basic ways: (a) Malignant tumors enlarge and extend into neighboring tissue. (b) Cancer cells break loose easily and are carried through blood vessels and lymphatic vessels to other parts of the body. (c) Dislodged cancer cells implant themselves in neighboring organs.

Malignant tumor A tumor that is cancerous and capable of spreading.

Neoplasm Also called a tumor, a new growth of abnormal cells that may be benign or malignant.

Benign tumor A tumor that is not malignant or cancerous.

Chromosomes Material in the nucleus of a cell that transmits genetic information. Abnormal chromosomes are common in cancer cells.

Metastasize The spread of cancer cells from one part of the body to another.

Carcinomas Cancer that originates in epithelial tissue (skin, glands, and lining of internal organs).

Sarcomas Cancers arising from bone, cartilage, or striated muscle.

Lymphomas Tumors originating from lymphatic tissue (neck, groin, armpit).

Leukemia Malignant disease of the blood-forming system.

Pap smear A scraping of cells from the cervix for examination under a microscope to detect cancer.

cancer cells enter either the lymph or the blood system, it is extremely difficult to stop their spread to other organs of the body. Cancer cells can ravage a formerly strong and healthy body with frightening speed, depending on the part of the body they invade. They may take over an artery, stopping the flow of blood to the kidneys, liver, and heart. Cancer cells growing in the pancreas or bone marrow may reduce the blood's ability to clot. If this happens, the victim may die from any ruptured blood vessel. Cancer in the lymph system weakens the body's ability to fight even the simplest infection (see discussion of the common cold in Chapter 22).

Exploring Your Emotions

You overhear the news that someone you know has either heart disease or cancer. Do you feel differently about these two diseases? Why? How might such feelings interfere with prevention?

Types of Cancer

Malignant tumors are classified according to the types of cells that give rise to them. The most common cancers are carcinomas, sarcomas, lymphomas, and leukemia (the suffix *-oma* means "tumor"). **Carcinomas** are the most common form of cancer. They arise from the skin; glands (breast, uterus, prostate); and membranes lining the respiratory (lungs, bronchial tubes), urinary, and gastrointestinal (mouth, stomach, colon, rectum) tracts. Carcinomas metastasize primarily via the lymph vessels.

Sarcomas occur less often than carcinomas. They arise from sources such as connective fibrous tissue: muscle, bone, cartilage, and membranes covering muscles and fat. Sarcomas metastasize primarily via the blood vessels.

Lymphomas are cancer of the lymph nodes, the body's infection-fighting structures.

Leukemia is cancer of certain tissues that form blood: an uncontrolled multiplication and accumulation of abnormal white cells.

How Many People Develop Cancer?

Although one person in three will develop cancer in his or her lifetime, many fewer will actually die from it. Cancer is second only to heart disease as a cause of death in the United States and is the leading cause of death among women aged 30 to 54 and among children aged 3 to 14. In 1900, 6 percent of the deaths in the United States were attributed to cancer; by 1984 cancer deaths had risen to 22 percent. More than 1,300 people a day die of cancer in this country.

Of the 950,000 people who were diagnosed as having cancer in 1987, about one-half will be "cured"; that is, they will be alive five years after treatment.

Who Is at Risk?

Who gets cancer and what kind? The answers to these questions depend on lifestyle, sex, age, occupation, and geography, and other things. Smoking is the most important known cause of cancer. Leukemia is the leading cause of death (from disease) among children aged 3 to 14. For men, the leading cancer sites are lungs, prostate, and large intestine. (See Table 18-1 and Figure 18-2.) More programs aimed at preventing and curing prostate cancer should be implemented. Early detection is the key to successful treatment of this neglected type of cancer.

For women the leading cancer sites are the lungs, breasts, and large intestine. (See Table 18-2 and Figure 18-2.) The success in the fight against cancer of the uterus is dramatic. Today it is a rare cause of cancer death. This decline is mainly attributable to the increasing use of the **Pap smear.** This simple procedure involves examining cells from the cervix and body of the uterus under a microscope. These cells can be taken by a physician as part of a pelvic examination. For the person not at risk, a Pap smear is recommended once every three years after two initial negative tests one year apart. Women at risk should have a tissue sample examined at menopause. (See Table 18-2 for factors that influence your risk of having breast cancer.)

Table 18-1 Leading Cancer Sites, 1987[a]

Site	Estimated New Cases 1987	Estimated Deaths 1987	Warning Signal: If You Have One, See Your Doctor	Safeguards	Comment
Breast	130,000	41,000	Lump or thickening in the breast.	Annual checkup; monthly breast self-examination.	The leading cause of cancer death in women.
Colon and rectum	145,000	60,000	Change in bowel habits; bleeding.	Annual checkup including proctoscopy, especially for those over 40.	Considered a highly curable disease when digital and proctoscopic examinations are included in routine checkups.
Lung	150,000	136,000	Persistent cough or lingering respiratory ailment.	80 percent of lung cancer would be prevented if no one smoked cigarettes.	The leading cause of cancer death among men and rising mortality among women.
Oral (including pharynx)	30,000	9,000	Sore that does not heal. Difficulty in swallowing.	Annual checkup.	Many more lives should be saved because the mouth is easily accessible to visual examination by physicians and dentists.
Skin	25,800[b]	7,800	Sore that does not heal or change in wart or mole.	Annual checkup; avoidance of overexposure to sun.	Skin cancer is readily detected by observation and diagnosed by simple biopsy.
Uterus	47,000[c]	10,000	Unusual bleeding or discharge.	Annual checkup, including pelvic examination with Pap test.	Uterine cancer mortality has declined 65 percent during the last 40 years with wider application of the Pap test. Postmenopausal women with abnormal bleeding should be checked.
Kidney and bladder	67,300	20,000	Urinary difficulty; bleeding—in which case consult doctor at once.	Annual checkup with urinalysis.	Protective measures for workers in high-risk industries are helping to eliminate one of the important causes of these cancers.
Larynx	12,100	3,800	Hoarseness—difficulty in swallowing.	Annual checkup, including laryngoscopy.	Readily curable if caught early.
Prostate	96,000	27,000	Urinary difficulty.	Annual checkup, including palpation.	Occurs mainly in men over 60; the disease can be detected by palpation and urinalysis at annual checkup.
Stomach	25,000	14,000	Indigestion.	Annual checkup.	A 40 percent decline in mortality in 25 years, for reasons unknown.
Leukemia	26,000	18,000	Leukemia is a cancer of blood-forming tissues and is characterized by the abnormal production of immature white blood cells. Acute leukemia strikes mainly children and is treated by drugs that have extended life from a few months to as much as 10 years. Chronic leukemia strikes usually after age 25 and progresses less rapidly.		
Other blood and lymph tissues	48,100	24,900	These cancers arise in the lymph system and include Hodgkin's disease and lymphosarcoma. Some patients with lymphatic cancers can lead normal lives for many years. Five-year survival rate for Hodgkin's disease increased from 25 percent to 54 percent in 20 years.		

[a]All figures rounded to nearest 100.
[b]Totals do not include nonmelanoma skin cancers (500,000 new cases annually).
[c]Totals do not include cases in which the carcinoma is confined to the epithelium (over 45,000 new cases).
SOURCE: Incidence estimates are based on rates from American Cancer Society, 1987, *ACS: Cancer Facts & Figures—1987* (New York: American Cancer Society).

in situ At the original site; has not spread.

Table 18-2 Factors that Influence Breast Cancer Risk

Increase in Risk	Decrease in Risk
Family history of breast cancer	Short number of menstrual years; early menopause
High-fat, high-calorie diet; obesity	Early pregnancy
Primary endometrial or ovarian cancer	Many children
Early onset of first menstruation (menarche); late menopause	Breastfeeding of infants
Late age for first pregnancy	Bilateral removal of ovaries early in fertile life
No children, unmarried	Low socioeconomic status
Live births with no nursing	Rural areas
Failure of ovulation	
Blood group O in young women; A in elderly women; S blood group	
Prolonged high-dose estrogen treatment	
Chest irradiation	
Low urinary estriol ratio; low androgen excretion	

SOURCE: Jay Roth, 1985, *All About Cancer* (Philadelphia: Stickley), p. 189.

Figure 18-2 Cancer incidence by site and sex, and cancer deaths by site and sex. Percentages shown are estimates for 1987.[a]

Male

INCIDENCE	Site	DEATH
3%	Skin	2%
4%	Oral	3%
20%	Lung	36%
14%	Colon and rectum	11%
3%	Pancreas	5%
20%	Prostate	10%
10%	Urinary	5%
8%	Leukemia and lymphomas	9%
18%	All other	19%

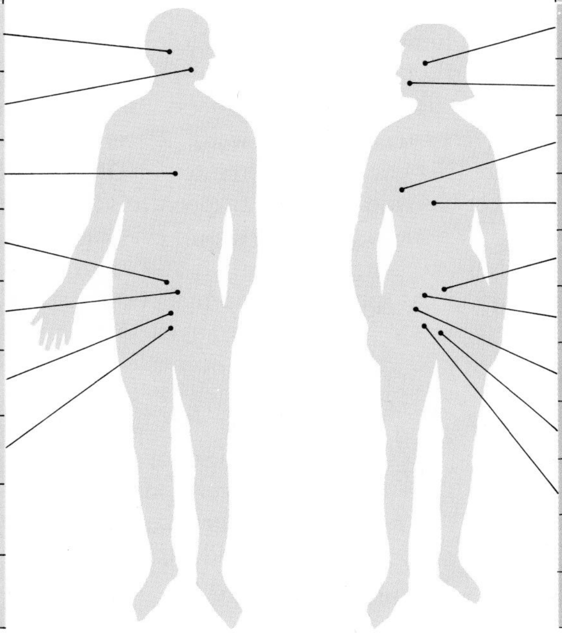

Female

INCIDENCE	Site	DEATH
3%	Skin	2%
2%	Oral	1%
27%	Breast	18%
11%	Lung	20%
16%	Colon and rectum	14%
3%	Pancreas	5%
4%	Ovary	5%
10%	Uterus	4%
4%	Urinary	3%
7%	Leukemia and lymphomas	9%
13%	All other	19%

[a]Excluding nonmelanoma skin cancer and carcinoma ***in situ***.

Malignant melanoma A highly malignant form of skin cancer.

DNA Deoxyribonucleic acid, a chemical substance that carries genetic information.

Oncogenes Genes that promote tumor growth.

Carcinogens Any substances that cause cancer.

The number of teenage and preteenage girls who smoke tobacco continues to rise. Therefore it is likely that women's incidence of lung cancer and cancer in other sites, such as the bladder, will continue to increase.

While stomach cancer has declined in the United States over the past fifty years, colon and rectum cancer has become more common. The warning signals include bleeding from the rectum, blood in the stool, and change in bowel habits. Risk factors include personal or family history of colon and rectum cancer, personal or family history of polyps in the colon or rectum, and inflammatory bowel disease. Evidence suggests that dietary habits are linked to this increase. A diet high in fat and/or low in fiber content may be a significant cause.

Who Survives Cancer?

In the United States, roughly 50 percent of people who are diagnosed as having cancer are alive five years after the diagnosis. This percentage continues to increase as technology improves and as the public becomes more aware of the importance of early diagnosis and treatment. For most forms of cancer, a person who shows no symptoms five years after treatment is considered "cured."

Only 13 percent of people with lung cancer live five years or more after diagnosis. The rate is 33 percent for cases detected early; but only 24 percent of lung cancers are found that early.

When colon and rectum cancer is found and treated early, the five-year survival rate is 87 percent for colon cancer and 77 percent for rectum cancer. This rate goes down to 40 and 30 percent after the cancer has spread to other parts of the body.

For breast cancer, the five-year survival rate is nearly 100 percent if it has not spread. If the cancer has spread, the rate drops to 60 percent.

The survival rate for ovarian cancer is only 38 percent. However, if ovarian cancer is diagnosed and treated early, more than 85 percent of such patients live five years or longer.

Survival rates for prostate cancer have improved steadily during the past twenty years. If the disease has not spread, about 83 percent of all patients are alive five years after treatment.

Smoking is the greatest risk factor for bladder cancer. When detected early, the five-year survival rate is 87 percent. The rate drops to 38 percent when detected at a later stage.

More than 500,000 cases of skin cancer are diagnosed each year, most of which are very curable. The most serious skin cancer is **malignant melanoma,** which strikes about 26,000 people each year. Even this perilous type of skin cancer has a survival rate of 89 percent when detected early. See Figure 18-3 for five-year cancer survival rates for selected sites.

Exploring Your Emotions

Your friend, who smokes, has been to the doctor for a chronic cough. You are waiting with her to find out about a shadow that appeared on her lung X-ray. In the waiting room, she lights up a cigarette. How do you react?

What Causes Cancer?

The causes of most cancers are essentially unknown. What is known is that cell growth becomes uncontrolled. But the reason for this loss of control can only be speculated on. Radiation, viral infections, chemical substances in the air or in your diet, and vitamin deficiencies have all been implicated. Some cancers develop in two or more stages, requiring exposure to a chemical "initiator" to start the process, then to a "promoter" to move cancer growth forward. Researchers think that the defect in cancer cells resides in **DNA (deoxyribonucleic acid),** the material that controls the genetics and hereditary part of each cell. Recent evidence points to genes (which are composed of DNA and are responsible for specific hereditary traits in normal cells) that have been shown to be altered or rearranged in such a way that encourages the growth of cancer cells. These **oncogenes** (*onco-*, "cancer") are being extensively studied to establish a link between them and specific cancers. Although we have yet to discover the causes of all types of cancer, researchers are making great strides in the race to uncover them. A few uncommon types, such as tumor of the retina, are inherited. And evidence suggests that families inherit tendencies toward one type of cancer rather than another.

Lifestyle is an important element in the incidence of cancer. Mormons and Seventh-Day Adventists, for example, are much less likely to develop cancer than the general population. Church doctrine of both groups forbids tobacco and alcohol use. The members also maintain a strong social support network that may influence both the prevention and outcome of disease.

Agents that cause cancer are called **carcinogens.** Some carcinogens occur naturally in the environment, such as ultraviolet rays from the sun. Others are manufactured or synthesized substances. Some are present in the home environment—in the food we eat, the drugs we take, or the tobacco smoke we inhale. Others are present in the work environment of certain industries (see Table 18-3). Most carcinogens are physical or chemical irritants. One general principle in carcinogenesis is that often much time elapses between (1) initiation and promotion and (2) the actual growth of cancer cells to form a tumor. This "latent" period may last anywhere from five to thirty years or more. Tobacco smokers, for example, seldom get lung cancer until they have been smoking for twenty years. Of course, the 4-year-old child who gets leukemia obviously has not had a long latent period. Many researchers think that short latency periods may be related to oncogenes or inherited tendencies to develop cancer, as discussed earlier.

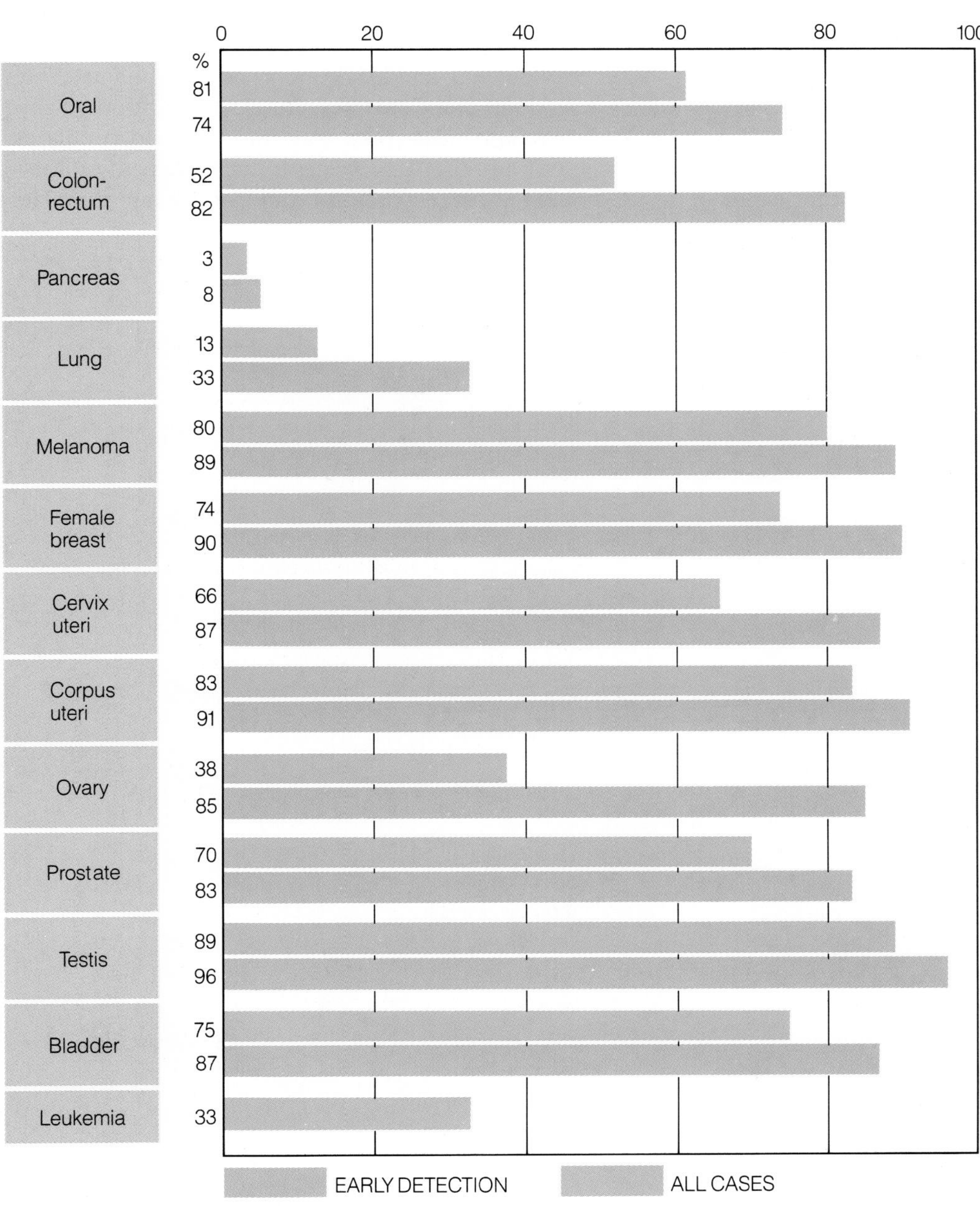

Note: This chart is based on cases diagnosed in 1974–1982.
[a]Adjusted for normal life expectancy.

Figure 18-3 Five-year Cancer Survival Rates[a] for selected sites.

Beta-carotene A vitamin-A precursor found in plants.

Provitamin A substance that can be converted into a vitamin.

Retinol A substance containing vitamin A.

Ingested Chemicals Some of the substances we eat, drink, or inhale are themselves carcinogenic. Others combine with chemicals present in the body to produce carcinogens. A great deal of money is invested in producing and marketing these substances, and debates over their possible dangers have been long and bitter. The position often taken by the manufacturer of a product suspected of being carcinogenic is that laboratory tests of the product were done on animals, not people, and that amounts of the substance given were much larger than a person would consume. The counterargument is that tests with laboratory animals have often been good predictors of results in people and that high doses are the best way we have of simulating the cumulative long-term effects of low doses.

Since World War II, new methods of marketing and distributing foods have greatly increased the length of time it takes food to travel from its source to the consumer. In the process, food may become stale and unappetizing or it may become spoiled and unsafe. The food industry has generally solved the spoilage problem by using preservatives and the staleness problem by using "cosmetic" additives—chemicals that disguise the look or the taste of staleness in food. Additives are, of course, used for many other reasons as well—as stabilizers, emulsifiers, fillers, or binders, for example. Some of the additives—such as salt, sugar, and saltpeter (potassium nitrate or sodium nitrite)—have been used for centuries; others such as BHA (butylated hydroxyanisole), BHT (butylated hydroxytoluene), and MSG (monosodium glutamate) are new products of the chemical industry. Dangerous chemicals may also make their way into the food supply as residues from insecticides and as traces of diethylstilbestrol (DES) or other synthetic hormones given to stimulate

Table 18-3 Cancer in the Environment: Ten Suspects

Agents	Where Found	Cancers They May Cause
Arsenic	Mining and smelting industries	Skin, liver, lung
Asbestos	Brake linings, construction sites, insulation, powerhouses	Lung, pleura, peritoneum
Benzene	Solvents, insecticides, oil refineries	Bone marrow
Benzidine (outlawed in Great Britain and U.S.S.R., still used widely in U.S.)	Manufacturing rubber, dyestuffs	Bladder
Coal combustion products	Steel mills, petrochemical industry, asphalt, coal tar	Lung, bladder, scrotum
Nickel compounds	Metal industry, alloys	Lung, nasal sinuses
Radiation	Ultraviolet rays from the sun, medical treatments	Bone marrow, skin, thyroid
Synthetic estrogens	Drugs	Vagina, cervix, uterus
Tobacco	Cigarettes, cigars, pipes	Lung, bladder, mouth, esophagus, pharynx, larynx
Vinyl chloride	Plastics industry	Liver, brain

Diet and Cancer

It has become clear that what we eat—or don't eat—for breakfast, lunch, and dinner may have profound effects on our chances of developing cancer. One estimate is that the death rate from all cancers in this country might be reduced more than a third by practical changes in our diet. These are some of the diet components that are believed to affect the cancer process:

Carotenoids and Vitamin A

Carotenoids are found in carrots, sweet potatoes, peaches, cantaloupes, and other yellow-orange fruits and vegetables, and in some dark green vegetables like broccoli, kale, and spinach. **Beta-carotene** and some of the other carotenoids are **provitamins**, or precursors, of vitamin A. When ingested, some of them are converted to vitamin A in the body.

Preformed vitamin A, or **retinol**, occurs only in foods of animal origin—chiefly whole milk, cheese, butter, egg yolks, and liver. Preformed vitamin A, in the form of retinyl acetate or retinyl palmitate, is also present in many multiple-vitamin pills and in some fortified foods.

In many cultures, carotenoids from fruits and vegetables are the source of most of the vitamin A, and particular plant foods often account for most of them. Dark green, leafy vegetables are the main source of beta-carotene among some Chinese, for example, as are carrots in this country, a red palm oil used for cooking in West Africa, and yellow-green vegetables in Japan.

Inverse associations have been found, in a number of studies, between dietary vitamin A or carotenoids and the incidence of a number of cancers—those of the oral cavity and pharynx, the larynx, and lung. These findings suggest that either or both of these substances may protect against cancer. A study of esophageal cancer has suggested that deficiencies of a number of micronutrients may increase risk for that cancer.

Vitamin C

Some studies show an inverse association between fresh fruit and vegetable consumption and some cancers, including stomach cancer, though no studies have implicated vitamin C deficiency in the etiology of this cancer. Animal studies show that ascorbic acid—vitamin C—can inhibit the formation of carcinogenic N-nitroso compounds from ingested nitrates.

Fats

Surveys of various populations in this country and in others have suggested a link between dietary fat intake and some cancers, particularly those of the breast, colon, endometrium, and prostate gland. Animal studies tend to confirm these associations. A link between per capita fat intake and breast cancer risk is also supported by a number of international studies, although case control studies do not, in general, support this link.

Animal studies have shown that high levels of fat in the diet enhance the development of both spontaneous and chemically induced mammary cancers in mice. This was true even if the fat was fed after tumor initiation, lending support to the hypothesis that dietary fat acts as a cancer promoter.

Correlations of international incidence and death rates with diet components indicate that colon cancer and, to a lesser extent, rectal cancer, are associated with total dietary fat intake. Some case control studies have also suggested a relationship between dietary fat intake and risk of colon and rectal cancers, but the evidence is not clear-cut.

Varying levels of fiber intake may help to explain some of the conflicting data on fat intake and colon and rectal cancers, because fiber is thought to protect against these cancers. Thus, fat intake—particularly milk fat—was found in one study to be about the same for individuals in rural Finland and in Copenhagen, Denmark, but the Finns, who eat large amounts of high-fiber, unrefined rye bread, had a much lower incidence of colon cancer.

An association between the incidence of prostate cancer and high dietary fat intake in humans has been seen chiefly in international surveys. Both prostate cancer incidence and fat intake are higher among Japanese living in Hawaii than among Japanese living in Japan. And prostate cancer incidence has been linked with the consumption of animal fat and protein among several ethnic groups in Hawaii.

Most population studies of dietary fat intake and cancer incidence have not been able to differentiate the effects of saturated and unsaturated fats, but consumption of the two often goes hand in hand. Total fat intake accounts for about 40 percent of total calories

(continued on next page)

Diet and Cancer (*continued*)

in the U.S. diet, compared with only 20 percent in the Japanese diet. Meat, eggs, dairy foods, and oils used in cooking and in salads are the chief sources of fat in the American diet.

Fiber

Dietary fiber appears to protect against some forms of cancer, particularly colon cancer. Which types of fiber, and how they may work, are not clear.

Fiber is found in fruits, vegetables, nuts, legumes (peas and beans), brown rice, and whole-grain breads and cereals. Some studies have shown an inverse association between the consumption of vegetables and the occurrence of colon cancers. But it has been difficult to single out the role of fiber in many of the studies that measure total fruit and vegetable intake. Individuals who eat diets high in fruits, vegetables, legumes, and whole grains usually eat less fat and protein and tend not to be overweight. And a diet high in fruits and vegetables is likely to be high in carotenoids and vitamin C.

Cured, Pickled, and Smoked Foods; Molds and Fungi

Studies in different parts of the world show an apparent link between frequent consumption of pickled, cured, and smoked foods and an increased risk of stomach cancer. This association could be due either to the curing agents or to molds and fungi toxins that may form in these foods if they are not refrigerated. The decrease in stomach cancer incidence in the United States since the 1930s has been attributed to the wide use of refrigeration, although there is no proof.

Vitamin E and Selenium

Both vitamin E and an enzyme that depends on selenium for its activity act as antioxidants, able to block damage to cellular DNA from some carcinogens. These substances can also keep cultured cells treated with chemicals from becoming cancerous. There is no evidence that "megadoses" of either of these substances help to protect humans against cancer. Selenium is known to be toxic in high doses, and vitamin E, which is fat-soluble, is potentially toxic.

SOURCE: Harriet S. Page and Ardyce J. Asire, 1985 (April), *Cancer rates and risks,* 3rd ed., NIH Publication No. 85-691 (Washington, D.C.: Public Health Service, National Institutes of Health, U.S. Department of Health and Human Services), pp. 44–48.

the growth of cattle or other animals. (The United States has now banned the use of DES.)

Nitrates and nitrites are a good case in point. Many food processing industries add sodium nitrate or sodium nitrite to ham, bacon, hot dogs, bologna, and other luncheon meats. The nitrates do two things: (1) they preserve a pink color, which has no bearing on taste but looks more appetizing to many people, and (2) they inhibit growth of bacteria that cause botulism, a disease that can be fatal. While nitrates are not carcinogenic in themselves, they may combine with amines in the body to form **nitrosamines,** which are highly potent carcinogens.

Some researchers suggest that nitrates added to smoked fish, a staple of the Japanese diet, are a factor in the high rate of stomach cancer in Japan. Other researchers claim that evidence linking nitrates and nitrites to cancer is inconclusive. They argue that nitrates and nitrites vaporize during cooking, that they occur naturally in saliva anyway, and that the formation of nitrosamines is blocked by vitamin C. Thus, according to these researchers a glass of orange juice will prevent your breakfast bacon from contributing to the manufacture of carcinogens in your body.

Diet Factors A "fatty diet" (high in saturated fats such as are found in red meats) appears to contribute to intestinal cancer and breast cancer. Scotland has the highest incidence of intestinal cancer in the world, and the Scots eat 20 percent more "fatty" meat than do their English neighbors. In Japan, fish, not fatty meat, is the staple, and intestinal cancer is uncommon. But Japanese who have emigrated to the United States, where fatty meats are a major part of the diet, are as susceptible to intestinal cancer as other Americans.

Some populations, particularly vegetarians, have little or no colon cancer. The vegetarian diet is typically high in fiber, which suggests that colon cancer may be related to lack of fiber in the diet. While fiber does not supply nutrition, it does provide the bulk needed to move other foods through the digestive tract. The shorter transit time afforded by a high-fiber diet may be an important factor in the low colon cancer rates of vegetarians. A diet high

Nitrosamines Chemical substances that can cause cancer.

Mammogram An X-ray of the breasts.

in meats, especially pork and beef, causes the digestive tract to work overtime to rid the body of material that is difficult to break down and excrete. Whether a diet high in both meat and fiber can result in a low incidence is still not known.

Breast cancer may also be linked to high fat intake. Scientists suspect that fats overstimulate hormone production or disrupt normal hormone balance. Recent evidence also suggests that calories by themselves may be linked to breast cancer, because many breast cancer patients are overweight.

Alcohol and Drugs High alcohol intake is correlated to cancer of the mouth, pharynx, esophagus, larynx, and liver. The risk is greatest among drinkers who smoke, which suggests that alcohol and tobacco may interact as carcinogens. Oral cancer deaths are two to six times greater among men who drink more than 1½ ounces of hard liquor a day than among teetotalers, depending on how much tobacco the drinkers smoke. For the heavy drinker and smoker, the risk is up to fifteen times greater than for the nondrinking nonsmoker.

Certain prescription drugs, especially estrogens (female sex hormones), are also suspected of being carcinogenic. Shortly after World War II, DES (the same drug used on cattle as discussed earlier) was prescribed for many infertile women. (DES mimics the effects of natural estrogen.) The drug worked—that is, the women conceived—but fifteen to thirty years later many of their daughters developed vaginal cancer.

Inhaled Chemicals Inhaling carcinogenic irritants over a long period of time triggers cancerous potentials in susceptible lung tissue cells. More Americans die of lung cancer (over 136,000, with the numbers increasing each year) than are killed in automobile accidents. Cigarette smoking is responsible for at least 80 percent of lung cancer cases, and perhaps more if you consider the incidence of lung cancer among those who inhale passive or sidestream smoke (see Chapter 9).

Smog is another source of carcinogens. Industrial smoke and other pollutants mix with fog to produce smog. The chemicals in this highly irritating mixture contribute to a higher rate of lung cancer among city dwellers than among rural dwellers. Los Angeles and Pittsburgh have the highest death rates from lung and other respiratory diseases—and the thickest smogs.

Many chemicals used in the rubber, plastics, paint and dye, cable, and petrochemical industries have serious consequences for workers and their families (see Table 18-3). Carcinogens such as asbestos, nickel, and arsenic, as well as dusts, gases, and tars, continually irritate the lung tissue and may eventually alter the cell structure. Coal tar and its derivatives account for the largest group of occupation-related cancers.

These chemicals are also a hazard to people living near factories that use them. New evidence shows that people who live near asbestos plants, copper-smelting facilities, and industries that use vinyl chloride have a significantly increased risk of cancer and other diseases.

Radiation Radiation can produce chemical changes in cells that eventually lead to cancer. All sources of radiation—including X-rays, radioactive substances, and sunlight—are potentially harmful. Uranium miners in Colorado, for example, have a very high incidence of lung cancer. Victims of the atomic bombs dropped on Hiroshima and Nagasaki continue to suffer radiation effects, in the forms of breast cancer and leukemia, more than forty years after the bombing. X-ray technicians also show a high incidence of leukemia. And children treated with radiation for tonsillitis and thymus gland diseases during the 1940s and 1950s have higher rates of thyroid cancer than those who were not treated. Radiation effects are cumulative through your lifetime.

Medical researchers cannot agree on the amount of risk involved in the use of diagnostic X-rays. Some researchers say that a single abdomen X-ray with the standard unit of dosage significantly ages the cells it strikes and thus increases the risk of leukemia. And some are convinced that irradiating men and women during their reproductive years increases the likelihood that offspring conceived thereafter will develop leukemia. The National Cancer Institute now recommends that people below the age of fifty avoid routine screening X-rays of all kinds, including dental X-rays and the low-dosage breast X-rays known as **mammograms**, except for a baseline mammogram after age 35–40.

Excessive exposure to ultraviolet radiation from the sun is the major cause of skin cancer, especially among fair-skinned people. Skin cancer has a 95 percent cure rate, but it is a common cancer and causes about 8,000 deaths a year. Melanoma, one type of skin cancer, has a

Exploring Your Emotions

Sunbathing is your favorite activity. How do you feel about the links that have been found between sunlight and cancer? Does that information affect your behavior?

Epidermis The outermost layer of the skin.

Basal cell carcinoma Cancer of the deepest layers of the skin.

Squamous cell carcinoma Cancer of the surface layers of the skin.

Melanoma A malignant tumor of the skin.

Nuclear magnetic resonance (NMR) A method for forming a visual image of the inside of the body.

---

75 percent higher death rate in the southeastern states than in the less sunny northern states. People with light skin, particularly the freckling type, are about ten times more likely to develop skin cancer after excessive exposure to sunlight than are dark-skinned people. Heavy pigment offers some protection against ultraviolet radiation. While skin cancer usually occurs in people over 50, people may receive half the ultraviolet radiation they will receive in their lifetimes by the time they are 30.

Viruses Viruses cause some types of cancer in animals and humans. Viruses survive by taking over living cells in the body. After the virus penetrates the cell, it sheds its protein overcoat, freeing its core to take over the functions of the plundered cell. The virus can then do one of several things. The virus can command the cell it has taken over to make more viruses like itself or to slow down its own self-multiplication. It can remain inactive for some time, all the while doubling its numbers with each division of the cells. Then, for reasons still unknown, it may suddenly infect the body. Although not a form of cancer, the "fever blisters" or "cold sores" caused by the herpes simplex virus seem to work this way. However it works, though, the virus robs the cell of its ability to make healthy cellular protein and to stick closely to other animal cells.

The National Cancer Institute and the Pasteur Institute in Paris have made substantial progress in identifying cancer-causing viruses in humans. Much of this progress was achieved from AIDS (see Chapter 21) research where viruses were identified that cause human leukemia and human lymphoma.

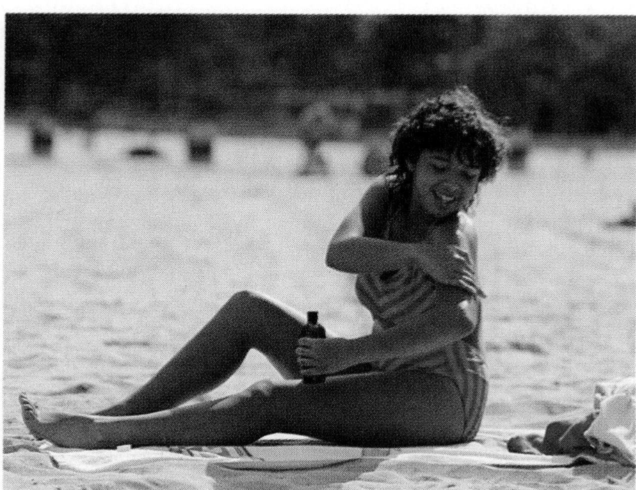

Richard Hutchings

Detection and Diagnosis

Detecting cancer at an early stage depends heavily on close self-monitoring. Unlike many other diseases, early signs of cancer are not apparent to anyone but the victim. Pain, for example, is seldom an early cancer signal, so if you wait until something hurts, it might be too late. The American Cancer Society recommends that people pay close attention to the following warning signs:

- **C**hange in bowel or bladder habits
- **A** sore that does not heal
- **U**nusual bleeding or discharge
- **T**hickening or lump in the breasts or elsewhere
- **I**ndigestion or difficulty in swallowing
- **O**bvious change in a wart or mole
- **N**agging cough or hoarseness

To this list could be added "unusual weight loss." Although none of these signs is a sure indication of cancer, the appearance of any one should send you to see your doctor.

Tests for Cancer

What tests should you have done to detect cancer? The American Cancer Society is probably the best authority on what tests should be done routinely. See Table 18-4 on p. 431 for their latest guidelines, intended only for people who have no symptoms of cancer. Remember that these recommendations change with time as new facts become available. The **nuclear magnetic reasonance (NMR)** scanner has made it easier to detect cancer as well as other diseases. This nonradiation device provides more detailed information of the body's soft tissues than X-rays or scanners that use X-rays. It works by surrounding the body with a powerful magnetic field and then, with radio waves, not only produces detailed computerized pictures of the tissue but also provides information about the complex metabolism going on within the cells. The NMR scanner is particularly effective in detecting brain cancers and cancers in other hard-to-reach places. It can detect liver and kidney disease as well as cancers of these organs in their early stages.

(Text continues on p. 431.)

Preventing Skin Cancer

Most skin cancers can be totally cured, especially if caught early, and the treatments are usually simple and nearly painless. Equally important and even more encouraging is the fact that some skin cancers can probably be prevented following a few simple suggestions.

Skin cancer is by far the most common form of cancer, with more than 400,000 new cases reported each year in the United States. Because most skin cancers can be readily treated, death from skin cancer is uncommon. Nonetheless, considerable deformity and scarring may occur if skin cancers are not found and treated early while they are small and relatively easy to remove. Learning to minimize your risk for developing skin cancer, and detecting possible skin cancers at an early stage can preserve much of your skin's function and appearance in later years.

As the human body's largest organ and chief protector against the outside environment, the skin is vulnerable to many cancer-causing influences. Although no one knows the exact mechanism(s) that lead to formation and growth of skin cancers, abnormal cellular changes in the most superficial layers of the skin known as the **epidermis** are consistently found. The role of sunlight in producing these abnormal changes has been well documented in animals, humans, and in laboratory cultures of skin cells. These changes can be temporary or permanent, and over time (months or years) can result in development of skin cancer. Both severe, acute sun reactions (sunburns) as well as chronic, low-level sun reactions (suntans) can lead to skin cancer later. People who have naturally fair skin pigmentation have a lower natural protection against sun-induced skin damage, and have a higher risk of developing certain skin cancers.

Although sunlight is probably the most important factor, chronic exposure to certain chemicals, including arsenic, coal tar, shale oil, and creosote oil can also increase the risk of developing skin cancers. Significant exposure to these chemicals is fortunately quite rare in the United States today. Smoking cigarettes, cigars, or pipes can increase the risk of developing skin cancers of the lips and mouth. Sites of previous severe injury such as burn scars, or areas of the body exposed to high doses of radiation (as for treatment of other forms of cancer) can also be more likely to develop skin cancer many years later. Members of families with a tendency to develop unusual moles or skin cancers can have an increased risk of developing skin cancer.

Three types account for more than 90 percent of all skin cancers: basal cell carcinoma, squamous cell carcinoma, and melanoma. These names are derived from the kind of skin cell from which the cancers develop.

- **Basal cell carcinoma** is the most common skin cancer and is usually found in chronically sun-exposed areas such as face, neck, arms, and hands. It usually appears as a small, shiny, pink, fleshy bump that grows slowly and persists beyond the time (several weeks) that usual skin inflammations and pimples take to resolve. Basal cell carcinoma is usually not painful, and occasionally may bleed or crust or form an open sore on the skin.
- **Squamous cell carcinoma** is the second most common type of skin cancer, and is seen most often on ears, face, lips, and mouth although it can occur anywhere on the skin. It may appear as a persistent, sharply outlined, red, scaly, platelike patch, open sore, or hard, rough bump.
- **Melanoma**, the third most common type of skin cancer, is the most dangerous, because it spreads so rapidly. It can occur anywhere on the body, but most common sites include the back, chest, abdomen, and lower legs. Melanoma can develop on normal-appearing skin, or it may occur at the site of a previous mole. It usually appears as a brown or black spot or bump that grows, has irregular borders, different colors (including black, blue, pink, white, and shades of brown) and may itch, burn, or bleed easily.

Anyone who develops an unusual growth, discoloration, or sore that does not heal should consult his or her regular physician or a dermatologist (a physician who specializes in skin diseases). It is sometimes possible, by a careful history and physical examination, to determine whether the skin lesion is benign, precancerous, or cancerous. In some cases, a skin biopsy will be necessary in order to definitely diagnose a possible skin cancer. This simple office procedure involves removing a small

(continued on next page)

Sunscreen Substance used to protect the skin from ultraviolet rays; usually applied as an ointment or a cream.

Biotechnology (genetic engineering) The commercialized techniques of cloning and expressing genes.

Cloning Identifying and isolating a piece of DNA that specifies a desired protein, such as interferons.

Preventing Skin Cancer (*continued*)

piece of skin tissue and submitting it for microscopic analysis.

The particular type, size, and location of a skin cancer will help determine which treatment is recommended. Often skin surgery is recommended and can almost always be performed in a dermatologist's office using local anesthesia. Occasionally, other forms of treatment may be used.

For optimal protection against developing skin cancer, people should avoid lifelong overexposure to sunlight. Sunburns should definitely be avoided, and although you may hear that a suntan is "healthy" or "protective against sun damage," clearly there is no such thing as a "safe" tan. Despite some advertising claims, artificial sun rays in tanning parlors are risky.

Active, outdoor lifestyles need not be curtailed, however, because selection of proper clothing and application of sunscreens can protect against most sun-induced skin damage. Loose, long-sleeved shirts made of closely woven cotton fabric can protect the forearms, chest and back. Beware of thin, white shirts and wet clothing that clings to the body, as these are only minimally protective. Hats with brims help deflect sun from ears, forehead, and upper cheeks. Hair styles that cover the tops of ears and/or neck can be helpful.

Lotions or creams known as **sunscreens** can also prevent sun-induced damage to skin cells. Because the ultraviolet portion of sunlight is the most damaging, currently available sunscreens are most effective at absorbing, reflecting, and scattering ultraviolet rays on the skin surface. They are rated according to effectiveness in blocking out damaging rays; higher numbers indicate more blocking action. For most people, a sunscreen with SPF-15 (sun protection factor 15) is recommended. For those with acne-prone skin, oil-free sunscreens are now available. Because these newer sunscreens are more resistant to loss through perspiration or swimming, they should be reapplied frequently during peak sun hours.

When possible, extensive sun exposure should be avoided between 10 A.M. and 3 P.M. when sun rays are most intense. Swimmers are not protected, because ultraviolet rays penetrate at least 3 feet in water. Locations close to the equator have more intense sunlight—as do high elevations, where there is less atmosphere to filter out ultraviolet rays. Snow and sand can reflect many sun rays, and up to 70 percent of ultraviolet light can penetrate clouds.

If someone in your family has had numerous skin cancers or melanoma, you may want to consult a dermatologist for a complete skin examination and discussion of your particular risk. It's always a good idea to examine your skin regularly and consult your physician early for any suspicious skin lesions. Remember that, with adequate protection, you can still enjoy the outdoors, and maintain healthy, vibrant skin now and in later years.

SOURCE: Judy Koperski, 1986 (March), Preventing skin cancer, *Healthline*.

Interferons The chemical factors made by body cells that can interfere with the growth of many viruses.

Interleukins Substances that carry messages from one lymphocyte to another.

Colony-stimulating factors (CSFs) Substances that promote the growth of red blood cells, lymphocytes, or macrophages.

Biotechnology and the Immune Response

The term **biotechnology** is used in many ways, but it most often refers to commercialized techniques of cloning and expressing genes (also known as **genetic engineering**). Without going into great detail, **cloning** a gene simply means identifying and isolating the piece of DNA that specifies a desired protein (such as interferon, an antiviral protein). This DNA fragment can then be inserted into an easily propagated species (such as the *E. coli* bacterium) in which the protein is made in large amounts. The value of this development is that many useful proteins occur in nature in only trace amounts, and are difficult and expensive to obtain in amounts sufficient for use in therapy. When they are made ("expressed") in an organism that we can control and grow easily, such as yeast or *E. coli,* then the desired protein can be obtained in limitless amounts.

Cells of the bone marrow and blood make proteins that defend against infection, injury, and the growth of cancer cells. Many of these genes have been cloned and expressed by genetic engineering techniques, and they represent only the first members of a new and diverse family of drugs, the immune response modifiers. Most important for our purposes are the interferons, interleukins, and colony-stimulating factors.

The **interferons** were the first of the immune response modifiers to be studied. The first interferon was discovered in 1959 by Aleck Isaacs, who showed that certain human cells produced factors capable of interfering with the growth of many different kinds of virus. In this way interferon differs profoundly from antibody molecules, which are specific for a single virus type. These early observations raised the hope that many viral diseases could be controlled by a single agent, and so interferon was one of the first human proteins to be cloned and expressed. This "recombinant" interferon has been shown to be effective against some virus infections, but many viruses are resistant to interferon, especially if the drug is injected when the infection is well under way. It does limit infections by viruses that are sensitive to its effects, and it hastens the immune killing of some leukemia (cancer) cells without excessively damaging normal cells. Many scientists feel that interferon will be most valuable when used together with other immune response modifiers. These combined therapies are achieving increasing success. One of the interferons has already been approved by the Food and Drug Administration (FDA) for use in treating leukemias, and other applications (such as treatment of AIDS symptoms), are being actively explored.

The **interleukins**—substances that carry messages from one lymphocyte to another—were the second set of factors to be cloned and studied by the molecular biologists. Interleukin 2, or T-cell growth factor, is the best studied of these, and has shown promise in cancer treatment, though it has been disappointing in AIDS trials. It is most effective against cancer when it is used to stimulate the patient's lymphocytes outside of the body. When the interleukin-2 stimulated cells are returned to the body, they often have a devastating and immediate effect on the tumor. Usually the improvement is only temporary, but—to be fair to the investigators and to the interleukins—it must be pointed out that much about the immune response remains obscure. Results of experimental treatments such as the one described are still difficult to predict. When more factors are isolated, and their function understood, it will be possible to plan more rational and more successful therapies.

Colony-stimulating factors (CSFs)—substances that promote the growth of red blood cells, lymphocytes, or macrophages in test tubes—are potentially very important, though still too new for their true value to be known. Potential uses of these factors fall into several broad categories: restoring blood cells when disease or chemotherapy slows their production, improving the patient's defenses against infection, and possibly increasing production of immune cells directed against cancer. One specific factor that seems especially promising is granulocyte-stimulating factor, which promotes the growth of the lymphocytes that defend against bacterial invasion. Probably the most important use of these factors will be to prevent infection in cancer patients who are immunosuppressed by the

(continued on next page)

Biotechnology and the Immune Response (*continued*)

toxic chemical therapy now used to kill cancer cells. CSFs may also be important in reconstituting the depleted immune system of AIDS patients, if the primary AIDS infection can be controlled by interferon and related drugs.

To appreciate the importance of molecular biology to the therapeutic use of these factors, we need only consider the amounts originally available. The mouse equivalent of one CSF factor was originally discovered by Dr. Donald Metcalf of Australia, who sacrificed 10,000 mice to harvest ten-millionths of a gram for his experiments. A hundred times that amount of the equivalent human factor would be required for a single adult dose! Fortunately, a few liters of *E. coli* now produce almost a gram. These factors are now undergoing clinical trial, and will probably be available for broad use in 1990.

A final category of important "biotechnology" molecules are the **monoclonal antibodies.** To appreciate the uniqueness of these molecules, you must remember that each B-lymphocyte makes only *one* type of antibody, and this antibody recognizes only a handful of amino acids in a single protein. However, until about ten years ago, this fact had no utility, since it was impossible to isolate and grow single lymphocytes. The serum of animals, of course, contains millions of different antibodies, from millions of different lymphocytes, directed against thousands of different proteins. It is also crucial to understand that monoclonal antibodies are not produced by the molecular cloning techniques used for genes, but rather by the "cloning" of individual antibody-producing B-lymphocytes.

If lymphocytes could grow indefinitely in the test tube (**in vitro**), monoclonal antibodies would have been available thirty or forty years ago. Unfortunately, unaided lymphocytes are incapable of dividing more than a few times *in vitro*. In 1975, two scientists in England discovered that fusing a cancerous lymphocyte (myeloma cell) with a normal lymphocyte resulted in a hybrid tumor cell (hybridoma) that could grow forever *in vitro,* but which still produced the antibody of the original normal lymphocyte. Once the hybrid cell was cloned (grown from a single cell), millions of such hybridoma cells could be propagated, all producing the antibody of the single original lymphocyte; these antibodies are termed "monoclonal" antibodies, since they are all produced from a single cloned lymphocyte.

The sudden availability of large amounts of these extremely specific antibodies has led to an explosion both in diagnosis of disease, and in experimental antibody therapies. A few examples should help make their usefulness clear. In life-threatening bacterial infection, a single bacterial molecule, **endotoxin**, is responsible for much of the fever and **morbidity** of the infection. A monoclonal antibody directed against endotoxin can be introduced into the body in large amounts to immediately neutralize its damaging actions; this treatment has already saved acutely ill patients from probable death, and will probably receive the FDA's blessing for broad use soon.

A second example comes from the use of a specific monoclonal antibody to control the immune response directed against transplanted organs. Often, after a heart or kidney transplant, the patient's cellular (helper T-cell) immune response threatens to destroy the transplanted organ. Older treatments that suppressed *all* immune response left the patient susceptible to overwhelming infections from bacteria or virus. Now a monoclonal antibody directed specifically against the T-helper cell protects the transplanted organ from harm, and leaves the other cells of the immune system (B-cells, suppressor T-cells, macrophages) free to pursue their own important business.

A rational use of the immune response modifiers, together with monoclonal antibodies will lead to successful treatment of a great many infectious diseases and tumors that are currently very damaging or incurable. However, because these molecules are so new, and their properties are still being explored, it may be some years before their full benefit is seen in medical practice.

Monoclonal antibodies Antibodies harvested from cloned lymphocytes.

In vitro In test tubes (*vitro* means glass).

Endotoxin The bacterial molecule that is responsible for the severity of the infection.

Morbidity Cell-killing effects.

Self-examinations (such as breast and testicle self-examination) and examinations by a physician of sites especially susceptible to cancer could save more lives than any other available means today. Men and women over the age of 50 should have a yearly rectal examination by a physician. Women of all ages should have a Pap smear test for cervical cancer at least once every three years. However, women who are sexually active, according to a consensus panel at the National Institutes of Health, should

(Text continues on p. 436)

Table 18-4 Summary of American Cancer Society Recommendations for the Early Detection of Cancer in Asymptomatic People

Test or Procedure	Population		
	Sex	**Age**	**Frequency**
Sigmoidoscopy	M & F	Over 50	Every 3–5 years after 2 negative exams 1 year apart
Stool guaiac test	M & F	Over 50	Every year
Digital rectal examination	M & F	Over 40	Every year
Pap test	F	20–65; under 20, if sexually active	At least every 3 years after 2 negative exams 1 year apart
Pelvic examination	F	20–40	Every 3 years
		Over 40	Every year
Endometrial tissue sample	F	At menopause; women at high risk[a]	At menopause
Breast self-examination	F	Over 20	Every month
Breast physical examination	F	20–40	Every 3 years
		Over 40	Every year
Mammography	F	Between 35–40	Baseline
		Under 50	Consult personal physician
		Over 50	Every year
Chest X-ray		Not recommended	
Sputum cytology		Not recommended	
Health counseling and cancer checkup[b]	M & F	Over 20	Every 3 years
	M & F	Over 40	Every year

[a]History of infertility, obesity, failure of ovulation, abnormal uterine bleeding, or estrogen therapy.

[b]To include examination for cancers of the thyroid, testicles, prostate, ovaries, lymph nodes, oral region, and skin.

Breast Self-examination

Early detection of breast cancer is possible through monthly self-examination. (a) Sit in front of a mirror, raise your arms, and check for unusual dimples in the skin or depression of the nipples. This check should also be done with your arms lowered. Then lie down and place a flat pillow or a folded towel under the shoulder of the same side as the breast to be examined. (b) Keep the left arm at the side while you examine your left breast. Check the outer side of the breast, moving your hand up into the armpit. (c) Using the flat part of your fingers, inspect the lower part of the breast and then (d) the upper part. Next (e–h) raise the left arm and repeat the procedure, beginning at the breast bone. Repeat with the right breast. If you detect a lump or unusual mass, you should contact a doctor immediately. (If you find a similar lump or mass in the same place in the other breast, it probably is normal tissue.) Breasts should be examined one week after the end of every menstrual period.

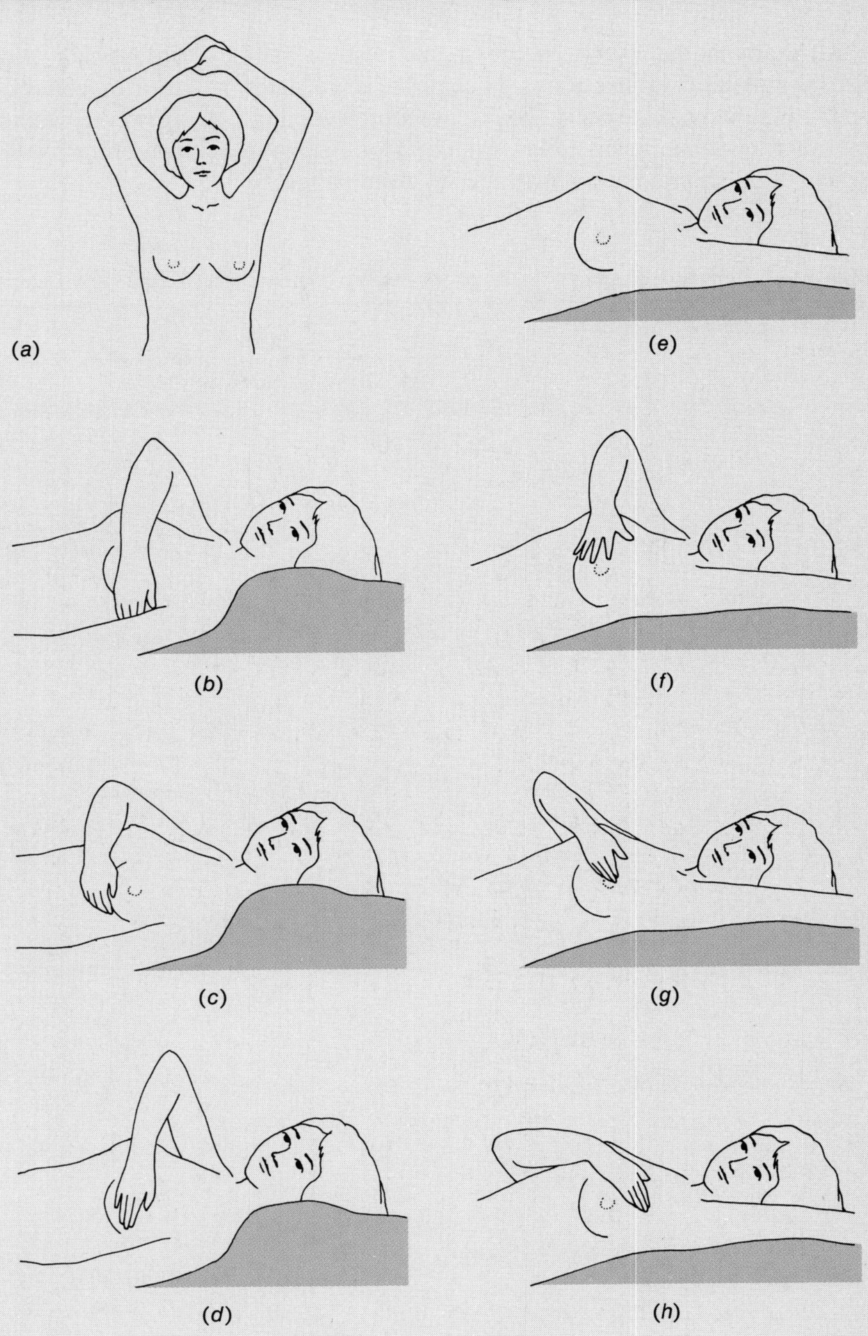

Breast Cancer: From Detection Through Treatment

The Biopsy

The lump is biopsied to see if it is cancerous. In many cases, this can be done with a needle in a doctor's office. In other cases, it must be surgically removed for biopsy.

If the Lump Is Benign Nine times out of ten, lump is found to be a cyst or other growth that is not a threat to health or a predictor of future cancer. No further treatment is needed.

If the Lump Is Malignant It contains cancer cells. Today, a two-stage procedure is used—biopsy first, surgery later. Decisions about how to further treat the cancer may be made over the next few days. No breast cancer patient need wake up from a biopsy with a surprise mastectomy.

Type of Surgery

Small Tumor If the tumor is very small, or small relative to the size of the breast, then breast-preservation surgery, such as a lumpectomy accompanied by radiation, is an option. Sometimes, if the tumor was removed for biopsy, additional tissue around it is taken in a second procedure.

Large Tumor If the tumor is large, or close to the nipple, a modified mastectomy—removal of the breast—is often indicated. (The modern mastectomy is less disfiguring than the old "Halsted radical" procedure and may be accompanied by immediate reconstruction.)

Removal of Axillary (Underarm) Lymph Nodes for Biopsy

This is the only way to determine if the cancer has already spread. A "positive" finding indicates the presence of cancer cells beyond the breast.

"Node-negative" Women who are node-negative show no evidence of cancer's spread. Probably no further treatment is necessary. But one in four node-negative women will die of a recurrence, so more tests should be performed to help predict which women are especially at risk. None of these tests is fool-proof, but better ones are under development.

"Node-positive" The cancer has spread. Depending on age, other risks and results of more tests, some type of additional therapy—cancer-fighting chemicals or hormones—is chosen.

Hormone-receptor Test

This test helps doctor and patient choose the right treatment. It is also a predictor of the course of the disease.

Estrogen or Progesterone-"rich" About one third of breast cancers fall into this relatively optimistic category—more in postmenopausal women. The cancer cells still resemble normal cells in their

(continued on next page)

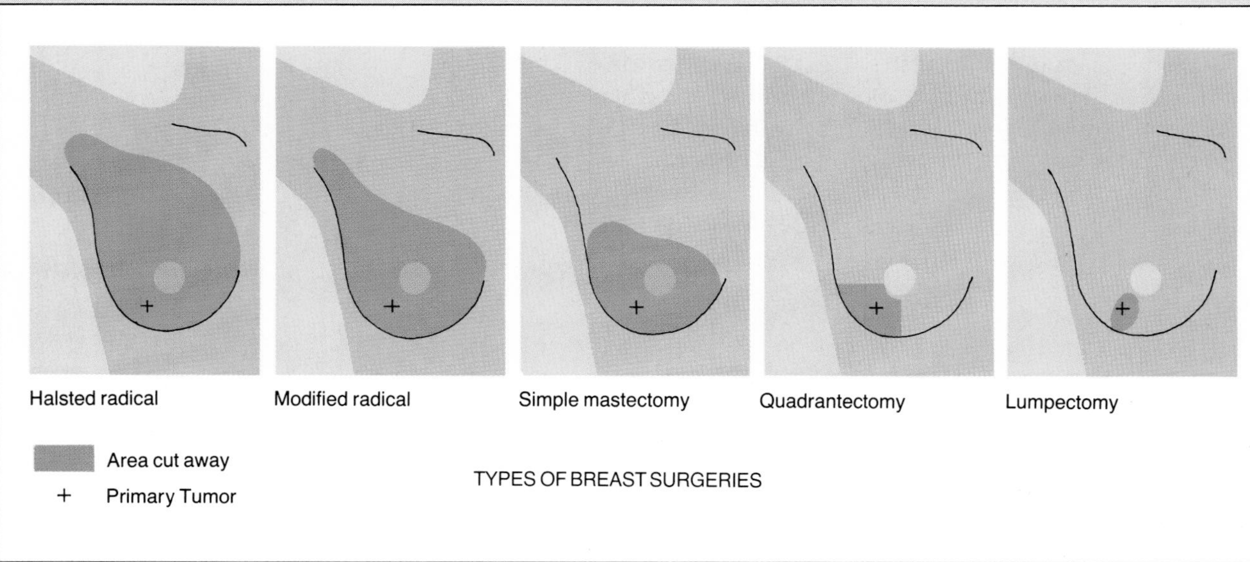

Types of Breast Surgeries

Breast Cancer: From Detection Through Treatment (*continued*)

response to the body's hormones, and cancer growth might be blocked by antihormone therapy like tamoxifen.

Estrogen or Progesterone-"poor" The cancer cells have "forgotten" their hormonal response. Other cell-killing, or cytotoxic, drugs may be needed.

The Outlook

Half of women diagnosed with breast cancer eventually die of it, but individual survival chances vary greatly. A postmenopausal woman whose tumor is discovered early—before it can even be felt—and who has no family history of breast cancer and no evidence of spread, has the best outlook—perhaps more than a 90 percent chance of surviving five years. The outlook is not as bright in the case, for example, of a young woman whose cancer has spread—but many of these patients also do well.

SOURCE: *The Washington Post,* March 17, 1987, p. 14 of health insert.

Testicle Self-examination

Self-examination can permit early detection of testicular cancer. Although this type of cancer accounts for only 1 percent of cancer in men, it is the most common type of cancer in those who are 29 to 35 years old. Males with undescended testicles are at high risk for testicular cancer, and for this reason the condition should be corrected in early childhood.

The American Cancer Society recommends the following:

1. Perform the examination after a warm bath or shower, when the scrotal skin is most relaxed. (*Scrotal* refers to the scrotum, the pouch in which the testicles normally lie.)

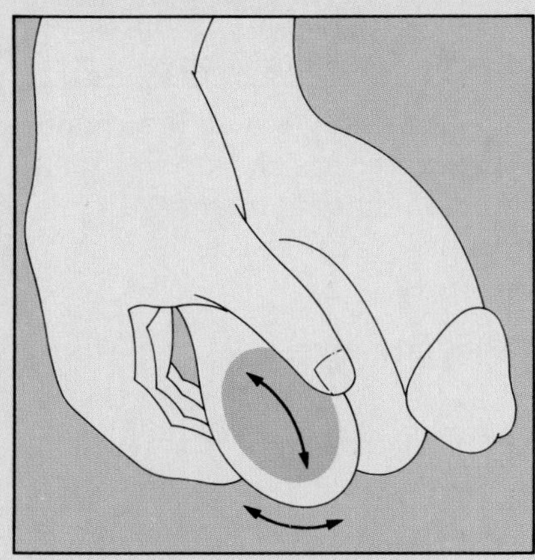

2. Cup each testicle in the palm of one hand and examine it by feeling with the fingers of your other hand. The normal testicle is smooth, egg-shaped, and somewhat firm to the touch.

3. At the rear of each testicle is a tube called the *epididymis,* which carries sperm away from the testicle. This is a normal part of your body; its presence does not indicate cancer.

4. If there is any change in shape or texture of the testicles—or any lumps, especially hard ones—consult a doctor immediately.

Repeat this examination every six or eight weeks. It is important that you know what your own testicles feel like normally so that you will recognize any changes.

Prevention

Primary prevention refers to steps that might be taken to avoid those factors that might lead to the development of cancer.

Smoking Cigarette smoking is responsible for 85 percent of lung cancer cases among men and 75 percent among women—about 83 percent overall. Smoking accounts for about 30 percent of all cancer deaths. Those who smoke two or more packs of cigarettes a day have lung cancer mortality rates 15 to 25 times greater than nonsmokers.

Sunlight Almost all of the more than 500,000 cases of nonmelanoma skin cancer developed each year in the U.S. are considered to be sun-related. Recent epidemiological evidence shows that sun exposure is a major factor in the development of melanoma and that the incidence increases for those living near the equator.

Alcohol Oral cancer and cancers of the larynx, throat, esophagus, and liver occur more frequently among heavy drinkers of alcohol.

Smokeless Tobacco Increased risk factor for cancers of the mouth, larynx, throat, and esophagus. Highly habit forming.

Estrogen For mature women, certain risks associated with estrogen treatment to control menopausal symptoms, including an increased risk of endometrial cancer. Use of estrogen by menopausal women needs careful discussion by the woman and her physician.

Radiation Excessive exposure to radiation can increase cancer risk. Most medical X-rays are adjusted to deliver the lowest dose possible without sacrificing image quality.

Occupational Hazards Exposure to a number of industrial agents (nickel, chromate, asbestos, vinyl chloride, and so on) increases risk. Risk factor greatly increased when combined with smoking.

Nutrition Risk for colon, breast, and uterine cancers increases for obese people. High-fat diet may be a factor in the development of certain cancers such as breast, colon, and prostate. High-fiber foods may help reduce risk of colon cancer, and can be a wholesome substitute for high-fat diets. Foods rich in vitamins A and C may help lower risk for cancers of larynx, esophagus, stomach, and lung. Eating cruciferous vegetables may help protect against certain cancers. Salt-cured, smoked, and nitrite-cured foods have been linked to esophageal and stomach cancer. The heavy use of alcohol, especially when accompanied by cigarette smoking or chewing tobacco, increases risk of cancers of the mouth, larynx, throat, esophagus, and liver. (See above.)

Secondary prevention refers to steps to be taken to diagnose a cancer or precursor as early as possible after it has developed.

Colorectal Tests The ACS [American Cancer Society] recommends three tests for the early detection of colon and rectum cancer in people without symptoms. The digital rectal examination, performed by a physician during an office visit, should be performed every year after the age of 40; the stool blood test is recommended every year after 50; and the proctosigmoidoscopy examination should be carried out every 3 to 5 years after the age of 50 following two annual exams with negative results.

Pap Test For the average-risk person, a Pap test is recommended annually until two consecutive satisfactory tests are negative, and then once every three years. The Pap test is highly effective in detecting cancer of the uterine cervix, but is less effective in detecting **endometrial** cancer.

Breast Cancer Detection The ACS recommends the monthly practice of breast self-examination (BSE) by women 20 years and older as a routine good health habit. Physical examination of the breast should be done every three years from ages 20–40 and then every year. The ACS recommends a mammogram every year for asymptomatic women age 50 and over, and a baseline mammogram between ages 35 and 39. Women 40 to 49 should have mammography every 1–2 years, depending on physical and mammographic findings.

SOURCE: American Cancer Society, 1987, *Cancer Facts & Figures—1987*. (New York: American Cancer Society), p. 18.

Endometrial Tissue lining the uterus.

Buccal smear Scraping of cells from the inside of the cheek for examination under a microscope.

have a Pap test either (1) yearly or (2) every three years after having two negative screenings one year apart (but more frequently if screening shows cancer or precancerous conditions).

Smokers should have annual examinations for lung and other cancers. Examination of saliva sometimes reveals the presence of precancerous cells. Tissues scraped from the inside of the cheek can also show the existence of cancer cells. This test is called the **buccal smear test.**

Reducing the Risk of Cancer

Can cancer be prevented? No person can guarantee another person that he or she will never get cancer. However, the facts clearly indicate that the risk of developing cancer can be significantly reduced by taking into account the things that cause cancer. We can speak of three kinds of prevention: primary, secondary, and tertiary. *Primary prevention* refers to behaviors that keep cancer from starting in the first place. For example, don't smoke! And if you do smoke, stop! *Secondary prevention* refers to detecting cancer at an early stage before it can do any harm. If you have a mole, for example, that changes its shape (and becomes cancerous), see a doctor immediately and have it removed before it becomes dangerous. *Tertiary prevention* refers to the effective treatment of cancer after it has been diagnosed by a qualified physician. Don't seek out unproven methods or unqualified people to treat cancer. Find a reputable source that you can trust and develop a therapeutic alliance that will be helpful.

Exploring Your Emotions

You find out that your best friend has cancer. How do you feel about this, and how will you express your feelings?

The American Cancer Society has compiled a list of ten practical steps to reduce the risk of cancer related to lifestyle:

1. Stop smoking.
2. Drink alcohol in moderation only.
3. Protect your skin against the sun.
4. Eat vegetables from the cruciferous family, such as broccoli, Brussels sprouts, cabbage, and cauliflower.
5. Eat high-fiber foods.
6. Choose foods that provide vitamin A (carrots, squash, melon, and so forth).
7. Choose foods with vitamin C (citrus fruits and juices).
8. Watch your weight and exercise regularly.
9. Trim fat from your diet by eating fish, lean meat, skinned poultry, and low-fat dairy products.
10. Eat fewer salt-cured, smoked, and nitrite-cured foods (bacon, hot dogs, ham, and luncheon meats).

Take Action

Your answers to the Exploring Your Emotions questions in this chapter and your placement level on the Wellness Ladder will, we hope, encourage you to begin a process of self-exploration and self-discovery that you will continue. Reflect on the entire chapter's content and ask yourself how each point relates to your own life. Then take action:

1. If you recently ate a hot dog or bacon, you probably ingested sodium nitrite, which has been shown to be a cancer-causing agent in animals. Contact the American Cancer Society for a list of other such agents. Then make a list of the potential cancer-causing agents you ingested during the past week. Which ones could you have easily avoided?

2. Write a letter to three insurance companies, asking them about the circumstances under which they would insure cancer patients.

3. During the next 30 days, keep track of periods of time of over 30 minutes during which you are exposed to the sun. If you feel you have been overexposed, show your records to your doctor and ask his or her opinion.

4. List the positive behaviors that may help you avoid cancer. How can you strengthen these behaviors? Also list the behaviors that tend to increase your risk of cancer. What can you do to change these behaviors?

5. Before leaving this chapter, review the Rate Yourself statements at the beginning of this chapter. Have your feelings or values changed? Are you now better equipped to handle the complex and very human problems associated with cancer?

Selected References

American Cancer Society. 1986 (September). Commonly asked questions about breast cancer. *Healthline*.

American Cancer Society. 1987. *Cancer Facts & Figures*. New York: American Cancer Society.

Baltrusch, H. J., and M. Waltz. 1985. Cancer from a biobehavioral and social epidemiological perspective. *Social Science & Medicine* 20:789–94.

Kupchella, C. E. 1987. *Dimensions of Cancer*. Belmont, Calif.: Wadsworth.

Maguire, P. 1985. The psychological impact of cancer. *British Journal of Hospital Medicine* 34:100–3.

Recommended Readings

National Cancer Institute Fact Book. 1987. Bethesda, Md.: Office of Cancer Communications.

Watson, M., and T. Morris, eds. 1985. *Psychological Aspects of Cancer*. New York: Pergamon Press.

Chapter 19

Contents

Rate Yourself

Your STD Risk Behavior Read the following statements carefully. Choose the one in each section that best describes you at this moment and circle its number. When you have chosen one statement for each section, add the numbers and record your total score. Find your position on the Wellness Ladder.

5 Refrains (or would refrain) from physical contact if infected
4 Refrains from sexual contact if infected
3 Uses contraceptives to prevent STDs
2 Takes few precautions to avoid STDs
1 Takes no precautions to avoid STDs

5 Seeks (or would seek) immediate treatment if infected
4 Seeks treatment if infected
3 Seeks treatment for an STD only after extensive symptoms
2 Doesn't voluntarily seek treatment for STDs
1 Deliberately avoids treatment for STDs

5 Discusses STDs openly with others
4 Discusses STDs openly with sexual partner(s)
3 Prefers not to discuss STDs openly
2 Rarely discusses STDs openly
1 Refuses to discuss STDs

5 Educates others about STDs
4 Is familiar with STD hotline
3 Is willing to be educated about STDs
2 Relies on friends for information
1 Has no sources of STD information

5 Knows sexual partner(s) very well
4 Knows sexual partners fairly well
3 Avoids one-night stands
2 Has occasional one-night stands
1 Prefers one-night stands

Total Score ______

Sexually Transmissible Diseases

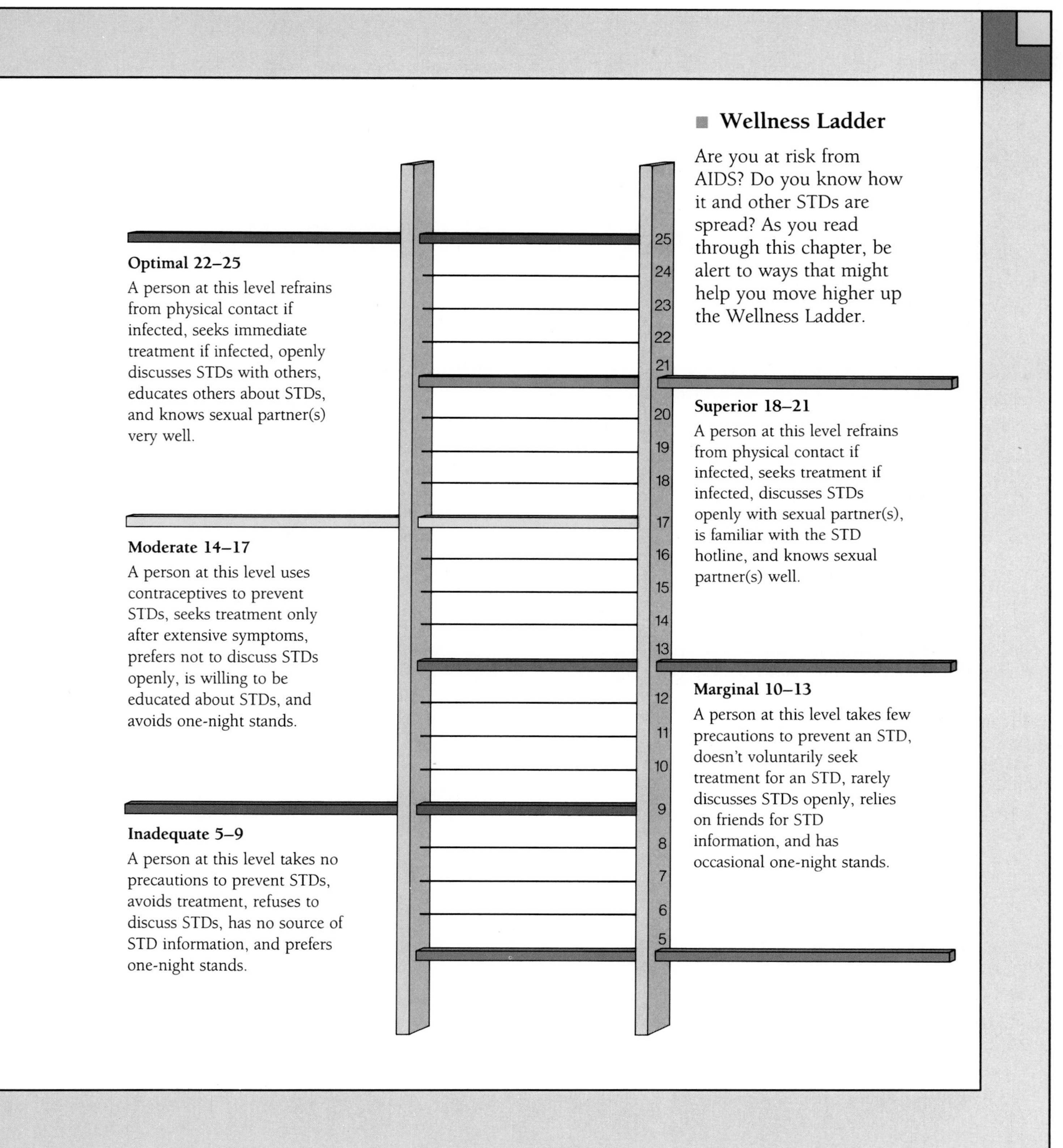

25
24
23
22
21
20
19
18
17
16
15
14
13
12
11
10
9
8
7
6
5
Optimal 22–25
A person at this level refrains from physical contact if infected, seeks immediate treatment if infected, openly discusses STDs with others, educates others about STDs, and knows sexual partner(s) very well.
Superior 18–21
A person at this level refrains from physical contact if infected, seeks treatment if infected, discusses STDs openly with sexual partner(s), is familiar with the STD hotline, and knows sexual partner(s) well.
Moderate 14–17
A person at this level uses contraceptives to prevent STDs, seeks treatment only after extensive symptoms, prefers not to discuss STDs openly, is willing to be educated about STDs, and avoids one-night stands.
Marginal 10–13
A person at this level takes few precautions to prevent an STD, doesn't voluntarily seek treatment for an STD, rarely discusses STDs openly, relies on friends for STD information, and has occasional one-night stands.
Inadequate 5–9
A person at this level takes no precautions to prevent STDs, avoids treatment, refuses to discuss STDs, has no source of STD information, and prefers one-night stands.

Wellness Ladder

Are you at risk from AIDS? Do you know how it and other STDs are spread? As you read through this chapter, be alert to ways that might help you move higher up the Wellness Ladder.

Sexually transmissible diseases (STDs) Diseases that can be transmitted by sexual contact; some can also be transmitted by other means.

Chlamydia trachomatis A sexually transmissible organism that produces a wide variety of sometimes acute infections; now reaching epidemic scale in the United States.

Until recently, the term *venereal diseases (VD)* was used to describe infections that were transmitted from person to person by direct sexual contact. The public health focus was on controlling and preventing first syphilis and then gonorrhea. Important advances in past decades, such as new antibiotics and diagnostic techniques, as well as public education, have brought about a decline in serious illnesses resulting from syphilis and gonorrhea.

During the 1970s, a major shift in thinking occurred as public health experts began to realize the complexity of diseases that can be transmitted sexually. An increased awareness of financial costs as well as long-term consequences such as infertility, ectopic (tubal) pregnancies, and even cancer broadened the perspective on these diseases. The term **sexually transmissible diseases** has replaced "venereal disease" and better represents the characteristics of this family of diseases. Today the expanded list of sexually transmissible diseases (STDs) includes acquired immune deficiency syndrome (AIDS), chlamydia, herpes, cytomegalovirus (CMV), hepatitis, vaginitis, and parasitic and enteric (small intestine) infections, in addition to the original five venereal diseases.

In the past decade alone, the STD field has grown in both scope and complexity. Over twenty organisms have been identified as being sexually transmissible. The STDs are no longer the sole domain of public health practitioners, but include medical specialists in internal medicine, pediatrics, obstetrics, gynecology, family practice, urology, opthalmology, and dermatology. In addition, with the advent of AIDS, research in hematology, oncology, immunology, and pharmacology is contributing to the search for control and prevention of the epidemic diseases of the 1980s and 1990s. The STDs are today considered among the national priorities in health care in the United States.

Exploring Your Emotions

In applying for your marriage license, you and your fiancé must take a screening test for sexually transmissible diseases. The results of your test are fine, but your partner's test is positive. How does this make you feel? Why do you feel this way? Will your feelings toward your fiancé be different?

Causes of STD Prevalence

The current high STD incidence may be traced to several factors. One of the most significant causes is the identification within the past ten years of sexually transmissible diseases other than syphilis and gonorrhea. Recognition and subsequent improved reporting of diseases through the Centers for Disease Control have prompted greater access to information and statistical data that were previously unavailable. In addition, diseases such as herpes are not reportable diseases but further increase the STD incidence by a figure that can only be estimated. Some diseases, such as the protozoal infection trichomoniasis ("trich"), were not even considered STDs a little over ten years ago. And in the current AIDS epidemic, prevalence is multiplied again by an exponential factor we are only learning about on a day-to-day basis.

Another factor may be the various changes in sexual attitudes that took place in the 1960s and 1970s. There was an apparent greater societal acceptance of premarital sex, greater accessibility of contraceptive information and services, and the influence of the women's movement on sexual freedom and marriage at an older age. Emphasis from the mass media on being "sexy" and being part of the "me generation" may have helped erode responsible behavior, as did abuse of drugs and alcohol. These various sociosexual changes dramatically influenced those people at risk of acquiring and transmitting STDs. More young people were becoming sexually active during the 1970s and were more sexually experienced than in the preceding generation. In addition, these young people also had more sexual partners, thereby also increasing the rate of STD transmission.

A third cause for the prevalence of STDs is the number of actual changes undergone by some of the organisms that cause the diseases. The best-known changes have been seen in antibiotic-resistant strains of gonorrhea. One of these strains developed in Southeast Asia during the Vietnam War. The self-administered weak dosages of penicillin obtained on the black market killed only the initial weakened bacteria, and allowed a stronger, more resistant strain of gonorrhea to take its place. (New antibiotics have been developed, however, to treat this particular strain of gonorrhea.)

A fourth factor is fear and guilt. Because the STDs are almost always contacted through intimate sexual contact with an infected person, sexual behavior itself is called into question. For a teenager, admitting such a disease

Myths about STDs and AIDS

Myth If you have syphilis or gonorrhea, you will know it.

Fact Some infected people show no signs of having syphilis or gonorrhea until many years later.

Myth STDs in the genitals cannot be transmitted to the mouth and the reverse.

Fact Transmission of STD infections from mouth to genitals and the reverse does occur.

Myth AIDS can be spread through casual contact.

Fact AIDS is transmitted only through clearly identifiable sexual activities and by blood-to-blood contact. There is no evidence that saliva, sweat, or tears transmits the AIDS virus.

Myth You cannot have more than one STD at a time.

Fact More than half of the women who visited one STD clinic had two or more STDs.

Myth There is a high risk of acquiring AIDS from a blood transfusion.

Fact The nation's blood supply is now screened for AIDS and is considered safe.

Myth Birth control pills protect you from STDs.

Fact Birth control pills may increase a woman's chances of contracting various STDs when exposed.

Myth Once you have been cured of an STD, you cannot get it again.

Fact You can get an STD infection any time you come into contact with it whether you have had it or not.

Myth AIDS cannot be prevented.

Fact Avoiding contraction or transmission of AIDS requires following the same precautionary steps as with other sexually transmissible diseases—do not allow semen, blood, urine, feces, or vaginal secretions to enter your body. Use condoms for all types of sexual intercourse. Avoid all forms of blood-to-blood contact, including the sharing of hypodermic needles, razors, and toothbrushes.

Myth Syphilis, gonorrhea, AIDS, and herpes can be contracted by contact with a toilet seat.

Fact The germs of these diseases cannot live in the open air.

SOURCE: Adapted from Knox, *Human Sexuality*, p. 357, and data from San Francisco AIDS Foundation.

may bring down parental wrath, or at least disapproval. For a single person, it may mean religious disapproval or an undesired admission of sexual activity. For a married person, it may signal infidelity. For these and other reasons, including ignorance, fear of an examination, and loss of confidentiality, some people resist seeking proper diagnosis and treatment. They thus risk serious medical complications and increased transmission of STDs.

The Most Common STDs

Over twenty different organisms are identified as causing sexually transmissible diseases. The nature of the organism, stage of disease, and certain sexual behaviors influence how common an STD is within the population.

Diseases can be categorized according to the type of causative agent. For example,

- *Bacterial infections:* chlamydia, NGU (nongonococcal urethritis), gonorrhea, syphilis
- *Viral infections:* herpes, warts, AIDS
- *Protozoal infections:* trichomoniasis
- *Fungal infections:* candida (yeast)
- *Parasitic infections:* lice and scabies

Chlamydia trachomatis ***Chlamydia trachomatis*** causes the most prevalent bacterial infection in the United States today. Each year an estimated three to four million Americans suffer from a chlamydia infection. Men, women, and infants are affected, but women particularly bear the greatest burden because of the possible consequences of this infection. STD clinics report a sharp increase in incidence since 1975 because of greater attention to the disease and improved laboratory diagnostic tests.

Chlamydia is a unique organism. Generally defined as a bacterium, chlamydia is also similar to a virus. Like a virus, chlamydia grows within the host cell's material, and like a bacterium, chlamydia has both DNA and RNA, divides by binary fission, and has cell walls. Chlamydia and gonorrhea are often mistaken for each other, because they produce similar symptoms. Unlike gonorrhea, however, chlamydia cannot survive outside the cell wall. Yet chlamydia is easily detectable and easy to treat with antibiotics.

In men, chlamydia is the leading cause of urinary tract infection, with an estimated incidence two and a half times greater than gonorrhea. Chlamydia is also responsible for approximately 50 percent of the estimated 500,000 cases of acute **epididymitis** (inflammation of the **testicle**) seen annually in the United States.

In women, the impact of chlamydia infections is more problematic. Most chlamydia infections in women produce no early symptoms. Chlamydia, if left untreated for two months or more, however, will likely lead to severe symptoms, such as inflammation of the **cervix** and **Fallopian tubes.**

Infants born to mothers with chlamydia infection can acquire the infection through contact in the birth canal. Over 150,000 babies are born each year to chlamydia-infected mothers. These newborns are often at high risk of developing eye infections, pneumonia, and occasionally ear infections. Chlamydia is the most common cause of newborn eye infections and pneumonia in infants under six months of age.

Sexually active women under 20 years old have chlamydia infection rates two to three times greater than women over 20 years of age. Similarly, teenage males have higher rates of chlamydia infection of the urinary tract than do adult males. Chlamydia is the most common STD among heterosexual whites, and increased risk of chlamydia infection has been seen in ethnic minority communities. Of gay men attending STD clinics, 4 to 8 percent have rectal chlamydia infections.

Symptoms Chlamydia symptoms in men are somewhat similar to those of gonorrhea. In fact, most men first believe they have been infected with gonorrhea and seek examination with this in mind. In men, chlamydia symptoms most commonly include a slight, watery discharge from the penis and painful urination. Symptoms generally occur two weeks after infection. Women may experience discharge from the cervix, painful urination, and inflammation of the Fallopian tubes. Most women, gay men with rectal infections, and up to 30 percent of heterosexual men infected with chlamydia have few or no symptoms.

Diagnosis Doctors often diagnose chlamydia only after they have excluded the presence of gonorrhea during examination. A definitive diagnosis is made after growing the chlamydia organism in tissue culture, which takes approximately one week, or from a microscopic antibody test that takes approximately one-half hour.

Treatment Once chlamydia has been diagnosed, the affected person and his or her sexual partner or partners must take prescribed antibiotics such as tetracycline and doxycycline. Erythromycin is substituted for those allergic to these drugs and for pregnant women. All sexual contacts to chlamydia require treatment to prevent reinfection and complications from untreated chlamydia infection. Untreated chlamydia infection can lead to reproductive consequences such as infertility or permanent sterility. Infected individuals should abstain from sexual relations until treatment is completed.

Great cost is associated with chlamydia infections. More than one billion in direct costs are spent on these infections each year in the United States. Most costs occur from the care of women with pelvic inflammatory disease (PID), and from the treatment of infants hospitalized with chlamydia pneumonia. These costs, however, do not reflect the human suffering experienced by those who are affected by this disease.

Nongonococcal Urethritis **Nongonococcal urethritis (NGU)** is one of the most common sexually transmissible diseases. Urinary tract inflammation is called *nongonococcal* if gonorrhea is not detected.

In 1972, NGU surpassed gonorrhea in number of patient visits to private physicians and public health clinics throughout the country. NGU is twice as common as gonorrhea, with an estimated 2.5 million Americans infected each year.

NGU is an infection of the urethra, which is believed to be caused by several different organisms. About 40 percent of all cases of NGU are caused by *Chlamydia trachomatis*. Less well known bacterial agents may cause NGU, and approximately 30 percent of men with symptomatic genital herpes infection suffer urinary tract discomfort.

It has also been suggested that some men become allergic to vaginal secretions of their sexual partners. Furthermore, it is possible that the urethra can become irritated by certain soaps, feminine deodorant sprays, contraceptive vaginal foams and jellies, and masturbation.

Symptoms In males, symptoms of NGU may resemble gonorrhea or chlamydia. Often in men, these symptoms do not occur simultaneously. Some men may only have a discharge, and others may only have urinary tract discomfort. Women who are infected by NGU do not get obvious symptoms because the urethra is not readily infected by the organisms that may cause NGU. However, vaginal discharge, pain, itching, and burning around the labia may signal NGU.

Diagnosis Diagnosis of NGU in men is made when their tests for gonorrhea are negative and they either show white blood cells (WBCs) on a smear of urethral discharge or have been exposed to a sexual partner with NGU. The diagnosis of this infection in women is often referred to as **nonspecific vaginitis (NSV)**. **Asymptomatic** (having no symptoms) men with negative gonorrhea tests are also presumed to have NGU when they display substantial

Epididymitis An inflammation of the small body of ducts that rests on the testes; part of the ducts that excrete sperm.

Testicle The male reproductive gland, the source of sperm and hormones that develop and maintain masculine characteristics.

Cervix The neck of the uterus; narrow outer end of the uterus that opens into the vagina.

Fallopian tubes The passages through which the egg leaves the ovary and passes to the uterus.

Nongonococcal urethritis (NGU) An infection in the urethra caused by a unspecified organism; is specifically not gonorrhea.

Nonspecific vaginitis (NSV) An inflammation of the vagina caused by an unspecified organism; often present in a woman who has been exposed to a male partner with NGU.

Gonorrhea A sexually transmissible disease caused by a type of bacteria that usually affects mucous membranes.

Asymptomatic Having no symptoms; no subjective evidence of disease.

---

numbers of WBCs microscopically on a urethral smear. Doctors often diagnose NGU solely on the basis of symptoms described by the patient, without laboratory confirmation.

Treatment NGU is usually treated with tetracycline or doxycycline. Pregnant women and those allergic to the tetracyclines are treated with erythromycin. Dosages may be prescribed for periods of seven, fourteen, or twenty-one days. Penicillin is of no value in treating NGU. Follow-up tests may be advisable after treatment. Infected individuals should abstain from sexual relations until treatment is completed. Sexual partners should also be referred for treatment to avoid reinfection and to prevent complications.

If left untreated—usually because of minimal symptoms and reluctance of individuals lacking severe symptoms to seek medical attention—NGU may lead to serious consequences. Among these may be sterility in both men and women, pelvic inflammatory disease in women, and serious infections in newborns of untreated mothers.

Gonorrhoeae Gonorrhea, also called "clap" or "drip," is one of the leading sexually transmissible diseases. Approximately one million people are infected each year in the United States. You can only get gonorrhea from an infected sexual partner.

Gonorrhea is caused by the bacterium *Neisseria gonorrhoeae*, one of the most sensitive disease-causing organisms. The bacteria grows well in mucous membranes, including the moist linings of the mouth, throat, vagina, cervix, urethra, and anal canal. Because these bacteria cannot live long outside the warm, moist environment of the human body (they die within moments after exposure to light and air), gonorrhea cannot be caught from toilet seats, door knobs, or towels.

A male during a single episode of vaginal intercourse with an infected partner has a 20 percent chance of developing the infection. A female, however, has a greater than 80 percent chance of developing gonorrhea from one encounter.

Symptoms The incubation period of gonorrhea in men is brief, generally averaging five days. Most men with gonorrhea (from 70 to 90 percent) experience discomfort on urination (urethritis) and a thick, yellowish-white or yellowish-green discharge. The lips of the urethral opening may become inflamed and swollen. In some cases, the lymph glands in the groin become enlarged and tender. From 10 to 30 percent of men infected with gonorrhea will have few or no symptoms.

Unlike men, women usually don't know when they are infected. Approximately 80 percent of infected women are asymptomatic carriers of gonorrhea. Furthermore, most women infected with gonorrhea cannot distinguish a normal vaginal discharge from a discharge caused by gonorrhea. When women do get symptoms, they are similar to symptoms in men. Pus may be discharged from the cervix, and a yellowish-white or yellowish-green discharge irritating to the vulva may occur. Discomfort on urination is also likely in many women.

Lower abdominal pain (cramping), fever, and vaginal bleeding are symptoms in women infected for a long period of time, generally two months or more. When an increased vaginal discharge and discomfort occurs—especially with a different, usually offensive odor—women should seek examination and laboratory testing for gonorrhea immediately.

Men and women who engage in oral or rectal sex can be infected with gonorrhea in the throat or rectum. Those with gonorrhea in the throat may develop pus on the tonsils or a sore throat, and those who have gonorrhea in the rectum may see mucus or pus in their feces or feel rectal irritation, pain, and itching, and have gas and runny stools. As with other infections, swollen glands often accompany the discomfort and fever may be present.

Diagnosis Gonorrhea is diagnosed through a culture and smear test in which samples of the discharge are taken and examined. A positive smear in men is generally sufficient to diagnose gonorrhea. Asymptomatic people who

Exploring Your Emotions

You have noticed symptoms that may indicate you have contracted gonorrhea, and your physician has just confirmed it. How do you feel about this? Do you feel different from the way you would if you had contracted influenza? If so, why?

suspect they may be infected can have cultures taken. If a woman suspects an infection, she should seek examination a week to ten days after sexual contact.

Although the incidence of gonorrhea has decreased since 1973, when a national control program began, problems with antibiotic-resistant strains of gonorrhea arose. **Penicillinase-producing *Neisseria gonorrhoeae* (PPNG)** was first isolated in the United States in 1976, most cases being linked to travel to Southeast Asia, including the Philippines, Thailand, Korea, Taiwan, and Singapore. Other biological changes in the gonococcal organism itself created additional outbreaks of resistant strains. Accurate diagnosis and proper treatment are thus a key to controlling infections, complications, and spread of disease.

Treatment Gonorrhea is easy to cure when treated early. It will become a chronic, sterility-producing disease, however, when it is treated late. Penicillin is the preferred drug for the treatment of acute, uncomplicated gonorrhea. For people who are allergic to penicillin, the tetracycline drugs are effective. It is very important to know that self-treatment with antibiotics found available on the street (black market) or around the home may be inadequate and even prove harmful if taken without medical supervision. Recently developed new antibiotics ensure effective treatment of penicillin- and tetracycline-resistant strains of gonorrhea.

A gonorrhea infection must be taken seriously. If left untreated for a prolonged period of time, it may cause serious inflammation of the Fallopian tubes in women (pelvic inflammatory disease), and inflammation of the testicles in men (epididymitis). Besides being a leading cause of infertility in men and women, gonorrhea can also cause arthritis and skin conditions **(dermatitis)**, as well as diseases in other organs of the body. An infant passing through an infected birth canal at the time of birth can also contract an eye infection **(gonococcal conjunctivitis)** which, if untreated, can result in permanent blindness.

Follow-up testing after all medication has been taken is important to be assured of cure. It is important not to resume sexual activity until the results of follow-up have been ascertained.

Figure 19-1 Infection from pelvic inflammatory disease can move from the vagina and cervix to the uterus, Fallopian tubes, and, finally, the pelvic cavity.

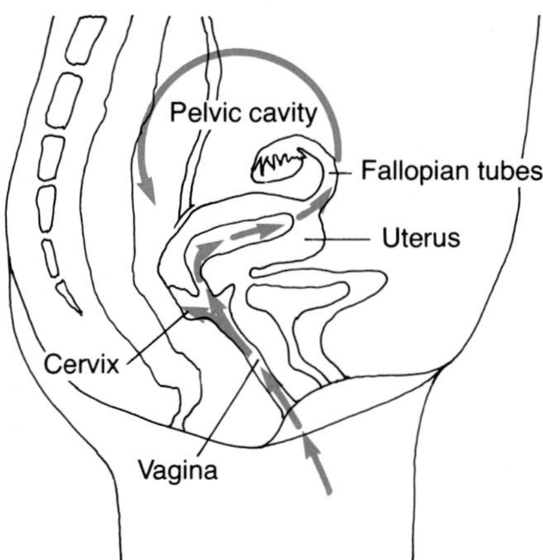

Pelvic Inflammatory Disease (PID) The major impact of gonorrhea is on women and their unborn children. About 10 to 15 percent of women infected with gonorrhea develop the complications of the disease, specifically **pelvic inflammatory disease (PID)**.

Pelvic inflammatory disease is an infection of the Fallopian tubes that may extend to the ovaries as well. An acute infection is often serious enough to require hospitalization and occasionally surgery. Even if the disease is treated successfully, the woman has a continuing susceptibility to recurrent infection and to tubal pregnancy, sterility, and chronic menstrual problems. PID is responsible for a majority of the economic costs, physical damage, and personal tragedy associated with gonococcal infection.

Gonococcal organisms are transmitted sexually to a woman from an infected partner. During or just after menstruation, these organisms appear to rise into the uterine cavity where they may cause inflammation, or they may pass directly into the Fallopian tubes. The organisms then invade the cells, which generate the discharge in a gonococcal infection. This discharge then enters the pelvic cavity to produce inflammation and possibly pelvic abscesses (see Figure 19-1).

Symptoms Following infection with gonococci that are capable of causing PID, most women remain asymptomatic for some time, usually until the next menstrual period. Once the organisms reach the Fallopian tubes, the rate of development of symptoms varies from one to seven days. Women with rapid onset of symptoms most often have chills, fever, loss of appetite, nausea, and/or vomiting. Most complain of abdominal pain on both sides, although the pain may be greater on one side than the other. The pain may be increased by sudden movements like sneezing or coughing. Some women may also have abnormal vaginal bleeding, prolonged menstruation, or abnormal vaginal discharge.

Diagnosis Diagnosis is usually made on the basis of clinical symptoms. Other diagnostic techniques are based on the relative severity of the illness and the need to identify the specific organism causing the disease. Laparoscopy, a surgical procedure that allows the physician to see into the Fallopian tubes, may be used to isolate the microorganism directly.

Penicillinase-producing *Neisseria gonorrhoeae* (PPNG) A strain of bacterial gonococci that produces an enzyme that inactivates or neutralizes the effects of penicillin, and is therefore resistant to penicillin treatment.

Dermatitis An inflammation of the skin evidenced by itching, redness, and various skin lesions.

Gonococcal conjunctivitis An inflammation of the mucous membrane lining of the eyelids, caused by the gonococcus bacterium.

Pelvic inflammatory disease (PID) An infection that progresses from the vagina and cervix to infect the pelvic cavity and Fallopian tubes.

Syphilis A sexually transmissible disease caused by a spiral-shaped, corkscrew bacteria called a *spirochete*.

Treponema pallidum The spiral-shaped organism that causes syphilis.

Chancre The sore produced by syphilis in its earliest stage.

Cultures from the cervix, rectum, and (when indicated) the Fallopian tubes are taken in order to identify the specific micro-organism. Gonorrhea is not the only causative agent. Increasingly, chlamydial infections and other agents are believed to be culprits in pelvic inflammatory disease.

Treatment Beginning treatment of pelvic inflammatory disease as quickly as possible is important in order to avoid severe damage. Antibiotics such as penicillin or tetracycline are started immediately. If there is no response within forty-eight hours, the specific drug can be changed. Periodic re-examination to detect abscesses is recommended, along with careful monitoring for complications. Repeat cultures are done to ensure that they are negative.

Of special importance is the treatment of all sexual contacts of a woman with PID. As high as 60 percent of male contacts of women with PID have been asymptomatic. Many men still believe that unless they have symptoms, they do not have the disease.

Complications of PID are serious and irreversible. Scarring of the Fallopian tubes, often as a result of abscesses, can result in adhesions, chronic pain, tubal pregnancies, and may well be responsible for premature sterility in young women.

Syphilis **Syphilis** has been called "evil pox, great pox, or the great imposter." It was a common disease only decades ago: 5 to 10 percent of the population died of syphilis or related causes. Widespread use of antibiotics has reduced the incidence of syphilis to manageable proportions, and it is no longer considered a fatal illness in adults.

Syphilis is caused by a bacterial organism called ***Treponema pallidum***, a thin, corkscrew-shaped organism that moves by rotating on its long axis. Warmth and moisture are essential to its survival, and the bacterium dies very quickly outside the human body.

The disease is usually acquired by sexual contact, although it can be acquired before birth. The bacteria can be transmitted through the placenta to the unborn child.

Transmission through sexual contact requires exposure to moist mucous membranes, or skin lesions. Therefore, a person can transmit syphilis during the early stages of the infection. The organism is transmitted through any opening or break in the skin or mucous membranes by means of kissing, or vaginal, oral-genital, or anal intercourse. Sores or lesions contain large numbers of the organism and make the disease highly contagious. In later stages, systemic and/or central nervous system damage presents no lesions to transmit the organism.

The incubation period for syphilis can range from 10 to 90 days, the average being about 21 days. An individual who goes untreated can remain contagious for as long as eighteen months.

Primary Syphilis In 10 to 90 days (on average, three weeks) a primary lesion, called a **chancre**, appears at the site where the organism entered the body, which is most commonly in the genital areas. Chancres, especially in the anal area, are increasingly common. Chancres can also appear on the mouth, tongue, tonsils, lips, breasts, armpit, umbilicus, and fingers. These sores are generally painless unless they become infected, and they generally heal in a few weeks.

Secondary Syphilis Approximately six weeks after a chancre first appears, an untreated person with syphilis will begin to show signs and symptoms of secondary syphilis. During this period, the bacteria have multiplied sufficiently to generate symptoms including malaise, fever, sore throat, headache, hoarseness, loss of appetite, swollen lymph glands, and loss of hair.

Among the symptoms of secondary syphilis is a rash that may appear anywhere on the body, particularly on the palms of the hands and the soles of the feet. The rash may also affect the mucous membranes of the lips, cheeks, tongue, tonsils, throat, and vocal cords. In these areas, grayish-white mucus patches appear, surrounded by dull-red borders. These sores break down and ooze a clear fluid that contains large numbers of the organism, making this a highly contagious stage.

Either with or without treatment, skin lesions of secondary syphilis usually heal in two to ten weeks. Recurrence of lesions of the skin or mucous membranes may occur in untreated or inadequately treated patients. Most relapses occur toward the end of the first year following infection. After two years they are rare, and after four years supposedly do not develop. Relapses are generally uncommon following adequate penicillin therapy.

Latent Syphilis By definition, people with historical evidence of syphilis but with no physical manifestations have latent syphilis. This category has been somewhat arbitrarily divided into *early latency* and *late latency* on the basis of the time when untreated people are likely to have relapses. The U.S. Public Health Service defines *early latency* (which is potentially infectious) as one year from the onset of infection, whereas others prefer a longer interval before designating the infection as *late latency*.

Syphilis in Pregnancy The *Treponema pallidum* organism can invade the placenta of an infected mother after the tenth week of gestation, although this generally takes place after the eighteenth week. If the mother is not treated before this time, stillbirth or congenital infection and deformities are probable. Possible damage includes crippling, blindness, deafness, and facial abnormalities. Children born with syphilis are contagious only while lesions are present. These children do not pass their syphilis on to the next generation because they are usually not infectious by the time they reach puberty.

Diagnosis A special microscopic examination, the **darkfield examination,** permits direct inspection of the organism itself, and remains the best tool for the diagnosis of primary syphilis. A specimen is obtained from the clean surface of the chancre and then examined under the microscope. In the case of secondary syphilis, diagnosis is made from blood tests and clinical observation. Two or three tests are used, the most usual being the **Venereal Disease Research Laboratory (VDRL) test** and the **fluorescent treponema antibody (FTA) reaction**.

Treatment Penicillin remains the drug of choice for the treatment of syphilis in all stages. Recommended treatment schedules have been prepared by the Centers for Disease Control (CDC) according to the stage of disease. Treatment also involves sexual partners.

For those people allergic to penicillin, tetracycline and erythromycin can be substituted effectively. Follow-up tests should be performed four weeks after completion of treatment and every three months thereafter for a year. A person who has had syphilis should not have sexual contact with others until at least one month after treatment is completed, and the partners must be participating in follow-up testing.

Exploring Your Emotions

You are a woman and realize that women frequently do not experience observable signs of a sexually transmissible disease. During a regular physical examination, you realize your doctor will not routinely test you for exposure. What do you say to the doctor? Will you be able to ask for appropriate tests? Why do you suppose your doctor does not make the inquiry?

Herpes The word *herpes* derives from the Greek word meaning "to creep," or "to spread." The word came into use because of the symptoms, long before the specific **herpes** viruses were ever identified.

Five viruses constitute the herpes virus family and include

- **Herpes Simplex, Type 1:** Generally cold sores and fever blisters
- **Herpes Simplex, Type 2:** Genital herpes
- **Cytomegalovirus (CMV):** Asymptomatic in adults, can cause serious problems for unborn children
- ***Varicella zoster:*** Chicken pox in children, shingles in adults
- **Epstein-Barr virus:** Mononucleosis or "kissing disease"

Of this family, Herpes Simplex 1 and 2, and cytomegalovirus appear to be sexually transmitted. Although the remaining two, *Varicella zoster* and Epstein-Barr, seem to be transmitted occasionally through sexual contact, they appear to play no significant role in STD incidence.

Researchers estimate that at least 20 million people in this country have genital herpes and that about 500,000 new cases occur each year. The complications and risks of herpes to newborn babies of mothers who have active genital herpes are very serious and not to be taken lightly. Herpes in newborns has been known to cause brain damage and in some instances can even be fatal to a newborn. Proper precautions can be taken before delivery to minimize risks. Newborns must be protected because their immune systems are immature, and they should not be exposed to family or friends who have facial lesions.

Symptoms Typically, a herpes infection appears two to twenty days after initial exposure. Symptoms can include one or more blisters (sores) on or around the mouth, the face, or sex organs. The sores are often painful, blisterlike lesions filled with fluid. They may be accompanied by swollen glands, general muscle aches and pains, fever, a mild burning sensation during urination in men, and in women, a vaginal discharge. Some women may have internal herpes lesions, with the cervix or vagina being the only site of infection. Because the cervix has no nerve endings, these women may be unaware of symptoms.

Although a direct relationship between the herpes virus and cancer is yet to be established, women with genital herpes are five to eight times more likely to develop cancer of the cervix. It is recommended that women who have

Darkfield examination The use of a special microscope to see organisms taken from a lesion suspected to be syphilis.

Venereal Disease Research Laboratory (VDRL) test A blood test to identify the presence of the syphilis-causing organism in the blood.

Fluorescent treponema antibody (FTA) reaction A laboratory test used to identify the presence of the antibody against the organism that causes syphilis.

Herpes A type of virus, or the disease produced by the virus, such as cold sores; is considered sexually transmissible.

Herpes simplex An infectious disease caused by the herpes virus.

Varicella zoster The virus that causes chicken pox in children, shingles in adults.

Cytomegalovirus (CMV) A virus in the herpes family, often present in salivary glands and commonly asymptomatic. CMV infections appear as a complication in people with AIDS.

Epstein-Barr virus A member of the herpes virus family associated with infectious mononucleosis.

Acyclovir A drug used in the treatment of recurrent herpes infection.

---

had genital herpes inform their doctor and be sure to have a Pap smear every six months. Although Type 1 is usually seen around the mouth and face, and Type 2 in the genital region, there have been increasing numbers of people with Type 1 virus in genital lesions, and Type 2 in oral lesions. It is presumed that the virus is transmitted through oral-genital sex. Both are equally contagious, and do not change types because of location.

Herpes infections can recur. Following an initial infection that may last three to four weeks, the virus lies dormant until it becomes active again as a result of many different "triggering" factors. Sun exposure, temperature extremes, high-level stress, illness, and reduced ability to fight infection may all play a role in reactivating the virus, which is a highly individualistic process. The major problem of recurrent genital herpes is contingent on its frequency, chronic nature, and its effects on the person's relationships and sexuality. Each time the person has symptoms, they are once again contagious and it is essential to avoid direct contact with lesions when symptoms are present.

Diagnosis Of the herpes cases seen by medical practitioners, 90 percent are diagnosed on the basis of sores or lesions present, medical history, and other characteristics such as swollen glands, muscle aches and pains, and fever. If doubt exists that the infection is caused by the herpes virus, a more definitive test is available at some clinics and other health care facilities. A sample smear is taken from the lesion, and grown on live tissue culture to determine the type of virus. At present, this test is relatively expensive and not available everywhere.

Treatment Treatment and care of herpes is directed at relieving pain, itching and burning, and at preventing the sores from becoming infected or spreading to other parts of the body. Bathing with soap and water, or other drying agents such as Epsom salts or Burow's solution is helpful in preventing secondary infection and speeds drying of the lesions.

Over the last ten years, significant research has been directed toward developing a drug to treat herpes infections. First introduced in 1977, **acyclovir** is now available in oral form for use by people with genital herpes infections. Until acyclovir was made available commercially, home remedies (such as Burow's solution) were used in addition to dietary supplements and food restrictions (no chocolate, nuts, seeds). These had varying degrees of effectiveness for different people and continue to be used even in combination with drug therapy. Most often, however, these treatments were unsuccessful in changing the frequency or severity of recurrences. Acyclovir has been proven to do the following:

1. Taken for five days, beginning at the outset of a recurrency of genital herpes, acyclovir shortens the episode.
2. Taken every day in doses ranging from two to five capsules per day, acyclovir can prevent most visible outbreaks. It reduces the severity of those that do occur.
3. Taken during the first episode of genital herpes, acyclovir shortens the episode by one week on the average. It has been shown to lessen the severity of urinary discomfort and swollen lymph nodes.

A word of caution is in order, however, because, although effective, acyclovir may not be for everyone. The decision to take oral acyclovir is one to make with your personal physician. Because the drug is new, long-term effects have yet to be determined and the question of drug resistance remains unanswered. In addition, once the drug is stopped, recurrences occur as frequently as before taking the drug. Acyclovir is not a cure for the disease, nor does it kill the latent virus. The ability to prevent herpes from becoming activated, however, is unquestionably a benefit to the herpes sufferer.

Other nonspecific treatments include ether, zinc, lysine, a variety of ointments, and ultrasound. None of these has stood the test of time nor careful clinical observation.

Where to Go for Help Information, recent research, and answers to more questions are available through the Herpes Resource Center in Palo Alto, California. Established by the American Social Health Association, this organization also publishes a newsletter for interested individuals. Information can be obtained by writing to the Herpes Resource Center, American Social Health Association, 260 Sheridan Avenue, Palo Alto, CA 94306.

Genital warts A sexually transmissible disease caused by a virus and characterized by the appearance of growths on the genital area of men and women.

Papilloma A raised growth of skin, or wart.

Podophyllin An acid used in the treatment of warts.

AIDS, acquired immune deficiency syndrome A fatal, incurable, sexually transmissible viral disease.

Human immunodeficiency virus (HIV) The AIDS virus. A virus that attacks white blood cells (T helper lymphocytes) in human blood.

Retrovirus An RNA virus that transcribes RNA into DNA through the manufacture of an enzyme, reverse transcriptase.

Ribonucleic acid (RNA) An acid present in all cells and is considered to be the genetic material of viruses.

Deoxyribonucleic acid (DNA) The carrier of genetic information in cells.

Helper T cells (lymphocytes) Blood elements that interact directly with foreign elements to fight off infection; important in the immune system's functioning.

Suppressor T cells (lymphocytes) Involved in the inhibiting of helper T cells and other blood elements for proper balance in the immune system.

Antibody A globular protein produced in the blood in response to a foreign substance with which it combines.

Genital Warts **Genital warts** have also been called "venereal warts," "fig warts," and "gonorrheal warts." Genital warts are an old disease and were apparently very common in the ancient world. The cause of these warts was initially thought to be syphilis. Not until 1949 were virus particles isolated as the cause of venereal warts, the same virus that also caused skin warts. Not until twenty years later, however, was the specific genital wart virus isolated and identified as the **papilloma** virus. Most genital warts are seen in young adults, age of onset usually between 16 and 25 in both men and women. The incubation period of genital warts has been estimated at 46 weeks, and it can be as long as two to three months before symptoms appear.

Symptoms Warts appear on the penis more commonly in circumcised males. They are usually multiple and can join together to form larger masses. Warts often involve the male urethra, appearing first at the opening of the urethra; then they may spread as a complication. This growth may lead to bleeding and irritation, which can cause a discharge and painful urination.

In women, warts may appear on the labia and vulva and may spread to the area between the vagina and the rectum. Despite the spread, warts are rarely seen on the thighs or trunk of the body. They may also appear on the cervix.

Large genital warts are uncomfortable and may be embarrassing to the person; however, if cared for properly, they are generally not very serious. Some researchers suspect a relationship between genital warts and cervical cancer, but this connection is not yet clear. Development of vaccines is also pending at the present time.

Diagnosis Genital warts should be differentiated from other lesions. The most important lesion to be differentiated is that of secondary syphilis. Sometimes both diseases may be present, and diagnosis should be made in order to begin appropriate treatment. Sexual partners should also be examined and treated if necessary.

Treatment No one method of treatment is completely superior to all others, and the decision should be made jointly with the physician.

The use of **podophyllin**, a toxic agent, is often recommended. Applying podophyllin causes the wart to dry up and fall off. This agent is not recommended for pregnant women. Other methods include electrocautery, cryosurgery (freezing), surgical removal, and laser therapy.

As with any treatment, the physician's instructions should be followed carefully and further sexual contacts avoided until healing has taken place.

AIDS This year **acquired immune deficiency syndrome (AIDS)** will kill about 14,000 Americans, car accidents will kill 42,000, cancer nearly 500,000, and heart disease nearly 800,000. Of the 2 million Americans who will die this year, AIDS will kill less than 1 percent. AIDS is a fatal condition that affects the immune system (the body's natural defense against disease), making an otherwise healthy person susceptible to a variety of infections, certain forms of cancer, and various neurological disorders. To date, there have been some 35,500 adult and child cases nationwide and over 20,500 deaths from AIDS. The number of new cases continues to double every seven to nine months. People with AIDS have been identified in all states and territories of the United States, and in at least twenty other countries. The largest group of patients (approximately 66 percent) is made up of homosexual and bisexual males. The second largest group of patients (17 percent) is intravenous drug abusers. Smaller percentages are found among people who have received blood or blood products donated by people infected with the virus, the sexual partners of those just described, infants born to infected mothers, and a few individuals with no apparent risk factor. Of all adult AIDS cases, 92 percent are male, and 7 percent are female.

The cause of AIDS is a virus variously termed (by different groups of investigators) *human T-lymphotropic virus type III* (HTLV-III), *lymphadenopathy-associated virus* (LAV), and *AIDS-associated retrovirus* (ARV). The internationally accepted term today is **human immunodeficiency virus (HIV)**. HIV is a **retrovirus**, so named because of its ability to convert **ribonucleic acid (RNA)** into **deoxyribonucleic acid (DNA)**, which is the chemical that constitutes the genes of human and animal cells. This virus uses the genetic machinery of the cells it infects to make the pro-

Intravenous Within or into a vein; as the injection of drugs or medication directly into the vein.

Hemophiliacs People who have a hereditary blood disease in which their blood fails to clot and abnormal bleeding occurs, which requires transfusions of blood with a specific factor to aid coagulation.

HIV antibody blood test A test currently being used to determine if an individual has been infected by the human immunodeficiency (HIV) virus.

Plasma The clear, colorless component of blood containing dissolved salts and proteins; blood minus the blood cells.

Opportunistic infections (diseases) "Runaway" infections that persist and resist healing due to poor functioning or failure of the immune system; often occurring in people with AIDS, and with cancer as a result of immune suppression.

Pneumocystis carinii An organism that causes a particular type of pneumonia present in people who develop AIDS.

Kaposi's sarcoma A form of cancer characterized by purple or brownish lesions that are generally painless and occur anywhere on the skin; usually appears in people who develop AIDS.

Dementia Deterioration of the mental state or reduction of intellectual functioning due to organic brain disease.

Meningitis An inflammation of the membranes of the spinal cord or brain.

---

tein it needs for survival. The virus only lives within the cells it invades, not outside the body. The virus does not live in the air, in swimming pools, on toilet seats, in food, or on objects such as knives, forks, or glasses.

All AIDS patients show a significant impairment of the immune system. Within this system, there are **helper T cells (lymphocytes)**, which marshall the defenses against infection; there are also **suppressor T cells**, which prevent the formation of **antibodies**. Generally, individuals with normal immune function have about twice as many helpers as suppressor T cells. In people with AIDS, however, this ratio is often reversed.

Blood and blood-contaminated fluids of the body and semen are the primary body fluids that carry the virus. Saliva has not been implicated in transmission of the AIDS virus. In homosexual and bisexual males—and to a lesser degree heterosexual males and females—transmission can occur through sexual activity that involves the exchange of these body fluids and their entry into the blood system. The route of transmission among **intravenous** drug users is the sharing of contaminated needles or syringes. **Hemophiliacs** who develop AIDS are probably infected by contaminated blood from a donor carrying the AIDS virus even though they are treated for their condition with a product prepared from the blood of as many as 1,000 donors.

The threat of transmitting the AIDS virus to hemophiliacs or others who need donated blood has been virtually eliminated with the advent of the **HIV antibody blood test** in early 1985. The antibody test is used to screen donated blood and **plasma** in all licensed blood banks and plasma centers in the United States. The test is also available through private physicians, most state or local health departments, and designated alternative test sites throughout the country. Presence of the HIV antibody means that a person has been infected with AIDS virus, and is most likely infectious. However, presence of the AIDS virus gives no indication of whether or not the person will develop AIDS in the future, although the likelihood of developing AIDS in the future is high. There is absolutely no danger of contracting the AIDS virus from *donating* blood.

Once a person is infected with the virus, the average incubation period for AIDS ranges from about four months to as long as five to seven years. Some researchers believe the incubation period may be longer. Fewer than 10 percent of people with AIDS have survived for more than three years following diagnosis, and few have recovered the ability to fight **opportunistic diseases** (ones that overcome the disabled immune system). It is therefore assumed that AIDS is a fatal disease.

Symptoms Signs and symptoms suggestive of AIDS include unexplained, persistent swollen glands, drenching night sweats, fever, chills, significant weight loss (unrelated to illness, dieting, or increased physical activity) of more than 10 pounds in less than two months, and immobilizing fatigue. Obviously, some of these signs and symptoms can occur with minor colds or stomach flu ailments.

The infection most commonly seen in people with AIDS is ***Pneumocystis carinii***, a protozoal infection that produces pneumonia and its symptoms, shortness of breath, a persistent dry cough, sharp chest pains, and (in severe cases) difficulty in breathing. **Kaposi's sarcoma** is the second most common problem seen in people with AIDS. This cancer produces purple or brownish lesions that resemble bruises but are painless and do not heal. They may occur anywhere on the skin or inside the nose, mouth, or rectum. New studies also show that HIV may exist in the brain, causing progressive neurologic disease. Unexplained **dementia** and **meningitis** also have been diagnosed in people with AIDS.

Candida infections in AIDS patients are considered one of the "opportunistic infections" in which the organisms proliferate as a result of the poorly functioning or nonfunctioning immune system. Uncontrollable candida infections may be seen in the mouth and throat of infected AIDS patients.

The risk of transmitting the AIDS virus to people not involved in high-risk behavior (male homosexual and bisexual activity, and sharing intravenous needles) is low. However, the AIDS virus can be transmitted to anyone, regardless of sexual preference, race, or ethnicity, if high-risk sexual behavior or needle sharing takes place.

Doctors and nurses and family members caring for

Azidothymidine (AZT) A drug used in the treatment of AIDS that inhibits reproduction of the AIDS virus.

people with AIDS for the past several years have not contracted this disease. Therefore, no one should fear being exposed to the AIDS virus through casual contact with people who have AIDS or people infected with the AIDS virus.

Diagnosis The most specific diagnosis of HIV infection is the detection of the virus in human tissues. The techniques for isolating the virus in tissue culture are costly and are not easily available.

For public health purposes, people who have repeatedly positive HIV antibody tests, supported by follow-up confirmatory antibody tests, should be considered both infected and infectious. There is a very strong correlation between the symptoms of AIDS and the presence of HIV antibody. Most people who show symptoms of the disease combined with a positive HIV antibody test meet the current diagnostic criteria established by the CDC.

A public health program, confronting a fatal incurable epidemic disease with sociomoral complications, cannot wait for scientific certainty before acting. Public health workers must make use of all clues, however ambiguous, that researchers have uncovered. Questions have been raised concerning the use of the HIV antibody test in diagnosing AIDS. It is not known if the presence of HIV antibody in people means they will inevitably develop AIDS. Yet all people positive for HIV antibody are advised about their being both infected with the virus, and capable of infecting others with whom they have sexual relations and exchange blood, particularly through needle sharing. Women who test positive for HIV antibody and who are considering pregnancy are advised to postpone pregnancy. Pregnant women who test positive for HIV antibody are counseled about abortion.

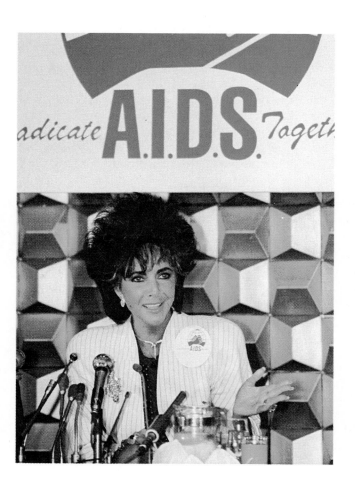

Reporting All cases of AIDS, as defined by the CDC, must be reported to public health authorities everywhere in the United States in order to determine the extent of the epidemic. Reporting requirements vary from state to state. Although reporting cases of AIDS is required, most states do not require the reporting of those people who test positive for HIV antibody.

The issue of ensuring confidentiality for individuals with AIDS and those who test positive for the antibody has provoked serious debate. Since misunderstanding of AIDS has produced so much fear, people with AIDS, or people suspected of having AIDS because they are associated with high-risk behavior, are often stigmatized and discriminated against. Therefore, physicians, hospitals, and public health departments have a duty to keep all facts about *individual* diagnosis, treatment, and HIV antibody positive tests confidential.

However, we feel that disclosure of facts about people who have AIDS or who are infected with the AIDS virus and test positive for the HIV antibody must be carefully reconsidered so that the best interests of both the individual patient and the public can both be served. In light of the AIDS epidemic, a re-examination of the process for controlling this epidemic is necessary so that humane measures can be developed and implemented that will achieve the proper balance between individual and public concerns.

Treatment Because the cause of AIDS has been identified, everyone hopes that a cure and a vaccine to prevent future infections will soon be forthcoming. Currently, no antiviral drugs anywhere have proven effective in curing AIDS, although researchers are actively pursuing such drugs. Some drugs have been found to inhibit the AIDS virus and can prolong life. **Azidothymidine (AZT)** has

Carefully into the Night

The sexual revolution may not be over, but things sure have changed. The deadly acquired immune deficiency syndrome (AIDS) and the prevalence of other sexually transmissible diseases such as herpes and gonorrhea have altered the game of recreational sex and slowed the initial sexual pace of potentially more serious relationships.

Fear of sexually transmissible diseases edged out war and peace as the subject most American women were concerned about in 1985, according to a national study of women's attitudes commissioned by *Glamour* magazine. When asked to cite those subjects that they worried about more in 1985 than the year before, 70 percent of the respondents cited sexually transmissible diseases, 69 percent cited war and peace (which was the Number One concern in 1984), and 65 percent said personal health.

In addition to changing people's attitudes, there's no doubt that sexually transmissible diseases—AIDS, herpes, gonorrhea, syphilis, and the recently recognized chlamydia—are changing the sexual climate in America. Some examples:

- Male dancers who entertain women at the Pulsations and Chippendales clubs in New York, Philadelphia, and Los Angeles gargle with antibacterial products before and after their performances, which include kissing women. Open-mouth kissing is prohibited.
- A New York therapist said a client told him that he hadn't had sex in two years so he "didn't have to think about dying."
- A "social card" that can be screened by a new sex partner is being sold at a Denver health clinic. It lists results of tests for sexually transmissible diseases.

Concern is particularly great among young adults who, traditionally, are more likely to be sexually active with more than one partner, experts said. "AIDS and herpes come up *daily* in conversations," said a recent Temple University graduate. In some college human sexuality classes, fear of herpes—which was the most feared sexually transmissible disease in the early 1980s—is already passé.

At Syracuse University, psychology professor Clive Davis conducted a three-part lecture series on human sexuality in October to 1,400 students and subsequently met with all of them in small groups. "The only questions related to sexually transmitted diseases were about AIDS," said Davis, who is president of the national Society for the Scientific Study of Sex and is studying the herpes virus.

In the sexually transmissible diseases discussion in his human sexuality course at American University this fall, "the only thing students wanted to hear about was AIDS," said Barry McCarthy, a clinical psychologist and sex therapist at the Washington Psychological Center, who teaches at AU. "That's an interesting myth, because gonorrhea and herpes are a much greater reality." Fear of AIDS apparently has reduced the fear and stigma of other sexually transmissible diseases, which infect many more people.

While concern about sexually transmissible diseases is cited as a major reason for recent shifts away from instant sexual relationships, some experts said that this is only partly responsible for new sexual attitudes.

"There's some disenchantment with the promiscuous lifestyle," said psychiatrist Quadland of Mt. Sinai hospital. "We had to go through the 1960s and 1970s, where people, especially gays and women, could express themselves as freely as they wanted to, but there are some costs to that. Now the general trend is toward seeing sex as most satisfying in a committed relationship."

"People are moving to a slightly more conservative stance about how sexually active they are, especially with relative strangers," said Dr. Martin Goldberg, director of the Marriage Council of Philadelphia and director of family study at the University of Pennsylvania. Longer courtships are in vogue, he said, for a variety of reasons, including the more conservative sociopolitical atmosphere and concern about sexually transmissible diseases.

"Psychologically, people have learned that quick physical intimacy does not establish real psychological intimacy, and is sometimes harmful to intimacy and can abort what might be a promising relationship," he said. The notion is most prominent among adults aged 21 to 35, Goldberg said, many of whom are divorced or separated and had once "thought there was no reason not to have sex immediately with someone you meet."

As for sexual diseases, "most people are taking the attitude that the more they can minimize the

(continued on next page)

Carefully into the Night (*continued*)

number of people with whom they have sexual contacts, the less risk," he said.

What is clear is the existence of a growing but irrational "AIDS hysteria"—the fear of having contracted the deadly disease from long-ago relationships, restaurants, door knobs and handshakes, several clinicians said. That reaction is typical when a new, widespread disease occurs, they said.

"We're certainly seeing a lot of people who are anxious anyway and believe themselves to be at risk," said Dr. Dolph Druckman, a research fellow at the division of infectious diseases at Johns Hopkins University Hospital. But, Davis said, "it will be some time," if at all, before any statistically recognizable change occurs throughout the population.

SOURCE: Janis Johnson, 1986 (January 8), Carefully into the night, *Washington Post*, pp. 10ff.

been recently approved for widespread use by the Food and Drug Administration (FDA). This drug will only be given to people diagnosed as having AIDS, not to those who are only infected with the AIDS virus. Problems are associated with the use of AZT. Significant side effects may occur, such as anemia that requires blood transfusions. Moreover, the cost of AZT is prohibitive—up to $10,000 per year. Eventually, a combination chemotherapy to combat the virus and restore the immune system may be the most effective therapy.

Other Services Other services include counseling and emotional support groups for people with AIDS, **AIDS-related conditions (ARC)**, individuals who test positive for HIV antibody, and their families and loved ones. In-home services, and hospice services for those dying from AIDS have also been developed. Legal services for people experiencing discrimination, and social services for people who need state and local financial support, are available in most areas.

Prevention If you engage in high-risk behavior, the most important action that you can take to prevent infection with the AIDS virus is to change your behavior so that you can avoid exchanging body fluids:

- Limit your sexual partners, preferably to one person who also prefers one sexual partner.
- Use condoms (rubbers) during sexual relations with people with AIDS, people who test positive for HIV antibody, and anyone known to be engaging in risk behavior, if you jointly decide to have sex.
- Do not abuse drugs, especially those known to significantly affect the body's immune system, such as cocaine, alcohol, and inhalant nitrites (poppers).
- Do not share intravenous needles or syringes, or razor blades, or toothbrushes, or anything that might have blood on it.
- Decontaminate needles and syringes with household bleach and water. Boiling needles and syringes will not guarantee elimination of the virus.
- If you or your partner is at high risk, avoid mouth contact with the penis, vagina, or rectum. Condoms (rubbers) may be effective if you or your partner decide to have oral (mouth to penis) sex.
- Avoid all sexual contact that could cause cuts or tears in the linings of the rectum, vagina, or penis.
- Remember that it is O.K. to say no to sex and drugs.
- Prefer "safer sex" activities that allow intimacy but prevent exposure to the AIDS virus. These activities are varied and pleasurable. Masturbation (individual or mutual), massage, touch, and fantasy are some examples.
- If you are at risk of being infected with the AIDS virus, do not donate blood, body organs, or semen.

In the immediate future, the number of cases will continue to rise at an alarming rate, threatening to produce economic and social chaos. Recent projections estimate 25 to 50 percent of those people who test positive for HIV antibody will develop full-blown AIDS. CDC estimates 1.5 million to 2 million Americans are now infected with the virus. According to the U.S. Surgeon General's report on acquired immune deficiency syndrome, by 1991 "an estimated 270,000 cases of AIDS will have occurred with 179,000 deaths. In 1991, an estimated 145,000 patients with AIDS will need health and supportive services at a total cost between $8 and $16 billion." The long incubation period makes it unlikely that preventive actions already undertaken will produce a decline in that rate within the coming years. However, research to find a vaccine and a cure will bring us closer to understanding the mysteries of the immune system, and possibly success with AIDS will also lead to some answers relating to cancer.

Education must be the cornerstone in preventing the spread of this disease. The Surgeon General's report emphasizes that "education about AIDS should start in

AIDS-related condition, or AIDs-related complex (ARC) A condition caused by the AIDs virus, with symptoms less severe than those of AIDS.

Trichomonas vaginalis The one-celled organism (protozoa) that causes a vaginal infection in women; may be carried by male sexual partners.

Candida albicans An infection, usually in the vagina, caused by a fungus.

Pubic lice Parasites that infest the hair of the pubic region.

early elementary school and at home." This education must focus on making children aware of which high-risk behaviors to avoid to prevent infection. The social and psychological implications of this disease make it necessary to tailor education programs very carefully so that misinformation and unnecessary anxiety within the general community are minimized and so that awareness of the seriousness of the disease in the affected communities is maximized.

Certain behaviors must change. This change must continue into the foreseeable future. It is well known that fear has a short-lived impact on behavior. Therefore, positive approaches to behavior change must be implemented to motivate people to continue safe and healthy practices. People must learn that they can prevent this virus's spread by modifying their risk-taking behavior. With intensified research into the cause, cure, and a vaccine for AIDS, and a comprehensive educational program, we may by the end of this decade be able to look back at AIDS as a past, tragic phenomenon.

Trichomoniasis Trichomoniasis, commonly called "trich," is one of the most common protozoal infections in North America. It is caused by a one-celled organism, ***Trichomonas vaginalis,*** a pear-shaped protozoa. The organism can remain alive on external objects for 60 to 90 minutes, in urine for three hours, and in seminal fluid for six hours. Because it thrives in warm, moist conditions, women are particularly susceptible to these infections in the vagina. Not all women will have symptoms of the infection, which contributes to transmission.

Symptoms For women who do become symptomatic, symptoms appear in about four days following sexual contact. For some, symptoms may not appear for twenty-eight days. Some women with trichomonas experience a greenish vaginal discharge and severe itching. In other cases, the discharge may be white or yellow and frothy, with an unpleasant odor, and it frequently irritates the vagina and vulva, which may become red and painful. In many women with "trich," bright red, slightly raised spots can be seen on the vaginal walls and cervix.

Although most males show no symptoms (the organism can survive under the foreskin of the penis without causing any symptoms), some males experience slight itching, clear discharge, and sometimes painful urination.

Diagnosis A simple diagnostic tool is available for immediate diagnosis. A slide is prepared from a sample of the discharge and examined under the microscope. The presence of the organisms determines the treatment.

Treatment If the organism is found, the drug of choice is Flagyl (generic name metronidazole). This drug should be taken as directed by the physician. In addition, all sexual partners are treated as well. This is to prevent the "ping-pong" effect of an untreated partner reinfecting the sexual partner and the potential for an infection being continually passed back and forth.

Candida albicans ***Candida albicans***, a microscopic yeastlike fungus, is present in the vaginal tract of most women. Several factors can make women more susceptible to increased fungal production and resultant symptomatic infection and discomfort. These include metabolic changes due to pregnancy, possible diabetes, use of birth control pills in some women, antibiotic therapy, and a general lowered body resistance to infection.

Symptoms Intense vaginal and vulval itching, and a thick, white, "curdy" vaginal discharge resembling cottage cheese are common. The vagina becomes red and dry, and sexual intercourse may be painful.

Diagnosis and Treatment Diagnosis of candida infection is made by microscopic examination of the discharge. The antibiotic mycostatin, in the form of vaginal tablets, is generally prescribed. Treatment usually lasts for four weeks, and further testing should be done if the condition persists or does not respond. Resistance may indicate a need to treat other coexisting medical problems, or to provide more extensive medical testing to identify causes of a persistent infection. As with any infection, following the prescribed form of treatment to completion is important in assuring that the infection is cured.

Pubic Lice Commonly known as "crabs," **pubic lice** are a type of parasite that has three claws in front and four pairs of small legs in back. They are a pest, not necessarily a disease. Called *pubic lice* because they are often attached to the pubic hairs of the body, they may be difficult to see. They are the color and size of small freckles until they have fed, and then become dark brown in color. Like mosquitoes, lice feed on human blood. Although usually found in pubic hair, lice can also attach themselves to hair of the head, underarms, eyelashes, and even moustaches and beards. Separated from their human hosts, lice are able to survive about twenty-four hours.

Scabies A contagious skin disease caused by a type of mite.

Easily transmitted from person to person, lice can also be transmitted via infested clothing, towels, bedding, sleeping bags, and even toilet seats. Sexual contact is not necessary to contract lice.

Symptoms Intense itching in response to the bites of the lice is the usual symptom. Self-examination might reveal red spots on the skin beneath the hair as a result of the bites. You can also see crabs directly.

Diagnosis You can generally confirm diagnosis by finding lice themselves, or lice eggs (nits) attached to your body hairs.

Treatment Lice are easily treated. Several over-the-counter drugs for lice infestation are available at the local pharmacy. These come in shampoo or lotion form and should come with a very fine-toothed comb for removing any remaining lice or nits from body hairs. Follow the directions carefully. Washing clothing and linen is essential to prevent reinfestation. For stubborn cases, other more potent drugs are available by prescription. You may need to repeat treatment in seven to ten days to kill any remaining nits that may have hatched.

Scabies Another fairly common infestation is caused by the **scabies** mite, *Sarcoptes scabiei*. The pregnant female mite burrows under the skin and deposits her eggs. These hatch in a few days, and the new mites congregate around hair follicles.

Symptoms Any burrowing parasite produces intense itching, especially at night. The usual sites of scabies infestation are between fingers, on wrists, in armpits, underneath breasts, along inner surfaces of thighs, penis, scrotum, and occasionally female genitals.

Scabies is easily spread from person to person, not only through sexual contact, but any direct or close contact. It can often infest an entire household.

Diagnosis Diagnosis of scabies is made by finding the actual mite, eggs, or larvae in scrapings taken from the burrows in the skin.

Treatment Standard treatment is a prolonged hot bath with vigorous scrubbing of affected areas, and the application of benzyl benzoate emulsion or Kwell lotion, available by prescription. Kwell is a toxic agent (a poison) and should be handled carefully and according to directions, especially around young children. Itching and inflammation that persist after treatment may be the result of secondary infection and should be checked by a health professional. Calamine lotion and starch baths may also help reduce itching and inflammation. Reinfestation can occur from any of the original sources, such as clothing, which should also be treated.

What Can You Do?

In three major areas, you can take responsibility for your health and contribute to a general reduction in the number of cases of sexually transmissible diseases: education, prevention, and diagnosis and treatment.

Education You must assume the responsibility of learning not only the causes and nature of STDs, but also their potential effects on you personally, your children, and on others with whom you share relationships. You must also take a share of the responsibility for passing on what you learn—for educating others.

Information and public awareness may, in fact, have already contributed a great deal to changing sexual behavior. For example, in a 1982 survey conducted by the Centers for Disease Control (CDC) in the United States, because of increasing concern with genital herpes, over half of unmarried people who believed themselves at risk reported changing their sexual behavior to avoid this disease. Evidence also shows that homosexual men are modifying their sexual behavior in response to concern about AIDS.

Students in colleges and universities are participating in courses on human sexuality, family life programs, and women's health. These courses encourage not only the gaining of knowledge, but also communicating among partners, which can help prevent and control STDs.

For specific questions about STDs, you can call the National VD Hotline, listed in local telephone directories, for free, confidential information and referral services to callers from anywhere in the country. Knowing where you can turn for STD diagnosis and treatment is vital in preventing transmission and avoiding complications.

In addition, you can get a number of relatively inexpensive, easy-to-read, and understandable books in the health sections of popular book stores. You can always pick up free literature about specific diseases in public health departments, Planned Parenthood agencies, health clinics, physicians' offices, and student health centers. The importance of learning about sexually transmissible diseases cannot be underemphasized. Every effort is being

The VD National Hotline

There appear to be four main reasons why young people remain at highest risk from venereal disease (now called sexually transmissible diseases, or STDs):

1. They don't realize how serious these diseases can be.
2. They don't know where to go for medical help.
3. They are afraid their parents will find out if they *do* go for help.
4. They don't know enough about the signs and symptoms that indicate they *should* seek help. (To make matters worse, most girls and women do not have symptoms, and an increasing number of males are also asymptomatic.)

For these reasons the VD National Hotline, sponsored by the Center for Disease Control and a core program service of the American Social Health Association, was established in October 1979.

Trained volunteers are available from 8 A.M. to 8 P.M. (Pacific time) Monday through Friday to provide free, confidential information and referral service to callers from the 48 continental states.

Anyone wishing to ask a question about VD (STD) or wanting to know where to go for diagnosis and treatment can call 800-227-8922; in California 800-982-5883. For information about AIDS only, call 800-342-AIDS (or 2437).

made to take the stigma out of open communication and make this kind of learning as "painless" as possible.

Diagnosis and Treatment Any sign such as unusual pain, sores, rashes, or discharge is a signal to get professional examination and testing. In addition, whether or not you have any symptoms, if your sexual partner has contracted an STD, you should get *immediate* testing. In some cases, partners are also treated, as a further preventive measure.

Testing can be done through private physicians, public health clinics, school health services, and other community health agencies across the country. Once a diagnosis is made, treatment should begin as quickly as possible. If you are infected, you should also inform your partner(s) as soon as possible in order to prevent further spread and/or delay in treatment, which could contribute to complications. If infected, you should also refrain from any further sexual activity until your treatment is completed and/or further testing indicates you are cured.

The available treatments are safe, effective, and generally inexpensive. As with any treatment, always remember to follow instructions carefully and to complete the prescribed course of medication. Do not stop taking your medication just because you feel better, or your symptoms have gone away. This doesn't mean you are cured, but simply that the initial doses of medication are working. It is *vital* to take all the medication prescribed as well as to return for follow-up testing to be sure the disease is completely gone.

Remember that being cured of an STD does not mean you can never get it again! Exposure to STDs does not provide lasting immunity, like some other diseases, nor does it prevent you from getting any other STD. All the more reason to be informed, to inform your partners, and to practice prevention.

Prevention All sexually transmissible diseases are preventable. The idea of preventing exposure to STDs, however, must first be included in the thoughts you have when you are about to engage in sexual relations. Thinking about STDs is something most people simply do not do, for many reasons. Some people believe that sex loses its spontaneity if they think of preventing disease. Others regard questions from a potential partner as a personal insult. But in fact, thinking—and talking—about STDs is an expression of caring for yourself, for your partner(s), and for all the people who make up your various communities, as well as for the children you may have. It is practical, courageous, and loving.

Everyone can reduce risk of infection by practicing safer sex, but it does require planning. Suggested methods

Exploring Your Emotions

A couple is about to engage in sexual intercourse. One of the partners asks the other, "Do you have a sexually transmissible disease?" How would you feel if someone asked you that in similar circumstances? Is it realistic to expect that such a question would be asked? Would you ask it?

Telling Your Partner Isn't Easy . . .

Telling your sexual partner(s) about exposing him or her to a sexually transmissible disease isn't easy. You have probably not been given any clear guidelines on how to do this, either in school or at home. Discussions about sexuality rarely stress open communication about sexually transmissible diseases. Somehow it is believed that you intuitively understand how to do this. Instead, you get stuck, and probably end up making bad decisions.

What are some of the reasons you might have difficulty telling your partners about possible exposure? How can you "tell" without risk of losing a spouse, a friend, or a lover?

First, you must understand that your failure to carry out the important ethical task of informing your sexual partner may result in serious medical complications from a disease if it is allowed to go undetected and untreated. Furthermore, if you don't tell your partner, he or she can spread the disease to yet others.

Secondly, sexually transmissible diseases cannot be controlled without your cooperation in preventive efforts. Individuals changing their own behavior, along with public health epidemiologic strategies, have proven effective in reducing the STD incidence. The best example is the significant reduction in cases of syphilis from the peak years of the 1950s. Today, syphilis incidence has stabilized at 25,000 cases yearly, and the consequences of late syphilis in adults are now rare.

Catching a sexually transmissible disease is a disturbing experience. The characteristic emotional responses can block communication with sexual partners. Nearly everyone infected with a sexually transmissible disease feels fear, embarrassment, shame, and anger. If you allow these feelings to dominate your behavior, you may make unwise decisions about informing your partners. You may lie about how you caught the infection—"I caught it from a toilet seat." You may tell your partner half-truths—"I have an infection, and no one seems to know how I got it, but you have to be treated also." Or worse, you may not tell anyone anything, using rationalizations as an excuse for avoiding the responsibility—"Serves them right for giving it to me in the first place, or they'll find out anyhow and get their own treatment in due time."

Honesty is still "the best policy." Being open, direct, and honest with your sexual partner(s) requires some risk taking, yet may result in the greatest benefit. People with sexually transmissible diseases fear rejection, loss, and retaliation. Certainly, you can expect emotional responses, but few actually lose their friendships or their marriage in the process. In fact, your relationships may take on new meanings as a result. The problems that may have led you to seek other sexual partners may be forced into the open to be dealt with. Many such episodes lead to positive resolution and a renewed commitment to the relationship.

Perhaps most importantly, when you act quickly, openly, and honestly you gain a great measure of self-respect. You feel more in control of preventing serious consequences and further transmission of the disease. Acting responsibly to inform your sexual partner(s), though not easy, will likely help prevent future infection.

for primary prevention include abstinence, monogamy, and condom use for those who are sexually active with multiple partners. Methods that are not effective are urination or douching following sexual intercourse, genital play without full penetration, ejaculation and oral sex, and depending on luck.

Condoms are very effective, especially when lubricated with a spermicide called non-oxynol-9, a common ingredient in spermicidal jellies and foams, in blocking the transmission of gonorrhea, syphilis, herpes, and the AIDS virus. Unless the condom breaks, or is improperly used, it is an effective barrier.

Other prevention activities are aimed at avoiding the development of complications from infections. In STD control, cure also means prevention. Proper treatment of infected people prevents transmission to others. Counseling people with infections also helps motivate them to assist in control efforts. To help control epidemics and the spread of infection, people must first have basic knowledge of STDs, their causes, symptoms, and treatment. If you recognize that whenever you are sexually active with another person you are at risk each time you have contact, you may be more willing to do something about it (see Figure 19-2). Men must take the lead in

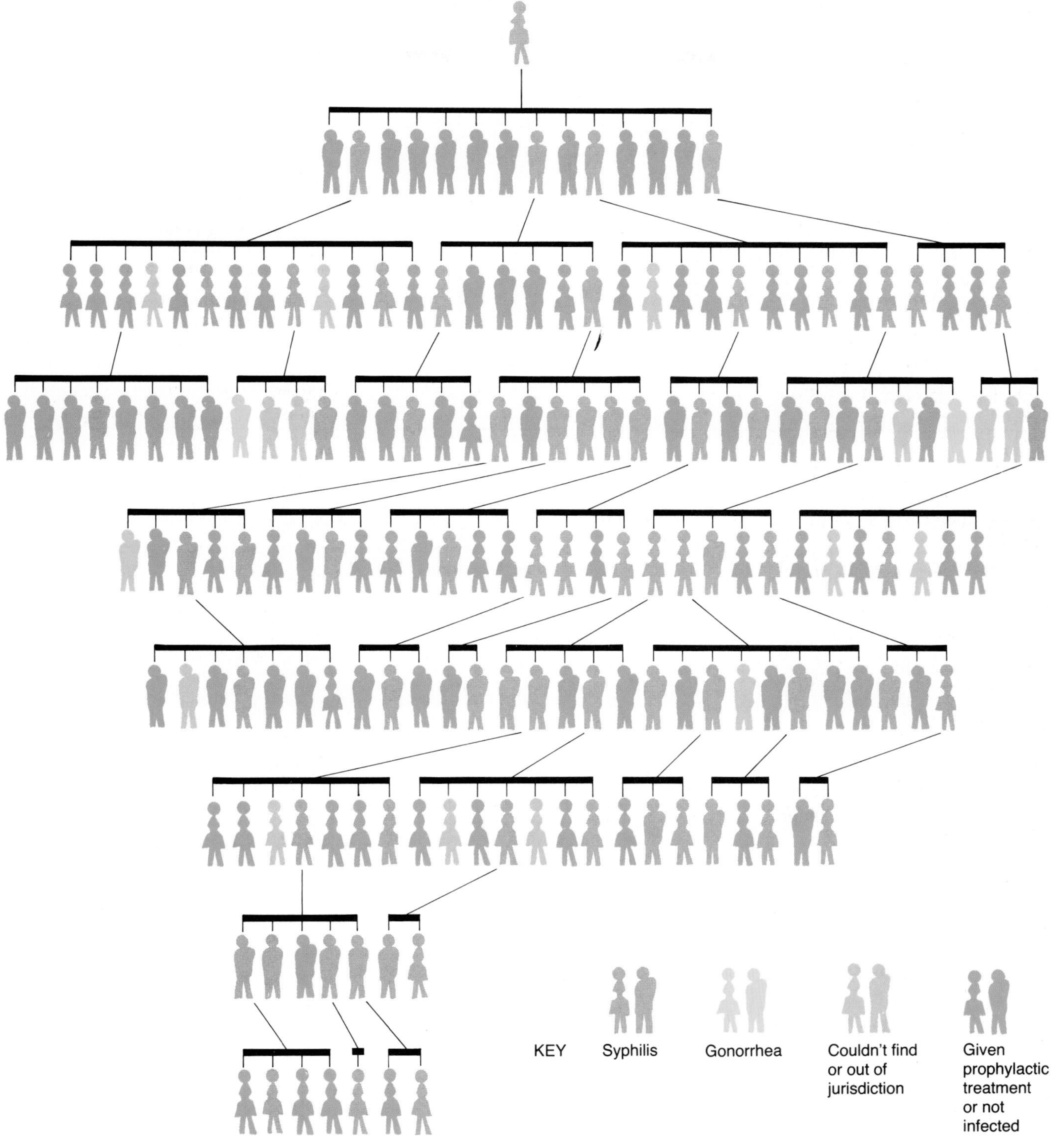

Courtesy of American Social Health Association.

Figure 19-2 This diagram shows how a sexually transmissible disease spread from a 17-year-old girl who had secondary syphilis. Investigators found and examined all but 15 of 141 people. Of the 126 examined, 34 were found to have syphilis or gonorrhea. The average age of those infected was 18.4 years; the youngest was only 6 years old.

secondary prevention, because they are generally the first to know and the first to get treated. The person, female or male, who is penetrated sexually will likely have no symptoms and therefore run the risk of rapid and severe complications. They may also unknowingly transmit their infection to others. This is particularly true for women.

People form relationships for many reasons: to have good times, avoid loneliness, develop intimacies, have sex, have families. And the decision to have a sexual relationship carries with it many uncertainties and risks—one of them being possible disease. You need mutual respect and open communication in making good decisions. Caring about yourself and your partner means asking questions and being aware of signs and symptoms. It may be a bit awkward, but the temporary embarrassment of asking intimate questions is a small price to pay to avoid contracting or spreading disease. If your partner thinks less of you for being concerned about and openly discussing such matters, perhaps that person is not really someone with whom you want a close relationship. Concern for STD is not an intrusion on a sexual relationship, but part of it, just as sex of any kind is not separate from life, but part of it.

Take Action

Your answers to the Exploring Your Emotions questions in this chapter and your placement level on the Wellness Ladder will, we hope, encourage you to begin a process of self-exploration and self-discovery that you will continue. Reflect on the entire chapter's content and ask yourself how each point relates to your own life. Then take action:

1. In your Take Action notebook, list the positive behaviors that help you avoid exposure to sexually transmissible diseases. Consider what additions you can make to this list or how you can strengthen your existing behavior. Reward yourself for these positive aspects of your life. Also list the behaviors that block your maintaining wellness. Consider each of these behaviors. Which ones can you most easily change? Start doing so.
2. Go to the drugstore and peruse the contraceptive section. Read the labels on various packages. What if anything do they tell you about STDs? Ask the pharmacist what he or she would recommend to prevent STDs.
3. Call the National VD Hotline. Ask the trained volunteer a question about something you would like to know or confirm about STDs.
4. Before leaving this chapter, review the Rate Yourself statements at the beginning of this chapter. Have your feelings or values changed? Are you now better equipped to handle the complex and very human problems associated with sexually transmissible diseases?

Selected References

Cates, W., Jr., and King K. Holmes. 1986. Sexually transmitted diseases. In King K. Holmes, Per Anders Mardh, P. Fredrick Sparling, and Paul J. Wiesner, eds., *Public Health and Preventive Medicine,* 12th ed. Atlanta, Ga.: U.S. Public Health Service, Department of Health and Human Services.

Chlamydia Trachomatis Infections, Policy Guidelines for Prevention and Control. 1985 (May). Atlanta, Ga.: Center for Prevention Services, Centers for Disease Control.

Corey, Lawrence. 1984. Genital herpes. In King K. Holmes, Per Anders Mardh, P. Fredrick Sparling, and Paul J. Wiesner, eds., *Sexually Transmitted Diseases.* New York: McGraw-Hill.

Holmes, King K., Per Anders Mardh, P. Fredrick Sparling, and Paul J. Wiesner, eds. 1984. *Sexually Transmitted Diseases.* New York: McGraw-Hill.

Knox, John M. 1984. Acquired infectious syphilis. In King K. Holmes, Per Anders Mardh, P. Fredrick Sparling, and Paul J. Wiesner, eds., *Sexually Transmitted Diseases.* New York: McGraw-Hill.

McGee, Zell A. 1984. Pelvic inflammatory disease. In King K. Holmes, Per Anders Mardh, P. Fredrick Sparling, and Paul J. Wiesner, eds., *Sexually Transmitted Diseases.* New York: McGraw-Hill.

Oriel, J. D. 1984. Genital warts. In King K. Holmes, Per Anders Mardh, P. Fredrick Sparling, and Paul J. Wiesner, eds., *Sexually Transmitted Diseases.* New York: McGraw-Hill.

Rapp, Fred. 1984. Herpes Simplex virus. In King K. Holmes, Per Anders Mardh, P. Fredrick Sparling, and Paul J. Wiesner, eds., *Sexually Transmitted Diseases.* New York: McGraw-Hill.

Sparling, P. Fredrick. 1984. Natural history of syphilis. In King K. Holmes, Per Anders Mardh, P. Fredrick Sparling, and Paul J. Wiesner, eds., *Sexually Transmitted Diseases.* New York: McGraw-Hill.

U.S. Surgeon General's Report on Acquired Immune Deficiency Syndrome. 1986. Washington, D.C.: U.S. Government Printing Office.

Recommended Readings

Hamilton, Richard. 1980. *The Herpes Book.* New York: St. Martin's Press.

This general volume is tailored to laypeople who want to learn more about what can be done to deal with the symptoms and how to communicate with potential or ongoing sexual partners.

Irvington Publishers. *Contraceptive Technology* 1986–1987. New York: Irvington.

An informational handbook that provides a scientific overview of reproductive health, including the integration of STDs.

Leishman, Katie. 1987 (February). Heterosexuals and AIDS. *Atlantic Monthly* 259(2): 39–58.

This article addresses concerns about AIDS in the heterosexual population.

Sacks, Stephen L., M.D. 1985 (Summer). Oral acyclovir—make up your own mind. *The Helper.* Palo Alto, Calif.: American Social Health Association.

This newsletter provides current medical and general information for those interested and concerned about herpes and its treatment.

Chapter 20

Contents

Rate Yourself

Your Infection Risk Behavior Read the following statements carefully. Choose the one in each section that best describes you at this moment and circle its number. When you have chosen one statement for each section, add the numbers and record your total score. Find your position on the Wellness Ladder.

5 Is well educated about causes of infection
4 Is informed about causes of infection
3 Knows that colds are caused by viruses
2 Is confused about causes of infection
1 Is totally ignorant about causes of infection

5 Washes hands vigorously before handling food
4 Washes hands before meals
3 Usually washes hands before meals
2 Occasionally washes hands before meals
1 Rarely washes hands before meals

5 Brushes teeth after eating
4 Brushes teeth at least once a day
3 Usually brushes teeth every day
2 Brushes teeth irregularly
1 Rarely brushes teeth

5 Recognizes spoiled food
4 Refrigerates perishable foods
3 Throws out moldy food
2 Eats food that has not been washed
1 Will eat moldy food

5 Keeps personal immunization history
4 Has been immunized against major diseases
3 Has been immunized against some diseases
2 Doesn't know own immunization history
1 Has never or rarely been immunized against disease

Total Score ______

Infection and Immunity

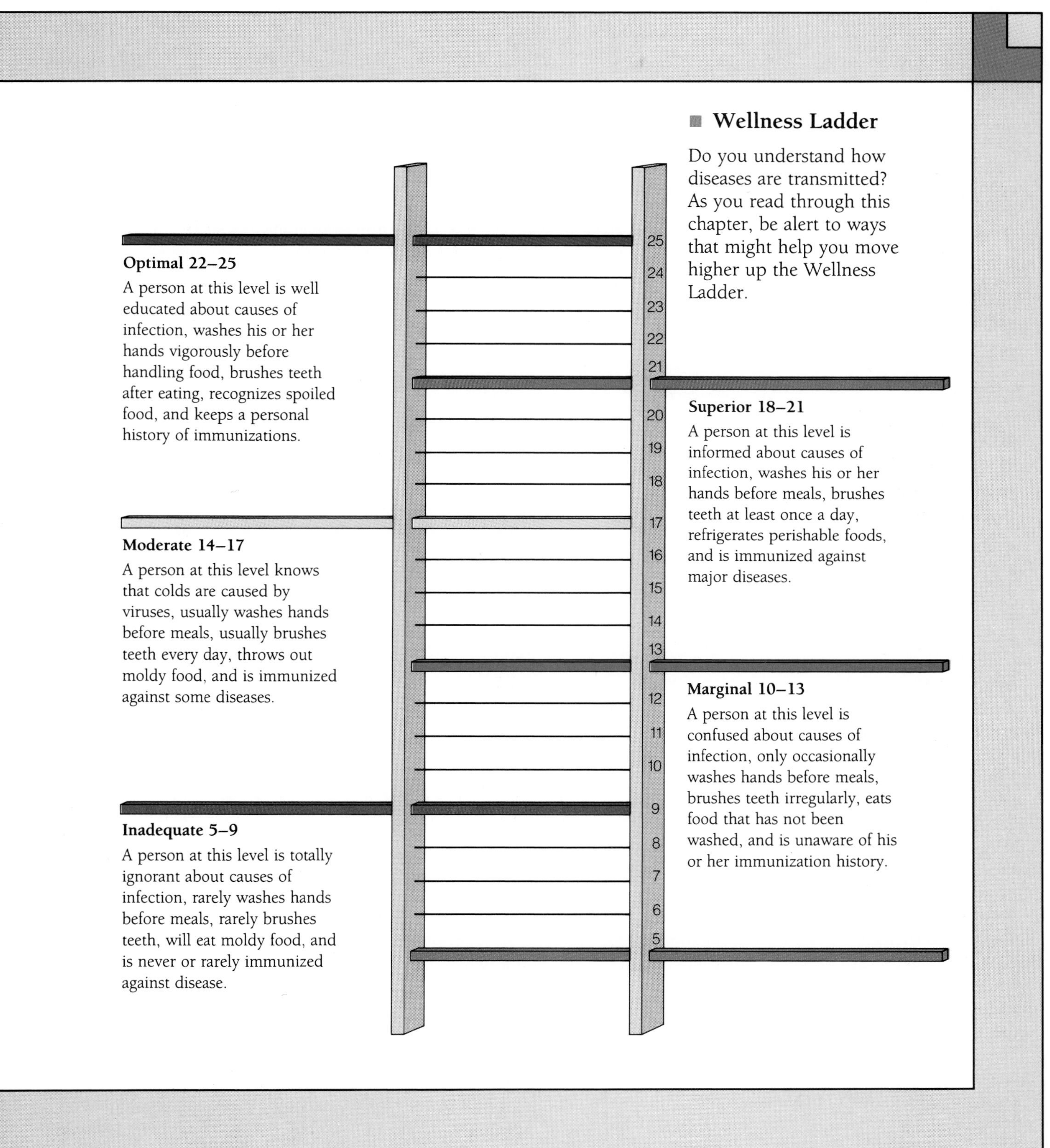

Wellness Ladder

Do you understand how diseases are transmitted? As you read through this chapter, be alert to ways that might help you move higher up the Wellness Ladder.

Optimal 22–25
A person at this level is well educated about causes of infection, washes his or her hands vigorously before handling food, brushes teeth after eating, recognizes spoiled food, and keeps a personal history of immunizations.

Superior 18–21
A person at this level is informed about causes of infection, washes his or her hands before meals, brushes teeth at least once a day, refrigerates perishable foods, and is immunized against major diseases.

Moderate 14–17
A person at this level knows that colds are caused by viruses, usually washes hands before meals, usually brushes teeth every day, throws out moldy food, and is immunized against some diseases.

Marginal 10–13
A person at this level is confused about causes of infection, only occasionally washes hands before meals, brushes teeth irregularly, eats food that has not been washed, and is unaware of his or her immunization history.

Inadequate 5–9
A person at this level is totally ignorant about causes of infection, rarely washes hands before meals, rarely brushes teeth, will eat moldy food, and is never or rarely immunized against disease.

Parasites Organisms that can invade and survive in the living tissue of other organisms.

Pathogens Organisms that cause disease.

Infection Disease caused by a pathogen.

Viruses The smallest pathogens; cannot grow or reproduce by themselves.

Enzymes Chemicals necessary for energy production and protein synthesis in normal animal cells.

Contagious disease Disease that can be transmitted from one carrier to another.

Herpes simplex virus The virus that produces sores around the mouth (Type 1); painful and sometimes damaging genital disease (Type 2); chickenpox and shingles; and mononucleosis.

We are surrounded and inhabited by a multitude of potential enemies, most of them much too small to be seen. We speak of these organisms, which can take up residence and survive in the living tissue of humans or animals, as **parasites.** When parasites cause a disease, they are known as **pathogens.** Disease caused by a pathogen is called **infection.** Who and what are these infective agents? How do you defend yourself from continuous infection? Under what conditions can pathogens breach your defenses and give rise to an infection? And how can you overcome infections once they have started?

Pathogens

In order of size, from smallest to largest, pathogens can be classified as follows:

- *Viruses:* subcellular, semiliving particles
- *Bacteria:* simple unicellular organisms
- *Fungi:* unicellular and multicellular plantlike organisms
- *Protozoa:* unicellular animals
- *Parasitic worms:* multicellular animals

Viruses **Viruses,** the smallest of the pathogens, are on the borderline between living and nonliving matter. They are visible only with an electron microscope. The pure virus particle appears to have no metabolism of its own. Viruses lack all the **enzymes** essential to energy production and protein synthesis in normal animal cells, and they cannot grow or reproduce by themselves. They must lead a parasitic existence inside a cell, borrowing what they need for growth and reproduction from the cells they invade. Once a virus is inside the host cell, it sheds its protein covering and its genetic material takes control of the cell and tricks it into manufacturing more viruses like itself. (See Figure 20-1.) The normal functioning of the host cell is thereby disrupted. Different viruses infect different kinds of cells, and the seriousness of the disease they cause depends greatly on which kind of cell is infected. The viruses that cause colds, for example, attack upper respiratory tract cells, which are constantly cast off and replaced. The disease is therefore mild. Polio virus, in contrast, attacks nerve cells that cannot be replaced, and the consequences, such as paralysis, are severe.

Exploring Your Emotions

As you arrive in class one morning, you learn that a friend has meningitis. Two days later he is dead. You are brutually reminded of our frail hold on life and of the sea of microorganisms surrounding us. Do you feel your life will be materially altered if you know about the processes of infection and immunity?

Over 150 viruses are known to cause disease in humans. Illnesses caused by viruses are the most common forms of **contagious disease.** They include most of the minor ailments that cause transitory illness and are rarely precisely diagnosed. Among these are the common cold, a variety of undiagnosed and short-lived respiratory infections, influenza, gastrointestinal upsets that cause diarrhea and can last for only twenty-four hours, and assorted aches and pains. More serious are the diseases that occur mainly in childhood and frequently cause a severe rash, such as measles, chicken pox, and mumps. Smallpox, which used to be the most severe of these diseases, has now been eliminated, thanks to a worldwide vaccination program carried out by the World Health Organization (WHO) in the 1960s and 1970s.

The herpes viruses are a large and important group of viruses. They are remarkable in that, once infected, the host is never again free of the virus. The virus lies latent within certain cells, and ventures forth from time to time to produce symptoms. Normally the immune system keeps these viruses in check. However, when the immune system is depressed—for instance, by drugs used to aid organ transplantation—the herpes viruses may cause life-threatening disease. The most familiar example of these infections is that caused by **herpes simplex virus** Type 1. This virus produces sores that last from a few days to a week or two and appear mainly on the face around the mouth. (Herpes of the eye can be extremely serious and can lead to loss of vision.) A second kind of herpes virus (Type 2), gives rise to a painful and recurring genital disease of similar duration. Another herpes virus causes both chicken pox and "shingles."

Infectious mononucleosis (or mono), is also caused by a herpes virus. This disease is spread by close contact,

(Text continues on p. 468.)

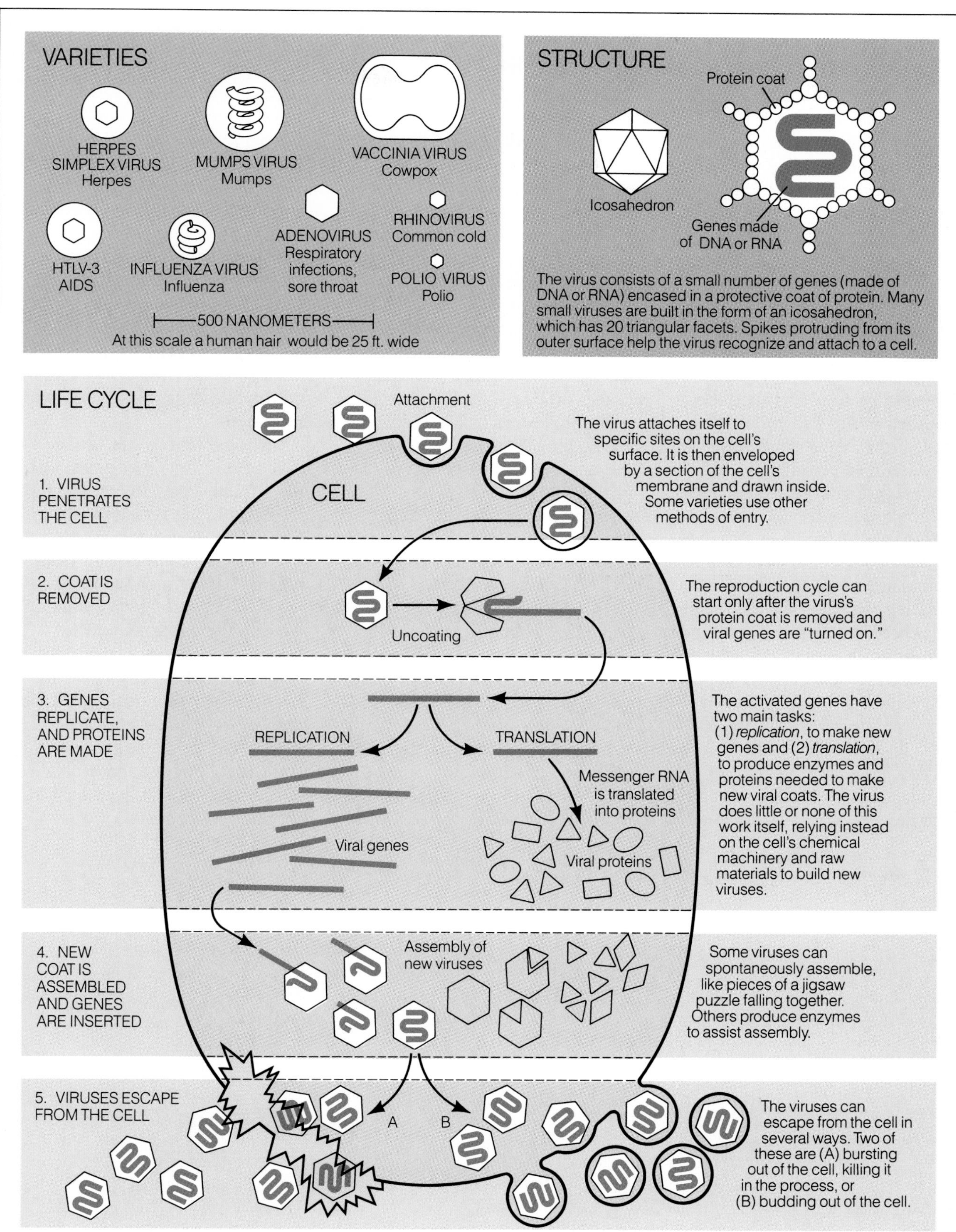

Figure 20-1 Viruses: (a) structure, (b) varieties, and (c) life cycle.

Epstein-Barr Virus and Mononucleosis

Epstein-Barr virus (EBV), a member of the herpes virus family, is possibly the most common human virus, affecting more than 95% of the world's population. Most primary infections occur during childhood; the virus is readily transmitted in saliva. In young children the infection may go undetected, but the severity of symptoms increases with age. Three to seven weeks after being exposed to the virus, adolescents and young adults can be expected to suffer fever, swollen lymph nodes, and an inflamed and painful throat for a period of two to four weeks. A blood smear taken at this time commonly shows an abundance of large mononuclear lymphocytes, thus the term infectious mononucleosis (IM) has been applied to this infection. IM can be mistaken for leukemia (lymphocyte cancer), but simple blood tests can identify antibodies to EBV, and so the diagnosis is usually accurate.

Infectious mononucleosis was first described in 1920, although it has undoubtedly existed as a human pathogen for hundreds, if not thousands, of years. The virus itself was not indentified until the 1960s, when the electron microscope and other tools of modern medicine made it possible to actually visualize the virus in infected lymphocytes. Reliable laboratory diagnosis has been possible since 1932 by using a test for antibodies produced during the EBV infection, known as *heterophile* antibodies. These antibodies are present only during the acute stage of the EBV infection. Oddly enough, they are not directed against the virus itself, but instead are directed against components of the red cells of both sheep and horses. Why these antibodies should be produced is a bit of a mystery. The probable explanation is that the EBV virus infects and stimulates division in millions of B lymphocytes, whose task normally is to produce antibodies against a great variety of antigens. Some of these lymphocytes apparently were previously directed against the sheep and horse red cell antigens. The immune system also produces antibodies directed against the virus, and these eventually control the infection. Once produced, these antiviral antibodies survive for years, while the heterophile antibodies are present only during the acute, active infection. Since the doctor is primarily interested in diagnosing current infection, the heterophile antibodies are usually measured.

The symptoms of IM usually disappear in time, but occasionally the infection may become more severe and long lasting. As the EBV-infected lymphocytes multiply, they can infiltrate important organs, leading to inflammation of the liver or to development of a large and fragile spleen. (The spleen is a soft, tennis ball-sized organ situated directly under the liver.) If the spleen ruptures, a life-threatening medical emergency results, requiring immediate surgery. Therefore rest and avoidance of sports are generally prescribed for acute IM patients.

Fatigue is a common complaint in IM, and it is a highly variable but troublesome symptom. A few patients don't regain their full energy until weeks or months after all other symptoms disappear. Cases of this kind have led to the concept that there exists a separate "chronic mononucleosis syndrome," characterized by long-lasting low-grade fever, muscle pains, depression, headache, recurrent sore throat, and, especially, persistent fatigue. Some sufferers have likened this condition to an endless bout of the flu, accompanied by mental confusion. This syndrome remains mysterious. At Lake Tahoe, Nevada, in 1984 to 1986, an epidemic of this syndrome was reported. It affected hundreds of people and was carefully investigated by the U.S. Centers for Disease Control. No definite conclusions have yet emerged from that study. In most cases a fatigue syndrome cannot be assigned with certainty to the Epstein-Barr virus, because there are many other potential causes of these symptoms, and the EB virus is present in almost everyone by the age of 25. The true cause of "chronic IM syndrome" may be a particularly unpleasant strain of EBV or a closely related but as yet undiscovered virus.

As with other herpes viruses, a primary EBV infection always leads to establishment of a latent infection, in which both lymphocytes and the cells that line the throat are permanently infected. These cells remain as a potential source of infectious virus for the remainder of the individual's life. Even after the immune response to the virus is well advanced and symptoms have vanished, perhaps 1 in 5 infected individuals continues to shed virus into the saliva. Because of this phenomenon of latency, any condition that interferes with an effective immune response, such as advanced cancer, organ transplantation, or AIDS, may reactivate an EBV infection. The EBV-infected lymphocytes, freed of the normal immune restraints, may then progress to become true cancers (lymphomas or leukemias), as happens in significant numbers of late-stage AIDS patients.

The association of EBV and tumors is not well understood, but it has become clear that EBV, together with environmental factors, is responsible for Burkitt's lymphoma, a cancer common to parts of Africa. Burkitt's lymphoma, a tumor of rapidly dividing lymphocytes, is primarily a disease of African children. It occurs only in those parts of Africa where malaria is common. It seems likely that the malarial parasite, which itself places an enormous burden on the immune system, may act together with the virus to produce the Burkitt's tumors. Exactly how this happens is not clear, but understanding the details of tumor development is of great scientific and medical interest. The EBV-Burkitt's connection is one of the clearest instances of the intimate relationship of viruses and human tumors.

AIDS (*A*cquired *I*mmune *D*eficiency *S*yndrome)

In 1980 no one had heard of AIDS, although a few cases of a puzzling immune deficiency disease had been described in the United States. By late February 1987, we had 31,000 cases of AIDS. The World Health Organization reports 50,000 AIDS cases worldwide but there may actually be more than 100,000.

The virus responsible for AIDS is the human immunodeficiency virus—HIV, for short. It originated in Africa, probably from a related monkey virus. It is passed from one person to another only by direct contact with bodily fluids, chiefly blood or semen. The modern increase in population and international travel have helped spread this virus throughout Africa and to the rest of the world.

The 31,000 cases of AIDS in the United States are only the tip of the iceberg—perhaps 50 people are infected for every one who is actually ill. We also have at least 150,000 cases of AIDS-related complex (ARC), an early stage of AIDS, and about 1.5 million Americans who are infected but have no symptoms. Within five years probably 20–30 percent of these will develop the disease—about 300,000 cases. Without much better therapies, most of these people can be expected to die within one to three years after developing symptoms. The costs of caring for this number of very sick people is staggering; estimates vary from $8 to $15 billion. And we have only about 400,000 hospital beds in the entire country!

How can you avoid AIDS? On this question, the evidence is very clear and education on this subject has been abundant. For those who aren't IV drug abusers, advice is very straightforward: short of abstinence from sex, one should practice safer sex; that is, using a condom for any sexual activity. While using condoms may seem inconvenient or unesthetic to some, it is the only practice that at this time is 100 percent safe.

What are the odds of remaining disease-free if you are infected with the AIDS virus? The data on this point are mixed and seem to depend in part on the lifestyle of the infected individual. A long-term study of a group of gay men in San Francisco showed that after six years of medical observation 80 percent had either AIDS, or the early symptoms of AIDS (AIDS-related complex, or ARC). About 30 percent had full-blown AIDS, 21 percent had severe ARC, and 27 percent had generalized swollen glands caused by the infection. Gay men may be particularly likely to develop symptoms, because of their high incidence of infection by non-AIDS agents, such as gonorrhea, chlamydia, and a variety of sexually transmitted viruses such as herpes and hepatitis. There is increasing evidence that a second virus infection may activate a dormant HIV infection, and thus push a person toward more rapid development of AIDS symptoms. In contrast, HIV-infected hemophiliacs who are relatively free of other infections remain AIDS-free much longer, and tend to have less severe disease at a given time after infection.

What cells are attacked by the AIDS agent? Formerly the HIV virus was thought to infect only the immune lymphocytes known as helper T-cells. However, more recent evidence indicates that cells other than lymphocytes have receptors for the virus, and may harbor HIV infection. These include cells of the brain, lungs, bowel, and even heart. These new findings help to explain unusual presentations of the AIDS infection, such as dementia and myocarditis (an inflammation of the heart). These findings complicate treatment and make much more difficult the already challenging task of developing drugs and vaccines to counter AIDS.

What therapies are available now? Current therapies are directed at slowing or stopping replication of the AIDS virus in infected lymphocytes. With most viral diseases, this would be a successful strategy, as the immune system would soon eliminate both remaining virus and infected cells from the body. The AIDS virus, however, enters into a latent or nondividing state in infected cells. These cells do not express virus-coded proteins, and so the normal immune mechanisms of antibody or cell-mediated killing have no effect. When the virus-infected lymphocyte does emerge from the latent state, perhaps because of an unrelated immune response to another infectious agent, more HIV virus is produced, with lethal damage to the cell. Additional cells are infected, and the cycle is repeated. After many such cycles, the immune system suffers damage it does not recover from, and the patient dies, often from infection by normally benign microbes.

Agents that interfere with virus replication, like interferon or azidothymidine (AZT), slow the development of the disease and thus preserve the immune system for a few more months. These drugs can't, however, eradicate the virus. Other experimental therapies include use of colony-stimulating factors, which are newly discovered and potent growth hormones that have been made available for therapeutic uses through modern genetic engineering techniques. These natural growth factors help the immune system repopulate the missing lymphocytes, by encouraging the growth of parental bone marrow cells. Combinations of these therapeutic agents may extend survival considerably for the AIDS patient, but they are expensive. For instance, a year's supply of AZT for a single patient presently costs the patient or his or her insurer about $10,000; with 300,000 patients using this drug, the bill would be $3 billion per year!

A vaccine may be the permanent solution to spread of AIDS, although it may not help those already infected. A great deal of ingenuity is presently being expended on designing a vaccine that will lead to immediate neutralization of AIDS virus, whenever it emerges from the infected cell. A vaccine of this kind should protect a normal individual from initial infection. For those already infected, a vaccine that will lead to killing of the infected cells may be necessary. However, it is not clear that we know enough about either the virus or the immune response to produce such a vaccine. Current favorites in the intense effort to devise a protective vaccine include vaccines based on modified vaccinia virus, and vaccines based on synthetic peptides.

Vaccinia virus has been used for years to immunize against smallpox, and is safe and well understood. Modified vaccinia viruses have been created, genetically engineered to include the genes for the surface proteins of the AIDS virus, but omitting other AIDS genes. Volunteers innoculated with this vaccine respond by making antibodies to both the AIDS virus and to vaccinia proteins. This vaccine appears to be quite safe, but it may not be able to prevent infection by latently infected donor cells, such as the lymphocytes in semen that may be passed during "unsafe sex." These cells are the usual pathways of the AIDS infection, and (as already described) they are very difficult for the immune system to eliminate. It is too early to say how successful the vaccinia vaccine approach may be.

An alternative approach, still highly speculative, is to use a carefully selected set of chemically synthesized peptides (small proteins), corresponding to a limited set of specific regions of AIDS virus proteins. These peptides would include only those regions of the virus that are known to be targets for neutralization by antibodies. Since the immune response in a natural AIDS infection is made up of antibodies that are for the most part not neutralizing, a directed response to selected peptides may result in more effective immunity.

These approaches are at the cutting edge of what is medically and scientifically possible. Neither was available ten years ago. Indeed, fifteen years ago the AIDS infection would have been a deep scientific mystery, almost unapproachable due to limitations of the then existing techniques and to our rudimentary knowledge of the immune system. We have reason to hope that the increasing scientific momentum directed at AIDS prevention and therapy will, during the next five years, lead to some solution of this otherwise tragic situation. Until then the best protection for individuals and society is a thorough understanding, and respect for, the mechanisms by which this deadly virus spreads.

Spleen Lymph organ that may rupture in infectious mononucleosis, permanently impairing resistance to infection.

AIDS, acquired immune deficiency syndrome A recently discovered, fatal, incurable, immune deficiency disease now reaching epidemic proportions in the United States and the world.

Poliomyelitis A disease of the nervous system, sometimes crippling; vaccinations now prevent most polio.

Hepatitis A severe liver inflammation: Type A, a less serious disease, can be transmitted through fecal matter; Type B through infected intravenous needles.

Bacteria Organisms about 100–1,000 times larger than viruses; about 100 species of which can cause disease in humans.

Toxins Poisons.

Staphylococci A group of bacteria, found on the skin, that can cause infection if allowed to multiply in food and then ingested.

Streptococci Bacteria that cause infections such as strep throat, which can lead to serious cardiac damage.

Impetigo A serious bacterial infection of the skin.

---

and usually affects children and young adults. The virus attacks white blood cells, and its symptoms may even look like leukemia. About three weeks after contact, the infected person has a severe sore throat with painful neck swelling, lethargy, and fever. Antibiotics have no effect on the disease process. With adequate rest, there are no long-term consequences; however, if the disease is neglected, the **spleen** may rupture. Loss of the spleen leads to a lifelong increase in susceptibility to infection.

More severe infections caused by viruses are **AIDS; poliomyelitis** (or polio), a disease of the nervous system; and **hepatitis,** a liver inflammation. There are two major kinds of hepatitis. One is mainly transmitted by blood transfusions or hypodermic injection and is common among drug addicts (Hepatitis B), and the other is transmitted through fecal matter and spread through infected food or drink (Hepatitis A). Hepatitis A causes a less severe disease, and is particularly prevalent in areas with poor hygienic conditions. It can also be spread readily wherever water is contaminated with sewage; for instance, in swimming areas close to sewage outlets. The disease is usually mild, although it is generally weakening and requires a long period of bed rest. Hepatitis B infection is generally more serious, and may lead to extensive liver damage, a chronic carrier state, and even liver cancer.

Certain viruses can also cause cell proliferation. The human disease clearly based on this property is warts, which generally is very mild but can become extremely severe if the resistance of the infected individual breaks down. There are many members of the human wart virus family, and some of them appear to be responsible for cancer of the uterine cervix in women. Another virus, called HTLV-I and distantly related to the AIDS virus, causes a rare leukemia in adults (T-cell leukemia). As our knowledge of the molecular biology of cancer increases, other tumors may turn out to be caused by viruses, but at present the majority of human cancers seem to be caused by other factors.

Figure 20-2 The three basic shapes of bacteria: (a) spirilla, (b) cocci, and (c) bacilli.

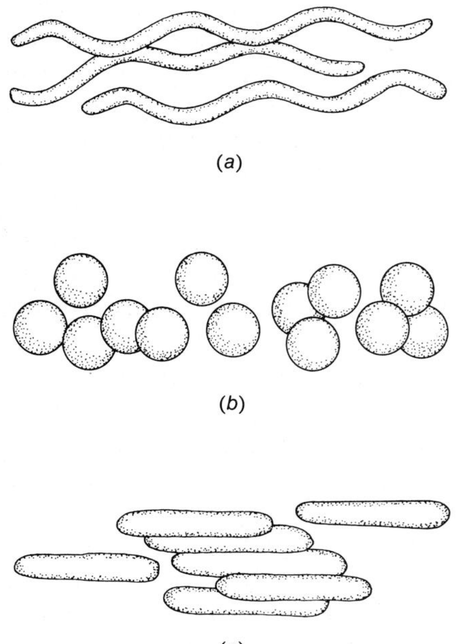

Bacteria **Bacteria,** which can be seen under a light microscope, are generally 100 to 1,000 times larger than viruses. But they are considerably smaller than mammalian cells, most of which can each hold 50 to 100 bacteria. Figure 20-2 shows the three basic shapes of bacteria.

Of several thousand species of bacteria, approximately 100 cause disease in humans. Most bacteria are neither parasites nor pathogens, however, and many are quite beneficial. Unlike viruses, many (but not all) disease-causing bacteria do not have to enter cells to cause infection. They generally thrive on, around, and between human cells and can cause harm through the **toxins** and poisonous enzymes that they produce. (Some bacterial toxins are among the most powerful poisons known. One-fourth of a teaspoon of a toxin released by the tetanus organism can kill over 10,000 people.)

Some of the toxins and poisonous enzymes bacteria produce work locally, killing and dissolving the cells near the site of the infection. The damaged cells become food for the bacteria. The infection then spreads deeper into the surrounding tissue, producing boils, abscesses, soreness, and the like. Other bacterial products are carried by the bloodstream, causing fever or affecting vital organs and systems (such as the nervous system in a tetanus

Acne A mild bacterial infection around hair follicles in the skin.

Sebum An oily secretion in the skin.

Strep throat Sore throat characterized by fever and pain; caused by streptococcus, can damage heart, and treatable with antibiotics.

Bronchitis Upper respiratory tract infection.

Pneumonia Lower respiratory tract infection; can lead to fluid in the lungs.

Tuberculosis Lung disease caused by an airborne bacterium.

Periodontal disease Bacterial infection of the gums.

Dental caries Tooth decay, caused by the byproducts of colonies of streptococci in the mouth.

Salmonella Infectious bacteria carried by fecal matter and transmitted through food; produces flulike symptoms.

Botulism Disease caused by botulinum organism, which grows in the absence of air, as in canned food. The toxin produces weakness, nausea, respiratory paralysis, and death.

---

infection). Some pathogenic bacteria have no specific toxic attributes. They grow to large numbers and cause damage by obstructing vital organs of the host—the lungs in pneumonia, for example—and by consuming materials needed by host cells for sustenance.

Generally speaking, bacterial infections require attention. Chief among these are skin infections such as small abscesses or boils, which, when unattended, can give rise to major complications. Such superficial skin infections are generally caused by bacteria known as **staphylococci** and **streptococci.** If the infection persists, it may cause a more serious disease known as **impetigo**, which requires a physician's attention. **Acne** is caused by relatively innocuous bacteria growing in hair follicles (pores that give rise to hair). These bacteria plug the pores and produce inflammatory substances that cause pus formation. Good hygiene often can remove **sebum** and other substances that such bacteria require.

Common respiratory diseases are **strep throat, bronchitis**, and **pneumonia.** These vary in severity. Because they generally respond rapidly to antibiotics, they should be treated early.

Tuberculosis, a disease of the lungs, is caused by a very resistant bacterium and was a major problem in the nineteenth and early twentieth centuries. Transmission from an infected individual to a new host almost always takes place by airborne bacteria. Sufferers once had to be isolated from the rest of the population during the infectious stage of the disease. The incidence of tuberculosis has significantly declined, in part because of better nutrition and living conditions, and in part through the use of antibiotics. Nonetheless, the disease is far from being eradicated in the United States (28,000 new cases in 1980), and it still presents a major problem in many countries of the world.

Women's urinary tracts are particularly accessible to bacteria, and urine presents a relatively good source of bacterial nutrient. Therefore, bladder infections occur fairly frequently in women. Although these infections are not necessarily severe, they can become so if they are not treated promptly. Such infections can also lead to an ascending infection of the kidneys, which can be extremely serious.

Periodontal disease, an infection of the gums, attacks over 50 percent of the population. It is caused by a variety of bacteria and if uncontrolled leads to abscesses and early loss of teeth. Probably the most common disease condition caused by bacterial infection is **dental caries,** a scourge known to almost everyone who has ever sat in a dentist's chair. It is caused by products of streptococci that are related to the organisms that cause strep throat.

Bacterial diseases of the stomach and intestines (gastrointestinal, or G.I., tract) are among the commonest infections, particularly among children, who have yet to develop immunity to the many bacterial pathogens that invade the G.I. tract. A common example of these is traveler's diarrhea, familiar to tourists in Latin America, which is usually caused by toxin-producing strains of such common bacteria as *Escherichia coli,* or *E. coli.* Although traveler's diarrhea is usually mild and self-limiting, such experiences can often be avoided by attention to personal hygiene (hand washing, drinking bottled drinks) and avoiding unwashed fruit and uncooked vegetables.

Food Poisoning Food poisoning is not always a consequence of direct infection. It can be caused by food that has been standing at temperatures that allow bacteria to grow. These bacteria produce toxins that can cause severe illness and high fever, and it is wise not to eat food that has been standing in a warm place for more than six hours. Among foods that can give rise to severe infection are insufficiently cooked poultry, unwashed eggs, and occasionally prepared meats, such as sausage. Infections arising from contaminated food are caused by organisms called **salmonella** and are therefore known as *salmonellosis.*

The most lethal bacterial poison carried by food is that of the botulinum organism. These organisms grow in the absence of air—for instance, in improperly canned food, which is a common cause of **botulism.** Home-canned foods are the chief offenders. The earliest symptoms of botulism—weakness, dizziness, and nausea—occur about twenty-four hours after eating contaminated food. If the person consumes enough toxin, these early symptoms may give way to respiratory paralysis, which can lead to death. Sterilizing foods by cooking before canning kills the organism. The toxin itself is broken down by boiling the canned food for ten minutes.

Rickettsiae Organisms that can reproduce only inside living cells; transmitted by insects, such as fleas.

Typhus fever Disease marked by high, disabling fever, transmitted by fleas and other parasites.

Trachoma Eye infection spread by poor hygiene, common in Asia and Africa.

Chlamydia trachomatis Organism that produces sexually transmissible disease, now reaching epidemic proportions in the United States. Especially damaging to infants (in childbirth) and to women.

Thrush A yeast infection of the mouth.

Plasmid A small segment of DNA carrying a few genes.

Fungi Molds, mushrooms, and yeasts—primitive plants.

Candidiasis A sexually transmissible disease caused by the fungus *Candida albicans;* producing vaginitis and infant thrush (mouth sores); an opportunistic infection often accompanying AIDS.

Athlete's foot Fungal skin infection of the feet.

Jock itch Fungal infection of scrotal skin.

Ringworm Fungal infection of the scalp.

Systemic Infecting large portions of the body.

Protozoa Microscopic single-celled animals, often producing recurrent, cyclical attacks of disease.

Malaria Severe, recurrent, protozoal disease. Insect-borne (mosquito).

African sleeping sickness Severe recurrent protozoal disease marked by lassitude. Insect-borne (tsetse fly).

Cryptococcosis Severe systemic fungal disease.

Coccidioidomycosis Valley fever; life-threatening systemic fungal disease.

Amoebic dysentery Protozoal infection of the intestines.

Trichomoniasis Protozoal vaginal infection; sexually transmissible.

Flukes Parasitic worms that can infest lungs and liver; can cause death.

Rickettsiae Some bacteria are like viruses in that they can reproduce only within living host cells. A group of these, called **rickettsiae,** are usually transmitted by insects such as fleas, lice, mites, and ticks. Diseases that are caused by rickettsiae include **typhus fever** and Rocky Mountain spotted fever. Another type of bacterium that needs the host cell causes an eye infection called **trachoma.** The trachoma organism is spread by poor hygienic conditions. It affects over 200 million people in Asia and Africa. In the United States, the chief infection due to the trachoma organism **(Chlamydia trachomatis)** is a sexually transmitted disease that may go unnoticed, but that can lead to sterility in women. This disease is difficult to diagnose. It has reached nationwide epidemic proportions, exceeding gonorrhea. (See Chapter 19.)

Fungi **Fungi** are primitive plants that may be multicellular (like molds) or unicellular (like yeasts). Mushrooms and the molds that form on bread and cheese are all examples of fungi. Only about fifty fungi of many thousands of species cause disease in humans, and these diseases usually are restricted to the skin, mucous membranes, and lungs. Curing fungal disease is extremely difficult. To defend themselves against treatments, some fungi form spores, which are an especially resistant dormant stage of the organism.

The most common fungal malady is **candidiasis,** a yeast infection of the vagina that can also occur in other areas of the body, especially in the mouth in infants (here it is known as **thrush**). Candidiasis, a relatively mild disease that causes itching, should be examined by a physician. When untreated and persistent, this disease can become severe and inflame the mucous membranes on which it normally exists. (See Chapter 19.)

Another common group of fungal diseases affect the skin, including **athlete's foot, jock itch,** and **ringworm,** a disease of the scalp. These three rather mild diseases, although difficult to treat, rarely give rise to major problems.

Fungi can also cause **systemic** (infecting large portions of the body) disease. Such disease is severe, life threatening, and extremely difficult to treat. Among the systemic forms of fungal disease are **cryptococcosis** and **coccidioidomycosis.** The latter disease is also known as "valley fever" because it is most frequently seen in the San Joaquin Valley in California.

Protozoa The **protozoa**, microscopic single-celled animals, are associated with such tropical diseases as **malaria, African sleeping sickness**, and **amoebic dysentery.** Many protozoa-based diseases are recurrent. The pathogen remains in the body, alternating between activity and inactivity. Hundreds of millions of Asians, Africans, and South Americans suffer from protozoal infections. The most common protozoal disease in the United States is **trichomoniasis**, a relatively mild vaginal infection. (See Chapter 19.)

Parasitic Worms The parasitic worms are the largest organisms that can enter the body to cause infection. The tapeworm, for example, can grow to a length of several feet. Worms, including such intestinal parasites as the tapeworm, hookworm, and pinworm, cause a great variety of relatively mild infections. Smaller worms, known as **flukes**, infect organs such as the liver and lungs and, in large numbers, can be deadly. Generally speaking, worm infections originate from contaminated food or drink and can be controlled by careful attention to hygiene.

Diagnosis of Pathogenic Diseases

Although most fungal and protozoal diseases are relatively easy to diagnose, it is frequently difficult to distinguish between viral and bacterial diseases. This is unfortunate, because most bacterial disease can be treated successfully

Antibiotic Overuse

Almost everyone has taken antibiotics at one time or another for strep throat, respiratory infections, or the like. However, evidence shows that these drugs are being misused and overused, and some serious medical problems may be in the making. The problems center around the possibility of creating antibiotic-resistant bacteria.

When bacteria are repeatedly exposed to small doses of antibiotics, they develop a resistance to the drug in order to survive when the drug is present. Not all the bacteria can do this, and many are readily killed by the drug. The bacteria that are not killed are the ones most resistant to the drug's effect, and they are the only ones left to reproduce. Soon, a whole colony of drug-resistant bacteria exists, able to cause illness.

To make matters worse, antibiotic-resistant bacteria that normally reside harmlessly in the digestive system can probably give up the drug-resistance portion of their genetic material, called a **plasmid,** to a more dangerous pathogenic strain of bacteria. That is, if a normal inhabitant of the gastrointestinal tract were to become resistant to antibiotics and then came in contact with, say, pneumonia bacteria, theoretically the plasmids that confer drug resistance could jump into the pneumonia bacterium. In this way, a strain of pneumonia might develop that would not respond to antibiotic therapy. It is a scientific fact that bacteria develop resistance to antibiotics upon repeated exposure; also a fact: they share resistance plasmids with other bacteria. The only missing link in the theory at present is the actual epidemic of drug-resistant diseases. Some people think that we are on the brink of disaster.

Misuse of the drugs may stem from a lack of understanding of what antibiotics can and can't do. For example, most virus-caused diseases, such as the common cold, do not respond to antibiotics. Repeatedly taking antibiotics for a cold is a waste of money and could set the stage for a much more serious problem.

Some people use illegally obtained antibiotics or leftover prescriptions to try to treat their own diseases without the aid of a physician. Not only do they take a shot in the dark at their own cure, but also they risk breeding and passing on bacterial superstrains to others because of improper doses and procedures that promote resistance. We now have among us antibiotic-resistant gonorrhea, as well as influenza bacteria, salmonella strains that cause digestive illnesses, and strep throat bacteria that no longer respond to the standard antibiotics.

Antibiotic misuse is responsible, though less directly, for other instances of these superinfections. Many people don't realize that agriculture routinely mixes antibiotics into daily animal feeds. It was discovered that not only do small daily doses of the drugs prevent infections when animals are crowded together, but that the drugs also promote extra growth in meat animals. There is strong evidence that animals may serve as breeding grounds for superinfection bacteria that can be served to the family at the dinner table, along with the hamburgers.

Not everyone agrees that the use of antibiotics in animal feed constitutes overuse. An example is the American Council on Science and Health (ACSH), an independent group that claims to evaluate consumer issues impartially and calmly. The ACSH points to the absence of epidemics caused by antibiotic-resistant bacteria as proof that such epidemics are not developing. We would be seeing pockets of such infection in the population already if such an epidemic were brewing, and until we do, the threat is only hypothetical. If antibiotics were prohibited from use in animal feed, more expensive farming methods would be necessary, fewer animals could be raised each year, and the consumer would foot the bill for the added expenses at the grocery checkout counter. The consumers must choose, the ACSH says, between paying higher meat prices and paying affordable prices but also taking a *hypothetical* risk of superbug infection.

At the opposite extreme stands the Center for Science in the Public Interest (CSPI), a consumer group that often takes an anti-industry view. They say that the consumers are bearing a great risk for the convenience of meat farmers. They point out that infections in animals can be prevented by good agriculture—that is, by less animal crowding and less stress for the animal population. Indeed, independent studies confirm that antibiotics make the biggest differences in the weight gains of animals that are under stress from overcrowding. The CSPI believes that these animals are suffering from infections caused by the

(continued on next page)

Antibiotic Overuse (*continued*)

stresses of their living conditions and that the antibiotics probably enhance growth because they wipe out the organisms of disease.

The CSPI concludes that the antibiotics should be discontinued and animals should be given healthy environments to live in. If higher meat prices are the result, then so be it.

Medical organizations, so far, tend to favor the latter argument, not out of concern for the quality of life of the animals, but because evidence of antibiotic-resistant infection is beginning to surface. Recently, there was an outbreak of disease caused by just such an infection of superstrain food bacteria. Eighteen people became ill, and one person died because the infection that was causing the illness could not be controlled. The drug-resistant strain of *Salmonella newport* was traced to a cattle herd in which animals were also falling ill with untreatable infections from the same bacteria. The antibiotics normally used to treat the salmonella infections were useless in these cases. Investigation revealed that the same drugs had been added to the animals' feed every day, and scientists concluded that the drug-resistant bacteria had developed in the animals' intestines and had been passed to people through normal grocery store meat products.

For the moment, science seems to be ahead of the game. New, stronger antibiotics, jokingly called "gorillacillins," have been developed that can deal with some resistant strains. Whether these, too, will lose their punch after years of overuse remains to be seen. For now, it's up to the FDA and the meat industry, as well as individual consumers, to acknowledge the danger and to curb overuse of antibiotics.

SOURCE: Frances S. Sizer, 1986 (January–February), *Antibiotic overuse, Healthline.*

with antibiotic drugs, while viruses are unaffected by antibiotics. If antibiotics are used indiscriminately for both conditions, the patient undergoes unnecessary risk (from side effects and drug allergies), and the development of drug-resistant bacteria is encouraged.

The most common viral diseases are relatively mild and of short duration. The symptoms they produce are usually caused by the reactions of the body's defense systems. Because this defense entails eliminating an invader that inhabits the body's own cells, some tissue destruction results, which contributes to such symptoms as fever, muscle aches, and lethargy. In addition, the mucus secretion and coughing that remove the invading organism, can be uncomfortable for the patient. The severity of the disease frequently depends on the extent of the body's own responses.

The more common bacterial infections, however, last longer and are usually accompanied by some marked symptoms. There are notable exceptions, however. The most important exception is **gonorrhea**, which (especially in women) may show no symptoms for long periods of time but which remains infectious and capable of causing severe problems, including sterility. (See Chapter 19.) The hallmark of bacterial infections, when they are localized, is the accumulation of pus, which is seldom present with viral infections.

The common fungal and protozoal infections, especially those prevalent in North America, are generally marked by their persistence and their mildness. However, any mild condition can become severe when neglected and allowed to spread, or when the defenses that keep it limited break down. Any persistent infection, even if only mildly disturbing to the individual, should be treated.

Infection

Infection breaches the defenses of your body in a variety of ways, depending on how strong your defenses are and how strong the organism is. Many circumstances affect how ill you will become.

Body Defenses Your body's primary lines of defense are the external barriers that prevent ready access to your more vulnerable interior.

In addition, your body has very sophisticated secondary defenses. Cells that can ingest and digest organisms are present in your mucous membrane surfaces and throughout your interior organs and bloodstream. Collectively, these cells are called "white cells," or **leukocytes.** As we explain later, these white cells have other functions that involve a learning process. They learn to recognize foreign materials and to produce **antibodies,** very specialized proteins that recognize the molecular elements of specific microbes, and neutralize them. This ability of immune system cells to remember previous infections is known as **adaptive** or **acquired immunity.** As

Gonorrhea A sexually transmissible bacterial disease that may show no symptoms for a long time, but that can cause sterility. Also called "the clap."

Leukocytes White blood cells that can eat and digest organisms.

Antibodies Specialized proteins, produced by white blood cells, that can recognize and neutralize specific microbes.

Adaptive or acquired immunity The body's ability to mobilize the cellular "memory" of an attack by a pathogen to throw off subsequent attacks. This ability can be acquired through vaccination.

Vaccination The injection of killed or weakened pathogens, arousing the body's natural adaptive immune system to produce specific antibodies.

Virulence The ability of a pathogen to cause serious or fatal disease.

Integrity Wholeness, intactness, or health.

Opportunistic organisms Organisms that take the opportunity presented by a primary (initial) infection to multiply and cause a secondary (additional) infection. For example, *Candida albicans* frequently infects people weakened by the AIDS virus.

Bubonic plague A virulent infectious disease carried by rodents and insects, marked by characteristic discolored swellings. One of the great plagues of the European Middle Ages.

Cholera A virulent infectious disease carried by food and water, marked by terrible fevers; periodically decimated city populations in all countries before this century.

Influenza The flu—a usually mild viral disease, highly infective and adaptable; the form changes so easily that every year new strains arise, making treatment difficult.

Endemic Disease that is localized in a regional population, producing either local epidemics or local immunity.

Epidemic Disease that breaks out of local stabilization and infects distant, less immune populations.

---

we shall see later, such immunity can be acquired either through natural infection by a particular disease agent, or through deliberate immunization with the pathogen or its components. When this immunization involves injection, it is called **vaccination.**

The defenses of your acquired immunity mechanisms are powerful and varied. Even in unimmunized people exposed to a particular disease agent for the first time, these mechanisms are rapidly mobilized as the infection advances. They constitute your body's ultimate means of eliminating invaders. Most of the time these defenses can protect the normal, healthy host from infection. So how do the potential invaders sometimes manage to break down your defenses? Their ability to do so depends on their **virulence**, the **integrity** of your defenses, and certain hereditary factors in your genetic makeup.

Scale of Infectivity Organisms can be ranked on a scale of infectivity. At the bottom of the scale are the so-called **opportunistic organisms,** those that need a great deal of circumstantial help in order to begin a disease process. These include a number of the organisms that normally survive in our gut and make up most of the fecal matter. In this group are a variety of organisms that rarely if ever cause infection by themselves but that can invade areas that are already infected by other organisms.

Midpoint on the infectivity scale are organisms that also normally inhabit your body but that become infective when they reach areas where they do not normally exist. Thus, for example, organisms that live on the surface of the skin can infect broken skin, particularly when dead tissue is present. Many agents that are not infective under normal circumstances become a threat when they are present in large numbers. It is mainly because of these agents that good hygiene is advisable. Many bacteria and some viruses and fungi fall in this category.

At the top of the scale are the very highly infective organisms. An organism's virulence—the severity of illness it can produce—does not go hand in hand with its level of infectivity, but does frequently parallel it. In this category are both the great plagues, **bubonic plague** and **cholera,** and minor ailments such as **influenza.** The agent causing such disease—and this is particularly true for bacteria—is frequently present in certain geographic areas where it persists in water sources and in animal reservoirs. Such bacteria give rise to local epidemics and are said to be **endemic** in that population or region. Their constant presence can cause immunity in the immediate population, and only their spread to more distant areas causes such organisms to become **epidemic** in nature.

How Body Defenses Break Down Whether or not an organism infects you depends both on its own infectivity and on how "together" your own defenses are. How do defenses break down? Skin and mucous membrane injuries or an obstructed urinary tract, scarred the heart valves, and so on can all let the few organisms normally present multiply to infective proportions before your white cells can reach them or before your acquired immunity comes into play. Physical stresses, such as extreme cold, exhaustion, and shock, can significantly depress your defenses. Psychological stress may lower resistance to disease, although scientific proof is still rather weak. Particular stresses that lead to depression can provoke infections, especially upper respiratory infections. Some medical treatments suppress the immune mechanism, especially X-rays or anticancer drugs. Cancer patients more often die of infection than they do of the tumor spreading. Treatment with cortisone, or corticosteroid derivates, which are used for arthritis and inflammation, can also significantly lower immune defenses. Such patients must be watched carefully for signs of infection.

Treating Infection The treatment of infection can include removing the disease agent from the environment, or using a vaccine to immunize the person. Environmental con-

DPT (diphtheria, pertussis, and tetanus) A triple vaccination for three major diseases, commonly given in childhood; has virtually wiped these diseases out in developed countries.

Immune gamma globulin Serum containing specific antibodies, injected to provide temporary immunity to specific antigens.

trols include personal and public hygiene, eradicating disease-carrying insects (and/or their sources of food), treating sewage, and controlling bacterial contamination of drinking water.

Vaccination has been extremely effective, and unwanted side effects are rare. Many common childhood diseases (measles, mumps, and rubella) have been significantly reduced, polio has been almost wiped out, and smallpox has been totally eliminated by means of vaccination. Triple vaccination in childhood for **diphtheria, pertussis (whooping cough) and tetanus (DPT)** is universal in developed countries, and these diseases have just about disappeared in the United States (see Table 20-1). Vaccination and available vaccines are discussed in the next section.

You can also become passively immune to infection, for a few months, by injection with **immune gamma globulin** from actively immune individuals. This material

Table 20-1 Immunizations Available in the United States

Type of Immunization	Who Should Be Immunized	Effectiveness of Immunization and Frequency of Booster Doses
Cholera	Foreign travelers	Only partial immunity; renew every 6 months for duration of exposure
Diphtheria	All adults in good health with no previous immunization; travelers	Highly effective; renew every 10 years
German measles (rubella)	Mainly for children	Highly effective; need for boosters not established
Influenza	All adults of any age, especially those with chronic disease of the heart, respiratory tract, or endocrine system	Renew every year (because viral strains change easily)
Measles	Mainly for children	Highly effective; usually produces lifelong immunity
Mumps	Most helpful to children and young adults who have not had mumps	Believed to confer lifetime immunity
Plague	Anyone exposed; travelers to Asia, Africa, and Tibet	Incomplete protection; boosters necessary every 3 to 6 months
Polio	All adults, particularly travelers, those exposed to children, and those in health and sanitation industries	Long-lasting immunity; no booster necessary unless exposure anticipated
Rabies	Only those bitten by rabid animal	A vaccination each day for 14 to 21 days beginning soon after the bite
Rocky Mountain spotted fever	—	Not very effective
Tetanus (lockjaw)	Everyone	Very effective; renew every 10 years or when treated for a contaminated wound if more than 5 years have elapsed since last booster
Tuberculosis	High-risk people; nurses and children in contact with active tubercular cases	Variably effective
Typhoid fever	Anyone exposed; travelers	About 80 percent effective
Typhus	Anyone exposed	Renew every year (if exposed)
Whooping cough (pertussis)	Essential for children by age 3 to 4 months	Highly effective
Yellow fever	Anyone exposed; travelers	Highly effective; provides immunity for at least 17 years

The Common Cold

Since the discovery of penicillin in 1928 more progress has been made toward preventing and treating infectious diseases than in all the rest of medical history combined. Smallpox has now been eradicated, typhoid fever has become a rarity, and pneumococcal pneumonia is both curable and, now, preventable. Yet no means has been found, to date, to eliminate or cure the common cold, which, it has been estimated, costs $5 billion each year in lost wages and medical expenses.

In fact, the common cold is not a simple matter; rather, it is a complex of symptoms. It is caused by any one of a group of viruses (more than 120 different viral strains that produce common cold symptoms in humans have been isolated). The common cold is primarily an infection of the lining membrane of your upper respiratory tract, including your nose, sinuses, and throat. This delicate membrane reacts to infection by swelling and by increasing its rate of mucus formation, leading to congestion, stuffiness, and a great deal of nose blowing. Because your nasal cavity no longer functions as a resonating chamber, a characteristic change in your voice quality also occurs. Increased mucus flow usually causes a postnasal drip, which is irritating and contributes to the familiar "scratchy" throat and cough.

Your sinuses, which normally empty into the nasal cavity, may become blocked by excessive swelling of the membranes. The resulting increase in sinus pressure may cause a headache. In similar fashion, swelling in the upper part of your throat can block your Eustachian tubes—the two narrow canals that lead to your ears. This blockage can cause accumulation of fluid and pressure in your middle ear, which may be painful. Less commonly, an unpleasant spinning sensation known as *vertigo* may result.

A cold is usually self-limited, lasting about one to two weeks. At any time during the course of a cold, bacteria (such as staphylococci or pneumococci) can be secondary invaders, bringing on painful infections of the sinuses and ears. However, the old warning that, if you don't take care, a cold will turn into pneumonia, is hardly ever true. Pneumonia and most other infections of the lower respiratory tract begin in the bronchi and the lungs rather than in the upper respiratory tract.

Most people stay home from work or school because of generalized symptoms—muscle aches, weakness, and fatigue. The extent of these symptoms varies from person to person. Although mild elevation of temperature can occur with the common cold, a rectal temperature above 101°F is usually a sign of a more serious viral or bacterial infection. If you have fever above 101°F, taken rectally, for more than two days, you should seek medical advice.

Americans spend more than $900 million a year for cold and cough remedies. Advertisers have claimed preventive and curative virtues for vitamins, alkalizers, lemon drinks, antihistamines, decongestants, timed-release capsules, bioflavenoids, nose drops and sprays, quinine pills, aspirin mixtures, laxatives, inhalers, aromatic salves, liniments, room air sprays, and a variety of other products. There are at least 300 over-the-counter (OTC) products —most of which are a combination of ingredients—marketed for treating symptoms of the common cold. Many of these drugs do neither good nor harm to the cold victim, but there is no doubt that they benefit the drug manufacturers.

Everyone has heard of sure-fire formulas for preventing a cold. Popular home methods include a cold shower, regular exercise, and a hot rum toddy. Some people swear by cod liver oil, tea with honey, citrus fruit juices (or massive doses of vitamin C), or keeping their feet dry. At one time, many large firms encouraged their employees to submit to inoculations with cold "vaccines." And splendid results from these programs were regularly reported. But such vaccines, like many other "scientific" (or folk) remedies, gradually have been abandoned as experience and controlled testing have proved their uselessness in preventing colds. Now, just as fifty years ago, Americans on the average will suffer two to three colds a year, the acute infectious stages of which will last about a week or two (although a cough or postnasal drip may linger), regardless of any physical measure, diet, or drug used to try to head off the colds. U.S. Public Health Service (PHS) studies show that, during the winter quarter of the year, 50 percent of the population experiences a common cold; during the summer quarter, the figure drops to 20 percent.

It is unfortunate that the name "cold" has been given to this common, but minor, malady. The name has led many people to infer that the common cold is somehow

(continued on next page)

The Common Cold (*continued*)

caused by walking bareheaded in the rain, not wearing enough winter clothing, or getting caught in a draft. There is as yet no evidence that the common cold ever occurs in the absence of an infecting organism. Moreover, studies have shown that chilling does not predispose one to infection with the cold virus (or viruses). The increased incidence of colds in winter reflects the fact that people spend more time indoors, thereby facilitating the transfer of viruses from person to person. In fact, one is less likely to catch a cold after exposure to the elements than after mixing with a convivial group of snifflers and sneezers at a fireside gathering.

The common cold, it is now reasonably certain, is not only spread by sneezing and coughing but also by shaking hands and handling contaminated articles. The home, office, classroom, bus, or any other place where people gather is a good spreading ground. But resistance seems to vary greatly among individuals, so that not everyone exposed to a common source of infection becomes ill. Moreover, the natural factors—whatever they are—that contribute to resistance in an individual may be operative at one time and not at another. Thus it is not uncommon for some unlucky person to have a "bad year," suffering from as many as five or six colds, and then remain in excellent health during the following year or two. These variations in resistance and the irregular pattern in the occurrence of colds make it extremely difficult to evaluate the effect of any medication on the course of the common cold.

SOURCE: Adapted from *The Medicine Show*.

is obtained from serum (the clear liquid residue that results when blood is allowed to clot) of people who are immune to a given disease, and it contains the protective antibodies. It is frequently given to travelers who may be exposed to hepatitis or cholera during their travels. Immune gamma globulin has also been used in hospitals, where patients whose immunity has been suppressed (by radiation therapy or burn wounds) risk getting infectious diseases from other patients.

Active drug therapy of infectious disease has become progressively more effective over the last seventy years. Such therapy is based on differences between parasites and the host. It is possible to produce substances that are toxic for parasites, but not or only mildly toxic for the host. Because the physiologies are not completely different, however, most drugs are slightly toxic for the host as well as for the pathogens, and should not be used indiscriminately. Into this category fall the antibiotics.

Antibiotics are substances produced by one micro-organism that are toxic to other micro-organisms. Antibiotics are important weapons used among competing microbes. The first important antibiotic was discovered by Alexander Fleming, an English researcher, who observed that a fungal colony, growing in a plate of bacteria, had produced a clear zone in which the bacteria had been killed. From this fungus he purified a substance that he called **penicillin.** This was the first of a long list of antibiotics that now includes such drugs as erythromycin, tetracycline, streptomycin, gentamicin, and the cephalosporins.

Antibiotics are effective only against bacteria and fungi; with almost no exception, they are ineffective against viruses. They may be used to prevent bacterial infection when a virus has weakened a person's immune defenses. There are also a number of excellent synthetic drugs, many of which are modifications of antibiotics. They can be very effective against bacteria as well as fungi.

Antibiotics and other antimicrobial agents act on a limited range of micro-organisms. The physician must choose the drug that best copes with the infecting organism. Equally important, the patient must tolerate the drug well. For example, penicillin kills streptococci, so it is the "drug of choice" for strep throat. Some patients, however, have allergic reactions to penicillin, so they must use erythromycin. Most gastrointestinal and urinary tract infections

Exploring Your Emotions

Suppose the grocer who supplied the food for a party you had given for 30 of your friends about to disperse for summer vacations is reported to be a hepatitis carrier, responsible for infecting many customers. Several weeks after the party one friend is severely ill from a virus to which all the others were also exposed. What is your immediate reaction? What should you do? Whose help should you enlist?

Penicillin An antibiotic substance produced by the fungus penicillium.

Mutation A rare, random change in the gene structure of an individual; because it is genetic, it can be inherited by that individual's offspring.

Immunity Mechanisms that defend the body against infection; or the status of those mechanisms in general; or specific immunity or defenses against specific pathogens.

are caused by organisms that resist penicillin; therefore, a number of other drugs, especially sulfa drugs and tetracycline, must be used instead.

Occasionally (about once in a million divisions), a **mutation** occurs. A mutant bacterium (slightly changed in some way) can occasionally resist a drug to which its parents were sensitive. When resistant bacteria appear in a bacterial infection that is being treated by the drug, they will soon take over because they soon have no competition for nutrients. The overuse of antibiotics has frequently produced resistant strains. This effect can be particularly disastrous in hospitals, where many drugs are used and susceptible patients abound. Many hospitals now have committees charged with preventing such abuse.

Viruses are considerably harder to kill than any bacteria and fungi, because they very closely resemble the human cell and lack any metabolic activity that drugs might block. Only two effective drugs are currently on the market, but several others are being tested. Because these drugs may interfere with the reproductive apparatus of the human cell itself, they are very toxic and potentially dangerous. At the moment, a substance produced by the human body itself—interferon—may be the best hope for treatment of viral disease.

Immunity

The one-celled organism copes with its environment mainly by trying to eat everything it meets. Its "universe" thus consists of two kinds of materials—those that are digestible and those that are not. In contrast, the many-celled organism is made up of different kinds of cells that have to live together in harmony, so it must be able to distinguish between itself and everything else, including other members of its species. In addition, the multicellular organism must also be able to recognize those portions of its own original structure that have become useless or harmful. To eliminate all harmful materials, multicellular organisms have evolved methods of protection, or immune mechanisms, together called the *immune system*. The immune system functions (1) to prevent entry of foreign and undesirable substances, living or dead, into the organism, and to remove any such substances that break through its barriers; and (2) to eliminate certain products of the organism itself—dead cells and cells that have changed and become lethal, such as cancer cells. Certain recognition systems, barriers, and toxic mechanisms have evolved within the organism to accomplish these purposes.

Sometimes, however, the recognition systems and toxic mechanisms themselves can be a problem, possibly a lethal one. For example, they can complicate or block blood transfusions and organ or tissue transplants. By attacking basically harmless substances like plant pollens with their full toxic power, they can cause a disease known as an *allergy*. They may even go totally awry and attack normal and necessary constituents of the body, causing autoimmune disease.

Immune mechanisms defend your body against infection. Nonspecific mechanisms keep out all foreign invaders, no matter what they are. Specific mechanisms recognize individual types of organisms and let your body focus on any single invader that might be the main threat of the moment. The word **immunity** is frequently used only to refer to specific mechanisms.

Nonspecific Mechanisms Nonspecific mechanisms include your physiological barriers, secretions and enzymes, and the phagocytic cells. The physiological defenses of your body include skin, mucous membranes, secretions such as tears and mucus, certain activities of enzymes, and some organisms, fluids, and biochemical processes of your gastrointestinal tract.

Your skin provides a multiple defense. It blocks the entry of micro-organisms both physically and chemically.

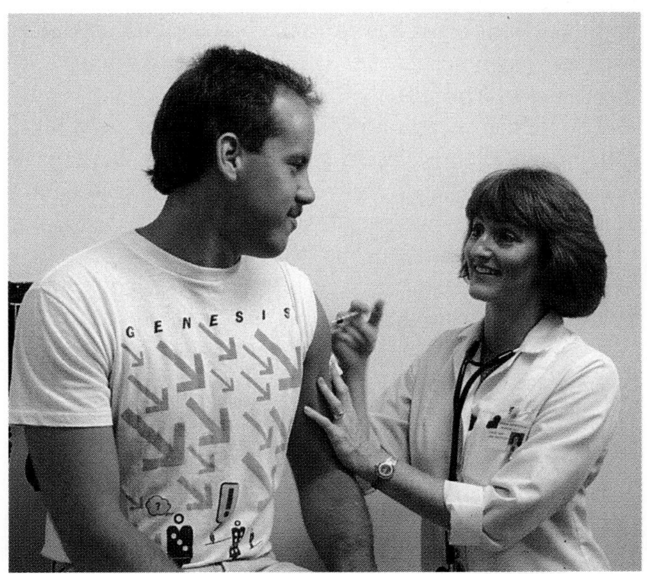

Kaiser

Cilia Microscopic hairlike structures that sweep mucus and foreign substances up out of the bronchial tubes.

Phagocytes White blood cells that specialize in eating undesirable matter.

Granulocytes Phagocytes that contain many granules, and that are the first line of defense against foreign particles in the bloodstream.

Macrophages Large phagocytes that especially guard the lungs by devouring foreign particles.

Lymphocytes White blood cells continuously made in lymphoid tissue as well as in bone marrow.

Platelets Blood particles that cause clotting.

Plasma The fluid portion of blood.

Lymphatic system The body system that traps pathogens and produces lymphocytes.

Antigen A molecule that marks an invading particle; can be recognized and neutralized by an antibody.

B-cells Lymphocytes that produce antibodies.

Helper T-cells Lymphocytes that stimulate other lymphocytes to increase.

Suppressor T-cells Lymphocytes that discourage the growth of other lymphocytes.

Neutralization The effect of an antibody that combines with an antigen to make it chemically harmless.

Agglutination The effect of an antibody that bundles bacteria together for ingestion by phagocytes.

Attentuated Weakened.

The normal weak acidity on the surface of your skin is a poor growth condition for bacteria and fungi. The non-disease-producing bacteria that do survive normal skin conditions are still another barrier. They occupy space needed by the attacking pathogens, they consume what little food is available, and sometimes they even secrete materials toxic to other bacteria.

Mucus membranes are also staunch defenders of your body. Located in the eyes, nose, sinuses, throat, windpipe, bronchial tubes, gastrointestinal tubes, and vagina, all have specific protective functions.

Tears keep the surface of your eyeballs from drying out. They provide a solution in which protective substances and cells can function. They wash away invaders from the mucous membranes of your eyes. And tears contain an enzyme that kills certain bacteria.

The mucus secreted by the membranes of the nose, throat, and bronchial tubes moistens, cleans, and regulates the temperature of the air that you breathe. This mucus coating, acting much like sticky flypaper, captures inhaled foreign substances. The membrane of your respiratory tract also has slender microscopic hairlike structures called **cilia.** These cilia gradually move the mucus up out of your bronchial tubes. When the mucus coating reaches your windpipe or voice box, you cough and spit it out or swallow it.

The mucus secretion of the vagina, which has a lubricating function, also helps prevent infection, perhaps by supporting the beneficial bacteria. When this secretion ceases, infections—especially those caused by fungi and protozoa—frequently occur.

Enzymes that exist in your blood act as defense agents by destroying some kinds of bacteria. (This process usually consists of rupturing the bacterium's outer membrane, causing its contents to spill out.) The clotting of blood around a wound is another form of defense. The scab physically blocks micro-organisms from entering your body.

Digestive enzymes, intestinal secretions, stomach fluids, and intestinal bacteria all protect your gastrointestinal tract. If you swallow a pathogen, your strongly acidic stomach fluids usually destroy it. Pathogens that survive your stomach must pass into the alkaline secretions of your small intestine, where they are attacked by your digestive enzymes. Still farther on lives a large army of intestinal bacteria whose density, living habits, and by-products discourage many pathogens.

Phagocytes are white blood cells that specialize in ingesting and digesting undesirable matter. The two kinds of phagocytes are **granulocytes** (so called because they contain many small granules) and **macrophages.** Both cell types circulate through the tissues and channels of your body, but specialized macrophages also line the walls of the blood vessels and form an integral part of their structure. Macrophages also predominate in your body cavities, especially in your lungs, where they immediately attack all particles that have managed to pass through your upper respiratory passages. Granulocytes predominate in the bloodstream and thus rapidly reach any area where a breach in the integrity of your body occurs. Granulocytes thus constitute a first line of defense. Phagocytes, which move along surfaces by changing their shape, travel rapidly through the two major traffic systems of your body: the circulatory system (bloodstream) and the lymphatic system (a network of extremely delicate, small vessels).

From one-third to one-half of your total volume of blood is made up of blood cells; these are continuously manufactured by bone marrow. Most of these are red cells, which give your blood its color and carry oxygen to the tissues. About 1 cell in 500 is a white cell, either a phagocyte or lymphocyte. **Lymphocytes** are a kind of white blood cell that is continuously made in lymphoid tissue as well as in bone marrow.) **Platelets,** which cause clotting, are also part of the solid constituents of blood. The fluid portion of your blood is called **plasma,** and the liquid that remains after clotting is called *serum.*

Your bloodstream carries white cells to areas of infection. White cells can move through the walls of your blood vessels and through tissue under their own power, sometimes in response to signals that originate at the breakdown site of local tissues. Pus is mostly made up of white cells.

Macrophages and lymphocytes travel through your **lymphatic system.** The liquid content of your lymphatic system resembles plasma. The lymphatic network serves and clears tissue spaces and organs; it ends in the main lymphatic vessel, the thoracic duct, which empties into your bloodstream. At major junctions in the lymphatic network are rice-grain-size to pea-size structures called lymph nodes. Lymphocytes and macrophages congregate here in great numbers. They enter these nodes directly from your bloodstream by passing through the two systems. The lymph nodes are traps for invading pathogens. If the invaders manage to multiply there, a lymph node becomes a major battlefield, aching and swelling. An infected cut on the hand can cause swollen lymph nodes in the armpit.

Your body's natural defenses can cope continuously with a small number of pathogens, but minor breakdowns in immune defenses lead to infection. Your defense barriers are also relatively ineffective in preventing viral infection, and viral diseases spread quite easily among us humans. The nonspecific defense mechanisms described so far are not adequate for coping with many infections. Highly specific mechanisms have evolved to fill the gap. These mechanisms can "learn" quickly to respond with vigor to a particular invader. The specific mechanisms can reproduce themselves rapidly; they have "memory"; and they can draw on other systems to increase their ability to defend. This specialized process is the adaptive immune system.

Specific Mechanisms Adaptive immunity and vaccination are essential weapons in your defense against infection. Thanks to recent research, our understanding of these weapons is increasing by leaps and bounds.

Adaptive Immunity Your lymphocytes provide you with adaptive immunity. You have two types of lymphocytes: **B-cells** and T-cells. The B-cells carry antibody molecules on their surfaces. More than a million different kinds of antibody molecules exist, each capable of recognizing and bonding to a slightly different molecular target. A single B-cell makes only one type of antibody, but it can make millions of copies of that one antibody. The antibody molecules are about one-twentieth the size of the smallest virus. Each kind of antibody molecule matches or recognizes an **antigen** molecule that has invaded your body (a particle, or parasitic organism, or a stray cancer cell). The recognition process works like a lock and key, or like two pieces of tape that stick to each other so that nothing else can stick to them. Like lock and key sets, antibodies are very specific to specific antigens.

T-cells also react to antigens, and like B-cells, they divide and proliferate in contact with them. The most important kinds of T-cells are helper and suppressor T-cells. **Helper T-cells** stimulate certain other B- or T-cells to increase, while **suppressor T-cells** discourage growth of specific cell types. These cells help mobilize for attack, and then *de*mobilize afterward.

A third important T-cell type is the so-called killer cell. Killer cells in some way recognize foreign cells, particularly tumor or virus-infected cells, and kill them. The importance of this mechanism may lie in defending the body from an occasional cancer cell that arises through mutation. T-cells may have evolved principally as a mechanism for removing altered cells, such as cancer cells, that could menace the body's integrity. They are not completely successful in doing so, however.

When they interact with antigens, T-cells directly secrete a number of important defensive substances. One such substance attracts macrophages and retains them in the needed area. In addition, T-cells, because they can identify changes in cell surfaces, can actually bind to areas of change caused by virus infection and destroy the altered cell before it finishes manufacturing complete viruses.

Antibodies and T-cells use several mechanisms to protect your body against infection. Antibodies, though smaller than viruses, can stop viral infection by binding to specific areas on the virus surface that the virus needs for attaching itself to the cell. This simple action prevents further infection, and so is called **neutralization.** Occasionally, antibodies prevent bacteria from multiplying by binding directly to their surfaces. More frequently, however, antibodies bind bacteria together in relatively large bunches, an action called **agglutination.** Phagocytes seem to prefer to ingest agglutinated bacteria.

Vaccination Late in the eighteenth century, Edward Jenner, an English physician, noticed that occasionally the hands of people who milked cows showed a pox infection similar to the dreaded smallpox. Jenner observed that victims of cowpox—a relatively mild disease—never contracted smallpox. He rubbed scrapings from infected cow udders into the skin and skin abrasions of people who had not had smallpox to see whether or not this procedure would protect them. It did. None of these people—the first to be vaccinated—contracted smallpox.

No one understood the process of vaccination in Jenner's time. We know now that cowpox and smallpox are caused by closely related viruses, called, respectively, *vaccinia* and *variola.* When the body successfully overcomes infection by one virus, it is then primed for a strong secondary response against the other, or against any sufficiently similar virus.

We can also breed viruses that are less virulent than the originals. In other words, we can breed mild disease organisms from severe ones. Such organisms are said to be **attenuated.** Oral polio vaccine is an attenuated virus. Attenuated organisms are generally the best possible means

CELL WARS

About one trillion strong, our white blood cells constitute a highly specialized army of defenders, the most important of which are depicted here in a typical battle against a formidable enemy.

VIRUS

Needing help to spring to life, a virus is little more than a package of genetic information that must commandeer the machinery of a host cell to permit its own replication.

MACROPHAGE

Housekeeper and frontline defender, this cell engulfs and digests debris that washes into the bloodstream. Encountering a foreign organism, it summons helper T cells to the scene.

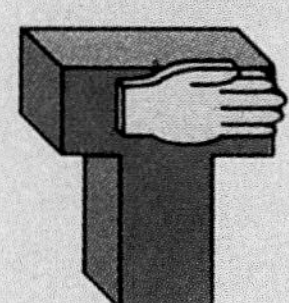

HELPER T CELL

As a commander in chief of the immune system, it identifies the enemy and rushes to the spleen and lymph nodes, where it stimulates the production of other cells to fight the infection.

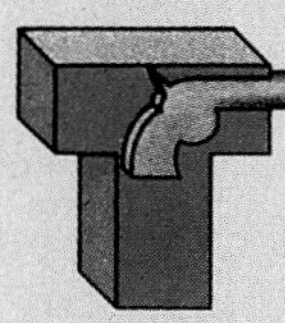

KILLER T CELL

Recruited and activated by helper T cells, it specializes in killing cells of the body that have been invaded by foreign organisms, as well as cells that have turned cancerous.

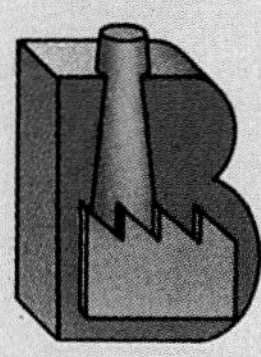

B CELL

Biologic arms factory, it resides in the spleen or the lymph nodes, where it is induced to replicate by helper T cells and then to produce potent chemical weapons called antibodies.

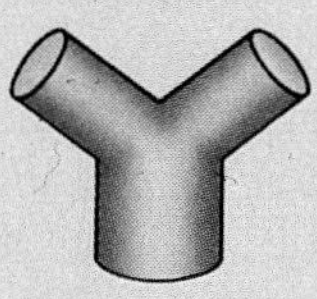

ANTIBODY

Engineered to target a specific invader, this Y-shaped protein molecule is rushed to the infection site, where it either neutralizes the enemy or tags it for attack by other cells or chemicals.

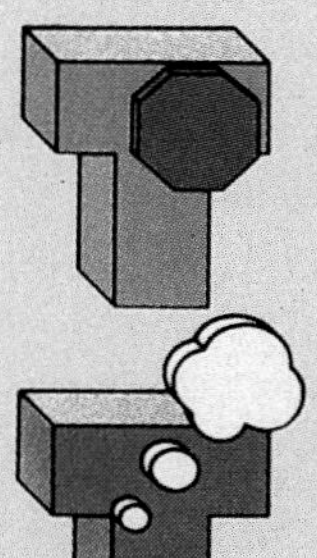

SUPPRESSOR T CELL

A third type of T cell, it is able to slow down or stop the activities of B cells and other T cells, playing a vital role in calling off the attack after an infection has been conquered.

MEMORY CELL

Generated during an initial infection, this defense cell may circulate in the blood or lymph for years, enabling the body to respond more quickly to subsequent infections.

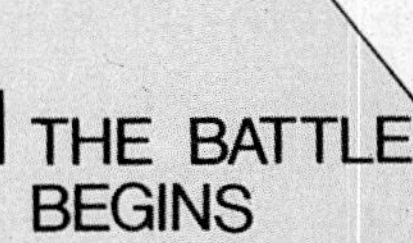

1 THE BATTLE BEGINS

As viruses begin to invade the body, a few are consumed by macrophages, which seize their antigens and display them on their own surfaces. Among millions of helper T cells circulating in the bloodstream, a select few are programmed to "read" that antigen. Binding to the macrophage, the T cell becomes activated.

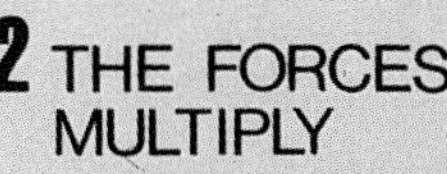

2 THE FORCES MULTIPLY

Once activated, helper T cells begin to multiply. They then stimulate the multiplication of those few killer T cells and B cells that are sensitive to the invading viruses. As the number of B cells increases, helper T cells signal them to start producing antibodies.

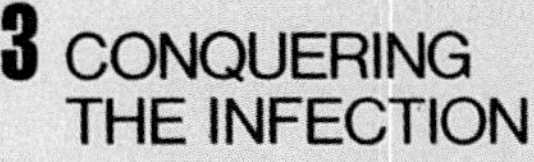

3 CONQUERING THE INFECTION

Meanwhile, some of the viruses have entered cells of the body— the only place they are able to replicate. Killer T cells will sacrifice these cells by chemically puncturing their membranes, letting the contents spill out, thus disrupting the viral replication cycle. Antibodies then neutralize the viruses by binding directly to their surfaces, preventing them from attacking other cells. Additionally, they precipitate chemical reactions that actually destroy infected cells.

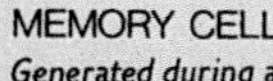

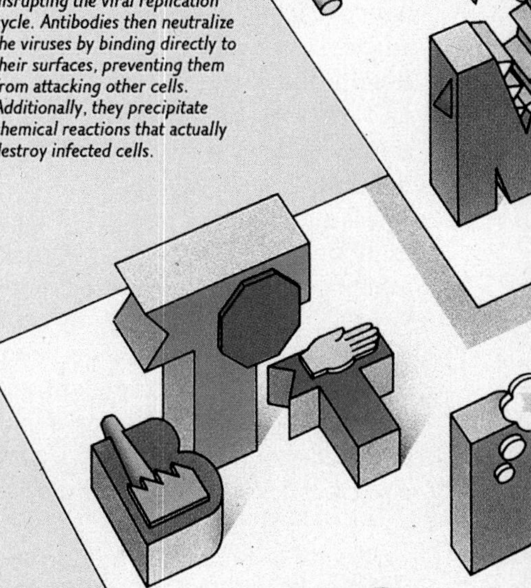

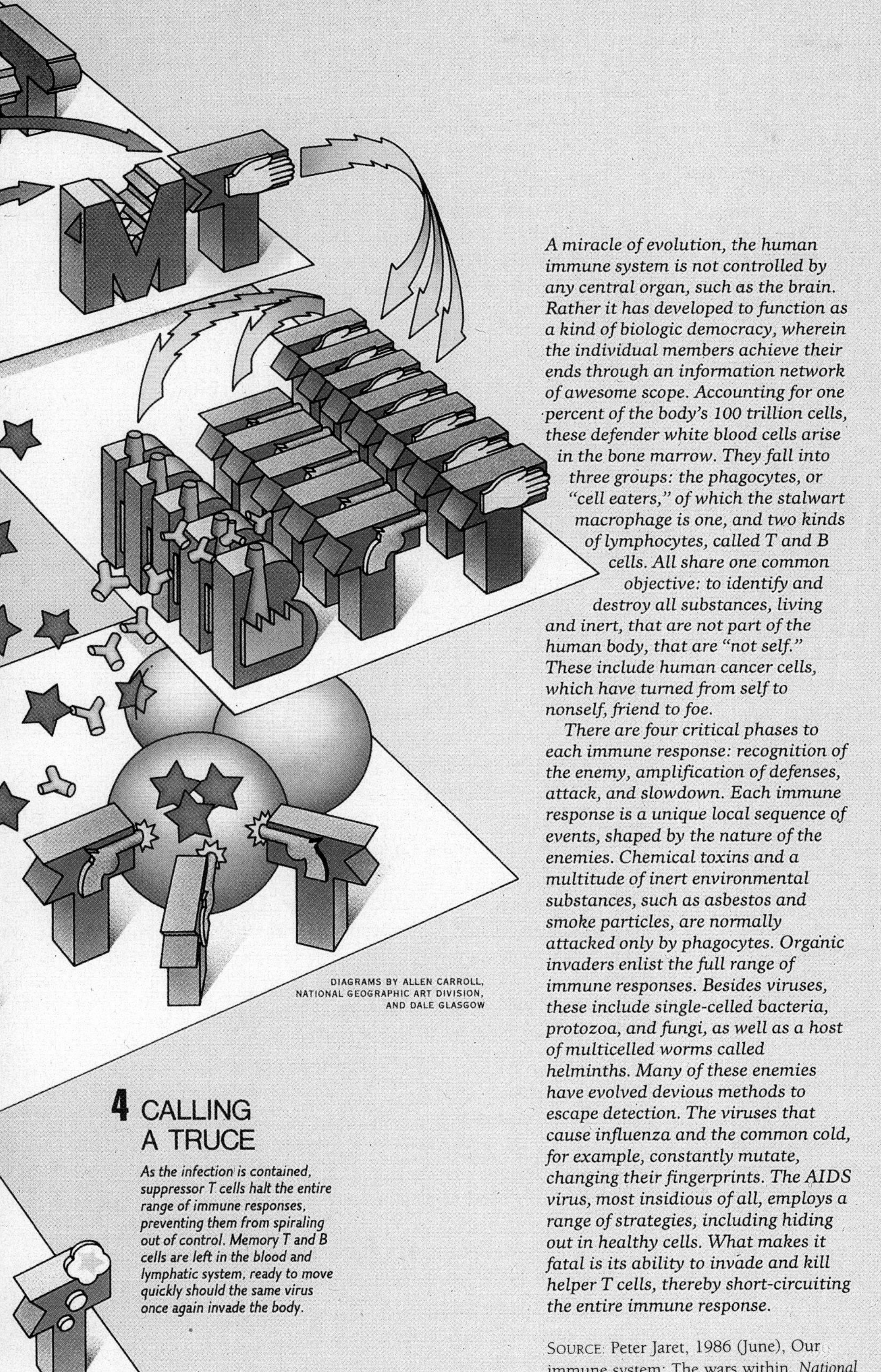

DIAGRAMS BY ALLEN CARROLL,
NATIONAL GEOGRAPHIC ART DIVISION,
AND DALE GLASGOW
4 CALLING
A TRUCE
As the infection is contained, suppressor T cells halt the entire range of immune responses, preventing them from spiraling out of control. Memory T and B cells are left in the blood and lymphatic system, ready to move quickly should the same virus once again invade the body.

A miracle of evolution, the human immune system is not controlled by any central organ, such as the brain. Rather it has developed to function as a kind of biologic democracy, wherein the individual members achieve their ends through an information network of awesome scope. Accounting for one percent of the body's 100 trillion cells, these defender white blood cells arise in the bone marrow. They fall into three groups: the phagocytes, or "cell eaters," of which the stalwart macrophage is one, and two kinds of lymphocytes, called T and B cells. All share one common objective: to identify and destroy all substances, living and inert, that are not part of the human body, that are "not self." These include human cancer cells, which have turned from self to nonself, friend to foe.

There are four critical phases to each immune response: recognition of the enemy, amplification of defenses, attack, and slowdown. Each immune response is a unique local sequence of events, shaped by the nature of the enemies. Chemical toxins and a multitude of inert environmental substances, such as asbestos and smoke particles, are normally attacked only by phagocytes. Organic invaders enlist the full range of immune responses. Besides viruses, these include single-celled bacteria, protozoa, and fungi, as well as a host of multicelled worms called helminths. Many of these enemies have evolved devious methods to escape detection. The viruses that cause influenza and the common cold, for example, constantly mutate, changing their fingerprints. The AIDS virus, most insidious of all, employs a range of strategies, including hiding out in healthy cells. What makes it fatal is its ability to invade and kill helper T cells, thereby short-circuiting the entire immune response.

SOURCE: Peter Jaret, 1986 (June), Our immune system: The wars within, *National Geographic*, p. 709.

ABO blood type system A blood classification scheme for antigen characteristics; helps ensure correct matching of blood in transfusions, to avoid inducing adverse reactions to the donor's blood.

Rh blood group system A blood classification scheme that describes the "rhesus factor" antibodies a human has. A mother who gives birth to a child who has an unlike Rh factor may produce antibodies that could kill a second fetus that had the same unlike factor.

Immunosuppression Suppression of the immune system through drugs and corticosteroid hormones.

of immunization. One of their major advantages is that immunization occurs at the same sites and in the same sequence as observed in the virulent organism.

Sometimes it isn't possible to breed attenuated organisms that retain enough of the original structure to confer immunity against their more dangerous ancestors. However, it is also possible to kill dangerous organisms and use them for vaccination. Each method has its advantages, and the polio vaccine is made in both attenuated and killed forms.

Adaptive immunity can also defend the body against fungi, protozoa, worms, and the like, but the process is more complex, because the pathogen is more complex, and vaccine development for diseases caused by these agents has been less successful.

Recognizing Foreign Cells

One of the oldest pursuits of medical science has been the search for ways to replace organs and limbs. Blood was the first "tissue" with which transfers were attempted—because the surgical procedure is simple. Failures in the effort to transfer animal blood to humans may be documented all the way back to the Middle Ages. Many attempts to transfer blood from one human to another were made at the end of the nineteenth century, but the results were unpredictable.

Karl Landsteiner, an Austrian-born American pathologist, solved the problem in 1900. He discovered that the surfaces of red blood cells contain antigen systems that vary from person to person. The major such system (and there are at least twelve others with about 100 different antigens), and the first one described by Landsteiner, is the **ABO blood type system.** Each letter stands for a different antigen on the cell surface. Each individual's blood contains one or two of these three antigens. A person with Type A blood cannot be given a transfusion of Type B blood—because his or her immune system will reject it. Military personnel and others who have a high risk of injury are routinely blood-typed and carry this information everywhere on their persons. Anyone would be well advised to do the same. Blood of the same ABO type is rarely rejected, and safe transfusion is usually ensured by cross matching the donor's and recipient's blood in a test tube.

One other blood group system of medical significance is the **Rh blood group system.** This system was first described by Karl Landsteiner and Alexander Wiener and independently by Paul Levine in 1940. The mother's immunization is believed to occur at the birth of her first child, when red blood cells from the fetus enter her bloodstream. If the fetus and the mother have different types within this group, the mother may become immunized to the fetus's blood. If in a later pregnancy, the new fetus also has an Rh type unlike the mother's, the mother's secondary response will cause Rh antibodies to cross the placenta and destroy the fetal blood cells. The resulting Rh disease can kill this fetus. The condition can be prevented by manipulating the mother's immune status at the time of the first delivery, using appropriate antibodies.

Although the immunology of blood cells has been understood for many years, similar insight into other kinds of cells is recent. For example, surgical techniques required for skin transplants have existed for some time. But (except in identical twins), the host body eventually recognizes transplanted skin as foreign, and so it rejects the skin by the sort of immune mechanisms already discussed. Inbred, or genetically identical mice, like identical human twins, have identical molecules at their cell surfaces, and so skin transplants among them are possible.

Surgical techniques for performing organ transplants were developed long ago, but physicians have not known how to control the immune response. Once researchers began to understand immune rejection, several kidney transplants between identical twins were successful. The next step, now widely practiced, was to suppress the immune response with a variety of drugs and corticosteroids (hormones that are produced by the adrenal cortex). This procedure is called **immunosuppression.** Immunosuppression is itself risky, however, and should be used only for a limited time. It weakens or blocks the natural defenses of the organism. The current techniques maximize interference with tissue rejection and minimize suppression of the body's defenses.

Greater success in organ transplants will come from increasing our ability to deceive the immune system into recognizing the transplanted organ as "self." The present method of achieving this deception involves using immunosuppression drugs to control the immune response. Dosage levels are gradually reduced as the transplant "takes hold." This approach has resulted in many successful kidney transplants. Some patients have survived for more

Stalking the Sneezemakers

If you are a hay fever sufferer, you may well feel that pollinating plants conspire against you personally. Or you may confer "culprit" status on dust, tobacco smoke, animal dander, lobster Newburg . . . any of a host of potential allergy triggers, or allergens.

Yet most allergens are harmless substances; the problem is a person's inappropriate *response* to them.

A key part of that response is the release of a chemical called *histamine*. Histamine can set off all the familiar symptoms of an allergy attack, ranging from the sniffling, tearing, and sneezing of hay fever to the itchy redness of hives or the wheezing and gasping of asthma.

Researchers have known about histamine's role in allergies since the turn of the century; antihistamines—drugs that counter its effects—have been the cornerstone of allergy treatment for some time. But a detailed understanding of what histamine actually does has only developed since the 1960s. In the last decade researchers have uncovered other crucial substances that conspire with histamine to trigger the allergic response.

Antigen Meets Antibody

No one knows precisely why some people get allergies and others don't. Since allergies tend to run in families, heredity must play some role. But genes cannot be the whole story.

To some degree, allergies may involve luck. As the immune system develops in the womb and during infancy, the genes in immune system cells undergo a random shuffling. As a result, no two people have precisely identical immune systems, and some may be more likely to spawn allergies than others.

Allergies arise when the immune system—so efficient at identifying and destroying disease-causing organisms like foreign bacteria and viruses—gets all worked up over basically benign invaders (a pollen particle, for example).

This oversensitivity involves an excess of one or more antibodies, which are proteins designed to latch onto unwelcome organisms and substances, marking them for destruction.

The antibodies that trigger allergic responses all belong to the broad class known as *immunoglobin E*, or IgE. IgE antibodies tend to take up residence on the surface of mast cells, which congregate in the soft tissue surrounding blood vessels in the lungs, sinuses, skin, and other areas. Among other things, mast cells contain reservoirs of histamine, which they stand ready to release on the proper signal.

If a person's mast cells are well stocked with IgE antibodies against a particular allergen, and if that allergen comes along and binds to them, the histamine floodgates open and the trouble begins.

Wide-ranging Effects

Histamine's main effect is to render nearby blood vessels more porous, allowing fluid and cells from the blood to flood the local tissue. Histamine also stimulates mucus production and, primarily in the lung, it can cause smooth muscle (the kind that functions without our awareness) to contract.

The precise symptoms that result depend on what part of the body is affected. In the nose, histamine causes flushing, congestion, and sneezing, mostly as a result of the influx of fluid from blood to tissue and the consequent blockage of airways. In the eyes, it can produce tearing, itching, and inflammation around the eyelids (conjunctivitis). In the skin, it can cause redness, swelling, and itching; and in the lungs, it can make breathing difficult by causing the muscles surrounding air passages to contract.

The most serious kind of allergic reaction, called *systemic anaphylaxis,* involves a widespread release of histamine throughout the body. Systemic anaphylaxis can cause a life-threatening loss of blood pressure known as *anaphylactic shock.* Although rare, this condition is most often brought on by bee stings or penicillin reactions in very sensitive individuals.

Allergic responses aren't the only way to cause the release of histamine. In some people, cold weather or heavy exercise can stimulate histamine release and bring on an asthma attack. In others, contact with ice can cause a skin rash.

The nervous system and emotions may also influence histamine release, by means not yet fully understood. One recent study even suggested that histamine release can be learned. In that study, guinea pigs were presented with a certain odor whenever they were exposed to a substance they were allergic to. Later, when presented

(continued on next page)

Stalking the Sneezemakers (*continued*)

with the odor but not the allergen, they still developed symptoms and had increased histamine in the blood.

Covert Co-conspirators

Although histamine clearly plays a major role in generating allergic symptoms, new research shows that it shares the stage with other, rarer cell products, such as *leukotrienes, prostaglandins,* and *platelet-activating factor (PAF).*

Unlike histamine, which is stored in mast cells awaiting release, these substances are manufactured on the spot, as they are needed. Like histamine, however, they contribute greatly to the inflammation of surrounding tissue, and molecule for molecule, they are considerably more potent.

Histamine and these other allergy mediators complement each other's actions in complex ways that researchers are only beginning to understand. In particular, it is hoped that further study of their interplay may lead to improved strategies for countering the "late-phase response" that affects many people with asthma or hay fever. In those individuals, an allergy or asthma attack often is followed several hours later by a milder repeat attack, which occurs even without further exposure to the offending allergen. It may be that the initial burst of mast cell products sets off a molecular chain reaction, which eventually comes full cycle and retriggers the release of histamine.

Pharmaceutical researchers are currently eyeing the possibility of drugs to block the action of the new-found mediators, the way antihistamines block histamine. So far, leukotriene blockers are showing the most promise. It seems to make sense that the more mediators we can block, the more allergy relief is in store.

And, just as the advent of antihistamines paved the way for new insights into histamine itself, leukotriene blockers and the like should help researchers refine their knowledge about which of these mediators does what, and when.

SOURCE: Adapted from Martha V. White and Ralph Bonheim, 1987 (March–April), Allergy research: Stalking the sneezemakers, R_x *Being Well,* pp. 38–42.

than fifteen years after such transplants. Heart transplants have also become increasingly successful, and survivals of ten years or longer are on record. Recent successes in this field are in large part due to the drug Cyclosporine A, which is somewhat selective in its suppression of the immune response, and leaves the host with adequate defenses against invading infectious organisms.

Allergies

As we have seen, the adaptive immune defenses cannot distinguish between potentially harmful materials and those that are harmless. Also, the adaptive system cannot distinguish between living and nonliving material. When the immune mechanism responds vigorously to an innocuous and common substance such as house dust or pollen, the defense may result in the complex of diseases called **allergies.**

Allergies are poorly understood. Their manifestations cover a wide range, from hives to respiratory difficulties to cardiac arrest (stopping of the heart). Allergies are roughly divided into two types: those caused by B-cell action (that is, antibodies) and those based on toxic materials released by T-cells. Which system predominates in the allergy depends to some extent on the antigen that causes it. The allergies related to T-cells are due to a specific set of compounds—for example, metals, oils present in plants such as poison oak, dyes, and the like. The chief causes of B-cell-related allergies are foreign proteins, such as those in plant pollens (ragweed and many kinds of grasses, for example), house dust (in which the active ingredient is probably some insect by-product), insect toxins such as those left by bee stings, and many foodstuffs.

Almost everyone can come into frequent contact with all these materials. Why, then, do only 10 to 15 percent of us suffer from allergies? The total answer is not known, but parts of it have become clear. The tendency to acquire allergies is hereditary. It may be directly related to an individual's ability to produce a particular kind of allergic antibody in large quantities.

A critical property of these allergic antibodies, which differentiates them from ordinary antibodies, is their ability to attach themselves to mast cells. **Mast cells** contain substances that are toxic when released. These substances cause spasms of certain lung, heart, and intestine muscles

Allergies Diseases caused by the body's own exaggerated response to foreign chemicals and proteins.

Mast cells Body cells that release histamine.

Histamine The toxic released by mast cells when the allergic antibody touches an allergen.

Antihistamines Drugs that interfere with histamine and its effects.

Autoimmune disease Disease in which an individual's immume system attacks the individual's own body or body parts.

and can increase the permeability of small blood vessels. The toxic substances (**histamine,** in particular) are released when the allergic antibody on the outside of the mast cell touches an allergenic material. The respiratory system is the principal entry for a number of allergenic materials, and many allergies have respiratory symptoms: coughing, mucus secretion, sinus congestion, and so forth. Toxic substances can travel from one part of the body to another, so even when the antigen enters through the skin, the eyes, or the gastrointestinal tract (after eating), respiratory symptoms frequently occur. Food allergies frequently result in hives, which can either be restricted to small areas or can cover the whole body.

A variety of treatments have been used for B-cell allergies. Drugs that interfere with histamine (called **antihistamines**) are well known and are fairly effective. Allergies based on T-cells have different symptoms from B-cell allergies, and are not relieved much by antihistamines. Certain of these allergies are referred to as "contact sensitivity," or "contact allergy." The most common is poison oak. Oils present in the poison oak plant attach to the skin components, modifying them and causing an immune response to the oil. No symptoms appear at first, because the immune response takes time to develop. On the second exposure, however, greatly increased numbers of T-cells bring about a toxic reaction that causes local inflammation. T-cell allergies are usually treated with corticosteroids, which directly suppress the immune response. Many allergies show both kinds of symptoms. Corticosteroids are often used to treat allergies in general, but they can have serious side effects that make prolonged use inadvisable.

Autoimmune Disease

The human immune system can recognize and attack an invading organism, but it also has the ability—usually carefully controlled—to attack a person's own tissues and organs. Fairly often, a body's self-recognition mechanisms break down. When such failures happen, the immune system may attack one of the body's organs. The thyroid gland is a frequent target, and some unfortunate people seem to have a genetic predisposition to autoimmune thyroid disease. One such disease is Hashimoto's thyroiditis. In this disease the organism produces both T-cells *and* antibodies that target the thyroid gland. The thyroid gland itself may eventually be destroyed. If so, the person must take thyroid hormone from animal sources, often for life. **Autoimmune** responses are suspected in many diseases, including rheumatoid arthritis and multiple sclerosis. Proof of the autoimmune origin of a disease is, however, extremely difficult to establish.

Controlling the immune response is clearly the key to controlling many diseases that still plague humankind. Recent studies have shown our ideas about the cellular interactions involved to be greatly oversimplified. The actual interactions are complex, specific, and full of feedback controls that have evolved over many millions of years. Unraveling this complexity is one of the chief preoccupations of medical research, and it is proceeding at an astounding speed. As these mechanisms are understood, it will be possible to prevent or cure many classes of disease, including infectious disease, autoimmune disease, and possibly cancer as well.

Exploring Your Emotions

Has anyone told you that a particular illness you have is "all in your mind," even though the symptoms (nausea, headache, running nose) are clearly real and uncomfortable? Can your mind trigger illness or predispose you to infection by lowering your natural resistance? If so, why has the medical profession expended so little effort in understanding the emotions, motivations, and thoughts of the "patient"?

Take Action

Your answers to the Exploring Your Emotions questions in this chapter and your placement level on the Wellness Ladder will, we hope, encourage you to begin a process of self-exploration and self-discovery that you will continue. Reflect on the entire chapter's content and ask yourself how each point relates to your own life. Then take action:

1. Find out what diseases you have been immunized against and list them in your Take Action notebook. Include the dates and note whether any further boosters are required.
2. Carefully observe the times you get a cold or cold symptoms. Note the date, time of day, actual symptoms, and your emotional state; for example, depressed, bored, and so forth. Also note how long it takes for the cold to run its course. Do you find any associations between your emotional state and the length of your colds?
3. List the positive behaviors that help you avoid or resist infection. Consider how you can strengthen these behaviors. List the behaviors that tend to block your positive behaviors. Consider which of these you can change.
4. Before leaving this chapter, review the Rate Yourself statements in this chapter. Have your feelings or values changed? Are you now better equipped to handle the complex and very human problems associated with infection and immunology?

Selected References

Kohler, G., and C. Milstein. (1974). Continuous cultures of fused cells secreting antibody of predefined specificity. *Nature* 256:495–97.

Springer, T. A., ed. 1985. *Hybridoma Technology in the Biosciences.* New York: Plenum Press.

Taylor-Papadimitriou, J., ed. 1985. *Interferon: The Impact in Biology and Medicine.* Oxford, England: Oxford University Press.

Unamue, E. R., and B. Benacerraf, eds. 1984. *Textbook of Immunology,* 2nd ed. Baltimore, Md.: Williams & Williams.

Recommended Readings

Cairns, J. 1978. *Cancer: Science and Society.* San Francisco: Freeman.
Excellent introduction to the general issue of cancer, and immunity to cancer. Still relevant and a pleasure to read, after 10 years!

Fields, B. N., and D. M. Knipe, eds. 1986. *Fundamental Virology.* New York: Raven Press.
A graduate-level text in human virology that is both challenging and highly readable.

Brown, T. A. 1986. *Gene Cloning: An Introduction.* New York: Van Nostrand Reinhold.
An introductory text for biology majors. The last chapter provides excellent examples of the medical and commercial applications of recombinant techniques.

Chapter 21

Contents

Rate Yourself

Your Awareness of Environmental Health Issues Read the following statements carefully. Choose the one in each section that best describes you at this moment and circle its number. When you have chosen one statement for each section, add the numbers and record your total score. Find your position on the Awareness Ladder.

5 Well educated about the environment's effect on health
4 Somewhat knowledgeable about the environment's effect on health
3 Can recall at least one recent issue about the environment and health
2 Very little interest in the environment and health
1 No interest in the environment and health

5 Picks up litter left by others
4 Complains to others about littering
3 Strictly observes the laws about littering
2 Occasionally throws litter on the ground
1 Frequently throws litter on the ground

5 Well educated about food storage
4 Knows how to avoid food poisoning
3 Refrigerates left over foods
2 Leaves foods at room temperature overnight
1 Occasionally eats bad food

5 Knowledgeable about the effects of noise pollution
4 Protects self from loud or persistent noise
3 Avoids loud or persistent noise
2 Occasionally exposes self to loud, persistent noise
1 Frequently exposes self to loud. persistent noise

5 Knows what agencies are responsible for environmental health
4 Knows how to get in touch with a public health agency
3 Vaguely familiar with the Environmental Protection Agency
2 Unfamiliar with environmental health agencies
1 Resistant to pursuing information about environmental agencies

Total Score ______

Environmental Health

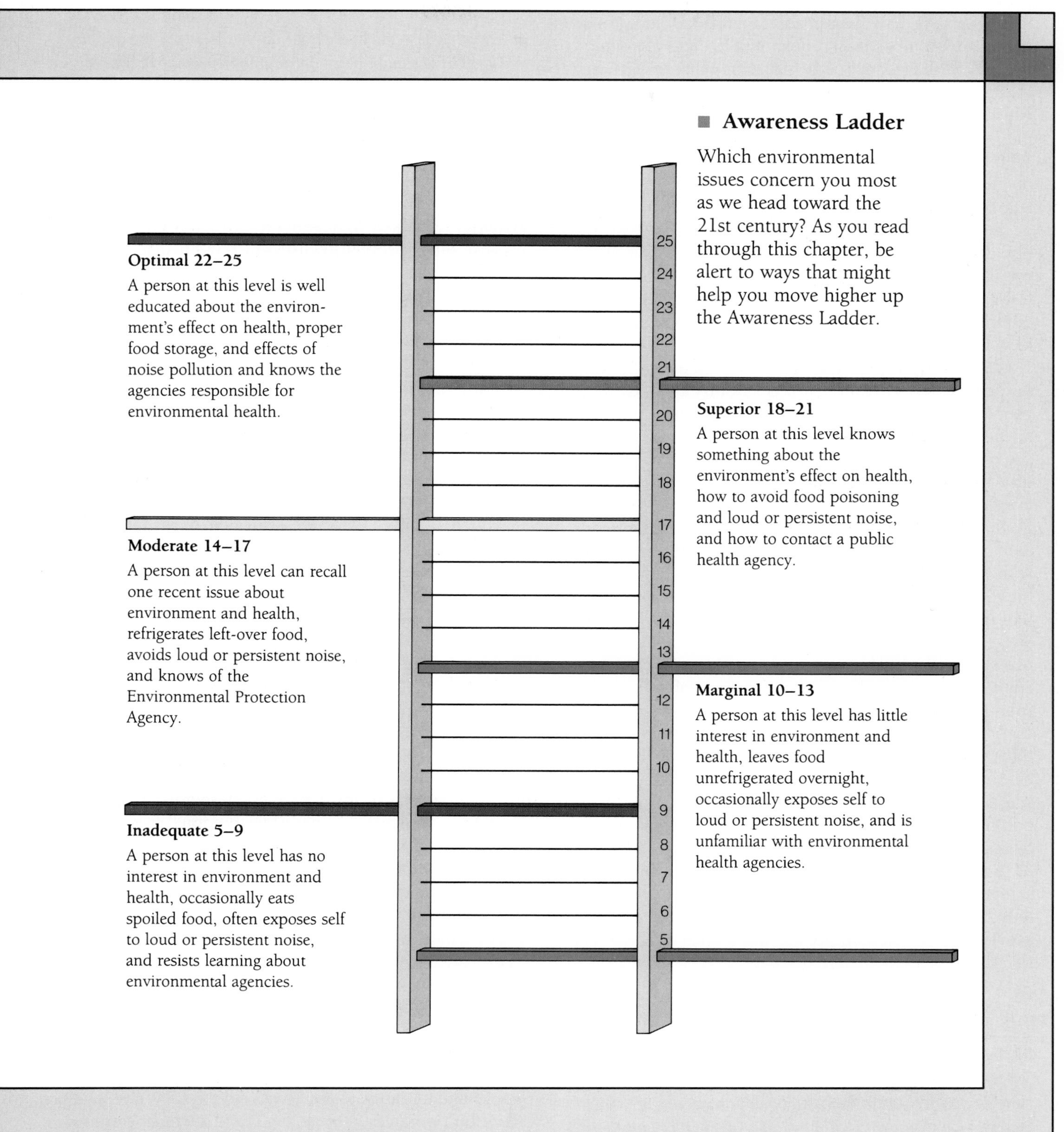

Optimal 22–25
A person at this level is well educated about the environment's effect on health, proper food storage, and effects of noise pollution and knows the agencies responsible for environmental health.

Superior 18–21
A person at this level knows something about the environment's effect on health, how to avoid food poisoning and loud or persistent noise, and how to contact a public health agency.

Moderate 14–17
A person at this level can recall one recent issue about environment and health, refrigerates left-over food, avoids loud or persistent noise, and knows of the Environmental Protection Agency.

Marginal 10–13
A person at this level has little interest in environment and health, leaves food unrefrigerated overnight, occasionally exposes self to loud or persistent noise, and is unfamiliar with environmental health agencies.

Inadequate 5–9
A person at this level has no interest in environment and health, occasionally eats spoiled food, often exposes self to loud or persistent noise, and resists learning about environmental agencies.

Awareness Ladder

Which environmental issues concern you most as we head toward the 21st century? As you read through this chapter, be alert to ways that might help you move higher up the Awareness Ladder.

We have always struggled against all that surrounds us—our environment. We have faced forces of nature, animals, and other humans, all of which have caused health problems and shortened the human life span. Since the mid-1800s we have begun to recognize additional and potentially more serious problems. The field of environmental health grew out of the realization that as we industrialize and move to cities in mass migrations, we also concentrate by-products of our activities. The list of examples seems endless, ranging from sewage to throwaway milk bottles, from wastes generated from industrial production that seep into groundwaters, to asbestos in insulation, from mosquito-transmitted diseases to the dangers of the chemicals used to control mosquitoes. And more than just the urban areas are affected. Acid rain, a by-product of generating power, threatens lakes hundreds of miles from the source of emissions. Thousands of acres of jungles are destroyed daily to provide wood and grow food for people in cities.

Although these problems are not new, they are far more serious than ever because of three reasons. First, far more people are living on the planet than ever before and they are much more concentrated in urban areas. This density places demands on resources that are not equally distributed throughout the environment. When people lived far from other groups, they usually lived in small, self-sufficient groups. Each group's environment could provide food, water, and take care of wastes without overlapping with another. Today, for example, one cannot even imagine each family in Los Angeles having its own well and a plot of land to grow food.

Second, our technology has allowed us to greatly increase our standard of living and even our life span. But this increase has costs. There are always tradeoffs. Some by-products of our technology are becoming concentrated in the environment in ways that are much more harmful than any naturally occurring hazard. With the exception of solar and water-generated electricity, our power sources—on which we have become so dependent—are not clean: they threaten the air with emissions ranging from sulfur dioxide to radiation. Our technology also allows us to make a far greater impact on the environment, in a shorter period of time, than ever before. Where it once took one worker a day to cut down a dozen trees to provide lumber, new equipment allows that same worker to clear more than an acre per day.

Exploring Your Emotions

How do you feel about human population growth in your lifetime? Do you want to limit it? How should growth limits affect the United States? third world countries?

Exploring Your Emotions

Do you feel human survival must take precedence over the survival of other species? Do you feel all human beings have an equal right to survival? How do you feel conflicts for limited resources should be resolved among people? Between humans and other species?

Third, a fundamental rule in environmental health is that "everything is related to everything else." All our activities are linked. We cannot dump sewage into a river, because other people downstream rely on that river for drinking water. We cannot allow mercury to enter water supplies because mercury concentrates in the food chain and will come back to affect our health. For example, the federal government warned in 1987 that we should not eat fish longer than thirty inches from Lake Superior—long thought to be not only the largest, but the cleanest of all freshwater supplies in the world.

Some environmental problems, such as the need for clean water, will always be with us. And new problems are and will be generated daily. The ecology movement of the 1970s increased our awareness of the fragile world in which we live. Once we struggled on a daily basis against the environment in order to survive; now we need to be conscious that we must protect the environment in order to protect ourselves. Our survival depends on making the right decisions and the right tradeoffs.

In this chapter we explore classical environmental health problems, which we still face on a daily basis, as well as new problems brought on by increased technological development and population growth. The classic, or historical, areas of environmental health include clean water, sewage and solid waste disposal, food and milk inspection, and rodent and insect control. Every time we camp in the wilderness or travel to a less developed area, these "historical" concerns immediately become important to us. Each time a flood, an earthquake, or a tornado damages a community, these areas become of prime importance. More modern concerns include air pollution, toxic wastes, radiation, and noise pollution.

A balance must always be reached. There is no doubt that today the environment is cleaner in most parts of the world than it has been since the Industrial Revolution. Since the 1960s, London has not had "killer smogs," nor have thousands been killed and disabled by a single-location mercury discharge in Japan. When we look carefully at environmental conditions of the past, very few of us would like to return to the "good old days." We've made significant progress in some areas, and we must continue to make progress as conservators of our planet for future generations. But at the same time, we need to keep in

Coagulate To cause separate molecules in a solution to be attracted to one another in large enough groups to settle out of the solution.

Sedimentation The process of allowing coagulated solids to settle out of water as part of filtering.

Coliform test A measure of the quantity of *E. coli* bacteria in water to determine if it has been contaminated with fecal matter and hence might be a vehicle for infectious disease.

Fluoridation The addition of fluoride to the water supply, which reduces tooth decay.

---

mind that the importance of environmental health is always relative to other health problems. Saving the lives of millions of people from starvation may be more important than the buildup of chemicals used in food production, at least in the short run. At each decision point, there is a tradeoff. That is the nature of the problem facing environmental health today. We cannot allow ourselves to become oriented to only one issue at a time, because most environmental issues are interrelated.

Clean Water

Few parts of the world have adequate quantities of safe, clean drinking water, and yet few things are as important to human health. Although water seems to be all around us, easily obtainable fresh water amounts to only 0.2 percent of the world's total supply of water. What we take for granted each time we turn on a faucet is really the product of a great revolution in the way we thought about disease transmission. In 1854, in London, John Snow showed a relationship between contaminated well water and cholera. Other researchers followed, proving that several infectious diseases could be transmitted by water. Until then, clean water wasn't a high priority. In the latter half of the 1800s in both Great Britain and the United States, governments and private companies began building complex water systems that brought clean water right into buildings. Instead of everyone having a well (as still occurs in rural areas), urban water came under governmental inspection, and in most instances the government provided it, too. As a result, disease rates for cholera, typhoid, and other water-borne diseases fell sharply by 1900 and are very rare today in areas that have municipal water supplies. As urban populations increased, cities often had to find lakes and rivers to supplement wells. Because such surface water is more likely to be "dirty"—containing both organic matter as well as disease organisms—water treatment plants purify the water before piping it into the community.

As water is pumped into a treatment facility from a river, lake, or well, workers add chemicals to **coagulate** the suspended solids. The water is then allowed to stand while the coagulated solids settle to the bottom in a process called **sedimentation**. The water is then filtered, disinfected, and (in many communities) fluoridated before being introduced into the water supply system. Filtering removes many of the odors and the remaining suspended solids. Disinfection is accomplished by adding chemicals such as chlorine in small quantities to kill disease-producing organisms. A **Coliform test** is frequently performed to determine if any of these organisms are still living. Instead of testing for all organisms, the *E. coli* bacterium, which is relatively easy to detect, is used as a marker. If all the *E. coli* are killed, then the water is generally considered to be free of disease-causing organisms. **Fluoridation** adds the fluoride ion to the water supply, which has been proven to reduce tooth decay by 60 to 65 percent.

As we move toward the year 2000, clean water, or the shortage of it, is once again becoming a matter of global concern. Many supplies of water, either on the surface or in groundwater, are becoming polluted with hazardous chemicals. Some parts of the United States are experiencing rapid growths of population that outstrip their ability to provide adequate amounts of water at all. Many proposals are being discussed to relieve these shortages, including diverting water from the Great Lakes to the Southwest.

Whatever the outcome of long-range proposals, two actions are now being implemented. One involves minimizing pollution of all waters with hazardous wastes. While many people might believe that this primarily is aimed at large manufacturing concerns, the total accumulated effect of hazardous household wastes is also important. All freshwater supplies must be treated as if they will be needed as a source of drinking water in the future. The second action involves a rethinking of our water distribution system. Most cities usually have just one system that provides "treated" water to homes, industry, and agriculture alike. However, not all that water has to be treated to the same level of purity and safety as your drinking water. The water you use to wash a car or water a lawn does not have to meet the same standards as the water you drink. As treatment becomes more expensive and as the cleanest water becomes more scarce, cities may have to develop several levels of distribution based on intended use, which may be less costly than treating *all* water.

Waste Disposal

Humans generate large amounts of waste, which must be handled in an appropriate manner if we are to live in a safe and sanitary environment. Some of this waste is sew-

Septic system A self-contained sewage disposal system for one family, used in rural areas.

Biochemical oxygen demand (BOD) A test done on waste water to determine the amount of dissolved nutrients. High amounts of dissolved nutrients compete with existing life forms in lakes and rivers for oxygen.

Polychlorobiphenyl (PCB) An industrial chemical used as an insulator in electrical transformers, among other uses, which is linked to cancers in humans.

Trichinosis A parasite-caused disease once commonly transmitted through poorly cooked pork.

age composed of human excrement, some is garbage from food materials, and some is solid waste, which is a by-product of our "throw-away" society. If proper attention is not paid to the disposal of these wastes, significant diseases can occur that could threaten entire populations.

Sewage One of the great advances in public health in the last one hundred and fifty years was the development of safe, and relatively inexpensive, ways in which human wastes could be disposed. Many of the great killing diseases, such as typhoid and cholera, and the disabling diseases, such as hookworm and some forms of hepatitis, are spread by contact with fecal matter, which was simply deposited at random. Until recently, very little regard was given to separating sewage from sources of drinking water or human habitation.

For example, the development of the outhouse, or privy, did much to control hookworm in the southern United States. This parasite can be transmitted by walking barefooted on grass or soil contaminated by fecal matter. Not only were people instructed how to build outhouses, they were also taught where to locate them—away from potential water sources. As plumbing moved indoors, sewage disposal became more complicated. In rural areas the **septic system**, which is a self-contained sewage disposal system for one family, has worked quite well.

As large numbers of people began to congregate in cities, the separation of sewage and drinking water became a critical element in the survival and growth of such urban areas. Many early cities developed on rivers. The inhabitants took their drinking water from upstream and dumped their sewage downstream. For small populations, this tended to work fairly well as long as the cities were sufficiently separated. Rivers and lakes can "clean themselves" if they are not overloaded by organic wastes that can be rendered harmless by naturally occurring bacteria and dilution.

Exploring Your Emotions

A neighboring city, one that has placed no limits on growth for the past decade, plans to release sewage into the river that flows past your home in a small rural community. How do you feel, and how will you handle your feelings?

City growth meant crowding, and since each city dweller could not drill a well and have his or her own septic system, government had to regulate water supplies and waste disposal for health reasons. Often that meant providing water and sewage hook-ups. So important to health are these services that in most states or large cities the health department supervises these functions, rather than just another utility such as a power company.

Most cities have sewage treatment systems that separate biologic matter from huge quantities of water and stabilize it so that it cannot transmit infectious diseases. This is done in huge separating tanks and stabilization ponds. A test for **biochemical oxygen demand (BOD)** is performed to measure the amount of organic matter in the waste water. This check assures that the water being released back into the environment will not overload the lake or river with nutrients, which leads to algal growths or blooms. Not only are these growths unsightly and smelly, but they also can "choke out" animal life such as fish. Once treated, the now biologically safe water can be released back into the environment. The remaining sludge may be spread on fields as fertilizer if free from heavy metal contamination, or may be burned or buried.

Many cities have now begun to further treat sewage to remove heavy metals and other hazardous chemicals. This is a result of many studies linking exposure to such chemicals as mercury, lead, and **polychlorinated biphenyls, or PCBs**, to long-term health consequences, including destruction of the central nervous system and cancer. Any system that collects and concentrates these chemicals from an entire city should not dump them back into the environment where they might contaminate a present or future water source. The technology to effectively remove heavy metals and chemicals is still developing, and the costs are immense.

Solid Waste Disposal Solid waste disposal in the United States has changed drastically in the last thirty years. Until recently, a primary component of household solid waste was garbage—food and cooking wastes. It had to be disposed of in a way that would not spread disease. Hence governments developed health regulations about feeding garbage to pigs, to prevent **trichinosis** (a worm disease transmitted to humans through poorly cooked pork), and regulations about garbage cans so as to minimize the number of insects or animals attracted. Usually garbage

Toxic Waste Clean-up

In the early 1970's, the public concern over clean air and clean water led Congress to establish the Environmental Protection Agency (EPA), which was designated as the primary agency to protect and clean up the environment. In its first fifteen years, the EPA was able to secure major legislation and funding to promote programs such as the Superfund bill of 1980, which allocated $1.6 billion in a five-year "crash" program to clean up thousands of leaking toxic waste dump sites.

The size of the problem is tremendous. For example, more than 66,000 chemicals are now in use in the United States, and the EPA has classified 60,000 of them as either potentially or definitely hazardous to human health. The EPA estimates that 247 million metric tons of hazardous wastes subject to governmental regulation are generated yearly. The EPA's Superfund data base lists more than 25,000 potentially hazardous waste sites in the United States. Of these, the Office of Technology Assessment contends that at least 10,000 sites pose a serious threat to human health. The General Accounting Office estimates that 378,000 waste sites may require corrective action. The cost may reach as much as $100 billion, or more than $1,000 per household.

In 1986, as the Superfund was being re-funded for a second five-year period, critics pointed out that the original appropriation of $1.6 billion only resulted in the complete clean-up of 13 sites and the beginning clean-up of an additional 500 sites. In other words, the task was barely begun. The legislative review did lead to several conclusions. First, it is difficult to start such an immense project from scratch. We are not finding simple ways to dispose of wastes currently being manufactured. We are also having to deal with those improperly disposed of since the start of the Industrial Revolution. In fact, there were no rules at all for the disposal of wastes in the United States until the Resource Conservation and Recovery Act of 1976. Second, there was mismanagement in the early days of the Superfund, which, when combined with an effort to limit government regulation, severely hampered progress in reaching even minimal goals. Third, basic technology such as how one might safely burn these wastes had to be developed. Fourth, and most important, until the EPA started to investigate the magnitude of the problem, no one realistically estimated the huge number of chemicals, sites, and costs involved. Therefore, the reauthorization of the Superfund in 1986 allotted $9 billion, or a five-fold increase over the second five-year-period of the Superfund. Even that will not be nearly enough.

Many of the chemicals involved have become familiar terms to the general public: dioxin, vinyl chloride, PCB, lead, mercury, and arsenic, to name just a few. The major concern is that toxic dump sites frequently leak into surrounding groundwaters that supply drinking water for humans and other animals. Up until now, the standard acceptable means of disposal has been to bury chemicals, often in metal drums. The drums would corrode and leak, records were not kept as to where they were buried, soil conditions were not determined to anticipate leaching into groundwaters, and surrounding groundwaters were not monitored for signs of contamination. This means that water for half of the U.S. population is threatened by poisons leaching into the ground. The EPA's new first priority is to protect the drinking water from seepage of toxic chemicals and then to worry about disposing both new and existing stockpiles.

The discussions surrounding the Superfund Amendments and Reauthorization Act of 1986 disclosed several new directions in toxic waste management. First, and most important, most experts now look at even the best of landfills as temporary solutions. Eventually all will leak over time. The options to landfills are not numerous. Some toxic wastes can be recycled. In fact, the majority of toxic wastes are now taken care of at the manufacturing site and are not transported. Other wastes can be chemically or biologically converted into stabilized solids. Some will have to be stored in secure deep wells. One of the most promising solutions is high temperature burning, either on land or at sea, with the resulting nontoxic ash buried in existing-technology landfills. Second, liability will become more important as sources of dumped wastes are traced back to companies or individuals to determine who should pay for clean-up. Third, states are mandated to have a twenty-year disposal capacity plan lined up by 1990. Most states currently do not even have a plan

(continued on next page)

Toxic Waste Clean-up (*continued*)

for the next year, and many rely on shipping wastes to other states—an option that will be even less available. None of this is going to be easy or inexpensive.

While various polls indicate that the U.S. population is increasingly concerned about hazardous wastes and a clean environment, it is also true that the biggest obstacle faced by public officials in their efforts to clean up the environment is the NIMBY (Not In My Backyard) syndrome. No one wants a hazardous waste disposal site, whether it be landfill or incineration, near their property. An additional worry is that many U.S. companies are finding manufacturing that involves paying for safe disposal of hazardous by-products too expensive to compete in the marketplace; they are moving these plants to other countries that have less stringent rules. Assuming that we all share the planet, environmentalist Barry Commoner's poignant assertion that "we are poisoning ourselves and our posterity" takes on an even more important meaning. We are either going to have to pay now or later.

was carted to the town dump, burned, and never thought about again. Technology has changed that practice.

The advent of the mechanical garbage grinder or disposal and the proliferation of disposable products, have changed the composition of the solid waste we throw away. The garbage often now ends up in the sewage treatment system, which may not be able to deal with the additional organic load. We are left with huge amounts of material that is not very hazardous from the standpoint of infectious disease, but does represent an enormous problem in terms of where to put it and how to protect the environment from chemical contamination.

The average U.S. citizen generates more than one ton of solid waste per year. This amount contains little food garbage and is now burned or buried. Both means of disposal present problems. Much of our solid waste contains chemicals, ranging from leftover pesticides to paints and oils, which should not be indiscriminately released into the environment. Burning reduces the bulk or mass, but may release hazardous materials into the air. Earth burial is expensive, requires huge amounts of space, may contaminate groundwater, and is socially unpopular—no one wants a disposal site near his or her home.

By the end of the 1800s, garbage and solid waste was being placed in a location at the edge of town called a *dump*. Very little attention was paid to what happened at the dump—it just had to be out of sight and away from homes. Then in the 1960s, **sanitary landfill** for earth burial of wastes became the next major development in solid waste disposal. Site selection and daily management become essential in a safe sanitary landfill. First, a thorough study is done on the site to make certain that it is not near groundwater, streams, or any other source of water that could be contaminated by leakage from the landfill. This includes looking at soil composition under and around the site to make certain that materials cannot leach, or seep, from the area. Sometimes protective liners are used, and most states are beginning to require monitoring wells. Second, layers of waste are covered with thin layers of dirt on a regular basis until the site is filled. Some communities then plant grass and trees and convert the site into a park.

Because of the expense and potential chemical hazards posed by any form of solid waste disposal, most communities encourage individuals and businesses to cooperate with recycling programs. Cities, businesses, and groups of citizens organize to encourage the separation of materials that can be "recycled" into new products. Some cities offer home pickup, and others require you to bring materials to recycling centers. These materials are not limited to paper, glass, and cans, but also include such things as discarded tires and used oils. By participating in recycling, we can slow the rate at which we use natural resources, reduce the cost of solid waste disposal, and gain time to develop more environmentally efficient methods of packaging and disposal.

Exploring Your Emotions

You discover that unmarked trucks carrying unmarked barrels of something are being routed through your residential area in the very early morning and dumping at a sanitary landfill site about a mile away from your home. How do you feel, and what will you do about your feelings? How would you feel and do about trains carrying nuclear waste through urban areas, headed for disposal sites in another state?

Sanitary landfill A special disposal site for solid wastes where there is some assurance that groundwater will not become contaminated.

Salmonella infection An often food-borne bacterial infection caused by eating food contaminated with fecal matter, such as improperly cleaned and cooked chicken.

Staphylococci A group of bacteria, found on the skin, that can cause food-borne infections if allowed to multiply in bland foods.

Miasma Bad-smelling air, which was thought to cause disease before germ theory became accepted.

Malaria A mosquito-borne disease marked by chills and fever. Malaria has killed more humans in history than any other cause.

Encephalitis An inflammation of the brain sometimes caused by insect-borne diseases.

Solid waste is not limited to household products. Manufacturing, cattle production, and mining all produce large amounts of materials that cannot simply be dumped. The experiences of communities such as Love Canal near Buffalo, New York, and Times Beach, Missouri, point out the dangers of careless disposal of toxic wastes. At Love Canal toxic wastes from industry had been dumped into a waterway for years until the 1970s when nearby residents began to suffer from associated birth defects and cancers. At Times Beach, oil contaminated with carcinogenic PCBs was spread on roads instead of being dumped in a landfill. In both cases, human health was affected, government had to step in, people had to move from homes, and huge costs were incurred.

Food and Milk Inspection

Today we take for granted that the food and milk we buy in grocery stores and in restaurants is safe to consume. This has not always been the case in the United States. At the turn of the century, tremendous pressure was put on the government to set minimum standards in all areas of food preparation and handling, resulting in the Pure Food and Drug Act of 1906. Illness and death associated with food-borne diseases, or toxic food additives, has decreased substantially ever since. However, we are now becoming more concerned with the long-term health consequences of the foods we eat, either because of chemical contamination or characteristics of the foods themselves.

Most people would be surprised at the number of agencies that inspect food at the various points of production. On the federal level, the Department of Agriculture inspects grains and meats, the Department of Commerce inspects some fish, and the Food and Drug Administration inspects most other food products. On the state level, inspectors examine dairy herds, milking barns, storage tanks, tankers that transport milk, and processing plants. Local health departments inspect and license restaurants.

Considering the number of meals eaten outside the home, and the number of meals prepared at home with purchased food, it is remarkable how few instances there are of food-borne illness or death. The food distribution system in the United States is very safe and efficient. Recalls of ice cream, cheese, and tuna in recent years have usually been based on a potential for illness because of a processing error, not on actual illness or death. In fact, most food-associated illnesses are caused by contamination in the home. For example, failing to wash a knife and cutting board after preparing raw chicken may lead to **salmonella infections**. Cooking the chicken will kill the salmonella bacteria, but the knife and board may contaminate other foods such as lettuce for a salad, which would not usually be cooked. Failure to refrigerate a bland food such as cold pasta salad or creampuffs may lead to a **staphylococci** poisoning. This common bacterium lives on the skin and can produce a toxin in foods left at room temperature. It is estimated that each person in the United States suffers an average of two to three episodes of food infection or poisoning every year. Rarely do they associate the discomfort with food they have eaten; instead, they call it a twenty-four-hour influenza (which is in fact a completely different disease with different symptoms).

Insect and Rodent Control

We have only known for a hundred years that insects and rodents could transmit disease. For most of history, people believed that bad odors, or **miasmas**, caused many diseases such as yellow fever and malaria (two diseases that may have accounted for more deaths in the history of the world than any other cause). In fact the very term **malaria** derives from the Greek for "bad air." This ignorance not only limited human life expectancy but also technological development. For example, several thousand people died of these two diseases while attempts were made to build the Panama Canal. Not until the role of mosquitoes was determined, and methods used to control them, could the canal be completed.

We now fully appreciate that continuous vigilance is necessary to minimize illness associated with insects and rodents. The number of diseases that can be transmitted to people from these sources is very large. In recent years we have seen outbreaks of **encephalitis** traced to mos-

Lyme disease A newly discovered disease that is spread by a deer tick and that can lead to fever and arthritis-like conditions if untreated.

Rocky Mountain spotted fever A wood-tick-borne disease causing high fevers and found primarily in the Southeast.

Typhus A louse-born fever disease associated with crowding and poor sanitation.

quitoes, **Lyme disease** from ticks in the Midwest, **Rocky Mountain spotted fever** from another type of tick in the Southeast, and even plague from fleas on rodents in the West. Rodents carry forms of **typhus**, salmonella, and even tapeworms.

Pollution

We often take for granted all the classic areas of environmental health just discussed. We don't realize that a huge, complex health system with a goal of prevention is at work behind the scenes. We are saved from countless illnesses and enjoy a longer life expectancy because daily attention is paid to the details of these traditional concerns. In addition, all these concerns are connected. For example, untreated sewage can attract disease-carrying insects and improperly treated sewage can contaminate water supplies.

Each of these areas continues to take on added significance as our technologies and our population growth contribute to new twists on old problems. For example, in cattle raising the antibiotics used to minimize bacteria that could be harmful for human consumption may foster the development of more resistant strains of bacteria, which may create more serious problems (see Chapter 20). At the same time, "new" areas of concern are being added to the environmental health field, which often are problems that have been around for a long time, but where public awareness is just now being raised.

Many of these modern problems are "pollution" problems. This term has taken on a general meaning for unsightly, noisy, smelly nuisances in our surroundings. The level of concentration becomes most important when we talk about health risks. In normal concentrations, very little evidence suggests that environmental pollutants harm our general health.

Air Pollution The air around us is constantly being "polluted" by nature with each forest fire, pollen bloom, and dust storm, as well as from countless other pollutants. To these natural sources, human beings have always contributed additional by-products of their activities. There-

(text continues on p. 499.)

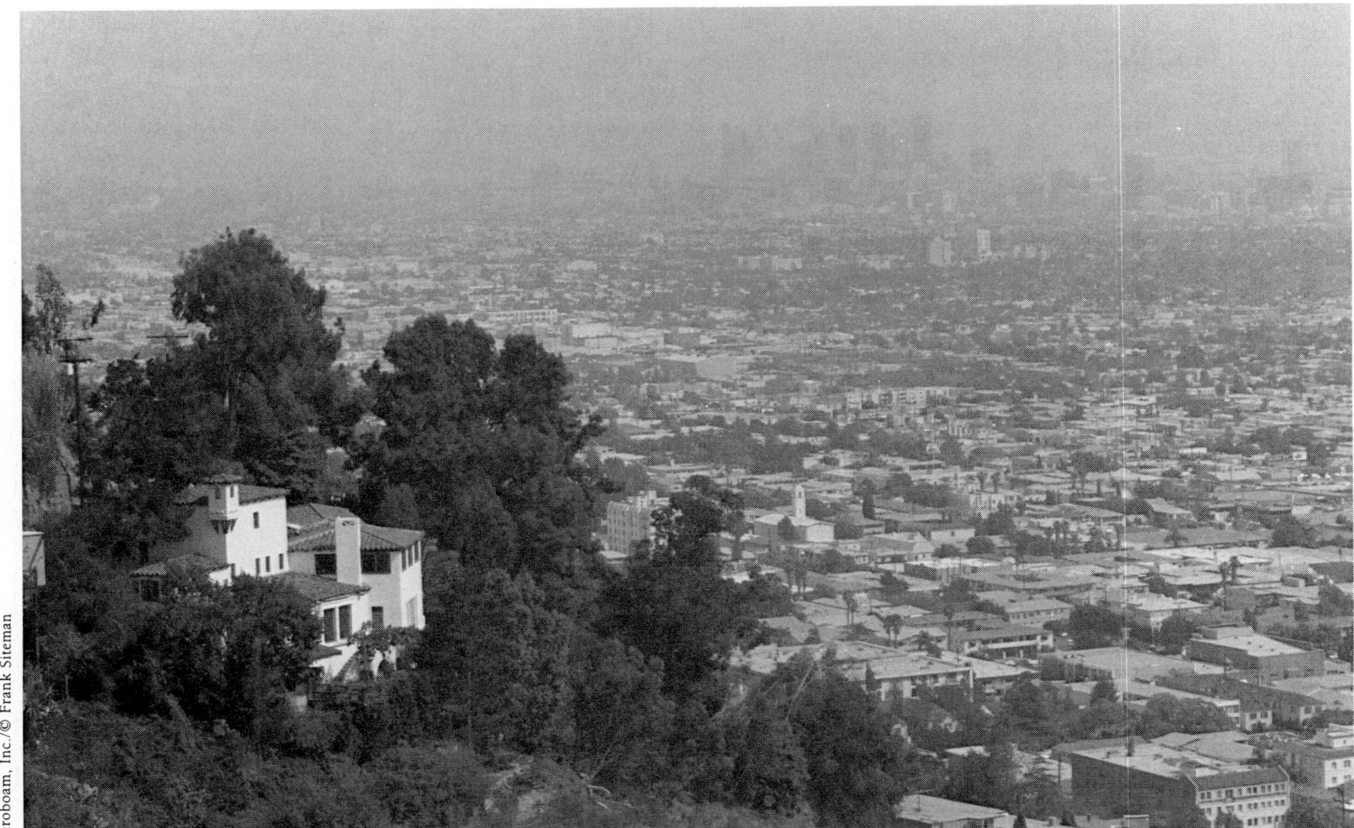

Jeroboam, Inc./© Frank Siteman

Indoor Air Pollution

If you think housework is killing you, you may be right. Your home could be harboring such potentially dangerous pollutants as asbestos, radon gas, benzene, and many more.

Some of these trigger allergic responses. Others have been linked to cancer in laboratory animals. Still others have been documented as causing human cancer. In fact, the U.S. Environmental Protection Agency has reported that toxic chemicals found in the home are three times more likely to cause cancer than outdoor airborne pollutants, even in areas near chemical plants.

In well-ventilated homes these indoor pollutants are found at very low levels. But as people try to save energy by adding insulation and weatherstripping to their homes, they are also trapping these unwanted hazards inside.

And chemical exposure can be cumulative: inhaling a single pollutant may not make you sick, but the more chemicals you are exposed to, the greater the chance of your health suffering.

You may bring some of these chemicals home with you. For instance, you are exposed to benzene vapors every time you fill up at a service station. The vapors get in your clothes and are later released into the air at home. Tetrachloroethylene follows you home from the dry cleaners, clinging to newly cleaned clothes.

Other indoor health hazards may be built into your home. One of the most widely publicized is asbestos. Commonly found in home insulation or wrapped around pipes in a basement or crawl space, asbestos is made up of tiny mineral fibers which, when released into the air and inhaled, can trigger cancer.

But the mere presence of asbestos insulation in your home does not necessarily put you at risk, according to Environmental Protection Agency scientist Terry Stanuch:

"If you do have asbestos in your home, it's not always a bad thing. Asbestos in your walls is no problem because it's sealed off from the living area. The same is true if it's wrapped around pipes in the basement. If the sheathing is in good shape, then leave it alone."

The danger, Stanuch explains, comes when asbestos fibers are exposed to the ambient air in the living area of your home. This can happen when the asbestos is damaged or worn.

"Look for areas of friable material in your home—that is, areas where the insulation is exposed and easily crumbled by hand. If the insulation is not obviously fiberglass, it's probably asbestos."

If you are unsure whether the material is asbestos, you can send a sample, about one inch on a side, to a lab for testing. Your local environmental agency can provide you with a list of labs that conduct such tests. The testing cost is about $25 to $40.

"Even if you find friable asbestos, it's not always necessary to have it removed," Stanuch says. "In many cases, if you're dealing with a small area, such as insulation wrapped around a pipe, you can seal the friable area yourself with a mastic paste or plaster."

If the area is too large to seal off, removal may be required. But, Stanuch warns, do not try to remove asbestos yourself. "Get in touch with contractors in your area and ask them if they are trained to remove asbestos. You can check with the EPA to confirm their qualifications."

Radon gas is another indoor pollutant that has received a lot of publicity recently. It is a colorless, odorless gas found in high concentrations in the soil in scattered areas throughout North America. It is a natural by-product of the decay of uranium and thorium, radioactive elements that occur naturally in the earth.

When radon gas is released into the atmosphere, it dissipates harmlessly. It only becomes a hazard when it seeps into a closed structure, such as a home, and then it can be a very real hazard indeed. The Centers for Disease Control estimate that as many as 5,000 to 20,000 excess lung cancer deaths each year are attributable to radon gas.

"The main route of seepage is through the soil around the foundation of a home, or through cracks in basement walls that expose the basement to the soil," says EPA health physicist Larry Jensen. "The gas can also seep into a home by coming up through the exposed earth in a crawl space."

Once inside an enclosed space, radon gas breaks down into tiny radioactive particles called "daughters," Jensen says. These particles, which have a radioactive half-life of 3.8 days, will cling to dust particles in your home, floating on air currents until they are inhaled. Then they irradiate the lung tissue, increasing your risk of cancer.

There are no safe levels of radon exposure, but the U.S. EPA has set the "level of concern" at .4 picocuries per liter of air. You can have

(continued on next page)

Indoor Air Pollution (*continued*)

your own air tested for about $12 to $50. The EPA or your local health or environmental agency can provide a list of firms that will conduct the test.

What do you do if you find higher-than-normal levels of radon in your home?

"Seal your basement—cracks, seams—cover the sump pump and cover the bare earth in the crawl space," Jensen says. "Then increase the ventilation, either with fans built into the block wall or by installing what is called an air-to-air heat exchanger. We find that the heat exchanger is an efficient and cost-effective means of ventilating your home."

While asbestos and radon are two of the better-known indoor environmental dangers, dozens of others may be lurking undetected in your home. Here are some you should be aware of.

Carbon monoxide is produced when carbon-bearing fuels—petroleum products and wood—are burned. Improperly vented gas appliances, woodburning stoves and kerosene heaters, as well as simple tobacco smoke, all raise indoor carbon monoxide levels. It can also enter your house when a vehicle is idling in an attached garage or near the house. At moderate levels, carbon monoxide can cause headaches and irregular heartbeat. At higher levels, it can cause loss of consciousness and death.

Formaldehyde gas seeping from resins used in manufacturing particle board, plywood paneling, and some carpeting and upholstery can cause headaches, dizziness, nausea, rashes, and eye and throat irritation. Some studies have linked formaldehyde exposure to cancer.

Found in some air fresheners and in moth ball crystals, **paradichlorobenzene** has been linked to cancer in laboratory animals.

Trichloroethane is an ingredient in some aerosol sprays. Prolonged exposure can cause dizziness and irregular breathing.

Removing the sources of these indoor air pollutants can sometimes be a costly and complicated business. Fortunately you can protect yourself to a large extent by using a little common sense.

- Be sure your house is adequately ventilated, including the basement. This will keep down levels of indoor airborne pollutants.
- Follow manufacturer's directions when using a product that emits pollutants. Use the proper protective equipment. Be sure your work space is very well ventilated—opening a window may not be adequate to safely work with some products. Install an exhaust fan, or, if possible, move the project outside. Note whether the product should be kept away from heat sources.
- Keep paints and cleaning solvents in the original, tightly sealed containers and store them in cool, well-vented areas. Discard partially empty containers unless you're sure you'll use the rest of the product soon.
- Clean air conditioners, air ducts, air filters, heat exchangers, and humidifiers regularly. They are all potential sources of allergens or disease-producing organisms.
- If you have gas appliances, check them regularly to make sure the pilot lights are burning with a clear blue flame. Burning gas produces small amounts of carbon monoxide and other harmful by-products, and when the pilots aren't burning cleanly, they give off even more pollutants. If you're buying new gas appliances, you might want to consider ones with spark ignition systems, which eliminate the need for pilot lights.

SOURCE: Mitch Coleman, 1986–87 (Winter), Air pollution: The inside story, *Family Safety & Health*, pp. 5–6.

Paradichlorobenzene A chemical found in some air fresheners and mothballs, linked to cancer formation in animals.

Trichloroethane A propellant in some aerosol spray cans that can cause dizziness, irregular respiration, and heartbeat.

Chronic obstructive pulmonary disease A general term for respiratory diseases such as emphysema and chronic bronchitis, which interfere with human oxygen intake.

Congestive heart failure One of the main results of heart diseases, where the heart cannot pump enough oxygenated blood because the system is overwhelmed with fluid.

Temperature inversion A weather condition whereby a cold layer of air becomes trapped by a warm layer, so that pollutants cannot be dispersed.

London-type smog An air pollution problem whose source is the result of industrial burning of coal.

Los Angeles-type smog An air pollution problem whose source is burning of transportation fuels in combination with sunlight.

Photochemical smog Another term for Los Angeles-type smog; caused by sunlight (hence "photo") reacting with transportation fuels (hence "chemical").

Greenhouse effect A theoretical warming of the earth due to a buildup of carbon dioxide.

---

fore, air pollution is not a new problem. During the Industrial Revolution, English cities had far more daily air pollution than we can observe or even imagine today. However, two things have happened to cause us to rethink our attitudes toward air pollution. First, we are living long enough to realize both the long-term and short-term health consequences. Second, increased population growth, combined with more industrialization using old technologies, concentrates problems and makes them more visible.

Air pollution can be more than just unsightly, it can cause illness and death if pollutants become concentrated for a period of several days or weeks. The first such situations came in the Meuse Valley in Belgium (1930) and Donora, Pennsylvania (1948). Public attention became focused when London (1952) and New York City (1963) experienced air pollution disasters that made thousands ill and caused hundreds of premature deaths, primarily among those who already had respiratory problems. Increased carbon monoxide and decreased oxygen, as well as airborne acids, all put excess strain on people suffering from **chronic obstructive pulmonary diseases**, such as chronic bronchitis or emphysema, and **congestive heart failure**.

In order to set the stage for an air pollution emergency such as the four just mentioned, three conditions must be present. First, there must be a source of pollution. Today, this is most frequently provided by the burning of fossil fuels, such as coal in industry or gasoline in cars. Second, there must be a topographical feature, such as a mountain range or a valley, that minimizes the possibility that prevailing winds could push stagnant air out of the region. Third, there must be a weather event called a **temperature inversion.**

A temperature inversion takes place when there is little or no wind and a layer of warm air traps a layer of cold air next to the ground. Normally, the sun heats the earth, making the air closest to the ground warmer than that just above it. Warm air rises and is replaced by cooler air, which in turn is warmed and rises, thereby causing a natural vertical circulation. This vertical circulation, combined with horizontal wind circulation, prevents pollutants from reaching dangerous levels of concentration. However, a temperature inversion prevents this replacement and cleansing action. The effect is like capping an area with a dome that traps all the pollutants. During an inversion, cool air at the earth's surface is trapped under a layer of warmer air, so vertical dispersion cannot occur. If this condition persists for several days, the buildup of pollutants may reach dangerous levels and public health advisories are issued. Most cities have plans for shutting down certain industries and even curtailing transportation if unsafe levels are approached. Most states also have "clean air" legislation, which has improved air quality in the last twenty years in U.S. cities.

The disasters just mentioned involve a humanmade form of air pollution called *smog*. There are two types of smog, London-type smog and Los Angeles-type smog, based primarily on the source of the pollution. **London-type smog** is the result of burning fossil fuels such as coal. At one time coal was the major source of heat for homes as well as the major energy source for factories. A very serious problem arose when a lengthy temperature inversion occurred in the winter months. Switching to oil, steam, gas, and electricity in many homes and factories has minimized this source.

Los Angeles-type smog (also known as **photochemical smog**) is a more complex phenomenon. Here the source of pollution is primarily transportation exhausts from cars, buses, and trucks that contain oxides of nitrogen. These products are acted on by sunlight (a photochemical reaction), and the result is a characteristic brown smog. Large cities with a high ratio of cars to people and with poorly developed public transportation are more likely to experience Los Angeles-type smog. The health effects are very similar to London-type smog.

Four additional air pollution concerns are developing among environmental scientists. The first is becoming known as the "**greenhouse effect**." One of the several byproducts of combustion is the gas carbon dioxide, which causes sunlight to generate more heat as it passes through the atmosphere. The level of carbon dioxide seems to be rising in the atmosphere and may eventually raise temperatures world wide. As polar ice caps melt, this rise may have implications for seacoasts as well as for the food-

Carbon monoxide (CO) A gas that is the by-product of combustion, will not support life, and combines with hemoglobin in human blood more readily than oxygen, which is necessary for life.

Ozone layer A layer of oxygen molecules in the upper atmosphere, that screen out ultraviolet rays from the sun.

Acid rain Precipitation with a low pH (acid) caused by rain forming with products of industrial combustion such as sulfur to form acids such as sulfur dioxide. Acid rain is harmful to forests and lakes, which cannot tolerate changes in acidity/alkalinity.

Radiation Electromagnetic rays such as light or particles given off from a source.

Radiation sickness An illness marked by low white blood counts, nausea, and death from an overexposure to nuclear radiation.

Nuclear generation of energy Use of controlled nuclear reactions to produce steam, which in turn drive turbines to produce electricity.

Chlorofluorocarbons (CFCs) Chemicals used as spray-can propellants, refrigerants, and industrial solvents.

---

producing areas of the world.

A second problem (and a related product of combustion) is **carbon monoxide (CO)**, which combines more readily with hemoglobin in blood than does oxygen. Less O_2 (oxygen) gets to the tissues, causing shortness of breath and other signs of oxygen deprivation. People suffering from respiratory and circulatory diseases are at risk in high-carbon-monoxide environments. The catalytic converter on cars significantly reduces CO emissions.

A third potential air pollution problem is the apparent reduction of the **ozone layer** of the atmosphere, which may be related to certain propellants in aerosols and some materials used in insulating materials such as insulation in homes, styrofoam cups, and fast food containers made of plastic. This concern first surfaced in the 1970s, but has taken on increased importance with better documentation in 1987 of a "hole" in the ozone layer over Antarctica. Ozone filters ultraviolet rays from the sun, and a reduction in the protective layer could result in more skin cancers and blindness.

A fourth problem is **acid rain**. This is a by-product of many industrial processes, especially when coal containing high amounts of sulfur is burned and chemicals such as sulfur dioxide, sulfur trioxide, nitrogen dioxide, and nitric acid are released into the atmosphere. These concentrations can be carried great distances by the prevailing winds and, when combined with rain, form a rather highly acid mixture containing sulfuric acid and nitric acid. Many trees, and some lakes, can tolerate only a very narrow range of acidity, and are either damaged or are killed. A "dead" lake is one that cannot support animal or plant life forms. The known risk at the moment is an esthetic one: we want to protect the environment from destruction. The potential health risk is that we might be endangering the food chain over the long run.

Concern about air pollution led to the establishment of the U.S. Environmental Protection Agency in the 1960s, which has the task of setting standards and monitoring pollution levels. The ten-year trend (trend considered for ten-year time periods) has been encouraging in that the EPA reports improved air quality as measured by decreased levels of smog and several airborne chemicals. How this improvement translates specifically into improved health status has yet to be determined.

Radiation Radiation is frightening to most people. They don't understand what it is in part because they can't see it. They don't recognize that there are various types, such as X-rays and ultraviolet light, and various sources, such as uranium or the sun. Basically, **radiation** is energy. The health effects of radiation can include **radiation sickness**, from a short but high-dose exposure, to various cancers from prolonged low-dose exposure. There are four major areas of current concern from a health point of view.

The first is the continued stockpiling of nuclear weapons. Most of the major public health associations have stated that in the event of an intentional or accidental discharge of these weapons, both "health" and "public" may well become meaningless words. In even the most conservative estimates of a "limited" attack, the casualties will run into the hundreds of thousands or millions.

The second concern is the safety of **nuclear-generation of energy**. As oil and coal became expensive sources of energy, nuclear power was promoted as being clean, efficient, inexpensive, and safe. In the short run, those predictions have largely been correct. Power systems in several parts of the world rely on nuclear generating plants. However, despite all the built-in safeguards and regulating agencies, accidents can happen with far more significant consequences than if a similar accident occurred in a coal-burning plant. The Chernobyl accident in the U.S.S.R. in 1986 is an excellent example for the potential for disaster. In addition, we face the enormous problem of the radioactive wastes these plants generate. They simply cannot be dumped in a sanitary landfill. The amount and type of soil used to cap a sanitary landfill is not sufficient to prevent radiation exposure. Because many of these landfills are converted into park land once they are filled, and because we might lose track of which ones have radioactive wastes, it is not reasonable to use these sites for even low concentrations of radioactive wastes. Deposit sites will have to be developed that will be secure for not just a few years, but for tens of thousands of years. Can

(Text continues on p. 506.)

What Is Destroying the Ozone?

In September 1986, fifteen scientists flew into McMurdo Station, Antarctica, to investigate a mystery: What causes a thinning in atmospheric ozone above the frigid continent, a phenomenon that has peaked each October since it was first observed in 1983? It was hardly an academic question; the ozone layer is a blanket of oxygen molecules that protects the earth's surface from the sun's harmful ultraviolet radiation, a form of light just beyond the human range of vision. Speculation on the reason for these "holes" has ranged from weather patterns and solar activity to the action of man-made **chlorofluorocarbons (CFCs)**, chemicals used as spray-can propellants, refrigerants, and industrial solvents.

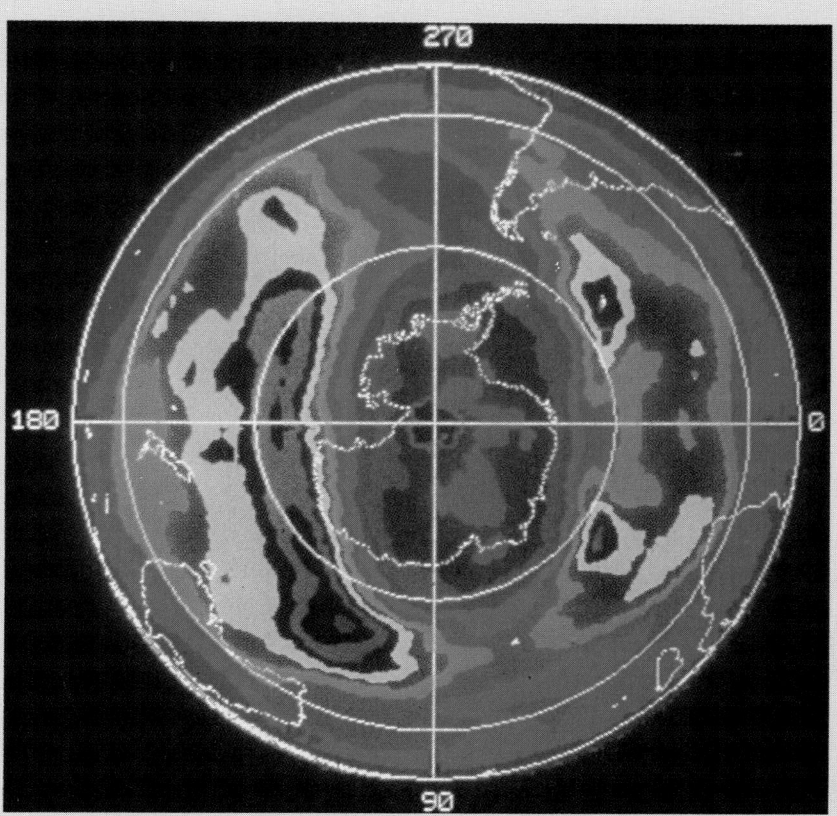

The purple in the center of the satellite image shows the ozone hole over Antarctica in September 1986.

Last week the team radioed Washington with its interim findings. Sure enough, the hole appeared in mid-September, right on schedule, and bloomed over the next twenty to thirty days, until the ozone content of the hole had dropped by about 40 percent. Says Team Leader Susan Solomon, a chemist with the National Oceanic and Atmospheric Administration in Boulder, Colo.: "We suspect a chemical process is fundamentally responsible," although atmospheric dynamics undoubtedly help shape it. The chemicals could be natural—volcanic perhaps—but CFCs might also play a role.

Antarctica is not the only spot where ozone levels are low, says Donald Heath, a NASA scientist. Tests over Arosa, Switzerland, since the 1920s have shown an average ozone loss of 3 percent, mostly in the past ten years. And Heath believes he has found another hole. Centered over Spitsbergen, Norway, 700 miles from the North Pole, it is one-third the size of the Antarctic hole. Heath claims the region's ozone loss has been 1.5 percent a year for the past six years and says this location fits models of CFC-caused loss.

The reason for concern is that without ozone, life on earth would be impossible. Ozone is oxygen but in an unusual form. Most oxygen comes in two-atom molecules, but external energy—in this case, the sun's ultraviolet radiation—can split some of them apart. The single oxygen atoms tend to attach themselves to the remaining molecules, forming an oxygen-atom triplet. The result: a layer, from six to 30 miles up, of ozone-enriched air. Once formed, an ozone molecule is a good absorber of ultraviolet. But when CFCs rise to the ozone layer, sunlight decomposes them, releasing the chlorine they contain. The chlorine is a catalyst, breaking ozone apart without itself being affected. At present, the ozone layer lets enough ultraviolet through to cause sunburn and, in some people, skin cancer. More ultraviolet would increase the effect: the Environmental Protection Agency estimates a 1 percent drop in global ozone could cause 20,000 additional skin cancers in the United States annually.

SOURCE: By Michael D. Lemonick, reported by Dick Thompson, 1986 (November 3), Washington *Time* 128(18):80.

Acid Rain

To date, a numbing 3,000 scientific papers and seven major government reports have weighed in on the causes and effects of acid rain, leaving little doubt about the basic alchemy that turns the emissions of electric plants and vehicles into the hard rain that damages lakes and soils. But opponents of mandatory emission controls seize on several unanswered questions to justify their opposition—one of the most divisive: where does the rain come from? Suspicions have long centered on the Midwest, where burning of high-sulfur coal creates millions of tons of the sulfur dioxide from which acid deposition forms. But some studies have shown that local sources might produce fully *half* the acid rain falling in the Northeast, suggesting that those states would do well to look to their own backyards before badgering the Midwest to clean up its act. Now, however, researchers at the University of Rhode Island have uncovered persuasive evidence that most of the Northeast's acid rain does indeed originate far away.

To trace acid rain, URI's Kenneth Rahn and Douglas Lowenthal identified chemical "fingerprints" in air masses. It happens that certain activities, such as smelting, and certain fuels, such as heavy oil, are concentrated in specific geographic areas. Since manufacturing and combustion spew characteristic pollutants into the air, this pattern is tailor-made for tracing air masses: the pollutants in them act like return addresses, indicating the air's origins. For instance, the Midwest burns more coal than the East, which burns more heavy oil. Coal combustion produces the elements selenium and arsenic; heavy oils generate vanadium. Identifying a high ratio of selenium in an air mass blowing over the Narragansett shore, then, tells scientists that it likely began its journey in the Midwest.

Air Mass

When the URI team applied the tracer system to air masses reaching Vermont and Rhode Island, they estimated that roughly 50 percent of the aerosol sulfates originated in the Midwest, and 50 percent came from local sources. But aerosols are, at best, a measure of the *precursors* of acid rain, not of acid rain itself. Extending the tracer system to actual precipitation yielded dramatic results. Rahn and atmospheric chemist Roy Heaton now find that roughly 80 percent of the sulfates in rain and snow falling on the Northeast probably come from the Midwest.

How can 80 percent of the acid rain originate in the Midwest while only 50 percent of its precursors bear that return address? The answer lies in meteorology. Rain forms high in the atmosphere; taking samples of rain, then, is tantamount to sampling high-altitude air. Because it requires time for air to rise after it has mixed with pollutants near the ground, the higher a sample of contaminated air, the longer it has been aloft. And the longer air has been aloft, the farther away it originated. Until now, scientists had only suspected, but had not demonstrated, that the altitude of air pollutants is tied to their regional origin. Says Rahn: "These results underscore the importance of emissions in the Midwest to acid rain."

The tracer technique has been criticized in the past, but this spring the Environmental Protection Agency accepted it in principle as a valid way to find the origin of pollutants. And this week Rahn and Lowenthal are being awarded a patent on the process. Still, the URI results will likely matter less to the lawmakers considering controls on acid rain than economics and politics do. Congress is now contemplating two bills addressing acid rain. The House version, with 169 cosponsors from both parties and all regions of the country, would reduce emissions of sulfur dioxide by 9 million tons a year by 1997; the Senate bill, with 21 cosponsors, would cut emissions by 12 million tons—about 50 percent—and would also control pollutants like ozone and carbon monoxide. Hearings on the Senate bill are set to start after Labor Day, and the bills' supporters already think they have enough science on their side; opponents, including the Reagan administration, call for still more study, seeking definitive answers to how acid deposition affects forests and how much cuts in sulfur emissions would cut acid rain. The URI results may not tip the balance toward controls, but they do add evidence to the case against the modern scourge.

Sharon Begley *with* Mary Hager, 1986 (August 11), Acid rain's fingerprints, *Newsweek*, p. 53.

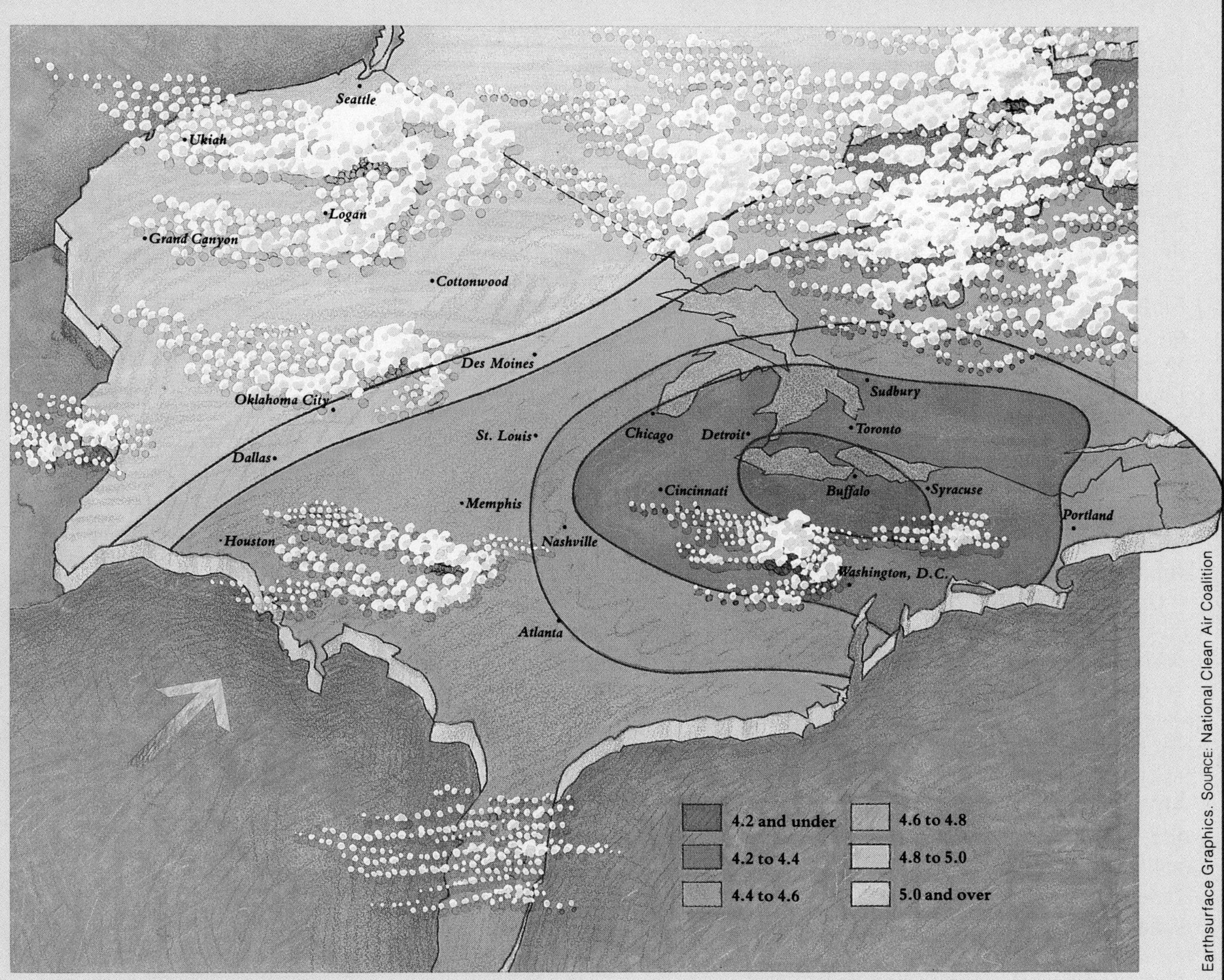

Earthsurface Graphics. SOURCE: National Clean Air Coalition

On the 14-point pH scale of acidity and alkalinity, a perfectly neutral sample of water would have a 7.0 rating. Unpolluted rainwater, which registers a pH of 5.6, may be described as slightly acidic because of the combination of carbon dioxide with water vapor.

A one-point increase in acidity on this logarithmic scale means a tenfold boost in that critical measurement, so a pH of 4.10—such as was recorded at Penn State University's monitoring station—shows that rainfall there is 31.6 times more acidic than normal.

Disposing of Nuclear Waste

The problem has been festering ever since the first commercial nuclear power plant went on line in 1957: How will we safely entomb the nuclear waste that remains radioactive for 10,000 years? All along it was to be a federal responsibility—but it wasn't until 1982 that Congress even set guidelines for selecting a burial site, and the final choice will not be made until 1991. The issue was a hot potato even before the Department of Energy (DOE) confirmed last month that Deaf Smith County (Texas), Nevada's Yucca Mountains, and Hanford (Washington) were finalists in the dubious sweepstakes.

Critics charge that severe technical or environmental problems exist at each of the three prospective sites. Even though ground water moves at a snail's pace through the Ogallala, a radioactive leak into the aquifer would be catastrophic for Panhandle agriculture. In Nevada, the proposed site is in an active seismic region and some citizens fear that weapons testing miles away could disrupt the underground tunnels. The DOE itself has stated that the basalt formations at Hanford would make it the hardest to mine, operate, and protect of any of the three sites.

Transporting the waste is an even more contentious issue, particularly since 85 percent of it is now stored in temporary facilities at power plants east of the Mississippi. DOE says it will take seventeen truckloads a day for twenty years to transport the waste to the burial site—a prospect that has galvanized opposition all along the various routes. Critics in Nevada, for example, say that waste brought to Yucca from the South would have to come across the Hoover Dam in Arizona, over a two-lane highway with a series of curves. Waste from the East would travel over Colorado's treacherous Loveland Pass. Critics aren't consoled that Sandia National Labs has conducted torture tests on nuclear-waste containers—running trains over them, slamming them into concrete walls at 80 miles per hour, and suspending them over pools of burning oil for hours—since the actual prototype casks have yet to be designed.

DOE officials are confident that the site will be chosen, constructed, and operating on schedule by 1998. But just in case opposition does make a difference, protest groups in all three states plan to keep on working and prove that the path of least resistance doesn't lead to their backyard.

The Disposal Alternatives

No one wants radioactive waste in, over, or under his backyard. But even if the United States builds no more commercial nuclear power reactors, the 95 already in operation will have produced some 100,000 metric tons of highly radioactive nuclear fuel waste by the year 2020. Already, the equivalent of 20,000 metric tons of solid and liquid waste produced by power plants and weapons factories is awaiting disposal.

No method for disposing of high-level waste has yet been implemented, and land burial, the method currently favored by the Department of Energy, will undergo years of study and testing as well as Congressional oversight before implementation.

One weapons laboratory has been disposing of middle-level waste for 20 years without causing measurable pollution of the environment. This is the Oak Ridge National Laboratory in Tennessee, which combines the waste with a liquid mixture of cement, fly ash, and clay and pumps the resulting fluid down through a drill pipe into a shale formation more than 1,000 feet underground. The fluid, under pressure, is forced into fractured, horizontally layered shale, opening up cavities in which the waste hardens into concrete.

For high-level spent fuel, the DOE is currently studying four kinds of underground mineral formations as repository candidates: salt, tuff, basalt, and crystalline rock, which includes the granite found beneath Hillsboro, N.H. Investigators say that salt formations, among their several advantages, are more plastic than others, tending to reseal any cracks that might form around an underground cavity.

Before burial, the DOE plans to encase high-level radioactive waste in several layers of protective shell.

Most high-level nuclear waste from the military is in liquid form. For that, the Departments of Energy and Defense plan to use a preliminary process called vitrification, in which waste uranium, plutonium and other dangerous substances are converted into salts and mixed with molten borosilicate (Pyrex-type) glass. After being cast into ingots and buried, the glass should remain waterproof indefinitely, thereby preventing the waste from dissolving in ground water and entering the environment. France has been using the process since 1978, with no known groundwater contamination.

The Soviet Union has proposed several methods of underground waste disposal. One would involve the excavation of huge underground caverns by means of nuclear explosions. The caverns would then be filled with radioactive waste and allowed to heat up to the point where the rock walls melted and sealed themselves. Western officials believe that currently some of the Soviet waste is in temporary storage and that a good deal more is buried.

The use of seabeds as disposal sites appeals to many scientists, in the United States and abroad. A system studied by experts at the Woods Hole Oceanographic Institution in Massachusetts would cast radioactive waste into heavy spikes, each about 10 feet long and a foot in diameter. These would be dropped into deep mid-ocean basins from special vessels. Oceanographers calculate that after a three-mile fall through sea water, a spike would acquire enough momentum to penetrate 100 feet below the ocean floor.

Many scientists agree that subseabed disposal, while more costly, would be significantly safer than land burial. But problems might arise from working in international waters, and it would be harder to meet the DOE's retrieval requirements. Thus, subseabed research is receiving less than the $365 million allotted to assessing terrestrial sites in 1986.

Still another idea is to rocket the most dangerous wastes into high earth or lunar orbits. The private American Institute of Aeronautics and Astronautics, for one, while acknowledging the risk inherent in the launch itself, has said that such disposal would probably pose less of a long-term hazard to humans than land or sea burial.

Paradoxically, nuclear waste may be so valuable that disposing of it would in itself be a waste. A British nuclear chemist, Dr. John Thornback, estimated recently that power plants in his country were producing more than $2 million worth of such valuable metals as rhodium, palladium, and ruthenium each year—as byproducts that wind up in the spent fuel.

Excerpted from "A nuclear burial ground," 1986 (June 16), *Newsweek*, p. 31; and from Malcolm W. Browne, The disposal alternatives, 1986 (May 11), *New York Times Magazine*, p. 24.

we assure safety for a projected period into the future that is longer than the total recorded history of human beings on this planet?

The third area of concern is the use of radiation in medicine, primarily the X-ray. The development of machines that could produce images of the internal bone structure, and now organs, has been a major advance in medicine. However, no advance is without risk. Much time passed before studies revealed that X-ray exposure is cumulative and that no exposure is absolutely safe. Early X-ray machines, which were used in mobile chest X-ray machines to screen for tuberculosis or to fit shoes in shoe stores would not be used today because of the high amounts of radiation they gave off. Each "generation" of X-ray machines has used less radiation more effectively. From a personal health point of view, you should never have a "routine" X-ray examination. Each X-ray exam should have a definite purpose where the benefit outweighs the possible risks. In addition, many health professionals are beginning to recommend that records be kept of all X-ray exposures, in a manner similar to that for vaccinations.

Exploring Your Emotions

The nurse at your doctor's office, where you have come for your yearly checkup, says they just want to get a routine chest X-ray for the files. How do you feel, and what do you say and do?

The fourth area of concern has just recently come to the public's attention. **Radon** is a form of ionizing radiation that is sometimes found in soils, rock, and some building materials. An unknown number of homes have been built on or with these substances. Well-insulated homes retain radon and allow higher concentrations to develop. Radon gas increases the incidence of lung cancer. Most state health departments can now test for radon gas concentrations, but we do not know what the short- or long-term health consequences will be.

Chemical Pollution Chemical pollution is by no means only a modern-day concern. The ancient Romans were plagued by lead poisoning, which damaged the central nervous system, because they stored sugar solutions in lead containers. Two hundred years ago in Europe, the term "mad as a hatter" came from the hatters' practice of cleaning felt hats with mercury—which also destroyed the central nervous system. Our problem today is that we have many more chemicals, in more concentrated forms and in wider use, and larger numbers of people are exposed and potentially exposed than ever before.

In Bhopal, India, in 1984, thousands were killed and injured when a powerful chemical used in manufacturing the insecticide Sevin was released from a plant. This catastrophe illustrates the short-term potential for disaster. The long-term exposure to many chemicals in our environment is seldom considered, but the health consequences may be just as deadly. The following are brief descriptions of just a few current problems.

Asbestos A mineral-based compound, asbestos was widely used up until the late 1960s for fire protection and insulation in buildings. It was often applied to pipes, metal supports, and ceilings. When first introduced, asbestos was hailed as a great advance in fire safety of buildings. As long as it stayed where it was applied and the protective coating was not disturbed, there was no problem. However, microscopic asbestos fibers are released into the air when this material is applied, or later damaged, that lodge in the lung, inflaming it. This condition, known as **asbestosis**, can result in lung cancer over a period of years. Similar conditions exist in the coal mining industry, from coal dust (black lung disease), and in the textile industry, from cotton fibers (brown lung disease).

Lead poisoning Modern concerns about lead poisoning focus on children in primarily urban settings. Concentrations of lead can damage the central nervous system, cause mental retardation, hinder oxygen transport by blood, and create digestive problems. Many people mistakenly think that this problem is past. Continuing studies by state health departments and the Centers for Disease Control point out that lead poisoning continues to affect children living in cities that have the greatest inner-city, low-income problems. Children are exposed to lead in two ways. The first is by chewing on surfaces, such as window sills, painted before 1960. Most paints used on older homes were lead-based. The second source comes from playing in dirt near heavily traveled roadways. One result of using leaded gasoline for so many years is that lead contaminates soil near highways. Legislation phasing out the use of leaded fuels will minimize this problem in the future.

Pesticides Pesticides are chemicals that are used to control insects and other pests, primarily for two purposes. The first is to prevent the spread of disease. Minimizing mosquito populations to control malaria is an example. The second is to maximize food production for people by attempting to reduce the amount of food eaten by insects. Both purposes have risks as well as benefits. The use of **DDT** to control mosquitos in the 1950s and 1960s dramatically decreased deaths from malaria, but this decrease has resulted in a tremendous population explosion in tropical countries. In addition, as Rachel Carson pointed out in her landmark book *Silent Spring,* DDT became concentrated in the food chain of large birds and possibly

Radon A naturally occurring radioactive gas that is emitted from rocks and natural building materials and that can become concentrated in insulated homes, causing lung cancer.

Asbestosis A lung condition caused by inhalation of microscopic asbestos fibers, which inflames the lung and can lead to lung cancer.

DDT A common insecticide now stringently controlled in the United States.

Dioxins Powerful chemicals found in herbicides and linked to human cancers.

Formaldehyde A powerful disinfectant gas often used in solution for germ control but also given off by some synthetic building materials.

Decibels A relative measure of the "loudness" or intensity of noise.

humans, although no direct evidence exists that DDT is toxic to humans. In the United States, DDT as well as many other pesticides have been banned or their use restricted. In the second case, it is clear that food could not become as plentiful, and as cheap, in urbanized countries without using pesticides. The cost may come in the yet-to-be-determined long-range health consequences of pesticide residues in food chains. Almost all the pesticide hazards to date have been a result of overuse or abuse.

The list of real and potential chemical pollution problems may well be as long as the list of known chemicals. To the preceding list we can add recent concern about **dioxins**, mercury, PCBs, **formaldehyde**, and other byproducts of our industrialized age. We seem to introduce a chemical, sing high praise about its contribution to our lifestyle, and then we discover a negative health consequence. After a period of time we either find a substitute, or we find a safer way of using that chemical. However, we usually don't retreat from the technological advance because we do not wish to give up the contribution to our way of living. The general opinion at this point in history is that benefits usually outweigh the perceived costs or risks.

Noise Pollution We are increasingly aware of the health effects of loud or persistent noise in the environment. Concerns focus on two areas, hearing loss and stress. Exposure to sounds above 80–85 **decibels** (a measure of the volume of sound) can cause temporary hearing loss, but prolonged exposure can cause permanently dulled hearing. The scream of an infant, certain music, and even freeway traffic sounds all can exceed the safe range. Some rock music, for example, is played at very high volume over prolonged periods of time. The danger is not in the type of music as much as it is in the volume at which it is played. The key is to minimize the quantity and frequency of exposure. The second area of concern is the relationship of noise to stress. Increased blood pressure is just one of many areas now being studied. (See Chapter 2.)

What Can You Do?

Every aspect of your health is influenced in some way by the environment around you. The great advances in disease reduction and increased life expectancy up to this point in time have been due to efforts in the classic areas of environmental health. However, as we now turn our attention to lifestyle concerns in an attempt to solve many of the chronic disease problems of today, we cannot let our past efforts lapse. A relatively minor disruption—a flood, for example—can put us right back to where we were one hundred years ago. And we must add new efforts to block potential new disasters.

Every decision requires balancing benefits with costs or risks. There are no zero risk situations. So we need to

Exploring Your Emotions

Your neighbors have been playing music so loudly that the pictures on your walls have been vibrating. How do you feel, and how will you handle your feelings?

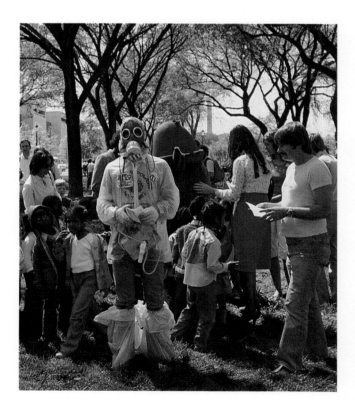

set levels of acceptable risk—but we must ask the question "acceptable to whom?" Advantages and disadvantages are not equally distributed across populations. What are we willing to live with, and at what cost? Who is to decide? It may be an unfortunate commentary on modern civilization, but most of these issues will be raised and determined based on underlying economic and political considerations instead of what is "right" or "proper."

The individual citizen is often overwhelmed. You may think you can do nothing about such global problems. But you *can* engage in two very important activities. First, you can practice behaviors that minimize your personal risk and the risk of those around you. You can be conscious of water supplies when you hike or camp, you can recycle, you can dispose of pesticides properly, and so on. Second, you can inform yourself about environmental issues and become involved in the political decision-making process; for example, by writing your representatives. For example, every community is involved in discussions about solid waste disposal. How do you feel about sanitary landfills in your neighborhood? How much are you willing to pay? Individuals can and do make a difference in these discussions where so few citizens participate.

The environment is no longer as threatening to humans as it was once. But we also realize that it is much more fragile than our predecessors ever imagined. We are also beginning to realize that we are not the only species with a right to inhabit the planet. We must view the environment as a trust for future generations and other forms of life. We must consider each action in terms of being able to pass on to the next generation an environment no worse, and preferably better, than the one we currently enjoy.

Take Action

Your answers to the Exploring Your Emotions questions in this chapter and your placement level on the Awareness Ladder will, we hope, encourage you to begin a process of self-exploration and self-discovery that you will continue. Reflect on the entire chapter's content and ask yourself how each point relates to your own life. Then take action:

1. Find out where drinking water comes from in your community (wells, lake, river) and how much it costs. Estimate the total cost in your household and figure savings that could be achieved using various conservation methods.

2. Find out how solid wastes are disposed of in your community. Estimate the total pounds and type of solid waste generated by your household in a month. Suggest methods of recycling that could reduce your contribution to the local landfill, etc., by 50 percent.

3. Call your local health department and ask what hazardous chemicals are of potential danger in your community (such as lead, mercury, PCBs) and where you are at most risk. Do an inventory of your household in terms of hazardous chemicals (such as lead-based paints, insecticides). Do you know how to properly dispose of each?

4. The next time you visit your physician, ask if a total cumulative record of your X-rays is kept in a manner similar to your immunization record. Do the same with your dentist. Maintain your own list of *all* X-ray exposures by type.

5. Before leaving this chapter, review the Rate Yourself statements that open the chapter. Have your feelings or values changed? Are you now better equipped to handle the complex and very human problems associated with environmental health?

Selected References

Freed, Virgil H. 1986. Hazards in the physical environment. In W.W. Holland, R. Detels, and G. Knox, eds., *The Oxford Textbook of Public Health,* Vol. 1. Oxford, England: Oxford University Press.

Okun, Daniel A. 1986. Water and waste disposal. In Maxcy-Rosenau, ed., *Public Health and Preventive Medicine,* 12 ed. Norwalk, Conn.: Appleton-Century-Crofts.

Revell, P., and C. Revelle, 1984. *The Environment: Issues and Choices for Society*. Boston: Willard Grant Press.

U.S. Council on Environmental Quality and the U.S. Department of State. 1981. *Global 2000 Report to the President*. Washington, D.C.: U.S. Government Printing Office.

U.S. Environmental Protection Agency. 1984. *Trends in the Quality of the Nation's Air*. Washington, D.C.: U.S. Government Printing Office.

Waldron, H. A. 1986. The control of the physical environment. W.W. Holland, R. Detels, and G. Knox, eds., *The Oxford Textbook of Public Health,* Vol. 2. Oxford, England: Oxford University Press.

Recommended Readings

Chiras, Daniel D. 1985. *Environmental Science: A Framework for Decision-Making*. Menlo Park, Calif.: Addison-Wesley, 1985.
Basic textbook in environmental health. Includes a good section on ethics.

Dubos, René. 1973. Health and environment. *American Lung Association Bulletin* (59), pp. 10–12.
Historic update on previous reference.

Dubos, René. 1986. *Man, Medicine, and Environment*. New York: Praeger.
A landmark book, written by a highly respected scientist, that started to focus scientific concern on environmental issues.

Ehrlich, Paul R. 1971. *The Population Bomb*. New York: Ballantine Books.
A landmark book calling attention to the problems associated with population growth.

Miller, G. Tyler. 1982. *Living in the Environment,* 2nd ed. Belmont, Calif.: Wadsworth.
A survey textbook in environmental health.

Murphy, E. M. 1983. *The Environment to Come: A Global Survey*. Washington, D.C.: The Population Reference Bureau.
A prediction of future trends in the environment.

Chapter 22

Contents

Rate Yourself

Your Attitudes about Aging Read the following statements carefully. Choose the one in each section that best describes you at this moment and circle its number. When you have chosen one statement for each section, add the numbers and record your total score. Find your position on the Awareness Ladder.

5 Considers aging a natural life process
4 Regards old age as another stage in life
3 Seldom thinks about old age
2 Worries about getting older
1 Finds the idea of becoming old painful

5 Views older people as valuable human resources
4 Feels older people can make significant contributions
3 Feels older people without resources should be subsidized
2 Feels older people burden the community
1 Views older people as hopeless burdens on society

5 Believes physical and mental decline can be avoided in old age
4 Believes mental decline can be avoided in old age
3 Believes severe physical and mental decline can be delayed
2 Believes severe physical decline is inevitable
1 Believes severe mental and physical decline is inevitable

5 Feels retirement age requirements should be eliminated
4 Feels retirement age requirements should be raised
3 Feels retirement age requirements are just about right
2 Feels retirement age requirements should be lowered
1 Feels older people should retire to make way for younger people

5 Enjoys older people
4 Likes spending time with older people
3 Doesn't mind spending time with older people
2 Reluctantly spends time with older people
1 Resents spending time with older people

Total Score ______

Aging

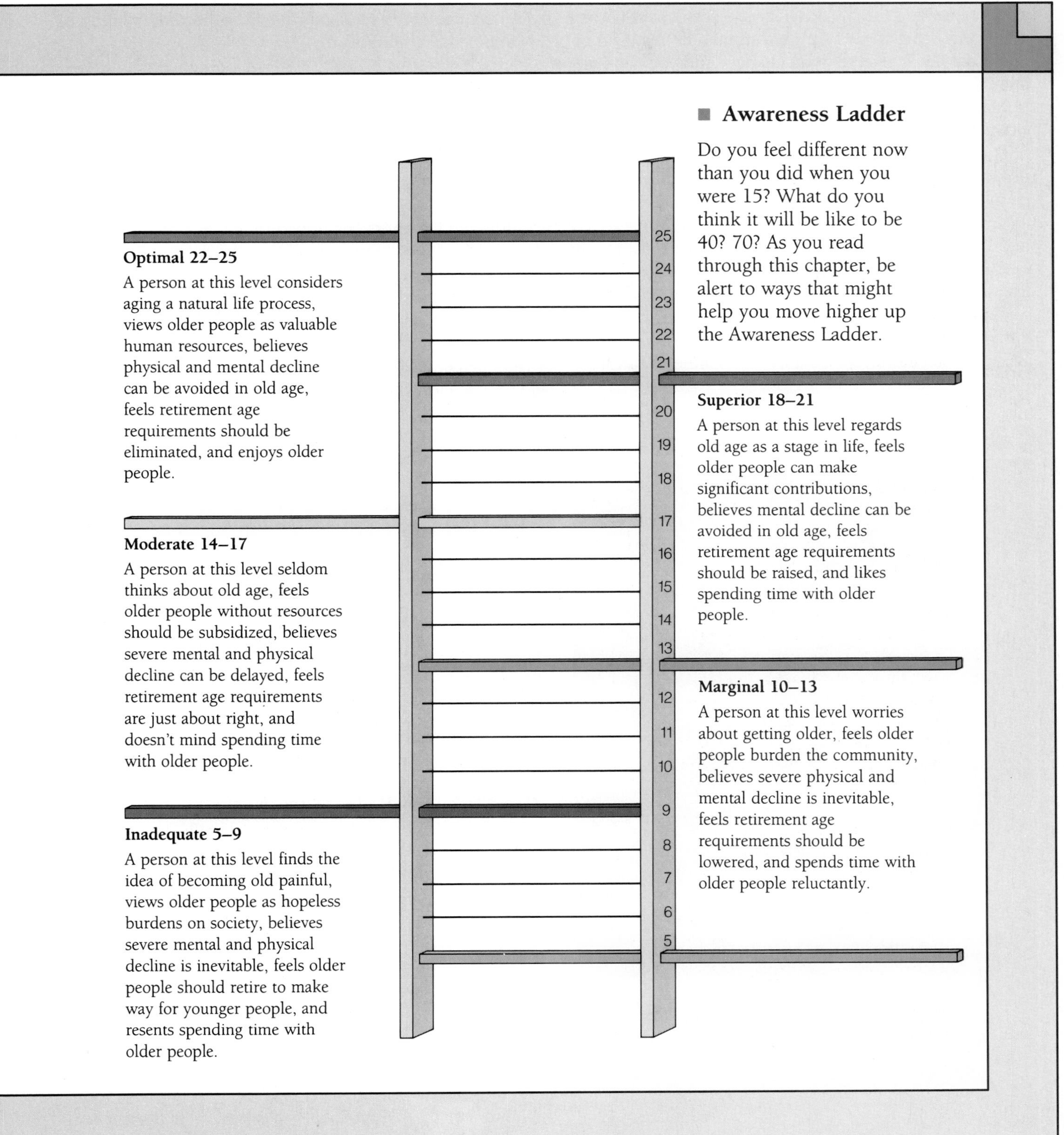
■ Awareness Ladder
Do you feel different now than you did when you were 15? What do you think it will be like to be 40? 70? As you read through this chapter, be alert to ways that might help you move higher up the Awareness Ladder.
Optimal 22–25
A person at this level considers aging a natural life process, views older people as valuable human resources, believes physical and mental decline can be avoided in old age, feels retirement age requirements should be eliminated, and enjoys older people.
Superior 18–21
A person at this level regards old age as a stage in life, feels older people can make significant contributions, believes mental decline can be avoided in old age, feels retirement age requirements should be raised, and likes spending time with older people.
Moderate 14–17
A person at this level seldom thinks about old age, feels older people without resources should be subsidized, believes severe mental and physical decline can be delayed, feels retirement age requirements are just about right, and doesn't mind spending time with older people.
Marginal 10–13
A person at this level worries about getting older, feels older people burden the community, believes severe physical and mental decline is inevitable, feels retirement age requirements should be lowered, and spends time with older people reluctantly.
Inadequate 5–9
A person at this level finds the idea of becoming old painful, views older people as hopeless burdens on society, believes severe mental and physical decline is inevitable, feels older people should retire to make way for younger people, and resents spending time with older people.
25
24
23
22
21
20
19
18
17
16
15
14
13
12
11
10
9
8
7
6
5

Most people would like to live long and never be old. When we see that old age grips us, we are stunned. "What has happened?" writes Aragon of ancient Greece. "It is life that has happened; and I am old." We have regarded old age as something alien, a foreign species: can I have become a different being while I still remain myself? Yes. And no. Life is a river. It changes; you change. And you can't step into the same river even once. Yet there is always continuity.

Many older people are happy, healthy, and self-sufficient. Changes that come with age, including negative ones, normally occur so gradually that the majority of people adapt, some even gracefully. Only 5 percent of people over age 65 in the United States are being cared for in institutions, and generally the rest continue to live meaningful and independent lives. Even so, most people in America do not happily anticipate growing old. They may dread it, feel that being old is somehow shameful or something to be regretted, and treat it with self-conscious humor to make themselves feel more comfortable about aging. Some cultures—notably the Chinese culture—venerate their elders and treat them with deep respect and deference. But culture in America is oriented toward youth, and it discriminates against the aged as mercilessly as it discriminates against other oppressed minorities. Yet we all age, and we are all likely to become victims of **"agist" discrimination.**

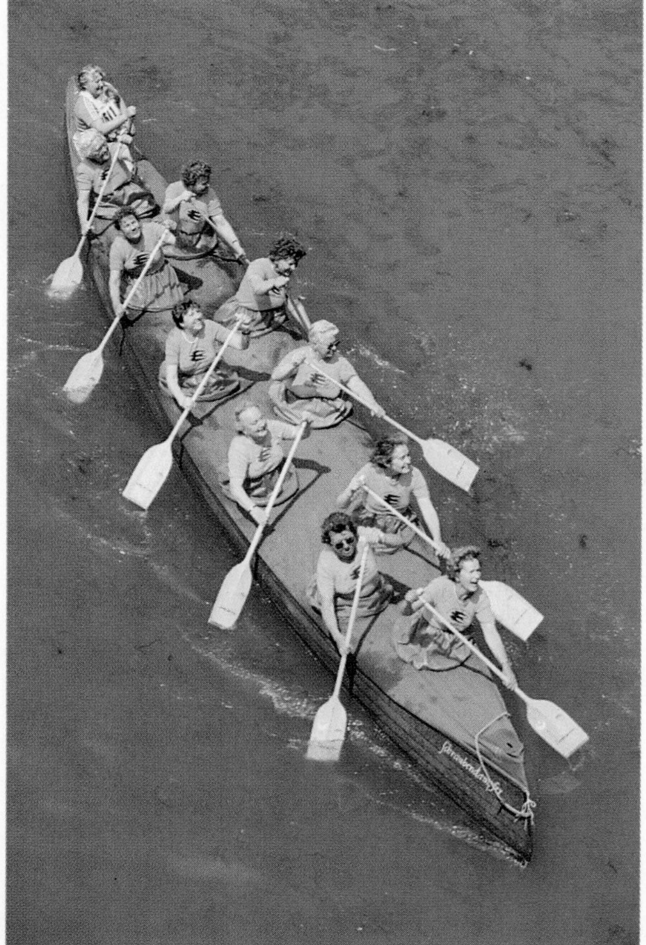
Karen S. Rantzman

America's Aged Minority

There is no precise age at which a person becomes "old." Some people are "old" at 25; others are still young at 75. Although Congress has upped the mandatory retirement age for nongovernment employees from 65 to 70, age 65 has formerly been taken as the dividing line between middle and old age. People 65 and older are a large minority in the American population—25 million people, 11 percent of the total population, in 1980. As birth rates drop, the percentage is increasing dramatically. Longer life expectancies will not contribute much to overpopulation, however, contrary to some thinking. Overpopulation results from too many babies who grow up to have too many babies—not from longer life expectancies. The greater numbers of older people who are often ill and dependent do, however, experience major social and economic problems. (See Figure 22-1 for age distribution trend.)

Whatever the American dream may have been, for some older citizens it has faded. Forced or persuaded into retirement, they find their income reduced to the point where they can barely subsist. They are also likely to feel worthless. Because many Americans are conditioned to value only what is shiny and new, objects lose value once they acquire a few scratches or scuffs or look worn around the edges. So, apparently, do people. In our youth-oriented culture, the changes in a person's appearance brought about by age are usually seen as negative. Urban life and the nuclear family intensify the effects of these attitudes on older people. In cultures that have **extended families,** older people stay active in society generally and help care for and teach the children. Here, they often face lonely isolation, or institutions, or geriatric ghettos: bleak downtown hotels or posh retirement cities.

Exploring Your Emotions

Look carefully at your parents and grandparents, or at pictures of them or of relatives. What changes has aging made in their appearance? How do you feel about these changes? How do you feel about the possibility that you may age in rather similar ways?

Agist discrimination Decisions against people made on the basis of their ages.

Extended family The nuclear family (parents and children) plus relatives by blood or marriage, sometimes living all together.

Biological aging Changes in body parts that result from the passage of time.

Illness sometimes makes the later years little more than a miserable prolonged wait for death. Medicare does not change the basic fact, although for some the wait may be eased a bit. Older people are like other people and need the same things. They have basic needs to be satisfied, and they need to feel their life has some meaning. More and more these needs are being considered basic human rights.

What Happens as You Age?

Circumstances, bodies, mental facilities change. Some changes occur gradually, over a lifetime. **Biological aging**, for example, includes all the normal, progressive, irreversible changes to one's body that begin at birth and continue till death. Changes of circumstance often occur more abruptly: retirement, relocating, changing homes, loss of a spouse and friends, lower income, switching roles and social status. Not all these things happen to everybody and even if they do occur, the time of life varies for people, partly depending on how well they have prepared for their later days. Some never have to leave their homes and can continue friendships in the same town; some appear to be in good health till the day they die. Others have tremendous adjusting to do in entirely new surroundings with fewer financial resources, new acquaintances, and increasing inability to get around, and possible loss of self-esteem and loneliness.

As with any other art, successful aging requires preparation. Taking stock of your mental and physical health habits right now in your teens or 20s may lead you to change strategies and practices that will allow you the best possible body and spirit 60 to 70 years down the road. By your mid 40s you will pretty well know your own lifestyle and how much money you need to support it. You will want to assess your financial status, perhaps begin setting aside savings to supplement a pension and Social Security. Later, maybe in your mid 50s you will need to decide on health plans and the type and location of housing after you retire. Right now, you have some control over most changes that occur during aging. They depend on what you do to and for yourself in your youth, as well as in your middle and old ages. You happen to yourself!

Changes in Physical Characteristics

Many characteristics we have assumed result from aging are not due to aging at all. They are due rather to neglect and abuse of our bodies and minds. These affronts lay the foundation for later mental problems and chronic diseases such as arthritis, heart problems, diabetes, hearing loss,

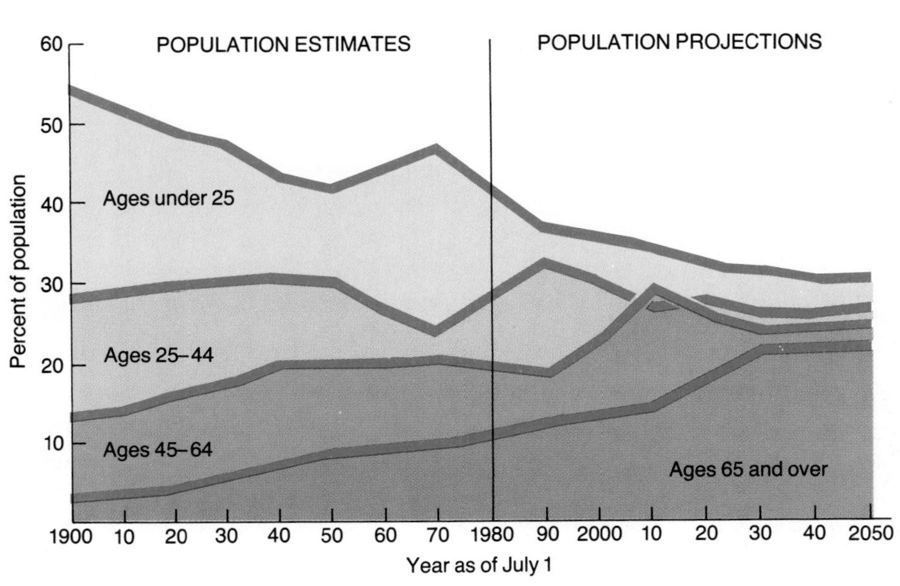

Figure 22-1 Trend in age distribution of United States population (including Armed Forces overseas), 1900–2050.

Aging and Changing: Your Body Through Time

Hair

- Thickest at age 20, our hairs shrink after that; by age 70, a person's hairs are as fine as when he was a baby.
- All people eventually turn gray. By age 50, one expert says, half of the population has a pronounced amount of gray hair.
- Twelve percent of men aged 25 are balding; 37 percent of men aged 35; 45 percent of men aged 45; and 65 percent of men aged 65.
- As a woman approaches menopause, she may get more body hair on the face, chest, or abdomen.

Brain

- Neuroscientists say that physical changes have little effect on cognitive functions. In fact, about 95 percent of all people, by most estimates, will never become senile, no matter how long they live.
- Still, almost everyone becomes slower in ability to learn and think, and memory almost always declines somewhat with age.
- Our sleep patterns change with age. According to one expert, an 80-year-old's typical pattern is 18 minutes to fall asleep, 80 percent of the night spent asleep, six hours of total sleep time, and one hour of REM sleep.

Face

- Cartilage begins to accumulate after age 30, so that by age 70, a man's nose has grown wider and longer, his earlobes have fattened, and his ears have grown a quarter-inch longer.

Height, Weight

- A woman's caloric needs drop 2 to 8 percent for each decade past age 20.
- In general, as we age, our shoulders narrow, our chest size grows and our pelvis widens. Such changes tend to occur 10 to 20 years later in women than in men. (For example, women's chest size tends to be largest from ages 55 to 64 and then starts to shrink; in men, it is largest between ages 45 and 54.)

Heart

- A person's resting heartbeat stays about the same all through life, but the heart pumps less blood with each beat. This is most pronounced during exercise, because his pulse can no longer rise as high as it once did.
- Although cardiovascular disease is more common in men, high blood pressure affects more women. Hypertension affects 30 percent of women in their late 50s and early 60s, compared with 28 percent of men; after 65, the sex gap widens: 36 percent of women have hypertension and 28 percent of men.

Lungs

- First, the good news: The respiratory system is one of the most resistant to change; also, the respiratory tract grows stronger with age in that after a lifetime of exposure to viruses, a person builds up immunity and catches fewer and less severe colds by middle age.
- However, a person's forced vital capacity (the amount of air that can be exhaled after a big inhalation, considered an accurate measure of vital capacity) decreases with age. Women in their 30s have an average FVC of 30 deciliters, for example, and that declines by about 3.1 deciliters every 10 years.

Abdomen

- Aging muscles in the gut tend to slacken, so it takes longer to digest a meal; cramps, gas, constipation, and a bloated feeling become more likely. Also, with age, the stomach secretes less acid, so some foods may become harder to digest. But the lower acid also makes heartburn less likely.

Eyesight

- Usually in the early 40s, our eyes begin having more trouble focusing on nearby objects and may need reading glasses.
- Also, as we age, our night vision weakens, we take longer to adjust to the dark, and we need

more light to see clearly (by age 80, a person needs three times more light than at age 20 to see with the same clarity); our depth perception weakens; we become more sensitive to glare because the lens is less elastic; and, because our eyes' cones deteriorate, we have more trouble distinguishing among colors, particularly blues, greens, and purples.

Hearing

- Our hearing begins to decline in our mid-30s. By age 35, for example, we may have a little more trouble hearing high-frequency sounds and we may need a sound to be about 10 decibels louder (about the level of a barely audible whisper) than we needed at age 25. By age 50, we may have trouble distinguishing among certain consonants—particularly *s, z, t, f,* and *g,* which are high-frequency sounds.

Mouth

- As we age, we get fewer surface cavities but more "cervical cavities," those that eat into the root of the tooth. Also, the gums recede.
- Also, a person's taste sensation diminishes.
- We begin to lose control over our vocal cords, so our voices begin to quaver. And as the vocal cords stiffen, our pitch rises.

Sexual Organs

- As time passes, a woman's menstrual periods tend to become shorter, with longer times in between. And women in their 30s and 40s, particularly those with children, tend to have fewer cramps.
- A woman's sexual responsiveness will reach a peak in her late 30s and remain on that plateau into her 60s (for example, women always retain the potential for multiple orgasm); men, however, reach their peak in the late teens and decline from there.
- Women's genitalia tend to decrease in size over the years. As a man ages, his scrotum hangs lower, the angle of his erections begins to decline in his 30s, his sperm production declines and the force of his ejaculations is less powerful.

Muscles, Bones

- The younger a person is, the more "trainable" his or her muscles. Aged muscles show under the microscope a loss and atrophy of cells, accumulation of fat and collagen, and loss of contractility. Aging muscles are less flexible and more susceptible to strains, pulls, and cramps.
- As we age, we shrink in height because the back muscles weaken and the discs between the bones in the spine deteriorate. If a man is 5 feet 10 inches at age 30, he will likely be 5 feet 8⅓ inches at age 70.
- A person's bones lose calcium with age, becoming more brittle and slower to heal. Joints become stiffer because cartilage around the joints is worn down and fluid around the joints is depleted. Also, ligaments contract and harden, making them more likely to tear.

Skin

- As skin ages, the oil glands that caused teenage skin breakouts quit, and the skin becomes drier; it also thins as it loses elasticity. Because a man's skin is more oily and thicker, he notices his aging skin about 10 years later than a woman does.
- Skin gradually becomes less and less sensitive to temperature changes. A young woman can detect a temperature drop of 1 degree Fahrenheit; after age 65, the temperature might need to drop 9 degrees before she feels it. But skin may concurrently become more sensitive to imaginary stimuli, like itchiness.

SOURCES: "How a Woman Ages," by Robin Marantz Henig and the editors of Esquire magazine, and "How a Man Ages," by Curtis Pesmen and editors of Esquire.

Osteoporosis Abnormal thinning and weakening of bones due to a loss of minerals.

Vital capacity The amount of air that can be expelled from the lungs.

Atrophy Waste away, diminish in size.

Neuron A nerve cell.

high blood pressure. We sacrifice our optimal health by smoking, eating a poor diet and overeating, abusing alcohol and drugs, bombarding our ears with excessive noise, and exposing our bodies to too much ultraviolet radiation from sun rays. We also jeopardize our bodies through neglect by sitting around most of the time, encouraging our muscles and even our bones to wither and deteriorate. And we endure much abuse from the toxic chemicals in our environment.

But even with the best behavior in the best environment, aging does occur. It results from biochemical processes that we don't yet understand.

Skin and Sensory Changes Tissues all over your body will lose elasticity. Your skin will not snap back so well when stretched, and your voice, after about 65, may begin to sound quavery because the collagen of your vocal cords will begin to lose elasticity. By your mid 40s you will probably become farsighted, unable to see things clearly up close, because your ocular lens no longer expands and contracts so readily. Changes in the pupil and the lens progress until by age 60 only a third as much light may reach the retina as at age 20, and the retina itself may become less efficient. The result is a loss of acuity, the ability to distinguish fine detail. Seeing in the dark becomes more difficult.

The ability to hear high-pitched tones declines for most people as they age, enough so that hearing loss is now the fourth most common chronic physical disability in the United States. This loss may be due to abuse rather than to aging, however. In less industrialized and quieter societies, hearing is almost as keen in old age as it is in youth.

Sensitivity to taste and smell appears to decrease with aging. About two-thirds of the taste buds in the mouth die by the age of 70, and a large proportion of sensory receptors in the nose have died by this age. Again it may be that such great taste and smell losses are not inevitable, but with stimulation can function at a high level.

Musculoskeletal System The effects of gravity appear in the form of jowls, drooping eyelids, and "growing" ears. Gravity wreaks havoc with bones, which normally act as a reserve for minerals in the body. Minerals are replenished through diet, but from the early 20s through the rest of life more minerals appear to be drawn out of the bones than are restored. The bones become porous, weak, and eventually fracture prone. At its extreme the condition deteriorates to **osteoporosis**, a devastating bone ailment that ends in multiple fractures of the vertebrae and pelvis. Right diet and exercise can help prevent such bone loss, or at least slow it.

Muscle strength and mass reduce only gradually in those who systematically continue to work and play hard physically. More protein is being broken down and less is being synthesized, so muscle fibers atrophy and some are lost. After the mid 40s, strength usually declines: a man may lose 10–20 percent of his maximum strength by 60, and a woman even more.

Without cartilage damage, your joints will withstand decades of hard use very well, with little or no deterioration evident. Joints become vulnerable to injury when supporting muscles lose their strength through disuse and can't support the joint properly. Bones weakened through inactivity can deform the joint surfaces and cause cartilage to erode. Joints can also be damaged by excessive pounding and stress and injury to the cartilage.

Your teeth, with proper care, will last a lifetime. Not aging, but disuse, abuse, and chronic degenerative disease cause teeth problems. Teeth and all their support systems respond to the stress and stimulation of chewing hard and crunchy foods. Periodontal disease begins in early life. Proper dental care can prevent it.

Cardiovascular System The efficiency of your heart can remain fairly steady with age, though your maximum heart rate will decline. You can roughly estimate maximum heart rate for any age by subtracting a person's age from 220. The decrease may be caused by infiltration of fatty and connective tissues in the heart's muscular wall, especially in people who sit around and eat fats.

The dramatic problems of the cardiovascular system associated with aging—heart attack and stroke—are actually caused by atherosclerosis and high blood pressure. You can do much to prevent them, just by eating right and walking briskly or exercising daily and avoiding smoking.

Respiratory System Decline in **vital capacity**—the amount of air that can be expelled from the lungs—is unlikely in those who keep fit and healthy and do not smoke. Otherwise, the rib cage becomes more rigid, cartilage calcifies, and joints about which the ribs rotate stiffen. Respiratory muscles weaken; capillaries atrophy and elastic fibers are lost, decreasing vital capacity. At 85 years, a person can inhale only half the volume of air that a 30-year-old can, though actual lung size doubles. Breathing becomes shallower and faster and more difficult as the number of alveoli decreases.

Cerebral cortex The outer layer of the brain that controls the behavior and mental activity of humans.

Dendrites A branched part of a nerve cell that transmits impulses toward the cell body.

Regular and vigorous exercise can increase vital capacity in young people and reverse losses in older ones. Swimming is most effective for this.

Digestive and Renal Systems With age, your stomach will secrete less acid and smaller amounts of the enzymes that aid digestion, but your small intestines won't lose power to absorb nutrients. Your kidneys will eventually filter wastes more slowly as they lose some of their filters. Kidneys deteriorate, not because of aging, but because of excessive protein in the diet. The stress of dealing with high daily intake of protein can lead to chronic degeneration. Excess calories and fat are also hard on the kidneys.

Immune System With age your defense system may become less efficient, predisposing you to infections and some chronic diseases. But the decline varies greatly among people. Only the progressive **atrophy** of the thymus gland seems invariably linked to advancing age.

Both good diet and exercise benefit the immune system. Undernutrition—not malnutrition—in animals has kept their immune systems younger for a longer period of time. (See theories of aging discussed later.) Vigorous physical activity can increase your body's response to antigens (foreign substances), while long periods of bed rest will reduce immunological efficiency. People in good physical shape rid themselves of respiratory infections much faster than those who are not.

Nervous System Only half as much blood travels to the brain of a 50-year-old as to that of a 10-year-old, most reduction occurring before 30 years of age. By age 85, your brain will have lost 10–20 percent of its weight, mainly through nerve cell atrophy. These **neuron** losses are selective: some sites show no decline, while in the **cerebral cortex,** the site of higher mental activities, loss is significant.

Your mental ability will not necessarily decline with the loss of neurons, partly because your brain will continue to sprout new **dendrites,** communication lines to other neurons. This may be one way the brain compensates for neuron loss.

Osteoporosis Risk Checklist

		YES	NO
1.	Do you have fair skin?	☐	☐
2.	Do you have a small frame?	☐	☐
3.	Are you past menopause?	☐	☐
4.	Did your family come from northern Europe?	☐	☐
5.	Do you drink more than 4 cups of coffee daily?	☐	☐
6.	Does your life involve much stress?	☐	☐
7.	Do you drink more than 4 oz. of alcohol daily?	☐	☐
8.	Do you exercise less than two days a week?	☐	☐
9.	Do you diet twice a year or more?	☐	☐
10.	Do you drink less than one glass of milk per day?	☐	☐
11.	Do you take thyroid, cortisone, or antacids regularly?	☐	☐
12.	Do you smoke?	☐	☐

Every "yes" you check increases your risk of osteoporosis. If you have checked yes more than six times you have an above average risk and you should take preventive measures.

SOURCE: *Healthline,* 1986 (October).

Life-extending Measures: Age Proofing

We create ourselves to some extent, and what you are aiming for now will influence who you are in your 50s, 60s, 70s, and 80s. Flabby muscles, loss of teeth, wrinkles, poor eyesight, stiff joints, failing memory, mental attitude, some chronic diseases—you can control. You can prevent, delay, lessen, even reverse the effects of some deterioration through good health habits. A few simple things you can do every day will make a vast difference in your looks, your health, your energy and vitality. The following suggestions have been mentioned throughout this text, but are profoundly related to health in later life, and are therefore highlighted here.

Develop Physical Fitness Exercise enhances both mental and physical health. Enough cannot be said for the positive effects of appropriate exercise throughout your life,

Is "Senility" Inevitable?

Both laypeople and physicians use the term *senility* loosely. Older people are often called "senile" when they forget something or seem to be confused. But small memory lapses in old age do not necessarily show intellectual deterioration. Slight confusion and occasional forgetfulness throughout life may only mean a temporary overload of facts in the brain. Or perhaps the person who exhibits such behaviors is merely tired and not functioning as well as usual. However, people also use the term *senile* to describe significant brain deterioration in elderly individuals.

Slowly losing one's mind was once considered an inevitable part of growing old. It was once thought that if people simply lived long enough, they became senile. However, we know that most elderly people in good health remain mentally alert. Well-designed studies suggest that although "response time" may slow down, many people become smarter as they become older and more experienced.

The current *medical* term for deterioration of intellectual capacity is *dementia*—which means "deprived of mind." Its earliest symptoms may appear as a slight disturbance in someone's ability to grasp the situations he or she is in—as illustrated in the movie *On Golden Pond* when the character portrayed by Henry Fonda lost his way in the long-familiar woods near his home. As dementia progresses, memory failure becomes apparent and the affected individual may forget conversations, events of the day, or the purpose of errands. Grooming usually decreases, confusion increases, and emotional outbursts may occur. The symptoms of dementia may have many possible causes, some of which are treatable, so it is vital that we not dismiss such symptoms as "just old age." Anyone exhibiting these symptoms should be given a thorough medical examination. Even if a person suffers from incurable dementia, appropriate treatment may greatly improve the quality of his or her life.

The two main incurable forms of dementia are Alzheimer's disease and multi-infarct dementia (formerly called "cerebral arteriosclerosis" which means "hardening of the arteries of the brain"). Alzheimer's disease involves progressive, diffuse atrophy of brain tissue. Multi-infarct dementia is caused by a series of minor strokes that result in death of brain tissue in different parts of the brain. However, many *reversible* conditions have similar symptoms—such as a minor head injury, high fever, poor nutrition, or reaction to a drug. Emotional problems, particularly severe depression, can also be confused with dementia. Thus a thorough mental and neurological evaluation should be obtained for anyone showing possible signs of deteriorating brain function. The National Institute of Aging estimated that 10 to 20 percent of dementias in the elderly are reversible.

Although they cannot be cured, people with irreversible brain disorders can often be helped. Carefully prescribed drugs can lessen agitation, anxiety, and depression and can improve sleeping patterns. Proper nutrition in the form of a well-balanced diet is desirable. The person should be encouraged to maintain daily routines, physical activities, and social contacts, and should not be overprotected or discouraged from trying new things. Supplying information on the time of day, place of residence, and what is going on in the immediate environment and in world events can stimulate the individuals to use those skills and information that remain.

Memory aids can also help people in their day-to-day living. Joseph D. Alter, M.D., Professor of Community Medicine at Wright State University School of Medicine, suggests posting a large calendar, lists of daily activities, written notes about simple safety measures, and labeling and directions for commonly used items. To help keep track of medications, he suggests making a chart or using a styrofoam egg carton with each day's pills arranged in a compartment in the order they are to be taken.

Maintaining constructive activity may help to slow down further deterioration of the brain. Of course as deterioration progresses, increased supervision and even institutionalization may become necessary.

SOURCE: Stephen M. Barrett, M.D., 1987 (May), *Healthline*.

Fluid intelligence Spontaneous decision-making ability.

Interleukin-1 An immune-enhancing protein produced in response to exercise.

Exploring Your Emotions

What kind of life will make you feel satisfied to have lived? How do you feel you could adjust your lifestyle to encompass such a life? What kind of person do you want to become?

particularly when weighed against the physical and mental deterioration of the elderly who have not kept their minds and bodies fit, who have not used, challenged, and stretched mind and body. The stimulus that exercise provides seems to protect against the loss of some **fluid intelligence**, our spontaneous decision-making ability. Fluid intelligence depends on rapidity of responsiveness, memory, and alertness. Contrary to former notions that this capability necessarily declined with age, studies reveal that older people who are highly fit score better on tests of intelligence than do their less fit counterparts. Also, older men who continue actively with racquet sports and running show faster response times than do their sedentary, age-matched control group opposites. Exercise also appears to have some power against depression, apathy, and boredom.

Exercise is the closest thing we have to a magic anti-aging pill and the fountain of youth: it slows the aging process and lessens chances of disease. So you need to find activities that you enjoy and can do on a regular basis. Read the exercise chapter for ideas. Alternate choices: swim and bike on alternate days. Walk instead of ride. Walk briskly and often. Climb stairs instead of taking the elevator.

You will reap the benefits of the active and vigorous lifestyle as you age:

- Increased resiliency and suppleness of arteries
- Better protection against heart attack and much increased chance of survival should one occur
- Sustained capacity of lungs and respiratory reserves
- Weight control through less accumulation of fat
- Maintenance of physical flexibility, balance, agility, reaction time
- Greatly preserved muscle strength
- Protection against ligament injuries, dislocation strains in the knees, spine, shoulders
- Sustained basal metabolic rates to a greater degree
- Improved peripheral resistance, blood cholesterol, blood pressure
- Protection against occurrence of bone fractures caused by bone brittleness, demineralization, and porousness
- Increased effectiveness of the immune system, perhaps through exercise-elevated temperature and related production of **interleukin-1**, an immune-enhancing protein
- Maintenance of mental flexibility, response time, memory, hand-eye coordination

Eat Wisely Health at every age is facilitated by a varied diet with perhaps special attention to lower calorie intake.

- Eat low-fat, high-complex carbohydrate meals. Concentrate on fresh fruits and vegetables, high-fiber, whole-grain cereals and breads, potatoes, brown rice, pasta.
- Eat dark-meat fish (salmon, tuna, mackerel, swordfish, rainbow trout) and poultry (no skin) instead of fatty meats and eggs. See the chapter on cardiovascular health.
- Use no-fat or low-fat dairy products. Substitute olive oil for other oils and fats. Say no to fatty, rich desserts.
- Control caloric intake so that it does not exceed your needs in maintaining an ideal weight.
- Use less salt, more calcium, and possibly more foods with iron.

Control Drinking Alcohol impairs both liver and kidney function. Heavy drinkers suffer brain damage too. Alcohol taken in excess directly destroys lives, both the drinker's and others: more than 25,000 traffic deaths each year involve drinking drivers and drinking pedestrians.

Maintain Normal Weight Obesity is not physically healthy. Obesity actually produces premature aging. The fat person deteriorates in the same way as the slim person, but earlier. The fatter people are, the more likely they are to die, but as people age, the risks become much greater. Adults who have been obese since infancy are not usually very successful in achieving normal weight, but their health risks seem to be less than those faced by people who become obese in adulthood. People can control their weight, although it takes time and is not easy. A sensible program of using more calories through exercise and perhaps cutting down on calories or a combination of both will work for most people who want to lose weight, but there is no magic formula.

Don't Smoke The average pack-a-day smoker can expect to live an average of 12 years fewer than those who don't smoke. Worse, smokers suffer more illnesses that last longer, and they are subject to respiratory disabilities that limit their total vigor many years before their death. Even young cigarette smokers suffer respiratory impairment, some within a year of starting to smoke. Premature balding and skin wrinkling have been linked to cigarette

Hypertension Abnormally high blood pressure.

Vascular system The heart and blood vessels.

Diabetes A chronic disease characterized by too much sugar in the blood and urine.

smoking. Smokers at age 50 have the wrinkles of a person of 60. More details (see Chapter 9) complete the picture: smoking is not part of the long or good life.

Detect and Control Hypertension and Diabetes The victim of **hypertension**, does not notice it in the early stages. It can take a terrible toll in premature disability and death, but it can be successfully controlled if the person will take medication and change some living habits. Without control, wear and tear and finally breakdown of **vascular systems** accelerate greatly. A simple check of blood pressure, which takes only a few minutes, will show if a person has hypertension. Blood pressure that is higher than 140/90 is abnormal for anyone, and even small increases in blood pressure can reduce life expectancy considerably.

Diabetes can escape detection for years. It accelerates the breakdown of body organs and systems, especially the circulatory system, and increases the risk of hypertension, heart attack, and stroke. When diabetes is diagnosed and treated early, however, the diabetic has an improved chance of living a full life span.

Recognize and Reduce Stress If you have to rush to meet work deadlines or catch yourself in a traffic jam or are continuously exposed to high noise levels, you are a victim of stress. Your blood pressure rises, your heart rate quickens, and your body chemistry changes. While early humans may have needed these responses to prepare them for "fight or flight," it appears now that these changes caused by stress increase wear and tear on our bodies. Cut down on the stresses in your life, perhaps by living within bicycling distance of work and shopping, choosing less stressful occupations and recreations, and avoiding noisy, frenetic environments.

If you contract a disease, you could consider it an attempt by your body to interrupt your life pattern to permit you to re-evaluate your lifestyle, perhaps to slow down. Someone once suggested, "Death is nature's way of telling you to slow down."

Confronting Social, Emotional, and Mental Changes of Aging

Although the practices just mentioned are useful throughout life, a cluster of events occurs around the 50s, 60s, and 70s that must be grappled with and resolved. These developmental tasks of aging are determined by biological and social changes and require significant adjustments. Although aging is unique for each person, these changes cut across ethnic and socioeconomic variables. If you have aging parents, grandparents, and friends, the following information may help you understand their behavior better and enable you to help them understand themselves better.

1. Decreased energy and changes in health require the aging to *develop priorities for how to use energy*. Energy level is psychologically related to life satisfaction. A boring, tedious, uneventful, or overscheduled, "dutiful" life tailored to meet someone else's expectations is exhausting.

Physical disabilities and chronic diseases drain and deplete energy. Time spent incapacitated is correlated with poverty. Also, much exhaustion attributed to aging actually is caused by depression, and may be directly related to poor health, poverty, poor adjustment to losses, or to a lack of preparation for aging. One common disability—hearing loss—particularly affects personality: depression and paranoia result from the sense of isolation that deafness can bring.

Rather than curtailing activities to conserve energy—a strategy that can actually perpetuate feelings of illness and depression—the aging need to learn how to stimulate themselves and to generate energy. That usually involves saying no to unenjoyable things as well as yes to enjoyable ones. It also requires close attention to needs for rest and to sleep schedules: each is unique and changes as people age.

2. Retirement may mean a severely restricted budget, possibly financial disaster. You need to *take stock of finances* and plan for the future while you are in your 40s and 50s. Estimate what you need to meet your standard of living, calculate your projected income, and perhaps begin a savings program.

The older person who is poor is likely to be unhappy. Some creative, energetic older people may live happily on very little money, but doing so is difficult in our society. Many pleasures, such as travel, must be purchased. In our culture we are taught to derive pleasure by consuming rather than to generate it. But there are alternatives. Europeans have been found to enjoy leisure time more, to need less money for their pleasure, and to take more vacations. They appear to enjoy simpler things: often they use a vacation for a walking tour, camping out at night. That's

(Text continues on p. 524.)

Selecting a Nursing Home

Afraid of entering a nursing home yourself? Grieving over a decision to place a spouse or family member in one? There is cause to feel more cheerful about such decisions these days. Considerable evidence suggests that the typical nursing home has improved in quality over the past several decades. In fact, the rapid increase in the number of nursing home beds has been traced to the improved image of this institution.

The chances of an aged person living in a nursing home at some point in a lifetime are currently estimated to be at least one in four. The risk of institutionalization is greater for women than for men because women tend to live longer and to reach an age where chronic disabilities are more common. Women are also more likely to be widowed and thus to lack a spouse—and a spouse is most often the person who takes care of a disabled elderly person living at home. Moving a family member into a nursing home can be very difficult for both the client and the family. It is wise to plan ahead for this possibility, for the best nursing homes usually have long waiting lists. A little forethought and planning help to ease this transition. Before making any decisions, two questions need to be addressed. First, is the placement really necessary? And second, how should one go about selecting a home?

Alternative Community Services

Many people who currently reside in a nursing home could actually be better cared for in the community if alternative services are available. Whether or not the nursing home is the right solution for you depends on two conditions: the availability of alternative community services (such as adult day health care, home health care, personal care, or congregate housing), and on the ability of the prospective client and caregivers to cope with the burdens imposed by illness. One way to determine the need for placement is by making a thorough assessment of the individual's and caregiver's resources. This type of assessment is becoming more available at hospital outpatient clinics or through other services for the elderly. One study has shown that evaluation by a team of physicians, psychiatrists, geriatric nurse practitioners, social workers, and rehabilitation therapists resulted in 80 percent of the clients being returned home after the evaluation. A good assessment service usually provides a case manager who can monitor the client's needs and the family's resources as they fluctuate over time. This person is a nurse or social worker who directly counsels and advises the client and his or her family. This worker can serve as a liaison and can lead families to the appropriate health and social services on an ongoing basis to meet these changing needs.

How to Select a Home

If placement in a nursing home is clearly in the best interests of the client and his or her family, they need to select a home best suited to their needs. Evaluating the quality of care these homes provide can be complicated. Does the home and its administrator have a current state license? If the client needs financial assistance and is eligible for government or other forms of assistance, select a home certified to participate in such programs. If the client needs a special diet or a specific treatment, be sure that the home can provide them. The location of the home also should be acceptable to the client, close to a general hospital, convenient for the client's personal physician, and not too distant for frequent visiting by family and friends. Once these criteria narrow the choices down to a few homes, both the client and his or her family need to visit each of them in person.

The actual quality of patient care is more difficult to assess, but your observations can be a useful guide. Start by checking the beds to make sure only those patients who *should* be in bed are actually there. Are patients unattended or unnecessarily restrained? Such problems may be indicative of poorly trained or too few staff.

Then check the overall standard of cleanliness, the quality of the amenities and furnishings, and the freedom from unpleasant odors. Check the rooms to see if many personal possessions have been brought from home. Encouraging the use of everyday objects brought from home fosters a more homelike setting and may ease adjustment to the new environment.

To evaluate the social environment, look for friendly interactions among residents, involvement in meaningful activities, and a supportive and friendly staff. The staff

(continued on next page)

Selecting a Nursing Home (*continued*)

should know the residents' names. From talking to staff members, one can see if they have positive attitudes toward the residents and toward their own work. Friends and relatives of other residents in the home, as well as other residents themselves, can give you some indication of the quality of care.

Financial worries may override other considerations. Understanding Medicare and Medicaid policies is a first step in finding out about any third-party payments to ease the financial strain. Become familiar with what services and supplies are covered in the basic daily rate, as well as what optional services are charged separately. Nursing homes are very expensive, and many residents exhaust all private sources of funds after admission. Those who are forced to seek Medicaid funds at some point after they have gained admission, however, do have the legal right to remain at the facility. According to federal law, it is illegal to discharge a patient for lack of funds.

Certain publications can serve as further guides in selecting a nursing home:

- Health Care Financing Administration, *How to Select a Nursing Home* (HCFA-30043 booklet), December 1980. The helpful checklist can be used to systematically compare different nursing homes.
- California Health Facilities Commission, *Choosing a Long-term Care Facility in California,* pamphlet (1984). It gives suggestions on how to use detailed cost and operational information about the 1,200 nursing homes in the state to compare selected features of these facilities. This information covers five areas: nursing services, nonnursing expenses, employee turnover, citations issued for noncompliance with regulatory standards, and the level of profitability. It is intended to help consumers make a more informed decision about which nursing home to select.

Many other states' departments of health services have similar reports. And your local Area Agency on Aging or your local Health Systems Agency may be able to give you information about the nursing homes and alternative community-based services in your area.

SOURCE: Leslie A. Grant and Colleen L. Johnson, 1986 (November), A family guide for selecting a nursing home, *Healthline.*

Abuse of Aged Parents

When her son walked out and left Sarah Clark to the mercies of his angry family, the 75-year-old widow kept her fears to herself. She didn't complain when her daughter-in-law, Nancy, began to shout drunkenly: "Since we can't take it out on your good-for-nothing bastard of a son, we'll just have to take it out on you." Nor did the frail old woman seek help even when Nancy made good on the threats: blackening her eyes, bruising her arms, and forcing her to grovel for food. The concern of a sharp-eyed Massachusetts neighbor and a persistent visiting nurse eventually ended Mrs. Clark's ordeal—but only after three years of repeated abuse. Her terrified rationale for silence, according to Boston elderly-rights advocate James Bergman: "No matter what, the daughter-in-law was her sole provider."

Now that Americans have finally faced the appalling realities of battered children and wives, a shocking new family secret is coming to light: the abused parent. Elderly and dependent, these long-silent victims are being physically assaulted and psychologically degraded by their own resentful children or even grandchildren, a problem geriatrics specialist Diana Koin calls "the King Lear syndrome" (after Shakespeare's aging monarch who fell afoul of his two scheming daughters). Like Mrs. Clark, many abused parents are reluctant to complain, fearing they will lose their source of support—or be shuttled off to an institution that could be still worse. Due to that reticence, their real numbers are not yet known. But at least one expert estimates that between

Abuse of Aged Parents (*continued*)

500,000 and one million aged parents are abused in any given year—and that number may well worsen as inflation drives more old people to move in with their families.

Some researchers say the abusers were once abused by these same parents, and now want their measure of vengeance. But many are not as monstrous as they seem. They may find tending to a senile, bedridden, bedwetting parent an unbearable financial and emotional burden just as their own children are growing up. Meanwhile, they are torn with guilt over the temptation to commit the invalid to a nursing home. "It may be a question of reaching a breaking point," says Marilyn Block, of the Center on Aging at the University of Maryland. "The children want to do right, but they find they can't cope."

Transferring the responsibility, however, is often impossible. "You can't divorce your parents," says sociologist Richard J. Gelles, co-author of *Behind Closed Doors,* a study of family violence. . . . "As stressful as it may get, this is not a relationship that society allows you to break." In her own study of the King Lear syndrome, Diana Koin discovered that the stresses usually grew out of long-term family conflicts. The tensions cut across socioeconomic lines, she discovered—and so did the resultant abuse. "Professional families did it, working-class families did it, black families did it, and white families did it," says Koin, who is chief of geriatric medicine at St. Luke's Hospital in Denver.

Pressured Few public counseling, financial aid, or day care programs are available to ease the pressure on children, and few laws adequately protect aged parents. Only eleven states now have laws requiring physicians and other professionals to report elderly abuse cases to legal authorities; another eleven are considering them. Where there are other legal remedies, moreover, they are often difficult to enforce. On the federal level, no abuse law specifically protects the elderly, although a domestic violence bill now pending before the Senate could provide assistance.

The state of Connecticut is a leading exception to the general rule of government neglect. Since 1978, anyone who regularly deals with the elderly must report suspicious occurrences or risk a $500 fine. Five ombudsmen from the Department of Aging check out complaints and arrange social services as needed; about one-third of the 1,000 cases reported in the first year involved physical abuse. In one chilling instance, a boy called police and said his grandmother was being beaten. When investigators arrived, they found the woman bruised and chained to a chair, but still refusing to give up her Social Security check. Her son was arrested.

Gray Power Even without much help from the government, the elderly are starting to fight back. Groups like the American Association of Retired Persons are lobbying for such services as senior citizen day care, and they expect to pick up power as the aged population continues to grow. But to rescue the victims, the law must first find them, and almost by definition, most are elderly shut-ins, hidden away from prying eyes. "Even a battered child is more protected," declares John Von Glahn, executive director for the Family Service Association of Orange County, California, which specializes in family abuse problems. "During the course of their activities they come in contact with all kinds of people—schoolteachers, nurses, and doctors. About the only place many of the elderly can call for help is the police department, and few will sign an arrest warrant for their own son or daughter." The ironic truth may be that, for all their fears, a nursing home could well provide a safer refuge for aged parents than the bosom of their own family.

SOURCE: *Newsweek*

Life expectancy The average length of life of members of a species.

Life span Theoretically projected length of life based on maximum potential of the human body in the best environment.

a sharp contrast to the American way of seeing how many miles can be driven in an air-conditioned car between luxury motels.

3. You need to *learn to enjoy yourself when you are alone.* Old age involves the problem of what to do with privacy. We know how to act in public; we hardly know what to do with ourselves when we are alone. In our culture, we are not encouraged to spend time alone. Taking pleasure in being alone with yourself may be considered antisocial.

People who enjoy time alone—reading, walking, doing genealogy, photography, quilting, keeping up with the news—are blessed. Loneliness is often felt by people who lack a sense of self and identity. One major problem for many older people today is that they have never established a personal identity independent from their social roles—which begin to break down in later years.

4. Loss of social roles and changes in status, retirement, loss of friends, spouse or peers, and problems of identity are linked problems. Our socialization process does not prepare us for living with the losses of retirement. Retirement means a new status, a new social definition, a new economic situation. And while it allows the advantages of leisure and freedom from deadlines, competition, and stress, many people do not know how to cope with free time. They do not know how "to leisure." Without work and "productivity," some fall prey to loneliness, boredom, depression.

With more free time, perhaps fewer friends, and increasing obstacles to getting around, you will need to *seek new sources of nurturance and stimulation* when your usual resources disappear. People who age best tend to be involved in various interests and with others; they are usually curious and flexible, and those who live in families fare better mentally than those who live alone. They may need to enroll in adult education courses, read and discuss more, travel, do volunteer work. They may have to reorder their values so that "productivity" and power are not the keys to their identity.

5. *Resolve grief and mourning.* We all have losses: friends, peers, physical appearance, and health. Grief is the work of getting through the pain of loss, and it can be one of the most lonely, intense, and intimate events in a person's life.

The griever must work through shock, disbelief, denial, and numbness. Usually within a year of a loved one's death, some resolution occurs: decreasing sadness, resumption of ordinary life, ability to recall the past with pleasure as well as pain. Unfortunately, most people endure grief alone in our society. But others can help by encouraging the mourner to express the grief and by being sympathetic.

Eventually we must relinquish grief. This is not a new experience: we have often said farewells to discarded self-images, broken dreams, friends who move away, parents who die. We all let go of illusions: we are not as brilliant, talented, famous, all-loving, or sensitive as we had dreamed. We lose people and possessions throughout life, not just in old age.

Death is a total loss—the loss of yourself. Adapting positively to the reality of your own death is a major task of aging. Older people need to discuss their feelings about death and dying, but rarely have an opportunity to do so because the subject is still taboo and because so many people are uncomfortable talking about death. Accepting future death can enrich your life now: Paul Keen has observed that "life is richest when we realize we are all snowflakes. Each of us is absolutely beautiful and unique. And we are here for a very short time."

6. Aging changes and slows down sexuality. Depending on the importance of sexual activity in your life, you will need to *adjust to sensory and sexual losses.* This adjustment can be difficult. Some people, grieving for the loss of this significant aspect of themselves, go through stages of mourning, especially depression.

Loss of interest in sex and impotence are often socially, rather than biologically, induced. Some people remain sexually active into their 80s. And when sexual problems do occur, usually counseling can help. Sexuality researchers and therapists William Masters and Virginia Johnson report that they are able to restore potency in about two-thirds of their elderly male patients. And older couples can free themselves from the "scoring" mentality of sex American style. They can learn to accept the idea that love play and pleasure can be enjoyed in themselves and do not always have to end in orgasm.

7. A major task of aging is to *adopt an appropriate attitude toward whatever life brings you.* Only the right mental attitude can stave off the negative effects of some circumstances. The attitude of youth is based on striving—for more knowledge, strength, capability, understanding of one's self. Its principle force is growth. But the proper mental attitude for a successful elder should be toward self-enjoyment rather than self-aggrandizement. Philoso-

pher George Santayana wrote, "To be interested in the changing seasons is in this middling zone, a happier state of mind than to be hopelessly in love with Spring."

To adapt, older people need to "stay open" to change. It takes some effort to be flexible, to go with the flow, to say yes more often, to open your mind to new experiences, new types of people, and new places.

Increased Life Expectancy: The Myth and the Reality

Human **life expectancy** is the average length of life we can expect to live. It is calculated by averaging the death ages of a group of people over a certain period of time. Life expectancy from birth in the United States has increased dramatically, from 49 years in 1900 to about 77 years in 1985. This does not mean that every American now lives twenty-eight years longer than in 1900. Rather, far fewer people die young now, because childhood and infectious diseases are much better controlled, and diet and sanitation have much improved since 1900. In 1900, only 30 percent of the population lived to be 70 years old. In 1980, 60 percent lived to 70. (For an even broader view of life expectancy through the ages, see Figure 22-2.)

The young benefit far more from modern medical and public health measures than do the elderly. As late as 1980, a person of 65 could expect to live only about six years longer than a person of 65 in 1900. In 1987, however, the U.S. Census Bureau reported a dramatic 3 percent decrease in death rates from the three preceding years: the life expectancy of women was raised to 78 years and that of men to 71 years. These all-time U.S. highs reflect new medical successes as well as health payoffs from early identification and treatment of high blood pressure, more prudent diets, and less cigarette smoking among middle-aged adults.

Another significant aspect of life expectancy is that as you age and survive the hazards to your life in younger years, you gain statistical life expectancy. For example, life expectancy for males born in 1980 is 70 years, but for men who were age 20 in 1980, the expected remaining number of years of life is 52.5, a total of 72.5 years (20 + 52.5). For a female born in 1980, life expectancy is 78 years, but for women who were age 30 in 1980, the expected remaining number of years of life is 50, or a total of 80 years. Statistically, you never run out of life expectancy. Even at age 85, men and women still have an expectation of 5.3 and 6.8 more years, respectively.

So how long can we humans expect to live in the best of circumstances? It now seems likely that genetically our maximum potential **life span** is from 100 to 120 years. Failure to achieve that span in good health results largely from destructive environmental and behavioral factors—factors we can exert considerable control over. Do not assume that prolonging life automatically prolongs old age disability. People often live longer because they have been well longer. A healthy, productive old age is almost always an extension of a healthy, productive middle age.

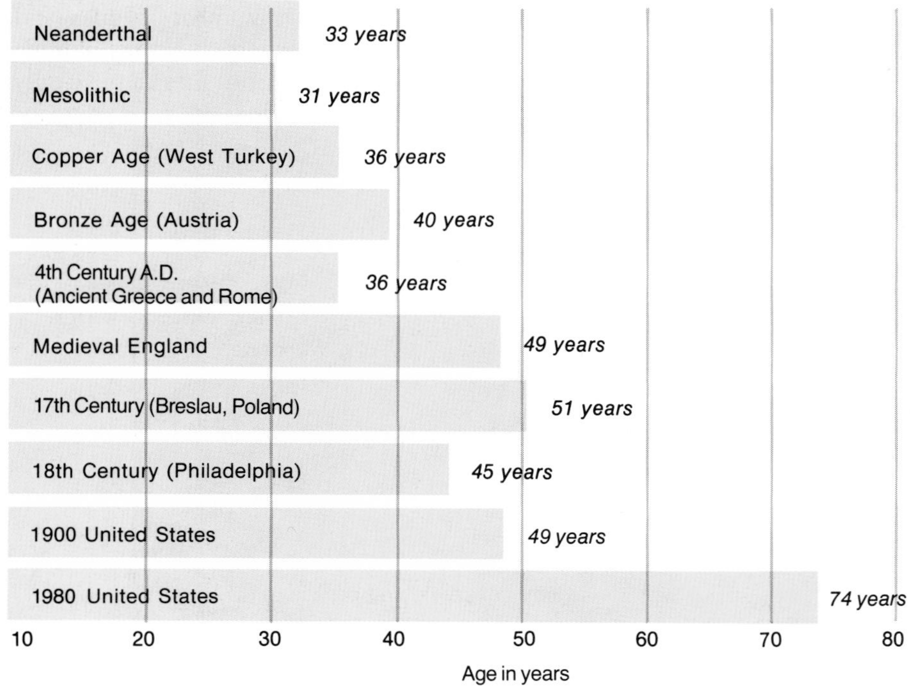

Figure 22-2 Estimated changes in life expectancy through history.

Increasing the average life span to 90-plus years would not affect maximum longevity. Few people would actually live to be 100. Only if science could unravel the biological mystery of aging and control the aging process would the picture be quite different. A greater number of people would live much longer lives. With some successes in studies of longevity, perhaps that is possible in this century.

Theories of Aging

Throughout history people have searched for and invented a great variety of "magic" preparations, devices, and practices for preserving youth. None works. More recently, science has entered the arena, directing research toward aging. Researchers would like to break through the riddles of cells and hormones to enable people to live longer and maintain much of their youthful vigor.

Some scientists believe aging is genetically programmed: a necessary process by which the older members of a species make way for the younger members. Like a spaceship designed to fly past Mars, but with no built-in instructions beyond that point, a human may be programmed to get to 85 or 90 years and to keep on going, but its various systems will begin to break down and continue until the breakdown is total.

What causes the breakdown, the decline in free energy production, the body's inability to function and maintain itself? (See Figure 22-3.) None of the existing theories of aging accommodates all the facts. Maybe aging is caused by a variety of different processes.

Environmental Factors As people lose their ability to withstand the stresses of the environment, they become more susceptible to certain diseases, particularly to the mass killers—heart attack and cancer. Environmental factors trigger many of these diseases.

One set of nutrition studies underscores its effects on aging. In the 1920s Clive McCay of Cornell concluded from an experiment that the 100- to 120-year barrier to the human life span can be surpassed. He fed white rats enough vitamins, minerals, and proteins to keep them alive, but he did not give them enough calories to grow normally. He fed another group of rats the same diet, but these rats were allowed to eat as much sugar and lard as they wanted. The animals on the diet with fewer calories did not grow as fast as the others, and they kept their youthful appearance even after the normally fed rats were dead (after about 1,000 days). Then he gave animals that had been "fasting" full rations. These animals developed to almost normal size, and some lived for as long as 1,400 days, or about 50 percent longer than the rats who ate the standard diet throughout their lives. This experiment is important because it was the first time the environment had been manipulated to change the "fixed" life span of an animal.

One implication of this study is that parents would be wise to avoid overfeeding infants and children during their developmental years, especially foods loaded with fat and sugar.

Genetic Factors Heredity also affects aging. Research on genetic factors has given rise to a variety of theories about aging.

Limited Replication Program in the Cell The genetic makeup of the cell largely controls aging. One theory is that a cell can duplicate itself only a limited number of times, and may have so-called aging genes that spell out the limiting number. This would explain why fruit flies can live only a maximum of about 100 days, dogs 30 years, humans

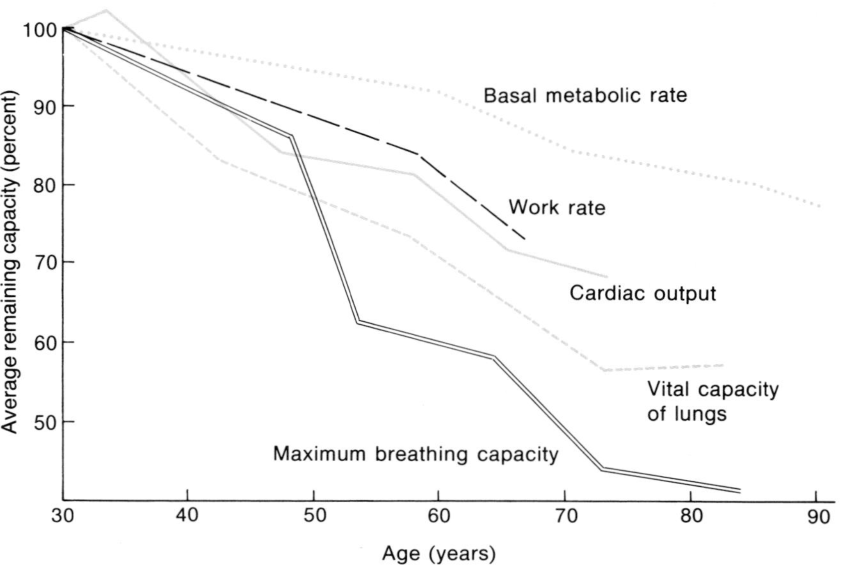

Figure 22-3 Decline of basic physiological capacities with age.

Neurotransmitter A substance that transmits nerve impulses.

Dopamine An important brain neurotransmitter.

Hypothalamus A part of the brain that controls functions such as eating and breathing.

Pituitary gland A master gland at the base of the brain that secretes hormones to control other glands.

Thyroid gland A gland in the neck that controls the rate of body metabolism.

Thymus gland A glandlike structure that aids in building resistance to disease in early childhood.

Dehydroepiandrosterone (DHEA) A hormone formed in the adrenal glands of the fetus and believed to influence the aging process.

---

120 years, and giant tortoises 180 years. Certain cells cultivated from the lung tissue of a four-month-old human embryo have multiplied only about 50 times before they died. In addition, about the thirty-fifth time they multiplied, these cells began to show signs of age.

Errors in DNA and RNA Duplication A change in DNA molecules may contribute to the aging process. DNA molecules contain the basic genetic instructions for the orderly behavior of the cell. In aging, the DNA may somehow become defective, and may consequently synthesize defective protein. This defect disables normal cell functioning, causing the cell to deteriorate.

Aged insects and experimental animals also show decreased amounts of RNA in their brain cells. If a similar condition occurs in aged human beings, preserving brain RNA might effectively slow aging. Drugs developed to improve memory by increasing RNA might also be applied to slow the aging process.

Destructive Immune System Responses Another theory suggests that for some unknown reason the aging body begins to err in synthesizing protein, and produces changed proteins that the person's immune system cannot recognize. The immune mechanism attacks them as it would any foreign substance, destroying cells and impairing body functions.

The increasing incidence of diseases among older people suggests that their immune systems may produce significantly fewer antibodies, increasing their vulnerability to disease. Researchers are testing drugs that would reinforce faltering immune systems.

Brain Chemistry Aging may be caused by a lack of coordination among the various tissues of the body, caused by faulty nerve impulse transmission. Chemical **neurotransmitters** in the brain transmit nerve impulses and are responsible for keeping the tissues of the body tuned as finely as the instruments of a symphony orchestra. In old age, the brain neurotransmitter **dopamine** is commonly greatly reduced. Insufficient dopamine prevents the **hypothalamus** from signaling the **pituitary gland** to produce the hormones necessary for the **thyroid** and **thymus glands** to function. Reduced thyroid impairs cell maintenance in the brain and elsewhere. Reduced thymus function lowers production of T cells—one type of lymphocyte—which are linked to immunity to cancer, among other disorders.

Takashi Makinodan at the National Institute on Aging has dramatically increased life spans of rats in two ways. One is by transplanting young thymuses into older animals. The other is by storing lymphocytes from young rats and transfusing those lymphocytes back into the same animals when they are older. Drug experiments aimed at maintaining certain levels of brain dopamine are being conducted to help slow down pathological aging.

Hormone Imbalance Some doctors have tried hormone therapy to prevent aging in both men and women. Men were given testosterone, the male sex hormone, to supplement their own production of testosterone. They experienced new vigor and better muscle tone, but because of its side effects it is not commonly used. Hormone therapy with estrogens is, however, often used with women to treat disturbances associated with menopause, including osteoporosis, a deterioration of the bones.

Gerontologists are enthusiastically watching experiments with the hormone **dehydroepiandrosterone (DHEA)**. Human production of DHEA falls sharply with age and is drastically reduced in women prone to breast cancer and in men who have heart attacks. In experimental animals, artificially administered DHEA has prevented decline in the immune system, lowered serum cholesterol, and blocked growth of induced cancer. Also, evidence shows that DHEA can control some weight gain and reduce blood-sugar levels in diabetics.

Should We Tamper with the Aging Process?

Significantly extended life spans would bring great social changes. Such extension appears to be inevitable, and the effects of slowing the aging process will vary depending on which diseases are eliminated. If, for example, diseases of the blood vessels now associated with aging were wiped out, people on the average might expect to live 11 years longer. With the most usual causes of death eliminated, however, more people would then die of remaining causes, and more would survive only to face long exposure to environmental hazards and accumulated stress. Some would suffer even greater disability and dependence during added years.

Scientific advances in lengthening lives must be matched with better control and understanding of environment and lifestyles. Researchers are aware of the problems, and they do not aim to prolong lives that are nothing more than living death. We can work, rather, toward adding productive and fulfilling years.

Realizing the Benefits of Aging

Research in aging today holds more hope and promise than in the past. People now in their 40s and 50s will probably benefit from new knowledge about the aging process. And the enormous increase in the over-55 population is markedly affecting our stereotypes of what it means to grow old. Being old is increasingly a state of mind rather than a biological marker. The misfortunes associated with aging—frailty, forgetfulness, poor health, isolation—occur to fewer people in their 60s and 70s, and have shifted instead to the very old, those over 85.

The "younger" elderly who are in good physical and mental health are being welcomed back into society; politicians are listening to them; advertisers have targeted them as a good market. The elderly are, in general, better off than they have been in the past. They have more money than they did twenty years ago. The median income today for those over 65 is $12,500 per year. Almost 75 percent of these people own their homes. Their living expenses are lower after retirement because they no longer support children and have fewer work-related expenses; they consume and buy less food. They are more likely to continue practicing their expertise for years after retirement and to be paid in cash. Thousands of retired consultants, teachers, technicians, and craftsmen work till their mid and late 70s. They receive greater amounts of in-kind assistance, such as Medicare; pay proportionately less in taxes; and have greater net worth from lifetime savings.

Yet for the most part the elderly are not a prosperous group. Tens of thousands of older Americans still live in poverty. These other elderly—the poverty-stricken, the disabled, and the lonely—are just as ignored as they ever were. How many of these unacceptable elderly there are is uncertain, but their numbers are increasing. One of seven subsists below the "official" poverty line of $5,000 per year. About half these poor elderly live in large cities, the other half in towns and rural areas. $5,000 does not go far in a city: maybe half for rent and half for food. Single black women fare worst: around 43 percent live in poverty. Of the country's 16.4 million elderly single white women, 17 percent are under the poverty line, and about 8 percent of elderly white males live in poverty. How would *you* live on $5,000 a year? Even $8,000?

Government Aid and Policies The government helps the elderly through several programs such as food stamps, housing subsidies, Social Security, and Medicare. Social Security, the life insurance and old age pension plan, has been a godsend for many, and it appears secure through the turn of the century. More help is needed, however—possibly a guaranteed annual income and guaranteed health care. Amid great controversy, health and Social Security planners are rethinking and reforming the government's role.

The future of government-subsidized health care is not clear. In 1984, the United States spent $387 billion on health, about 11 percent of the **gross national product (GNP)**. About one-third of these personal health care expenditures went to care for aged people. The average expenditure for personal health services for those over age 65 was $3,140 in 1981, compared with $828 for those under 65.

The government picks up a substantial share of the health expenses of the elderly—primarily through the Medicare program, which finances acute health services for the elderly and disabled, and through Medicaid, which finances acute and long-term care services for the poor, including aged poor. Federal expenditures for Medicare have been projected to rise from $74 billion in 1985 to $120 billion in 1989, a 60 percent increase in 4 years.

Medicare is essential, paying about 45 percent of medical costs for the elderly. And almost 40 percent of Medicaid expenditures goes for the care of 3.5 million elderly people. But serious gaps in Medicare coverage require the elderly to pay for health care expenses out of their own pockets. Chronic diseases, for example, affect over half of those over 75 years old and force 22 percent to alter their lives to some extent. One-third of those over 85 need help walking, bathing, or eating. Over a million live in nursing homes, and 15 years from now when there are 2 million people over 85, the nursing home business will boom. But Medicare now pays less than 2 percent of the total nursing home bills, and private insurers pay less than 1 percent for nursing home costs. The financial burden on individuals and families is enormous, often sending them into poverty.

The question is, "What is the proper proportion of public resources that should be devoted to the elderly?" Can we continue to spend 11 percent of the GNP on health care of the entire population without inhibiting economic growth, especially when some other developed nations spend only half as much per capita while apparently enjoying equally good health?

Many health planners believe that instead of adding

Gross national product The total market value of all goods and services produced by a nation during a specific time period.

Gerontologists Medical doctors who specialize in studying and treating the elderly.

stop-gap measures to Medicare and Medicaid, we should reform the entire system of financing and delivering health service in the United States, not just those that serve the elderly. Because most health services are provided privately, and are financed by a mix of public programs, private insurance plans, and direct patient payments, we have no explicit means for controlling the health care quality and resources. Patients are largely free to choose their own physicians and health service providers. The government does not establish budgets for health services, and only a few states regulate rates charged by hospitals. Physicians charge patients whatever fees they choose and make virtually unchallenged decisions about which health services patients need and receive. As a result, the United States lacks both effective market control and governmental regulation of health expenditures.

As our population ages—and it is aging rapidly as fewer babies are born and people live longer—we shall either have to limit the public resources devoted to health care or be prepared to divert ever increasing economic resources for that purpose. Unfortunately, projections show that by the year 2000 the trust fund that pays Medicare's bills will be $150 billion in debt. Radical changes in the system are mandatory.

Exploring Your Emotions

How do you envision your old age? How will it resemble the life of old people you know now, and how will it differ? What worldwide events may affect your control of your old age lifestyle?

Politicians usually ignore this awkward problem. But perhaps the increasing numbers of the elderly will soon force us to change this attitude. The political clout of the elderly is increasing. In 1900 only 123,000 people were over age 85; now there are about 2.2 million. In 60 years there will be about 16 million people over 85 (5 percent of the population) and about 20 million people aged 75–84 (7 percent of the population). They are beginning to mobilize themselves.

Health policy planners hope that rising medical costs for the elderly will dwindle dramatically through education and preventive medicine. Health professionals, including **gerontologists** (medical doctors who study aging and minister to the elders in our society), are beginning to practice preventive medicine, just as pediatricians do. They advise the aging how to avoid and, if necessary, how to manage disabilities. They aim to instill an ethic of bodily and mental maintenance that would prevent chronic disease and allow the elderly to live long and vigorous lives until they arrive at death's doorstep.

Changing the Public's Idea of "Aging" Aging people may be one of our least used resources. How can we harness and use the knowledge and productivity of our growing numbers of older citizens, particularly of those we are now losing through mandatory early retirement?

Exploring Your Emotions

Before you yourself become old, your parents may die or need nursing care. How can you begin to prepare now for the feelings these events may evoke in you?

First we must change our thinking about what aging means. The public must learn to judge productivity rather than age. Capacity to function should replace age as a criterion for usefulness; statutory senility would end. Instead of singling out 65 as a magic number, we could consider ages 50 to 75 as the third quarter of life. Changes occur around 50 that signal a new era: children are usually grown and gone; a person has reached the maximum level of advancement in employment and highest real earnings. It is often the time of some restlessness, time for "repotting" the plant that has outgrown its container. The upper end of the quarter is determined by the fact that most people today are vigorous, in good health, mentally alert, and capable of making a productive contribution until they are at least 75 years old. That age estimate may be a bit high for some, but not for most. About 20 percent of the population—50 million people—falls within the third quarter. But twenty-five years from now, about 85 million will be in their third quarter.

Other formulas have been suggested for drawing the boundary line between middle and old age. Rather than counting from birth, we could count back a fixed number of years from the expected age at death. Using a current life table, we could calculate the age at which the average number of remaining years of life is 15. That would place old age around 67 today and 72 in the year 2030. Another way to decide who is old would be to limit the group to the most elderly 10 percent of the population, which would fix the age at 75 in 2030.

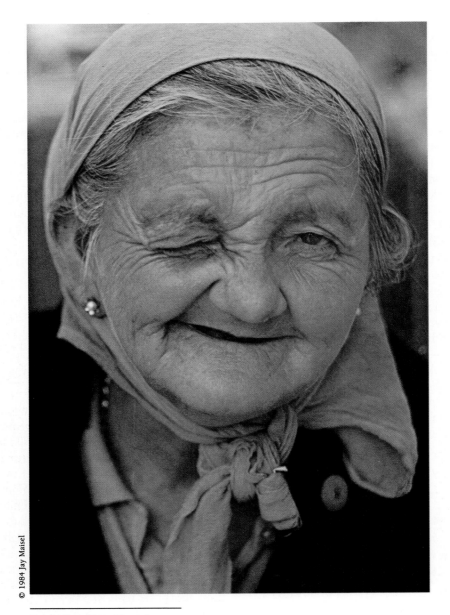

Exploring Your Emotions

Suppose you were sharing a long bus ride sitting beside this woman. What do you imagine she might tell you about her adaptation to aging? What questions would you like to ask her that might help you age gracefully?

Aging and Health: An Anthropological Point of View

Aging should be just another word for growing, for we are designed to grow (increase in amplitude) and develop (increase in complexity) all the days of our lives. When I say "designed," I mean precisely that, for the scientific evidence clearly shows that just as we have evolved physically, retaining our neotenous (or childlike) traits—for example, the large brain, the high forehead, the flatness of the face, and small teeth—so we are designed behaviorally by retaining the behavioral potentialities of the child. Those childlike traits are

The need for love	Speech
Friendship	Fantasy
Sensitivity	Self-esteem
The need to think soundly	Trust and honesty
The need to know	Openmindedness
To learn	Flexibility
To work	Experimental-mindedness
To organize	Explorativeness
Curiosity	Resiliency
Wonder	Sense of humor
Play	Joyfulness
Exercise	Laughter and tears
Imagination	Optimism
Creativity	Compassionate intelligence
Enthusiasm	Dance
Spontaneity	Song
Touch	

These are our inbuilt system of values which tell us what we ought to do: to grow young, to grow in health, to die young (as late in life as possible), and to live as if to live and love were one. To grow young means to grow and develop in the spirit of the child, in the childlike basic behavioral traits. To grow in health means to develop the ability to love, work, play, and use one's mind as a fine instrument of precision. If one will do these things one will certainly grow older with time, but one will never grow old.

The quality of life is a matter of the spirit, and all the evidence indicates that where the spirit is happily realized, the body will be too, for spirit, mind, and body are simply various faces of the same organism that is the human being. Certainly physical and physiological changes will occur during our life, but many of these are avoidable. Unfortunately the mythology that surrounds aging has resulted in a self-fulfilling prophecy which has deceived many, nay, almost everyone, into believing that growing older is a descent into senility and decrepitude. The old are expected "to act their age," to retire into nonentityism and anecdotage. Older people are made to feel old, to believe that they *are* old, and to fulfill only those requirements that are expected of them, to walk, talk, sit, think, rise and move as old people should. Dr. Gay Luce in her inspiring book, *Your Second Life* (New York: Delacorte, 1979), has listed the stereotypes of our culture relating to "old age":

- Old people should be dignified and circumspect.
- Old dogs cannot learn new tricks.
- Old people are close-minded, set in their ways, slow, senile.
- Old people are ugly.
- There is no future for old people. Why teach them?
- Old people don't want to use or touch their bodies.
- Old people like to sit still and be quiet.

These myths about old people are all false and very damaging. Nevertheless, our culture has forced millions of wonderful human beings into the tragedy of acting out the stereotypic roles expected of them, much of the time not altogether unwillingly, for the old have come to accept the mythology of aging quite as much as the young. In this way too many people have been shipwrecked by "old age" simply because they have never learned to navigate the waters in which they suddenly find themselves. They find themselves in unfamiliar territory, traumatically displaced persons consigned to the very outskirts of the society in which they were once full members; forced into a lifestyle for which they have not been prepared, a lifestyle of unstructured time and reduced input from the world with which they were once familiar.

The results are abandonment, rejection, and a kind of exile or excommunication.

Those who retain their youthfulness into the later years are the biologically elite, not simply because they have survived, but because they have attained that weathered wisdom that only they can possess. The truth is that age is in no way connected with feeling old, but in every way with feeling young. There is an untouched freshness that comes to us when we are old, which need not for a moment ever waver, but keep us buoyant all the days of our lives,

(continued on next page)

Aging and Health: An Anthropological Point of View (*continued*)

bringing to others that wisdom and that other gift which is the true vocation of the "old," love.

The whole of life is a journey toward youthful old age, toward self-contemplation, love, gaiety, and in a most fundamental sense, the most gratifying time of our lives. Growing older should mean reaching one's full behavioral potential, a completeness.

Our preoccupation with youth has made us forget that people considered "too old" often have the youngest ideas of all. "Old age" should be a harvest time when the riches of life are reaped and enjoyed, and shared, while it continues to be a special period of self-development and expansion, instead of a half-life waiting to die. And in that connection, one needs a special strength to die, rather than a special weakness, and that strength can only come to us by dying young, at whatever age that may be, neither surprised by time nor attenuated by it.

And finally: always remember that the fountain of youth resides in yourself.

SOURCE: Ashley Montagu, *Healthline*

Exploring Your Emotions

How do you feel about spending time with old people? How do you think they feel about you? How might you begin to open up communications with them?

Whatever way we define old age, the costs of losing these people to our national productivity is too high. We lose likewise their contribution to our quality of life, and we forfeit through their early retirement substantial income tax and Social Security tax revenues on their earnings. Those who retire at 62 start using their Social Security benefits earlier than otherwise.

A far better arrangement would be to make available full- and part-time volunteer and paid employment. We would benefit by providing retraining programs for both occupational and leisure time training. We need a greater number of community-sponsored classes in remunerative activities such as real estate selling and management, horticulture, library work, and classes for leisure time in the arts and music and writing, health maintenance, and genealogy. Volunteer jobs could include preparation of audiotapes and records for the blind, help with the retarded, doing textile design. At the same time we could possibly change both public and private pension programs to make partial retirement possible. In such cases we could allow people to borrow against their Social Security benefits to finance their retraining or enrollment in wholly new educational programs. One octogenarian, Russell Lee, founder of a medical clinic in California, suggests some potential advantages of aging: "The limitations imposed by time are compensated by the improved taste, sharper discretion, sounder mental and esthetic judgment, increased sensitivity and compassion, clearer focus—which all contribute to a more certain direction in living. . . . The later years can be the best of life for which the earlier ones were preparation."

Take Action

Your answers to the Exploring Your Emotions questions in this chapter and your placement level on the Awareness Ladder will, we hope, encourage you to begin a process of self-exploration and self-discovery that you will continue. Reflect on the entire chapter's content and ask yourself how each point relates to your own life. Then take action:

1. Imagine yourself as elderly. You have just made the decision to live in a retirement or nursing home. Visit such a home. Interview the manager and one or more residents. Write down you reactions in your Take Action notebook. Would you eventually want to live in such a home? Would you recommend it to an elderly relative or friend?

2. At what age should people retire? Survey five college students in their late teens or early twenties and five older people. Did the answers of the two groups vary?

3. What are the most pronounced differences between a 20-year-old and a 70-year-old? List the differences you perceive in your Take Action notebook, and ask your grandmother or some other older person if he or she agrees. What are the similarities between a 20-year-old and a 70-year-old?

4. Before leaving this chapter, review the Rate Yourself statements that open the chapter. Have your feelings or values changed? Are you now better equipped to handle the complex and very human problems associated with aging?

Selected References

Dickinson, Peter A. 1984. *The Complete Retirement Planning Book: Your Guide to Happiness, Health, and Financial Security*. New York: Dutton.

Lee, Russell V., M.D. 1976. *No Gravy on the Vest.* Corte Madera, Calif.: Omega Books.

Lieberman, Morton A., and Sheldon S. Tobin. 1983. *The Experience of Old Age*. New York: Basic Books.

Myers, Albert, and Christopher P. Andersen. 1984. *Success Over Sixty: How to Plan It; How to Have It; How to Live It.* New York: Summit Books.

Oberleder, Muriel, Ph.D. 1982. *Avoid the Aging Trap at 30, 50, 70 . . . .* Washington, D.C.: Acropolis Books.

Rosenfeld, Albert. 1985. *Prolongevity II*. New York: Knopf.

Walford, Roy L., M.D. 1983. *Maximum Life Span*. New York: W. W. Norton.

Recommended Readings

Dangott, Lillian R. and Richard A. Kalish. 1979. *A Time to Enjoy: the Pleasures of Aging*. Englewood Cliffs, N.J.: Prentice-Hall.
Introduction to the psychological aspects and developmental tasks of aging; warm and supportive tone.

Fromme, Allen, Ph.D. 1984. *60+: Planning It, Living It, Loving It.* New York: Farrar, Straus & Giroux.
Advice on senior life: practicing for retirement; better sex after 60; impact of inflation; art of living alone; making friends after 69.

Hallowell, Christopher. 1985. *Growing Old, Staying Young*. New York: Morrow.
A highly readable and sympathetic account of most aspects of aging, with a particular look at Alzheimer's.

Ogle, Jane. 1984. *Ageproofing*. New York: American Library.
Detailed and excellent description of physiological changes throughout life. Nutrition and fitness guides for aging gracefully.

Chapter 23

Contents

Rate Yourself

Your Attitudes about Dying and Death Read the following statements carefully. Choose the one in each section that best describes you at this moment and circle its number. When you have chosen one statement for each section, add the numbers and record your total score. Find your position on the Awareness Ladder.

5 Accepts death as a part of life
4 Recognizes that everyone must die
3 Seldom thinks about death
2 Feels that death is something that happens to others
1 Denies that everyone must eventually die

5 Feels and expresses grief unashamedly
4 Cries openly at funerals
3 Is somewhat inhibited about expressing grief
2 Holds back feelings of pain and loss
1 Is embarrassed to show feelings of loss and mourning

5 Feels the dead human body is a valuable source of organ transplants
4 Encourages people to donate organs after death
3 Agrees to permit own organs to be used after death
2 Is uncomfortable about donating organs after death
1 Feels people should be buried intact

5 Feels that funerals should celebrate life
4 Feels that funerals help the survivors
3 Feels that funerals provide a chance to honor the dead
2 Feels that funerals are useless
1 Uses funerals to impress others

5 Knows the costs of and how to plan funeral arrangements
4 Knows the options for appropriate disposition of the body
3 Is willing to learn about planning for death
2 Is not interested in learning about planning for death
1 Is unwilling to consider planning for death

Total Score ______

Dying and Death

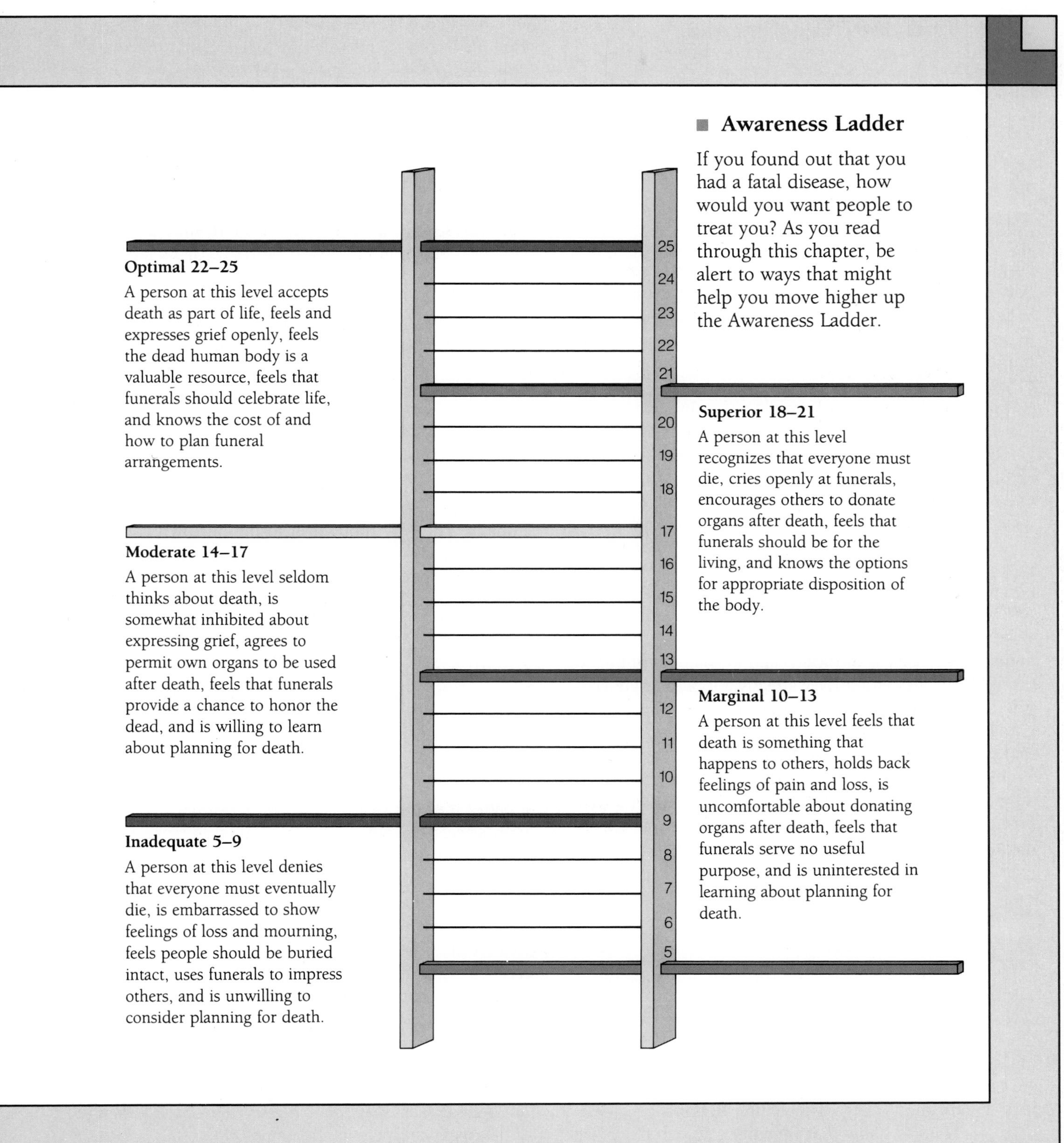

■ Awareness Ladder
If you found out that you had a fatal disease, how would you want people to treat you? As you read through this chapter, be alert to ways that might help you move higher up the Awareness Ladder.
25
24
23
22
21
20
19
18
17
16
15
14
13
12
11
10
9
8
7
6
5
Optimal 22–25
A person at this level accepts death as part of life, feels and expresses grief openly, feels the dead human body is a valuable resource, feels that funerals should celebrate life, and knows the cost of and how to plan funeral arrangements.
Superior 18–21
A person at this level recognizes that everyone must die, cries openly at funerals, encourages others to donate organs after death, feels that funerals should be for the living, and knows the options for appropriate disposition of the body.
Moderate 14–17
A person at this level seldom thinks about death, is somewhat inhibited about expressing grief, agrees to permit own organs to be used after death, feels that funerals provide a chance to honor the dead, and is willing to learn about planning for death.
Marginal 10–13
A person at this level feels that death is something that happens to others, holds back feelings of pain and loss, is uncomfortable about donating organs after death, feels that funerals serve no useful purpose, and is uninterested in learning about planning for death.
Inadequate 5–9
A person at this level denies that everyone must eventually die, is embarrassed to show feelings of loss and mourning, feels people should be buried intact, uses funerals to impress others, and is unwilling to consider planning for death.

A man hiking on a high mountain suddenly lost his footing and found himself hurtling toward certain death. As he plummeted past a small bush growing out of the sheer rock wall, he caught a berry in his hand and ate it. It was the most delicious berry he had ever eaten.

In this short story, the man's condition is the same as yours or mine or anyone else's. Each of us is hurtling toward certain death, and how we deal with it has a lot to do with how freely and rewardingly we live our lives.

What Is Death?

Death, like life, is change. Matter and energy are never destroyed. They merely change from one form to another. When the body can no longer resist unhealthy changes in itself, or is mechanically broken beyond repair, or is poisoned by the environment, it ceases to function and dies.

Traditionally, death has been defined as occurring when the heart stops beating and the person stops breathing. However, the brain continues to function for a short time (less than 10 minutes) after the heart stops beating. Scientists now agree that the brain, not the heart, is the key to human life. Four characteristics describe brain death, according to a Harvard Medical School committee: unreceptivity and unresponsivity, no movements or breathing, no reflexes, and a flat electroencephalogram for 10 minutes.

Brain death is most reliably shown by a flat tracing on an **electroencephalogram.** Once the brain stops functioning, the person is medically, and in some states legally, dead. Most states either have already adopted or are considering legislation that redefines death in this way. There are a few exceptions, however. Overdoses of some depressant drugs can produce a flat electroencephalogram trace. Some people have shown no brain life after such overdoses, yet they have recovered. A stilled heart is not always final, either. Some patients recover when their hearts are directly massaged or otherwise manipulated.

Why Is There Death?

There is no totally mind-satisfying answer to the question, "Why is there death?" We can say, "there is death because there is life; nothing dies that hasn't lived." That's not much comfort, however. Knowing that matter and energy are never destroyed but are simply changed, is also not very comforting. We want that little light of consciousness. We want to know that we will be able to recognize ourselves. Being alive in some other form without the same ego is not enough to satisfy most of us.

Exploring Your Emotions

Think back to your childhood. Can you remember the first time someone close to you died? Was it a person? A pet? How old were you? How did you feel about it at the time? How does recalling it make you feel right now?

But death does allow variety: death permits the renewal and evolution of the human species. The normal life span is long enough to ensure that we reproduce ourselves and that our species continues. It is short enough to allow new genetic combinations to be tested. This fact means that we, as a species, can adapt better to changing conditions in the environment. Seen from the viewpoint of species survival and improvement, the arrangement makes sense. Unnecessary and wasteful death, however, is another matter.

How Do People Feel about Death?

How *do* people feel about death? Outraged and pained initially. The very thought of losing our own consciousness of this world goes against everything we have ever known. We prefer not to think about it, because we have no proof that any good thing happens to a person after he or she dies. People are thrust involuntarily and unwillingly into the dilemma of having to choose an explanation of what happens to us when we die. Some controversial issues, such as the likelihood of an afterlife, can be avoided, but death cannot.

Consequently, theories abound concerning what happens when we die. Most religions build their philosophies on the issue of death and its consequences. Some promise a better life after death, in a wonderful place—a heaven with streets of gold and pearls for some Christians and Jews, a land of green meadows and running water for desert Muslims—if adherents behave according to the rules of their group and their god(s). Other religions teach that everyone is growing toward godhood in this life, and that we are born again and again until we reach that perfection. Some philosophers say that we cannot possibly know what happens after death, and that we can only judge whether life is or is not worth living according to the rewards we find or make in this life.

Regardless of the explanations we choose to believe, death is painful, both to the dying person and to the ones left behind. The dying person grieves both the loss of self and leaving the people and things he or she has loved. Young children, particularly, know death as an interruption and an absence, but lacking a time perspective, they

Electroencephalogram Record of fluctuating electrical potentials of the brain (brain waves) as recorded from electrodes on the scalp.

do not fathom death as final separation. Then from about age 5 to age 9 the child's view of death matures considerably. Now the child understands that death is final, but only for others, not for himself or herself. He or she will escape somehow. From about age 10 upward, the child begins to adjust to the inevitable: death comes to be seen as inevitable and universal and irreversible. Again in later life, worries about the deaths of loved ones may be particularly gnawing, if a person fears he or she will be left alone after a lifetime with another person.

Some People Appear to Welcome Death Some people never accept death. But people who have suffered great depression or a painful terminal disease often eventually find the idea of death a relief and a release. That attitude is understandable to most of us, particularly if the person is old and has lived a full life. But others—over 30,000 annually in the United States—feel death, even if repulsive, is preferable to living, and end their lives before nature takes its course.

Forty percent of suicides are over age 60, and the rate among 15- to 24-year-olds has increased over the last twenty years: 20 percent of male suicides are among this age and 14 percent of female suicides. Among the immediate motives for suicide, despair is the most common. In one study, a high level of hopelessness was the strongest sign that a person who has attempted suicide will try it again.

Adolescents do not necessarily commit suicide for the same reason as adults. Because they lack experience and long time patterns of grappling with and working through problems, they may overreact to and surrender easily to frustrations: failure on a final exam may be interpreted to mean failure in life; a disappointing relationship can be translated to mean permanent loneliness. Suicidal adolescents, like suicidal adults, are likely to be deeply depressed, but the signs may be hard to recognize, because their sadness and hopelessness are often masked by boredom, apathy, hyperactivity, or physical complaints.

Anxiety about schoolwork and exams is an important cause of suicide among college students. Some investigators believe that many young people have an emotionally lifeless relationship with their parents and defend themselves from it by overemphasizing the importance of their schoolwork. Suicidal high school students are more likely to be defiant and delinquent, and reckless drivers. They have a high rate of antisocial behavior. They are often at odds with their parents and may have been victims of child abuse and neglect. The disturbing rise in adolescent suicide over the last thirty years has not been well explained. Increasing family and social disorganization and rising teenage unemployment may all have something to do with it.

When someone commits suicide, it is scary to almost everyone involved, even to those on the fringes, and it is very difficult to explain and justify to yourself. For one thing, it means someone you may have loved dearly has chosen to relinquish you, and chosen to relinquish this life. You may feel betrayed. It also may make you feel guilty, as though you have failed and as though you should have done more to help the person. And you may be anguished that the suicide must have suffered great pain to have made such a horrible decision alone, and angry

Exploring Your Emotions

What feelings does this picture evoke in you? Put together a collage of images cut from magazines that expresses or evokes your own feelings about death.

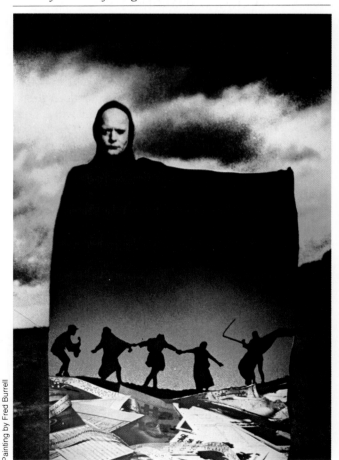

Painting by Fred Burrell

Emphysema Irreversible lung disease marked by loss of tissue elasticity and breakup of air sacs in the lungs; usually results from smoking.

Exploring Your Emotions

Consider your own death for a few minutes. Is this difficult for you to do? What emotions are you experiencing?

that he or she could have decided without yelling for help. You may also be angry that the person didn't care enough about us to have hung on longer. How could he or she have been so rude and thoughtless! A suicide has used death as a weapon in our death-denying culture: the suicide reminds us that we too will die, that we have the ability—and perhaps some of us, sadly, even the desire—to kill ourselves. And we do not want suicide to be an option for people we love. We want them to stick it out and fight their problems, and prevail over them.

Most societies have considered suicide an attack. On what? On the government, certainly. Until 1961 it was a felony in England, and it is still a crime in the United States. One hundred fifty years ago, suicides in England forfeited property and good name. By committing suicide, people were considered to have broken their contract with society, because suicide disintegrates the fabric and structure of society. Suicides have judged society, recognized its limitations, and rejected its values, usually expressing a hope of some better life. Society has treated suicides as though they were deluded or were in such deep despair that they couldn't think straight. Western law has found all sorts of reasons for justifiably killing others, but no reason for killing oneself.

Religious groups and theologians consider it an attack on God, saying that the suicide tries to usurp God's place by taking power over something that God has created. For Aquinas, an influential medieval theologian, suicide is the most fatal of sins because it cannot be repented of, and consequently the suicide forfeits any future life in heaven.

Denying Death in America In the United States we try to deny that death occurs. We have practiced this denial for several generations. Some people still can't bring themselves to say "die," so they describe their relatives as having "passed away," "gone to glory" or "to the great beyond." Families segregate children from the elderly if the older ones are sick, in hospitals or nursing homes. A grandparent's death is rarely a home event. We make sure it takes place in a hospital. Children are not likely to be around. They usually do not see what happens when a person dies, and they often are not told the details—or the details are hedged—because the subject is distasteful and difficult for the parents to deal with. Many Americans, both adult and children, have never seen someone die. Death happens to someone else—not to you or me.

Besides "protecting" children from the actual, physical fact of the dead body, we present false ideas of it. Death, the real thing, its finality, its aftermath of grief, is largely taboo. But fake death is a game that is played all over TV and movie screens, and it is always reversible. Children playing war or cops and robbers or cowboys and Indians play the game, mimicking the actors, suddenly gasping and sprawling on the ground, "dead." In a minute, they get up and play the same scene over again. Our death taboo, like our sex taboo, is distorted for the public. In both cases, natural events are either presented out of context or are hidden, especially for children.

Perhaps these are some of the reasons why people refuse to use safety belts in cars, even though they know that safety belts save lives. Perhaps these reasons also explain why people continue to smoke cigarettes even after developing **emphysema** or some other possibly fatal disease.

Coming to Terms with Dying

Most people have definite ideas about when and how they want to die. Usually we do not get to choose the time or the means. But if you have a terminal illness that lasts a while, you will have to cope with specific issues in facing the "end game." Doing so may be the most difficult experience you ever have. You may have to adjust to becoming dependent; your activities may be reduced drastically; you may be very depressed. But there is no question that the dying benefit from having others around them—to listen, to share, to care. Most people can adapt and learn and grow if they have enough time and help, but it is a gradual process.

It should not be surprising that one of the best ways to learn to cope with the reality of your own death is to participate in the deaths of your loved ones, even from childhood. With the pain of experiencing each death, you work through some of your fears and resolve some of your questions about the unknown.

Coping with Dying How can you come to terms with the prospect of your own death? Responses vary greatly. One author, John Hinton in his book *Dying* (1967), observed that about half of dying people openly acknowl-

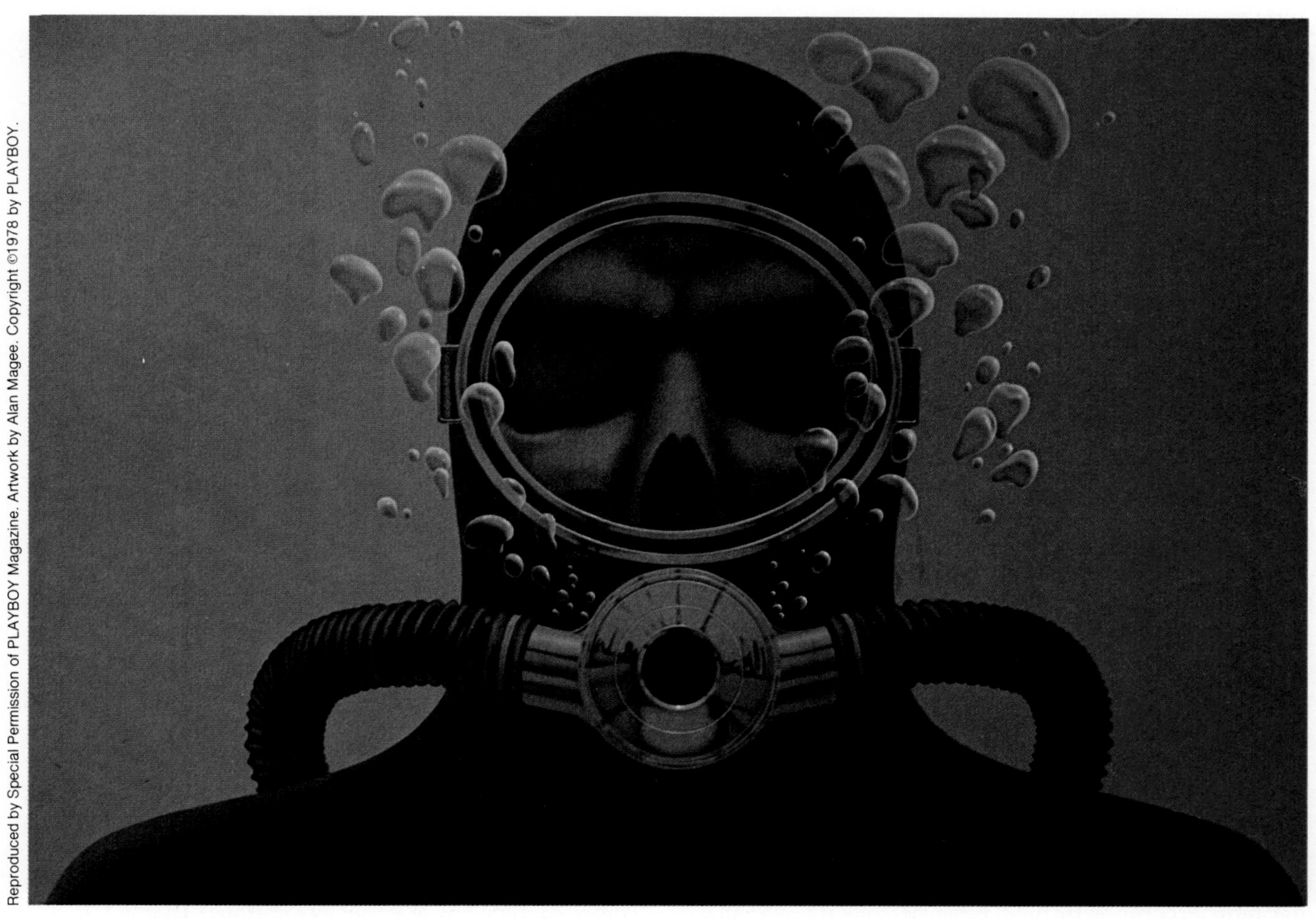

Exploring Your Emotions

What is the artist suggesting in this picture? How do you feel about the image? Write a caption for it.

edge their death and accept it. About a quarter of them speak with undisguised anguish about their death, and a quarter deny it entirely and do not speak about it at all.

After observing and interviewing hundreds of dying people, Dr. Elisabeth Kübler-Ross identified and generalized several common—though not inevitable—psychological stages people experience in coming to terms with their own deaths, and published these in her book *On Death and Dying* (1969). Not everyone experiences every stage of emotions, nor in the same order, nor for the same duration. Some reactions may be experienced simultaneously.

Stage One: Denial and Isolation Stage One is a temporary state of shock in which people deny the fact and isolate themselves from further confrontation with it. They say, "Not me" and "You're wrong" and insist, "It can't be!" Denial is a useful stage because it acts as a buffer against shocks and gives people time to collect themselves and mobilize other defenses.

Stage Two: Anger When people can no longer deny the truth, anger often follows. They ask, "Why me?" and tend to lash out at family, physicians, the hospital, blaming them for the situation. Anger at this stage is also a normal response to disability and losing control over one's life and situation.

Stage Three: Bargaining As a means of marshalling remaining hope, people may work to discover a way out: a common tack is to make promises to God in exchange for a prolonged life. Grasping at any straw of hope—any new treatment—makes one especially vulnerable to quackery and to charlatans.

Stage Four: Depression At this stage people accept their fate, and often become depressed about problems they are leaving behind and unfinished work. Depression is also a kind of grief that they experience to prepare themselves for the final separation from this world. While this stage is often emotionally painful, it is an appropriate step in the process and is eased considerably when people are allowed to express sorrow in an atmosphere of nonjudging support and care.

Stage Five: Acceptance Finally people may reach a point at which they are no longer angry, nor hoping for a miracle, nor depressed. They just accept that nothing is certain until it happens, and are willing to live as much as is possible in the time that remains; and to wait, and watch. They appear both to suspend judgment about their future and to appreciate the present. They acknowledge that they are powerless over the future and appear somewhat content to make the best of it. They may choose not to talk with visitors, even family, in preparation for departing. It is part of the letting go.

Other observers have mapped quite different response patterns to the dying process. One suggests that there is no predictable sequence to the way people live their final days; their predicament tosses them from one emotion to the next. Another suggests that people die in a fashion that most accords with their basic personality, and that the given disease affects the way people die. Dr. Edwin Schneidman observes a continual seesaw effect, dictated somewhat by the person's personality: "a waxing and waning of anguish, terror, acquiescence and surrender, rage, and envy, disinterest and ennui, pretense, taunting and daring and even yearning for death—all these in the context of bewilderment and pain."

Seemingly contradictory theories that do not match every situation are not necessarily right or wrong. They merely underline the variety of human situations and responses, and they point out what has been said by others about death: that it is a mountain with many paths to the top, and that each observer will see only those paths and that part of the mountain that experience and perspective allow him or her to see. The point is not to expect that any dying person will or should behave predictably, but rather that each person's needs should be discovered, so that we can help ease the last days most efficiently.

Being with a Dying Person Modern medicine can now predict earlier and more accurately whether illnesses are **terminal.** Increasing numbers of people know in advance that they or others will die in weeks or months. More than ever before, people have a chance to help others experience dying gracefully and with dignity. Establishing and maintaining physical and emotional closeness with the dying person is an important part of the process. Allowing them to speak and act honestly and openly about the experience that is foremost on their mind is crucial, even though talking about death may be painful for you and others who will need to spend time with the dying person.

There is no rule about who tells people they are dying. Sometimes the doctor does it, a family member or a friend. Sometimes the dying figure it out themselves and ask if their suspicions are true. Then the task is to support and help people take care of their unfinished business and to deal with the array of emotions that will confront them.

The dying person's needs are not so different from anyone else's, but they are more urgent. Dying people need to know that they are valued, that they are not alone, that they are not being judged, and that those around them care and are trying to understand and to learn about this final hard place just as they are. Dying people often need someone to listen to them while they talk their way through the experience. Friends are as important to dying people as they are to the living. As with any friendship, there are opportunities for growth on both sides.

Besides friends and family, the dying person should have access to other sources of support. These might be the family physician, psychological counselors, organizations for group-oriented self-help work with the dying and their families, and religious counsel. Not all therapists are equally effective and helpful. It pays to shop around.

To be effective with the dying, a counselor must be compassionate, have some professional training in the principles of caring for the dying, be comfortable with the idea of death, and have a nonjudgmental philosophy. As a benevolent outsider, the counselor can run interference for patients and serve as liaison between patients and their families and doctors. The therapist can help patients in a number of ways toward accepting death, by working through specific fears such as that their families may not be able to cope without them, by finding purpose in their past and a pattern to their existence, and by resolving negative feelings they may have held toward themselves and others.

Some hospitals and health organizations run group programs for the dying. They are usually chaired by a professional counselor, and are designed to help patients voice their worries. Discussion is usually voluntary, and mutual support is encouraged, along with honest, open discussion. You can contact these groups by inquiring of social workers, doctors, medical services, other patients, and by checking local bulletin boards and newspapers.

Terminally ill people often testify that they have had the most significant experiences of their lives after they found out they were soon to die. Aware of their limited time, they are sometimes enabled to delight and to find greater meaning in life experiences that are still open to them. They become more aware of what they will lose

Terminal Term used to describe a disease that shortly will end in death.

Hospice Community-oriented, long-term treatment facility for chronic and dying patients; provides social and psychological support as well as medical care.

and are able to appreciate small events that might have seemed insignificant before. Some people find a deep meaning in putting their business affairs in order and finally saying to loved ones important things they may have been too inhibited to say before.

Planning for Death

Once people discover their days are numbered, many decisions will occupy their time. Will they spend their last days at home tended by relatives and friends, or would dying in the hospital improve the quality of life? Dying at home involves receiving considerable time and energy from relatives, and may require money for hired nurses. Only about 2 percent of Americans die at home. Dying in the hospital may be more appropriate if small children in the home need care, if the patient needs intravenous feedings, if the patient cannot afford private nurses, or if a person plans to donate organs for transplant.

If you decide to die at home, many good books can guide your caregivers about every facet of tending a patient. Such books get right down to the details of instructing how to give injections and teaching other practical home care techniques; they list medical supplies that may be needed; they discuss how to deal with morale, how to handle visitors, and other practical issues. They discuss financial considerations in hiring nurses and aides. And they are a mine of resources for help: they suggest how to get financial aid from city, county, and state services; Social Security and survivor benefits; Medicaid, Veterans Administration aid; legal help from legal aid services, state board of health, medical examiner, and county coroner; medical supplies through rentals; specific disease-oriented groups such as the American Cancer Society; and medical supply companies and hospital pharmacies.

The Hospice The **hospice** is an alternative to both home care—when relatives need some relief—and hospital care for the dying. The special needs of dying people are usually not well served by regular hospitals because the primary objectives of hospitals are short-term intense medical treatment, not long-term maintenance care. The professional staff is geared toward short-term treatment, and the social mix of patients does not lend itself to the special problems of the dying. Hospital costs are very high.

To better serve the needs of dying patients, their families and their friends, the hospice philosophy was suc-

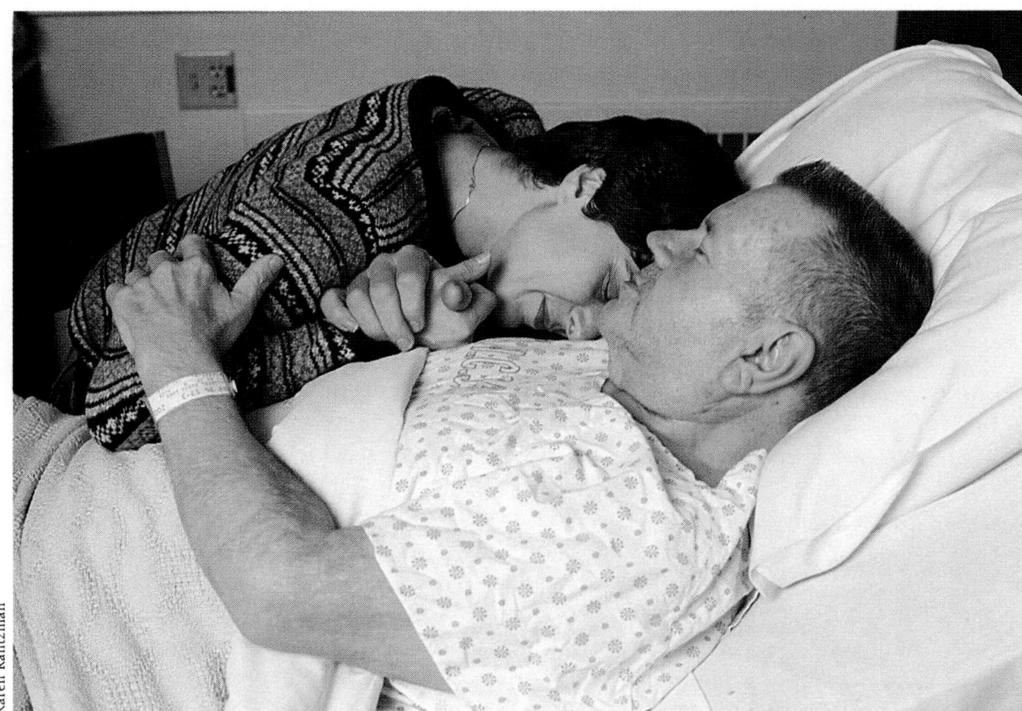
Karen Rantzman

Elements of a Hospice Program

Hospice programs aim to meet a wide range of physical, social, psychological, and spiritual needs of people who require sustained medical attention. While they are known to be effective in treatment of the terminally ill, they are also open to other chronically ill patients as well. About 40 percent of cases use the hospice program to give respite to relatives; 20 percent of admissions are social isolates with no one able or willing to care for them. At the same time, 60 percent of admissions need help with better control of their pain. So hospice patients represent a mix of social and clinical needs.

Hospice programs vary from one facility to another. Some are entirely home care oriented, while others are exclusively institutional, with no home care services. Some have very limited bereavement follow-up service, while others offer extensive bereavement service. Many have services available on a 24-hours-a-day, seven-days-a-week basis, while some operate fewer hours.

The following list represents the ideal program toward which hospice administrators strive:

1. Service availability to home care patients and inpatients on a 24-hours-a-day, seven-days-a-week, on-call basis with emphasis on availability of medical and nursing skills
2. Home care service in collaboration with inpatient facilities
3. Knowledge and expertise in the control of symptoms (physical, psychological, social, and spiritual)
4. The provision of care by an interdisciplinary team
5. Physician-directed services
6. Central administration and coordination of services
7. Use of volunteers as an integral part of the health care team
8. Acceptance to the program based on health needs, not on ability to pay
9. Treatment of the patient and family together
10. A bereavement follow-up service

cessfully developed some years ago in England. Hospices are now being established in the United States. They are usually administered by a team of medical, social work, mental health, legal, and spiritual practitioners who provide support, comfort, and resources for dealing with the problems of dying. The hospice philosophy discourages inappropriate treatment and expensive life-extending medical services. Since volunteers are used widely, costs are greatly reduced. In the past they have ministered mainly to cancer patients and the terminally ill, but programs vary among the hospices.

What to Do with the Body Dying people will probably want to decide how their bodies should be disposed of: whether embalmed or not, buried, cremated, given to medicine for research, or prepared for donating organs. They can indicate whether they want a funeral or a memorial service, a wake or a party, and they can plan the agenda. Some people prefer no services.

A dead human body is a valuable resource. Many of its parts can be used to help the living. Eye corneas can be transplanted to give sight to the blind. Kidneys can be used to give years of vigorous life to people who have kidney disease. Human skin is the best dressing for wounds of burn victims. Bones can be used for grafting. Pituitary glands are desperately needed to enable some children to grow normally. In some parts of the world, undiseased blood from dead bodies is used for transfusions. Jaws are needed for dental training. People who may be horrified at the thought of this "mutilation" often change their minds when they learn how routine autopsies are performed and how bodies are usually prepared for burial.

The simplest and most widely used plan for donating body parts is through the **Uniform Donor Card** (see Figure 23-1), available from the National Kidney Foundation. The Uniform Anatomical Gift Act, or its equivalent, has been adopted in all states, and permits you to bequeath your body for immediate use after death. Several steps are involved, so you need to look into this possibility early and to read the fine print about costs and requirements.

Exploring Your Emotions

Suppose a friend of yours suggests that you both sign cards stating that on your deaths you wish to donate your bodies and organs to allow someone else to see or hear or have a new heart, or to help medical research. What would be your immediate reaction to this request?

Uniform Donor Card A consent form authorizing use of the signer's body parts upon his or her death.

Memorial societies Nonprofit groups of consumers that guide members toward simple, economical burials or cremations.

Cremation Burning a body to its bones at very high temperatures.

Embalming Treating a dead body to retard decomposition.

In some states, permission to "harvest" usable tissues after death is communicated by a card signed and attached to the driver's license.

Burial The tradition of this country has been burial, and still is in many places. However, recent exposés of the funeral industry have documented the industry's inflated costs and hard sell of unnecessary options. In response, **memorial societies** have sprung up: they are nonprofit groups of consumers who help members prearrange simple, economical burials. Because they are nonprofit, they'll give you straight information about legal requirements, costs, and arrangements. About 175 memorial societies are now operating in the United States and Canada. Membership usually runs $5 to $15, and anyone can join. You can join these societies at any time, preferably before the need is urgent so that you can decide options while you are not grieving.

Because of adverse publicity and the rise of memorial societies, the funeral industry has attempted to tone down its tough tactics with people made vulnerable by grief.

Cremation Burning a body to its bones—**cremation**—is a clean, simple, economical way of returning earth to earth. The entire job of picking up the body, cremating, and preparing the death certificate may cost around $300. As the population increases and land prices rise, more people may prefer cremation.

Ceremonies The bereaved can benefit from participating in a ceremony. Traditionally, the American funeral ceremony has involved **embalming** the corpse; friends viewing the body in the funeral home before the funeral service; friends and fellow church members supplying flowers and food to the bereaved for entertaining the people at a religious ceremony a few days later; a processional to the graveside; and a final ceremony there.

Other ceremonies are evolving. Anyone can create a new one. Some people dispose of the body immediately, so that neither embalming nor viewing of the body takes place. A celebration can grow in whatever way is appropriate for all involved. Choose a place that's meaningful—indoors or outside in nature. Allow the participants to decide whether they wish to speak about their feelings for the person, or to be silent. Do they want a minister? a leader? Do they want to share food or dancing or song? A prayer circle?

The dying can also choose a cemetery plot and gravestone, or if cremated, indicate whether they want their ashes kept somewhere or scattered in a garden or at sea. In choosing a cemetery plot, be sure to compare advice from several sources, and to consider such things as dis-

UNIFORM DONOR CARD

OF__________________________

Print or type name of donor

In the hope that I may help others, I hereby make this anatomical gift, if medically acceptable, to take effect upon my death. The words and marks below indicate my desires.

I give: (a) ____ any needed organs or parts

(b) ____ only the following organs or parts

____

Specify the organ(s) or part(s)

for the purposes of transplantation, therapy, medical research or education;

(c) ____ my body for anatomical study if needed.

Limitations or special wishes, if any:____________________

Signed by the donor and the following two witnesses in the presence of each other:

Signature of Donor | Date of Birth of Donor

Date Signed | City & State

Witness | Witness

This is a legal document under the Uniform Anatomical Gift Act or similar laws.

For further information consult your physician or

National Kidney Foundation
116 East 27th Street, New York, N.Y. 10016

Figure 23-1

Intestate Having made no legal will.

Probate To establish the validity of a will.

Surety bond Guarantee—usually an amount of money—put up by a person who assumes responsibilities and debts of another, to insure against loss or damage.

Age of majority When one is legally responsible for oneself.

Power of attorney A legal document that confers authority to do things in another person's name.

Life-support technology Machinery and artificial body parts used to keep alive patients who would otherwise die.

Euthanasia Helping a terminally ill person die quickly, easily, and painlessly.

---

tance from the homes of the relatives, costs, religious denomination, how well the graves are maintained, and the reputation of the cemetery. The gravestone can be a separate consideration.

Paying for the Funeral Arranging how to pay for the funeral is a significant decision, because it can be quite costly. Social Security insurance allows several hundred dollars toward it. Veterans Administration also allots around $400 to honorably discharged veterans for funeral and cemetery costs, which may be claimed. Other ethnic groups, fraternal societies, and unions sometimes provide lump sum benefits to pay funeral costs. A special bank account can be earmarked for funeral expenses, so that relatives will not be strapped by paying them. Or the money can come out of the estate's assets, if the estate is large enough to cover them. And other plans are possible, including prepayment plans.

Making a Will Fewer than one-fourth of all Americans get around to drawing up a will. Unfortunately, even in the case of those who feel their estate is very modest, dying without a will usually causes difficulties for the survivors. And if there is any substance to the estate, the complications can be tremendous.

A will is a document drawn up during your lifetime that declares your intentions of how you want your estate—everything you own—distributed when you die. Until you die it can be changed, replaced, destroyed. When you die, it is a binding legal instrument that governs the redistribution of your property. Only property jointly owned—such as automobiles, bank accounts, stocks, real estate, life insurance proceeds and death benefits—bypasses the law of **intestate** succession. So besides considering a will, you may want to transfer titles of property or add names for joint ownership to avoid having your estate pass through **probate.**

If you die without a will—intestate—your property will be distributed in any case. The court appoints an administrator to supervise the distribution and awards him or her a commission that is taken directly out of your estate. Usually the administrator is the closest inheriting next of kin, who must post a **surety bond,** which is costly (in some states $10 per $1,000 of the estate assets, renewable annually until the estate is settled). There will also be commissions (as high as 10 percent of the estate's worth) for the attorney suggested by the administrator, and for an appraiser.

If you die intestate, the benefits of your children and those of your spouse are considered as separate and not necessarily compatible with each other. A fairly rigid and predetermined formula, based on marriage and blood relationships, determines who inherits what. Anyone who is close to you in spirit only—perhaps living with you or taking care of you—if not related by blood or marriage, will get nothing. Although the distribution may be just the way you would have done it, chances are that it will not be.

Everyone should make out a will on reaching the **age of majority.** You can have an attorney draw it up for you for a fee, or you can get some do-it-yourself books—usually written by attorneys—that will show you how. Every will includes some standard elements. Your will should contain specific language canceling any previous will. Give your full name and where you live. Name your personal representative (the person you choose to take charge of your financial affairs and distribute property after your death), and lay out general directions for that person to follow, and specific instructions on how you want your property disposed of. You may specify general policy guidelines for the executor, perhaps regarding your children, and regarding any ongoing business or property investments. Finally, designate who is to receive what's left.

Asking for Help Perhaps so many things must be decided that the dying person will ask for help. It is possible to delegate authority to someone else whom you trust. You can grant that person your **power of attorney**—a legal document that confers authority to do things in another person's name. It can be general or for a specific project only, and it can set a time limit. A dying person will want to acquaint someone with survivor benefits (Social Security, pension benefits, life insurance), and should gather all official documents in one place. Here is a partial list:

- Last will and testament
- Birth and adoption certificates
- Marriage and divorce papers
- Citizenship papers

- Military service papers
- Social Security numbers
- Organization memberships and benefits
- Life and accident insurances
- Bank accounts, stocks, bonds, savings bonds
- Safe deposit box
- Real estate papers

Letting People Die

Thousands of people are alive today under conditions that would have been fatal if nature had taken its course. Anyone who uses a heart pacemaker or an artificial kidney is benefitting from advanced **life support technology.** Even severely disabled people, such as those who cannot use any of their limbs, are helped to continue living.

In spite of some apparent successes, there are serious objections to the medical tradition of keeping people alive by all means and at any expense. Should a patient be kept alive who cannot possibly recover, one who is not capable of knowing a meaningful life, and who may have even requested *not* to be kept alive for a long time in a coma? Some families are emotionally and financially ruined while a loved one (or any dependent) is maintained in a seemingly endless coma or in a vegetative state.

Is Euthanasia Moral? Several issues are involved. One is the morality of **euthanasia,** also called "mercy killing" or "aid in dying." Some people believe that life itself is sacred, and that under no circumstances should we kill

Exploring Your Emotions

How do you feel about "pulling the plug" on life support systems for the dying?

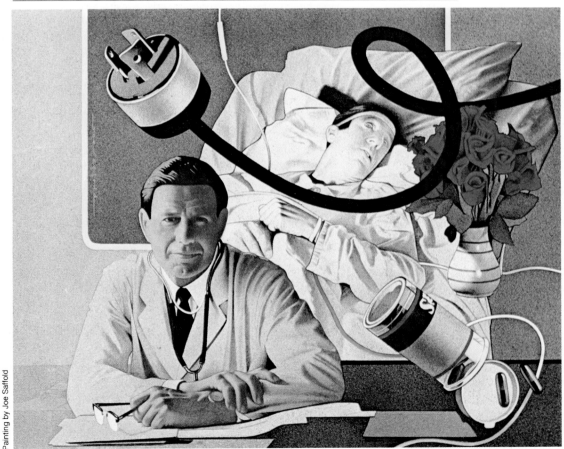

Painting by Joe Saffold

When Life and Death Are in Your Hands

If you look only at his face, eyes closed and mouth slightly open, he looks as if he's just taking an afternoon nap. But the people standing around the bed are wearing yellow paper gowns, gauze masks and rubber gloves. There's an air tube through a hole in his throat and IV tubing from a drip bottle taped to his wrist.

A motor whines as it rocks the bed slowly; the respirator wheezes rhythmically, pushing into his lungs. On a shelf above the bed, a monitor's spiked tracing shows that his heart is beating regularly.

Above their masks, the eyes of two family members meet, asking silently the question the doctor put to them a few minutes before:

"I'm wondering whether it makes any sense to go on with the treatment. What do you think?"

Every day in intensive-care units, families, friends and physicians stand at such bedsides and ask that question.

With improvements in life support technology and medical treatments, the chances are increasing that you too will be one of the actors in such a scene. And if you're like most of the others, under stress and emotionally spent, you'll appreciate all the help you can get in making the decision.

With that in mind, here are some of the questions I suggest to clients, to help them sort out the issues and make their own decision:

A. Questions about the medical treatment.

When treatment is clearly futile, physicians are authorized to stop giving it. That's true whether it's a headache pill or kidney dialysis. It's a medical decision. These are some of the questions the doctors will have been mulling over:

1. *If the treatment continues, to what extent—being very realistic—can health be restored? Over how long a time?*

2. *To what extent can the symptoms be relieved, including pain and suffering?*

3. *Is the treatment in question truly therapeutic—"serving to cure or heal or to preserve health," as the New World Dictionary puts it?*

Many times, it's not necessary to go beyond the medical questions. But in the new medicine, there's almost always one more thing to try; the question moves from "What to do next?" to "Ought we do anything more?"—and from medicine into ethics.

And even when it's a clear medical decision, most physicians hesitate to move without consulting the patient and family. Therefore, these other questions arise:

B. Questions about the patient's wishes.

This is the most crucial area. Courts increasingly are saying that the patient's autonomy and the historic right to refuse treatment have priority, even if refusing treatment would hasten death.

4. *Is the patient mentally competent and able to communicate?*

or shorten anyone's life, especially since God created life. Some of these same people might not fight in a war, support the death penalty, or allow abortions. They draw the line against killing where it makes the most sense to them, or they follow the suggestions of their church. They frequently also support punishment for anyone who helps someone die.

Others believe that quality, rather than quantity, of life is the issue, and that under certain conditions it is an act of compassion to help a person die. The most radical acceptance of euthanasia in the world is found in the Netherlands. There, a physician who meets strict criteria can give a lethal injection to a dying person who has requested death, and the physician will not be punished. A landmark case in the evolution of Dutch euthanasia occurred in 1981 when the criminal court in Rotterdam set standards for noncriminal aid in dying and laid out these rules:

1. There must be physical or mental suffering that the sufferer finds unbearable.
2. The suffering and the desire to die must be lasting, not temporary.
3. The decision to die must be the voluntary decision of an informed patient.
4. The person must have a correct and clear understanding of his or her condition and of other possibilities (treatments); he or she must be capable of weighing these options and must have done so.
5. There is no other reasonable (acceptable to the patient) solution to improve the situation.
6. The time and manner of death will not cause avoidable

5. *If the answer is yes, what does he or she want done?*

6. *If the answer is no, has the patient named a surrogate to represent his or her wishes, by filling out a Durable Power of Attorney for Health Care? Or a "Directive to Physicians," or any other form of living will?*

7. *If not, did the patient ever express an opinion orally or in a letter about what people should do in such situations?*

8. *Has the patient or the surrogate been fully informed of the possibilities, limits and possible consequences of proposed treatment?*

C. Questions about quality of life.

These have to be asked with one principle in mind—only the patient really can judge whether the quality of his or her life is such that further fighting is worthwhile.

9. *Is there physical discomfort or pain? To what extent can it be fully relieved?*

10. *Is there loss of mobility?*

11. *Is the patient able to communicate? To hear?*

12. *Is there suffering—despair, emotional pain—caused by the situation and its limitations?*

13. *How does the patient feel about all these? Or how would the patient feel if he or she could communicate with us?*

D. External factors.

These are not as important as the medical and patient's wishes questions, but may help in the overall decision.

14. *Do the family members agree on what the patient probably would want?*

15. *All other things being equal, would continued treatment put an intolerable psychological burden—or a financial one—on the relatives?*

16. *Would agreeing to withdrawal of treatment create too much guilt for the kin?*

How to get your questions answered.

Find out who, of the several doctors involved, is the physician of record or the case manager. Ask that doctor or one of the hospital social workers to set up a family conference. If you wish, ask that your pastor, priest, rabbi, or guru be present.

The hospital can also put you in touch with its ethics committee or a clinical ethicist. These people are trained to help you sort out the questions, so you can make a decision that's best for you and the patient.

The futurologists tell me that by the end of the century, eight out of ten of us will be dying in intensive care units, supported by one technological device or another that requires a decision to turn off.

With that in mind, you may want to save these questions. Let's hope it's a long time before you need them.

SOURCE: Bruce Hilton, 1986 (July 2), When life and death are in your hands, *San Francisco Examiner*, Section C, p. 5.

misery to others; that is, if possible, the next of kin should be informed beforehand.

7. The decision to give aid in dying should not be a one-person decision. Consulting another professional (medical doctor, social worker, psychologist, according to the circumstances of the case) is obligatory.
8. A medical doctor must be involved in the decision to prescribe the correct drugs.
9. The decision process and the actual aid must be done with the utmost care.

Will Euthanasia Be Legalized? Another issue concerning euthanasia is its legality. In most countries, helping someone die is against the law and punishable by prison, perhaps even death. The charge can be murder or manslaughter. Although some people know that they are doing the right thing in helping a loved one to die, they also know that they can be prosecuted and punished. The most compassionate of crimes must also be the most secret of crimes. Few cases of euthanasia are reported. And it is

Exploring Your Emotions

How would you feel if someone you loved were terminally ill and in pain and asked to be allowed to die, not to be kept alive by artificial means such as a respirator? What would you say to this person? What would you do? What would be your response to a friend who told you he (or she) wished to die if he was not terminally ill, but depressed and unable to come to grips with life's problems?

Churches' Beliefs about Euthanasia*

Religion	Passive	Active
Assemblies of God	individual decision	individual decision
The Baha'is	individual decision	oppose
Baptist	accept	oppose
Buddhism	accept	oppose
Christian Church (Disciples of Christ)	individual decision	individual decision
Christian & Missionary Alliance Church	oppose	oppose
Christian Scientist†	individual decision	individual decision
Church of the Brethren†	accept	oppose
Church of Christ (Christian)	oppose	oppose
Church of the Nazarene	oppose	oppose
Episcopal† (Anglican)	accept	individual decision
Evangelical	oppose	oppose
Greek Orthodox	accept	oppose
Hindu†	individual decision	individual decision
Humanists	accept	accept
Islam†	oppose	oppose
Jehovah's Witnesses	accept	oppose
Judaism†	accept	oppose
Krishna†	accept	oppose
Lutheran	accept	oppose
Mennonite†	accept	oppose
Mormon	oppose	oppose
Moravian	accept	oppose
Quaker Religious Society	accept	individual decision
Reformed Church of America	oppose	oppose
Roman Catholic	accept	oppose
Russian Orthodox	accept	oppose
Seventh-Day Adventist†	accept	oppose
Sikh Dharma†	individual decision	individual decision
Swedenborgianism	accept	oppose
Theosophical Society	individual decision	individual decision
Unitarian Universalist	accept	individual decision
United Church of Christ	accept	individual decision
United Methodist	accept	individual decision
United Presbyterian	individual decision	individual decision

*Where churches have no stated official position on this topic, it is assumed that the decision is one of individual choice. Individual decision usually implies a matter of concern between patient, family, and doctor.

†"No official statement": In such cases, spokespersons form their conclusions based on religious rationale and opinion.

Passive: allowing a hopelessly ill person to die by not imposing extraordinary measures.
Active: taking one's own life or helping another to die.

SOURCE: Derek Humphry and Ann Wickett, 1986, *The Right to Die: Understanding Euthanasia* (New York: Harper & Row), p. 295.

County coroner A public official authorized to investigate unexpected deaths and deaths in unusual circumstances.

Autopsy Medical examination of a body after death.

not always possible to tell exactly the cause of death, because dying patients are often heavily dosed with drugs.

Some people who cannot justify active administration of lethal drugs to help others die, do accept the practice of passive euthanasia: withdrawing life support systems such as respirators and intravenous feeding tubes when the dying no longer have any chance of recovery. Whether such practices are legal has not been finally decided. When it is possible, though, more and more doctors are letting families of patients make this decision, and patients themselves, when they are able.

People are beginning to realize that we each have the right to determine the nature of our own death. Between 1976 and 1985, thirty-six states enacted living will laws that protect our right to refuse medical procedures that only prolong the dying process. They also protect doctors from liability for acting in accordance with our wishes. The laws allow anyone to sign a document, known as a living will, stating that if they are suffering from a terminal illness that is certified by one (or two) doctors, their life should not be sustained by medication, artificial means, or heroic measures. Figure 23-2 shows an example of a living will.

After a Death

Regardless of the time spent preparing for a death, some tasks cannot be completed until afterward.

Things for the Family to Do after the Death To prevent legal complications, you'll need a death certificate signed by a physician, medical examiner, or **county coroner** (see Figure 23-3). If a person dies unexpectedly, though of natural causes, or from a rare or highly researched disease, the doctors may request an **autopsy.** This means that the body will be opened, the organs of interest examined, and perhaps certain parts removed for study. In cases of a natural death, family permission is required to

TO MY FAMILY, MY PHYSICIAN, MY LAWYER, MY CLERGYMAN
TO ANY MEDICAL FACILITY IN WHOSE CARE I HAPPEN TO BE
TO ANY INDIVIDUAL WHO MAY BECOME RESPONSIBLE FOR MY HEALTH, WELFARE OR AFFAIRS

Death is as much a reality as birth, growth, maturity and old age—it is the one certainty of life. If the time comes when I, ______________________ can no longer take part in decisions for my own future, let this statement stand as an expression of my wishes, while I am still of sound mind.

If the situation should arise in which there is no reasonable expectation of my recovery from physical or mental disability, I request that I be allowed to die and not be kept alive by artificial means or "heroic measures". I do not fear death itself as much as the indignities of deterioration, dependence and hopeless pain. I, therefore, ask that medication be mercifully administered to me to alleviate suffering even though this may hasten the moment of death.

This request is made after careful consideration. I hope you who care for me will feel morally bound to follow its mandate. I recognize that this appears to place a heavy responsibility upon you, but it is with the intention of relieving you of such responsibility and of placing it upon myself in accordance with my strong convictions, that this statement is made.

Signed ______________________

Date ______________________

Witness ______________________

Witness ______________________

Copies of this request have been given to ______________________

____

____

____

Figure 23-2 Euthanasia Educational Council's "living will" can clarify your wishes in case of terminal illness or trauma. (Copies can be obtained by writing the council at 250 W. 57th St., New York, NY 10019.)

CERTIFICATE OF DEATH

STATE FILE NUMBER

STATE OF CALIFORNIA

LOCAL REGISTRATION DISTRICT AND CERTIFICATE NUMBER

DECEDENT PERSONAL DATA

1A. NAME OF DECEDENT—FIRST	1B. MIDDLE	1C. LAST	2A. DATE OF DEATH (MONTH, DAY, YEAR)	2B. HOUR
John	Peter	Doe	1-28-87	

3. SEX	4. RACE/ETHNICITY	5. SPANISH/HISPANIC	6. DATE OF BIRTH	7. AGE	IF UNDER 1 YEAR MONTHS	DAYS	IF UNDER 24 HOURS HOURS	MINUTES
M	W	NO ☒	11/3/37	49 YEARS				

8. BIRTHPLACE OF DECEDENT (STATE OR FOREIGN COUNTRY)	9. NAME AND BIRTHPLACE OF FATHER	10. BIRTH NAME AND BIRTHPLACE OF MOTHER
PA	Henry M. Doe, PA	Mary Jones, PA

11A. CITIZEN OF WHAT COUNTRY	11B. IF DECEASED WAS EVER IN MILITARY GIVE DATES OF SERVICE.	12. SOCIAL SECURITY NUMBER	13. MARITAL STATUS	14. NAME OF SURVIVING SPOUSE (IF WIFE, ENTER BIRTH NAME)
USA	19__ TO 19__	000-00-0000	Married	Jane Smith

15. PRIMARY OCCUPATION	16. NUMBER OF YEARS THIS OCCUPATION	17. EMPLOYER (IF SELF-EMPLOYED, SO STATE)	18. KIND OF INDUSTRY OR BUSINESS
Lawyer	25	Self-employed, CA	Law firm

USUAL RESIDENCE

19A. USUAL RESIDENCE—STREET ADDRESS (STREET AND NUMBER OR LOCATION)	19B.	19C. CITY OR TOWN
300 Elm St.		Palo Alto

19D. COUNTY	19E. STATE	20. NAME AND ADDRESS OF INFORMANT—RELATIONSHIP
Santa Clara	CA	Jane S. Doe, wife

PLACE OF DEATH

21A. PLACE OF DEATH	21B. COUNTY
Palo Alto General Hospital	Santa Clara
21C. STREET ADDRESS (STREET AND NUMBER OR LOCATION)	**21D. CITY OR TOWN**
2000 El Camino Real	Palo Alto

CAUSE OF DEATH

22. DEATH WAS CAUSED BY: (ENTER ONLY ONE CAUSE PER LINE FOR A, B, AND C)

IMMEDIATE CAUSE — CONDITIONS, IF ANY, WHICH GAVE RISE TO THE IMMEDIATE CAUSE, STATING THE UNDERLYING CAUSE LAST.

	Cause	APPROXIMATE INTERVAL BETWEEN ONSET AND DEATH
(A)	Acute anterior myocardial infarct	3 days
	DUE TO, OR AS A CONSEQUENCE OF	
(B)	Thrombosis of l.a.d. coronary artery	3 days
	DUE TO, OR AS A CONSEQUENCE OF	
(C)	Generalized atherosclerosis	20 yrs

24. WAS DEATH REPORTED TO CORONER? No
25. WAS BIOPSY PERFORMED? No
26. WAS AUTOPSY PERFORMED? Yes

23. OTHER SIGNIFICANT CONDITIONS—CONTRIBUTING TO DEATH BUT NOT RELATED TO CAUSE GIVEN IN 22A: Diabetes Type II

27. WAS OPERATION PERFORMED FOR ANY CONDITION IN ITEMS 22 OR 23? TYPE OF OPERATION: Coronary bypass — DATE: 2-10-86

PHYSICIAN'S CERTIFICATION

28A. I CERTIFY THAT DEATH OCCURRED AT THE HOUR, DATE AND PLACE STATED FROM THE CAUSES STATED.

I ATTENDED DECEDENT SINCE (ENTER MO. DA. YR.)	I LAST SAW DECEDENT ALIVE (ENTER MO. DA. YR.)	28B. PHYSICIAN—SIGNATURE AND DEGREE OR TITLE	28C. DATE SIGNED	28D. PHYSICIAN'S LICENSE NUMBER
2-6-75	1-27-87	William Osler, MD	1-29-87	G 000000

28E. TYPE PHYSICIAN'S NAME AND ADDRESS: William Osler, M.D., 5000 Welch Rd., Palo Alto, CA

INJURY INFORMATION / CORONER'S USE ONLY

29. SPECIFY ACCIDENT, SUICIDE, ETC.	30. PLACE OF INJURY	31. INJURY AT WORK	32A. DATE OF INJURY—MONTH, DAY, YEAR	32B. HOUR

33. LOCATION (STREET AND NUMBER OR LOCATION AND CITY OR TOWN)	34. DESCRIBE HOW INJURY OCCURRED (EVENTS WHICH RESULTED IN INJURY)

35A. I CERTIFY THAT DEATH OCCURRED AT THE HOUR, DATE AND PLACE STATED FROM THE CAUSES STATED. AS REQUIRED BY LAW I HAVE HELD AN (INQUEST-INVESTIGATION)	35B. CORONER—SIGNATURE AND DEGREE OR TITLE	35C. DATE SIGNED

36. DISPOSITION	37. DATE—MONTH, DAY, YEAR	38. NAME AND ADDRESS OF CEMETERY OR CREMATORY	39. EMBALMER'S LICENSE NUMBER AND SIGNATURE
Burial	1-31-87	Peaceful Meadows, Palo Alto, CA	0000 E.M. Baumer

40A. NAME OF FUNERAL DIRECTOR (OR PERSON ACTING AS SUCH)	40B. LICENSE NO.	41. LOCAL REGISTRAR—SIGNATURE	42. DATE ACCEPTED BY LOCAL REGISTRAR
D. Odell		A. Clark	1-30-87

STATE REGISTRAR	A.	B.	C.	D.	E.	F.

VS-11 (1-85)

Figure 23-3

perform an autopsy. If causes of death are unnatural, questionable, unexplained, accidental, or bizarre, the coroner will require an autopsy.

Otherwise, if the person has signed a Uniform Donor Card, find it and call the closest medical school. The school will generally pick up the body, or you may have to pay transportation costs. You will need to state what you want done with the body after the school is finished with it.

Advising friends and relatives of the death and burial plans should be done promptly to allow them time to plan to be there. A list of phone numbers and addresses should be ready beforehand. You might find volunteer friends who could help with the calls.

In his book *A Manual of Death Education and Simple Burial,* Ernest Morgan provides this checklist of things to be done shortly after the death. It may take you and friends weeks or months to finish.

- Take care of yourself first.
- List immediate family, close friends, employer, business colleagues. Notify each by phone.
- If flowers are to be omitted, decide on appropriate memorial or charity to which gifts may be made.
- Write obituary. Include age, place of birth, cause of death, occupation, college degrees, memberships held, military service, outstanding work, lists of survivors in immediate family. Give time and place of memorial services. Deliver in person or by phone to newspapers.
- Notify insurance companies, including automobile insurance, for immediate cancellation and refund of premium.
- Arrange for family members or close friends to take turns answering door and phone. Keep a record of the calls.
- Arrange appropriate child care.
- Coordinate the supplying of food for the next several days.
- Consider special household needs, such as cleaning, that might be done by friends.
- Arrange hospitality for visiting relatives and friends.
- Select pall bearers and notify. Choose sturdy people who can carry a heavy load.
- Notify lawyer and personal representative.
- Plan for disposition of flowers after funeral.
- List people to be notified by letter or printed notice.
- Prepare message for printed notice, if needed.
- List people to receive acknowledgments of flowers, calls, and so forth. Send appropriate written or printed notes.
- Check carefully all life and casualty insurance policies and death benefits, including Social Security, fraternal, military, credit, and trade unions. Check also on income for survivors from these sources.
- Check promptly on debts, mortgages, and installment payments. Some may carry life insurance clauses that cancel the debt. If payments must be delayed, consult creditors to ask for more time.
- If the deceased lived alone, notify utilities and landlord. Tell post office where to send mail. Take precautions against thieves.

Grieving It is a deep loss when someone close to you dies, and it is emotionally very painful. If you can allow yourself to feel and express anguish, you will be better able to accept the loss and free yourself to continue with your life. Grieving is a way to heal yourself.

If your loved one dies after a long illness, you will probably have mixed feelings of relief that it's over, and pain as you try to adjust. You may feel anger over unresolved issues in the relationship. And you may have feelings similar to those the person had while dying: denial, isolation, guilt, anger, bargaining, depression, and acceptance. You will have so many different feelings—perhaps conflicting—and such intense feelings that you will need to find some resolution through talking and crying, maybe yelling. Do not try to hold back feelings and be strong and brave; no one should expect you to. However, you need not pretend to grieve if you do not have strong feelings of grief. Only be sensitive to the pain around you.

Although there is no universal pattern of stages to the mourner's grief, certain tendencies repeat themselves in mourning. First you will probably feel some shock and numbness in the few days after death and through the funeral. One valuable aspect of a funeral is that it provides activities to occupy thoughts and time.

When the immediate bustle of activities following the death ends, a letdown and some silence may begin. Friends may not be as accessible as they had been while they were seeing you through the crisis. You begin to face the fact that you are really alone, and then you may experience throbbing emotional pain.

The second stage can last a long time. During this period you may feel disorientation, despair, bewilderment, unreasonable worry, fear for your own survival. A feeling of malaise and "Why bother to go on?" may take over, and you may feel drained of energy so that you can barely make yourself do anything. Thoughts of the dead person may seem obsessive. This depression often manifests itself as a series of physical symptoms such as insomnia, impotence, midnight sweats, anxiety attacks, lack of appetite, and physical inertia, and you may become more accident prone. Usually these feelings and symptoms disappear within a period of months, certainly within a year. If they continue longer, it may indicate that the natural self-healing process of grief has given way to a more serious depressive illness.

Eventually, you notice that the pain lets up for periods of time. Terrible lamenting turns more and more into quiet sadness. Sleep patterns, appetite, and energy grad-

How to Cope with Grief

- Realize and recognize the loss.
- Take time for nature's slow, sure, stuttering process of healing.
- Give yourself massive doses of restful relaxation and routine busy-ness.
- Know that powerful, overwhelming feelings will lessen with time.
- Be vulnerable, share your pain, and be humble enough to accept support.
- Surround yourself with life: plants, animals, and friends.
- Use mementos to help your mourning, not to live in the dead past.
- Avoid rebound relationships, big decisions, and anything addictive.
- Keep a diary and record successes, memories, and struggles.
- Prepare for change, new interests, new friends, solitude, creativity, growth.
- Recognize that forgiveness (of ourselves and others) is a vital part of the healing process.
- Know that holidays and anniversaries can bring up the painful feelings you thought you had successfully worked through.
- Realize that any new death-related crisis will bring up feelings about past losses.

SOURCE: The Centre for Living with Dying

ually return, and you can face forays into the outside world. Most people do come to terms with bereavement pain and somehow accommodate the grief: they do not forget, but they regain the capacity to remember peacefully.

Beyond Death

Most religions spell out beliefs concerning death, and provide comfort for those who believe them. They usually are based on the hope that people transcend death. The Judeo-Christian traditions are the most widely held in the United States. These fundamental beliefs about death are that the body is a temporary house, a cocoon, for the soul. The body dies, but the soul is immortal and lives forever.

Other religions hold to the idea of reincarnation, the rebirthing of the spirit in a different body. This idea negates some aspects of death, and encourages people to do good so that they can return in a better body and situation. It is related to another belief based on the idea of a common cosmic consciousness shared by all people. For these believers, it is an illusion to think of each person as a separate self with an individual ego. When a person dies, his or her consciousness lives on. The further we live from nature, the more difficult it is for us to be aware of this continuity and to accept our part in it.

The Walking Dead All who live, die. No one can control the process, so the best that anyone can do is to live fully. This course does not mean clutching at life in a frantic effort to squeeze out the last ounce of pleasure or meaning or accomplishment. It does mean being aware, open, sensitive, and able to experience the pain and joy of existence. Unfortunately, many people turn themselves off from life when they are quite young, perhaps because of some pain or fears they have endured. They live only in a technical sense, controlling every emotion so that they do not risk getting too close to anyone or letting anyone know they are vulnerable. Compare the fixed faces and bodies of a crowd of adults on their way to work with the faces and bodies of 2- and 3-year-olds, revealing intense, spontaneous, and unrepressed delight, anger, fear, surprise. The real tragedy in life is to die without ever having lived.

Facing Death as a Way to Renew Life A confrontation with death makes us aware of the preciousness of life. European writers expressed this theme over and over again after World War II. Many of them had been condemned to death and forced to await execution. Without exception, these people found that the confrontation with death liberated them from many former fears. Why? Once death is upon us, we somehow begin to see how trivial our other fears are. Facing the fear of death allows one to place these other fears in some perspective and to reorder one's priorities. We can dare to feel compassion and affection and to express it to others without great fear of rejection. We might be able to risk a job by speaking up to an oppressive boss, or to risk relationships by being truer to ourselves, less self-effacing, bolder. Knowing that life is short on this earth can help people value themselves and others more, and to cut through the red tape of our fears and society's rites and forms when they interfere with more humane values.

Take Action

Your answers to the Exploring Your Emotions in this chapter and your placement level on the Awareness Ladder will, we hope, encourage you to begin a process of self-exploration and self-discovery that you will continue. Reflect on the entire chapter's content and ask yourself how each point relates to your own life. Then take action:

1. Write to the National Kidney Foundation at 116 East 27th Street, New York, NY 10016, requesting a Uniform Donor Card. When you receive it, consider the advantages and disadvantages of an after-death donor plan.
2. Find out what resources are available in your community to counsel the dying. Write an evaluation of the service.
3. Find out what resources are available in your community for counseling the bereaved. If none is locally available, find out where this service is offered and inform the appropriate local community agency.
4. Write an ethical will. Tell what kind of person you are and what traits or values you would like to bequeath to your children or best friends or siblings: loyalty? perseverance? honesty? humor? good education? a way with your fellow humans? What impact would you like to make in this world and what goals would you want for your children?
5. Write your own obituary as it would appear thirty years from now, noting your best qualities. What would you like to have accomplished? Then write one as it might appear for you now.
6. What would be your feelings if your very close friend died suddenly? or if he or she committed suicide?
7. Develop and write up a preplanned burial. List the steps and duties to carry through.
8. Before leaving this chapter, review the Rate Yourself statements that open the chapter. Have your feelings or values changed? Are you now better equipped to handle the complex and very human problems associated with death and dying?

Selected References

Carroll, David. 1985. *Living with Dying: A Loving Guide for Family and Close Friends.* New York: McGraw-Hill.

Hemphill, Charles F., Jr. 1980. *Wills and Trusts: A Legal and Financial Handbook for Everyone.* Englewood Cliffs, N.J.: Prentice-Hall.

Krementz, Jill. 1981. *How It Feels When a Parent Dies.* New York: Knopf.

Maguire, Daniel. 1974. *Death by Choice.* New York: Doubleday.

Moffat, Mary Jane. 1982. *In the Midst of Winter: Selections from the Literature of Mourning.* New York: Random House.

Morgan, Ernest. 1980. *A Manual of Death Education and Simple Burial.* 9th ed. Burnsville, N.C.: Celo Press.

Tatelbaum, Judy. 1982. *The Courage to Grieve: Creative Living, Recovery and Growth through Grief.* New York: Harper & Row.

Wilcox, Sandra Galdieri, and Marilyn Sutton. 1985. *Understanding Death and Dying: An Interdisciplinary Approach.* Palo Alto, Calif.: Mayfield.

Recommended Readings

DeSpelder, Lynne Ann, and Albert Lee Strickland, 1987. *The Last Dance: Encountering Death and Dying,* 2nd ed. Palo Alto, Calif.: Mayfield.
Wide selection of readings arranged by topics: death in children's lives; survivors; medical ethics; the law and death; and eleven others.

Duda, Deborah. 1982. *A Guide to Dying at Home.* Santa Fe, New Mexico: John Muir.
A practical and positive manual for caring for and tending the terminally ill and planning for death. It provides mental, emotional and spiritual support. Lists hospices and memorial societies in the US and Canada.

Humphry, Derek and Ann Wickett. 1986. *The Right to Die: Understanding Euthanasia.* New York: Harper & Row.
A dispassionate attempt to explain euthanasia against the historical, cultural and legal backgrounds. It reports court cases, the legal and religious status of euthanasia in different states and countries.

Schneidman, Edwin S., ed. 1984. *Death: Current Perspectives,* 3rd ed. Palo Alto, Calif.: Mayfield.
Thoughtfully selected essays concerning wide variety of issues: the legal and ethical aspects of death, quality of life during dying, fresh views about suicide, personal statements of grief.

Chapter 24

Contents

Rate Yourself

Your Awareness of Safety and First Aid Read the following statements carefully. Choose the one in each section that best describes you at this moment and circle its number. When you have chosen one statement for each section, add the numbers and record your total score. Find your position on the Wellness Ladder.

5 Accidents are mainly the result of poor prevention planning
4 Accidents are caused mainly by unsafe behavior
3 Accidents are caused mainly by the inability to react quickly
2 Accidents are mainly the results of unseen hazards
1 Accidents are mainly the result of chance

5 Speed limits are used to enhance safety
4 Speed limits establish the safest maximum speed
3 Speed limits reduce fatal accidents
2 Speed limits infringe upon driving rights
1 Speed limits cause accidents

5 I always use a seat belt when driving
4 I usually use a seat belt when driving
3 I often use a seat belt when driving
2 I sometimes use a seat belt when driving
1 I rarely use a seat belt when driving

5 Well prepared in case of accidental poisoning
4 Familiar with procedures in case of accidental poisoning
3 Knows how to reach the nearest poison control center
2 Unfamiliar with appropriate response to accidental poisoning
1 Disinterested in learning how to respond to accidental poisoning

5 Encourages others to be safety minded
4 Rarely if ever takes unnecessary risks
3 Occasionally takes unnecessary risks
2 Frequently takes unnecessary risks
1 Prefers to live dangerously

Total Score ______

Safety and First Aid

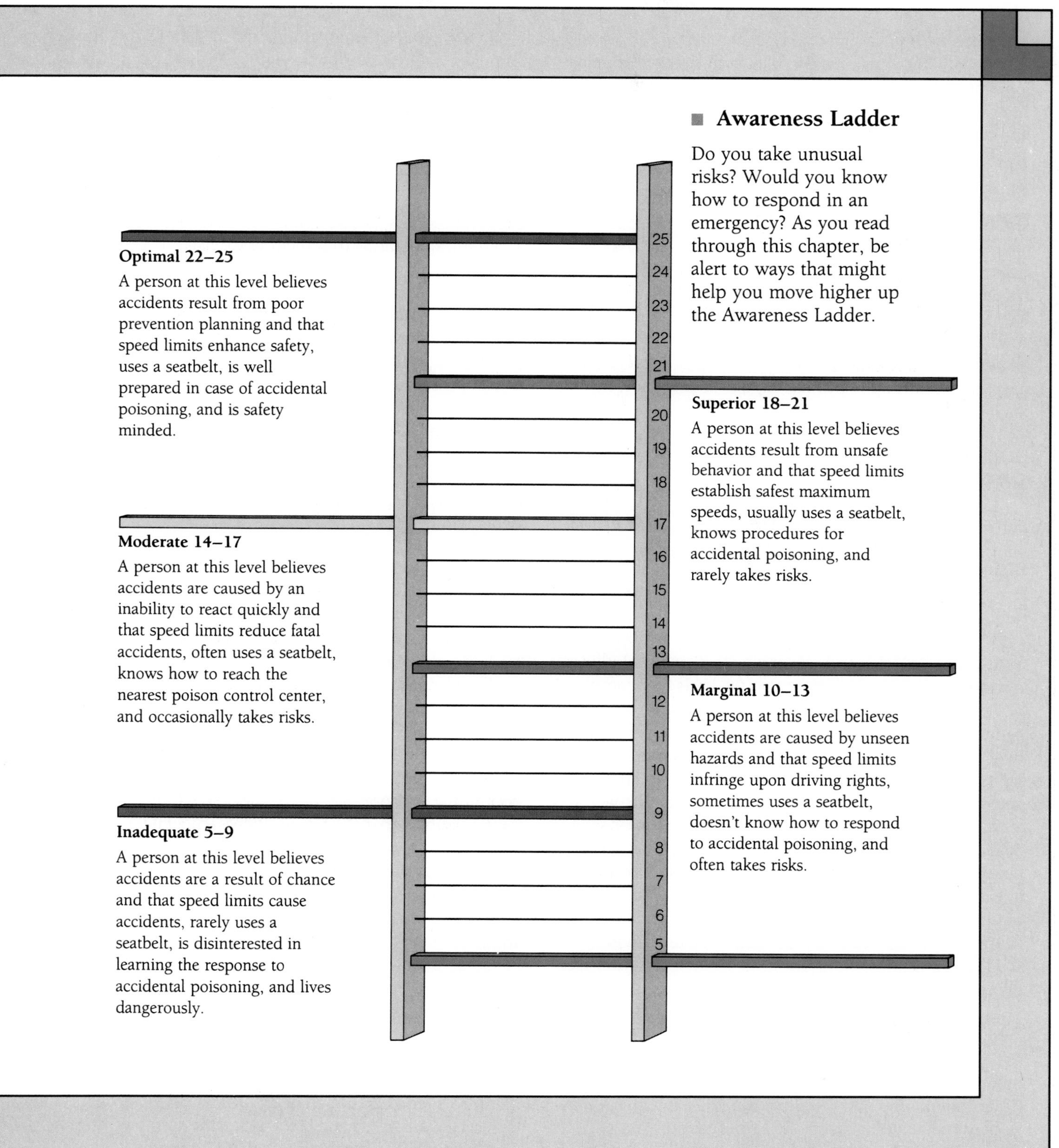

Awareness Ladder
Do you take unusual risks? Would you know how to respond in an emergency? As you read through this chapter, be alert to ways that might help you move higher up the Awareness Ladder.
Optimal 22–25
A person at this level believes accidents result from poor prevention planning and that speed limits enhance safety, uses a seatbelt, is well prepared in case of accidental poisoning, and is safety minded.
Superior 18–21
A person at this level believes accidents result from unsafe behavior and that speed limits establish safest maximum speeds, usually uses a seatbelt, knows procedures for accidental poisoning, and rarely takes risks.
Moderate 14–17
A person at this level believes accidents are caused by an inability to react quickly and that speed limits reduce fatal accidents, often uses a seatbelt, knows how to reach the nearest poison control center, and occasionally takes risks.
Marginal 10–13
A person at this level believes accidents are caused by unseen hazards and that speed limits infringe upon driving rights, sometimes uses a seatbelt, doesn't know how to respond to accidental poisoning, and often takes risks.
Inadequate 5–9
A person at this level believes accidents are a result of chance and that speed limits cause accidents, rarely uses a seatbelt, is disinterested in learning the response to accidental poisoning, and lives dangerously.
25
24
23
22
21
20
19
18
17
16
15
14
13
12
11
10
9
8
7
6
5

Social pathology theory The notion that accidents reflect a person's attitude toward life.

Accident proneness theory The idea that personality characteristics predispose an individual toward having accidents.

Accident repetitiveness Result when an individual is placed at greater risk because of given occupational hazards or chosen lifestyle.

Accidents are the leading cause of death among all people aged 1 to 37. Yet you need not rush to prepare yourself for a premature death. You *can* take steps to reduce the possibility of becoming the victim of a serious accident, and this chapter can help you.

Causes and Effects of Accidents

Contrary to common belief, accidents are *not* the end result of some mysterious game of chance. It is important to realize that accidents do *not* "just happen." In fact, any combination of five basic ingredients can conspire to cause an accident. Those five ingredients are inadequate knowledge, unsafe attitudes and habits, unsafe behavior, insufficient skill, and environmental hazards.

Exploring Your Emotions

Have you ever had a serious accident? What caused it? Did you contribute to it? How did it change your feelings and behavior about safety?

Knowledge is critical. You need to know what is safe and what is unsafe, and, surprisingly, that is *not* always obvious. Sometimes people act on the basis of incomplete or unreliable information. For example, someone who believes that safety belts trap people in cars when an accident occurs and who consequently decides not to wear a safety belt is acting on an inaccurate belief. No study has shown a higher incidence of injury for accident victims wearing safety belts than for those who don't wear safety belts, yet this misconception persists. Safety belts actually help a person retain control of the vehicle and reduce the likelihood of being thrown out of the car or against an object inside the vehicle and knocked unconscious. Knowing the facts can help us make safe decisions.

Unsafe attitudes can also lead to accidents. One example is the belief that accidents happen to "the other guy." This kind of thinking contributes to increased and usually inappropriate risk taking. For example, many people speed so they can get someplace a few minutes earlier, while others drink several alcoholic beverages and are willing (if not necessarily able) to drive home. Such drivers may or may not arrive safely at their destination. And even if they do, what about the next time?

Unsafe behavior can include careless actions by people who lack enough skill or strength, or who do not realize they no longer have the required ability to do something. Many people have accidents because they try to do something beyond their capabilities, such as riding a bicycle on a busy street, performing gymnastic feats on a parallel bar, or swimming across a lake. A key factor in accident prevention is knowing your own limitations and capabilities.

Environmental factors include external forces, which account for about 15 percent of all accidents. Technological advances create potentially dangerous situations, but the safety movement has not kept pace to maintain human control. However, safety devices that are comfortable, convenient, and easy to use are beginning to be readily available. Yet people often fail to take necessary precautions to protect themselves. Accidents *will* happen eventually if you do not control your environment. You must realize you have the ability and the opportunity to control yourself and to avoid hazardous conditions most of the time. When people learn to do so, the number of accidents will drop.

What Causes Accidents? Theorists have offered different hypotheses about the physiological, psychological, social, and environmental causes of accidents. Among the explanations are social pathology, accident proneness, and multiple causation.

Social pathology theory is based on the notion that accidents reflect your attitude toward life. Observations reveal that accidents tend to decrease as you take more responsibility for your own actions. You can also expect more accidents if you guide your behavior by a set of rules condoning irresponsibility. Studies have found a significant relationship between accidents and characteristics that are often associated with social deviance, such as hostility, aggressiveness, lack of self-control, and disrespect for others and/or regulations. Rejecting social constraints is associated with higher incidence of accidental injuries.

Some people seem to have more than their fair share of accidents. Society often labels such people "**accident prone.**" This term is often confused with the notion of "**accident repetitiveness.**" The label "accident prone" implies they are born with a disease or related condition that cannot be changed and that inflexibly predisposes them to accidents. On the contrary, accident proneness reflects a person's life and behaviors, which can be changed. The personality characteristics that predispose someone

The Risk Game

Crashing an automobile at 30 mph is like diving headfirst off a three-story building. As the car stops, you slam with about the same force into the windshield, steering wheel or dashboard—or, if you're lucky, the protective arms of a seat belt. Traffic accidents are the leading cause of death for people between the ages of 5 and 34; last year nearly 45,000 people died in auto collisions, the equivalent of a fully loaded passenger jet crashing with no survivors every day. If everybody wore seat belts, more than half of these deaths could have been avoided. . . .

Despite millions of dollars spent on advertisements urging people to "buckle up for safety," only about one out of seven American drivers wears a seat belt.

Paul Slovic, a psychologist and former president of the Society for Risk Analysis, thought he might be able to persuade people to take better care of themselves. . . .

"We make about 50,000 automobile trips in a lifetime," says Slovic, "and the probabilities add up to a risk that is not trivial." About one out of every 140 people dies in a car accident; one out of three is injured seriously enough to be disabled for at least a day. If motorists would think in terms of a lifetime of driving rather than single trips, says Slovic, then perhaps they would decide once and for all to buckle up.

Slovic and co-worker Norman Schwalm produced new seat belt messages emphasizing the lifetime risks of automobiles. Several hundred volunteers watched the ads and answered questionnaires about which ads they found most effective. Though the results seemed to indicate that the approach showed promise, one thing did not: Slovic and his colleagues, surreptitiously watching their volunteers drive away from the parking lot, noted with dismay that there was no increase in seat belt use. The advertising effort, says Slovic, added "one more flop to an impressive list of failures." He now supports laws, recently passed in New York, California, and several other states, that make wearing seat belts mandatory.

Imagine how the apparent irrationality of Slovic's subjects frustrated him. His subjects were, after all, drawn from the general public, the same general public that smokes billions of cigarettes a year while banning an artificial sweetener because of a one-in-a-million chance that it might cause cancer; the same public that eats meals full of fat, flocks to cities prone to earthquakes, and goes hang gliding while it frets about pesticides in foods, avoids the ocean for fear of sharks and breaks into a cold sweat on airline flights.

In short, we, the general public, are irrational and uninformed. We don't understand probability, are biased by the news media and have a fear of some technologies that borders on the primeval. But a few scientists are beginning to ask if technical savvy is the only qualification needed to be a legitimate worrier. They are finding that, while our behavior often appears irrational and confused, perhaps we're not so dumb after all. We may be lousy with mortality statistics, but our fears may tell us a lot about how a risk affects society as a whole. . . .

Amos Tversky and Daniel Kahneman . . . discovered the fundamentals of our flip-flops about risks: "When it comes to taking risks for gains, people are conservative. They will take a sure gain over a probable gain," says Tversky. "But we are also finding that when people are faced with a choice between a small, certain loss and a large, probable loss, they will gamble."

If we can't be certain about the risks we face, we at least want to have some control over the technologies and activities that produce them. It has long been known, much to the frustration of some risk experts, that we may be much more willing to accept higher risks in activities over which we have control, such as smoking, drinking, driving, or skiing, than things over which we have little control, such as industrial pollution, food additives, and commercial airlines.

A feeling of control can actually make a risky technology even more dangerous. That's because we often have inflated opinions of ourselves. Most of us consider ourselves above-average drivers, safer than most when using appliances and power tools, and less likely to suffer medical problems such as heart attacks. "Such confidence is dangerous," says Slovic. "It indicates that we often do not realize how little we know and how much additional information we need about the risks we face."

When we think about risk, says Slovic, we are not only concerned that technology has the potential to cause deaths, we also worry about more subtle aspects: How well do we understand the risk?

(continued on next page)

The Risk Game (*continued*)

How will it affect society? Could it wipe out an entire community? Make a particular area uninhabitable for a long time? Would it affect future generations or some members of society more than others?

Slovic and his colleagues found that when people were asked to apply these societal concerns to the risks of some 90 different activities and technologies, each took on a profile that was broader than a simple death statistic. Some items, like dynamite, were considered deadly, but also fairly controllable. Others, like microwave ovens, were thought to involve risks that were delayed in their effects and not well known, but were also voluntary and unlikely to cause catastrophes. The respondents overwhelmingly regarded the risks of nuclear power as involuntary, uncontrollable, unknown, inequitably distributed, likely to be fatal, potentially catastrophic and evoking feelings not just of fear but of dread. Automobiles, which kill far more people per year, evoked few of these concerns.

According to Slovic, we are also concerned about the inherent riskiness of assessing risks. Part of our worry about technologies such as nuclear power, toxic wastes and genetic engineering, for example, stems from the knowledge that the assessments of these risks are based not so much on the experience of a proven track record as on scientific analysis that, like some scientific analyses, might be in error.

The fact that the public is keenly aware that scientists can be wrong is at the root of the concern about the nuclear accident at Three Mile Island. Before the accident, scientists had said confidently that the chances of a serious reactor breakdown were quite remote. But when a potential disaster occurred relatively early in the history of nuclear power, even though the safety systems worked and the disaster never materialized, the mishap sent out a signal that the overall assessment of the risks of nuclear power might be in error. . . .

SOURCE: Adapted from William F. Allman, The risk game: Why we gamble with our own safety, *Science 85*.

toward having accidents are shown in Table 24-1. Whether you are Type Y (accident prone) or Type X (not accident prone) is not as important as the fact you can change your behavior.

Often people try to identify a single cause of an accident, such as faulty brakes, inadequate visibility, or a broken switch. In reality, it is very difficult to pinpoint one particular cause for any type of accident. **Multiple causation theory** suggests that human and environmental factors dynamically interact to produce an accident.

Human factors in accidents are intrinsic factors that lead to an unsafe state or unsafe act (see Table 24-2). The unsafe state may be physical, emotional, and/or psychological distress. When you cannot perceive events objectively as clearly as possible, or cannot control your anger, you are in an unsafe state induced by stress. Your unsafe acts are your own behavioral responses. For example, someone may mow a lawn carelessly in order to finish on time to watch a television program. When you are tempted to engage in unsafe behavior, ask yourself whether negative consequences are worth the risk.

Environmental factors are extrinsic factors that surround unsafe conditions or an unsafe event. The unsafe conditions are the environmental circumstances. For example, low visibility and snow-packed roads are unsafe conditions. Unsafe events are unexpected or unanticipated occurrences, such as a child running into the street or a baseball being hit toward a person.

The antecedents interact to produce an unsafe situation. At a critical moment, you must make a decision that influences the outcome of the situation. If you avoid the accident, you may learn from the experience. Unfortunately, some people learn nothing from a near-miss event because they are unaware of what happened. Even worse is when the potential for an accident exists, but the person does not even recognize the danger. For example, a person who rides a motorcycle without wearing a helmet may believe it is unnecessary to wear such protective equipment simply because he or she has never been involved

Exploring Your Emotions

Do you know anyone who seems to be accident prone? What kinds of feelings do this person's accidents arouse in you?

Multiple causation theory The idea that accidents are caused by several factors that dynamically interact.

in an accident. Consequently the unsafe behavior is reinforced. The person develops a false sense of security and the bad habit pushes the person toward taking even higher risks in the future.

How Do Accidents Affect Our Lives? Accidents are the fourth leading cause of death in the United States, following heart disease, cancer, and stroke. (For people between the ages 1 and 37, as already mentioned, accidents *are* the leading cause of death.) We can classify accidents into four major categories—motor vehicle, home, work, and public. In at least the past decade, the highest number of deaths have occurred in motor vehicle accidents, and the highest number of disabling injuries have resulted from home accidents. These rates occur even though people often feel safe when they are driving a motor vehicle or are in their homes.

Accidents now account for nearly $100 billion in costs in the United States every year. Motor vehicle accidents comprise nearly 50 percent of that total, followed by work accidents at 33 percent, home accidents at 10 percent, and public accidents the remaining 7 percent. Such financial costs include wage loss, insurance administration, property damage in motor vehicle accidents, indirect loss from work accidents, medical expenses, and fire loss. There are many other less tangible factors to consider in the costs of accidents, the most obvious of which is the human life lost, either in terms of death or disability. Not only is the victim affected, but significant others as well. (See Table 24-3.)

No one is immune to accidents. According to the National Safety Council, about 69 percent of all accidental deaths involve males. Extended exposure rates (such as number of miles driven annually), high risk-taking jobs (such as construction), and risk-taking behaviors (such as more drinking and driving incidents) all contribute. The figures are changing slightly as more women enter new

Table 24-1 Personality Traits that Predispose Toward Accidents

TYPE X Not Accident Prone	TYPE Y Accident Prone
Has conventional goals	Holds unconventional values
Is goal oriented	Has no clearly defined goals
Is satisfied with life	Is dissatisfied with life
Respects rights and opinions of others	Is insensitive to rights and opinions of others
Relates to others	Does not relate easily or warmly to others
Is noncombative	Has difficulty in controlling hostility
Shows concern for others	Is self-oriented

Table 24-2 Human and Environmental Factors in Accidents

Human Factors	Environmental Factors
Physical incapability	Imperfect weather conditions
Poor visual acuity	Overcrowded conditions
Stress and fatigue	Defective equipment
False sense of security	Inadequate law enforcement
Distractibility	Nonsupportive social environment
Lack of knowledge	Poor attitudes
Poor attitudes	Inadequate legislation
Bad habits	Lack of safety education programs

Table 24-3 Accidental Deaths and Injuries in the United States in 1985

	Deaths	Change from 1984	Deaths per 100,000 People	Disabling Injuries
Motor Vehicle	45,600	−1%	19.1	1.7 million
Work	11,600	−1%	4.9	2.0 million
Home	20,500	−2%	8.6	3.1 million
Public	19,000	+3%	8.0	2.4 million
All Classes	92,500	−1%	38.7	9.0 million

SOURCE: National Safety Council, *Accident Facts*, 1986 (Chicago: National Safety Council), p. 3.

Accident Proneness Inventory

Following are twenty items designed to indicate your tendency to be accident-prone. If you feel a statement is true for you, circle T. If you feel a statement is false for you, circle F. The scoring instructions will enable you to examine the extent to which you may be accident prone.

	TRUE	FALSE
1. When buying a car, economy is more important to me than safety.	T	F
2. I often smoke more than one pack of cigarettes a day.	T	F
3. I am extremely impatient with slow drivers.	T	F
4. I often burn myself when working in the kitchen.	T	F
5. It doesn't bother me to eat things that are dropped on the floor.	T	F
6. I have had two or more broken bones during my life.	T	F
7. When driving, I usually do not buckle my seat belt.	T	F
8. I often drop things for no apparent reason.	T	F
9. I am usually in a hurry.	T	F
10. I often drive faster than the speed limit.	T	F
11. Many times I will discover bruises on myself without knowing how they happened.	T	F
12. I often leave tools lying about the house.	T	F
13. I tend to be a sloppy housekeeper.	T	F
14. Rather than wait for a green light, I sometimes run across the street in heavy traffic.	T	F
15. I sometimes throw razor blades in the wastepaper basket.	T	F
16. I will sometimes pass a slow driver on a two-lane road when I can't see if a car is coming.	T	F
17. I frequently cut myself.	T	F
18. I can walk on high ledges without feeling frightened.	T	F
19. I get extremely irritated by people who are slow.	T	F
20. I will do almost anything "on a dare."	T	F

Scoring Instructions To find out the degree to which you are accident prone, add up all items you have circled T. The following table indicates the degree to which you are accident-prone.

15–20 Extremely accident prone
10–14 Moderately accident prone
5 – 9 Average
0 – 4 Low tendency toward accident proneness

occupations and begin taking similar risks. The inconsistency and unpredictability of human nature plays a major role.

How Can Accidents Be Prevented?

It would be unrealistically hopeful to try to eliminate all accidents, but you can take positive preventive measures to reduce your risk of accidents. It is important that you become more aware of your own risk taking and how it can influence the outcome of risky situations.

Education is primary in preventing accidents. A comprehensive approach to safety education involves cognitive (knowledge), affective (attitude), and psychomotor (behavior and skill) domains. You need information in order to make responsible decisions. Direct and indirect information can help you recognize that safety *does* affect your life every day and that potential hazards *do* exist. Those hazards need not become reality, because you can change your behavior.

Attitude is an educational factor that involves your values and priorities. You must not only believe that safety is important, but you must also realize you are not "immortal" and are just as likely as "the other guy" to be involved in accidents. With that thought in mind, you are in a better position to avoid injury and/or death from an accident.

According to the **health belief model**, your preventive behavior depends on your perceptions. Your perceived susceptibility might vary from one extreme (denying the problem totally), to a more moderate acceptance of probability, to the other end of the continuum (realizing that

Health belief model Model based on the premise that preventive health behavior is an attempt to avoid negative outcomes, such as disease or accidents. The preventive behavior depends on the perceptions of that individual, so the person must believe there is a risk in order to take action to avoid disease or injury.

Reaction time The time it takes for a person to react to what he or she has seen or heard. In a driving situation, the time required for the driver to release the accelerator and apply the brake.

Second collision When the occupants of a motor vehicle collide with the car interior and/or are ejected from the vehicle. At the time of crash, occupants experience a deceleration force equal to their weight multiplied by the speed of the vehicle.

the danger exists for you personally). The perceived seriousness involves your feeling threatened by an accident situation. Seriousness and threat are usually perceived in terms of medical, psychological, social, and/or economic consequences.

Your perceptions are influenced by cues to action, which may be passive or active in nature. To be effective, the cues must also be relevant to you. You are more likely to act safely if the cues to safe action occur more frequently, come from a variety of sources, are more recent, have some emotional appeal, and represent an existing belief of yours. In the final analysis, the benefits must usually outweigh the barriers in order for you to take the safer course of action.

In the end, safe behavior is your goal. By increasing your knowledge and level of awareness, you can motivate yourself to act in the safest way possible. Probably you will not eliminate all risk-taking behaviors, but you will make more responsible and intelligent decisions that are reflected in your safety precautions. Such behaviors should have long-term consequences and become habits for a safer life.

What Can You Do to Prevent Accidents?

You can prevent many accidents from occurring by evaluating each situation. The action you take can mean the difference between injury or death and no accident at all.

Motor Vehicle Accidents Nearly three-fourths of all motor vehicle accidents are caused by bad driving; speeding is the most often recorded error. Most people do not truly understand the safety implications of speeding. As speed increases, the motor vehicle's momentum and force of impact increase; simultaneously, the driver's **reaction time** *decreases.* A car traveling at a speed of 30 miles per hour is in reality traveling at a speed of 44 feet per second! As the driver, you must be able to react within three-fourths of a second *and react correctly* in order to stop that vehicle within the minimum distance of 80 feet. Moreover, these figures assume that conditions are ideal; wet pavement, decreased visibility, driving under the influence of drugs or when half asleep, and additional passengers in your car increase the stopping distance significantly.

Exploring Your Emotions

Do you feel that everything that happens to a person is somehow deserved? Or fated? How might these feelings (whether vague feelings or firm beliefs) influence your safety behavior?

Speed limits are posted to establish (1) the safest *maximum* speed limit (2) for a given area (3) under *ideal* conditions. Such laws are meant to enhance safety, not infringe on your driving rights. If you consistently find yourself in driving situations that seem to require speeding, allow more time for traveling. By leaving ten or fifteen minutes earlier, you can relieve a lot of the pressure and compulsion to speed. Reduced speed also gives you control of your vehicle and increased time to react to any emergency situation.

A second factor that contributes to injury and death in motor vehicle accidents is the decision not to wear safety belts. Most people understand that restraint systems such as safety belts offer protection in an accident. What most people do not realize is that failure to wear them doubles your chances of being hurt in a crash! Using safety belts could reduce the number of serious injuries by at least 50 percent and the number of fatalities by 60 to 70 percent in motor vehicle mishaps. If you use a system that combines a lap and shoulder belt, your chances of survival are three to four times better than a person who rides beltless.

Most people who don't use safety belts don't understand their value. Safety belts work at the time of the "second collision." If a car is traveling at 55 mph and hits another vehicle, first the car must stop and then the occupants must stop because they are also traveling at the same speed. The "**second collision**" occurs when you hit some-

Exploring Your Emotions

How do you feel when you are trapped in a traffic jam or in slowly moving traffic? How do you feel about drivers who cut in and out of line to gain an advantage? How do your feelings affect your driving style in general?

Blood alcohol concentration (BAC) The amount of alcohol found in the blood.

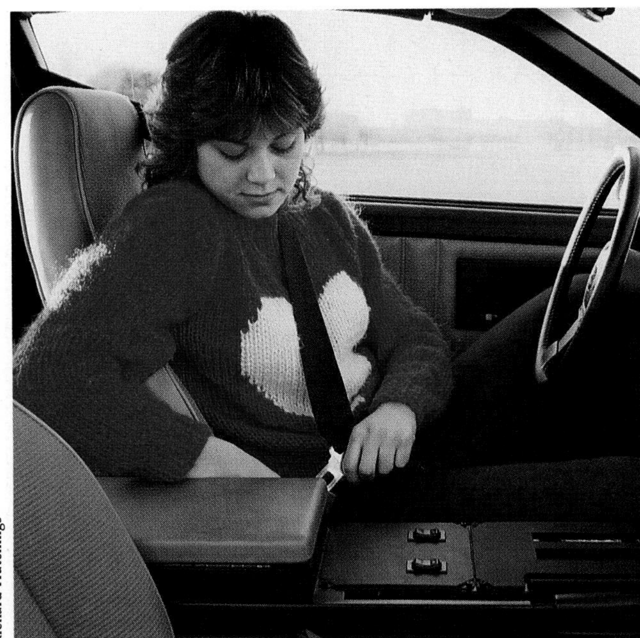
Richard Hutchings

Some Accident Facts

Did you know that . . .

- On the average there are 11 accidental deaths and about 1,030 disabling injuries every hour during the year.
- A motor vehicle death occurs every 12 minutes.
- Work deaths on the job occur every 45 minutes, as compared to off the job, which occur every 15 minutes.
- An injury occurs in the home every 10 seconds.
- Nearly 75 percent of all motor vehicle accidents cite improper driving as the error, with speeding being the type most often recorded.
- Use of safety belts can reduce the number of serious injuries by at least 50 percent and the number of fatalities by 60 to 70 percent.
- Drinking alcohol is identified as a factor in at least 50 percent of all fatal motor vehicle accidents.

SOURCE: National Safety Council, *Accident Facts,* 1986, Chicago: National Safety Council.

thing inside the car, like the steering column, dashboard, or windshield. Using a safety belt helps prevent that second collision from occurring and the safety belt spreads the stopping force over your body to reduce the likelihood of injury. (It also keeps you from being thrown out of the car.)

People give lots of reasons for not wearing their safety belts. Typical responses include discomfort, lack of mobility, wrinkling of clothes, fear of getting trapped in the car, believe that safety belts do not work, and the admission that safety belt use has not become a habit for them. All those answers can be easily countered by the facts. It would be wonderful if you could know in advance when you were going to be involved in an accident situation, whether a collision with another car or just stopping suddenly to avoid hitting a child who has run into the street to retrieve a ball. But you can't know in advance. Developing the habit of buckling up puts you one step ahead. Taking three seconds for that one click can mean the difference, but you must take *responsibility* for that decision. Safety belts save lives—it's as simple as that.

Another major cause of motor vehicle accidents is the unsafe behavior of drinking and driving. Alcohol is identified as a factor in at least half of all fatal motor vehicle accidents. Alcohol-impaired driving is illegal in all states because it threatens the health and safety of many people, both directly and indirectly. People who have a few drinks at a party may feel relaxed and less inhibited initially, but alcohol is a depressant that slows down body functions. The effect is the same after drinking a 12-ounce can of beer, a 3-ounce glass of wine, or a 1-ounce shot of distilled spirits, as long as the amount of alcohol content in the drink is the same.

A person is not considered alcohol impaired or alcohol intoxicated until the **blood alcohol concentration (BAC)** level is between 0.05 and 0.10 percent (acceptable levels vary from state to state). Alcohol is a drug that first affects the brain in terms of reason and caution, followed by judgment and then motor skills. Unfortunately, most people do not realize what is happening to them until they reach the third phase of motor skill impairment. The impaired person who continues to drive is not in control and is taking a major risk. The safest thing to do is not to drive if at all possible. Your options are either to wait and allow the alcohol to oxidize at a rate of about one drink per hour, call a cab, or to let a designated sober driver help you get home. If you are the host of a party, you should take responsibility for your guests needing assistance and make sure that they are delivered home safely.

Myths about Safety Belts

Myth If I wore a seat belt, I might get trapped in my car if it caught on fire or were submerged in water.

Fact In reality, only one-half of 1 percent of motor vehicle accidents involve fire or submersion. If that does happen, safety belts will help prevent you from being knocked unconscious, so you will be able to escape from your car.

Myth I would be better off if I were thrown clear of the car in a crash.

Fact The chances of being killed are twenty-five times greater if you're thrown out of the vehicle. Hitting a tree or the pavement causes severe injuries, which wouldn't occur if you stay buckled inside the car. Also, people who are thrown out of their cars are sometimes crushed or hit by their own vehicles or those of others.

Myth I can brace myself in an accident, so I don't need to bother with a safety belt.

Fact The force of an impact at just 10 mph can be equivalent to catching a 200-pound bag of cement thrown from a 10-foot ladder. At 35 mph the force of impact is even more brutal. There's no way your arms and legs can brace against that kind of force—even if you could react in time.

Myth A safety belt couldn't possibly hold me in place during a sudden stop or accident. When I yank it by hand, it doesn't work.

Fact Most safety belts are designed to automatically lock when the car stops suddenly or changes directions quickly. Belts normally expand and contract to allow freedom of movement.

Myth I'm not going far or driving fast, so I don't need to wear a safety belt.

Fact It is wise to wear a safety belt no matter where you are going since 75 percent of all crashes occur within 25 miles of home. Most deaths and injuries (80 percent) occur in automobiles traveling less than 40 mph. People have been killed in accidents at crash speeds of less than 12 mph.

Myth Pregnant women are not supposed to wear safety belts.

Fact According to the American Medical Association, both a pregnant woman and her unborn child are much safer with belts than without, provided the lap belt is worn as low as possible on the pelvic area.

Myth I am a good driver, so I will never be in an accident. I don't need to wear a safety belt.

Fact Safety belts are the most effective defense against a drunken driver. No matter how well you drive, you can't control what other drivers are going to do. A typical American is almost certain to be involved in a traffic crash during his or her lifetime, according to the University of Michigan's Transportation Research Institute. Regardless of driving skills, everyone faces a one-in-fifty chance of dying and a 50 percent probability of suffering a disabling injury from an auto accident.

SOURCE: "Buckle up," 1987, a publication of Traffic Safety Now, Inc., Detroit, Michigan.

In recent years, social acceptability of the drinking and driving behavior has decreased. People now realize the dangers associated with such behavior, not only for the drinking driver, but for others as well. National groups such as Students Against Drunk Driving (SADD) and Mothers Against Drunk Drivers (MADD) have also raised public awareness of the problem and have helped create a social stigma against impaired driving. Their efforts have resulted in stronger drunk driving legislation and stricter enforcement of the laws, although the problem has not been overcome. Each person must now assume a greater responsibility for unsafe drinking and driving behaviors, because society as a whole is affected by the outcome.

The environment is another factor that affects motor vehicle accidents. Weather is an obvious problem, because of its unpredictability. When weather deteriorates, you must drive more defensively. You need to increase the distance at which you follow another car in traffic, and reduce speed to compensate for hazards. Of course, you also need to have your car in good working order. People typically take care of the obvious needs like tires, gas, and oil, but it's easy to forget the simple things like replacing windshield wipers, at least until it starts to rain and you find out they don't work! Regular inspection and maintenance checks make sense if you expect your vehicle to perform well.

Road type and location also influence the likelihood of injury or fatality in an accident. Many people travel on rural highways because they think they can drive at faster speeds without getting caught. Consequently, the fatality rates on rural highways are much higher. Contrary to common belief, interstates are much safer for a number of reasons; for example, visibility is increased, all travel is in one direction, and fewer incidents require driving adjustments. If you have a choice, it makes more sense to travel on the interstate. Moreover, about 75 percent of all motor vehicle accidents occur within twenty-five miles from home, where the driver is probably more familiar with the driving terrain and on roadways with speed limits of less than 40 miles per hour. Often the driver mistakenly believes that safety measures are not warranted for a quick trip to the store, or for a short ride of a few blocks to a friend's house. The facts prove otherwise.

Pedestrian Safety Pedestrian safety is another area of personal concern. Each year about 18 percent of all motor vehicle deaths involve pedestrians and another 100,000 people are injured each year as a result of such accidents. As would be expected, most pedestrian accidents occur in urban settings. The young and the elderly are involved most often, but it is important to note that alcohol contributes to nearly 25 percent of the adult pedestrian deaths. The most unsafe pedestrian behavior is crossing between streets or intersections, whether walking or darting into traffic. Poor decision making accounts for the biggest problem, not the traffic situation itself. Simple actions such as increasing your visibility, crossing at the corner in designated walk areas, not hitchhiking, and not darting into traffic could greatly improve the overall traffic situation as well as your own safety.

Home Accidents Contrary to common belief, one of the most dangerous places to be is at home. One obvious reason is because people spend a major portion of their day at home, often alone. The majority of deaths in the home involve accidents classified as falls, fires and burn-related accidents, poisoning by solids and liquids, and suffocation by ingested objects.

Falls are second only to motor vehicle accidents in terms of causing deaths. About 85 percent of the fatal falls involve people 45 years of age and older, but note that falls are the fifth leading cause of accidental death for all people under 25 years of age. Most falls occur as a result of common activities in the home, with nearly two-thirds of the deaths occurring from falls at floor level rather than at a height. In most cases, it is the person's difficulty in adjusting to different degrees of traction, rather than the slipperiness of the surface, that makes a person fall. A rug, a bathtub, or the floor itself is a common problem in the home; icy, snowy, or rough ground are common factors outside. Ladders and stairs are also common sources of accidents.

Fires pose another safety problem in the home. Most people do not really appreciate or understand the dangers associated with fires. To burn a fire requires (1) a source of ignition, (2) fuel, and (3) oxygen. If any one component can be eliminated, fire can be prevented. Each year approximately 80 percent of fire deaths and 65 percent of fire injuries occur in the home. Fire ignition of furniture, combustible liquid or gas, and bedding account for 60 percent of the cases. Two-thirds of all home fires begin in the living room and bedroom. Many are caused by careless actions such as leaving a burning cigarette in an ashtray or smoking in bed.

Exploring Your Emotions

You have rented an apartment and can't get the landlord to put in smoke detectors. How do you feel, and how do you handle your feelings?

Most people are inadequately prepared to handle fire-related situations, especially those in the home. Such preparation includes planning escape routes, locating fire and smoke detection devices at every floor level of the home, and practice using fire-extinguishing devices. You should not wait until the time of a fire emergency to consider such actions. When a fire does occur, the important point to remember is to get out of the house as quickly and safely as possible.

Since smoke is the largest single cause of death and injury in fires, you should also know how to avoid smoke inhalation. The simplest method is to crawl along the floor away from the heat and smoke and cover your mouth, ideally with a wet cloth. If trapped in a burning building, you should also know how to signal for help with a white cloth. If you must try to extinguish a fire, you should be aware that fires are classified into four categories—Class A (wood, cloth, and paper), Class B (flammable liquids such as greases, gasoline, and lubricating oils), Class C (electrical equipment), and Class D (combustible metals). All these preventive efforts, coupled with an increased understanding of fire and the burning process, are positive measures to counter the home fire situation and the needless number of deaths and injuries each year.

Accidental poisonings pose another health and safety threat in the home. Statistics reveal that the home is the site for about 80 percent of the deaths by poisonous solids and liquids and over 60 percent from poisonous gases and vapors. A majority of the cases involve children under

Managing Poisonings

ABCs

With all serious injuries maintain an open Airway. Restore Breathing and Circulation if necessary.

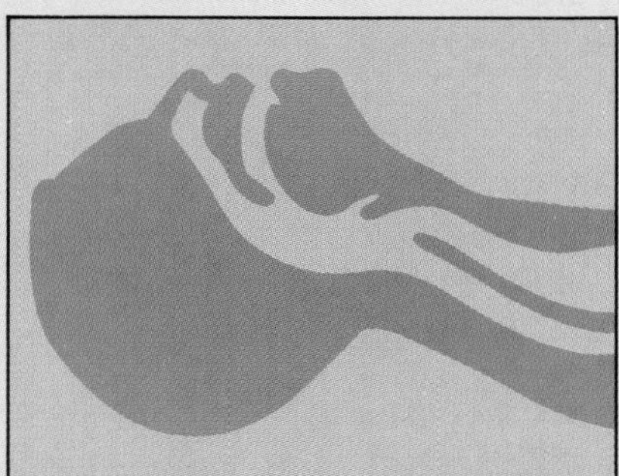

Tilt head backward to maintain an open airway.

Poisoning from Household Products That Are Swallowed

It is extremely important to call a Poison Control Center (if available), a hospital emergency room, a doctor or paramedics for instructions if someone has swallowed a poison. When calling, be sure to give the following information:

1. Victim's age
2. Name of the poison
3. How much poison was swallowed
4. When poison was swallowed
5. Whether or not the victim has vomited
6. How much time it will take to get the victim to a medical facility

Emergency treatment for victims of swallowed poisons consists of

1. Diluting the poison with water or milk as quickly as possible. *Do not* give fruit juice or vinegar to neutralize the poison.
2. Getting the poison out of the victim by induced vomiting (on medical advice only—preferably from the staff at a Poison Control Center)
3. Seeking prompt medical attention

Beware

Never give liquids to dilute the poison or induce vomiting if the victim is unconscious or is having convulsions. Also, *do not induce vomiting* if you do not know what the victim has swallowed.

Do not induce vomiting if the victim has swallowed,

1. A strong ACID such as toilet bowl cleaner, rust removers, chlorine bleach, dishwasher detergent or clinitest tablets.
2. PETROLEUM PRODUCTS such as kerosene, gasoline, furniture polish, charcoal lighter fluid or paint thinner.

Give water, not milk, with these products.

Strong acids and alkalis, if vomited, may cause further damage to the throat and esophagus. Petroleum products, if vomited, can be sucked into the lungs and cause a chemical pneumonia. It is important to note, however, that Poison Control Centers may recommend induced vomiting for some of the above-mentioned products (particularly the petroleum products) because of other, more harmful effects to the body.

Always follow the instructions of the Poison Control Center.

If the victim vomits, whether induced or spontaneous, keep the victim's face down with head lower than the rest of the body so that he will not choke on the vomit. Place a small child face down across your knees. *Be sure* to take the poison container and any vomited material to the hospital for inspection.

Note: Antidotes on labels of poisonous substances are not always correct, particularly if the container is old. It is always best to consult a Poison Control Center if possible.

Immediate Treatment Options

A. If the victim is *not* breathing,

1. Maintain an open airway.
2. Restore breathing.
3. Seek medical attention immediately. Call paramedics, ambulance, fire department, or other rescue personnel for transportation to the hospital.
4. Take the poison container and any vomited material to the hospital with the victim.

B. If the victim is *unconscious* or *having convulsions,*

1. Maintain an open airway if possible. Restore breathing if necessary.
2. Loosen tight clothing around the victim's neck and waist.
3. Seek medical attention immediately. Call paramedics, ambulance, fire department or other rescue personnel for transportation to the hospital. Victim should be transported lying on his or her side.
4. Take the poison container and any vomited material to the hospital with the victim.
5. *Do not* give any fluids to the victim.
6. *Do not* try to induce vomiting. If the victim vomits, turn his or

(continued on next page)

Managing Poisonings (*continued*)

her head to the side so that he or she will not choke on the vomit.

C. If the victim is conscious,

1. Immediately give the victim at least one 8-ounce glass of water or milk (give only water with gasoline products) to dilute the poison. *Do not* give fruit juice, vinegar, carbonated drinks, or alcohol to neutralize the poison.

2. Have someone else (if possible) call the Poison Control Center, hospital emergency room or doctor for further instructions while you continue to care for the victim.

3. Induce vomiting *only* if told to do so by one of the just listed medical personnel. If no medical advice is readily available, induce vomiting only if the swallowed poison is *not* an acid, alkali, or petroleum product. Vomiting may be induced by giving an adult (over 12 years of age unless low weight) 2 tablespoons of syrup of ipecac; a child, 1 tablespoon of syrup of ipecac; an infant under 1 year of age, 2 teaspoons. Follow with one to two glasses of water or milk. If vomiting does not occur within 15 to 20 minutes repeat dosage of ipecac *only* once.

4. *Do not* give mustard or table salt to the victim to induce vomiting.

5. If syrup of ipecac is not available, induce vomiting by tickling the back of the victim's throat with your finger or a spoon.

6. If vomiting does not occur, seek medical attention immediately.

7. If vomiting occurs, keep the victim face down with head lower than the rest of the body so that he or she will not choke on the vomit. Place a small child face down across your knees.

8. Seek medical attention immediately. Take the poison container and any vomited material to the hospital with the victim.

SOURCE: *The American Medical Association's Handbook of First Aid and Emergency Care,* 1980, New York: Random House, pp. 190–93.

age 5, although the 15–24 and 25–44 age groups have shown increased death rates in recent years. Common causes include analgesics, cleaning substances, poisonous plants, and drug-related overdoses. Over two million poisonings occur every year, with about 90 percent due to accidental exposures. It is important to note that poisons come in many forms and are not harmful in every case. For example, medications are safe when used as prescribed, but overdoses and incorrectly combining medications with another substance may result in accidental poisoning.

Your home may contain a multitude of potentially poisonous substances. Solid and liquid forms include medications (aspirin, prescriptions, vitamins and minerals, and over-the-counter drugs), cleaning agents (furniture polish, oven cleaner, bleach, toilet bowl cleaners, and detergents), petroleum-based products (kerosene, gasoline, and antifreeze), insecticides (pesticides and herbicides), and toxic plants (avocado leaves, iris, marijuana, potato sprouts, rhubarb leaves, tulips, mushrooms, and tomato vines), and other household items (cosmetics, nail polish and remover, room deodorizers, and floor polishes). The most common type of poisoning by gases is due to carbon monoxide poisoning, such as that emitted by motor vehicle exhaust. Other types commonly result from improper ventilation and incomplete combustion involving furnaces, kerosene heaters, and cooking appliances.

Poisons enter the body through four primary avenues—inhalation, injection, oral injestion, and absorption through the skin. You must be able to recognize the characteristic signs and symptoms, identify the poisonous substance, and then take appropriate action. Action includes calling the nearest Poison Control Center and then giving first aid. Preventive measures to help avoid such problems include proper storage of poisons, proper use of the substances, and proper supervision.

Work Accidents Since the earliest industrial records of 1912, the work site has become a much safer place, as evidenced by a reduction in the accidental death rate by nearly 76 percent. That figure becomes even more impressive when one realizes that the size of the work force has more than doubled and produces more than ten times as much as the work force did in 1912. One very significant factor to account for such a marked decline has been the Occupational Safety and Health Act of 1970. As a result of that act, the Occupational Safety and Health Administration (OSHA) was created within the U.S. Department

Date rape Also known as "acquaintance rape" because the rape may involve people who know each other or who may even be dating at the time.

of Labor to assure workers a safer and healthier working environment. Inspections, more detailed recordkeeping, and penalties for noncompliance have probably been most responsible for the changes.

Laborers have the occupation with the highest risk of injury or illness. Although laborers make up less than half of the work force, they account for over 75 percent of all work-related injuries and illnesses. Such jobs usually involve extensive manual labor and lifting, both of which are not addressed in OSHA safety standards. Consequently, back problems are the most frequently cited injury and account for over 20 percent of work injuries. As far as occupational illnesses are concerned, skin disorders account for nearly 40 percent of the recorded cases. These disorders are becoming an increasing concern due to the introduction of more chemicals and hazardous materials at the work site. A third area of concern is the worker's experience. Data show that more than 40 percent of work-related injuries and illnesses involve workers on the first year of a job. Intensifying technology raises demands on job performance, and the influx of more workers, many of whom are women, into work force situations, also increases the need for more training and educational programs for all laborers.

Statistics compiled by the National Safety Council reveal that about 75 percent of the deaths and more than 50 percent of the injuries suffered by workers occur off the job. Regardless of where the injury occurred, industry must still compensate for time the worker loses from the job. And a good safety program is not just the responsibility of management, but the worker as well.

Public Accidents The number of public accidents has demonstrated a marked reduction of 73 percent in the death rate since 1912. Falls are the primary cause of death in public accidents, followed by drownings. The highest number of drownings occur in the 15–44 age group, with rates higher than average for all age groups under 25 years of age. Over 80 percent of all public drowning victims are males and involve swimming or playing in the water. Most drownings can be attributed to a person's lack of swimming skill, being chilled by water whose temperature is less than 70°F, and/or excessive consumption of alcohol. Swimming alone is irresponsible, and can obviously lead to problems if you need help. All these factors can be countered by education, increased awareness of the associated dangers, and increased individual responsibility for taking precautions.

Another recreational activity that deserves attention is jogging. Several million joggers exercise every day in this country. Jogging has a variety of associated risks from heat illnesses (cramps, exhaustion, and the serious condition known as heat stroke), but the greatest danger facing a jogger is motor vehicles. Surprisingly, most jogging accidents involve more "experienced" runners, many of whom believe they deserve to be part of the traffic flow and have equal rights to share the roadway.

A safe jogger should try to avoid busy roadways whenever possible, but if that is the only option, at least run against the traffic rather than with the traffic flow. Other suggestions include making eye contact with all drivers, not running during times of decreased visibility, increasing your visibility with bright and light-colored clothing, and not using equipment that might distract from your attention, such as stereo headsets.

Rape

Rape has been identified as the most underreported crime in the United States. It is estimated that for every rape, ten others are never reported. Rape is not always a sexually motivated crime, although the sexual act usually gets most of the attention. Rape is usually a crime where hostility or aggression are directed toward the victim. Criminal profiles show that the rapist is someone who has low self-esteem and little control over his life. By dominating the other person who eventually becomes the rape victim, the rapist tries to regain some self-esteem and control. Statistics reveal that a majority of rape victims are under 25 years of age, single women between the ages of 17 and 24 representing the largest percentage.

Although most people believe rapes usually involve strangers, a new type has become acknowledged, known as "acquaintance rape" or **"date rape."** Statistics reveal that as many as 75 percent of all rapes may involve people

Exploring Your Emotions

Has anyone you know been raped? How do you feel about the possibility that you may be raped at some point in your life? Do your feelings about rape affect the way you behave? How?

First aid Emergency care given to an ill or injured person until medical care can be obtained.

Cardiopulmonary resuscitation (CPR) Emergency first aid procedure that combines artificial respiration and artificial circulation. It is used in first aid emergencies where breathing and blood circulation have stopped.

Heimlich maneuver A maneuver developed by Henry J. Heimlich, M.D., to help force an obstruction from the airway. If the victim is standing or sitting, you should (1) stand behind him and wrap your arms around his waist, (2) grasp your wrist with your other hand and place the fist against the victim's abdomen, slightly above the navel and below the rib cage, and (3) press your fist forcefully into the victim's abdomen with a quick upward thrust. The procedure should be repeated several times if necessary.

---

who know each other and who may even be dating at the time. What may start out as a date or other leisure activity may turn into something more seriously dangerous. Although the full extent of acquaintance rape and sexual exploitation is not known, studies have suggested that a high amount of sexual aggression falls into these categories.

In any rape, the victim bears the task of documenting the assailant's actions. This may be difficult because guilt, whether actual or perceived, is such an overwhelming emotion in rape cases. A person who believes he or she has been the victim of a rape should contact the police immediately. Other support resources include a friend or crisis center. The victim needs to preserve any evidence because it is critical for the sake of convicting the offender.

People can often protect themselves from attack, whether or not rape is involved. Studies have shown that women who do physically resist an attacker initially are twice as likely to escape rape. This resistance may mean running, screaming, or being verbally aggressive, and therefore is not limited to fighting. Both physical and psychological skills should be developed to deal with an assailant. In some situations, passive methods of resistance may be your only viable option. The victim may have to plead, persuade, and possibly submit to the demands of the attackers. In such cases, the victim must try to stay emotionally stable, using good judgment to go along with the assailant until safer action can be taken. The goal in any case of violence is survival. The course of action may not be under the victim's control, but may actually be dictated by the situation. Of course, the best advice is to avoid potentially dangerous situations.

First Aid

Finally, you should be trained in **first aid, cardiopulmonary resuscitation (CPR)**, and the **Heimlich maneuver**. These skills can help you live a safer and healthier life. Many accident situations do not result in major trauma, but even the simplest accident can cause problems for the untrained person. One important aspect of first aid training is that training helps you assess your capabilities and limitations in responding to an accident. Sometimes little can be done or a technique may not be recommended under the circumstances. A good example is that a person with a suspected neck or back injury should not be moved unless other life-threatening conditions exist. A person trained in first aid learns how to assess a situation before acting. First aid training opens up many opportunities to help others, as well as volunteer and paid jobs in the helping professions.

Take Action

Your answers to Exploring Your Emotions in this chapter and your placement level on the Awareness Ladder will, we hope, encourage you to begin a process of self-exploration and self-discovery that you will continue. Reflect on the entire chapter's content and ask yourself how each point relates to your own life. Then take action:

1. In your Take Action notebook, keep track of any accidents you are involved in for the next two weeks. For each accident, determine the factors that contributed to its occurrence, decide whether or not the accident could have been avoided, and list any preventive measures that would be beneficial to avoid such incidents in the future.
2. Reread the list of characteristics and classify yourself as a Type X or Type Y individual. What do you believe has influenced you the most toward characteristics typical of Type X or Y? What factors are you able to change that would decrease your degree of accident proneness? Which ones are you willing to change? Justify your decisions.
3. Develop a survey to find out what other people think about accidents. Be sure to include questions relevant to home, work, public, and motor vehicle (especially the use of safety belts) situations. Survey twenty-five people and tabulate the results. What did you find out? Even though this is a small sample, what does this information indicate to you regarding the public's general attitude and knowledge about safety? What would you recommend to improve the situation?
4. How "safe" is your community? What kind of safety services does your community provide? Make a list of those services and the telephone number of each. Find out the appropriate course of action to notify authorities of an accident or emergency situation in your community.
5. If you came upon a motor vehicle accident, what would you do? Would you know what to do if you were alone and first aid was required? Contact the Emergency Medical Services unit for your community and find out the legal requirements for aiding the victims of a motor vehicle accident in your state. If you are not trained in first aid, think about enrolling in such a course to learn the basic procedures. Such action is good for others, as well as for your own health and safety.
6. What would you do if you suspected someone had been poisoned? Where is the nearest Poison Control Center for your community or state? What are the basic procedures for dealing with poisoning by ingestion, inhalation, injection, and absorption? What is the phone number for that center? Call and request any needed information.
7. Contact your local fire department and obtain a checklist for fire safety procedures. What would you do if your home caught on fire? What types of safe evacuation procedures are critical? Practice your own fire drill at home and note any potential problems or concerns.
8. Before leaving this chapter, review the Rate Yourself statements that open the chapter. Have your feelings or values changed? Are you now better equipped to handle the complex and very human problems associated with personal safety?

Behavior Change Strategy

None of us are immune to accidents. However, many people put themselves into dangerous and untenable situations, creating the inevitable "accident searching for somewhere to happen."

Freud suggested that people who have tendencies to be "accident repeaters" are accident prone. Many of us can be temporarily accident prone because of physical illness, insomnia, hunger, boredom, excitement, drug or alcohol intoxication, or other factors that cause an increase in distractibility and preoccupation. Emotional problems, such as depression and feelings of hostility, induce carelessness in some people or an attitude of "I don't care what happens to me or anyone else." In these cases automobiles sometimes provide convenient weapons to express unrelieved emotions.

Psychologists have identified many accident repeaters as restless, easily distractable, highly impulsive, aggressive, hurried, and unable to tolerate tension and frustration. They are inclined to trust to luck and take chances to prove their abilities "just for the fun of it." These individuals tend to develop an "accident habit" and often have a history of minor mishaps before a major accident is incurred.

The psychological study of accidents has been particularly fruitful in explaining why accidents occur despite caution warnings and otherwise safe conditions. An estimated 88 percent of industrial accidents are caused by human factors, including unsafe operating procedures, poor attitudes, and stress. Younger workers have a consistently higher accident rate than older workers. Studies of traffic accidents show that many people have dangerous attitudes, which increases the probability of an accident: overconfidence about their driving ability, a tendency to blame others, and the conviction that, "it can't happen to me."

Diary (Self-monitoring) The first step in your behavior change strategy is to collect baseline information about any behavior that increases your risk for accidents. Begin by making a daily record of the following events: each time you cut yourself, burn yourself, fall down, run into someone—any accident no matter how trivial. Also note each time you fail to wear your seat belt or someone reminds you to wear your seat belt. Specify the time of day or night and your mood, if possible. Record this information in a diary for at least seven days. Plot the number of events you recorded for each day on the graph provided.

Stimulus Control You can change your personal environment in many ways that will encourage you to follow through with an accident prevention program. For example, if you find you frequently are having accidents in the kitchen, you could post your graph on the refrigerator door or an equally obvious place you can't miss when working in the kitchen. This will stimulate you to think about the possibility of an accident. This use of stimulus control is similar to the way in which an alarm clock is used to help us awaken at the desired hour. Another useful strategy would be to make yourself a checklist of behaviors that can prevent accidents, such as turning off the stove, wiping up wet spots on the floor, putting away knives and sharp objects, and unplugging electrical appliances when not in use.

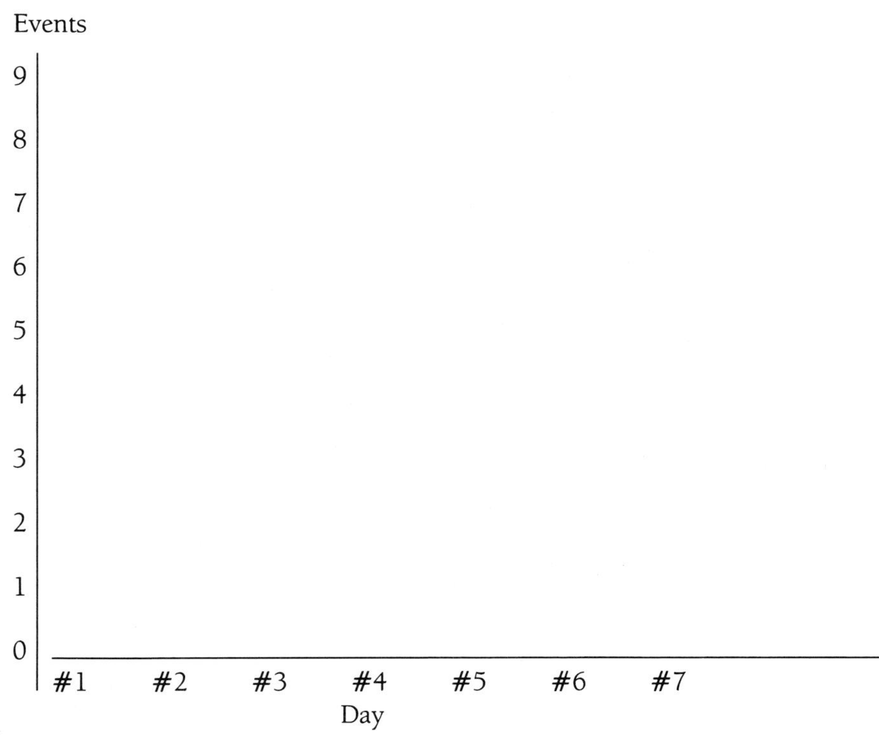

Self-Contracts and Reward Systems Personal contracts can provide an added incentive to an accident prevention program. A typical contract specifies in detail the target behaviors of concern, such as fastening your seat belt or keeping objects out of common walking paths. A reward system can provide more immediate positive consequences and can be related to the target behaviors you hope to achieve. For example, if all accident prevention behaviors are checked off by a specified time in the evening, a payment of money or points is "earned." Points can be turned into money or some other tangible reward.

This behavioral approach to achieving desired behaviors, which is more fully described in Chapter One, can help you reduce accidents and engage in more healthful safety behaviors.

Selected References

Bateman, P. 1982. *Acquaintance rape: Awareness and prevention.* Seattle, WA: Alternatives to Fear.

Bart, P. B. 1980. *Avoiding Rape: A Study of Victims and Avoiders.* Rockville, Md.: National Center for the Prevention and Control of Rape.

Bergeron, J. D. 1982. *First Responder.* Bowie, Md.: Brady.

Bever, D. L. 1984. *Safety: A Personal Focus.* St. Louis: Times Mirror/Mosby.

Bullard, J. A. 1981 (June). Death in sports and recreation. *The Physician and Sports Medicine* 9(6):124–28.

Florio, A. E., W. F. Alles, and G. T. Stafford. 1979. *Safety Education,* 4th ed. New York: McGraw-Hill.

National Highway Traffic Safety Administration. 1982 (May). *The Automobile Safety Belt Fact Book.* Washington, D.C.: U.S. Department of Transportation.

National Research Council. 1985 (May). *Injury in America: A Continuing Health Problem.* Washington, D.C.: National Academy Press.

National Safety Council. 1986. *Accident Facts.* Chicago: National Safety Council.

Sleet, D., et al. 1984. Automobile occupant protection: An issue for health educators? *Health Education* 15(5):54–56.

Recommended Readings

Baker, S. P., and S. P. Teret. 1981 (March). Freedom and protection: A balancing of interests. *American Journal of Public Health* 71(3):295–97.

Jackson, T., R. Quevillon, and P. Petretic-Jackson. 1985. Assessment and treatment of sexual assault victims. In P. Keller and L. Ritt, eds., *Innovations in Clinical Practice: A Sourcebook.* Florida: Professional Resource Exchange.

McIntyre, J. J. 1980. *Victim Response to Rape: Alternative Outcomes.* Rockville, Md.: National Center for the Prevention and Control of Rape.

Perin, M. J., W. L. Stohler, and W. G. Faraclas. 1984. *None for the Road.* Dubuque, Iowa: Kendall/Hunt.

Root, N., and D. McCaffrey. 1980 (January). Targeting worker safety programs: Weighing incidence against expense. *Monthly Labor Review,* pp. 3–8.

Shaw, L., and Sichel, H. S. 1971. *Accident Proneness.* Oxford, England: Pergamon Press.

Suchman, E. A. 1970. Accidents and social deviance. *Journal of Health and Social Behavior* 11:6.

U.S. Fire Administration. 1982. *Fire in the United States.* Washington, D.C.: U.S. Fire Administration.

Index

Boldface numbers indicate pages on which glossary definitions appear.

(continued from copyright page)

Page 301 From William L. Scheider, "Evaluating a Fad Diet," *Nutrition: Basic Concepts and Applications,* reprinted by permission of McGraw-Hill Book Company. Copyright © 1983 by McGraw-Hill Book Company.

Page 306 Reprinted by permission from *Understanding Normal and Clinical Nutrition,* 2e, by Whitney, Cataldo and Rolfes. Copyright © 1981 by West Publishing Company, pages 84–87. All rights reserved.

Pages 330–31 From *Rating the Exercises* by Charles T. Kunzleman and the Editors of *Consumer Guide.* Copyright © 1978 by Publications International Limited. Reprinted by permission of William Morrow & Co.

Page 338 Reprinted from *USA Today Weekend,* January 31, 1986.

Page 463 "Viruses" from *Time,* November 3, 1986. Copyright © 1986 by Time, Inc. All rights reserved. Reprinted by permission from TIME.

Page 501 "What Is Destroying the Ozone?" from *Time,* November 3, 1986. Copyright © 1986 by Time, Inc. All rights reserved. Reprinted by permission from TIME.

Page 502 From "Acid Rain's Fingerprints," *Newsweek,* August 11, 1986. Copyright © 1986 by Newsweek, Inc. All rights reserved.

Pages 504–505 From "A Nuclear Burial Ground," *Newsweek,* June 16, 1986. Copyright © 1986 by Newsweek, Inc. All rights reserved. Reprinted by permission.
From the "Disposal Alternatives," *Time,* May 11, 1986. Copyright © 1986 by Time, Inc. All rights reserved. Reprinted by permission from TIME.

Page 522 From "Unveiling a Family Secret," *Newsweek,* February 18, 1980. Copyright © 1980 by Newsweek, Inc. All rights reserved. Reprinted by permission.

STUDY NOTES

STUDY NOTES

STUDY NOTES

STUDY NOTES

STUDY NOTES

STUDY NOTES

STUDY NOTES

STUDY NOTES